KU-733-672
SGH000517

CORE TECHNIQUES IN
OPERATIVE NEUROSURGERY

CORE TECHNIQUES IN OPERATIVE NEUROSURGERY

Rahul Jandial, MD, PhD
Assistant Professor
Division of Neurosurgery
City of Hope Comprehensive Cancer Center
Los Angeles, California

Paul C. McCormick, MD, MPH, FACS
Herbert and Linda Gallen Professor of Neurological Surgery
Director, Spine Center
Columbia University Medical Center
New York, New York

Peter M. Black, MD, PhD
Founding Chair, Department of Neurosurgery
Franc D. Ingraham Professor of Neurosurgery, Harvard Medical School
Brigham and Women's Hospital
Department of Neurosurgery
Boston, Massachusetts

ELSEVIER
SAUNDERS

ELSEVIER
SAUNDERS

1600 John F. Kennedy Blvd.
Ste 1800
Philadelphia, PA 19103-2899

Core Techniques in Operative Neurosurgery ISBN: 978-1-4377-0907-0

Notices

Knowledge and best practice in this field are constantly changing. As new research and experience broaden our understanding, changes in research methods, professional practices, or medical treatment may become necessary.

Practitioners and researchers must always rely on their own experience and knowledge in evaluating and using any information, methods, compounds, or experiments described herein. In using such information or methods, they should be mindful of their own safety and the safety of others, including parties for whom they have a professional responsibility.

With respect to any drug or pharmaceutical products identified, readers are advised to check the most current information provided (i) on procedures featured or (ii) by the manufacturer of each product to be administered to verify the recommended dose or formula, the method and duration of administration, and contraindications. It is the responsibility of practitioners, relying on their own experience and knowledge of their patients, to make diagnoses, to determine dosages and the best treatment for each individual patient, and to take all appropriate safety precautions.

To the fullest extent of the law, neither the Publisher nor the authors, contributors, or editors assume any liability for any injury and/or damage to persons or property as a matter of products liability, negligence or otherwise, or from any use or operation of any methods, products, instructions, or ideas contained in the material herein.

Library of Congress Cataloging-in-Publication Data
Core techniques in operative neurosurgery / [edited by] Rahul Jandial, Paul C. McCormick, Peter McLaren Black.
p. ; cm.
Operative neurosurgery
Includes bibliographical references and index.
ISBN 978-1-4377-0907-0 (hardcover : alk. paper)
1. Nervous system–Surgery. I. Jandial, Rahul. II. McCormick, Paul, 1956- III. Black, Peter McL. IV. Title: Operative neurosurgery.
[DNLM: 1. Neurosurgical Procedures–methods. 2. Central Nervous System Diseases–surgery. 3. Orthopedic Procedures–methods. WL 368]
RD593.C67 2011
617.4′8–dc22
2011009300

Acquisitions Editor: Julie Goolsby
Developmental Editor: Taylor Ball
Publishing Services Manager: Anne Altepeter
Senior Project Manager: Cheryl A. Abbott
Design Direction: Louis Forgione
Marketing Manager: Cara Jespersen

Printed in the United States of America

Last digit is the print number: 9 8 7 6 5 4 3 2 1

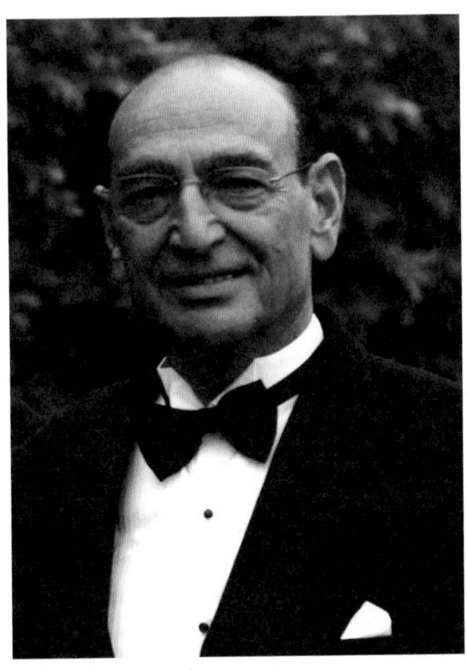

To my life's greatest and most lasting formative influence
To my best teacher, confidant, and mentor
To my father, Satya Pal Jandial

Rahul Jandial

To Dodi

Paul C. McCormick

I dedicate this book to our world neurosurgery family—faculty, residents, practitioners, and supporters—who work so hard to make neurosurgery the most dynamic surgical enterprise on the planet

Peter M. Black

Section Editors

Christopher P. Ames, MD
Associate Professor
Director of Spine Tumor and Deformity Surgery
Department of Neurosurgery
University of California, San Francisco
San Francisco, California

Kim Burchiel, MD, FACS
John Raaf Professor and Chairman of the Department of Neurological Surgery
Oregon Health and Science University
Portland, Oregon

Joseph D. Ciacci, MD
Program Director, Neurosurgery Residency
Academic Community Director, School of Medicine
Associate Clinical Professor of Surgery
Division of Neurosurgery
University of California, San Diego;
Chief of Neurosurgery, Veterans Administration Hospital, San Diego
San Diego, California

Steven Giannotta, MD
Chair, Neurological Surgery
Professor of Neurological Surgery
Keck School of Medicine
University of Southern California
Los Angeles, California

George I. Jallo, MD
Professor of Neurosurgery
Director, Clinical Pediatric Neurosurgery
The Johns Hopkins University School of Medicine
Baltimore, Maryland

Michael L. Levy, MD, PhD
Professor of Neurosurgery
Chief, Pediatric Neurosurgery
Division of Neurological Surgery
University of California, San Diego;
Rady Children's Hospital of San Diego
San Diego, California

Alfred Ogden, MD
Department of Neurological Surgery
Neurological Institute
Columbia University
New York, New York

Jon Park, MD, FRCS(C)
Chief, Spine Neurosurgery
Associate Professor
Stanford University School of Medicine
Stanford, California

Andrew T. Parsa, MD, PhD
Brain Tumor Research Center
Department of Neurological Surgery
University of California, San Francisco
San Francisco, California

Alfredo Quiñones-Hinojosa, MD
Associate Professor of Neurosurgery and Oncology
Neuroscience and Cellular and Molecular Medicine
The Johns Hopkins University School of Medicine;
Director, Brain Tumor Surgery Program
The Johns Hopkins Bayview Medical Center;
Director, Pituitary Surgery Program
The Johns Hopkins Hospital
Baltimore, Maryland

Contributors

Rick Abbott, MD
Professor of Clinical Neurosurgery
Department of Neurosurgery
Albert Einstein College of Medicine
Bronx, New York

Frank Acosta, MD
Assistant Professor
Department of Neurosurgery
Cedars-Sinai Medical Center
Los Angeles, California

R. Todd Allen, MD, PhD
Assistant Clinical Professor
Department of Orthopaedic Surgery
University of California, San Diego
San Diego, California

Jorge E. Alvernia, MD
Senior Resident
Department of Neurosurgery
Tulane University Medical Center
New Orleans, Louisiana

Vijay K. Anand, MD
Clinical Professor
Department of Otorhinolaryngology
Weill Cornell Medical College
New York, New York

Carmina F. Angeles, MD, PhD
Clinical Instructor
Department of Neurosurgery
Stanford University Medical Center
Stanford, California

Henry E. Aryan, MD, FACS
Associate Clinical Professor of Neurosurgery
University of California, San Francisco
San Francisco, California;
Chief, Spine Service
Sierra Pacific Orthopedic and Spine Center
Fresno, California

Issam Awad, MD, MSc, FACS, MA (hon)
Director of Neurovascular Surgery
Professor of Surgery, Neurosurgery
University of Chicago Pritzker School of Medicine
Chicago, Illinois

Behnam Badie, MD
Professor and Chief
Division of Neurosurgery
City of Hope Medical Center
Los Angeles, California

Neil Badlani, MD
Orthopaedic Surgery Resident
Department of Orthopaedic Surgery
University of California, San Diego
San Diego, California

Lissa C. Baird, MD
Chief Resident, Division of Neurosurgery
University of California San Diego Medical Center
San Diego, California

H. Hunt Batjer, MD
Department of Neurological Surgery
Northwestern University Feinberg School of Medicine
Chicago, Illinois

Allan J. Belzberg, MD
Associate Professor of Neurological Surgery
Department of Neurosurgery
The Johns Hopkins University School of Medicine
Baltimore, Maryland

Bernard R. Bendok, MD
Department of Neurological Surgery
Northwestern University Feinberg School of Medicine
Chicago, Illinois

Edward C. Benzel, MD
Department of Neurosurgery
Neurological Institute
Cleveland Clinic
Cleveland, Ohio

Chetan Bettegowda, MD, PhD
Neurosurgery Resident
Department of Neurosurgery
The Johns Hopkins University School of Medicine
Baltimore, Maryland

William E. Bingaman, MD
Vice Chairman
Neurological Institute;
Professor of Neurosurgery
Department of Neurosurgery;
Richard and Karen Shusterman Chair in Epilepsy Surgery
Epilepsy Center;
Cleveland Clinic
Cleveland, Ohio

Markus Bookland, MD
Neurosurgery Resident
Department of Neurosurgery
Temple University School of Medicine
Philadelphia, Pennsylvania

Kim Burchiel, MD, FACS
John Raaf Professor and Chairman of the Department of Neurological Surgery
Oregon Health and Science University
Portland, Oregon

Mohamad Bydon, MD
Resident
Department of Neurosurgery
The Johns Hopkins University School of Medicine
Baltimore, Maryland

Peter G. Campbell, MD
Neurosurgery Resident
Department of Neurosurgery
Thomas Jefferson University Hospital
Philadelphia, Pennsylvania

Kaisorn L. Chaichana, MD
Neurosurgery Resident
Department of Neurosurgery
The Johns Hopkins University School of Medicine
Baltimore, Maryland

Saad B. Chaudhary, MD, MBA
Department of Neurosurgery
Neurological Institute
Cleveland Clinic
Cleveland, Ohio

Mike Yue Chen, MD, MS, PhD
Assistant Professor
Department of Surgery
Division of Neurosurgery
City of Hope National Medical Center
Los Angeles, California

Tsulee Chen, MD
Epilepsy Surgery Fellow
Department of Neurosurgery
Neurological Institute
Cleveland Clinic
Cleveland, Ohio

Dean Chou, MD
Associate Professor of Neurosurgery
Associate Director of Spinal Tumor Surgery
Department of Neurological Surgery
University of California, San Francisco
San Francisco, California

Joseph D. Ciacci, MD
Program Director, Neurosurgery Residency
Academic Community Director, School of Medicine
Associate Clinical Professor of Surgery
Division of Neurosurgery
University of California, San Diego;
Chief of Neurosurgery VASDHS
San Diego, California

Steven R. Cohen, MD, FACS
Director, Craniofacial Surgery
Rady Children's Hospital;
Clinical Professor
Department of Plastic Surgery
University of California, San Diego
San Diego, California

Geoffrey P. Colby, MD, PhD
Resident
Department of Neurosurgery
The Johns Hopkins University School of Medicine
Baltimore, Maryland

E. Sander Connolly, Jr., MD
Bennett M. Stein Professor and Vice-Chair
Department of Neurological Surgery
Columbia University
New York, New York

James E. Conway, MD
Neurosurgeon
Baltimore Neurosurgery and Spine Center
Baltimore, Maryland

Ralph G. Dacey, Jr., MD
Henry G. and Edith R. Schwartz Professor and Chairman of Neurological Surgery
Department of Neurosurgery
Washington University School of Medicine
St. Louis, Missouri

Mahua Dey, MD
Neurosurgical Resident
University of Chicago Pritzker School of Medicine
Chicago, Illinois

Michael J. Dorsi, MD
Chief Resident
Department of Neurosurgery
The Johns Hopkins University School of Medicine
Baltimore, Maryland

Matthew J. Duenas
Bachelor of Science Candidate, Biology
Stanford University
Stanford, California

Gavin P. Dunn, MD, PhD
Resident
Department of Neurosurgery
Massachusetts General Hospital
Harvard Medical School
Boston, Massachusetts

Christopher S. Eddleman, MD, PhD
Department of Neurological Surgery and Radiology
University of Texas Southwestern Medical Center
Dallas, Texas

Mohamed Samy Elhammady, MD
Resident
Department of Neurosurgery
University of Miami School of Medicine
Miami, Florida

Azadeh Farin, MD
Resident
Department of Neurological Surgery
Keck School of Medicine
University of Southern California
Los Angeles, California

Richard G. Fessler, MD, PhD
Professor
Northwestern University Feinberg School of Medicine
Chicago, Illinois

Howard W. Francis, MD
Associate Professor
Division Otology-Neurotology
Department of Otolaryngology, Head and Neck Surgery
The Johns Hopkins University School of Medicine
Baltimore, Maryland

Ryan C. Frank, MD
Craniofacial Fellow
Department of Plastic Surgery
University of California, San Diego
San Diego, California

Justin F. Fraser, MD
Chief Resident
Department of Neurological Surgery
Weill Cornell Medical College
New York, New York

Takanori Fukushima, MD, DMSc
Professor of Neurosurgery
Duke University Medical Center
Duke Raleigh Community Hospital
West Virginia University Medical Center
Morgantown, West Virginia

Gary Gallia, MD
Assistant Professor
Department of Neurosurgery
The Johns Hopkins University School of Medicine
Baltimore, Maryland

Julio Garcia-Aguilar, MD, PhD
Professor and Chair
Department of Surgery
City of Hope National Medical Center
Los Angeles, California

Ira M. Garonzik, MD
Neurosurgeon
Baltimore Neurosurgery and Spine Center
Baltimore, Maryland

Melanie G. Hayden Gephart, MD, MAS
Neurosurgery Resident
Department of Neurosurgery
Stanford University Hospital and Clinics
Stanford, California

Anand V. Germanwala, MD
Assistant Professor
Department of Neurosurgery
University of North Carolina School of Medicine
Chapel Hill, North Carolina

Christopher C. Getch, MD
Professor of Neurosurgery
Department of Neurological Surgery
Northwestern University Feinberg School of Medicine
Chicago, Illinois

Steven Giannotta, MD
Chair, Neurological Surgery
Professor of Neurological Surgery
Keck School of Medicine
University of Southern California
Los Angeles, California

Paul Gigante, MD
Resident
Department of Neurological Surgery
Columbia University Medical Center
New York, New York

Giuliano Giliberto, MD
Nuovo Ospedale Civile of Modena
Department of Neurosurgery
Modena, Italy

David Gonda, MD
Resident
Division of Neurosurgery
University of California San Diego Medical Center
San Diego, California

Jorge Alvaro Gonzalez-Martinez, MD
Staff, Department of Neurosurgery
Neurological Institute
Epilepsy Center
Cleveland Clinic
Cleveland, Ohio

Robert E. Gross, MD, PhD
Associate Professor
Department of Neurological Surgery
Emory University
Atlanta, Georgia

James S. Harrop, MD
Associate Professor
Chief of Spine and Peripheral Nerve Surgery
Departments of Neurological and Orthopedic Surgery
Thomas Jefferson University Hospital
Philadelphia, Pennsylvania

Adam O. Hebb, MD, FRCSC
Assistant Professor
Department of Neurological Surgery
University of Washington School of Medicine
Seattle, Washington

Juha Hernesniemi, MD, PhD
Professor and Chairman
Department of Neurosurgery
Helsinki University Central Hospital
Helsinki, Finland

Roberto C. Heros, MD
Professor, Co-Chairman, and Program Director
Department of Neurosurgery
University of Miami School of Medicine
Miami, Florida

Sebastian R. Herrera, MD
Resident
Department of Neurosurgery
University of Illinois at Chicago
Chicago, Illinois

Girish K. Hiremath, MD
Staff Neurosurgeon
Riverside Methodist Hospital
Columbus, Ohio

Allen Ho, BS
Harvard Medical School
Boston, Massachusetts

Samuel A. Hughes, MD, PhD
Chief Resident
Department of Neurological Surgery
Oregon Health and Science University
Portland, Oregon

Daniel S. Hutton, DO
Oregon Neurosurgery Specialists
Sacred Heart Medical Center, RiverBend Campus
McKenzie-Willamette Medical Center
Springfield, Oregon;
Sacred Heart Medical Center, University District
Eugene, Oregon

Robert E. Isaacs, MD
Director of Spine Surgery
Associate Professor
Department of Surgery
Division of Neurosurgery
Duke Medical Center
Durham, North Carolina

Jennifer Jaffe, MPH, CCRP
Clinical Research Associate
Hemorrhagic Stroke Trials Unit
Section of Neurosurgery
University of Chicago Pritzker School of Medicine
Chicago, Illinois

George I. Jallo, MD
Professor of Neurosurgery
Director, Clinical Pediatric Neurosurgery
The Johns Hopkins University School of Medicine
Baltimore, Maryland

Jack I. Jallo, MD
Professor and Vice Chair for Academic Services
Director, Division of Neurotrauma and Critical Care
Department of Neurological Surgery
Jefferson Medical College
Philadelphia, Pennsylvania

Rahul Jandial, MD, PhD
Assistant Professor
Division of Neurosurgery
City of Hope Comprehensive Cancer Center
Los Angeles, California

Pawel Jankowski, MD
Department of Neurosurgery
University of California, San Francisco
San Francisco, California

Vijayakumar Javalkar, MD
Fellow
Department of Neurosurgery
Louisiana State University Health Sciences Center
Shreveport, Louisiana

Brian Jian, MD, PhD
Resident
Department of Neurological Surgery
University of California, San Francisco
San Francisco, California

J. Patrick Johnson, MD, FACS
CEO and Chairman
The Spine Institute Foundation;
Director
California Association of Neurological Surgeons;
Co-Director
Stem Cell Research Program, The Spine Center
Cedars-Sinai Medical Center
Los Angeles, California

James M. Johnston, Jr., MD
Fellow, Pediatric Neurosurgery
Department of Neurosurgery
Washington University School of Medicine
Saint Louis Children's Hospital
St. Louis, Missouri

Michael G. Kaiser, MD
Assistant Professor of Neurological Surgery
Department of Neurological Surgery
Columbia University
New York, New York

Adam S. Kanter, MD
Assistant Professor of Neurological Surgery
University of Pittsburgh;
Director
Neurosurgical Biomechanics Research Lab
Pittsburgh, Pennsylvania

Christopher P. Kellner, BA, MD
Resident
Department of Neurological Surgery
Columbia University Medical Center
New York, New York

Sassan Keshavarzi, MD
Division of Neurosurgery
University of California, San Diego
San Diego, California

Bong-Soo Kim, MD
Assistant Professor of Neurosurgery
Director, Minimally Invasive and Complex Spine Fellowship Program
Temple University School of Medicine
Philadelphia, Pennsylvania

Kee D. Kim, MD
Associate Professor
Chief, Spinal Neurosurgery
Department of Neurological Surgery
School of Medicine
University of California, Davis
Davis, California

Ryan M. Kretzer, MD
Neurosurgery Resident
Department of Neurosurgery
The Johns Hopkins University School of Medicine
Baltimore, Maryland

Giuseppe Lanzino, MD
Professor of Neurologic Surgery
Mayo Clinic
Rochester, Minnesota

Michael T. Lawton, MD
Professor of Neurosurgery
Chief, Vascular Neurosurgery
Tong Po Kan Endowed Chair
Department of Neurological Surgery
University of California, San Francisco
San Francisco, California

Marco Lee, MD, PhD
Assistant Professor
Department of Neurosurgery
Stanford University School of Medicine
Stanford, California

Martin Lehecka, MD, PhD
Consultant Neurosurgeon
Department of Neurosurgery
Helsinki University Central Hospital
Helsinki, Finland

Michael L. Levy, MD, PhD
Professor of Neurosurgery
Chief, Pediatric Neurosurgery
Division of Neurological Surgery
University of California, San Diego
Rady Children's Hospital of San Diego
San Diego, California

Jason Liauw, MD
Resident
Department of Neurosurgery
The Johns Hopkins University School of Medicine
Baltimore, Maryland

Michael Lim, MD
Assistant Professor of Neurosurgery and Oncology
The Johns Hopkins University School of Medicine
Baltimore, Maryland

Timothy Link, MD
Department of Neurological Surgery
The Neurological Institute
Columbia University Medical Center
West Long Branch New Jersey Office
West Long Branch, New Jersey

John C. Liu, MD
Associate Professor
Department of Neurological Surgery
Northwestern University Feinberg School of Medicine
Chicago, Illinois

Richard A. Lochhead, MD
Senior Resident, Neurosurgery
Barrow Neurological Institute
Phoenix, Arizona

Jaliya R. Lokuketagoda, MD, MS, FRCSEd
Instructor
Department of Neurological Surgery
Emory University
Atlanta, Georgia

Daniel C. Lu, MD, PhD
Assistant Professor
Department of Neurosurgery
University of California, Los Angeles
Los Angeles, California

Dzenan Lulic, MD
Department of Neurosurgery
University of South Florida
Tampa, Florida

Ricky Madhok, MD
Chief Resident in Neurological Surgery
Department of Neurological Surgery
University of Pittsburgh Medical Center
Pittsburgh, Pennsylvania

Geoffrey T. Manley, MD, PhD
Professor and Vice-Chairman
Department of Neurological Surgery
University of California, San Francisco
San Francisco, California

Joseph L. Martinez, MD
Department of Neurosurgery
University of Miami Miller School of Medicine
Miami, Florida

Virgilio Matheus, MD
Department of Neurosurgery
Neurological Institute
Cleveland Clinic
Cleveland, Ohio

Nnenna Mbabuike, MD
Resident
Department of Neurosurgery
Tulane University Medical Center
New Orleans, Louisiana

Michael W. McDermott, MD
Professor of Neurosurgery
Department of Neurological Surgery
University of California, San Francisco
San Francisco, California

Vivek Mehta, BS
The Johns Hopkins University School of Medicine
Baltimore, Maryland

Hal Meltzer, MD
Clinical Professor of Neurosurgery
Division of Neurologic Sciences
University of California, San Diego
Rady Children's Hospital of San Diego
San Diego, California

Jayant P. Menon, MD
Division of Neurosurgery
University of California, San Diego
San Diego, California

Edward A. Monaco, III, MD, PhD
Resident
Department of Neurological Surgery
University of Pittsburgh Medical Center
Pittsburgh, Pennsylvania

Praveen V. Mummaneni, MD
Associate Professor of Neurological Surgery
Co-Director, Spinal Surgery and Spine Center
University of California, San Francisco
San Francisco, California

Valli P. Mummaneni, MD
Associate Clinical Professor
Department of Anesthesiology
University of California, San Francisco
San Francisco, California

Anil Nanda, MD, FACS
Professor and Chairman
Department of Neurosurgery
Louisiana State University Health Sciences Center
Shreveport, Louisiana

Mika Niemelä, MD, PhD
Associate Professor
Head of Section
Department of Neurosurgery
Helsinki University Central Hospital
Helsinki, Finland

Shahid M. Nimjee, MD, PhD
Neurosurgery Resident
Division of Neurosurgery
Duke University Medical Center
Durham, North Carolina

Christopher S. Ogilvy, MD
Director of Endovascular and Operative Neurosurgery
Robert G. and A. Jean Ojemann Professor of Neurosurgery
Department of Neurosurgery
Massachusetts General Hospital
Boston, Massachusetts

David O. Okonkwo, MD, PhD
Chief of Neurotrauma
University of Pittsburgh Medical Center
Pittsburgh, Pennsylvania

Alessandro Olivi, MD
Professor of Neurosurgery and Oncology
Director
Division of Neurosurgical Oncology
Department of Neurosurgery
The Johns Hopkins University School of Medicine
Baltimore, Maryland

John E. O'Toole, MD
Assistant Professor of Neurosurgery
Rush University Medical Center
Chicago, Illinois

Alexander M. Papanastassiou, MD
Epilepsy Surgery Fellow
Department of Neurosurgery
Yale University School of Medicine
New Haven, Connecticut

Jon Park, MD, FRCS(C)
Chief, Spine Neurosurgery
Associate Professor
Stanford University School of Medicine
Stanford, California

Andrew T. Parsa, MD, PhD
Brain Tumor Research Center
Department of Neurological Surgery
University of California, San Francisco
San Francisco, California

Mick Perez-Cruet, MD, MS
Vice Chairman
Professor of Neurosurgery
Department of Neurosurgery
Director, Spine Program
Oakland University William Beaumont Medical School
Michigan Head and Spine Institute
Royal Oak, Michigan

Erika Anne Peterson, MD
Department of Neurological Surgery
University of Texas Southwestern
Dallas, Texas

Randall W. Porter, MD
Director Interdisciplinary Skull Base Program
Co-Director CyberKnife
Co-Director Acoustic Neuroma Center
Department of Neurosurgery
Barrow Neurological Institute
Phoenix, Arizona

Mathew B. Potts, MD
Resident
Department of Neurological Surgery
University of California, San Francisco
San Francisco, California

Alfredo Quiñones-Hinojosa, MD
Associate Professor of Neurosurgery and Oncology
Neuroscience and Cellular and Molecular Medicine
The Johns Hopkins University School of Medicine;
Director, Brain Tumor Surgery Program
The Johns Hopkins Bayview Medical Center;
Director, Pituitary Surgery Program
The Johns Hopkins Hospital
Baltimore, Maryland

Ivan Radovanovic, MD, PhD
Clinical Fellow in Cerebrovascular Surgery
Division of Neurosurgery
Toronto Western Hospital
University Health Network and University of Toronto
Toronto, Ontario, Canada

Ahmed Raslan, MD
Neurosurgical Resident
Department of Neurological Surgery
School of Medicine
Oregon Health and Science University
Portland, Oregon

Shaan M. Raza, MD
Neurosurgery Resident
Department of Neurosurgery
The Johns Hopkins University School of Medicine
Baltimore, Maryland

Pablo F. Recinos, MD
Neurosurgery Resident
Department of Neurosurgery
The Johns Hopkins University School of Medicine
Baltimore, Maryland

Matthew R. Reynolds, MD, PhD
Resident
Department of Neurological Surgery
Washington University Medical School
St. Louis, Missouri

Alejandro Rivas, MD
Otology and Neurotology Fellow
The Otology Group of Vanderbilt
Vanderbilt University Medical Center
Nashville, Tennessee

Nader Sanai, MD
Director, Neurosurgical Oncology
Division of Neurological Surgery
Barrow Neurological Institute
Phoenix, Arizona

Matthias Schulz, MD
Neurosurgeon
Pediatric Neurosurgery
Charité Universitätsmedizin Berlin
Campus Virchow Klinikum
Berlin, Germany

Theodore H. Schwartz, MD, FACS
Professor of Neurosurgery
Departments of Neurosurgery, Otolaryngology, Neurology, and Neuroscience
Weill Cornell Medical College
New York Presbyterian Hospital
New York, New York

Stephen S. Scibelli, MD
Institute for Spinal Disorders
Cedars-Sinai Medical Center
Los Angeles, California

Daniel L. Silbergeld, MD, FACS
Arthur A. Ward, Jr., Professor
Department of Neurological Surgery
University of Washington School of Medicine
Seattle, Washington

Konstantin V. Slavin, MD
Professor
Department of Neurosurgery
University of Illinois at Chicago
Chicago, Illinois

Matthew D. Smyth, MD, FACS, FAAP
Associate Professor of Neurosurgery and Pediatrics
Washington University
Saint Louis Children's Hospital
St. Louis, Missouri

Volker Sonntag, MD
Vice Chair of Neurological Surgery
Alumni Chair for Spinal Surgery
Barrow Neurological Institute;
Clinical Professor, Department of Surgery
University of Arizona;
Vice Chairman, Barrow Neurosurgical Associates
Phoenix, Arizona

Dennis D. Spencer, MD
Harvey and Kate Cushing Professor
Chair, Department of Neurosurgery
Yale University School of Medicine
New Haven, Connecticut

Gary K. Steinberg, MD, PhD
Bernard and Ronni Lacroute Professor of Neurosurgery and the Neurosciences
Director, Stanford Institute for Neuro-Innovation and Translational Neurosciences
Chief, Department of Neurosurgery
Stanford University School of Medicine;
Chief, Department of Neurosurgery
Stanford University Hospital and Clinics
Stanford, California

Shirley I. Stiver, MD
Assistant Professor
Department of Neurological Surgery
University of California, San Francisco
San Francisco, California

Sathish Subbaiah, MD
Assistant Professor
Department of Neurosurgery
Mount Sinai Hospital
New York, New York

Michael E. Sughrue, MD
Brain Tumor Research Center
Department of Neurological Surgery
University of California, San Francisco
San Francisco, California

Patrick A. Sugrue, MD
Resident Physician
Department of Neurological Surgery
Northwestern University Feinberg School of Medicine
Chicago, Illinois

Omar N. Syed, MD
Chief Resident
Department of Neurological Surgery
Columbia University Medical Center
New York, New York

Rafael J. Tamargo, MD, FACS
Walter E. Dandy Professor of Neurosurgery
Director, Division of Cerebrovascular Neurosurgery
The Johns Hopkins University School of Medicine
Baltimore, Maryland

Ramesh Teegala, MD
International Spine Fellow
Spinal Surgery and Spine Center
University of California, San Francisco
San Francisco, California

Charles Teo, MD
Director, Center for Minimally Invasive Neurosurgery
Sydney, Australia

Nicholas Theodore, MD
Chief, Spine Section
Division of Neurosurgery
Barrow Neurological Institute;
Adjunct Professor School of Life Sciences
Arizona State University
Phoenix, Arizona

Ulrich W. Thomale, MD
Consultant Pediatric Neurosurgeon
Pediatric Neurosurgery
Charité Universitätsmedizin Berlin
Campus Virchow Klinikum
Berlin, Germany

Andrew P. Thomas, BS
Northwestern University
Feinberg School of Medicine
Chicago, Illinois

B. Gregory Thompson, MD
Professor and J.E. McGillicuddy Chair
Departments of Neurosurgery, Radiology, and Otolaryngology
University of Michigan
Ann Arbor, Michigan

William D. Tobler, MD
Department of Neurosurgery
Neuroscience Institute
College of Medicine
University of Cincinnati
Mayfield Clinic
Cincinnati, Ohio

Nestor D. Tomycz, MD
Department of Neurological Surgery
University of Pittsburgh Medical Center
Pittsburgh, Pennsylvania

Matthew J. Tormenti, MD
Resident in Neurological Surgery
Department of Neurological Surgery
University of Pittsburgh Medical Center
Pittsburgh, Pennsylvania

Timothy D. Uschold, MD
Senior Resident, Neurosurgery
Barrow Neurological Institute
Phoenix, Arizona

Prasad Vannemreddy, MCh, MBBS
Fellow
Department of Neurosurgery
University of Illinois at Chicago
Chicago, Illinois

Ram R. Vasudevan, MD
Resident
Department of Neurosurgery
Cedars-Sinai Medical Center
Los Angeles, California

Shoshanna Vaynman, PhD
Research and Education Administrator
The Spine Institute Foundation
Los Angeles, California

Kenneth P. Vives, MD
Associate Professor of Neurosurgery
Director, Section of Stereotactic and Functional Neurosurgery
Department of Neurosurgery
Yale University School of Medicine
New Haven, Connecticut

M. Christopher Wallace, MD, MSc, FRCSC, FACS
Professor, Department of Surgery
University of Toronto
Head, Division of Neurosurgery
Toronto Western Hospital, University Health Network
Toronto, Ontario, Canada

Michael Y. Wang, MD, FACS
Associate Professor
Departments of Neurological Surgery and Rehabilitation Medicine
University of Miami Miller School of Medicine
Lois Pope LIFE Center
Miami, Florida

Vincent Y. Wang, MD, PhD
Clinical Instructor
Department of Neurosurgery
University of California, Los Angeles
Los Angeles, California

Marcus L. Ware, MD
Assistant Professor
Department of Neurosurgery
Tulane University Medical Center
New Orleans, Louisiana

Chad W. Washington, MD, MS
Resident
Department of Neurosurgery
Washington University School of Medicine
St. Louis, Missouri

J. Dawn Waters, MD
Resident
Division of Neurosurgery
University of California San Diego Medical Center
San Diego, California

Louis Anthony Whitworth, MD
Associate Professor
Department of Neurological Surgery
Department of Radiation Oncology
University of Texas Southwestern Medical Center
Dallas, Texas

Kamal R.M. Woods, MD
Department of Neurosurgery
Loma Linda University Medical Center
Loma Linda, California

Graeme F. Woodworth, MD
Neurosurgery Resident
Department of Neurosurgery
The Johns Hopkins University School of Medicine
Baltimore, Maryland

Zilvinas Zakarevicius, MD, PhD
Fellow
Department of Neurosurgery
University of Illinois at Chicago
Chicago, Illinois

Gregory J. Zipfel, MD
Assistant Professor of Neurological Surgery and Neurology
Department of Neurosurgery
Washington University School of Medicine
St. Louis, Missouri

Benjamin M. Zussman, BS
Jefferson Medical College
Philadelphia, Pennsylvania

Preface

Core Techniques in Operative Neurosurgery was conceived with clear recognition of the evolving pedagogical landscape. The presentation of medical information is undergoing a renaissance, and the pressing need and unparalleled opportunity to develop digital medical textbooks are upon us. Soon the concepts of "book editions" and "page length" will become obsolete, as information is continually updated and infinitely linked from digital sources that coalesce. In this transition, neurological surgery—the most challenging and complicated of medical endeavors—should be at the forefront.

The structure of this text consists of two main sections: Cranial and Spinal. Specific design elements have been included to allow for quick reference in preoperative considerations regarding "Indications," "Contraindications," and "Planning and Positioning." Further, thoughtful "Tips from the Masters" and "Bailout Options" are included, which present condensed and accessible pearls that have been distilled from more exhaustive texts, as well as senior author experience. Both for neophyte students of neurological surgery and for established neurosurgeons seeking a targeted review of operations that may have become an infrequent aspect of their practices, this text intends to serve both as a reference and a conduit to further learning.

My intention is for *Core Techniques to Operative Neurosurgery* to function as a bridge between the best of conventional paper textbooks and the transition toward discrete quanta of information that facilitate delivery through the digital milieu. Indeed, the last punctuation within methods and models of didactic delivery was the printing press, adding accessibility and reproducibility of knowledge previously impossible. Similarly, the transition of paper texts to digital texts will add another indelible exclamation mark in the advancement of didactic methods. My hope is that *Core Techniques in Operative Neurosurgery* will lead that evolution.

Rahul Jandial

Acknowledgments

I would like to thank the Elsevier team that has helped bring this project to fruition: Adrianne Brigido, Julie Goolsby, Cheryl Abbott, and most of all, Taylor Ball.

Rahul Jandial

Contents

PART ONE · CRANIAL

Section 1 GENERAL

Section Editor: Alfredo Quiñones-Hinojosa, with Shaan M. Raza

Section 2 SKULL BASE

Section Editor: Andrew T. Parsa

Section 3 VASCULAR

Section Editor: Steven Giannotta, with Azadeh Farin

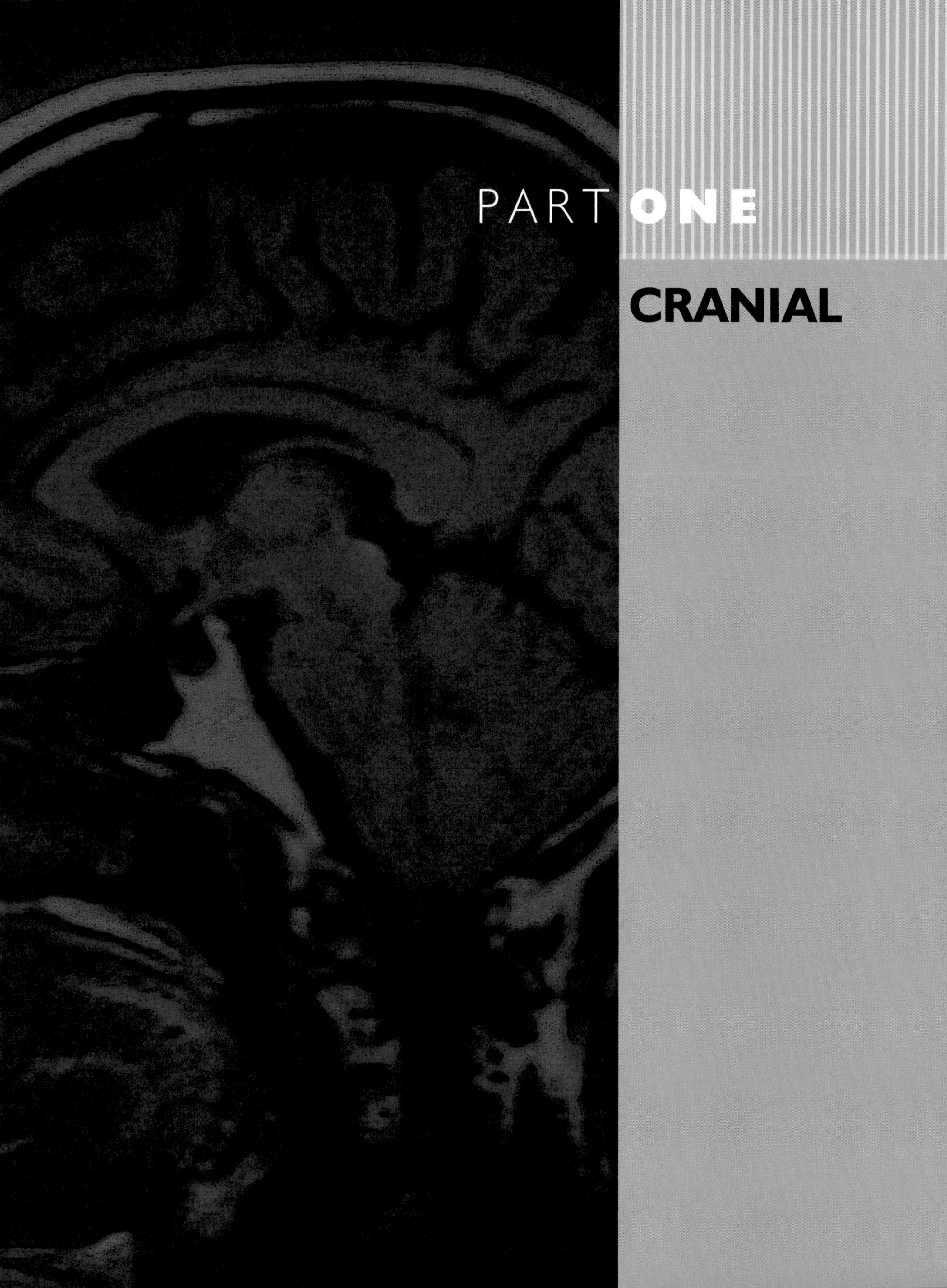

PART ONE

CRANIAL

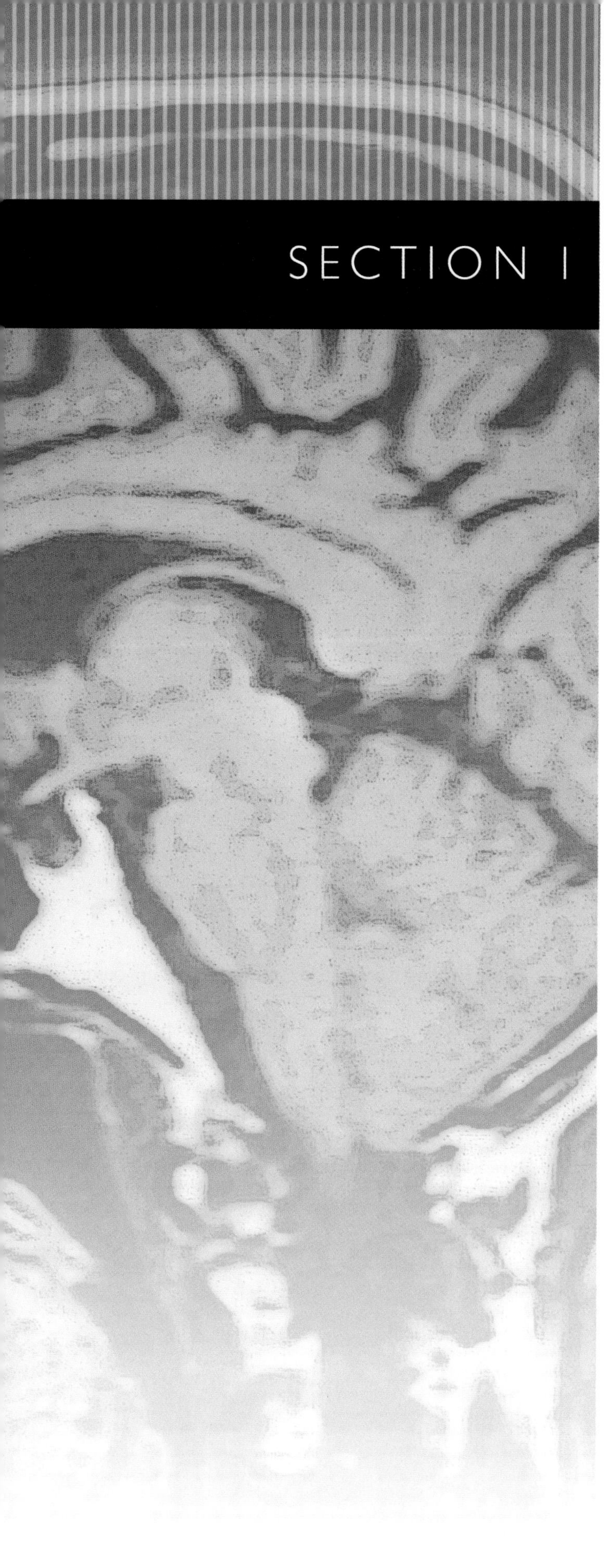

SECTION I General

SECTION EDITOR — ALFREDO QUIÑONES-HINOJOSA, WITH SHAAN M. RAZA

Procedure I

Pterional (Frontosphenotemporal) Craniotomy

Geoffrey P. Colby, Mohamad Bydon, Rafael J. Tamargo

INDICATIONS

- Surgical approach for clipping aneurysms of the anterior and posterior circulation (upper basilar and its proximal branches)
- Surgical approach for tumors of the anterior and middle cranial fossa, including sphenoid, parasellar, and cavernous sinus regions
- Resection of arteriovenous malformations of the perisylvian frontal and temporal regions

CONTRAINDICATIONS

- High-riding basilar aneurysms with the aneurysm neck significantly above the posterior clinoid are not amenable from this approach because the rostral angle is insufficient.
- Large parasellar or sellar tumors with significant superior extension are not amenable from this approach because the rostral angle is insufficient.

PLANNING AND POSITIONING

- Before initiating a surgical procedure, the patient should have had all the appropriate imaging studies, blood tests, and medical and cardiac clearance.
- The anesthesia team should have adequate peripheral or central access.
- Additional operative equipment (e.g., microscope) should be properly set up before beginning the surgery to reduce delay at critical points during the operation.
- Antibiotics are given to all patients before skin incision, and repeat doses are given as appropriate. Depending on the case, steroids, antiepileptics, and mannitol are also used.
- **Figure 1-1:** Positioning the patient and head. The patient is placed supine on the operating table with the ipsilateral shoulder elevated as needed to facilitate head rotation toward the contralateral side. The skull clamp is fixated with the paired posterior pins at the equator in the occipital bone and the single anterior pin at the equator in the contralateral frontal bone superior to the orbit. The head is positioned

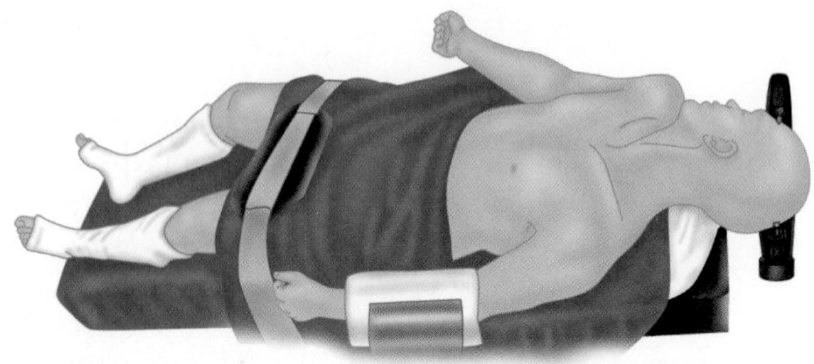

FIGURE 1-1

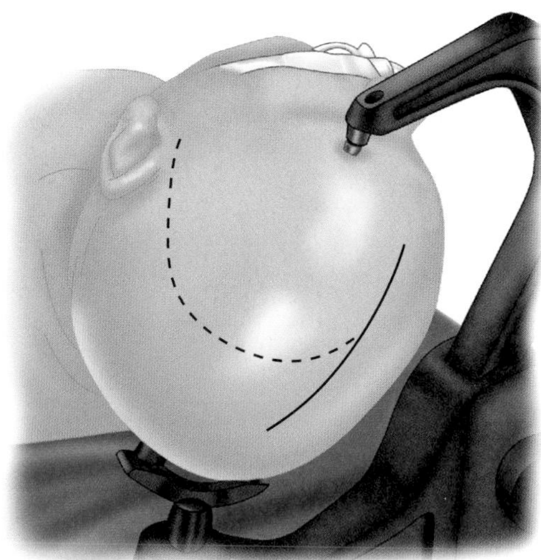

FIGURE 1-2

by first elevating the head above the heart in the "sniffing" position. Second, the head is rotated up to 60 degrees to the contralateral side depending on the intended operation. Third, the neck is extended so that the vertex is angled down 10 to 30 degrees, allowing for self-retraction of the frontal lobe off the anterior cranial fossa floor. When the head is ideally positioned, the malar eminence of the zygomatic bone should be the highest point in the operative field.

- **Figure 1-2:** Planning and marking the incision. Before drawing the incision, the midline is identified and marked. The incision for a pterional craniotomy is curvilinear and courses from the root of the zygoma to the anterior midline. The incision is divided into two segments. The first segment starts at the root of the zygoma (1 cm anterior to the tragus of the ear) and extends to the linea temporalis. This section can be angled anteriorly or posteriorly for varied exposure. The second segment extends anteriorly and superiorly from the linea temporalis to the midline just behind the hairline.

PROCEDURE

- **Figure 1-3:** Elevation of the skin flap. Starting at the anterior, midline portion of the marked incision and extending to the linea temporalis, the scalp is cut full-thickness (including galea aponeurotica and pericranium) down to the bone with a No. 10 blade. Raney clips are applied to the scalp edges for hemostasis. Plastic and towel

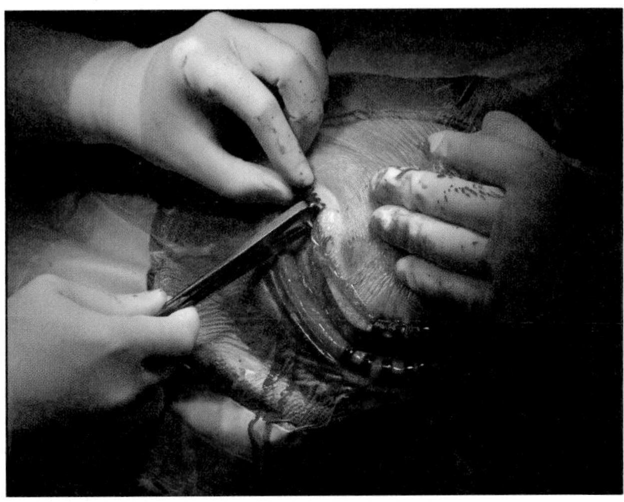

FIGURE 1-3

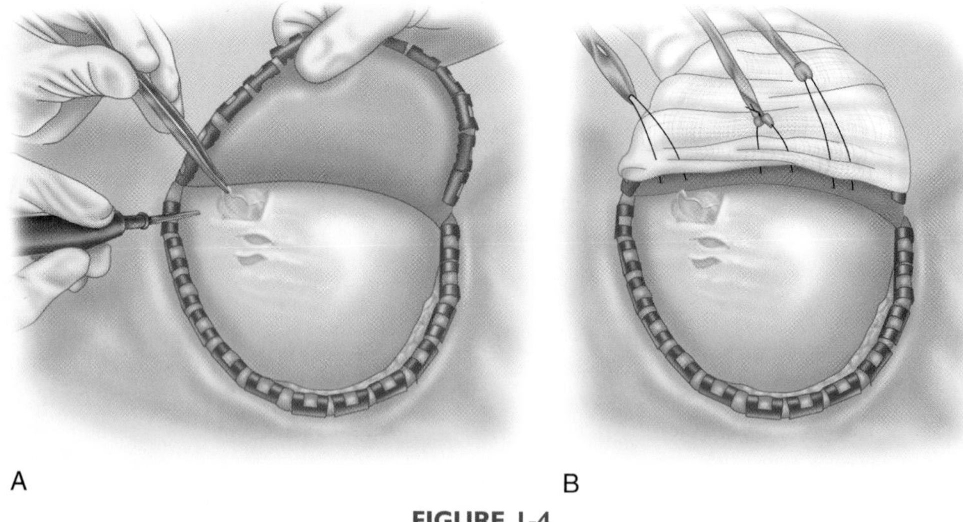

FIGURE 1-4

drape edges are included in the applied Raney clip when possible to secure the drapes in position; this maneuver also helps hold the clip in position when the scalp is thin. After Raney clips are applied to this section, the next section of the incision is addressed. Before making a cut, the remaining scalp is bluntly dissected from the temporal fascia with an instrument (e.g., fan-shaped periosteal elevator). The skin is incised down to the level of the temporal fascia, using blunt dissection when necessary to preserve the superficial temporal artery, and Raney clips are applied.

- **Figure 1-4:** Preservation of the frontalis branch of the facial nerve. The frontalis branch of the facial nerve is found in the fibrofatty tissue ("fat pad") deep to the superficial temporalis fascia. The scalp flap is reflected anteriorly until the fat pad is visualized, at which point the fascia is incised and the frontalis branch is elevated via the interfascial dissection of the skin flap (**A**). The scalp flap is wrapped in a moist gauze sponge and anchored anteriorly by suture retraction (**B**).
- **Figure 1-5:** Elevation of the temporalis muscle. Starting approximately 1.5 thumb widths posterior to the frontozygomatic process and along the linea temporalis (**A**), a cuff of temporalis muscle is preserved (**B** and **C**). The remaining temporalis muscle is elevated off the skull using a subperiosteal dissection (**B**) to preserve the deep temporal arteries and nerves. The temporalis muscle is reflected anteriorly and inferiorly, and it is anchored in place with suture retraction (**C**).
- **Figure 1-6:** Drilling burr holes and preparation of the craniotomy flap. Five burr holes are made with a self-arresting perforator drill in the following locations: *1* at the keyhole; *2* above the root of the zygoma; *3* inferior to the linea temporalis, approximately 1 cm above the temporal squamosa, in line with the zygomatic root (under the muscle cuff); *4* anterior to the coronal suture; and *5* in the anterior frontal bone above the orbit and frontal sinus (**A**). The keyhole burr hole is best made with a 5-mm high-speed drill. At each burr hole site, the dura is freed from the bone using a Penfield No. 3, and the inner table is undermined in the direction of neighboring burr holes using a Kerrison punch (**B**) so that a Lahey retractor can be passed with ease. A trough is drilled with a 5-mm cutting bit in the sphenoid and temporal bone between the burr holes at the keyhole and zygomatic root (**B**).
- **Figure 1-7:** Removal of the bone flap. The Gigli saw is used to connect the burr holes and complete the craniotomy. The Gigli saw makes a thin, beveled cut that eventually results in a superior cosmetic appearance. After the burr holes are properly undermined, the Gigli guide is passed between adjacent burr holes, and the Gigli saw is set up. Before using the saw, the assistant stabilizes the head and the bone flap by placing his or her fingers at burr holes, similar to gripping a bowling ball (**A**). The cut is made with the Gigli saw by using a fluid back-and-forth motion (**A**). The craniotomy flap is freed by a controlled fracture of the greater wing of the sphenoid. The final bone flap with attached muscle cuff appears as shown (**B**).

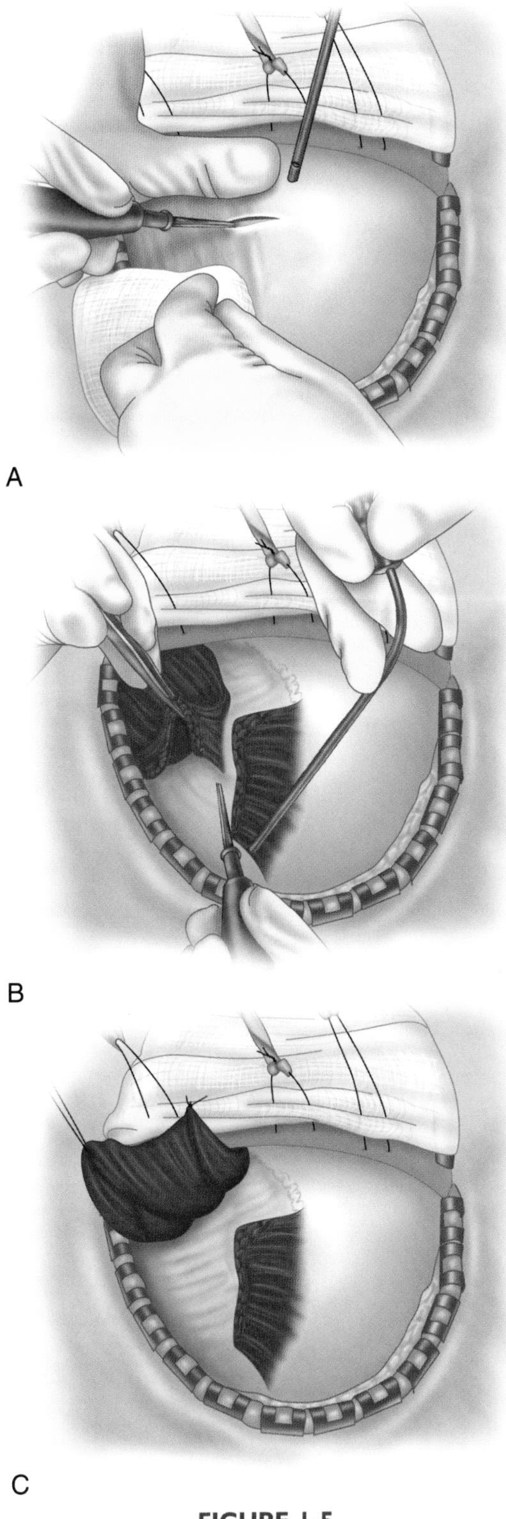

FIGURE 1-5

- **Figure 1-8:** Subtemporal exposure and drilling of frontal and sphenoid bones. Temporal bone is removed with a rongeur (as low as the floor of the middle cranial fossa) to achieve the desired subtemporal decompression (**A**). Further bony work is done to connect the anterior and middle cranial fossa. This is accomplished by first flattening the orbital roof and the inner table of the frontal bone with a high-speed drill. Special care is taken to avoid entering the orbit or the frontal sinus (see Bailout Options section for repair). Second, the lesser wing of the sphenoid is removed using a drill

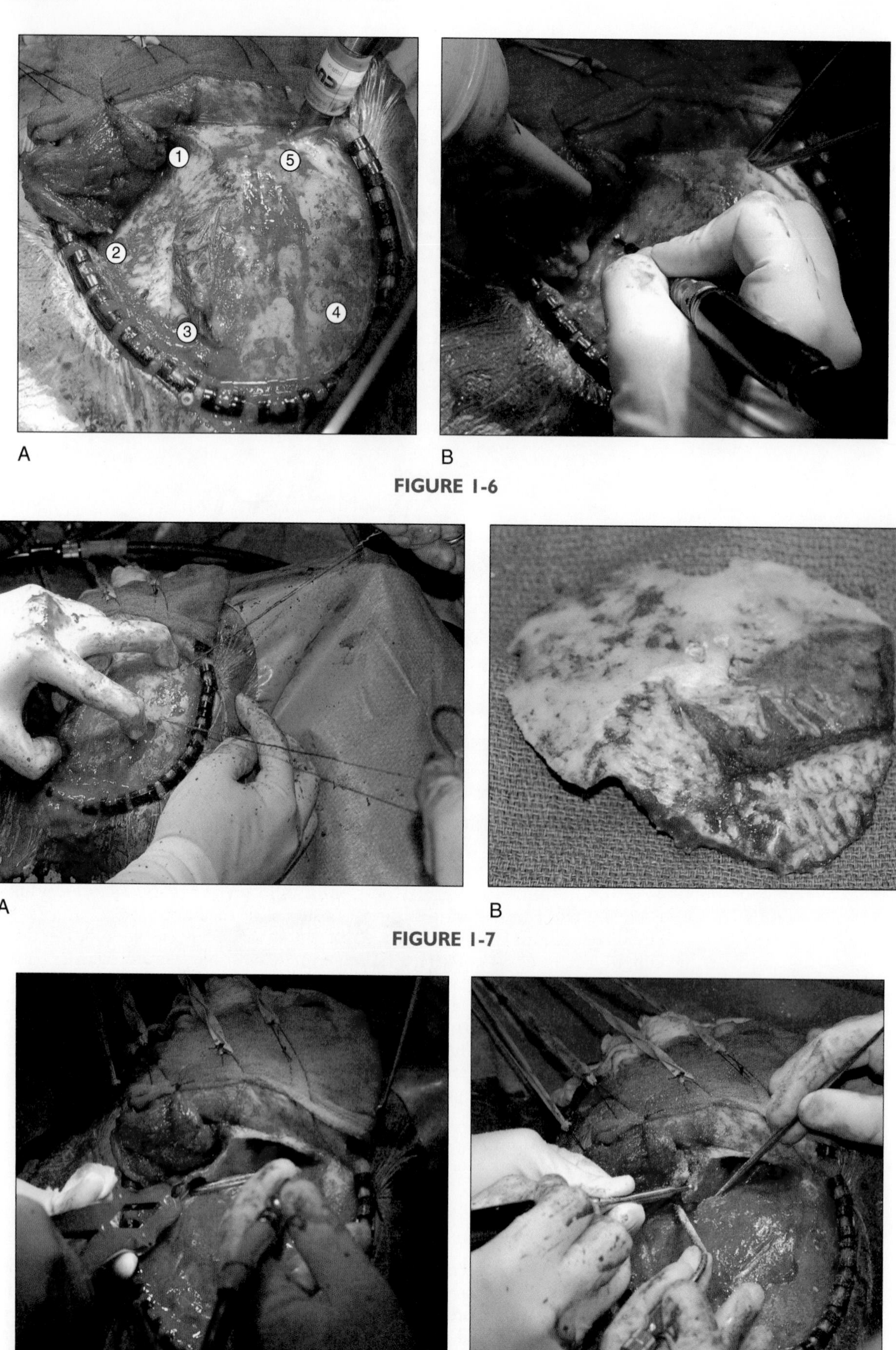

FIGURE 1-6

FIGURE 1-7

FIGURE 1-8

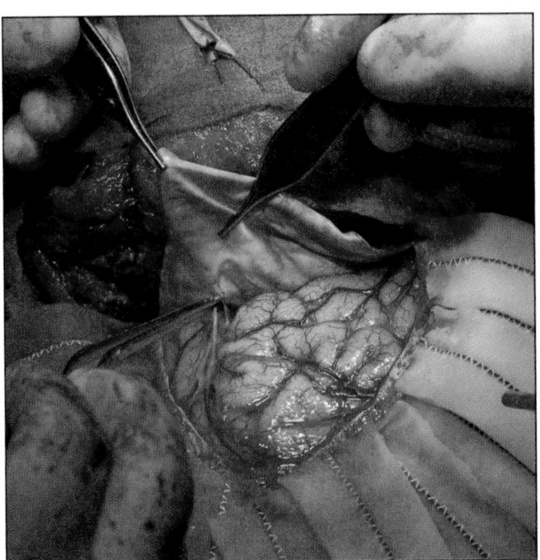
A

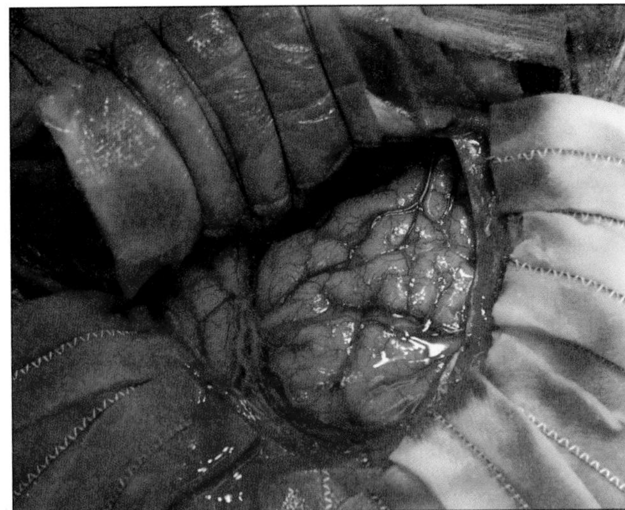
B

FIGURE 1-9

(**B**) and bone rongeurs until the orbitomeningeal artery is exposed. The assistant helps to reflect the dura and protect the brain during these steps (**B**). After these steps, dural tacking sutures are placed (not illustrated) to prevent extension of a postoperative epidural hematoma.

- **Figure 1-9:** Elevating the dural flap. Before opening the dura, cottonoids are placed at the bone flap edges to wick any bleeding. The dura is opened to create a semicircular flap and is reflected anteriorly. The initial dural cut should be done away from the sylvian fissure, and special care should be taken to dissect any bridging veins and other adhesions when reflecting the dura (**A**). To prevent desiccation of the dura (which makes closure more difficult), one should cover the dura with wet Telfa pad and then anchor it anteriorly with suture retraction (**B**). The bony work should be sufficient such that the dura rests flat on the anterior margin of the bony opening, and the stitches placed for suture retraction should be as low as possible on the dural flap to prevent the flap from falling into the field and obstructing the operator's view.
- **Figure 1-10:** Anterior clinoidectomy: bony exposure. After the pterional craniotomy is complete and the sylvian dissection is accomplished, the intradural anterior clinoid is visualized. Under special circumstances, it is advantageous to remove the anterior clinoid. The dura covering the anterior clinoid is devascularized with bipolar coagulation (**A**) and incised with a No. 11 blade in a semilunar fashion with the base above the optic nerve. This dural flap is reflected down toward the optic nerve (**B**) and cut sharply with microscissors (**C**). Some surgeons prefer to leave this flap reflected downward to help protect the optic nerve while drilling the anterior clinoid. The authors prefer to remove this dural flap, however, so that it does not get caught in the drill bit and secondarily injure the nerve or rupture the aneurysm.
- **Figure 1-11:** Anterior clinoidectomy: drilling. The anterior clinoid is drilled using a 3- and 2-mm cutting bur (**A**) with constant irrigation to prevent thermal injury to the optic nerve and to improve visualization in the field. A diamond drill bit is avoided because it generates too much heat and can cause a thermal injury of the optic nerve. When the appropriate amount of drilling is complete, the falciform ligament is cut sharply (**B**), and the optic nerve can be mobilized.
- **Figure 1-12:** Closure. After the dura is adequately closed with 4-0 braided nylon suture, and a central tack-up stitch is placed, the bone flap is reapproximated and fixed to the skull with titanium burr hole covers and a titanium mesh (**A**). The frontozygomatic fossa is covered with a titanium mesh. The temporalis muscle is sutured to the titanium mesh (**B**) and the remaining muscle cuff on the bone flap (**C**) using nonabsorbable sutures. The scalp is realigned using the perpendicular etch marks from Figure 1-3 and closed in two layers, galea and skin.

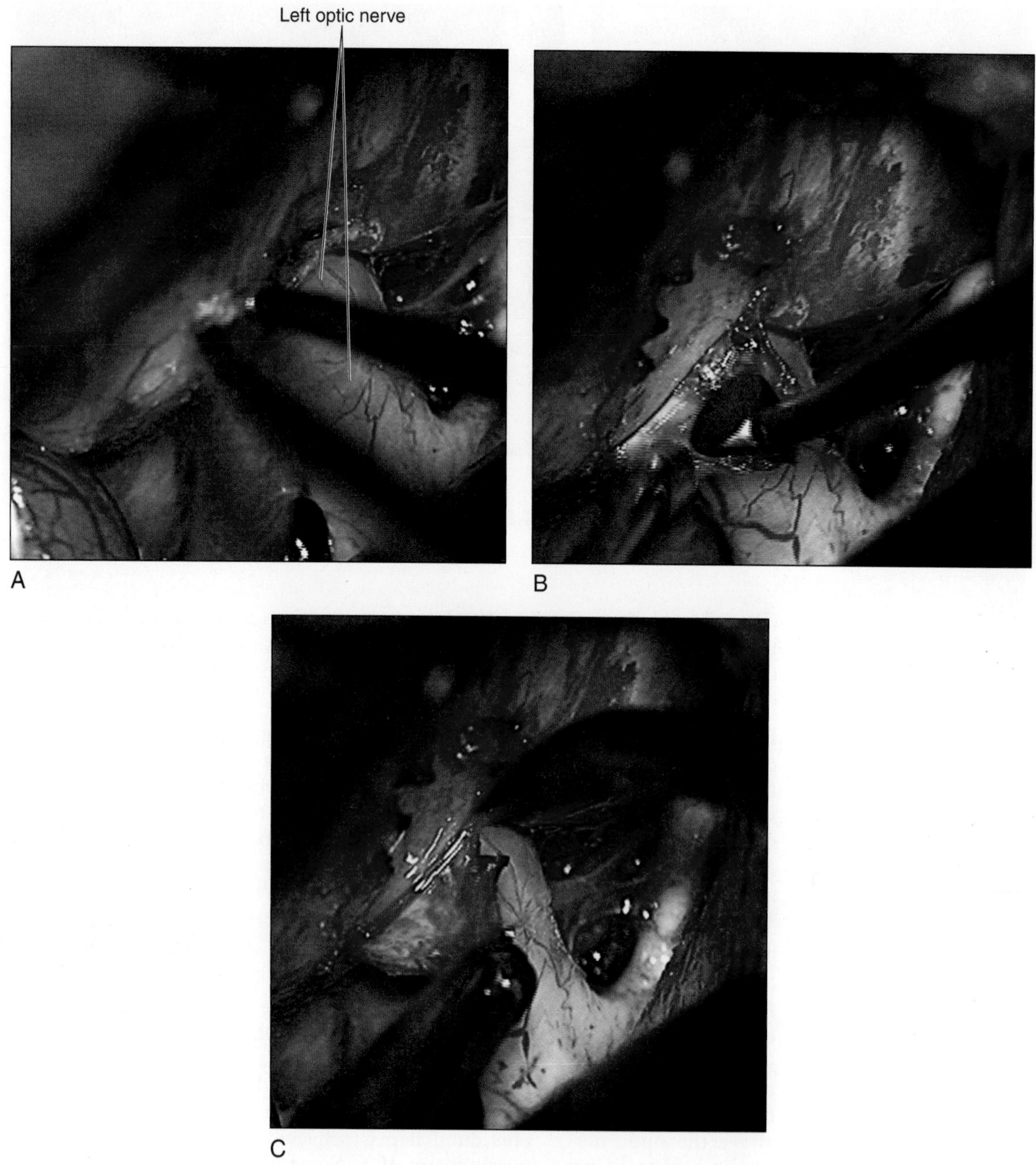

FIGURE 1-10

TIPS FROM THE MASTERS

- The Gigli saw is preferred for the craniotomy cuts for several reasons. The cuts are thinner than with other available craniotomes, which facilitates reapproximation of the bone flap and allows for superior esthetic results. Gigli saw cuts are beveled, creating a powerful, more natural bony barrier to depression of the flap that allows patients to participate in contact sports if they choose. With proper undermining of the burr holes, the Gigli guide and saw can be passed with excellent protection of the dura.
- When brain relaxation and cerebrospinal fluid drainage are indicated, such as in a craniotomy for aneurysm clipping, a maneuver can be performed to achieve early relaxation. Before turning a full dural flap, a small opening in the dura is made, and the sulcal subarachnoid space visible through this hole is opened sharply. This opening

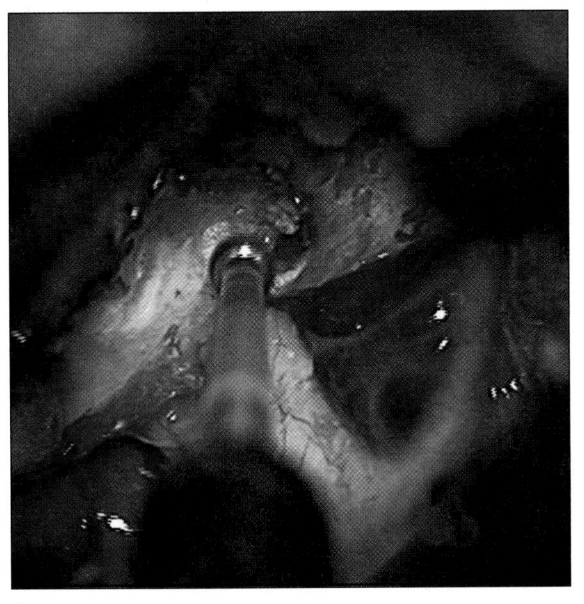

A

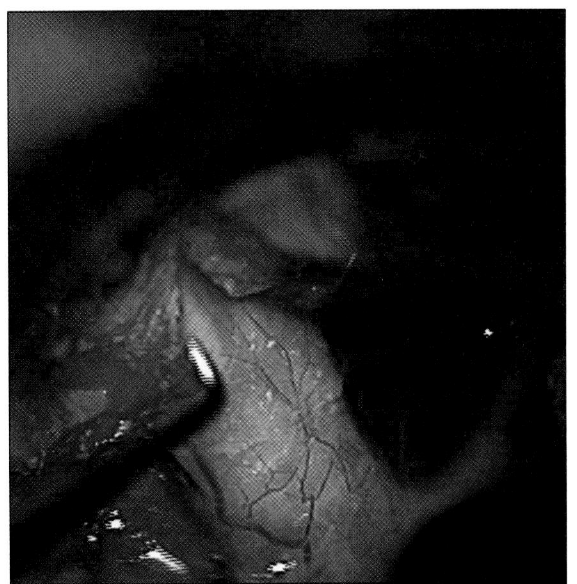

B

FIGURE 1-11

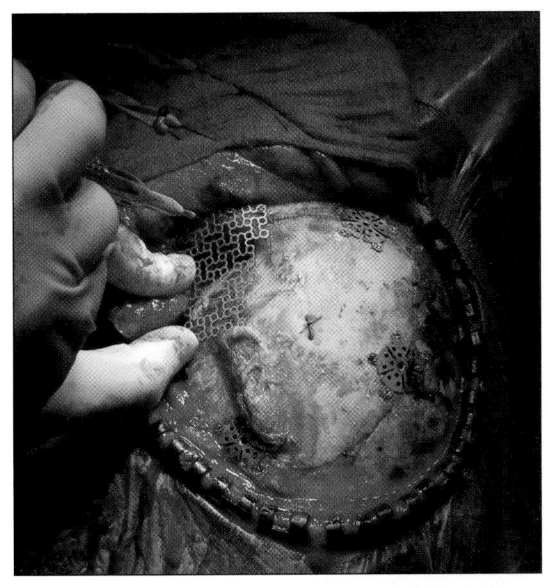

A

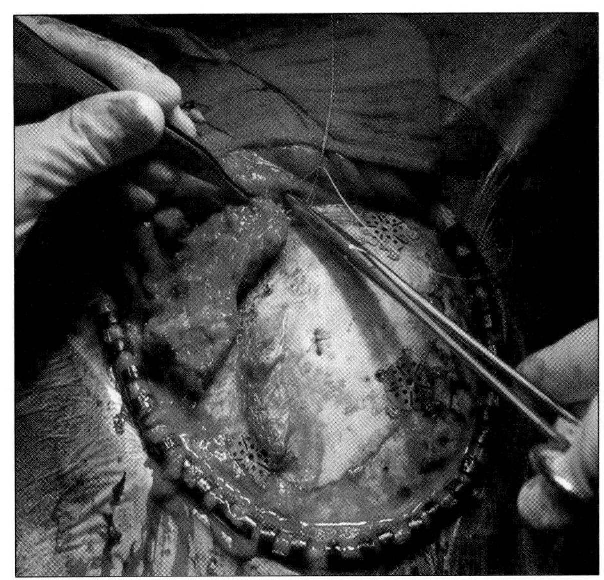

B

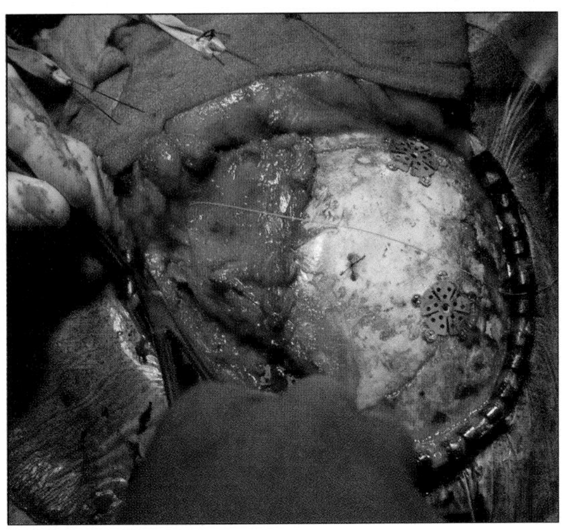

C

FIGURE 1-12

allows continuous cerebrospinal fluid (CSF) drainage to occur while the full dural flap is turned and the field is prepared for cisternal dissection.

- Superior cosmetic results are obtained with titanium cranioplasty over the frontozygomatic fossa. This approach reduces the incidence of long-term postoperative muscle depression and cosmetic defects in this region.
- The pterional craniotomy is used in conjunction with various extensions (e.g., orbitozygomatic) to increase the working area, increase the angle of attack, and minimize brain retraction.
- During anterior clinoidectomy, copious irrigation should be used while drilling to prevent thermal injury to the optic nerve.

PITFALLS

Breach of the frontal sinus can cause higher rates of CSF leak, pneumocephalus, and infection.

Large lesions require additional bone removal to decrease the amount of brain retraction required.

BAILOUT OPTIONS

- If the frontal sinus is entered, it should be fully cranialized, exenterated, and filled with hydroxyapatite.
- When the orbit or periorbita is violated, care should be taken to minimize intraorbital bleeding by inserting oxidized cellulose into the opening and bipolaring any obvious bleeding vessels.
- In the event that the Gigli guide is passed subdurally, it is left in place, and a separate guide is passed over it in the opposite direction.

SUGGESTED READINGS

Andaluz N, Beretta F, Bernucci C, et al. Evidence for the improved exposure of the ophthalmic segment of the internal carotid artery after anterior clinoidectomy: morphometric analysis. Acta Neurochir (Wien) 2006;148:971–5.

Gonzalez LF, Crawford NR, Horgan MA, et al. Working area and angle of attack in three cranial base approaches: pterional, orbitozygomatic, and maxillary extension of the orbitozygomatic approach. Neurosurgery 2002;50:550–5.

Kadri PS, Al-Mefty O. The anatomical basis for surgical preservation of temporal muscle. J Neurosurg 2004;100:517–22.

Raza SM, Thai QA, Pradilla G, et al. Frontozygomatic titanium cranioplasty in frontosphenotemporal ("pterional") craniotomy. Neurosurgery 2008;62:262–4.

Yasargil MG, Reichman MV, Kubik S. Preservation of the frontotemporal branch of the facial nerve using the interfascial temporalis flap for pterional craniotomy. Technical article. J Neurosurg 1987;67:463–6.

Procedure 2

Occipital Craniotomy

Jorge E. Alvernia, Nnenna Mbabuike, Marcus L. Ware

INDICATIONS

- The occipital craniotomy is a versatile approach that provides access to the occipital lobes; tentorium; torcular Herophili; transverse sinus; sigmoid sinus; and tumors, vascular malformations, or other lesions that may be associated with these structures.

CONTRAINDICATIONS

- Cervical spine pathology that would oppose flexion of the neck
- Persistent foramen ovale (echocardiogram should be performed if the sitting or semisitting position is considered)

PLANNING AND POSITIONING

- Three positions may be used for the occipital craniotomy.
  - Prone position
  - Concorde position

    Secure the head in a head holder before turning the head. The head is flexed, and the bed is tilted, elevating the head above the heart.

    Advantages include lower incidence of air embolism than sitting (10% vs. 25%) and increased comfort for the surgeon.

    Disadvantages include venous air embolism and injury to cervical spine.
  - Park bench position

    This is also known as the three-quarter prone position.

    The head is secured in the head holder before turning. The patient's torso is brought to the side opposite of which the patient is turned so that when turned, the patient's backside rests at the edge of the bed.

    A roll should be placed under the dependent axilla to protect the brachial plexus. The dependent arm is placed over the end of the table, and the upper arm is supported on a pillow or roll and flexed at the elbow.

    Advantages include optimal access to lesions of the median parafalcial, occipital, and pineal region, and the occipital lobe falls away from the falx, allowing for less retraction.

    Disadvantages include venous congestion possibly resulting from the head turn and possible cervical injury.

PROCEDURE

- **Figure 2-1:** Incision for an occipital craniotomy extends through the median of posterior cranial fossa. The skin flap ensures that the blood supply of the occiput is spared. A semicircular or arcuate incision extending downward toward the transverse sinus is made depending on how far infratentorial the field may need to be extended.
- **Figure 2-2:** Craniotomy. Burr hole is made 1 to 2 cm lateral to midline and 2 cm below the external occipital protuberance and superior nuchal line representing the plane of

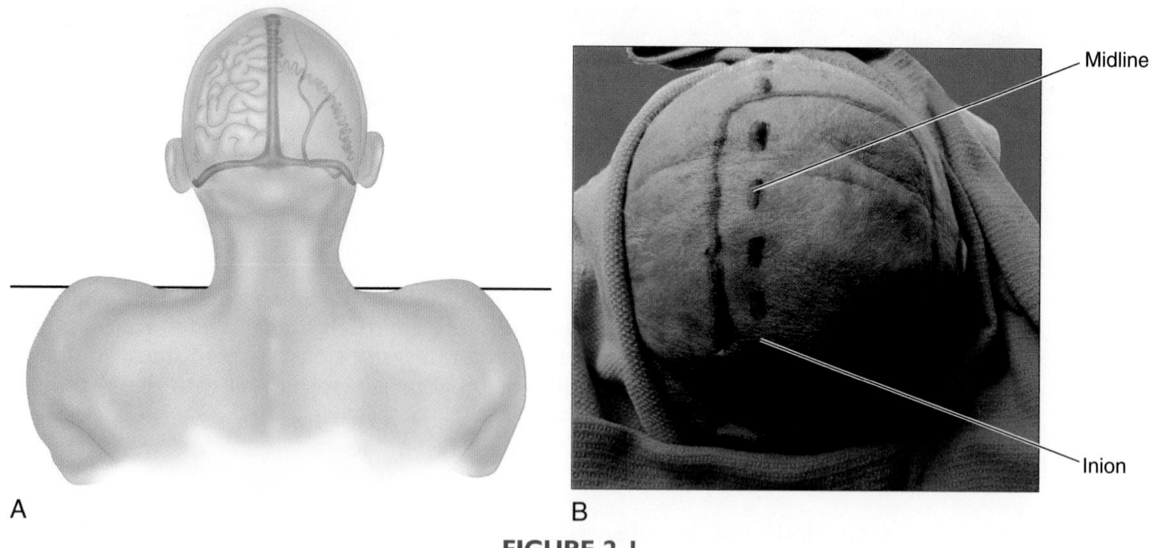

FIGURE 2-1

transverse sinus. The craniotomy stops 2 cm short of the sagittal sinus in the case of transcortical approaches; however, partial or complete exposure of the superior sagittal sinus or the transverse sinus may be needed with posterior interhemispheric or suboccipital approaches. The cranial flap is made with the transverse sinus in the inferior border and the sagittal sinus in the medial border. Occipital V. = occipital vein; Rolandic V. = rolandic vein; S.S.S. = superior sagittal sinus.

- **Figure 2-3:** Supratentorial approach. Dural incision is made with a broad base in the direction of the sagittal sinus or the transverse sinus. The occipital lobe may be lifted off the tentorium and falx for access to the pineal region and supratentorial and infratentorial surface. Bridging veins from the occipital lobe into the superior sagittal sinus may be seen, and if necessary they can be sacrificed. Special care must be taken when lifting up the occipital lobe to prevent tearing of the vein of Labbé mainly when working on the left dominant hemisphere. Post. occ. v. = posterior occipital vein; Post. temp. v. = posterior temporal vein; S.S.S. = superior sagittal sinus; Tent. = tentorium; Tent. s. = tentorial sinus.
- **Figure 2-4:** Occipital transcortical approach. Dural incision at the base includes the sagittal sinus. Direct access to the occipital lobe is now possible. A transventricular

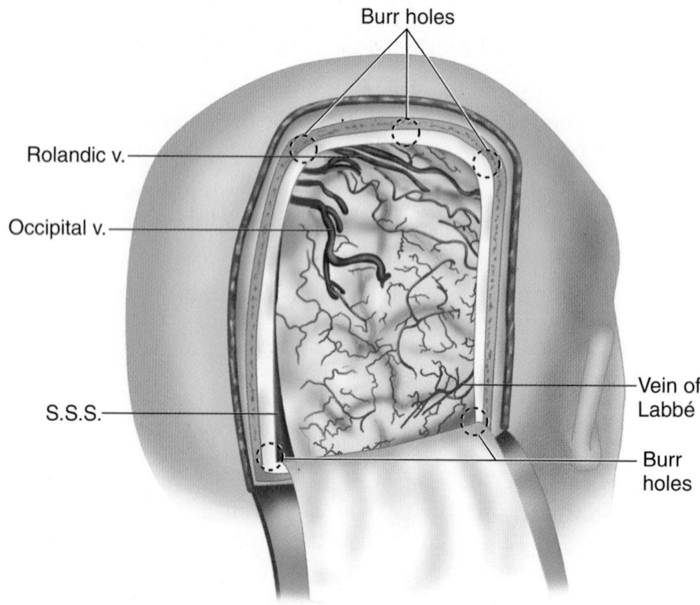

FIGURE 2-2

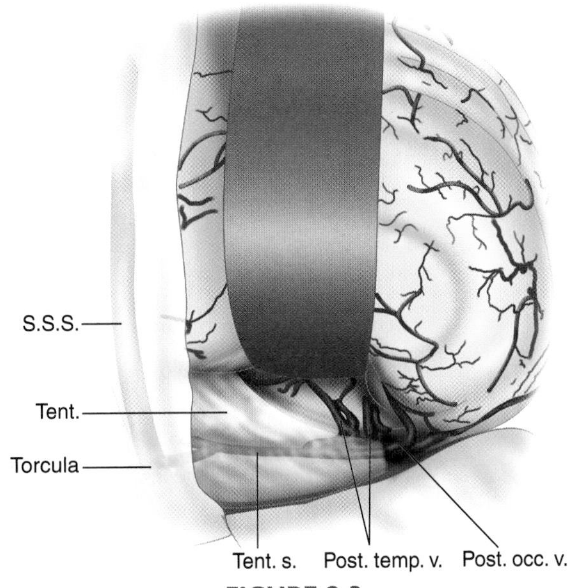

FIGURE 2-3

approach is accessible. Lat. Atr. V. = lateral atrial vein; Occipital v. = occipital vein; Post. lat. chor. a. = posterior lateral choroidal artery; S.S.S. = superior sagittal sinus.

TIPS FROM THE MASTERS

- To decrease the likelihood of air embolism in the sitting position, continuous irrigation with water over the surgical field and close end-tidal CO_2 monitoring with a central line in place to remove air if needed is recommended.
- In the case of large lesions located bilaterally on the notch of the tentorium, the unilateral view of the occipital transtentorial approach is aided by cutting through the falx and tentorium on the other side to achieve complete resection of the lesion.
- The occipital transtentorial approach provides a good working angle along the anterior aspect of the cerebellum within the precentral cerebellar fissure (Moshel et al, 2009).
- It is recommended to limit the interhemispheric occipital transtentorial approach to lesions of the upper part of the precentral cerebellar fissure with primarily superior

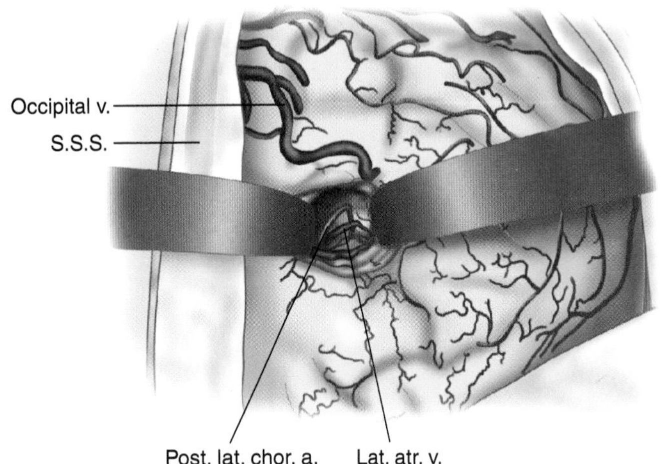

FIGURE 2-4

exterior extension into the posterior incisural space, which decreases the need for occipital lobe retraction and the incidence of transient visual loss.

PITFALLS
Air embolism
Injury to the brain as a result of overzealous brain retraction
Injury to the dura or sinuses during craniotomy
Cerebrospinal fluid leak secondary to lack of a watertight closure
Postoperative epidural hematoma because of inadequate elevation of the dura on closure
Avulsion of bridging veins

BAILOUT OPTIONS

- Temporary control of bleeding from the sinus may be achieved by holding pressure on the sinus for 5 minutes. Gelfoam with fibrin glue may also be used to patch temporarily small injuries to the sinuses. Venous reconstruction may be performed using patches or bypasses with postoperative anticoagulation to avoid venous thrombosis.
- In the case of mastoid cell opening, plug and closure with fat is recommended. Bone wax may be used for very small openings.

SUGGESTED READINGS

Kawashima M, Rhoton AL Jr, Matsushima T. Comparison of posterior approaches to the posterior incisural space: microsurgical anatomy and proposal of a new method, the occipital bi-transtentorial/falcine approach. Neurosurgery 2002;52:1208–21.

Kurokawa Y, Uede T, Hashi K. Operative approach to mediosuperior cerebellar tumors: occipital interhemispheric transtentorial approach. Surg Neurol 1999;51:421–5.

Moshel YA, Parker EC, Kelly PJ. Occipital transtentorial approach to the precentral cerebellar fissure and posterior incisural space. Neurosurgery 2009;65:554–64.

Sato O. Transoccipital transtentorial approach for removal of cerebellar haemangioblastoma. Acta Neurochir (Wien) 1981;59:195–208.

Shirane R, Kumabe T, Yoshida Y, et al. Surgical treatment of posterior fossa tumors via the occipital transtentorial approach: evaluation of operative safety and results in 14 patients with anterosuperior cerebellar tumors. J Neurosurg 2001;94:927–35.

Tymowski M, Majchrzak K. Surgical treatment of tentorial and falco-tentorial junction meningiomas. Minim Invas Neurosurg 2009;52:93–7.

Procedure 3

Temporal and Frontotemporal Craniotomy

Shaan M. Raza, Alfredo Quiñones-Hinojosa

INDICATIONS

- Treatment option in temporal lobe epilepsy for patients in whom anticonvulsant medications do not control epileptic seizures
- Techniques for removing temporal lobe tissue, such as in anterior temporal lobectomy, and for more restricted removal of only the medial structures, such as in selective amygdalohippocampectomy
- Treatment of temporal brain tumors, including intraventricular tumors in the anterior temporal horn or intraaxial temporal lobe tumors such as intrinsic glioma
- Treatment of temporal lobe lesions of unknown etiology, such as an infection
- Treatment of trauma to the middle meningeal injury with epidural hematoma, subdural component, and temporal lobe contusions
- Treatment of vascular lesions, such as aneurysms, arteriovenous malformations, and cavernomas

CONTRAINDICATIONS

- If lesions go above the sylvian fissure, a limited temporal craniotomy may not be enough to reach the lesion components above the fissure, and the craniotomy may need to be extended.
- If the lesion is in the dominant hemisphere, special consideration should be given to obtaining functional magnetic resonance imaging (MRI) or doing an awake craniotomy with speech mapping.

PLANNING AND POSITIONING

- Plan to give steroids and antibiotics depending on the lesion.
- Plan to give 0.5 to 1.0 g/kg of mannitol for brain relaxation if necessary.
- If the patient is to be awake during the procedure, ensure that the face is clear of any obstruction for the speech or motor mapping. Also ensure enough local anesthetic is administered at the site of pin insertion of the fixation device.
- **Figure 3-1:** The patient is placed in the supine position with a small roll under the ipsilateral shoulder. The head is rotated 30 to 75 degrees away from the lesion, and it can be declined 15 to 20 degrees depending on the location of the lesion. Special care should be taken to ensure that all areas of the body are properly padded to avoid skin injuries, especially if the case is long.
- Surgical navigation can be registered at this point per the preference of the surgeon and depending on the likely pathology. Tumors are more likely to require surgical navigation than vascular lesions in general.
- After the patient is given antibiotics, the patient is prepared in a sterile fashion, and local anesthetic is placed on the skin, one can proceed with incision of the skin.
- **Figure 3-2:** Skin incision is performed after the patient is placed in position. Care must be taken with the superficial temporal artery. If this artery is not properly cauterized, it can be a potential source of a postoperative epidural hematoma.

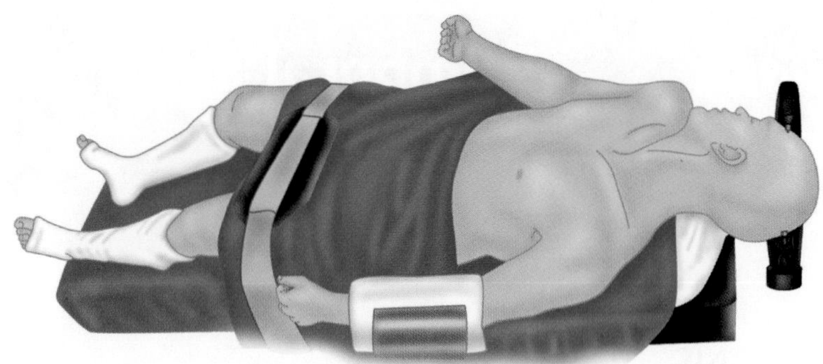

FIGURE 3-1

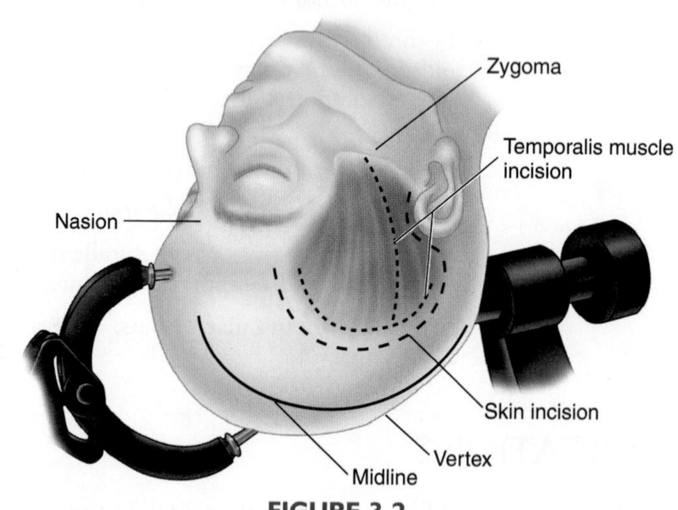

FIGURE 3-2

- Sometimes a hair-sparing technique can be used that requires shaving only a ¼-inch-wide area along the proposed incision.

PROCEDURE

- **Figure 3-3:** When the scalp flap is reflected anteriorly, a selective temporal or a larger frontotemporal craniotomy is performed depending on the extent of resection or the location of the lesion. Ideally, the burr holes are made under the muscle for good cosmetic outcomes. A temporalis muscle cuff should be preserved for closure. Selective temporal craniotomy is performed by connecting the keyhole (*1*), inferior temporal (*2*), and posterior temporal (*3*) burr holes. If a frontotemporal craniotomy is needed, the craniotomy extends into the frontal region using the same burr hole sites.
- **Figure 3-4:** The dura is reflected anteriorly exposing the surface of the brain. Moist Telfa pads should be used to prevent desiccation of the dura and to cover the surrounding craniotomy site. During dural opening, one must preserve not only the sylvian veins, but also the vein of Labbé (at the posterior margin of the dural incision). In addition, the surgeon must pay attention to the temporal veins draining into the sphenoparietal sinus. If necessary, these veins should be sacrificed in a controlled fashion as close to the temporal lobe as possible to prevent uncontrolled bleeding from the sinus.
- **Figure 3-5:** For an anterior temporal lobectomy, one has to appreciate the lateral view of the left hemisphere. A distance of 4 to 5 cm is measured over the middle temporal gyrus from the anterior wall of the middle fossa of the dominant side; this distance can be up to 5 to 6 cm for the nondominant side.

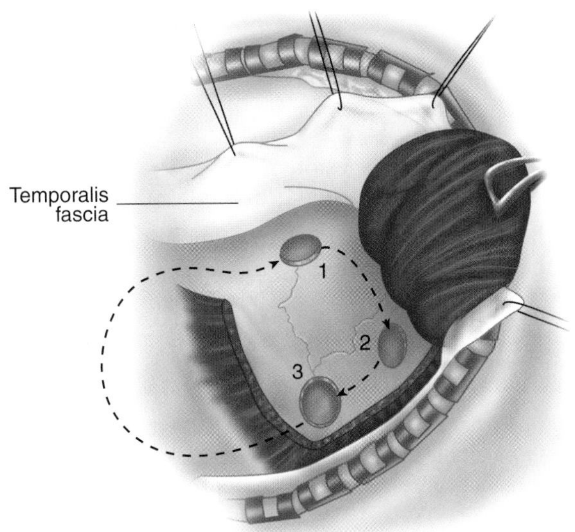

FIGURE 3-3

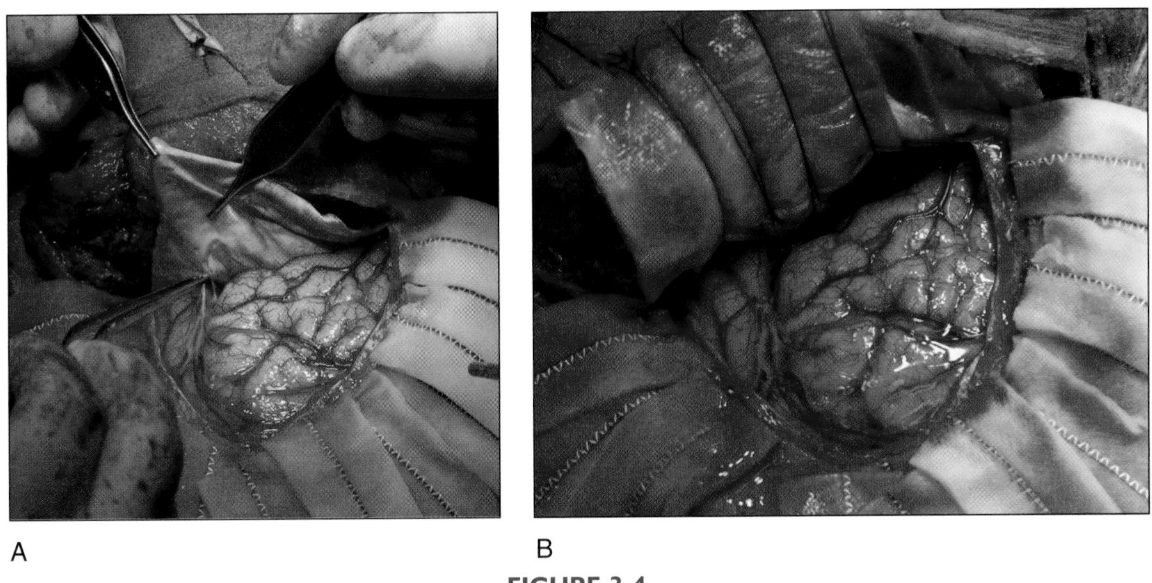

FIGURE 3-4

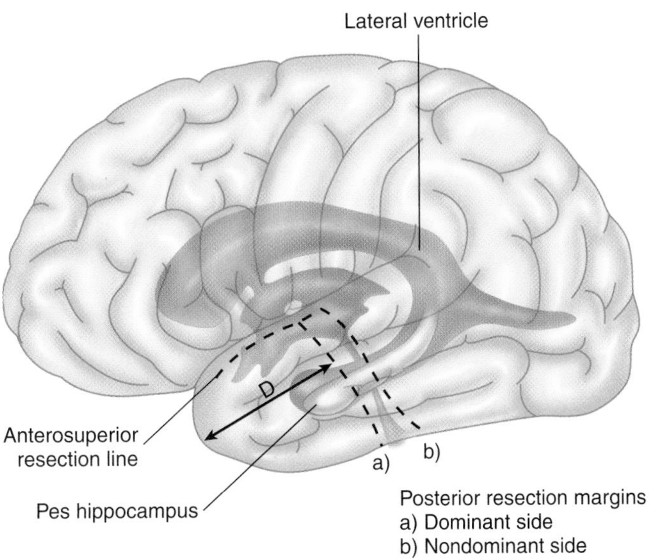

FIGURE 3-5

TIPS FROM THE MASTERS

- The reconstruction should be done well to avoid suboptimal cosmetic results.
- Special care should be taken when opening the dura to avoid injuring a large draining vein.
- If the lesion is very mesiotemporal, extraaxial, or high up in the incisura, sometimes it is better to perform more aggressive bone removal to minimize brain retraction.
- In the dominant hemisphere, to minimize speech damage, one must be constantly aware of the superior temporal gyrus and use speech mapping as needed.

PITFALLS

This approach may not work well for extraaxial lesions and lesions that are in the mesiotemporal lobe incisura region. Also, if lesions are suprachiasmatic, this approach may present difficulties in regard to appropriate exposure.

BAILOUT OPTIONS

- Orbital rim, zygomatic arch, and orbitozygomatic osteotomies can be useful adjuncts to the classic frontopterionotemporal craniotomy in facilitating the exposure of deep-seated skull base lesions, sparing brain retraction injuries.

SUGGESTED READINGS

Campero A, Tróccoli G, Martins C, et al. Microsurgical approaches to the medial temporal region: an anatomical study. Neurosurgery 2006;59(4 Suppl. 2):ONS279–307.

Rhoton AL Jr. The temporal bone and transtemporal approaches. Neurosurgery 2000;47(Suppl. 3):S211–65.

Yasargil MG, Krayenbühl N, Roth P, et al. The selective amygdalohippocampectomy for intractable temporal limbic seizures. J Neurosurg 2010;112:168–85.

Procedure 4

Subtemporal (Intradural and Extradural) Craniotomy

Shaan M. Raza, Graeme F. Woodworth, Alfredo Quiñones-Hinojosa

INDICATIONS

- This technique is preferred for lesions of the middle fossa (i.e., cavernous sinus, medial temporal lobe, tentorial region, petrous bone, incisura) and posterior fossa (i.e., extraaxial lesions in the petroclival region, intraaxial lesions in the anteromedial region of the superior cerebellum).
- It is ideal for lesions that can be approached via a right-sided craniotomy.
- Surgical adjuncts such as division of the tentorium, zygomatic osteotomy, and anterior petrosectomy can provide additional working space and versatility to this approach.

CONTRAINDICATIONS

- Left-sided approaches owing to the risk the approach places on the vein of Labbé
- Preoperative imaging showing the vein of Labbé to be in the path of the planned surgical trajectory
- Lesions extending below the internal auditory meatus (where tentorial sectioning, superior petrosal sinus ligation, or resection of petrous bone [Kawase triangle] no longer enable sufficient exposure)

PLANNING AND POSITIONING

- Preoperative planning includes assessment of the patient's cardiopulmonary status, evaluation of comorbidities, and basic laboratory tests, including a basic metabolic panel, complete blood count, coagulation profile, and type and screen. Baseline chest x-ray and electrocardiogram are also useful.
- Preoperative magnetic resonance venography is obtained to determine the caliber of and the location of the vein of Labbé. In addition, its drainage entrance into the transverse sinus can be determined.
- Within 60 minutes of skin incision, perioperative antibiotics are administered.
- Brain relaxation can be achieved by administering mannitol, dexamethasone, and mild hyperventilation.
- For all patients, a lumbar subarachnoid drain is inserted before pinning to facilitate temporal lobe retraction.
- **Figure 4-1:** The patient is positioned supine with a shoulder roll under the ipsilateral shoulder. After pinning, the head is angled 90 degrees from the vertical plane and then tilted approximately 20 degrees toward the floor such that the zygoma is the highest point in the field. This position allows for the temporal lobe to fall with gravity in addition to providing a line of view flush with the tentorium.

PROCEDURE

- **Figure 4-2:** A horseshoe incision is made beginning anteriorly at the zygomatic root extending superiorly to the superior temporal line and turning posteriorly to end at the asterion. During this process, an effort is made to preserve the superficial temporal

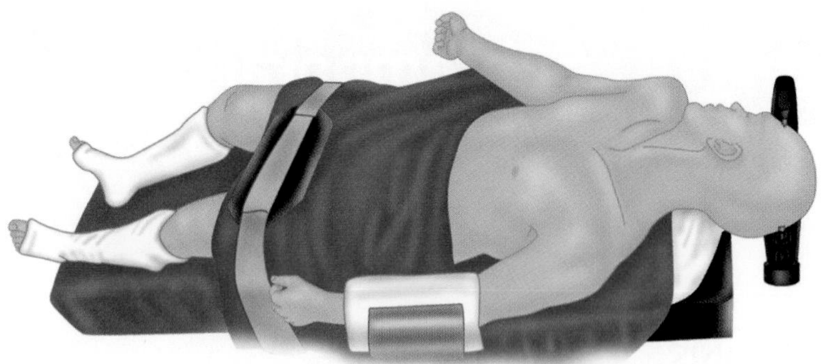

FIGURE 4-1

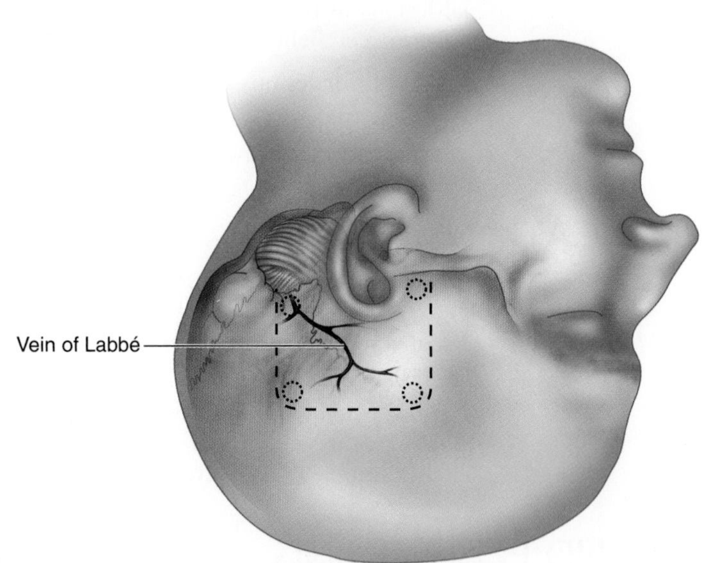

FIGURE 4-2

artery and its branches in case of the need for vascular bypass. A myocutaneous flap is raised with periosteal elevators and retracted inferiorly. In this process of dissection, the surgeon must be cognizant of the cartilaginous portion of the external auditory meatus because this can be inadvertently entered. The burr holes for the temporal craniotomy are placed at the following locations: squamosal temporal bone at the zygomatic root, superior temporal line, asterion flush with the middle fossa, and the remaining burr hole superiorly and behind the insertion of the vein of Labbé into the transverse sinus. A craniotome is used to create a flap flush with the floor of the middle cranial fossa. Approximately two thirds of the craniotomy is placed anterior to the external auditory meatus to maximize the middle fossa floor visualized for any drilling. Either a rongeur or a cutting drill is used to remove bone down to the floor of the middle fossa. Mastoid air cells are thoroughly waxed as they are encountered.

- **Figure 4-3:** If necessary, drilling of the middle fossa floor is performed before dural opening. Landmarks exposed after extradural dissection along the floor of the middle cranial fossa: arcuate eminence corresponding to the superior semicircular canal; greater superficial petrosal nerve delineating the lateral and medial aspects of the Kawase and Glasscock areas, and critical to safe removal of bone adjacent to the petrous carotid artery; mandibular branch of the trigeminal nerve, exiting through the foramen ovale.
- **Figure 4-4:** Inferiorly based U-shaped dural incision is made. In this process, extreme caution must be exercised to preserve the vein of Labbé. After incision, the vein of Labbé is identified and traced. As the subtemporal dissection proceeds, infratemporal veins draining into the tentorial dural lakes and transverse sinus are typically encountered. These venous structures often have a reciprocal relationship with the

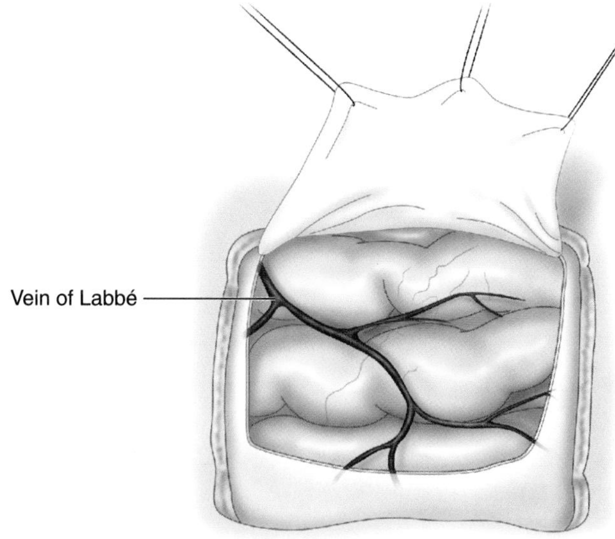

FIGURE 4-3

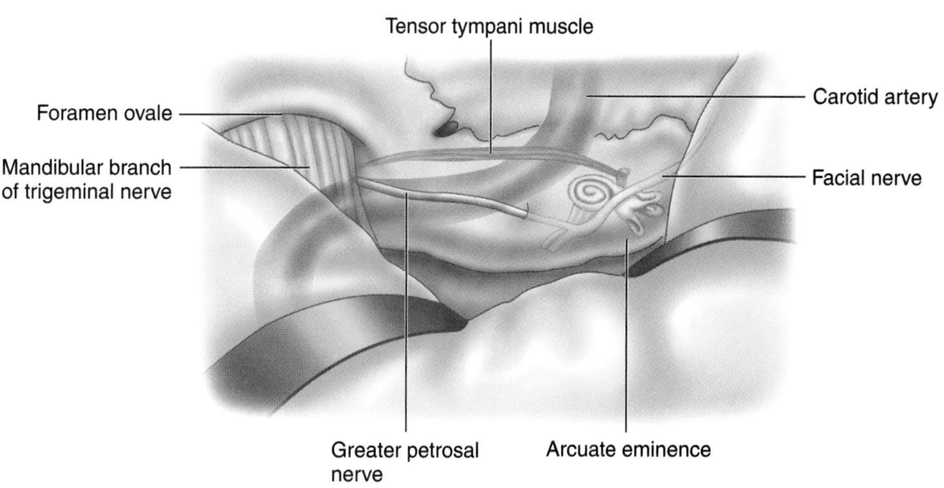

FIGURE 4-4

vein of Labbé with regard to flow. Surgical judgment must be practiced in deciding to sacrifice these veins in a controlled fashion.

- **Figure 4-5:** At this point, subtemporal dissection begins to permit elevation of the temporal lobe. This is done with the use of a malleable brain retractor. To facilitate this process, adequate brain relaxation must be obtained with the use of cerebrospinal fluid drainage from the lumbar drain, hyperventilation, and diuresis through use of mannitol and furosemide (Lasix). The subtemporal dissection proceeds until the brainstem and surrounding vasculature are visualized.
- **Figure 4-6:** The tentorial edge can be divided in a lateral-to-medial direction to access the posterior fossa. The trochlear nerve must be traced as it courses around the mesencephalon and enters the tentorial edge. Bipolar cautery is used on the tentorium along the proposed incision, which is ultimately made with a No. 11 blade. As the incision is made, the bipolar cautery is used to control bleeding from the tentorial venous sinuses and arteries of Bernasconi and Cassinari. The anterior and posterior flaps of the tentorium are retracted with 4-0 Surgilon sutures. At this point, further dissection proceeds according to the target lesion.
- Dural closure and bone reconstruction are performed according to standard practice; a titanium cranioplasty may be necessary to reconstruct the gap created by removal of bone down to the floor of the middle fossa. The lumbar drain is removed at case completion.

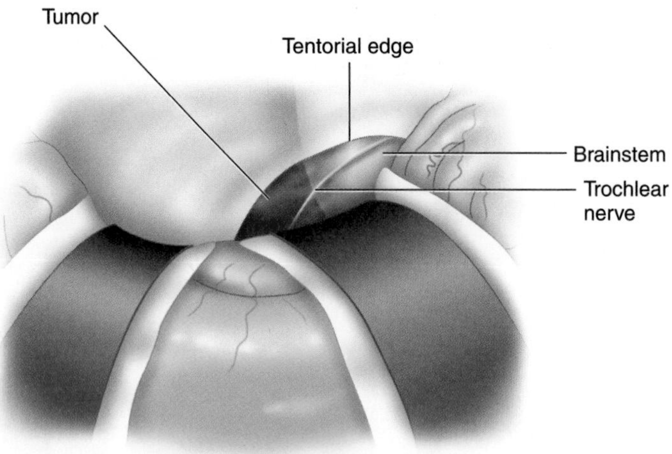

FIGURE 4-5

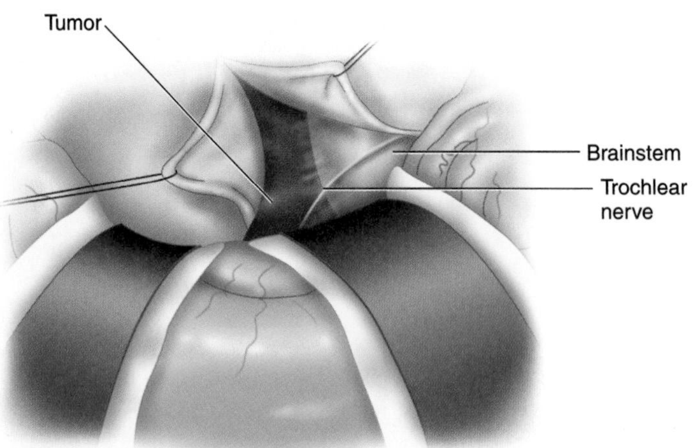

FIGURE 4-6

TIPS FROM THE MASTERS

- The primary risk is for injury of critical venous structures with subsequent temporal lobe venous infarcts or edema. Extreme caution and surgical judgment are needed in the management of these structures. Preoperative magnetic resonance venography must be carefully studied to determine the drainage of the vein of Labbé.
- Adequate brain relaxation and proper positioning are of paramount importance to provide enough temporal lobe retraction to facilitate dissection.
- Lesions in the medial temporal lobe of the nondominant hemisphere can also be approached transcortically through the inferior temporal gyrus if the brain is full and adequate relaxation is not accomplished or the vein of Labbé is near and retraction may lead to injury.

PITFALLS

The primary limitation or risk of this approach is the potential for venous injury. This approach is rarely used for dominant hemisphere approaches.

BAILOUT OPTIONS

- If the vein of Labbé obstructs dissection, a portion of the inferior temporal gyrus can be resected.

SUGGESTED READINGS

Drake CG. The treatment of aneurysms of the posterior circulation. Clin Neurosurg 1979;26:96–144.

Kawase T, Toya S, Shiobara R, et al. Transpetrosal approach for aneurysms of the lower basilar artery. J Neurosurg 1985;63:857–61.

Mortini P, Mandelli C, Gerevini S, et al. Exposure of the petrous segment of the internal carotid artery through the extradural subtemporal middle cranial fossa approach: a systematic anatomical study. Skull Base 2001;11:177–87.

Osawa S, Rhoton AL Jr, Tanriover N, et al. Microsurgical anatomy and surgical exposure of the petrous segment of the internal carotid artery. Neurosurgery 2008;63(4 Suppl. 2):210–38.

Tanriover N, Abe H, Rhoton AL Jr, et al. Microsurgical anatomy of the superior petrosal venous complex: new classifications and implications for subtemporal transtentorial and retrosigmoid suprameatal approaches. J Neurosurg 2007;106:1041–50.

Procedure 5

Suboccipital Craniotomy

Shaan M. Raza, Alfredo Quiñones-Hinojosa

INDICATIONS

- Most lesions in the posterior fossa
- Developmental anomalies such as Chiari malformations
- Brain tumors such as meningiomas, ependymomas, astrocytomas, and medulloblastomas
- Vascular lesions such as aneurysms, cavernous malformations, and arteriovenous malformations
- Posterior fossa infections
- **Figure 5-1:** Cavernous malformation.

CONTRAINDICATIONS

- If lesions extend rostral to the tentorium, consideration should be given to a combined supracerebellar and supratentorial approach.
- If the lesion extends from the posterior fossa to the middle fossa, consideration should be given to a combined middle and posterior fossa approach.

PLANNING AND POSITIONING

- Preoperative antibiotics are given, and mannitol is given for brain relaxation.
- Depending on surgeon preference, lumbar subarachnoid drain placement for cerebrospinal fluid drainage can help with brain relaxation. This drain is particularly useful in situations in which the location of the lesion may prohibit early access to critical cisterns (i.e., cisterna magna).
- **Figure 5-2:** Patient position is prone for a straight midline posterior fossa approach. The prone position is optimal for lesions located caudally and at the craniocervical junction. For midline lesions, it is important to translate the head posteriorly and flex as much as possible to open the foramen magnum–C1 interval as much as possible, facilitating any bone work. Surgical navigation can be registered at this point per the preference of the surgeon and depending on the likely pathology. Tumors are more likely to require surgical navigation than vascular lesions in general.
- **Figure 5-3:** Linear skin incision is made in the midline extending from 4 to 5 cm above the inion down to the spinous process of C2. The midline attachments of the paraspinal musculature should be preserved. Lateral dissection on the posterior arch of C1 should be performed with a lower cautery setting and with microinstruments to avoid inadvertent injury to the vertebral artery. The length of the incision allows for wide lateral exposure of the posterior cervical fascia. In all posterior fossa cases, a Dandy burr hole is included in the field in case of an intraoperative catastrophe or when preoperative hydrocephalus exists.

PROCEDURE

- **Figure 5-4:** Craniotomy is done with care to preserve underlying dura. Burr holes can be placed close to the transverse sinus or the sigmoid sinus to complete a craniotomy.

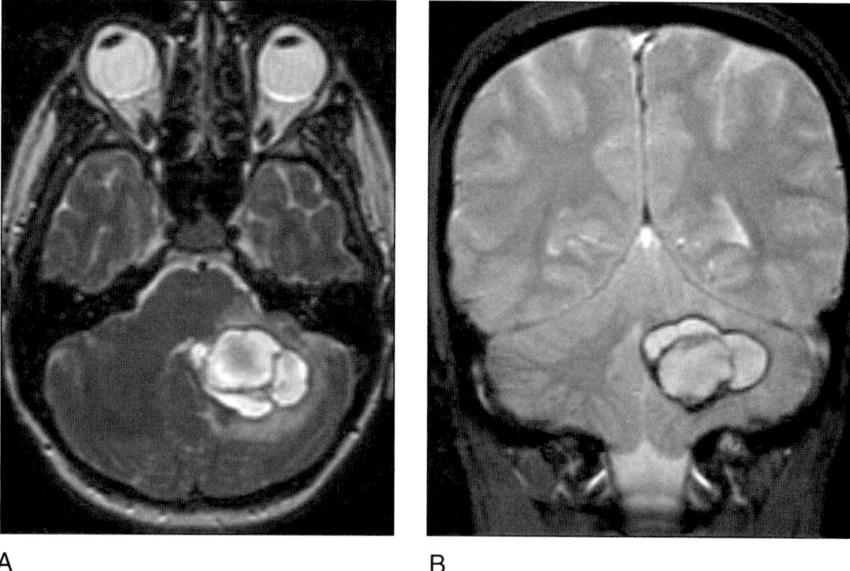

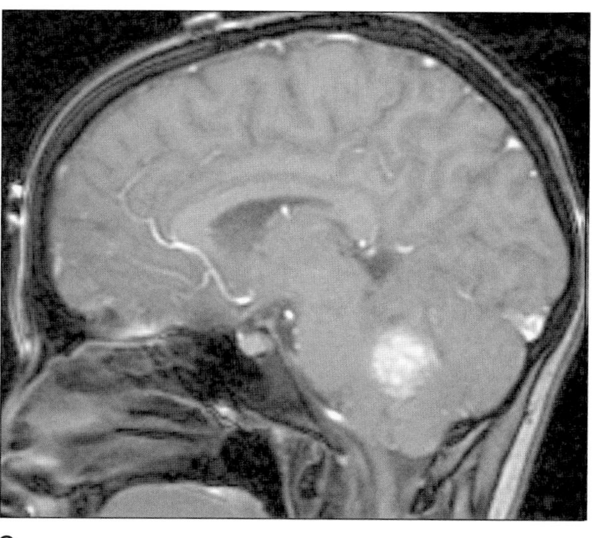

FIGURE 5-1

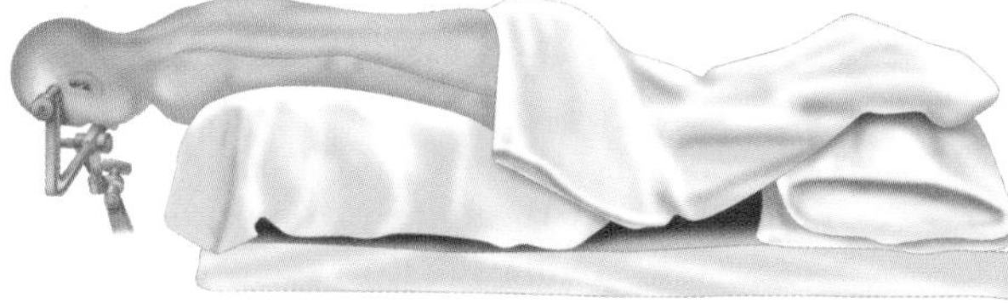

FIGURE 5-2

- A laminotomy at C1 allows for a wider dural opening, with a more inferior extension and more lateral mobilization of the dural flaps. In young patients, the craniotomy begins on one side of the foramen magnum, extends up to the transverse sinuses, and finishes on the other side of the foramen magnum, without requiring an initial burr hole.
- **Figure 5-5:** The rim of the foramen magnum is cut with a rongeur to extend the opening laterally to the occipital condyles (**A**), which exposes laterally to the cerebellar tonsils (**B**).

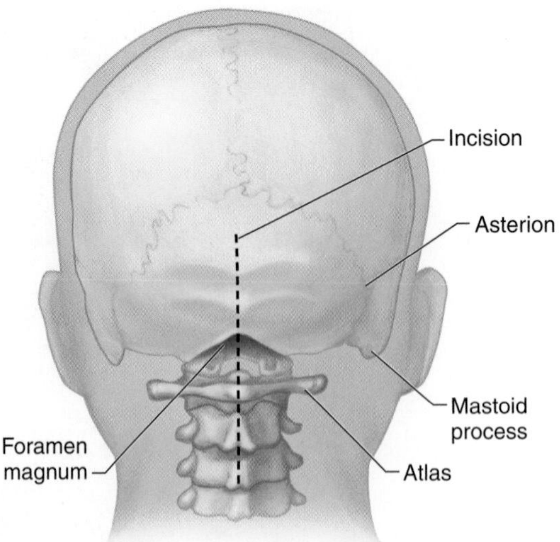

FIGURE 5-3

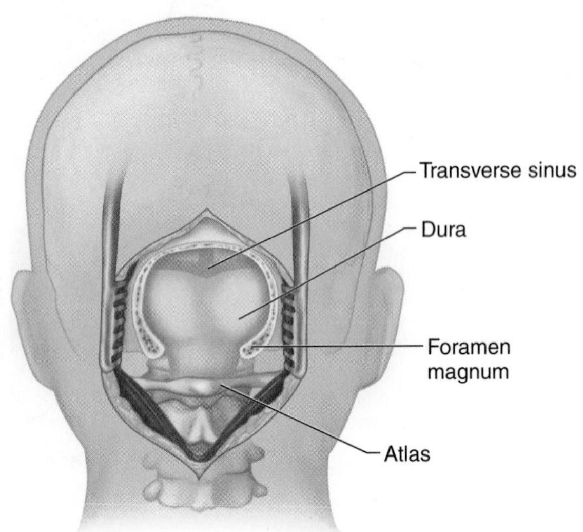

FIGURE 5-4

- **Figure 5-6:** Depending on the extent of resection or the location of the lesion, the dura can be opened in a Y-shaped fashion in the suboccipital craniotomy. The superior limb of the dura extends to the inferior aspect of the transverse sinus. The ring of C1 can be left intact as depicted here or taken out depending on the pathology. Removal of C1 is necessary for pathology resulting in tonsillar herniation; in addition, a C1 laminectomy is done for tumors in the fourth ventricle—this permits the surgeon to angle the instruments upward. The cisterna magna can be opened at the bottom to visualize the tonsils fully or to be able to release cerebrospinal fluid for decompression.
- The dura is primarily closed with 4-0 Nurolon running or interrupted sutures; often a dural graft is sutured to ensure watertight dural closure. A piece of dural substitute or a sealant can be placed over the dura to decrease postoperative cerebrospinal fluid leaks. The bone flap is replaced and secured with a titanium plate system. The muscle fascia galea is closed with interrupted 3-0 polyglactin 910 (Vicryl) sutures. The skin is closed with a nonabsorbable suture.

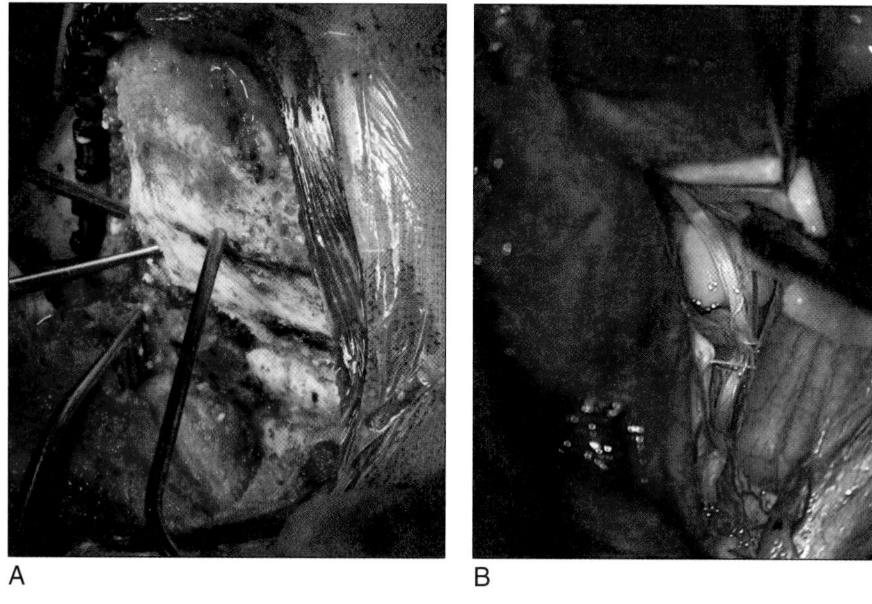

A B

FIGURE 5-5

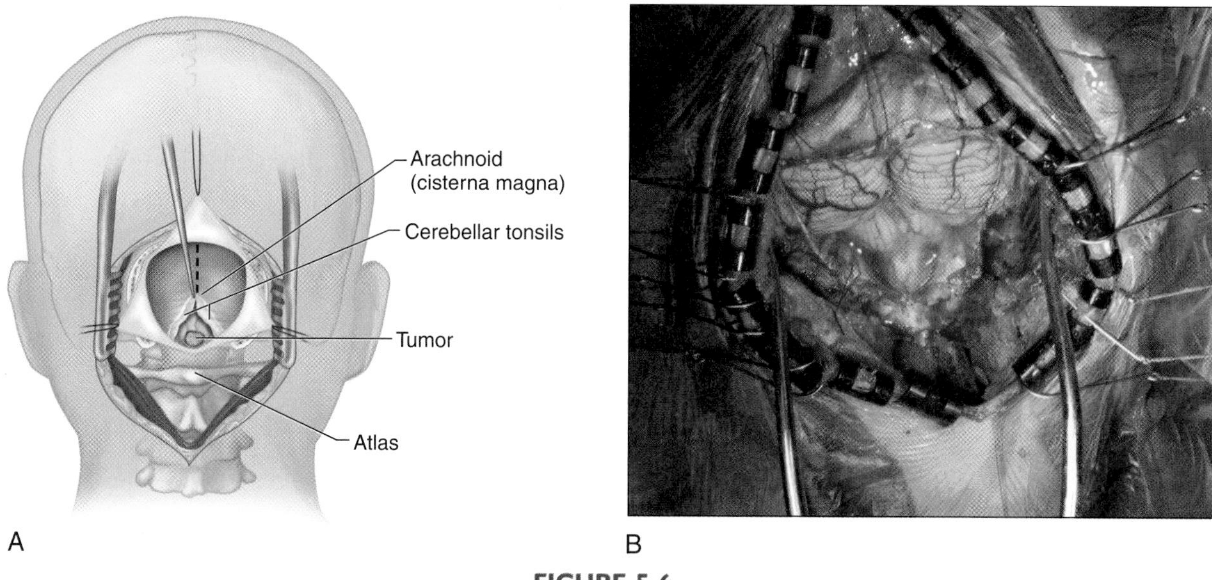

A B

FIGURE 5-6

TIPS FROM THE MASTERS

- During paraspinal dissection and exposure of the occipital bone, brisk bony bleeding is best managed with bone wax.
- Cerebellar retractors placed on the superior aspect of the incision help provide retraction during periosteal dissection.
- Using fish hooks for retraction of the inferior aspect of the incision eliminates the need for an inferior cerebellar retractor, the handles of which can be bulky and unnecessarily raise the depth to the operative field.
- Appropriate head flexion during positioning facilitates craniotomy and the trajectory into fourth ventricle.

PITFALLS

During suboccipital craniotomy, a patent circular sinus can be encountered leading to brisk sinus bleeding. This bleeding should be controlled with Gelfoam and bipolar cautery.

When dissecting laterally to the occipital condyle, injury to the vertebral artery may occur and can be avoided with less traumatic dissection techniques. A good preoperative understanding based on imaging of the vertebral artery anatomy is recommended.

BAILOUT OPTIONS

- If the lesions are large and the planes of dissection are suboptimal, particularly against the brainstem or peduncles, one can decide to do a subtotal resection depending on histology of lesion, clinical context, and adjuvant treatment options.
- If the posterior fossa is tight, an external ventricular drain can be placed in the occipital horn. This area needs to be prepared in a sterile fashion before starting the case.

SUGGESTED READINGS

Lawton MT, Quiñones-Hinojosa A, Jun P. The supratonsillar approach to the inferior cerebellar peduncle: anatomy, surgical technique, and clinical application to cavernous malformations. Neurosurgery 2006; 59(4 Suppl. 2):ONS244–51.

Quiñones-Hinojosa A, Chang EF, Lawton MT. The extended retrosigmoid approach: an alternative to radical cranial base approaches for posterior fossa lesions. Neurosurgery 2006;58(4 Suppl. 2):ONS208–14.

Procedure 6

Extended Retrosigmoid Craniotomy

Shaan M. Raza, Alfredo Quiñones-Hinojosa

INDICATIONS

- Lesions in the cerebellopontine angle and petroclival region can be surgically challenging to resect because of surrounding vascular and eloquent neural structures (i.e., brainstem) that have zero tolerance for retraction. Numerous surgical approaches, such as translabyrinthine, transcochlear, and presigmoid approaches, are part of the surgeon's armamentarium. Retrosigmoid craniotomy allows for easy and rapid access to the cerebellopontine angle.
- The extended version of the traditional retrosigmoid craniotomy is characterized by bony skeletonization of the sigmoid and transverse sinuses with an optional additional mastoidectomy. This modified version permits access to areas that are difficult to access with the classic approach—ventral to the brainstem and near the tentorium. This technique can often serve as a safe alternative to more radical cranial base approaches.
- This approach can be employed for extraaxial lesions in the cerebellopontine angle and intraaxial lesions arising along the petrosal surface of the cerebellum, cerebellar peduncles, or brainstem.

CONTRAINDICATIONS

- Patients must have patent contralateral transverse and sigmoid sinuses before manipulation of the sinuses ipsilateral to the approach.
- This approach is relatively contraindicated in older patients with poor-quality dura mater; in these patients, a craniectomy as opposed to a craniotomy should be performed.

PLANNING AND POSITIONING

- Preoperative planning includes assessment of the patient's cardiopulmonary status, evaluation of comorbidities, and basic laboratory tests, including a basic metabolic panel, complete blood count, coagulation profile, and type and screen. Baseline chest x-ray and electrocardiogram are also useful.
- In addition to standard magnetic resonance imaging (MRI) for intraoperative guidance, magnetic resonance venography is also obtained to ensure that the venous sinuses contralateral to the approach are patent before manipulation of the transverse and sigmoid sinuses ipsilaterally.
- Within 60 minutes of skin incision, perioperative antibiotics are administered.
- Brain relaxation can be achieved by administering mannitol, dexamethasone, and mild hyperventilation. For moderate-to-large lesions, a lumbar subarachnoid drain is also placed for intraoperative drainage; this drain is removed at case completion before extubation.
- After anesthesia induction, a multichannel central line and precordial Doppler is placed for early intraoperative detection and management of air embolism.
- Surgical navigation can be used as an adjunct depending on availability and complexity of the case. Surgical navigation can aid in the precise location of the transverse and sigmoid sinuses and in the placement of the burr holes before making the craniotomy flap.
- **Figure 6-1:** The patient is placed supine on the operating table with the ipsilateral shoulder elevated as needed to facilitate head rotation toward the contralateral side. The skull clamp is fixated with paired posterior pins at the equator in the occipital bone and single anterior pin at the equator in the contralateral frontal bone superior

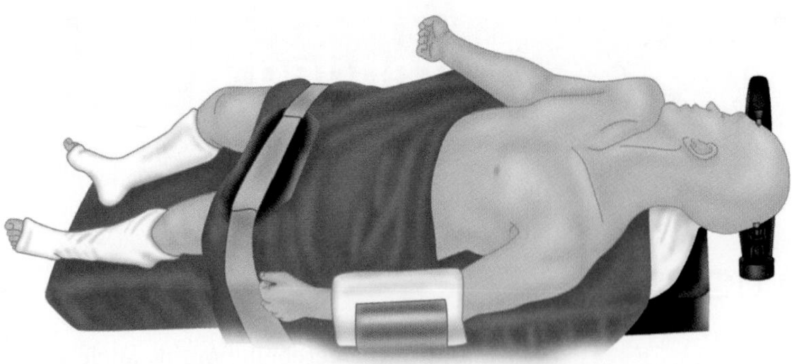

FIGURE 6-1

to the orbit. The head is positioned by first elevating the head above the heart in the "sniffing" position. Second, the head is rotated up to 60 degrees to the contralateral side depending on the intended operation. Third, the neck is extended so that the vertex is angled down 10 to 30 degrees, allowing for self-retraction of the frontal lobe off the anterior cranial fossa floor. When the head is ideally positioned, the malar eminence of the zygomatic bone should be the highest point in the operative field.

PROCEDURE

- **Figure 6-2:** C-shaped incision is made extending from 2 cm superior to the pinna and ending two fingerbreadths below the mastoid tip. A soft tissue dissection is performed so that bone is exposed from superior to the asterion down to the foramen magnum and from the mastoid process to several centimeters posterior to the sigmoid sinus. Osteotomies consist of two conceptual components:
- Retrosigmoid craniotomy with skeletonization of the venous sinuses
- Limited posterior mastoidectomy (if needed) for exposure of the jugular bulb
- **Figure 6-3:** Four burr holes are placed in the following order: inferiorly over the cerebellar hemisphere *(A)*, over the transverse sinus proximal to the transverse-sigmoid junction (placed slightly supratentorial so that the entire sinus can be exposed) *(B)*, over the sigmoid sinus as it enters the jugular foramen *(C)*, and over the transverse-sigmoid junction but slightly supratentorial *(D)*. With a Penfield No. 3, careful epidural dissection is performed to separate the dura and the venous sinuses. A craniotome is used to connect all the burr holes and create a free bone flap. The lumbar drain is optional; if placed right at this point, it is used to drain cerebrospinal fluid and to relax the brain slowly to facilitate the dissection of the epidural space.

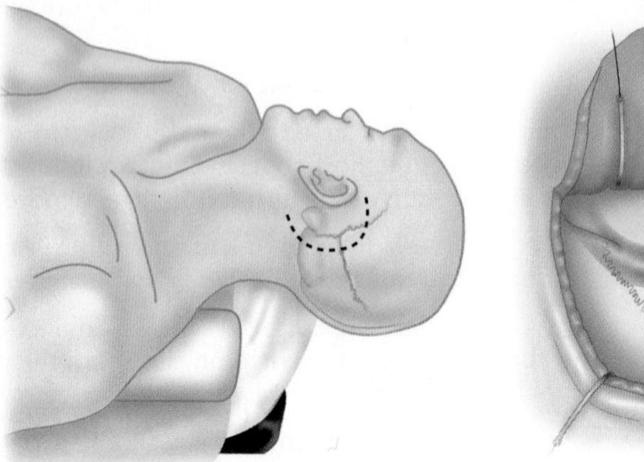

FIGURE 6-2

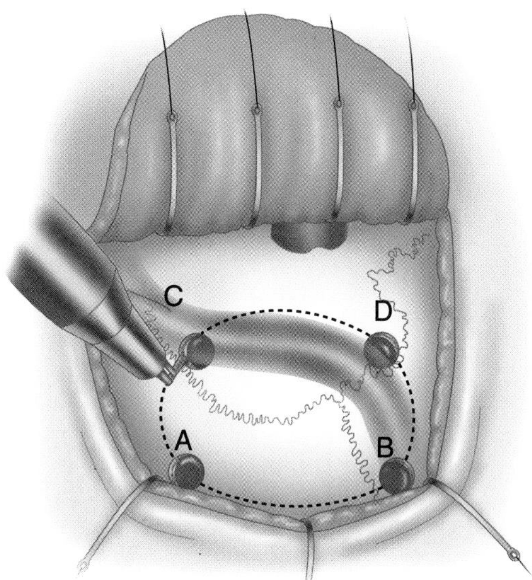

FIGURE 6-3

The bone overlying the sigmoid sinus transitions from compacted bone to a more trabeculated quality as the sinus enters the jugular foramen. Although the craniotomy can effectively unroof the compacted bone, a limited posterior mastoidectomy must be done to skeletonize the sinus as it drains into the jugular.

- **Figure 6-4:** Process of the limited posterior mastoidectomy begins with a cutting bur but then transitions to a diamond bur as the veil of blue to visualize through a thin eggshell rim of bone. In this process, the mastoid emissary vein may be encountered; hemostasis can be obtained here with cauterization.
- **Figure 6-5:** Cruciate dural opening is performed with pedicles based on the sigmoid and transverse sinuses. The flap based on the sigmoid sinus allows for the sinus to be reflected anteriorly and provide unobstructed access to the cistern lateralis and cerebellopontine angle. The flap pedicled on the transverse sinus allows for access between the cerebellum and tentorium.

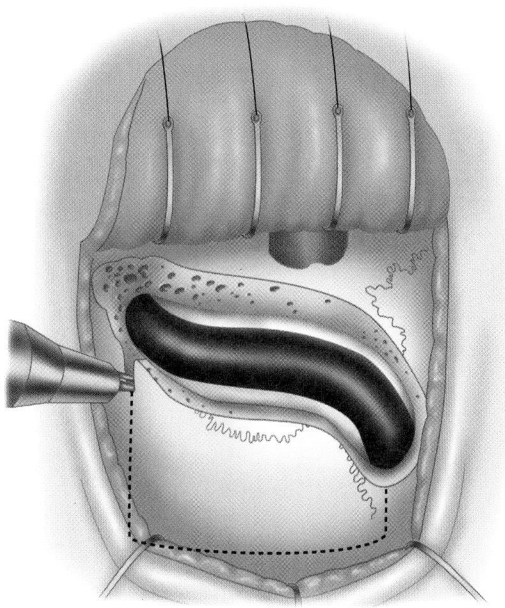

FIGURE 6-4

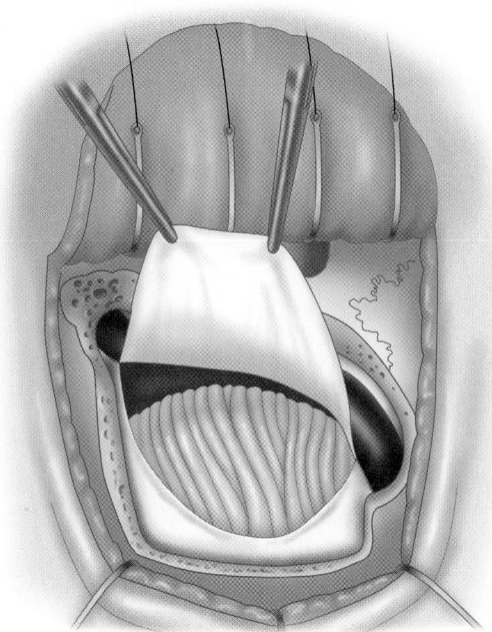

FIGURE 6-5

- At this point, intradural dissection proceeds per the target lesions. A lumbar drain can be used to facilitate cerebellum relaxation for larger tumors.
- The dura is primarily closed with interrupted sutures. Of key importance, in light of performing a mastoidectomy, the mastoid air cells must be thoroughly waxed to circumvent a potential route of cerebrospinal fluid egress.
- **Figure 6-6:** Bone flap is secured with titanium plates and screws.

TIPS FROM THE MASTERS

- This approach is a safe and effective alternative to more radical cranial base approaches to the cerebellopontine angle and to the petroclival region. Skeletonization of the venous sinuses provides the advantage of increased working angle—especially providing a line of sight parallel to the petrous surface of the cerebellum.
- A lumbar subarachnoid drain should be considered in cases in which early access to cerebrospinal fluid cisterns may be challenging.

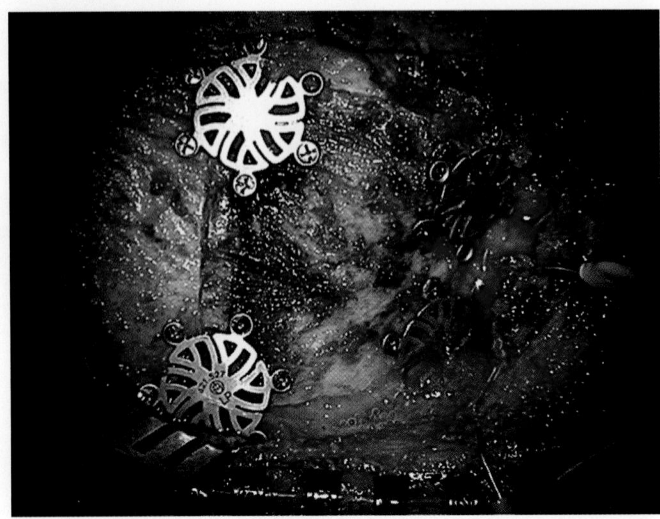

FIGURE 6-6

PITFALLS

The primary limitation or risk of this approach is the potential for venous injury. This potential highlights the importance of confirming that the patient has patent contralateral venous drainage in case intraoperative sinus injury occurs and sacrifice becomes necessary.

BAILOUT OPTIONS

- For older patients with poor-quality dura (which can be assessed after initial burr hole placement) and to prevent inadvertent sinus injury, a craniotome should not be used for skeletonization. In these patients, a standard retrosigmoid craniotomy or craniectomy should be performed. The sinuses can be subsequently unroofed with a series of cutting and diamond drill bits.
- The management of venous sinus injury depends on the extent of the defect and the presence of contralateral drainage. Small injuries can often be managed by packing. In situations of larger injury in which contralateral flow is not patent on preoperative imaging, a patch (muscle or dural substitute) can be sutured to repair the defect.

SUGGESTED READINGS

Katsuta T, Rhoton AL Jr, Matsushima T. The jugular foramen: microsurgical anatomy and operative approaches. Neurosurgery 1997;41:149–201.

Lang Jr J, Samii A. Retrosigmoidal approach to the posterior cranial fossa: an anatomical study. Acta Neurochir (Wien) 1991;111:147–53.

Quinones-Hinojosa A, Chang EF, Lawton MT. The extended retrosigmoid approach: an alternative to radical cranial base approaches for posterior fossa lesions. Neurosurgery 2006;58:ONS208–14.

Rhoton AL Jr. The cerebellopontine angle and posterior fossa cranial nerves by the retrosigmoid approach. Neurosurgery 2000;47:S93–129.

Shelton C, Alavi S, Li JC, et al. Modified retrosigmoid approach: use for selected acoustic tumor removal. Am J Otol 1995;16:664–8.

Figures 6-1 through 6-6 adapted from Quiñones-Hinojosa A, Chang EF, Lawton MT. The extended retrosigmoid approach: an alternative to radical cranial base approaches to lesions in the posterior fossa. Neurosurgery 2006;58:ONS208–14.

Procedure 7

Presigmoid Approaches to Posterior Fossa: Translabyrinthine and Transcochlear

Alejandro Rivas, Howard W. Francis

There are multiple variations of the presigmoid approach to the posterior fossa: retrolabyrinthine, transcrusal, translabyrinthine, transotic, and transcochlear. Each variation increases the amount of temporal bone resected, which increases the surgical freedom at the expense of increased surgical morbidity of cranial nerves VII and VIII. In this chapter, we focus on the translabyrinthine and transcochlear approaches (retrolabyrinthine is described in Procedure 20).

PLANNING AND POSITIONING

- Management of some cerebellopontine angle lesions is best accomplished between interaction of the neurosurgeon and the neurootologist.
- The role of each surgeon in the procedure, potential complications, and realistic postoperative goals are discussed preoperatively with the patient.
- The extension of the surgical approach is determined preoperatively based on lesion location, tumor size, preoperative facial nerve function, and serviceable hearing.
- Serviceable hearing includes a pure tone average threshold better than 50 dB, speech discrimination greater than 50%, or both (50/50 rule).
- The patient lies supine, with the head at the end of the table and rotated to the contralateral side.
- The patient is strapped to the table to allow tilting of the table safely during the procedure.
- Facial nerve monitoring electrodes are placed in the orbicularis oris and oculi muscles.
- In hearing preservation cases, auditory brainstem responses are monitored by placing an acoustic ear insert in the external auditory canal, a recording electrode on the vertex, a reference electrode in the ipsilateral ear lobule, and a ground electrode.
- Preoperative steroids and antibiotics are used. Before opening the dura, mannitol (0.5 to 1 g/kg) is given.
- **Figure 7-1:** Contrast-enhanced T1-weighted magnetic resonance image of a large vestibular schwannoma shows a straight route to access the posterior fossa.
- **Figure 7-2:** The retrolabyrinthine (RL) approach provides access to the presigmoid posterior fossa dura between the sigmoid sinus and the labyrinth. The translabyrinthine (TL) approach entails sacrificing the labyrinth to give direct access to the internal auditory canal (IAC) and cerebellopontine angle without cerebellar retraction. Bone drilling occurs extradurally, limiting subarachnoid exposure to bone dust and associated headache. The transcochlear (TC) approach extends the translabyrinthine approach anteriorly, by sacrificing the entire inner ear and rerouting the facial nerve to provide access to the anterior cerebellopontine angle, petrous apex, and ventral brainstem.
- **Figure 7-3:** Proper positioning for the translabyrinthine/transcochlear approach.

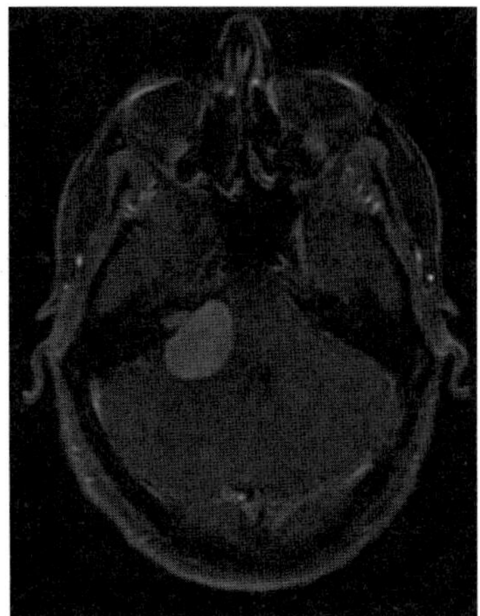

FIGURE 7-1

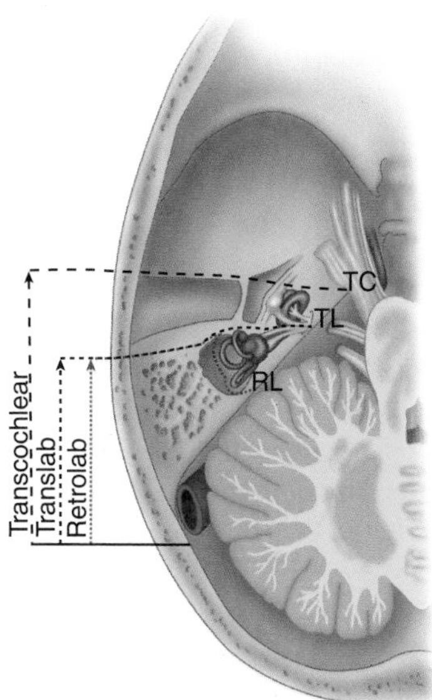

FIGURE 7-2

TRANSLABYRINTHINE APPROACH

Indications

- The rationale for this approach includes exposure of the posterior fossa and 320-degree exposure of the IAC circumference while sacrificing any residual hearing.
- Indications include removal of cerebellopontine angle lesions with preoperative unserviceable hearing, regardless of lesion size (e.g., vestibular schwannoma, meningioma, epidermoid, dermoid).

Contraindications

- Lesions extending anteriorly to prepontine cistern
- Ipsilateral chronic otitis media (relative)
- Only hearing ear

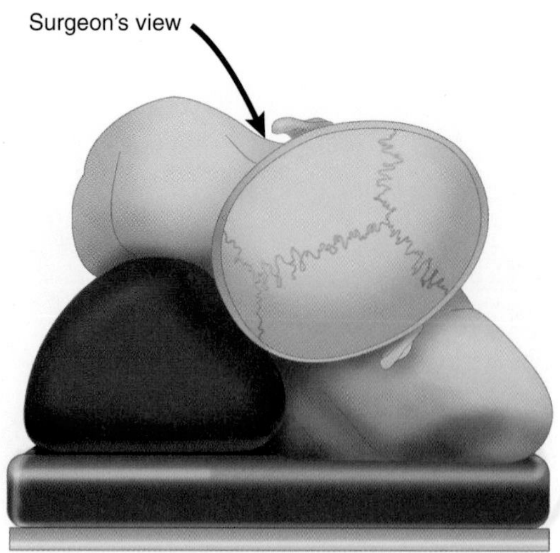

FIGURE 7-3

Procedure

- **Figure 7-4:** Because the translabyrinthine approach is an extension of the retrolabyrinthine approach, the same steps are used to identify the facial nerve and lateral and posterior semicircular canals and to skeletonize the posterior and middle fossa dura (see Procedure 20). A labyrinthectomy is then performed. It is started by blue lining and opening the lateral semicircular canal from anterior to posterior. The posterior semicircular canal is located posterior and perpendicular to the lateral canal. Attention must be paid to the facial nerve as this dissection is performed because it lies parallel to the lateral canal in the tympanic segment and parallel to the posterior canal in its vertical segment.
- **Figure 7-5:** The lumen of the posterior semicircular canal is followed superiorly to its junction with the superior semicircular canal at the common crus. The superior canal is opened toward its ampulla anteriorly. The subarcuate artery is identified in the center of the arch of this canal and can be cauterized as the dissection is carried medially.

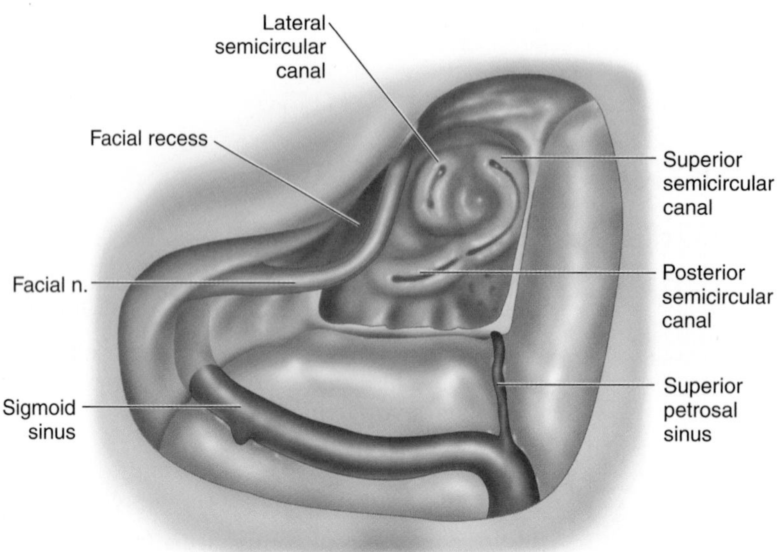

FIGURE 7-4

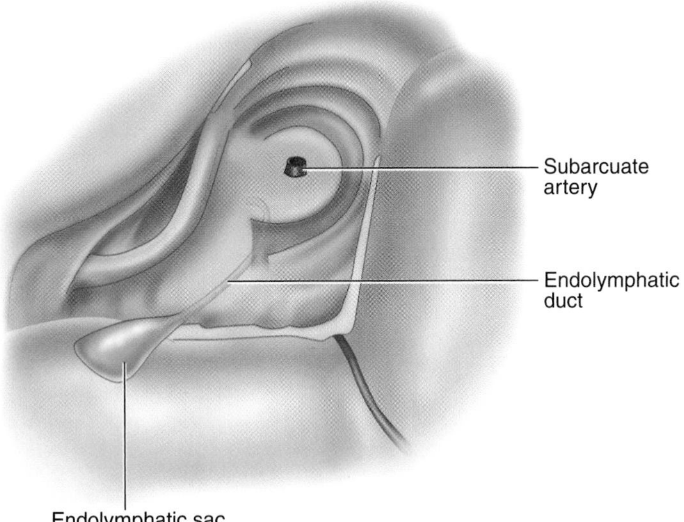

FIGURE 7-5

Leave the superior ampulla unopened because it serves as a valuable landmark for the lateral-superior limit of the IAC fundus.

- **Figure 7-6:** The common crus is followed until the vestibule is opened. The facial nerve is skeletonized further at the second genu to widen access to the vestibule. The spherical recess of the saccule is localized in the anterior portion of the vestibule, and the elliptic recess of the utricle is localized in the posterior portion. The ampullated end of the superior canal and the ampullated end of the posterior canal provide the expected superior and inferior limits of the IAC.
- **Figure 7-7:** The IAC dissection is started in the mid-portion and extended posteriorly toward the porus. Superior and inferior troughs are created and deepened parallel to the identified path of the IAC dura. Bone is removed from two thirds of the circumference of the IAC using a diamond bur. All presigmoid bone is removed from underlying posterior fossa dura. The jugular bulb is defined medial to the facial nerve and serves as the inferior limit of the labyrinthine portion of the dissection. Wider access to larger lesions in the cerebellopontine angle require complete removal of

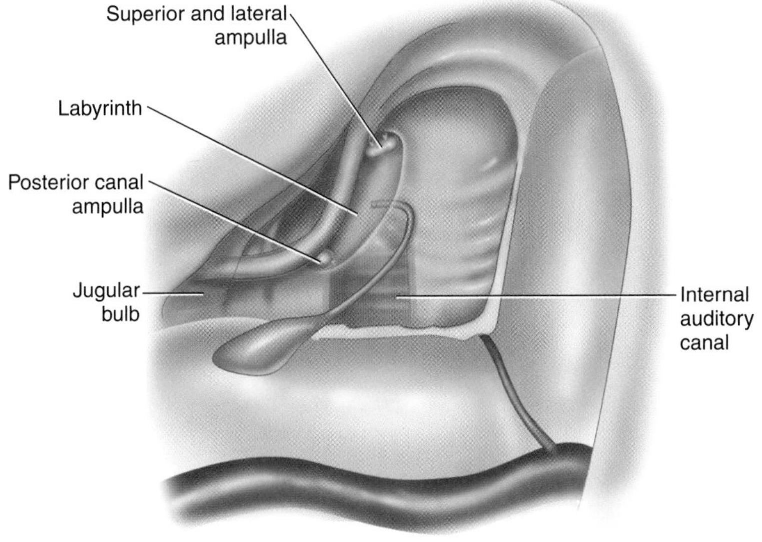

FIGURE 7-6

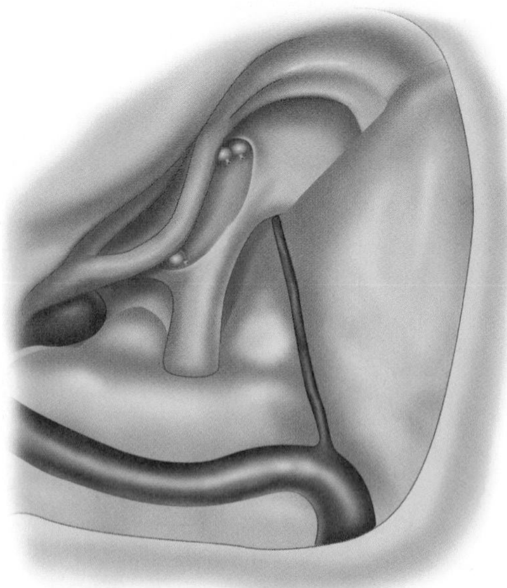

FIGURE 7-7

bone inferior and superior to the IAC with extensions anterior to the porus acusticus. The middle fossa dura and superior petrosal sinus should also be cleared of bone to facilitate this access.

- **Figure 7-8:** The proximal eggshelled bone over the porus is removed using a small round knife. The IAC is skeletonized in the fundus. The transverse crest is identified as it divides the superior and inferior vestibular nerves entering into the vestibule. Superior to the superior vestibular nerve, the vertical crest is identified next to the facial nerve in its labyrinthine segment.
- **Figure 7-9:** A dural flap is delineated, and bipolar cautery is used on the dura before opening it. This provides a wide exposure to the posterior fossa. Minimal retraction of the cerebellum allows visualization of the pons and upper medulla.

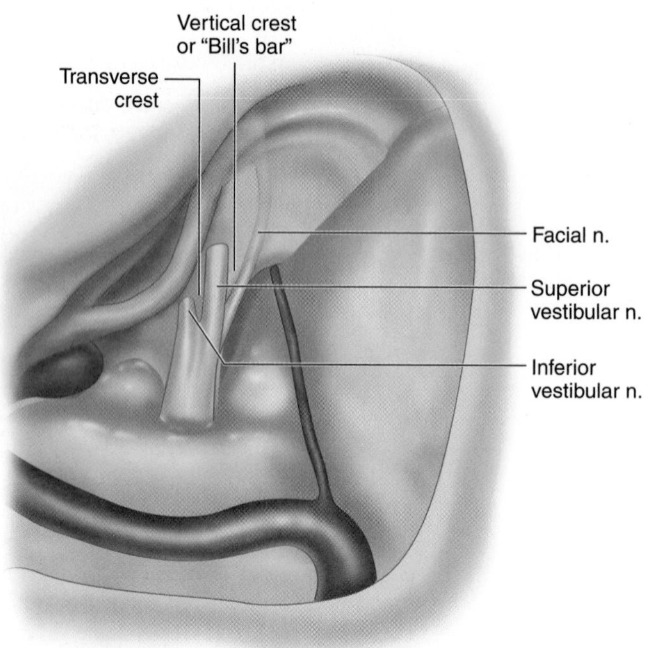

FIGURE 7-8

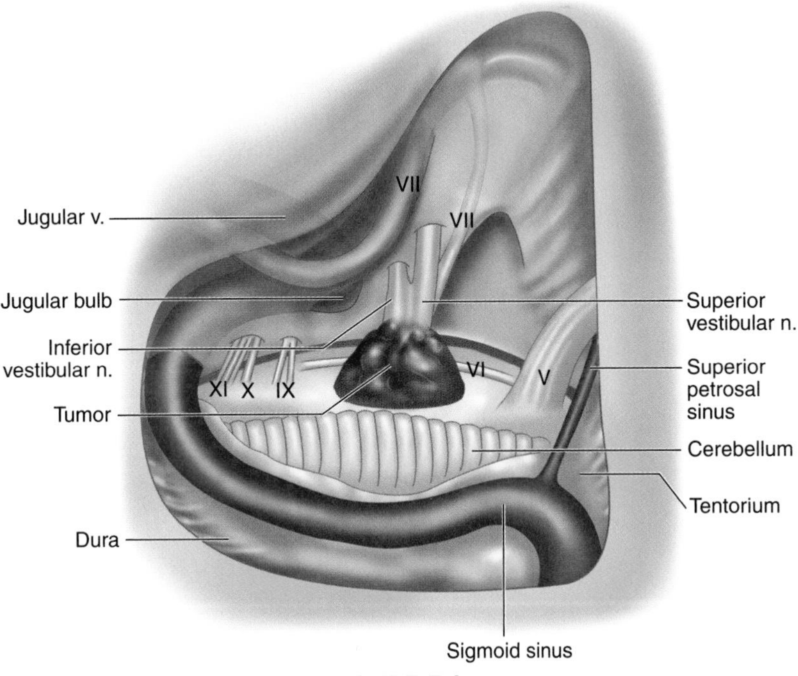

FIGURE 7-9

TRANSCOCHLEAR APPROACH

Indications

- This approach is an extension of the translabyrinthine approach, which includes drilling the posterior and superior external auditory canal and sacrificing middle ear structures and cochlea. It also entails mobilizing the facial nerve, which can produce some degree of facial nerve weakness.
- Cerebellopontine angle tumors with anterior extension and unserviceable hearing, such as extensive vestibular or cochlear schwannomas.
- Extensive petrous apex lesions with inner ear compromise such as petrous apex cholesteatomas or facial nerve tumors.
- Petroclival lesion with extension ventral to the brainstem.
- Temporal bone and clival lesions with extension to the posterior fossa, such as chordomas and chondrosarcomas.

Contraindications

- Ipsilateral chronic otitis media (relative)
- Only hearing ear (relative)

Procedure

- The transcochlear approach is an extension of the translabyrinthine approach. Similar actions are taken, including an extended mastoidectomy, removal of bone over the sigmoid sinus and posterior fossa, and identification of the facial nerve. At this point, the skin of the external auditory canal is separated from the bony canal and closed in a blind pouch. The bony posterior and superior external auditory canal is drilled down, and the tympanic membrane and ossicles are removed. Labyrinthectomy is performed, and the IAC is skeletonized as previously described.
- **Figure 7-10:** Using a diamond bur, the facial nerve is skeletonized from the geniculate ganglion to the stylomastoid foramen. The cochlea is drilled to a mid-modiolar section,

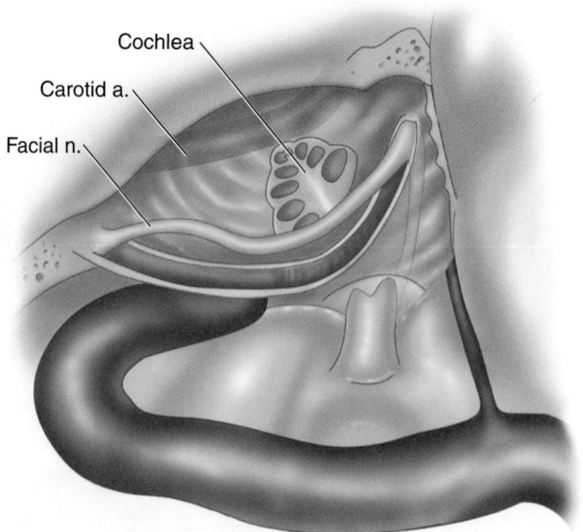

FIGURE 7-10

taking as limits the genu of the petrous carotid artery and eustachian tube anteriorly, the facial nerve posteriorly and superiorly, and the jugular bulb inferiorly. The eggshelled bone over the facial nerve and its attachment to the stapedius muscle are removed with a sickle knife.

- **Figure 7-11:** The middle fossa dura is gently retracted, and the bone over the labyrinthine segment of the facial nerve is gently drilled. Using a sickle knife, the nerve is decompressed in this portion, and the greater superficial petrosal nerve is transected distal to the geniculate ganglion. The dura of the IAC is opened. The cochlear and vestibular nerves are transected, and the facial nerve transposition is performed.
- **Figure 7-12:** The remnant cochlea is drilled down through the apical petrous bone and into the clivus. Dura lining the posterior face of the petrous bone is exposed anterior to the porus acusticus as the jugular bulb is uncovered. Location of the carotid artery immediately anterior to the cochlea and inferior to the opening of the eustachian tube

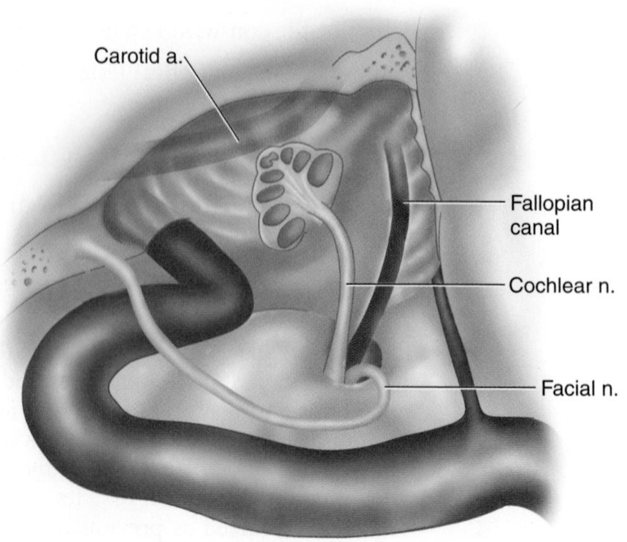

FIGURE 7-11

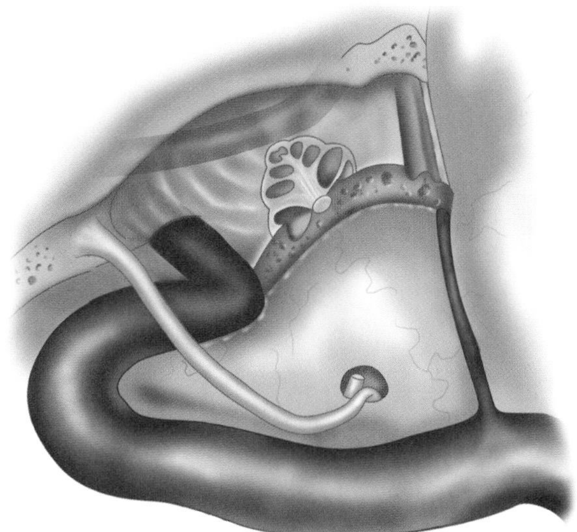

FIGURE 7-12

must be considered. The superior petrosal sinus and middle fossa dura are uncovered in a similar manner.

- **Figure 7-13:** Thickening of the dura is encountered anteriorly, which corresponds to the posterior face of the clivus and represents the deep limit of the dissection. The dura is opened, and the posterior fossa and petroclival region are visualized.
- **Figure 7-14:** Closure in all presigmoid approaches is performed similarly to prevent cerebrospinal fluid leak. The eustachian tube is packed with temporalis fascia or temporalis muscle, followed by pieces of fat graft harvested from the abdominal wall. Temporalis fascia and subcutaneous tissue are closed in a watertight fashion, followed by skin.

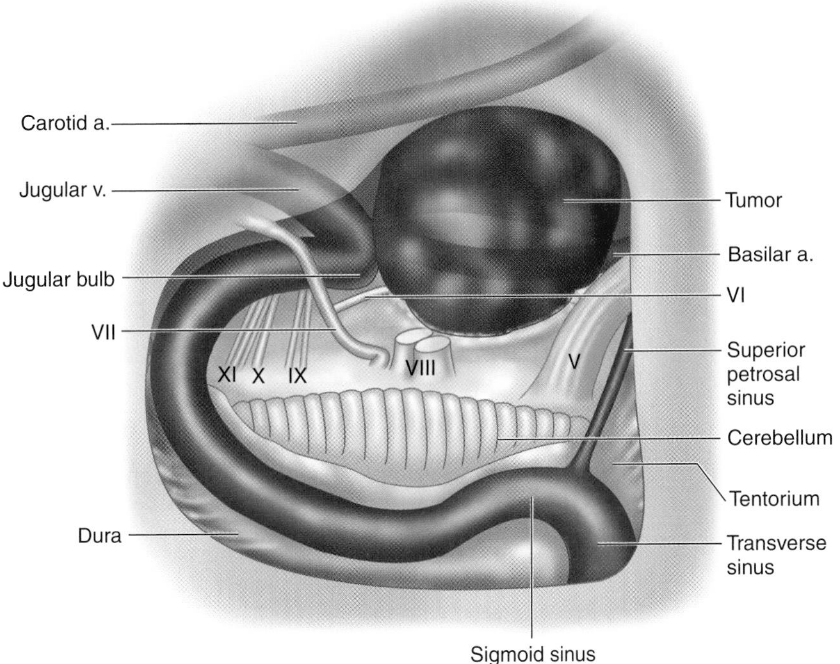

FIGURE 7-13

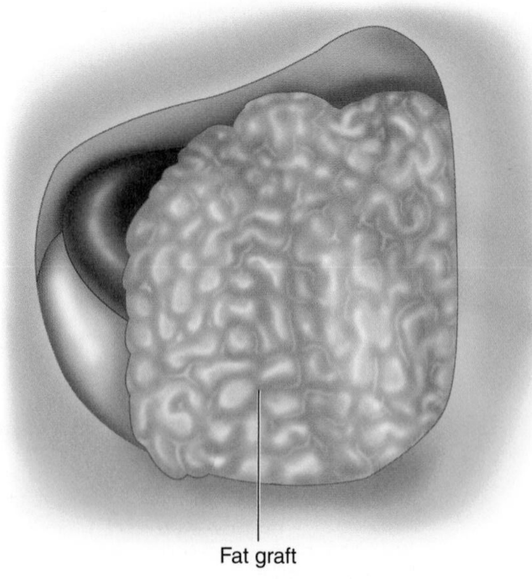

FIGURE 7-14

TIPS FROM THE MASTERS

- Retracting the sigmoid sinus as the posterior fossa plate is skeletonized provides an efficient and safe way to perform the approach.
- To localize the facial nerve in its vertical segment without injury, the posterior wall of the external auditory canal must be drilled razor-sharp thin.
- Circumferential removal of bone around the vertical segment of the facial nerve including the stylomastoid foramen reduces injury related to mobilization of the nerve. Maintaining soft tissue around the nerve at the stylomastoid foramen, including the digastric muscle, as the nerve is mobilized reduces ischemia-related paresis.
- Large pieces of Gelfoam can be used over the facial nerve, after it is transposed, to protect it when drilling the remnant cochlea and petrous apex in the transcochlear approach.
- When the bone from the posterior and middle fossa is removed and dura is exposed, use bipolar cautery from medial to lateral over the dura for it to retract and provide a wider plane of dissection.
- After opening the dura, the lateral cistern must be opened first to allow decompression of cerebrospinal fluid and prevent cerebellar herniation, particularly in large tumors.
- In the transcochlear approach, the jugular bulb must be completely uncovered. If a prominent bulb obstructs anterior access, it can be decorticated, elevated intact from remaining jugular fossa, and compressed out of the way with the help of bone wax.

PITFALLS

The facial nerve is located immediately lateral to the vestibule. Care must be taken to visualize it and prevent its injury when opening the vestibule.

In the transcochlear approach, all bone must be removed in the geniculate ganglion to prevent injury during transposition.

When separating the facial nerve from the fallopian canal, circumferential removal of bone is necessary to minimize traction injury, which is helped further by cutting fibrous attachments sharply.

When closing with fat graft, the fat must be located as deep as the craniotomy opening and not fill the intracranial cavity to allow expansion of the compressed brainstem.

BAILOUT OPTIONS

- Small sigmoid sinus tears can be closed using bipolar cautery. Medium tears can be managed by placing Gelfoam (Pfizer, Inc., NY, NY), Surgicel (Ethicon, Inc., Cornelia, GA), or Avitene Flour MCH (Davol, Inc., a subsidiary of C.R. Bard, Inc., Warwick, RI) over the opening followed by a wet cottonoid until bleeding stops. Larger tears can be sutured over a muscle plug.
- Cerebrospinal fluid leaks can be prevented by packing the middle ear and eustachian tube with fascia, or muscle, and a watertight fat graft mastoid obliteration.
- In cases of facial nerve injury with perineurium exposure and edema, the facial nerve must be decompressed, and the perineurium must be opened.

SUGGESTED READINGS

Angeli SI, De la Cruz A, Hitselberger W. The transcochlear approach revisited. Otol Neurotol 2001;22:690–5.

Becker SS, Jackler RK, Pitts LH. Cerebrospinal fluid leak after acoustic neuroma surgery: a comparison of the translabyrinthine, middle fossa, and retrosigmoid approaches. Otol Neurotol 2003;24:107–12.

Bennett M, Haynes DS. Surgical approaches and complications in the removal of vestibular schwannomas. Neurosurg Clin N Am 2008;19:331–43.

Brackmann DE, Green JD Jr. Translabyrinthine approach for acoustic tumor removal. Neurosurg Clin N Am 2008;19:251–64.

De la Cruz A, Teufert KB. Transcochlear approach to cerebellopontine angle and clivus lesions: indications, results, and complications. Otol Neurotol 2009;30:373–80.

Pitts LH, Jackler RK. Treatment of acoustic neuromas. N Engl J Med 1998;339:1471–3.

Russell SM, Roland JT Jr, Golfinos JG. Retrolabyrinthine craniectomy: the unsung hero of skull base surgery. Skull Base 2004;14:63–71.

Sanna M, Bacciu A, Pasanisi E, et al. Posterior petrous face meningiomas: an algorithm for surgical management. Otol Neurotol 2007;28:942–50.

Steward DL, Pensak ML. Transpetrosal surgery techniques. Otolaryngol Clin North Am 2002;35:367–91.

Figures 7-1 through 7-11 are modified with permission from Jackler RK. Atlas of Skull Base Surgery and Neurotology, 2nd ed. New York: Thieme; 2008.

Procedure 8 Transcallosal Approach

Jason Liauw, Gary Gallia, Alessandro Olivi

INDICATIONS

- Tumors of the lateral and third ventricles

CONTRAINDICATIONS

- This approach is contraindicated if the patient is medically unstable and would not tolerate surgery.
- The transcallosal approach, although it provides exposure to tumors in the lateral and third ventricle, is limited in providing satisfactory access to tumors in the posterior trigone, temporal horn, or superior frontal horn. Patients with these tumors are best approached by the transcortical route, with its own set of indications and complications.
- Although a partial callosotomy (usually anteriorly located) generally does not lead to significant neurologic deficit, serious impairment may arise because of poor patient selection, inattentive consideration of the vascular anatomy, or inadequate techniques.
- Crossed dominance, wherein the hemisphere controlling the dominant hand is contralateral to the hemisphere controlling speech and language, is a contraindication. Crossed dominance can arise after cerebral injury during childhood that resulted in cortical functional reorganization. These patients may develop writing and speech deficits postoperatively. Special consideration should be given to cases in which a more posterior callosotomy (splenium) is required, increasing the risks of cognitive dysfunction (e.g., alexia), particularly in patients with established preoperative visual field cuts (e.g., homonymous hemianopsia).

PLANNING AND POSITIONING

Patient Selection

- Patients who present with symptoms of cognitive impairment, such as memory deficits, should have preoperative neuropsychologic evaluation owing to potential risk of injury to the fornices.
- A preoperative vascular anatomy study is often helpful to assess the cortical and deep venous drainage and the relative risk of venous engorgement associated with a protracted hemispheric retraction and a meticulous surgical manipulation.

Patient Positioning

- For a parasagittal approach, the patient can be positioned in a neutral supine position or alternatively in a lateral decubitus position.
- **Figure 8-1:** For supine positioning, the vertex is elevated 45 degrees from the horizontal.
- The lateral decubitus position allows for gravity to help pull down the hemisphere away from the falx, allowing for greater midline exposure with less retraction on the hemisphere. Some surgeons prefer lateral positioning because the greater exposure allows access to a greater portion of the corpus callosum. The disadvantage of lateral positioning compared with supine positioning is the greater amount of midline distortion caused by gravity. Maintenance of a midline reference plane helps with operative orientation.

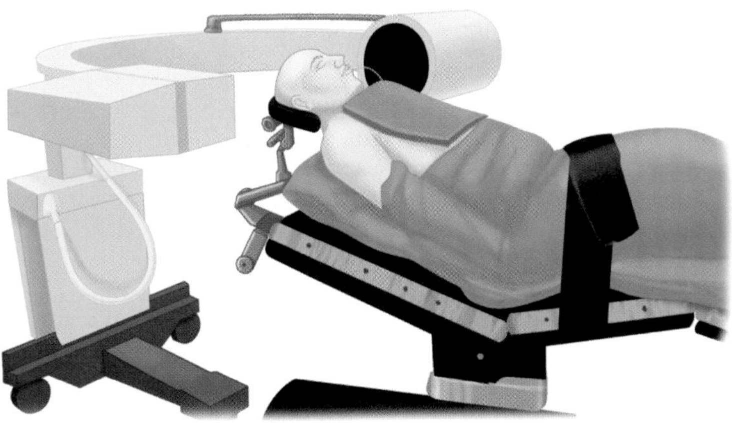

FIGURE 8-1

PROCEDURE

Craniotomy

- The location of a given lesion is an important factor in planning the positioning of craniotomy. For better visualization of a lesion in the posterior lateral ventricle, a more anterior craniotomy is used. Most often, a craniotomy is made paramedian to the sagittal sinus along the nondominant (right) hemisphere. Preservation of draining veins takes priority, and consideration should be given to a left hemisphere approach if preservation of veins can be accomplished. A modified bicoronal incision (usually shorter and centered on the midline) is used to create a skin flap that can be distracted in the anteroposterior dimension.
- Exposure of the interhemispheric region requires the use of an anterior parasagittal craniotomy extending to or encompassing the midline. The midline craniotomy is over the superior sagittal sinus. The bone flap is positioned in relation to the coronal suture. To minimize the chances of injuring the sinus or parasagittal veins feeding the sinus, care should be taken to position the posterior margin of the bone flap no more than 2 to 3 cm posterior to the coronal suture. This is done to avoid venous tributaries, which often enter the sinus approximately 2 to 3 cm behind the coronal suture. The anterior-most edge of the bone flap can be made up to 4 to 5 cm in front of the coronal suture depending on the extent of exposure needed. For definitive understanding of individual variations in venous tributary anatomy, obtaining preoperative computed tomography (CT) venography or magnetic resonance venography is recommended.
- On exposure of the parasagittal region, we make a rectangular craniotomy using a variable number of burr holes according to the condition of the underlying dura. It is of paramount importance to dissect free the dura of the superior sagittal sinus, and this can be done by placing two burr holes on the paramedian ipsilateral edge of the sinus or three burr holes (two ipsilateral and one contralateral) on each side of the sinus. In each case, the interhemispheric region is generously exposed with a covered sinus in the first case and a visualized sinus in the second. Time should be taken to dissect the dura carefully from the inner table working away from the sagittal sinus. The burr holes are then connected with either a craniotome or a Gigli saw.

Interhemispheric Dissection

- A semicircular or trapezoidal dural dissection is made based on the lateral edge of the sagittal sinus. As the flap is retracted, an effort should be made to preserve bridging veins. The objectives of the interhemispheric dissection are to prevent venous infarction and to ensure minimal retraction on the brain. To prevent venous infarction secondary to overretraction, one must be cognizant to limit retraction to no more than 2 cm along any part of the corridor. Pauses of 2 to 3 minutes should be observed after every advancement of the retractor blade down the interhemispheric fissure. This pause allows for the ventricular pressures to equilibrate in the face of forces exerted by the retractor itself.

- Initially, arachnoid granulations along the medial hemisphere are opened with sharp dissection. A combination of blunt dissection with the blunt end of a No. 1 Penfield and advancement of the retractor blade should enable for adequate dissection down the midline. Before arriving at the corpus callosum, the inferior falx, inferior sagittal sinus, cingulated gyri, callosomarginal arteries, and pericallosal branches of the anterior cerebral arteries should be identified. The corpus callosum can be identified easily because of its glistening and relatively hypovascular aspect.

Collosotomy

- The length and site of the callosotomy incision depend on the location of the lesion one is trying to approach. The corpus callosum should be split down the midline with the use of microinstruments and microirrigators. With ventricular masses, there may be midline distortion of the corpus callosum. It is important to anticipate asymmetry by thoroughly reviewing preoperative imaging. After the trunk of the corpus callosum is split, the callosotomy is widened with bipolar coagulation and a microsuction (5F) tip. Care must be taken at this stage to ensure proper hemostasis to prevent intraventricular hemorrhage.
- After the callosotomy is made, the retractor can be advanced to expose the lateral ventricular anatomy. If the foramen of Monro is open, a physical barrier should immediately be placed at its entry to prevent blood from pooling into the third ventricle. If the contralateral ventricle is entered, fenestration or excision of the septum pellucidum can open access into the ipsilateral lateral ventricle. Fenestration of the septum also allows for the alternative pathway of cerebrospinal fluid flow. The fornices travel across the base of the septum and must be preserved. Identification of normal ventricular anatomy should reveal the septal vein, septum pellucidum, fornices, thalamostriate vein, internal cerebral veins, choroid plexus, and head of the caudate. Following the thalamostriate vein, septal vein, fornices, or choroid plexus reliably guides the surgeon to the foramen of Monro.

Approach Options to the Third Ventricle

- **Figure 8-2:** Numerous approaches exist to gain access to lesions within the third ventricle. Selection of one approach over another is determined by the size, position, and intrinsic characteristics of the lesion within the third ventricle and the drive to prevent postoperative deficits.
- **Figure 8-3:** Because intraventricular dissection involves a small space with a target far from the brain surface, orientation to reliable anatomic landmarks is imperative. The fornix, thalamus, and septum pellucidum can be localized to the course of the choroid plexus and thalamostriate vein to the foramen of Monro, where it is joined by the caudate and septal vein to form the internal cerebral vein. At all times, the plane between the tumor and ependymal surface should be maintained.

Transforaminal Approach

- **Figure 8-4:** Lesions in the anterior portion of the third ventricle are often easily accessible through the foramen of Monro and sometimes even expand and protrude through the foramen.

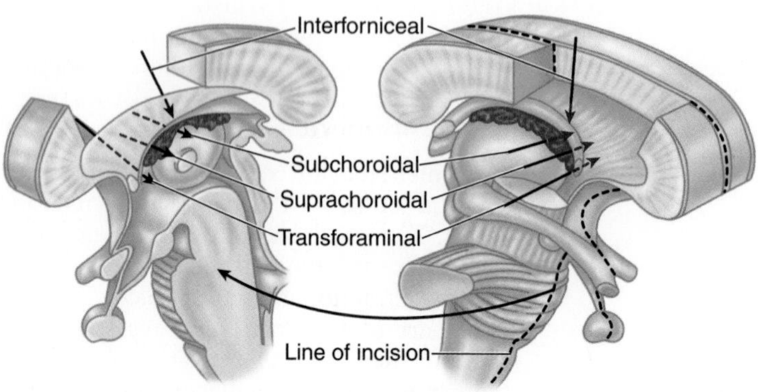

FIGURE 8-2

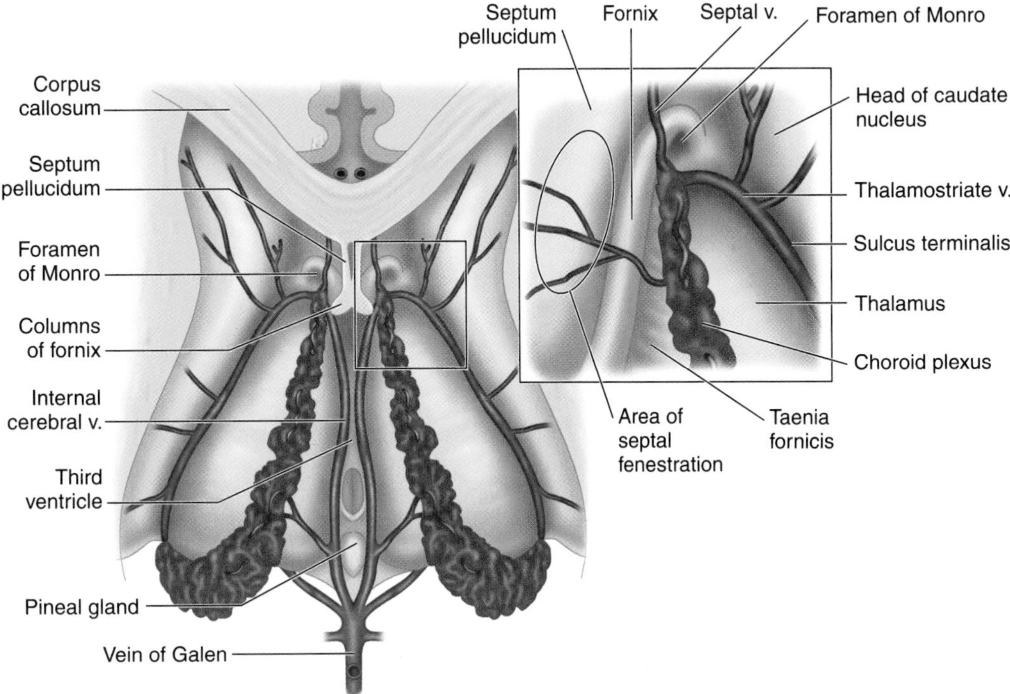

FIGURE 8-3

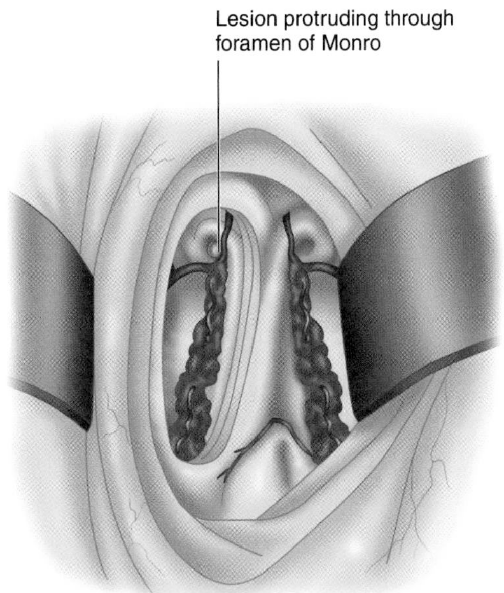

FIGURE 8-4

- For lesions that are soft or cystic, it is often appropriate to resect and deliver the lesion through the foramen of Monro. Lesions with significant mass effect sometimes already have caused dilation of the foramen, facilitating the surgical approach. The foraminal patency can be assessed with the use of forceps or with probing with a Silastic shunt tube. Given that the foramen is bordered by the forniceal column at the anterosuperior margin, further dilating the foramen can lead to postoperative memory deficits. Dilation of the foramen, which can lead to forniceal damage, is often not a viable option, especially in cases where the third ventricular mass impinges on the contralateral fornix. Such lesions require an alternative method of exposure.
- The transchoroidal (subchoroidal or suprachoroidal) approach is a preferred method for access into the third ventricle through the velum interpositum, which serves as the roof

for the third ventricle. In the subchoroidal approach, an incision is made in the taenia choroidea, and the choroid plexus is reflected upward. In the suprachoroidal approach, an incision is made above the choroid plexus in the taenia fornicis, and the choroid is deflected inferiorly. The suprachoroidal approach offers an approach that requires less manipulation of the superficial thalamic and caudate veins and has been regarded to be safer. If a subchoroidal approach is taken, it may be necessary to cauterize one of the thalamostriate veins, which may be a limiting factor in the untethering of the choroid. Potential consequences of sacrificing a unilateral striate vein include hemiplegia, mutism, and drowsiness. These postoperative morbidities may not occur, however, because of collateralization by superficial cortical, posterior medullary, and galenic venous systems.

- Given the high morbidity of the interforniceal approach, in which bilateral forniceal injury can occur through manipulation, this approach is generally reserved for cases in which there is significant mass effect that distends the roof of the third ventricle. During development of a dissection plane in the interforniceal approach, the surgeon must remain cognizant of the hippocampal commissure in the posterior component of the fornices. Damage to the fornices may lead to devastating memory impairment. Care must also be taken to preserve and retract gently the internal cerebral veins.
- **Figure 8-5:** The transchoroidal approach can be accomplished by entering either above or below the choroid plexus in the body of the lateral ventricle. The interforniceal approach involves the midline division of the forniceal bodies.

Closure

- After resection of the tumor, it is imperative to ensure complete hemostasis and to prevent delayed ventricular obstruction. First, the entire ventricular system should be irrigated with body-temperature Ringer lactate solution to removed pooled blood, trapped air, or debris.
- All natural pathways of cerebrospinal fluid flow and alternative routes of exit (callosotomy, septal window, and possibly hypothalamic floor defect) should be inspected to prevent delayed ventricular obstruction. To ensure hemostasis, layer-by-layer inspection of each exposed surface, from the ependymal lining in the third ventricle to the cortical pial surface, must be performed.

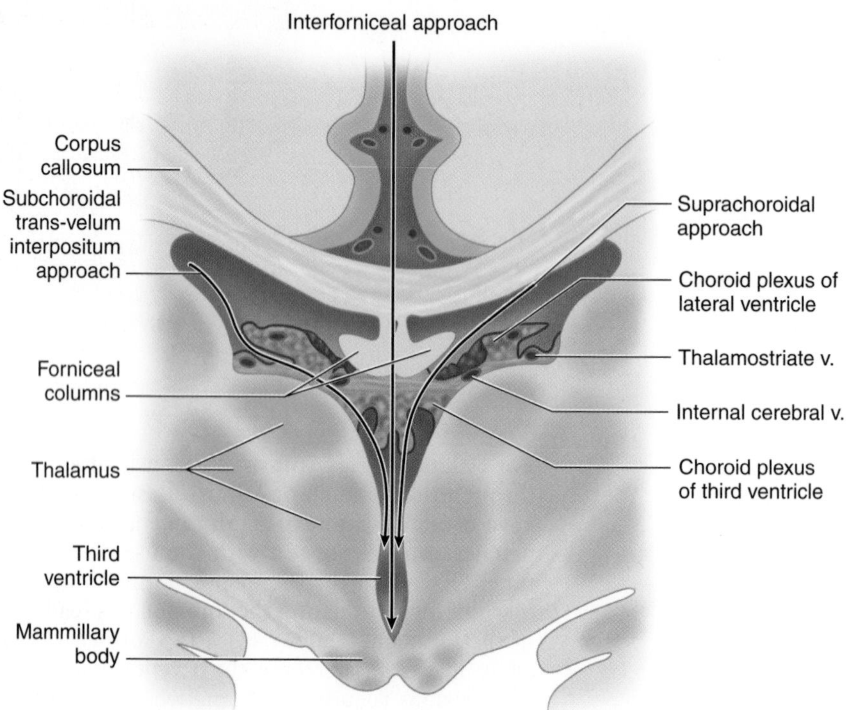

FIGURE 8-5

- Special attention should be paid to the ependymal surface adjacent to the callosotomy and abraded medial and paramedial cortical surface because these areas are particularly susceptible to postoperative hemorrhage.
- A ventricular catheter should be left in the lateral ventricle for about 48 hours postoperatively to monitor intraventricular pressure and to ensure patency within the ventricular system. A CT scan should be obtained on the 1st postoperative day to rule out obstruction and to evaluate the extent of tumor resection.

TIPS FROM THE MASTERS

- Although preoperative ventriculomegaly might facilitate a transcortical route, the transcallosal approach is equally effective in reaching the area of the foramen of Monro with large or small ventricles.
- Because tumors within the ventricles can become quite large before detection, the surgery must be planned to reach and decompress the lesion to remove it via a relatively small opening. Control of arterial supply is also essential.
- Because choroid plexus tumors, such as papillomas and meningiomas, receive their blood supply from the choroidal vessels, early identification and ligation of these vessels reduce bleeding.
- Tumors arising from the ependymal surface and septum pellucidum, such as gliomas and neurocytomas, are supplied by small vessels of the ventricular walls. Although these small vessels create less intraoperative blood loss, they are often numerous and small and require meticulous microscopic dissection.

PITFALLS

Although dissection of the lesion within the third ventricle may lead to complications, including alteration of consciousness, endocrinopathy, visual loss, mutism, and other signs of diencephalic injury, the major complication of the transcallosal approach is the development of hemiparesis and memory loss. With minimization of midline retraction and with care during midline entry with regard to cortical venous structures, the incidence of permanent paresis can approach zero, whereas incidence of transient paresis is less than 10%.

The most commonly encountered postoperative problem is transient amnesia of recent events, which was seen in about 30% of cases in a personal series, but this usually resolves completely within 21 days. The amnesia is most striking 24 to 72 hours postoperatively, with most patients recovering within 7 days, and all patients reaching preoperative baseline status within 3 months postoperatively.

The transcallosal approach can also lead to damage of adjacent structures. During initial interhemispheric exposure and subsequent retraction, manipulation of the parasagittal veins may lead to cortical injury and venous infarcts. Although some surgeons argue that bridging veins anterior to the coronal suture can be sacrificed, others believe in absolute preservation of these venous structures. Experimental evidence also points to a higher risk of venous infarct when injury to a bridging vein is combined with brain retraction than either manipulation alone.

Limited incision of the callosal trunk usually leads to minimal physiologic complications. An acute syndrome of decreased speech spontaneity, ranging from mild slowness of speech initiation to frank mutism, with onset in the hours and days after surgery and possibly persisting for several months, has been described after transcallosal injury. Although longer callosal incisions (2 to 3 cm compared with 0.8 to 2 cm) may be associated with this syndrome, other manifestations of this acute syndrome, including lower extremity paresis, incontinence, emotional disturbance, and seizures, suggest that additional neural structures are likely involved. Mutism may also be caused either by direct retraction of the anterior cingulate gyrus, septum pellucidum, and fornix or by circulatory disturbances of the supplementary motor area, thalamus, and basal ganglia.

Continued

PITFALLS—cont'd

Disorders of interhemispheric transfer of information, which can include visuospatial and tactile information and bimanual motor learning, are another potential complication. Although the exact deficits depend on the topographic relationship within the corpus callosum, several studies have suggested that interhemispheric transfer should be preserved as long as the splenium is intact.

Although severe amnesia secondary to injury to the hippocampus and mammillary bodies has been convincingly documented, there have been contradictory reports regarding memory deficit resulting from isolated injury to the fornix. In many cases, memory loss erroneously attributed to injury to the fornix probably resulted from inappropriate transmission of pressure gradients to structures of the limbic system.

SUGGESTED READINGS

Amar AP, Ghosh S, Apuzzo ML. Ventricular tumors. In: Winn RH, editor. Youmans Neurological Surgery, vol. 1. Philadelphia: Saunders; 2004. p. 1237.

Apuzzo ML, Chikovani OK, Gott PS, et al. Transcallosal, interforniceal approaches for lesions affecting the third ventricle: surgical considerations and consequences. Neurosurgery 1982;10:547–54.

Apuzzo ML. Surgery in and around the anterior third ventricle. In: Brain Surgery: Complication Avoidance and Management. New York: Churchill Livingstone; 1993. p. 541.

Bogen JE. Callosotomy without disconnection? J Neurosurg 1994;81:328–9.

Clatterbuck RE, Tamargo RJ. Surgical positioning and exposures for cranial procedures. In: Winn RH, editor. Youmans Neurological Surgery, vol. 1. Philadelphia: Saunders; 2004. p. 623.

Geffen G, Walsh A, Simpson D, et al. Comparison of the effects of transcortical and transcallosal removal of intraventricular tumours. Brain 1980;103:773–88.

Jeeves MA, Simpson DA, Geffen G. Functional consequences of the transcallosal removal of intraventricular tumours. J Neurol Neurosurg Psychiatry 1979;42:134–42.

Kasowski H, Piepmeier JM. Transcallosal approach for tumors of the lateral and third ventricles. Neurosurg Focus 2001;10:E3.

Levin HS, Rose JE. Alexia without agraphia in a musician after transcallosal removal of a left intraventricular meningioma. Neurosurgery 1979;4:168–74.

Long DM, Chou SN. Transcallosal removal of cranio-pharyngiomas within the third ventricle. J Neurosurg 1973;39:563–7.

Nakasu Y, Isozumi T, Nioka H, et al. Mechanism of mutism following the transcallosal approach to the ventricles. Acta Neurochir (Wien) 1991;110:146–53.

Piepmeier JM, Sass KJ. Surgical management of lateral ventricular tumors. In: Paoletti P, Takakura K, Walker MD, editors. Neuro-Oncology. Boston: Kluwer Academic Publisher; 1991. p. 333.

Sakaki T, Kakizaki T, Takeshima T, et al. Importance of prevention of intravenous thrombosis and preservation of the venous collateral flow in bridging vein injury during surgery: an experimental study. Surg Neurol 1995;44:158–62.

Shucart WA, Stein BM. Transcallosal approach to the anterior ventricular system. Neurosurgery 1978;3:339–43.

Tanaka N, Nakanishi K, Fujiwara Y, et al. Postoperative segmental C5 palsy after cervical laminoplasty may occur without intraoperative nerve injury: a prospective study with transcranial electric motor-evoked potentials. Spine 2006;31:3013–7.

Tanaka Y, Sugita K, Kobayashi S, et al. Subdural fluid collections following transcortical approach to intra- or paraventricular tumours. Acta Neurochir (Wien) 1989;99:20–5.

Wen HT, Rhoton Jr AL, de Oliveira E. Transchoroidal approach to the third ventricle: an anatomic study of the choroidal fissure and its clinical application. Neurosurgery 1998;42:1205–17.

Winkler PA, Ilmberger J, Krishnan KG, et al. Transcallosal interforniceal-transforaminal approach for removing lesions occupying the third ventricular space: clinical and neuropsychological results. Neurosurgery 2000;46:879–88.

Winkler PA, Weis S, Buttner A, Raabe A, et al. The transcallosal interforniceal approach to the third ventricle: anatomic and microsurgical aspects. Neurosurgery 1997;40:973–81.

Winkler PA, Weis S, Wenger E, et al. Transcallosal approach to the third ventricle: normative morphometric data based on magnetic resonance imaging scans, with special reference to the fornix and forniceal insertion. Neurosurgery 1999;45:309–17.

Procedure 9

Transnasal Transsphenoidal Approach to Sellar and Suprasellar Lesions

Kaisorn L. Chaichana, Alfredo Quiñones-Hinojosa

INDICATIONS

- The transnasal transsphenoidal approach is employed for various pathologies involving the sella, suprasellar space, and sphenoid bone, including pituitary adenomas, Rathke pouch cyst, and craniopharyngiomas. Other indications include clival chordomas, meningiomas, metastatic lesions, and medial temporal lobe lesions such as encephaloceles.
- This approach is minimally traumatic to the brain, avoids brain retraction, does not create visible scars, provides excellent visualization of the pituitary, and is thought to cause less surgically related morbidity than transcranial approaches.
- This approach can be augmented with the use of an operative microscope and an endoscope. The operative microscope affords magnification, illumination, and three-dimensional viewing, and the endoscope expands the surgeon's field of view. Both tools can be used simultaneously to complement each other.

CONTRAINDICATIONS

- A classic transnasal approach is relatively contraindicated in cases of sphenoid sinusitis or ecstatic midline carotid arteries. Other relative contraindications include relatively small sellae, tumors with firm consistency, lesions with extensive intracranial invasion into the anterior cranial fossa or lateral or posterior extension, and asymmetric sellae. For these types of lesions, an expanded endonasal approach must be considered to maximize the visualization of lesions and to minimize potential vascular or neural complications.

PLANNING AND POSITIONING

- The sella can be approached by three transsphenoidal approaches: direct transnasal, submucosal tunnel via an anterior mucosal incision, or sublabial. The direct transnasal approach provides adequate visualization of the sella with minimal tissue dissection.
- Magnetic resonance imaging (MRI) provides the most useful preoperative imaging. T1-weighted images with and without gadolinium are useful for defining sellar anatomy and the relationship of sellar lesions to surrounding structures, including the optic chiasm, cavernous sinus, and internal carotid artery. T2-weighted images are useful for identifying cystic structures. Computed tomography (CT) scans are also helpful for defining sellar bony anatomy and identifying different subtypes of sphenoid sinus (i.e., conchae) that would be encountered intraoperatively.
- Special care should be taken in cases in which there is a suspicion of a vascular lesion with aneurysms in the cavernous carotid and cases in which surrounding vascular structures can be similar on imaging to pituitary lesions.
- Intraoperatively, surgical navigation with MRI or CT as an adjunct can be used in cases in which the anatomy is distorted by either the tumor or prior surgeries. Some authors have also reported the use of intraoperative real-time MRI, which can be considered if available for complex cases.

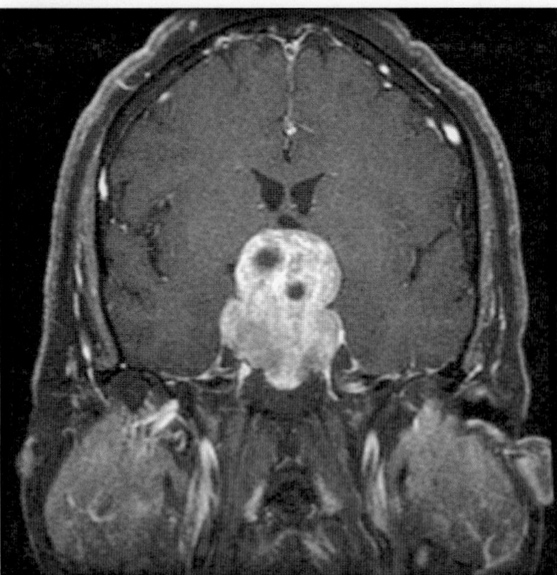
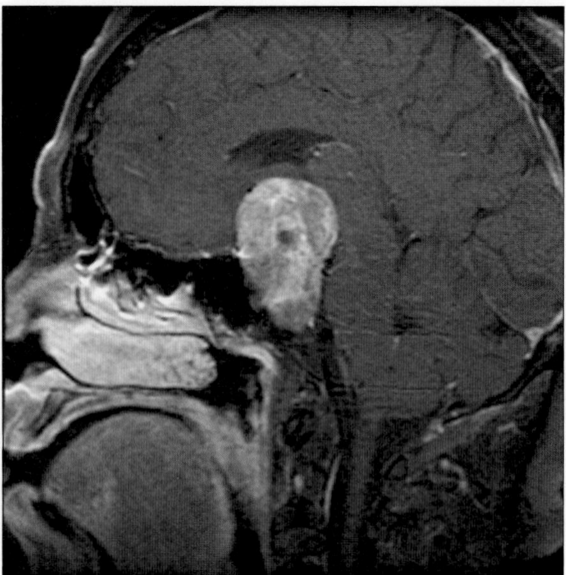

FIGURE 9-1

- Preoperative endocrine evaluation by an endocrinologist helps identify conditions of hormone excess or deficiency. This evaluation is especially critical for patients with hypoadrenalism or hypothyroidism, which pose surgical and anesthetic risks if not corrected before surgery. In addition, patients with prolactinomas may be sufficiently treated with dopamine agonist therapy, obviating the need for surgery. An evaluation by a neuroophthalmologist helps identify and define a patient's preoperative visual acuity and visual field ability.
- **Figure 9-1:** Preoperative T1-weighted contrast MRI defines sellar anatomy and the relationship of sellar lesions to surrounding structures.
- **Figure 9-2:** The patient is positioned supine with the head elevated above the right atrium. The head is placed in a three-pin fixation device, with the neck flexed and turned toward the right shoulder so that a midline axis of approach is aligned with the surgeon's field of view. The fluoroscope is positioned to give a coplanar view of the sella, and navigational devices are positioned for ease of view. An orogastric tube should be used to prevent drainage of blood products into the esophagus, which can result in immediate postoperative emesis or aspiration pneumonia. Some surgeons place a role of Kerlex gauze into the oropharynx as an alternative.
- **Figure 9-3:** The patient's nose and facial structures are prepared with povidone-iodine (Betadine) solution, and the nasal mucosa is prepared with cotton-tip applicators soaked with Betadine solution. After preparation, the nose is packed with pledgets soaked with oxymetazoline (Afrin). Most patients are given ceftriaxone before beginning the surgery,

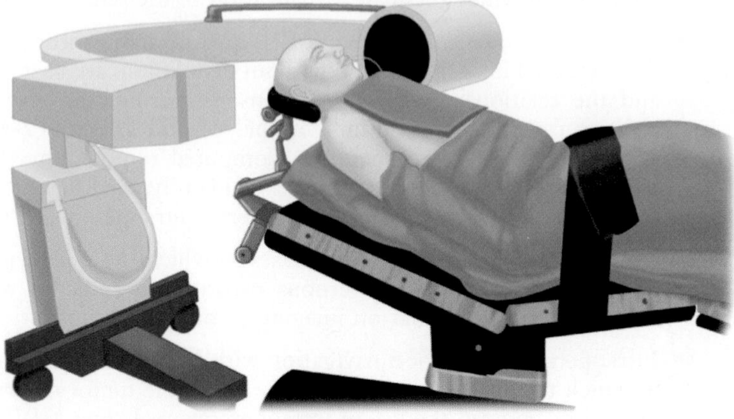

FIGURE 9-2

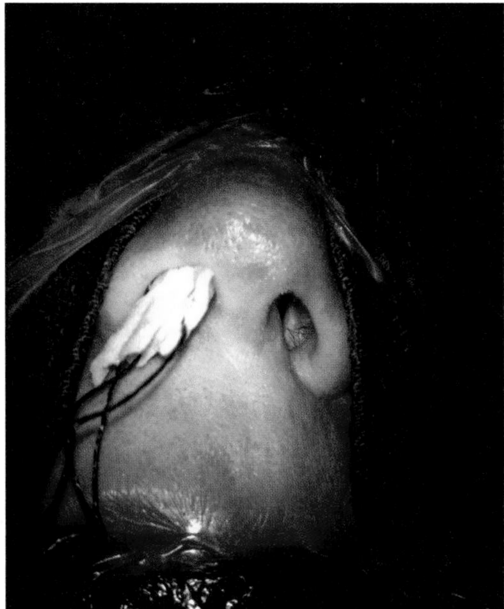
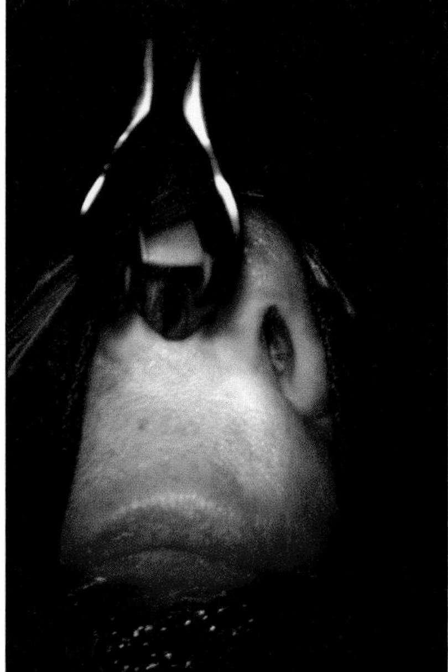

FIGURE 9-3

and patients with Cushing syndrome are given preoperative stress dose steroids. The right lower abdominal quadrant, above the waste line, or the right thigh is prepared for harvesting of a fat or fascia lata graft. Also, a lumbar drain can be placed preoperatively if the tumor has suprasellar extension; a drain is optional if the lesion abuts the sellar diaphragm.

PROCEDURE

- **Figure 9-4:** A long hand-held nasal speculum and endoscope are used to visualize and infiltrate the mucosa overlying the nasal septum and turbinates with 0.25% lidocaine and epinephrine (1:200,000) for local anesthesia and hemostasis. A linear incision is made in

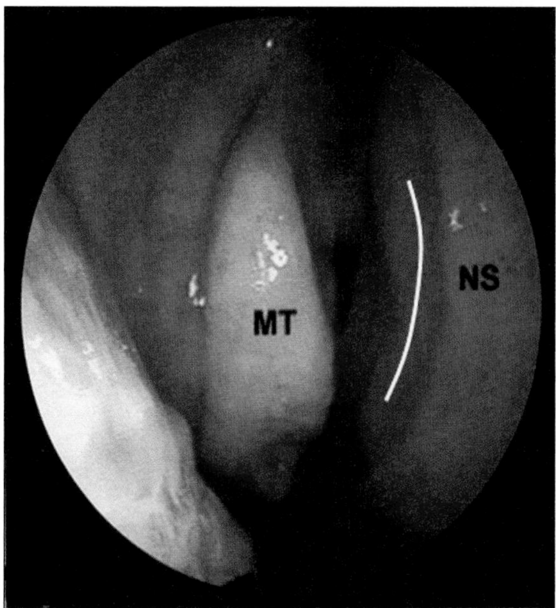

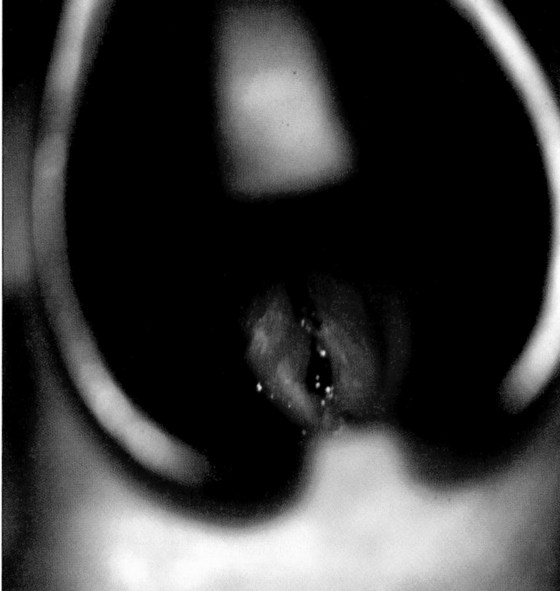

FIGURE 9-4

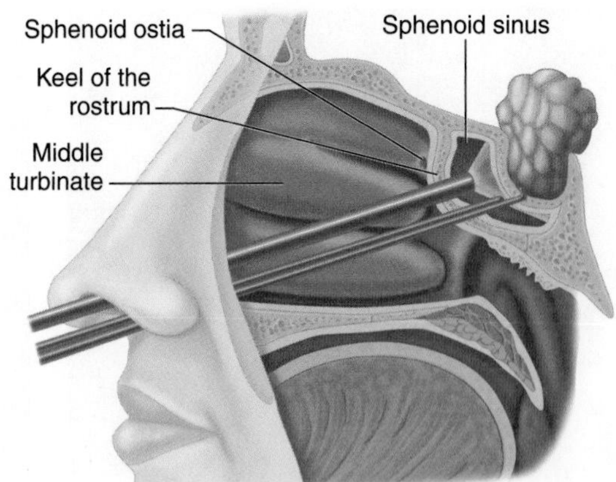

FIGURE 9-5

the mucosa overlying the posterior septum, and the septum is fractured and deviated to the opposite side with the use of a No. 2 Penfield dissector. A self-retaining speculum is placed on either side of the remnants of the fractured septum to allow visualization of the sphenoid ostia and keel of the rostrum. *MT*, medial turbinate; *NS*, nasal septum.

- **Figure 9-5:** Orientation in the sagittal plane is confirmed with use of an intraoperative fluoroscope if necessary, or surgical navigation can be used if available as a complement, provided that the registration is accurate. Anatomic landmarks, including the sphenoid ostia, orientation of the middle turbinate, and location of the keel of the rostrum, can help confirm a midline trajectory to the sphenoid sinus. A midline approach is essential to prevent inadvertent damage to the cavernous sinus, carotid artery, optic canal, and other perisellar structures.
- **Figure 9-6:** The sphenoid is entered by drilling through the rostrum of the sphenoid with the use of a high-speed diamond-tipped drill to the dura. Bone removal is carried back to the edges of the speculum. This can also be accomplished with rongeurs. The dura is typically opened with a cruciate incision using a No. 11 blade, and bipolar cautery is used on the dural leaves for hemostasis.
- **Figure 9-7:** With large macroadenomas, the tumor typically is seen immediately after opening the dura. The tumor is entered at its inferior margin using ring curets and

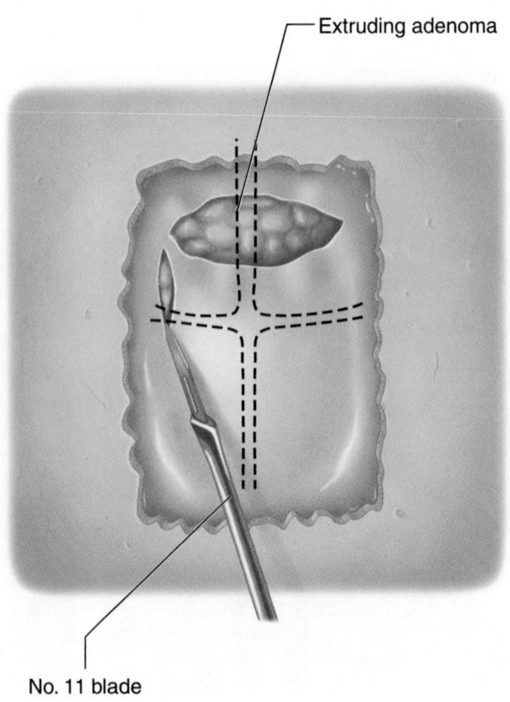

FIGURE 9-6

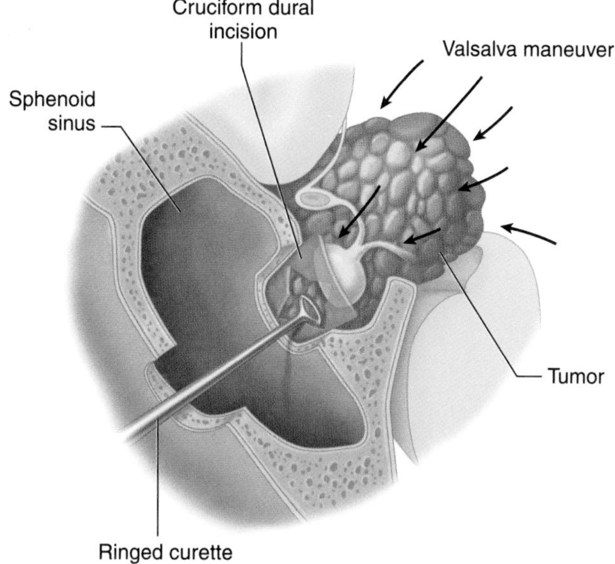

FIGURE 9-7

removed in a piecemeal fashion. Dissection is continued superiorly and laterally until the diaphragm sella prolapses into the field. With microadenomas, the normal pituitary gland is typically encountered first. Microadenoma is typically approached by dissecting through the gland with a blunt probe and then removed with a small ring curet.

- Valsalva maneuver can be used to increase intracranial pressure, which may cause the tumor to descend into the suprasellar space. Alternatively, a lumbar drain can be used at this point if the tumor or the diaphragm or both are not visualized and if there is suspicion of residual tumor in the suprasellar space. To complement the Valsalva maneuver and to increase intracranial pressure in an effort to bring the tumor down, 1 to 3 mL of preservative-free saline can be injected through the drain. Another option is to use an expanded exposure by removing more bone superiorly to visualize the sellar diaphragm and beyond to accomplish a gross total resection if necessary.
- **Figure 9-8:** With macroadenomas and cerebrospinal fluid (CSF) leaks, the tumor resection cavity is supported with the use of a fat graft, which can be harvested from the abdomen or

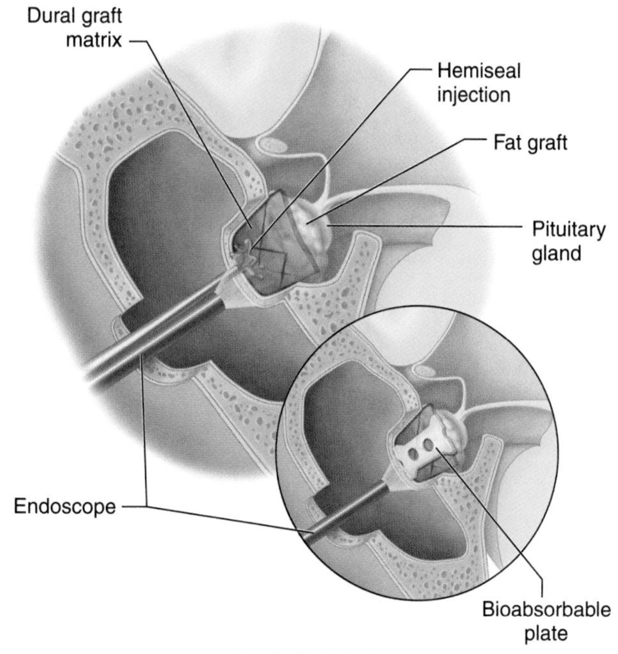

FIGURE 9-8

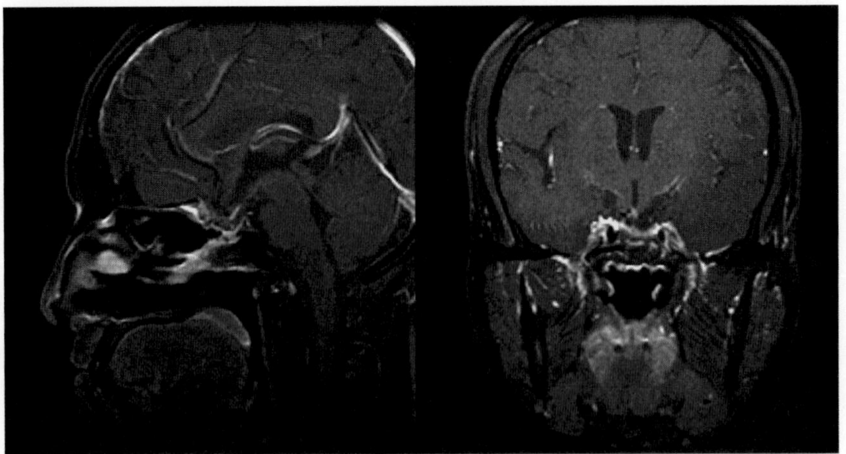

FIGURE 9-9

leg. The anterior wall of the sella is reconstructed using dural graft matrix and a bioabsorbable plate. Titanium plates, muscle, fascia lata, or lyophilized dura can also be used to reconstruct the sella. With microadenomas and the absence of CSF leaks, a fat graft is typically unnecessary. The construct can be coated with a fibrin sealant if needed, and a lumbar drain can be placed at the end of the case to decrease intracranial pressures.

- Hemostasis must be achieved after the procedure. Transient packing with Surgicel, injecting a slurry of Avitene, or placement of Floseal may help with achieving hemostasis. When hemostasis is achieved, the septum can be returned to the midline. A nasal stent can be used if extensive mucosal dissection occurred. We recommend at the end of the procedure to pack the nose again with oxymetazoline-soaked pledgets to aid with mucosal hemostasis. These pledgets are removed just before patient extubation.
- **Figure 9-9:** Patients should be monitored closely in the postoperative period. Serum sodium and urine specific gravity should be monitored every 6 hours to monitor for the possible development of diabetes insipidus or syndrome of inappropriate antidiuretic hormone secretion. This monitoring should be done in conjunction with an endocrinologist. In addition, visual fields and acuity should be monitored in conjunction with a neuroophthalmologist. Patients are typically given maintenance doses of steroids immediately in the postoperative period. MRI should be performed within 48 hours to evaluate extent of resection.

TIPS FROM THE MASTERS

- Sometimes during the transsphenoidal approach, the suprasellar portion of the tumor may be difficult to access. Delivery of the suprasellar portion can be aided by injecting 2 to 3 mL of preservative-free saline via a lumbar subarachnoid catheter or Valsalva maneuvers. Sometimes a staged resection may be necessary for suprasellar tumors that do not descend during the initial procedure, when CSF pulsations over time would help deliver the tumor. Additionally, the suprasellar portion can be exposed with the use of a 30-degree lens endoscope or with further removal of the bone at the tuberculum sella or planum sphenoidale.
- It is important during the transnasal approach to maintain orientation. Disorientation can occur easily and lead to injury of perisellar structures. Horizontal orientation can be maintained with the use of intracranial navigation (identifying the optico-carotid recess (OCR) and carotid groove is paramount to avoid going too far lateral), whereas vertical orientation can be maintained with the use of intraoperative fluoroscopy.
- For tumors with suprasellar extension, the thinned pituitary tissue is often identified rostrally when the suprasellar portion of the tissue is removed. This tissue can be severely thinned and appears to be a transparent membrane similar to the arachnoid membrane. If this tissue is penetrated, a CSF leak can occur.

PITFALLS

Lost of orientation can lead to catastrophic injury. A too superior orientation can lead toward the cribriform plate, which can lead to central nervous system injury, CSF leak, or meningitis. A too horizontal orientation can lead to injury to the cavernous sinus or carotid arteries.

It is important during closure to avoid overpacking, which can cause pressure against the optic nerves and chiasm.

CSF leakage is a known complication and can occur intraoperatively or in a delayed fashion. If patients have continuous CSF leakage, the leak must be repaired expeditiously to minimize the risk of meningitis.

It is probably safer if the surgeon decides to leave a suprasellar tumor unscathed than manipulate the tumor only to avoid resecting it. The reason is that the residual tumor can bleed or become edematous, leading to significant optic nerve compression (residual tumor can be adherent to suprasellar structures—basal frontal veins, arterial structures, and chiasm). A gross total resection is always associated with better outcomes, however.

BAILOUT OPTIONS

- If the surgeon loses orientation during the approach, despite using surgical navigation and fluoroscopy, it is probably safest to stop the procedure and resume at a later time to avoid catastrophic injury to perisellar structures.
- A transcranial supraorbital or classic pterional craniotomy approach can be used especially when the sellar lesion is too fibrous or tough, the suprasellar tumor fails to descend, or the lesion extends above the optic chiasm.
- If injury to the carotid artery occurs, the operative field should be packed with Surgicel, Gelfoam, or moist Telfa cotton pads, and gentle pressure should be applied. The mean arterial pressure should also be lowered; however, some surgeons would argue to increase mean arterial pressure to promote cross-filling. A cerebral angiogram should be performed to identify possible fistula (and rule out dissection), which may be able to occluded with the use of endovascular coils or with open craniotomy and trapping the carotid artery. Brisk bleeding intraoperatively can occur with a breach in McConnell's capsular artery, which arise from the cavernous carotid that often supply vascularized sellar tumors.

SUGGESTED READINGS

Cappabianca P, Cavallo LM, Colao A, et al. Surgical complications of the endoscopic endonasal transphenoidal approach for pituitary adenomas. J Neurosurg 2002;97:293–8.

Chang EF, Zada G, Kim S, Lamborn KR, et al. Long-term recurrence and mortality after surgery and adjuvant radiotherapy for nonfunctional pituitary adenomas. J Neurosurg 2008;108:736–45.

Jho HD, Alfier A. Endoscopic endonasal pituitary surgery: evolution of surgical technique and equipment in 150 operations. Minim Invasive Neurosurg 2001;44:1–12.

Rhoton AL Jr. The sellar region. Neurosurgery 2002;51:S335–74.

Sanai N, Quiñones-Hinojosa A, Narvid J, et al. Safety and efficacy of the direct endonasal endonasal transphenoidal approach for challenging sellar tumors. J Neurononcol 2008;87:317–25.

Procedure 10

Supracerebellar Infratentorial Approach

Shaan M. Raza, Alfredo Quiñones-Hinojosa

INDICATIONS

- This approach provides excellent exposure for lesions of the pineal region, posterior third ventricle, and posterior mesencephalon.

CONTRAINDICATIONS

- The angle of the tentorium is an important consideration; this approach is not suitable for patients with a steeply angled tentorium. For such situations, alternative approaches such as the occipital transtentorial approach should be considered.

PLANNING AND POSITIONING

- Preoperative planning includes assessment of the patient's cardiopulmonary status, evaluation of comorbidities, and basic laboratory tests, including a basic metabolic panel, complete blood count, coagulation profile, and type and screen. Baseline chest x-ray and electrocardiogram are also useful. A preoperative bubble cardiac Doppler study is recommended to rule out any possible cardiac shunting or patent foramen ovale.
- Preoperative magnetic resonance imaging (MRI) including magnetic resonance venography is obtained; particular attention is paid to the relationship of the deep venous structures (vein of Galen, basal vein of Rosenthal, internal cerebral veins, and straight sinus) in relation to the trajectory and tumor. Imaging is also assessed for degree of tumor infiltration into surrounding critical neural structures (e.g., midbrain, thalamus).
- A preoperative surgical navigation image is recommended as a surgical adjunct.
- For patients with preoperative hydrocephalus, an intraventricular catheter is placed before soft tissue dissection; this can be placed at the mid-pupillary line on the lambdoid suture.
- We prefer to use the sitting position for this approach. The upright positioning permits the cerebellum to fall with gravity away from the tentorium, in addition to preventing pooling of venous blood in the operative field. The prone position is the only recommended position if the patient has a patent foramen ovale, given the risk of pulmonary air embolism with the sitting position. An intraoperative discussion should be held with the anesthesia team to perform cardiac Doppler during the procedure to prevent a venous air embolism. Precordial Doppler ultrasonography is the most sensitive of the generally available monitors capable of detecting intracardiac air. Placement of a central venous catheter with multiple orifices is strongly recommended as a means of aspirating air from the circulation should a venous air embolism occur.
- **Figure 10-1:** The patient is first placed supine on the operative table (with reverse orientation) (**A**). After application of Mayfield holder, the bed is maneuvered to raise the patient's back and flex the legs. The head is flexed to place the tentorium parallel to the floor (**B**).
- **Figure 10-2:** The skin incision is marked from above the inion down to approximately C2. Registration with surgical navigation can be performed at this point.

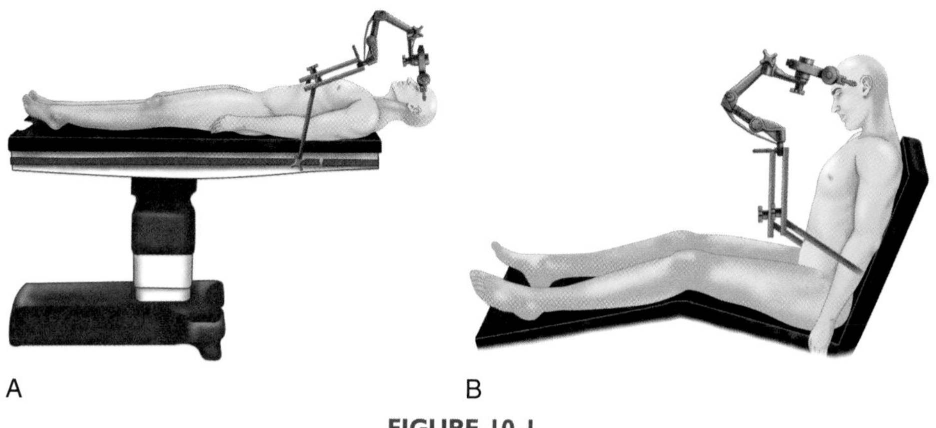

FIGURE 10-1

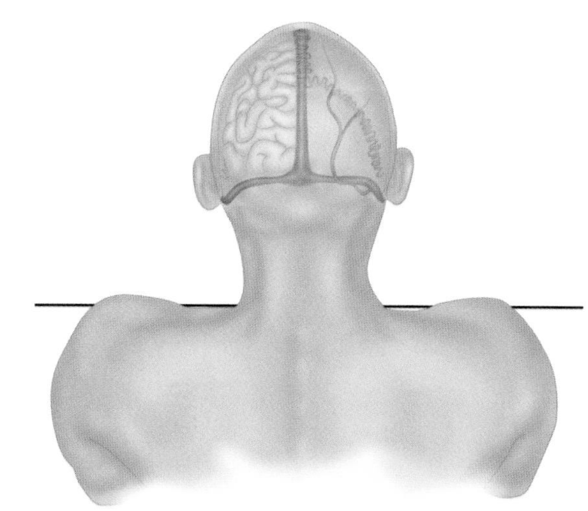

FIGURE 10-2

PROCEDURE

- **Figure 10-3:** Suboccipital exposure is performed with dissection of the suboccipital musculature; the musculature is not detached and is preserved from the spinous processes of C1-2. A craniotomy is performed. Burr holes are placed on each side of the superior sagittal sinus (right above the torcular Herophili), and superior and inferior to each transverse sinus a few centimeters distal to the torcular Herophili. A craniotome is used to connect the burr holes to create a bone flap. If there is evidence of preoperative tonsillar descent, the foramen magnum can be removed in addition to a C1 laminectomy. A semilunar or cruciate dural incision is made based on the transverse sinuses and torcular Herophili and reflected superiorly with tenting sutures. The surgeon should be cognizant of the retraction placed on the venous sinus when reflecting the dural flap.
- **Figure 10-4:** Arachnoid adhesions and bridging veins between the cerebellum and tentorium are divided to open the supracerebellar infratentorial corridor. These bridging veins should be divided close to the cerebellum to prevent retraction of inaccessible bleeding sources back into the tentorium. As this process of dissection proceeds, the cerebellum falls with gravity, and a retractor can be placed on the tentorium if necessary.
- **Figure 10-5:** Thickened arachnoid overlying the pineal gland and quadrigeminal cistern is exposed and sharply dissected open. In this process, the precentral cerebellar vein is

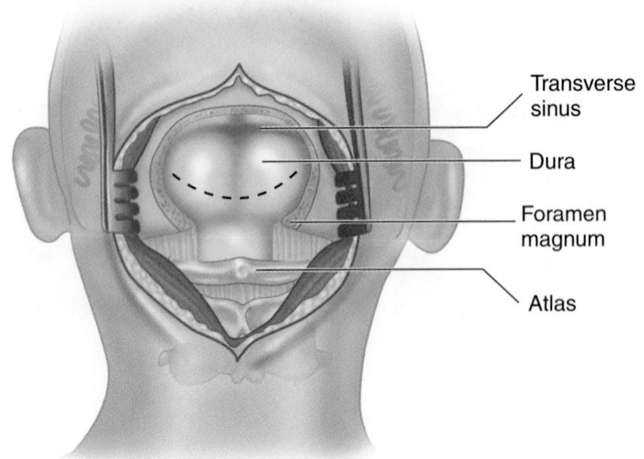

FIGURE 10-3

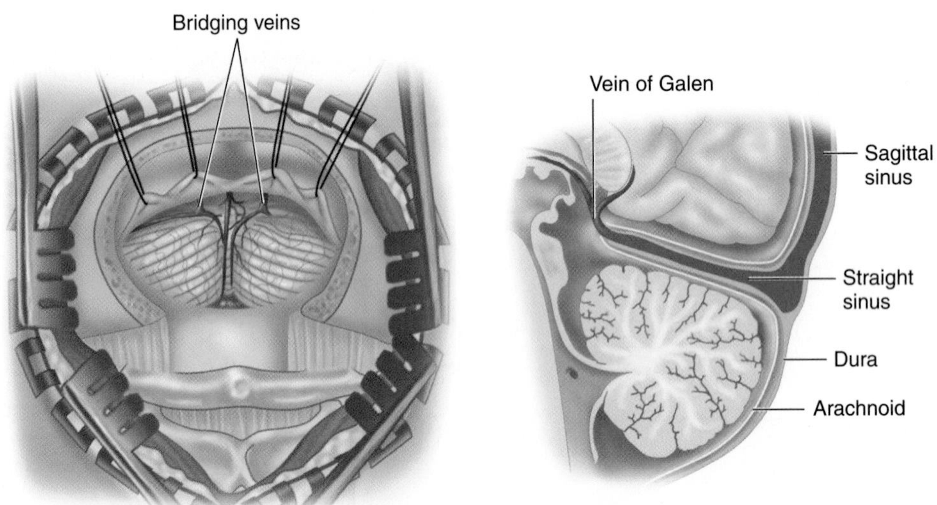

FIGURE 10-4

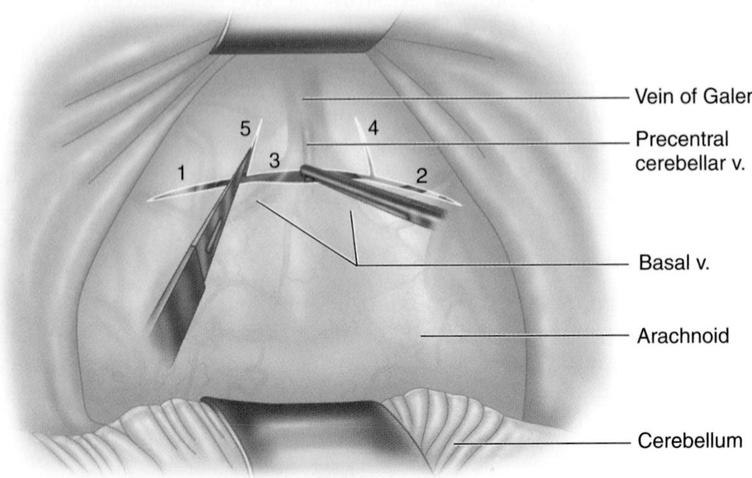

FIGURE 10-5

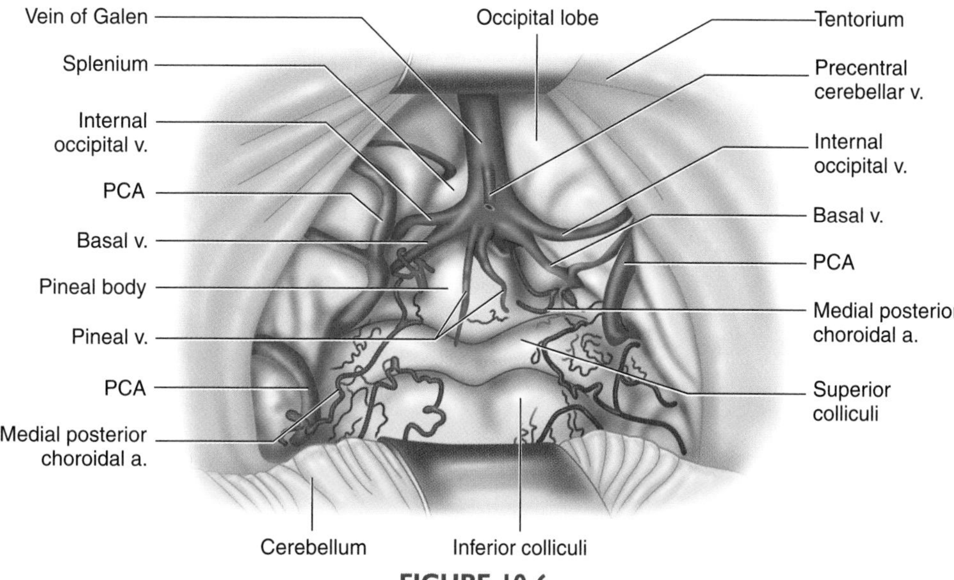

FIGURE 10-6

visualized draining into the vein of Galen—this is the only deep venous structure that should be cauterized and divided.

- **Figure 10-6:** Normal anatomy when exposure is achieved and cerebellar retraction occurs. Depending on the pathology for which this approach is chosen, the vascular structures and neural structures are shifted to nonanatomic positions.

TIPS FROM THE MASTERS

- The angle of the tentorium and relationship of venous structures to the tumor are crucial to the success of this approach versus other alternatives.
- The placement of an intraventricular catheter is not only useful for treatment of preoperative hydrocephalus, but also facilitates brain relaxation and decompression of posterior fossa.
- Special preoperative cardiac work-up and planning should be considered if the sitting position is to be used. Communication with the anesthesia team should occur regarding the need of a cardiac Doppler examination intraoperatively with a multiple-channel central line for dealing with a potential air embolism.
- In the event of an intraoperative air embolism, the transverse torcular Herophili sinus area should be covered with laparotomy pads, and the field should be flooded with irrigation.

PITFALLS

The primary limitation of the sitting position is the risk for air embolism. All patients should have intraoperative monitoring via end-tidal CO_2 monitoring and Doppler ultrasound. Formation of emboli is halted by flooding the field with irrigation and lowering the patient's head. A central venous catheter can be used to retrieve any large emboli.

BAILOUT OPTIONS

- If the angle of the tentorium is too steep, the craniotomy can be extended for an occipital transtentorial approach, or the tentorium can be cut and retracted via the supracerebellar approach.

SUGGESTED READINGS

Abla AA, Turner JD, Mitha AP, Spetzler RF. Surgical approaches to brainstem cavernous malformations. Neurosurg Focus 2010;29(3):E8.

de Oliveira JG, Lekovic GP, Safavi-Abbasi S, et al. Supracerebellar infratentorial approach to cavernous malformations of the brainstem: surgical variants and clinical experience with 45 patients. Neurosurgery 2010; 66(2):389–99.

Lozier AP, Bruce JN. Surgical approaches to posterior third ventricular tumors. Neurosurg Clin N Am 2003; 14(4):527–45.

Jittapiromsak P, Little AS, Deshmukh P, et al. Comparative analysis of the retrosigmoid and lateral supracerebellar infratentorial approaches along the lateral surface of the pontomesencephalic junction: a different perspective. Neurosurgery 2008;62(5 Suppl. 2):ONS279–87.

Sanai N, Mirzadeh Z, Lawton M. Supracerebellar-supratrochlear and infratentorial-infratrochlear approaches: gravity dependent variations of the lateral approach over the cerebellum. Neurosurgery 2010;66(6 Suppl. Operative):264–74.

Ulm AJ, Tanriover N, Kawashima M, et al. Microsurgical approaches to the perimesencephalic cisterns and related segments of the posterior cerebral artery: comparison using a novel application of image guidance. Neurosurgery 2004;54(6):1313–27.

Procedure 11

Occipital Transtentorial Approach

Nader Sanai, Michael W. McDermott

INDICATIONS

- An occipital transtentorial craniotomy can provide excellent exposure for falcitentorial meningiomas and any lesion arising from the precentral cerebellar fissure, posterior incisural space, and adjoining structures.

CONTRAINDICATIONS

- Standard medical contraindications for prone positioning
- Patent foramen ovale with positive bubble study for sitting position, owing to risks arising from venous air embolism

PLANNING AND POSITIONING

- Standard preoperative magnetic resonance imaging (MRI) is needed as well as magnetic resonance venography or angiography to confirm patency of the straight sinus. Preoperative visual field testing is required as a baseline for all patients with larger tumors and greater risk of transient cortical blindness.
- **Figure 11-1:** For small tumors (<3 cm), a unilateral approach with the ipsilateral lobe down is sufficient. For most patients, a lateral or semilateral position is adequate. An approach from the right is preferred because a right hemianopsia, resulting from a left-sided approach, produces greater difficulty with reading. For the lateral position, using arm extension allows the shoulder to drop down avoiding collision of the chin with the clavicle. For larger patients, a modified park bench position is necessary.
- **Figure 11-2:** For larger tumors (>3 cm), a bilateral occipital transtentorial approach is needed. Patients can be placed prone or in the sitting position. Patients with a large body habitus benefit from the sitting position because high intrathoracic pressures in the prone position can complicate exposure.
- Preoperative embolization is safe if the blood supply arises from external branches and the meningohypophysial branches of the internal carotid arteries.
- The operating room setup may include bipolar cautery and bovie cautery, operating microscope (foot pedal for focus and zoom, mouthpiece for fine adjustments), chair with arm rests and floor wheels, and neurophysiologic monitoring with somatosensory evoked potentials.

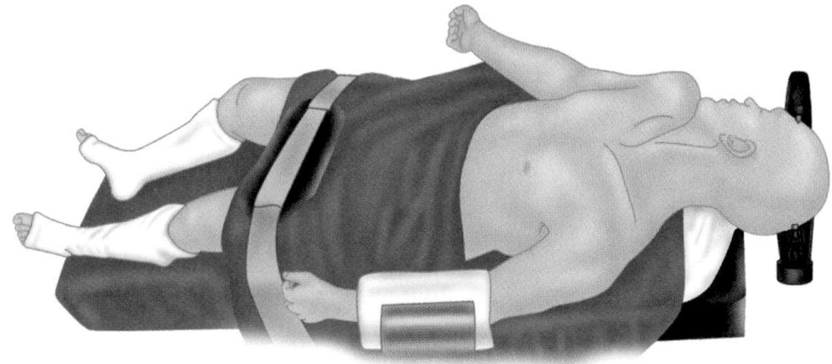

FIGURE 11-1

- Anesthesia includes 1 g of ceftriaxone, 10 mg of dexamethasone (Decadron), and 1 g/kg of mannitol on skin incision. Cerebral perfusion pressure should be maintained at greater than 70 mm Hg to prevent ischemia from brain retraction. Severe hypertension should be treated aggressively (e.g., propofol, thiopental, vasoactive drugs).

PROCEDURE

Positioning for Occipital Transtentorial Craniotomy

- Patient prone or sitting with head fixed in Mayfield head holder
- Prone position: neck extended on the chest, head flexed on the neck
- Armored endotracheal tube to prevent kinking
- Bilateral kidney rests to allow operating table to be laterally rotated

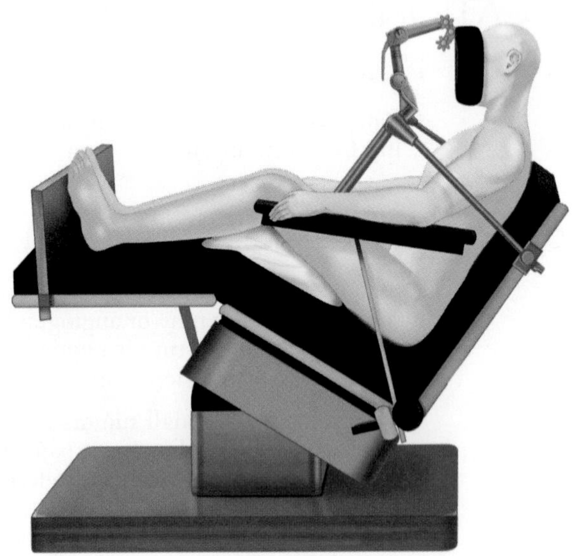

FIGURE 11-2

Occipital Transtentorial Craniotomy

- An external ventricular drain via a parietooccipital trajectory or a lumbar drain should be placed.
- **Figure 11-3:** After adequate positioning, a U-shaped, inferiorly based incision is made extending supratentorially and infratentorially. This flap provides excellent exposure to both occipital lobes and both cerebellar hemispheres.
- **Figure 11-4:** Burr holes facilitate the craniotomy with preservation of the superior sagittal and transverse sinuses. Two burr holes are placed on both sides of the superior sagittal sinus at the rostral extent of the desired bone flap. Four burr holes are placed above and below the lateral transverse sinus on both sides at the lateral extent of the desired bone flap. The dura is carefully dissected before craniotomy and elevation of the bone flap.
- **Figure 11-5:** Dural flaps are created based away from the venous structures. The occipital dural flaps are based laterally and retracted with sutures. The cerebellar flap is based on the inferior transverse sinuses and torcular Herophili. When completed, the dural opening should expose above and below the tentorium and beyond the lateral margins of the tumor.
- **Figure 11-6:** For tumors that involve the torcular Herophili, resection is based on knowledge of venous drainage from the preoperative work-up. If the torcular Herophili and one or both transverse sinuses are patent, the tentorium is incised from lateral to medial in front of the torcular Herophili. If the sinuses are occluded, they are suture ligated at the lateral margins of the tumor.

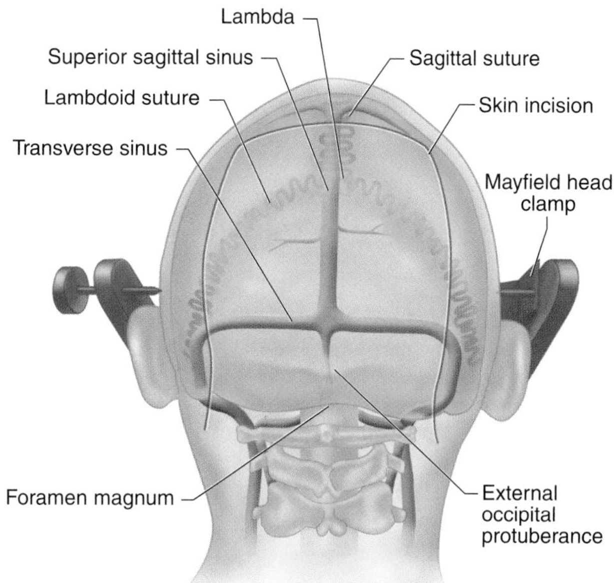

FIGURE 11-3

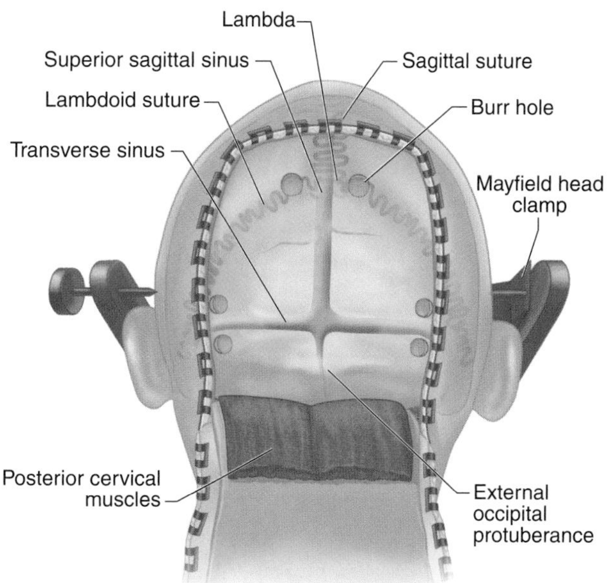

FIGURE 11-4

- **Figure 11-7:** In cases in which the tumor results in occlusion of the superior sagittal sinus, the venous structures in the region can be secured and ligated. This along with falcine and tentorial incisions allows for complete resection of the tumor.

TIPS FROM THE MASTERS

- For larger tumors, a two-surgeon team is recommended for efficient tumor removal and minimal surgeon fatigue.
- The foramen magnum is opened at the surgeon's discretion with significant infratentorial components.
- The infratentorial portion is more often the exophytic component of the tumor.

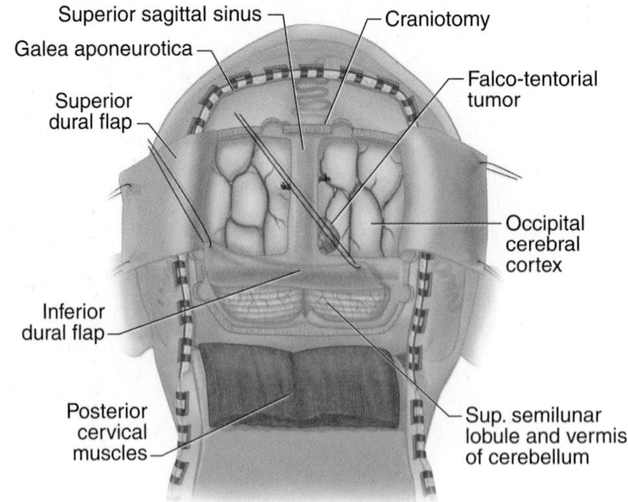

FIGURE 11-5

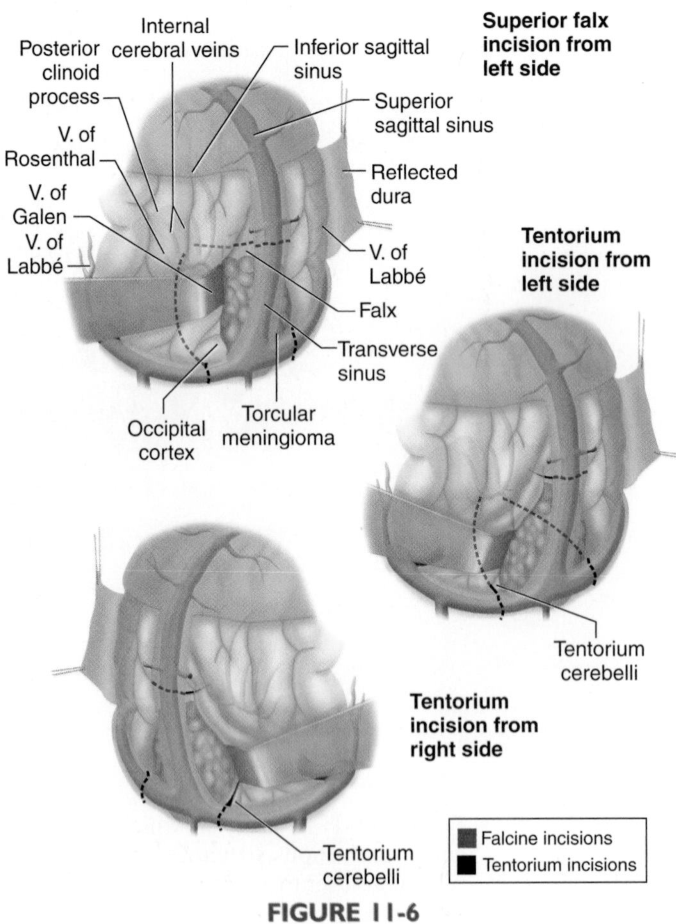

FIGURE 11-6

- Patience is necessary when dissecting the vein of Galen.
- The pial surface is covered with rubber dams during the procedure to minimize retraction injury.
- Patients and families should be counseled preoperatively regarding the risks of transient cortical blindness. Several days of transient cortical blindness should be expected after larger tumor resections.

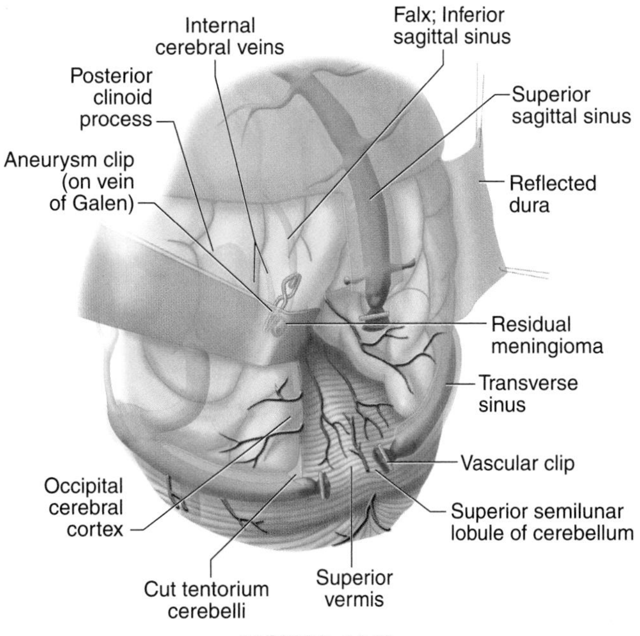

FIGURE 11-7

PITFALLS

Retraction edema can be minimized by careful placement of the initial retractor, brain relaxation with release of cerebrospinal fluid, and intermittent placement and replacement of the retractors.

Avoidance of venous infarction requires extensive preoperative vascular imaging, including magnetic resonance venography or formal angiography or both to ascertain patent and occluded structures.

The most difficult portion of the case is finding and preserving the straight sinus when it is patent.

Dural leaflets may be expanded by tumor and create false walls within the tumor.

BAILOUT OPTIONS

- Uncontrolled external cerebral herniation after decompression can risk primary closure of the scalp. If this possibility is suspected in advance, it is wise to obtain hemostasis and be prepared to close before the dura is opened.
- In especially urgent cases, such as cases with recent development of anisocoria and an underlying subdural hematoma, making a cruciate opening in the dura through the first burr hole may provide some relief of intracranial hypertension during the craniotomy.

SUGGESTED READINGS

Kawashima M, Rhoton AL Jr, Matsushima T. Comparison of posterior approaches to the posterior incisural space: microsurgical anatomy and proposal of a new method, the occipital bi-transtentorial/falcine approach. Neurosurgery 2008;62(6 Suppl. 3):1136–49.

Reid WS, Clark WK. Comparison of the infratentorial and transtentorial approaches to the pineal region. Neurosurgery 1978;3:1–8.

Shirane R, Kumabe T, Yoshida Y, et al. Surgical treatment of posterior fossa tumors via the occipital transtentorial approach: evaluation of operative safety and results in 14 patients with anterosuperior cerebellar tumors. J Neurosurg 2001;94:927–35.

Shirane R, Shamoto H, Umezawa K, et al. Surgical treatment of pineal region tumours through the occipital transtentorial approach: evaluation of the effectiveness of intra-operative micro-endoscopy combined with neuronavigation. Acta Neurochir (Wien) 1999;141:801–8.

Procedure 12

Trauma Flap: Decompressive Hemicraniectomy

Michael E. Sughrue, Mathew B. Potts, Shirley I. Stiver, Geoffrey T. Manley

INDICATIONS

- Elevated intracranial pressure (ICP) is one of the most common causes of death and disability following severe traumatic brain injury and ischemic stroke.
- There have been no new medical treatments for elevated ICP in more than 90 years. A decompressive craniectomy may be a useful surgical option in ICP that is refractory to medical treatment. Decompressive craniectomy is also performed as a prophylactic measure in the emergency setting during evacuation of a traumatic subdural or epidural mass lesion when the bone is not replaced in anticipation of postoperative elevated ICP as predicted by computed tomography (CT) scan or the appearance of the brain at surgery.
- Decompressive craniectomy, when performed correctly, can reduce ICP and prevent cerebral herniation and death. Successful decompressive craniectomy allows the brain to swell, reducing the risk of neurologic injury from elevated ICP. In most instances, decompressive craniectomy also reduces the intensity of medical management in the intensive care unit.

CONTRAINDICATIONS

- Decompressive craniectomy is most often performed in the setting of life-threatening, impending cerebral herniation. It is important that the surgical and critical care teams and the family members know the dire prognosis of many of these cases to avoid unrealistic expectations. Decompressive craniectomy is well established to treat elevated ICP, but it is less certain which patients are most likely to benefit from this procedure.
- Older patients and patients with limited brainstem reflexes and a low Glasgow Coma Scale score from the time of injury may be at greatest risk for a poor outcome.

PLANNING AND POSITIONING

- **Figure 12-1:** For unilateral decompressive craniectomy, the patient is positioned supine with a small towel roll under the ipsilateral shoulder and the head turned to the contralateral side. In the setting of trauma, it is important to position the patient with cervical spine precautions. Care should be taken not to compress the jugular veins, which can lead to decreased venous return and further increase in ICP. The head can be rested on a foam headrest; this allows for repositioning of the head intraoperatively if venous outflow obstruction is suspected. We generally prefer not to use a rigid head holder with pins unless we are certain that there are no skull fractures.

PROCEDURE

- **Figure 12-2:** Skin incision. After the head is shaved and prepared, a large reverse question mark incision is made, beginning at the zygoma extending far behind the ear, then curving a few centimeters lateral to the sagittal suture, anteriorly to the hairline. If possible, the superficial temporal artery should be protected to preserve the blood supply to the flap.
- **Figure 12-3:** Muscle and soft tissue dissection. The incision is carried through the subcutaneous tissue, including the temporalis, down to the cranium. The

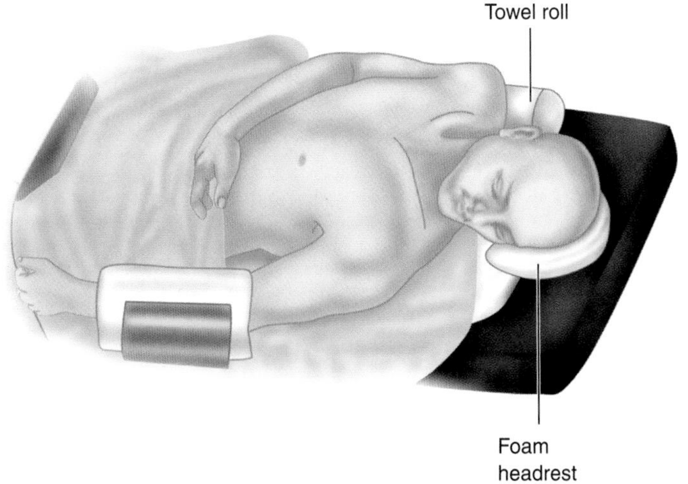

FIGURE 12-1

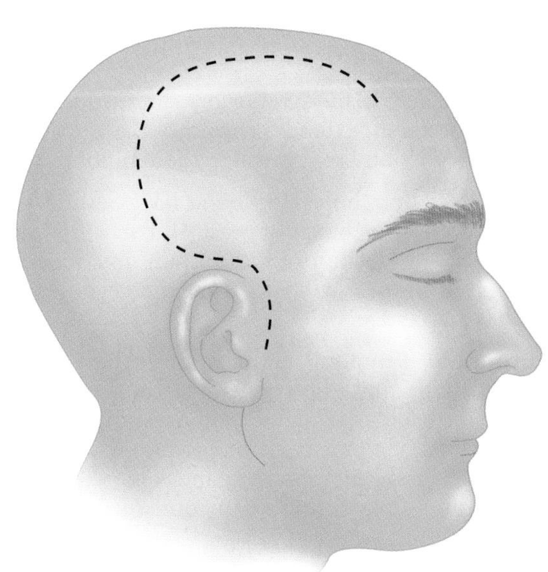

FIGURE 12-2

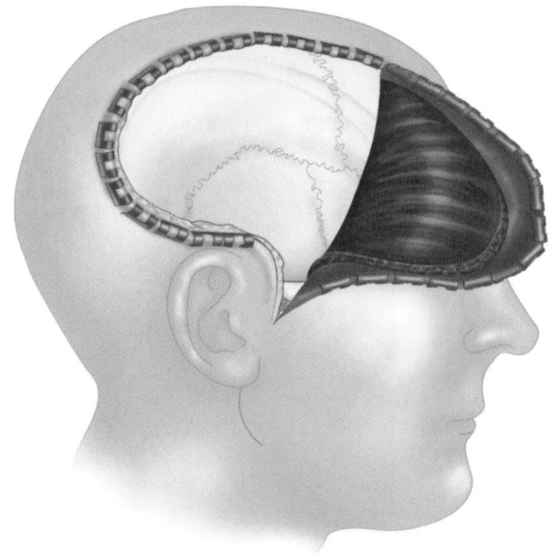

FIGURE 12-3

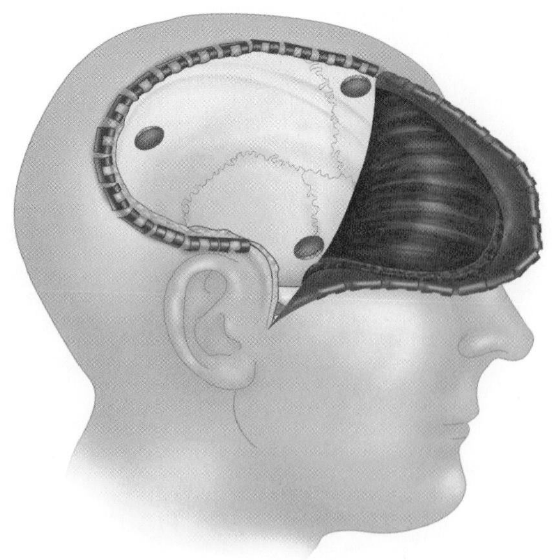

FIGURE 12-4

musculocutaneus flap is reflected anteriorly and fixed with scalp hooks. Ideally, this muscle dissection extends down to the root of the zygoma and as far below the keyhole as possible, to maximize the temporal decompression achieved.

- **Figure 12-4:** Burr holes and bone flap. Several burr holes (at least three) are made to create a bone flap that is at least 10 cm × 15 cm. Bone flaps smaller than this would not sufficiently decompress the brain and reduce ICP. When possible, a small ruler can be used to measure back from the keyhole to ensure the anteroposterior extent of the bone flap is 15 cm.
- **Figure 12-5:** Temporal craniectomy. After removal of the bone flap, the remaining temporal bone must be cut with a rongeur down to the floor of the middle cranial fossa to provide maximal decompression of the lateral brainstem. Care should be taken to bite, and not twist or torque, with the rongeur during bone removal low in the middle fossa. Aggressive maneuvers with the rongeur can open or displace skull base fractures and precipitate uncontrolled bleeding.
- **Figure 12-6:** Dural opening. After achieving hemostasis, there are several choices for the durotomy. Our preferred method is to open the dura slowly with multiple radial incisions (in a stellate fashion) to provide maximal cerebral decompression (**A**).

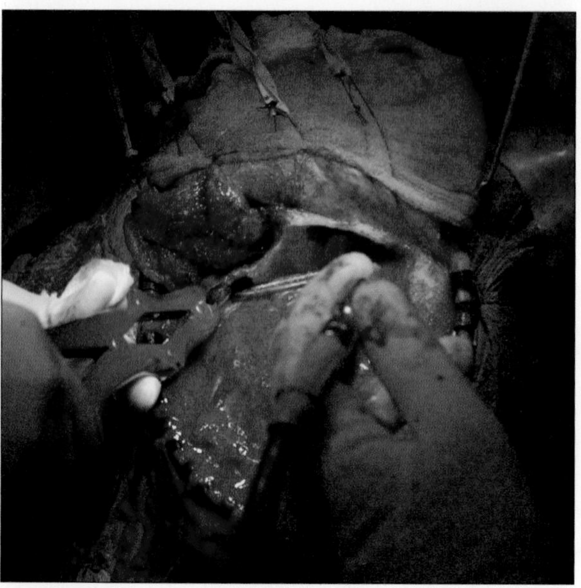

FIGURE 12-5

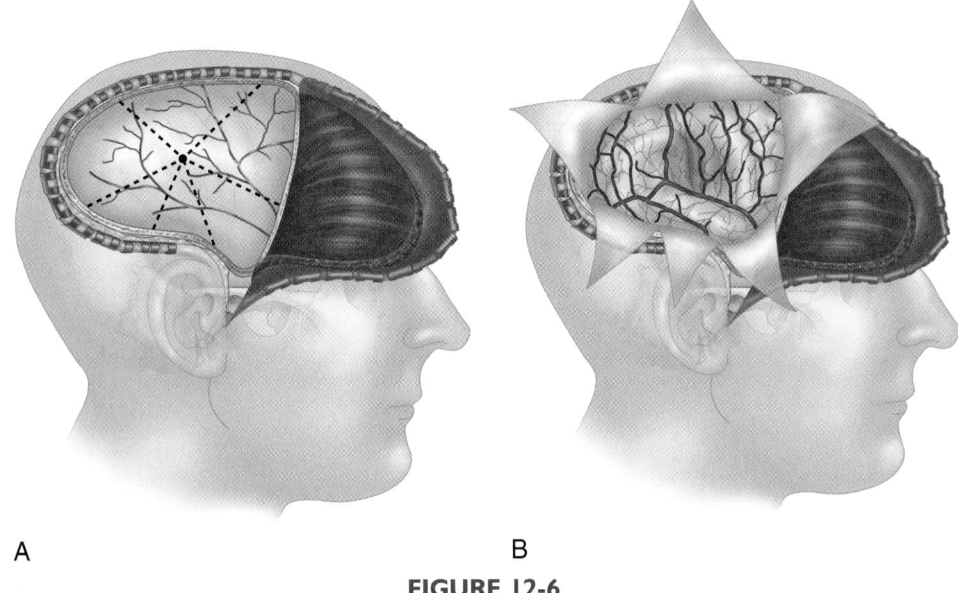

FIGURE 12-6

Associated hematomas can be removed, and hemostasis can be obtained (**B**). When the dural opening is completed, closure can be undertaken. Although some surgeons perform a duraplasty, we prefer to leave the durotomy open and simply to cover the brain with a dural substitute or similar material to protect the brain surface and reduce adhesions. The leaves of the dura are folded over the dural substitute. Unless there is an urgent need to leave the operating room, drains are placed over the surface of the dural substitute and tunneled externally. The galea should be closed with numerous, closely spaced interrupted 2-0 absorbable braided sutures. The skin is closed with a running 4-0 absorbable monofilament suture. To ensure a watertight closure, the sutures are placed very close together.

TIPS FROM THE MASTERS

- With the rare exception of bifrontal extraaxial mass lesions, we have found that good ICP control can be obtained with unilateral decompressive surgery, even in cases of bifrontal contusions. Unilateral decompressive surgery on the side of the larger intraparenchymal injury is technically more straightforward than bifrontal decompression, and a larger decompression can be obtained without manipulation or exposure of the sagittal sinus. Unilateral hemicraniectomy also enables a more extensive decompression low in the temporal region compared with a bifrontal procedure. In addition, with attention to the size of the frontal sinuses on CT scan, opening into the frontal sinuses can be more easily avoided in a unilateral decompression. Cranioplasty repair of the skull defect after unilateral decompression is simpler and safer, making it preferable.
- It is crucial to avoid the midline when turning the bone flap. It is easy to get off midline in an emergency setting, however, wherein technical maneuvers and details need to be streamlined. It is a good idea to mark the midline rapidly and place the drapes up to midline so that you are always oriented to the midline, especially if the head is not pinned. The location of the sagittal suture can also be used to determine midline.
- Preparing the contralateral Kocher point for invasive neuromonitoring with a ventricular catheter during the head shave can save some time after the case.
- Arterial blood exiting from the middle fossa in large amounts warrants exploration and often arises from the middle meningeal artery or the sphenoid wing. If this bleeding is seen, a slightly more conservative temporal craniectomy provides bone to which the temporal dura can be tacked, which may stop the bleeding.

PITFALLS

In experienced hands, wound complications are the most common source of surgical morbidity with this procedure. These complications largely result from either traumatic injury to the skin in the region of the incision or cerebrospinal fluid egress caused by a combination of the widely open dura and the resultant cerebrospinal fluid absorption problems many patients develop. Diligent attention to closure, including multiple, closely spaced inverted galeal stitches; the routine prolonged use of drains; and skin closure with running absorbable monofilament suture have nearly eliminated these problems at our institution.

Leaving at least two Jackson-Pratt drains in the surgical cavity is highly recommended because these patients often do not clot properly, and without the tamponading effect provided by the bone flap, the risk of symptomatic epidural hemorrhage is high.

Although it is tempting to rush the dural opening, given the urgency of these cases, we recommend a slower dural opening because we have seen sudden cardiovascular collapse and profound hypotension resulting from sudden reversal of elevated ICP and the loss of the catecholamine support that comes with the Cushing response. Adequate resuscitation by anesthesia can also prevent this complication. In most cases, a central line can facilitate a successful resuscitation.

The dura over the anterior frontal lobe is commonly torn, typically in emergencies and older patients. It is a good practice to assume that the dura may be incompetent in the frontal area and to begin to strip the dura and elevate the bone flap away from this site.

A skull fracture contralateral to the side of decompression is a significant risk factor for a postoperative epidural hematoma. A routine CT scan early after decompressive hemicraniectomy should be considered in patients who harbor a skull fracture remote to the site of decompression. Precipitous external herniation can rarely occur intraoperatively, soon after decompression. Especially in the setting of a contralateral skull fracture, empiric surgical exploration on the other side, without an interim CT scan, may be considered.

BAILOUT OPTIONS

- Uncontrolled external cerebral herniation after decompression can make primary closure of the scalp difficult. If this possibility is suspected in advance, it is wise to obtain hemostasis and be prepared to close before the dura is opened.
- In especially urgent cases, such as cases with recent development of anisocoria and an underlying subdural hematoma, making a cruciate opening in the dura through the first burr hole may provide some relief of intracranial hypertension during the craniotomy.

SUGGESTED READINGS

Bullock MR, Chesnut R, Ghajar J, et al. Guidelines for the surgical management of traumatic brain injury. Neurosurgery 2006;58(Suppl. 3):s2-1–62.

Coplin WM, Cullen NK, Policherla PN, et al. Safety and feasibility of craniectomy with duraplasty as the initial surgical intervention for severe traumatic brain injury. J Trauma 2001;50:1050–59.

Munch E, Horn P, Schurer L, et al. Management of severe traumatic brain injury by decompressive craniectomy. Neurosurgery 2000;47:315–22.

Schneider GH, Bardt T, Lanksch WR, et al. Decompressive craniectomy following traumatic brain injury: ICP, CPP and neurological outcome. Acta Neurochir Suppl 2002;81:77–9.

Valadka AB, Robertson CS. Surgery of cerebral trauma and associated critical care. Neurosurgery 2007;61:203–20.

Procedure 13 Parasagittal Approach

Pablo F. Recinos, Michael Lim

INDICATIONS

- Parasagittal approaches are used to treat lesions located near the falx, corpus callosum, or other deep midline structures. These lesions include parasagittal and falcine meningiomas; midline gliomas; cavernomas and arteriovenous malformations (AVMs) located in the thalamus; paraventricular masses; and lesions located in the medial frontal gyrus, cingulate gyrus, or corpus callosum.
- Surgical intervention should be considered for tumors that exhibit growth, cause neurologic deficit, or cause uncontrolled seizures.
- Surgical treatment of AVMs in this area is a challenge because the risk of hemorrhage is greater than in other cortical locations; however, surgery itself can carry a high morbidity.

CONTRAINDICATIONS

- Conservative management should be considered in patients who are older, have multiple medical comorbidities, have poor baseline neurologic function, or have a poor Karnofsky score.
- AVMs involving the posterior limb of the internal capsules should be treated nonsurgically because of the extremely high risk of permanent neurologic deficit.
- Pathologies that affect eloquent structures should be approached with caution.
- The vasculature needs to be carefully studied preoperatively; complete obliteration of the sinuses can increase the risk of venous infarcts.

PLANNING AND POSITIONING

- Preoperative magnetic resonance imaging (MRI) with intraoperative, frameless neuronavigation has become widely used in approaching parasagittal lesions. For lesions located posterior to the coronal suture, incorporating data from functional MRI into the neuronavigation system can help the surgeon avoid eloquent areas of the brain. Evaluation of functional MRI preoperatively may decrease morbidity.
- Preoperative four-vessel catheter angiography is imperative for the diagnosis and planning of treatment of AVMs and can provide crucial information regarding the vascularity of tumors. Before treatment of an AVM, it is important to understand the arterial supply and venous drainage of the lesion. Angiography can dramatically change the approach in complex midline tumor resections by visualizing arterial feeders and draining veins, identifying whether the superior sagittal sinus (SSS) is patent and whether significant collateralization has occurred in areas where the SSS is occluded, and determining whether there is a role for preoperative embolization.
- Preoperative staged embolization in the appropriate setting may decrease the risk of hemorrhage and decrease lesion volume before surgery.
- Magnetic resonance venography can also be useful for imaging meningiomas to better understand the involvement of the sagittal sinus and anticipate potential bridging or draining cortical veins. When the sinus is occluded, particular attention should be paid to surrounding cortical veins because there is an increased risk of venous infarcts from surgery.

- Intraoperative monitoring is an important tool in resection of midline lesions. Typically, somatosensory evoked potentials of the upper and lower extremities bilaterally, motor evoked potentials, and cortical mapping can direct the surgical approach and resection and decrease morbidity.
- The operative position chosen depends on the location of the lesion. For lesions involving the SSS or deep to the anterior third of the SSS, the patient is positioned supine. Lesions located in the area of the middle third of the SSS can be approached with the patient supine and the neck and head of bed flexed or with the patient in the semisitting position. Lesions located in the area of the posterior third of the SSS can be approached with the patient in the park bench or prone position. If prolonged retraction is planned, sometimes placing the patient's head with one side down allows gravity to retract the brain naturally.
- Intraoperative medications need to be discussed with the anesthesiologist before initiation of the operation. Antiepileptic medication (e.g., levetiracetam, phenytoin) is useful for seizure prophylaxis if the patient is not already receiving an antiepileptic. Administration of mannitol or furosemide before skin incision and mild hyperventilation produce brain relaxation and minimize the need for excessive brain retraction. We prefer to give a dose of 10 mg of intravenous dexamethasone before skin incision with redosing every 4 hours during the case, especially in cases in which there is significant edema surrounding the lesion. A single dose of intravenous antibiotics (e.g., cefazolin, clindamycin, vancomycin) should be administered within 60 minutes of skin incision with redosing as appropriate during the operation.
- Monitoring for development of air embolism is especially important in cases performed with the patient in the semisitting position. Precordial Doppler ultrasound equipment is often placed to screen for development of air embolism. Monitoring and maintaining adequate central venous pressure via a central venous catheter is also imperative during cases performed with the patient in the semisitting position.
- Placement of the Mayfield head clamp should ensure that the three pins are not in the operative field but are appropriately engaged to prevent pin slippage during the case. Delineation and marking of the tumor location and borders using intraoperative navigation is recommended as a guide to ensure the ideal position and trajectory and to mark out the skin flap. A bicoronal incision is preferable in patients with a receding hairline or for anterior frontal lesions. A trapdoor incision that crosses the midline or linear incisions for smaller lesions can also be considered. Clipping of the hair is done according to the surgeon's preference. Infiltration of the incision line with bupivacaine and epinephrine before patient preparation maximizes hemostasis.
- **Figure 13-1:** Lesion location and trajectory that is taken for midline (*1*) frontal, (*2*) parietal, and (*3*) occipital lesions.
- **Figure 13-2: A,** For the frontal interhemispheric approach, the patient is positioned supine with slight translation and flexion of the neck so that it lies above the heart.

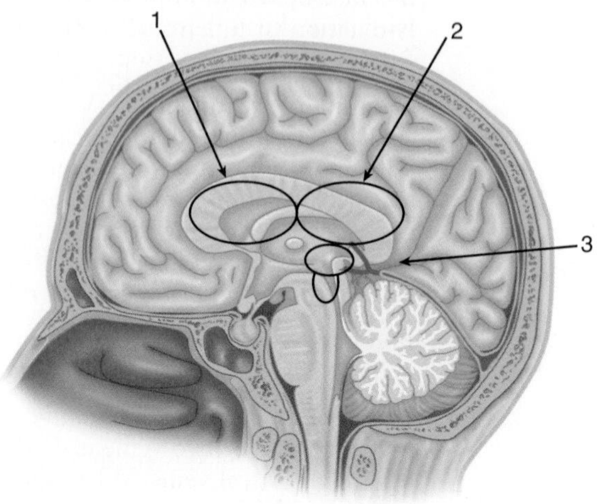

FIGURE 13-1

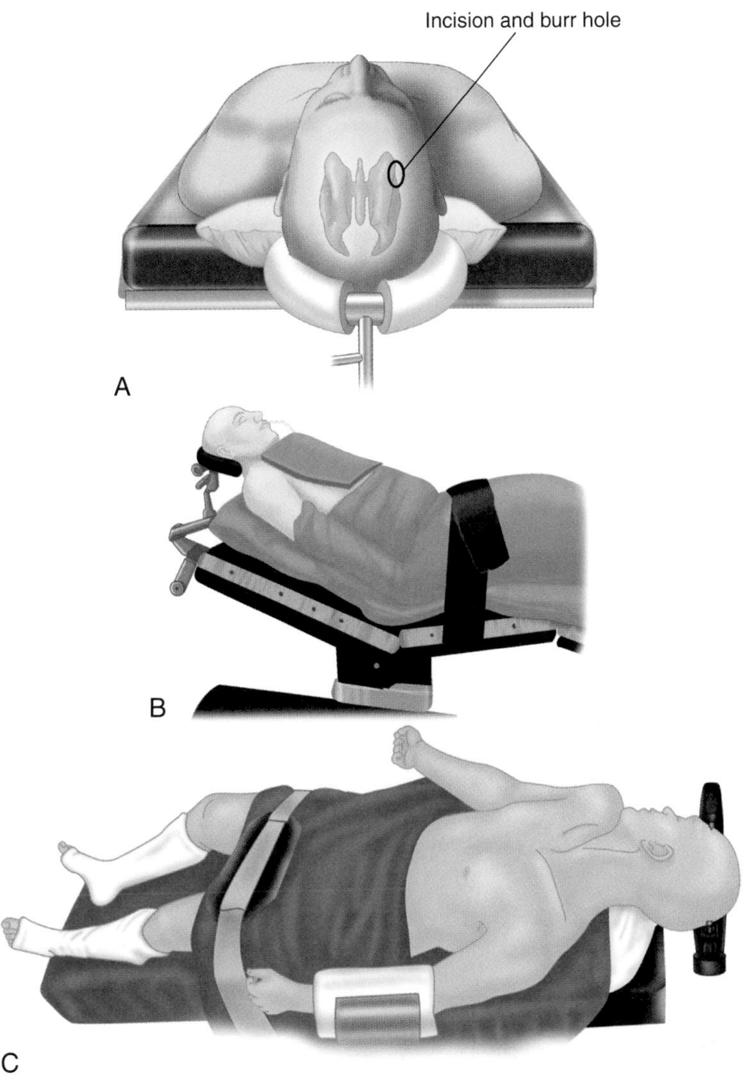

FIGURE 13-2

B, For the middle parietal interhemispheric approach, the patient can be placed in the supine position with the head flexed or in the semisitting position. **C,** For the posterior parietooccipital approach, the patient can be placed in the supine position with the head tilted 90 degrees using a shoulder roll for additional elevation. Alternatively, the patient can be placed in the park bench position with the head turned laterally toward the floor.

PROCEDURE

- **Figure 13-3:** Using intraoperative navigation, the tumor borders and SSS are marked out on the skull. The craniotomy limits are marked out to ensure adequate exposure. The lesion size and depth dictate the number of burr holes needed. Typically, two burr holes are placed 1 cm lateral to the contralateral side of the SSS, and two to three burr holes are placed on the ipsilateral side. A No. 3 Penfield dissector is used to strip the dura off of the inner table.
- **Figure 13-4:** The craniotomy flap is made using the craniotome. The last cuts of the craniotomy should be those crossing the sinus. When the bone flap is elevated, long strips of Gelfoam wrapped in Surgicel are placed over the SSS and then covered with a cotton strip. Any bleeding from dural lakes should be controlled with

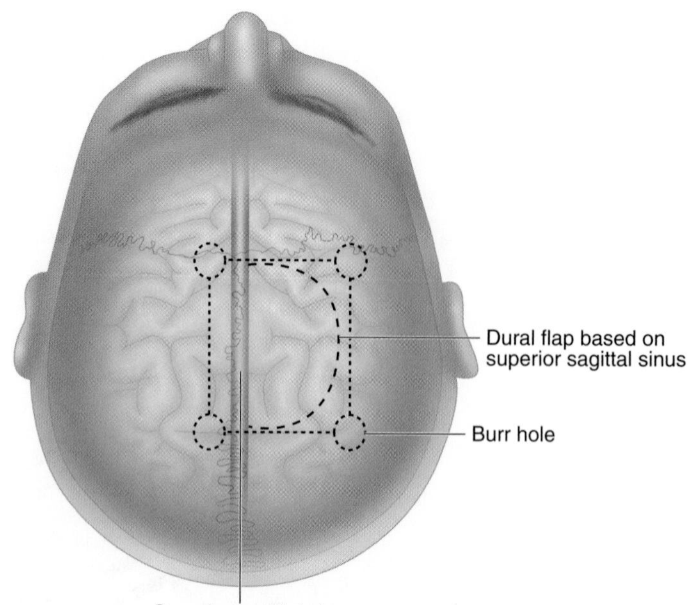

FIGURE 13-3

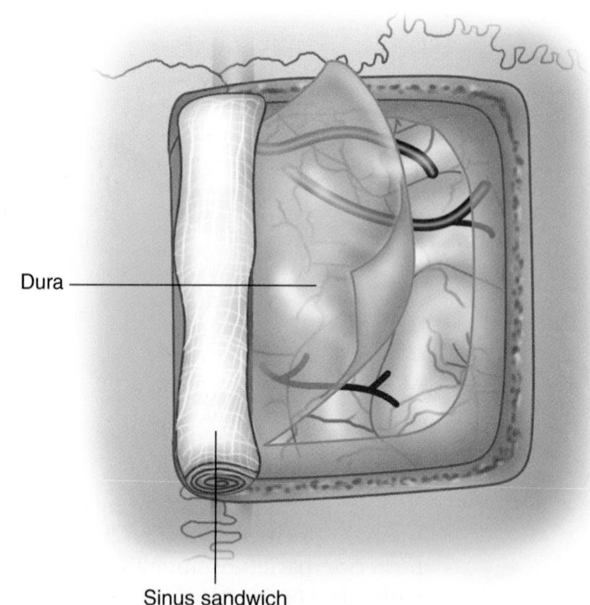

FIGURE 13-4

thrombin-soaked Gelfoam, and coagulation should be minimized. The dura is incised in a trapdoor fashion with the SSS forming the medial border of the dural attachment. Small snips with Metzenbaum scissors are made on the medial edge to avoid entering the SSS. Also, this ensures that one does not cut aggressively into dural lakes. Dural stitches are placed to reflect the dura off.

- **Figure 13-5:** For anterior or frontal tumors, the first third of the SSS may be taken. This is done by ligation of the sinus using silk suture and placement of small vascular clips.
- For anteriorly located parasagittal meningiomas involving the SSS, resection of the anterior third of the SSS is needed to prevent tumor recurrence. For parasagittal meningiomas involving the middle or posterior third of the SSS, incomplete tumor resection is favored with subsequent treatment with stereotactic radiosurgery unless the SSS is completely occluded.

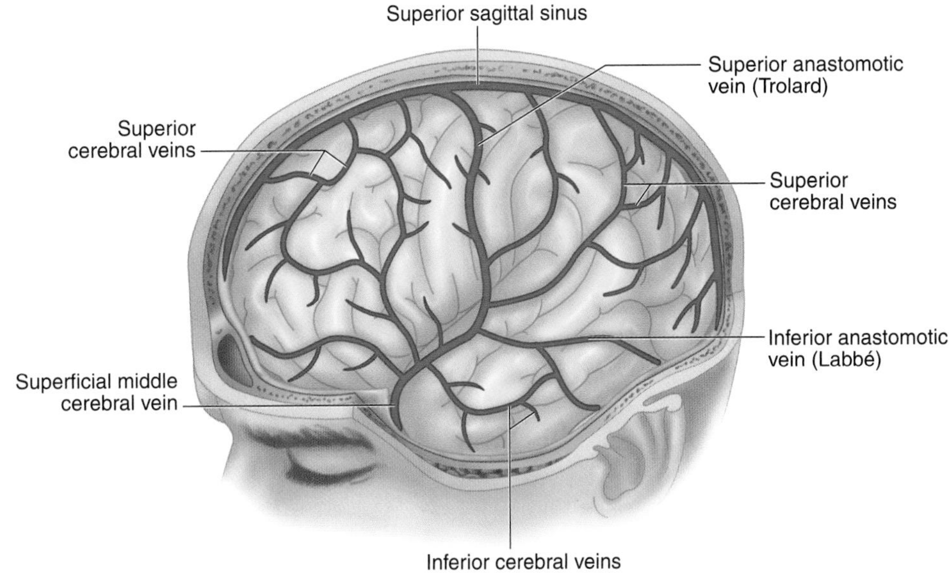

FIGURE 13-5

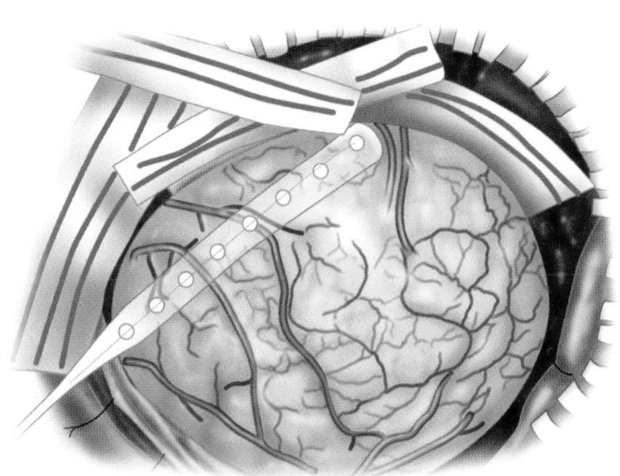

FIGURE 13-6

- The superior anastomotic vein of Trolard delineates the posterior margin of the anterior third of the SSS.
- **Figure 13-6:** For lesions located near or in eloquent areas, critical areas are identified using preoperative functional MRI. Alternatively, the motor strip may be mapped out using the Ojemann cortical stimulator (Integra LifeSciences Corp., Plainsboro, NJ) or using phase reversal.
- **Figure 13-7:** Placement of Bicol collagen sponges (Codeman, Raynham, MA) or Telfa strips on the exposed brain protects the brain from desiccation. Veins draining into the SSS are identified, and dissection around them is performed to avoid venous infarction. The lobe is retracted laterally taking great care to apply pressure slowly. The surgeon also needs to be cognizant of the deeper structures (i.e., anterior cerebral arteries, corpus callosum). If the lesion is superficial, a plane is dissected around it and the surrounding brain. Parasagittal meningiomas may strip off of the SSS or be adherent, depending on the characteristics of the tumor. Reconstruction of the SSS may be required. The operating microscope is draped and brought into the field. Care must be taken to not retract on the anterior cerebral arteries or on draining veins.
- After the lesion is resected, meticulous hemostasis is obtained. A tight dural closure should be attempted but is not required in these locations. The bone flap is replaced with burr hole covers placed over each burr hole. For lesions that involve the skull, the inner table should be drilled off. Alternatively, if a large portion of the skull was involved, the defect is covered with a cranioplasty, and the bone flap is left off.

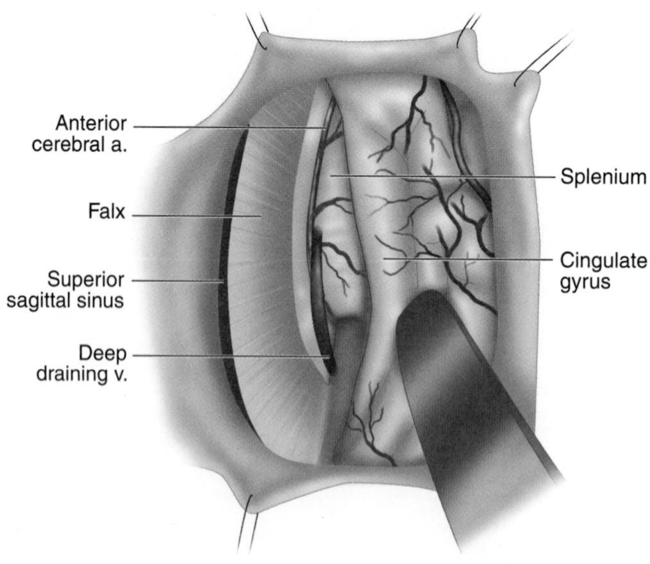

FIGURE 13-7

TIPS FROM THE MASTERS

- Make every effort to understand the venous anatomy, particularly the draining veins, when planning the dural opening.
- Be patient when initially retracting the brain and look for important vessels such as the anterior cerebral arteries.
- If you need to remove tumors, such as a meningioma, that may have invaded the lateral aspect of the sagittal sinus, consider reconstructing the sinus as you take the tumor out.

PITFALLS

Taking draining cortical veins, especially those that drain into the posterior two thirds of the sagittal sinus, can lead to venous infarcts. This possibility is a particular concern when the sinus is occluded because the brain may depend on these veins. Also, avoid stretching the veins in surgery.

Make sure you carefully visualize the course of the retractors during surgery to avoid injuring the branches of the anterior cerebral arteries.

Anticipate injuries to the sagittal sinus.

BAILOUT OPTIONS

- "Sinus sandwiches" should be created before drilling near the sagittal sinus or when manipulating the sagittal sinus. The "sandwich" is a piece of Gelfoam that is cut in a 0.75 cm × 3 cm strip that is wrapped with Surgicel, which can be immediately placed on top of the sinus should it start bleeding or over an arachnoid granulation.
- If the sinus is cut from the side during the dural opening, 4-0 Nurolon nylon sutures (Ethicon, Inc., Somerville, NJ) or small vascular clips are usually effective in stopping the bleeding.
- In cases in which bleeding over the sagittal sinus cannot be controlled with pressure and Gelfoam and Surgicel, a piece of dura should be mobilized laterally and sewn over the defect. Putting a piece of the "sinus sandwich" between the leaf and defect also helps to promote hemostasis.

SUGGESTED READINGS

Giombini S, Solero CL, Lasio G, et al. Immediate and late outcome of operations for parasagittal and falx meningiomas: report of 342 cases. Surg Neurol 1984;21:427–35.

Kondziolka D, Flickinger JC, Perez B. Judicious resection and/or radiosurgery for parasagittal meningiomas: outcomes from a multicenter review. Gamma Knife Meningioma Study Group. Neurosurgery 1998;43:405–13.

Nakamura M, Roser F, Michel J, et al. The natural history of incidental meningiomas. Neurosurgery 2003;53:62–70.

Simpson D. The recurrence of intracranial meningiomas after surgical treatment. J Neurol Neurosurg Psychiatry 1957;20:22–39.

Sindou MP, Alaywan M. Most intracranial meningiomas are not cleavable tumors: anatomic-surgical evidence and angiographic predictability. Neurosurgery 1998;42:476–80.

Procedure 14

Supraorbital (Keyhole) Craniotomy with Optional Orbital Osteotomy

Chetan Bettegowda, Shaan M. Raza, George I. Jallo, Alfredo Quiñones-Hinojosa, Behnam Badie

INDICATIONS

- Supraorbital craniotomy allows for relatively easy and rapid access to structures in the anterior cranial fossa and sellar and parasellar regions. This minimally invasive technique provides a subfrontal approach with minimal disruption of normal anatomy, excellent cosmetic results, shorter operation times and hospital stays with faster recovery, and less morbidity.
- This approach can be used to treat many different intraaxial and extraaxial pathologies in or near the frontal lobes, including extraaxial lesions (i.e., anterior skull base meningiomas, craniopharyngiomas, epidural abscesses) and intraaxial lesions (i.e., gliomas, metastatic lesions) of the frontal lobe.
- The decision to use this technique versus other approaches to the frontal lobe (e.g., bicoronal or pterional craniotomy) is based on the desired anatomic and operative trajectory (i.e., subfrontal vs. anterolateral approach). The decision requires detailed preoperative examination of the location of the lesion, its relationship to other vital structures, the size of the lesion, edema and mass effect of the lesion, the planned angle of dissection, and the patient's comorbidities and overall health.
- The supraorbital approach can be combined with an orbital osteotomy to provide additional visualization of structures and lesions above the level of the anterior communicating artery complex.

CONTRAINDICATIONS

- Supraorbital craniotomy is not ideal for lesions with significant middle fossa or cavernous sinus involvement.
- Lesions with significant edema and associated hydrocephalus are relative contraindications. We have placed preoperative lumbar subarachnoid drains in situations in which the lesion may restrict early intraoperative access to the cisterns that would otherwise be fenestrated to facilitate brain manipulation.
- Superior and more posterior frontal lobe lesions are difficult to access from this approach.
- A large frontal sinus is a contraindication.
- Lesions requiring significant vascular manipulation and dissection are contraindications.

PLANNING AND POSITIONING

- Preoperative planning includes assessment of the patient's cardiopulmonary status, evaluation of comorbidities, and basic laboratory tests, including a basic metabolic panel, complete blood count, coagulation profile, and type and screen. Baseline chest x-ray and electrocardiogram are also useful.
- Preoperative magnetic resonance imaging (MRI) with fiducial markers is obtained for intraoperative navigation.
- Within 60 minutes of skin incision, perioperative antibiotics are administered. If the surgery is to entail significant manipulation or violation of the frontal cortex, an antiepileptic is administered before the start of surgery.

- Brain relaxation can be achieved by administering mannitol and dexamethasone, mild hyperventilation, and preoperative lumbar drain placement.
- After anesthesia induction and Mayfield clamp fixation, the head is elevated and extended to allow the frontal lobe to fall away from the floor of the anterior fossa. Thereafter, the head is rotated to the contralateral side from 15 to 60 degrees depending on the anatomic location of the lesion. The orientation of the head is of paramount importance—considering the relative limited working space, ideal rotation maximizes the surgeon's view of the lesion in relation to surrounding structures. The extent of rotation performed is as follows: 15 degrees for ipsilateral sylvian fissure, 20 degrees for lateral suprasellar, 30 degrees for anterior suprasellar, and 60 degrees for olfactory groove and cribriform plate region.
- The focus here is on the traditional supraorbital craniotomy without orbital osteotomy. The planned eyebrow skin incision is drawn where the medialmost extent of the incision extends to the supraorbital neurovascular bundle, preserving the nerve. The incision typically extends laterally to the edge of the eyebrow; if necessary, it can be extended posteriorly to one of the patient's facial creases. The patient is prepared and draped in usual sterile fashion.

PROCEDURE

- **Figure 14-1:** A 4- to 5-cm incision is made through the eyebrow along the direction of hair follicles.
- **Figure 14-2:** The frontalis muscle is divided, and the supraorbital nerve is dissected using sharp scissors.
- **Figure 14-3:** Although the supraorbital nerve can be preserved and retracted medially for smaller lateral craniotomies (**A**), it is freed from the supraorbital notch and cut in most cases to obtain a larger corridor (**B**). The periosteum is freed from the orbital ridge and the frontal bone. This plane is extended into the orbit by carefully dissecting the periorbita from the orbital roof.
- **Figure 14-4:** After the anterior aspect of the temporalis muscle is dissected over the keyhole area, a small burr hole is placed laterally using a 3-mm drill attachment, and the dura is freed from the bone using a blunt dissector.
- **Figure 14-5:** A high-speed drill is used to perform the superiormost aspect of the craniotomy starting from the burr hole and stopping medially at the edge of the frontal sinus.

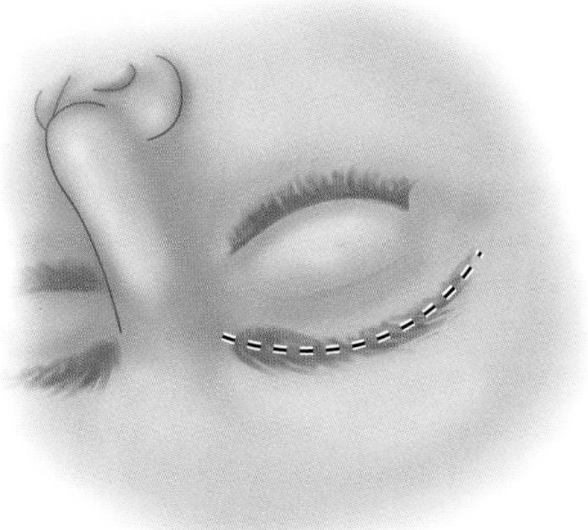

FIGURE 14-1

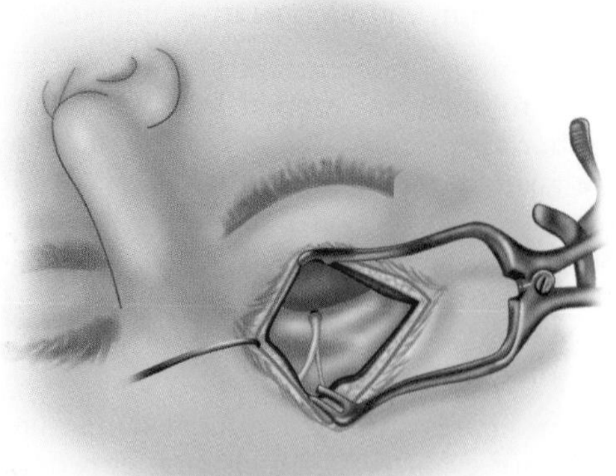

FIGURE 14-2

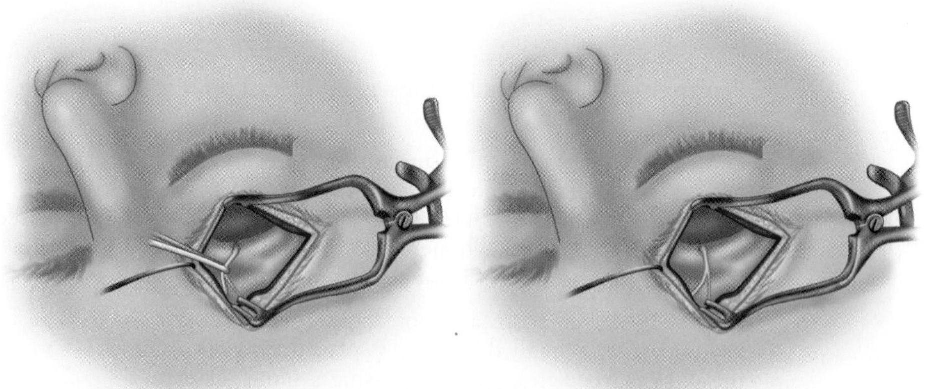

FIGURE 14-3

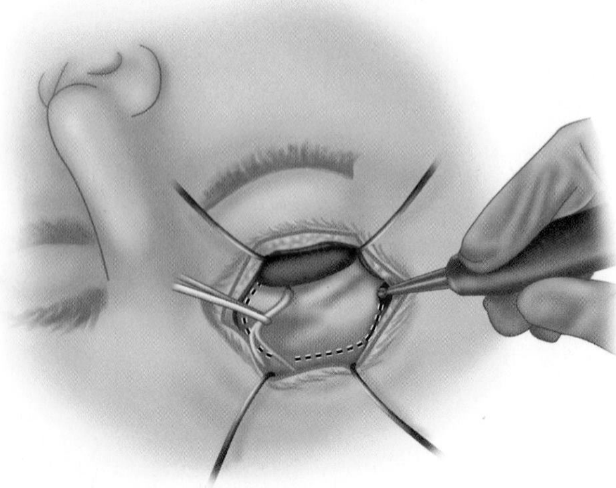

FIGURE 14-4

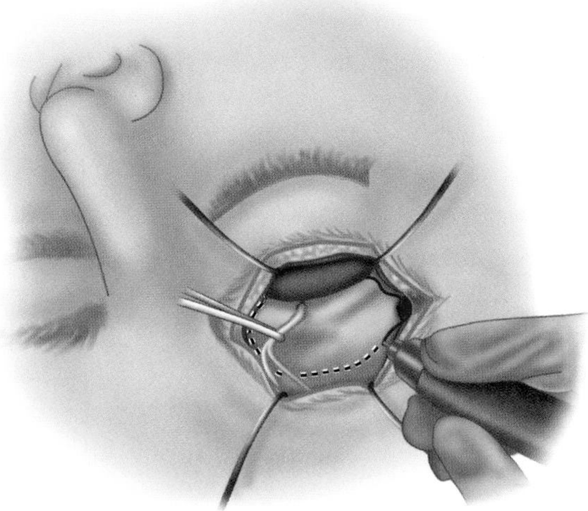

FIGURE 14-5

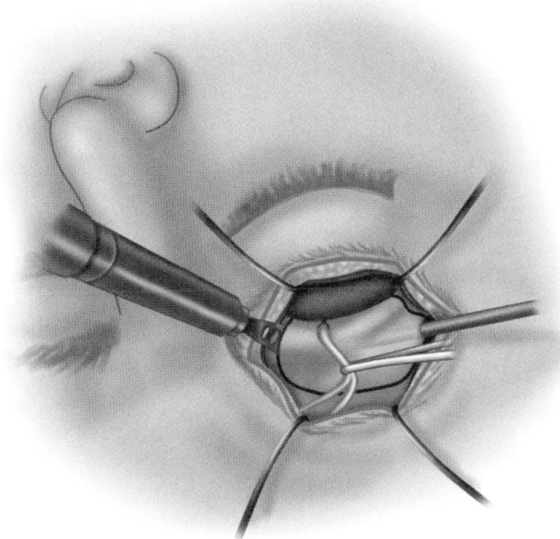

FIGURE 14-6

- **Figure 14-6:** While protecting the dura through the burr hole and the eye through the orbit, a limited orbitotomy that extends into the frontal sinus medially and through the burr hole laterally is performed using an oscillating saw.
- **Figure 14-7:** As the dura is protected through the burr hole, a small osteotome is used to fracture the roof of the orbit to free a single bone flap consisting of the orbital ridge and the orbital roof.
- **Figure 14-8:** The mucosa of the frontal sinus is removed completely, and the sinus is packed with pieces of Gelfoam, bone wax, and sometimes abdominal fat. The dura is opened in a curvilinear fashion.
- **Figure 14-9:** The eyelid is closed in a single layer with (**A**) small absorbable monofilament or (**B**) nonabsorbable monofilament that is removed 4 to 5 days postoperatively.

TIPS FROM THE MASTERS

- This approach should be selected primarily on the angle of dissection. Supraorbital craniotomy (with the optional orbital ridge osteotomy) provides an anterior subfrontal approach and is a replacement for the larger craniotomy and soft tissue dissection that

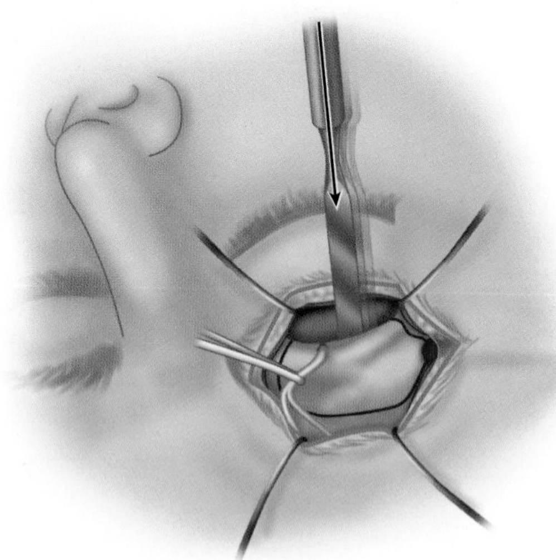

FIGURE 14-7

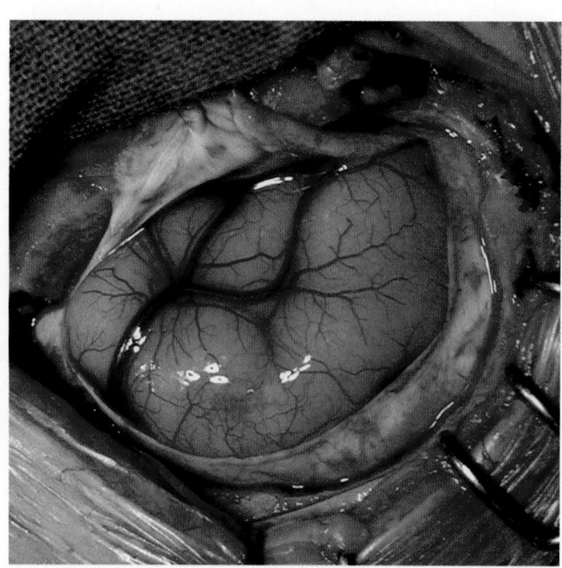

FIGURE 14-8

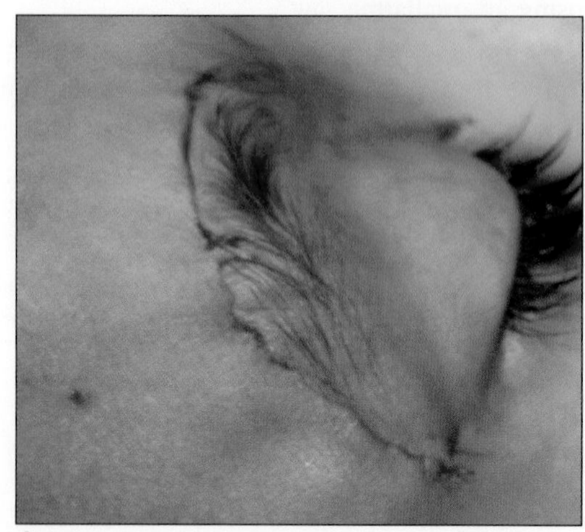

A

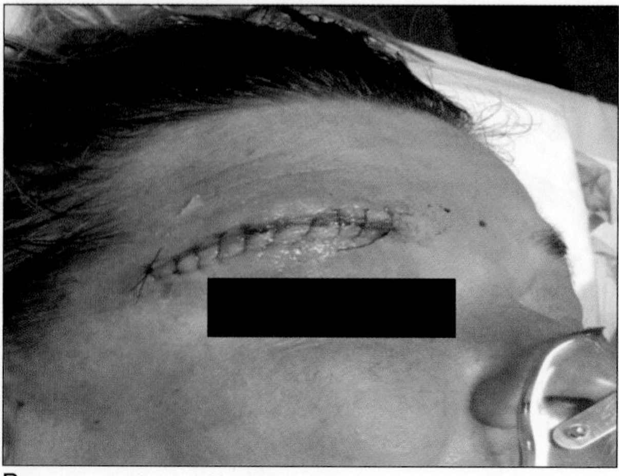

B

FIGURE 14-9

has been traditionally employed for this trajectory. We selectively use this technique (without the orbital osteotomy) for smaller (<3 cm) extraaxial lesions in the anterior cranial fossa and sellar region that are primarily in the midline and would traditionally be approached through a subfrontal approach.

- A lumbar drain should be considered in cases with significant edema or where early access to cerebrospinal fluid cisterns may be challenging.
- The use of angled surgical instruments—similar to the instruments used for transsphenoidal resection of pituitary tumors—permits the surgeon to work around corners and angles.
- After performing the craniotomy, drilling the osseous ridges of the orbit allows for decreased retraction of the frontal lobe when going subfrontal.
- If performing the supraorbital craniotomy with the orbital osteotomy, the eyelid incision, also referred to as the upper blepharoplasty or supratarsal approach, is preferred because it provides direct access to the orbital rim.
- Skin should be closed with 6-0 nylon sutures, which are removed on the 5th postoperative day to minimize scar formation.

PITFALLS

Entry into the frontal sinus can lead to increased rates of postoperative infection and pneumocephalus.

Given the narrow corridor within which to work, vital structures may be obscured from view and difficult to manipulate.

This approach is unsuitable for repair of dehiscence within the cribriform plate or midline anterior cranial fossa defects.

Patients can develop severe hypoesthesia over the forehead, but these symptoms typically improve over 6 to 8 months.

Excessive brain swelling may limit exposure of ruptured aneurysms through this approach. Standard pterional craniotomy (with or without orbitotomy) may be more appropriate for such cases.

Removal of the orbital roof should be minimized, and tears in the periorbita should be repaired to avoid postoperative pulsatile exophthalmos.

BAILOUT OPTIONS

- If the frontal sinus is violated, great care must be taken to exonerate the sinus completely. Muscle can be packed into the portion of the exposed frontal sinus. A vascularized pericranial flap can be placed over the defect to help prevent future infection.
- In case of excessive brain swelling, the perichiasmatic cistern should be accessed to drain cerebrospinal fluid.
- Angled instruments such as those used during an endoscopic transsphenoidal procedure are helpful when working in tight spaces. In addition, an endoscope can be used to enhance visualization.
- We perform a one-piece orbital osteotomy in combination with a supraorbital craniotomy through an eyelid incision to expand our effective working space. This additional maneuver provides a direct view of not only the sellar and parasellar region, but also the suprachiasmatic and anterior communicating complex region. Removal of the orbital rim and roof provides additional working room, while minimizing the need for frontal lobe retraction.

SUGGESTED READINGS

Andaluz N, Romano A, Reddy LV, et al. Eyelid approach to the anterior cranial base. J Neurosurg 2008;109:341–6.

Bognar L, Czirjak S, Madarassy G. Frontolateral keyhole craniotomy through a superciliary skin incision in children. Childs Nerv Syst 2003;19:765–8.

Czirjak S, Szeifert GT. The role of the superciliary approach in the surgical management of intracranial neoplasms. Neurol Res 2006;28:131–7.

Delashaw JB Jr, Tedeschi H, Rhoton AL. Modified supraorbital craniotomy: technical note. Neurosurgery 1992;30:954–6.

Jallo GI, Bognar L. Eyebrow surgery: the supraciliary craniotomy: technical note. Neurosurgery 2006;59(1 Suppl. 1): ONSE157–8.

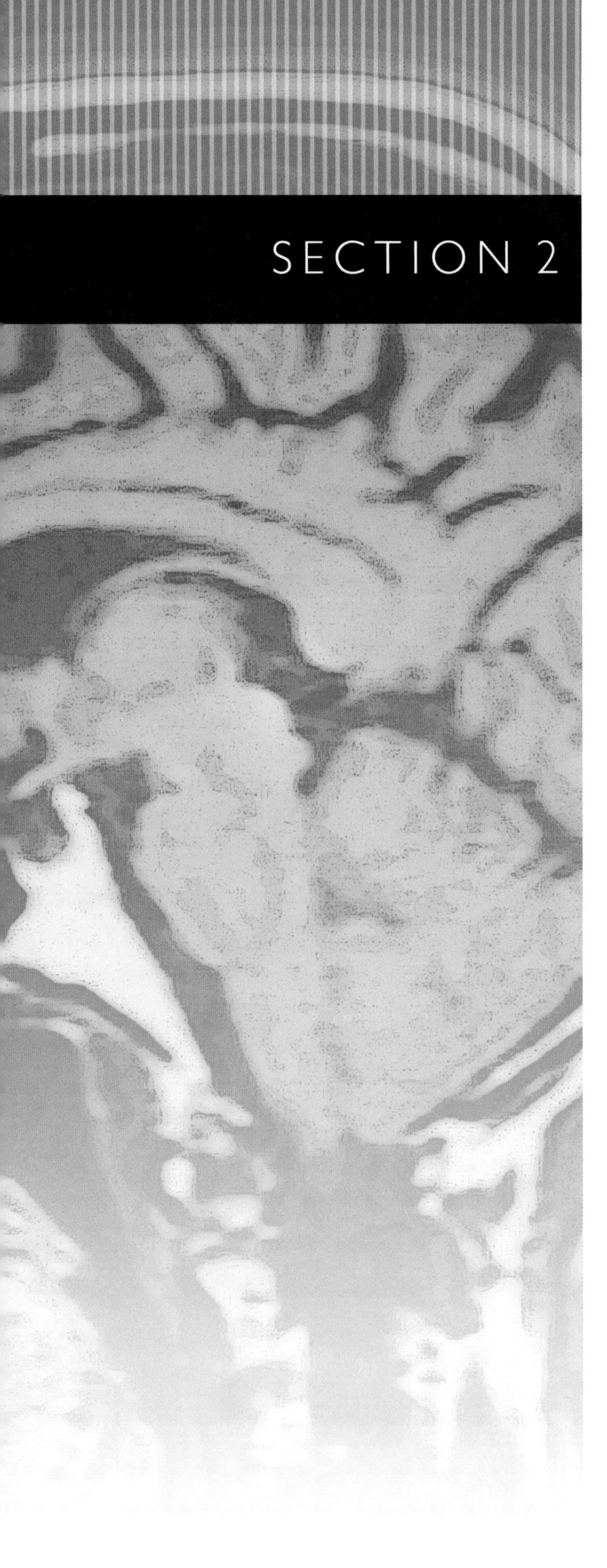

Skull Base

SECTION EDITOR — ANDREW T. PARSA

Procedure 15

Frontotemporal Craniotomy with Orbitozygomatic Osteotomy*

Michael E. Sughrue, Andrew T. Parsa

INDICATIONS

- Frontotemporal craniotomy with orbitozygomatic osteotomy is an adjunct to pterional craniotomy that allows greater rostral trajectory to midline structures. By removing the superior and lateral bony orbit, one gains a more anterior and inferior starting point for the approach than would be possible with a conventional pterional craniotomy.
- Removal of the zygomatic arch enables inferior displacement of the temporalis muscle, allowing for a lower starting point for subtemporal visualization.

CONTRAINDICATIONS

- If a midline view of the suprasellar region is needed, a bifrontal craniotomy may be a better approach.
- Access to the petrous apex and retrosellar space is limited and requires a long reach.

PLANNING AND POSITIONING

- The exact positioning needs vary by case. The patient generally is placed supine on the operating table.
- The head is placed in a Mayfield head holder with two pins placed in the occiput just off the midline. The single pin is placed in the contralateral forehead, in the mid-pupillary line ideally behind the hairline.
- After pinning, the head is usually positioned such that the lateral orbital ridge and keyhole region is the highest point on the patient's head. This position is achieved by about 5-1 degrees of contralateral head rotation and a slight degree of neck extension and head elevation.
- **Figure 15-1:** Positioning the patient and head. The patient is placed supine on the operating table with the ipsilateral shoulder elevated as needed to facilitate head rotation toward the contralateral side. The skull clamp is fixated with the paired

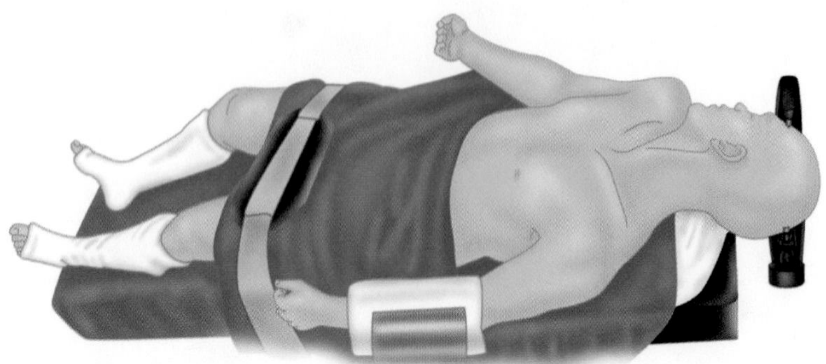

FIGURE 15-1

*See also Procedure 1.

posterior pins at the equator in the occipital bone and the single anterior pin at the equator in the contralateral frontal bone superior to the orbit. The head is positioned by first elevating the head above the heart in the "sniffing position." Second, the head is rotated up to 30 degrees to the contralateral side depending on the intended operation. Third, the neck is extended so that the vertex is angled down 10 to 30 degrees, allowing for self-retraction of the frontal lobe off the anterior cranial fossa floor. When the head is ideally positioned, the malar eminence of the zygomatic bone should be the highest point in the operative field.

PROCEDURE

- **Figure 15-2:** Skin incision. Various skin incisions can be used depending on the needs of the particular case. For most cases, particularly cases focused at the parasellar skull base and circle of Willis, a simple C-shaped incision beginning at the widow's peak and extending posterolaterally back to the root of the zygomatic arch suffices.
- **Figure 15-3:** Soft tissue elevation and identification of landmarks (petrous apex approach). The frontalis branch of the facial nerve runs in a posteroinferior to anterosuperior direction in a large subcutaneous fat pad that sits on the outside of the temporalis fascia and connects the skin to the temporalis fascia just behind the lateral orbital rim. To expose the lateral orbit and maxillary buttress safely and adequately, the scalp and fat pad must be separated from the temporalis muscle. The scalp and fat pad must be reflected anteriorly over the bone; this can be achieved by either a suprafascial or a subfascial approach.
- In the suprafascial approach, sharp dissection is used to create a plane beneath the fat pad and above the temporalis fascia. Blunt dissection is used to reflect the fat pad and scalp over the lateral orbit and maxilla until adequate exposure is obtained.
- In the subfascial approach, as soon as the fat pad is visualized, the temporalis fascia is elevated off the superficial surface of the muscle with scissors and is separated from the bone of the lateral orbit, maxillary buttress, and zygomatic arch with a small periosteal dissector. The scalp and fat pad are reflected anteriorly with the temporalis fascia to enter the lateral orbit.
- **Figure 15-4:** Temporalis elevation. Regardless of how the frontalis nerve is removed from the muscle, two cuts are made in the temporalis muscle to elevate the muscle

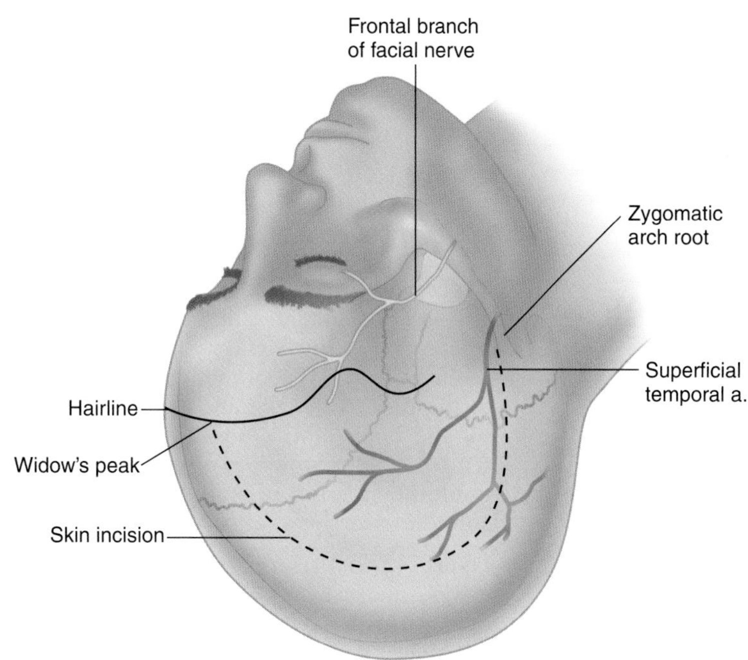

FIGURE 15-2

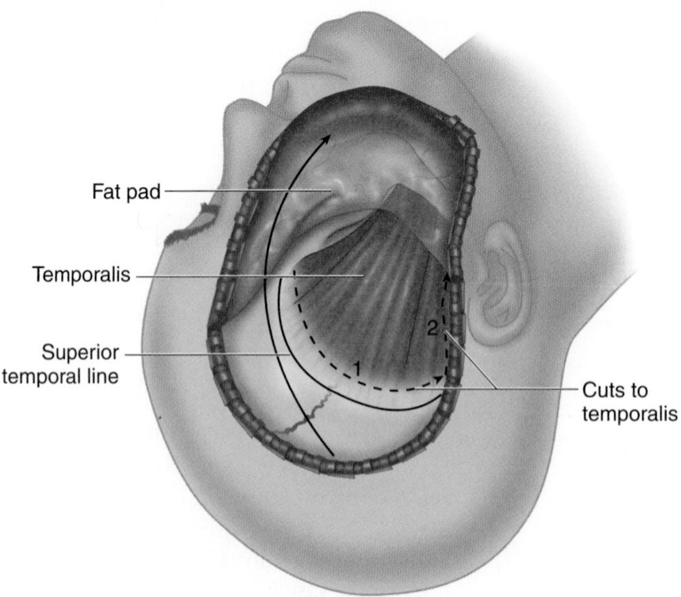

FIGURE 15-3

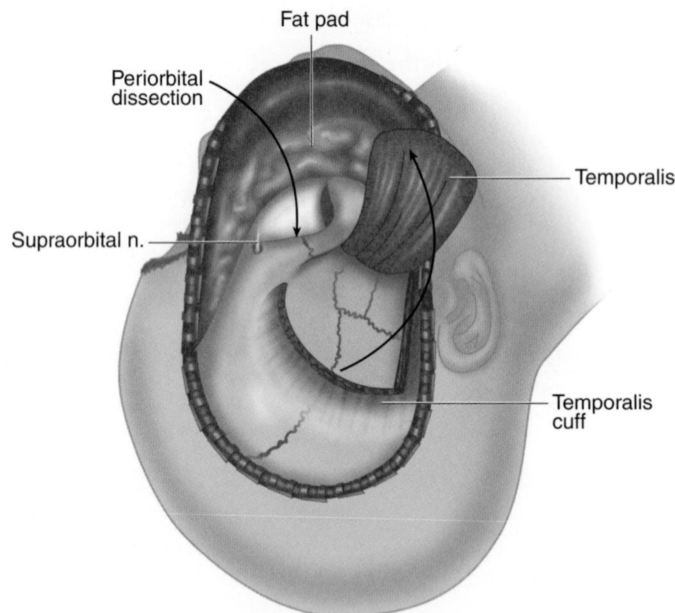

FIGURE 15-4

and leave a fascial cuff to reattach the muscle during the closure. One cut runs parallel and inferior to the superior temporal line, from the posterior surface of the lateral orbital rim at the McCarty keyhole, back about 1 cm in front of the posterior edge of the incision. The second cut is made perpendicular to the first and is continued down to the root of the zygoma. Monopolar electrocautery is used to dissect the temporalis off the bone of the posterior face of the lateral orbital rim and off the squamous temporal bone down to the zygomatic arch. The dissection should be carried down until the inferior orbital fissure can be palpated with a No. 4 Penfield dissector anteroinferiorly.

- **Figure 15-5:** Periorbital dissection and bony exposure. A small dissector is used to elevate the scalp off of the orbital rim from just medial to the supraorbital rim, down over the frontozygomatic suture, onto the maxilla and zygomatic arch. Dissection continues anteriorly until the zygomaticofacial branch of the maxillary nerve is encountered exiting the anterior surface of the maxilla. Soft tissue is also elevated off

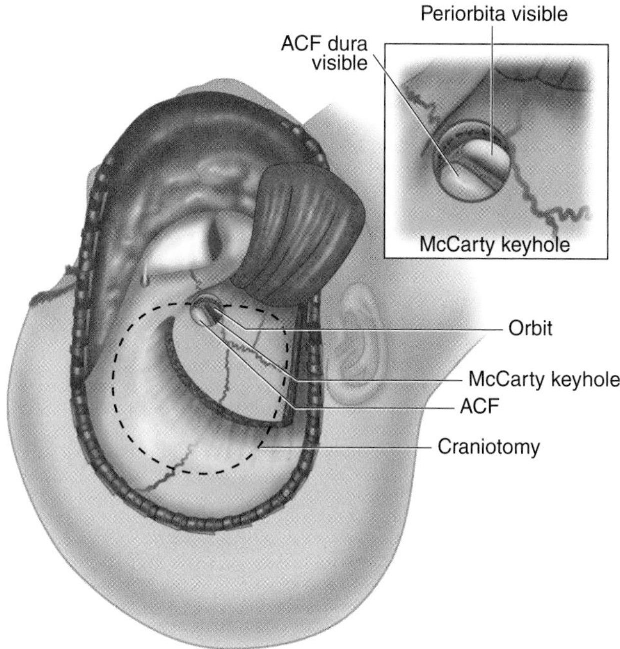

FIGURE 15-5

the zygomatic arch on all surfaces; this typically requires sharp dissection at points of dense attachment of the temporalis fascia. After releasing the supraorbital nerve, the periorbita is gently dissected away from the inner bony surface of the superior and lateral orbit. Dissection continues in the orbit in a lateral and inferior direction until the inferior orbital fissure is able to be palpated with a No. 4 Penfield. Although the inferior orbital fissure is identified by blind feel, ideally the probe should be visualized exiting the fissure in the subtemporalis space.

- **Figure 15-6:** Frontotemporal craniotomy. The burr hole placed at the McCarty keyhole should be placed slightly more anterior than is typical. Ideally, the burr hole should expose the lateral orbit because two cuts involved in the orbitozygomatic osteotomy terminate in this burr hole. Also, it is important that the craniotomy cuts on the

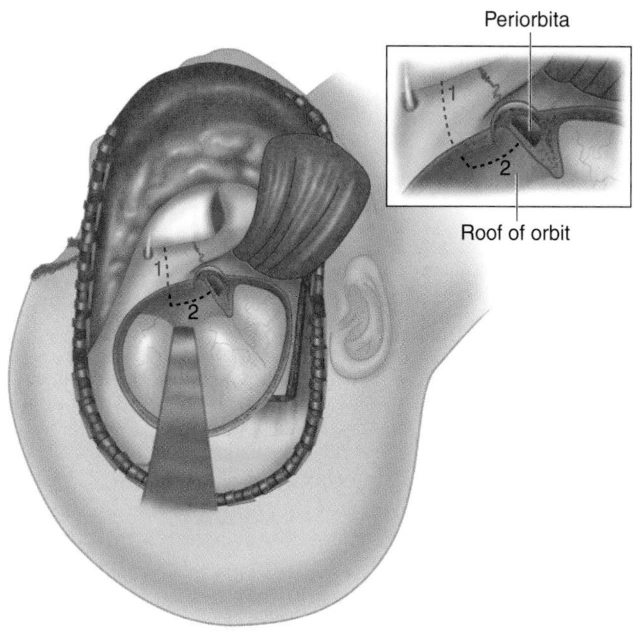

FIGURE 15-6

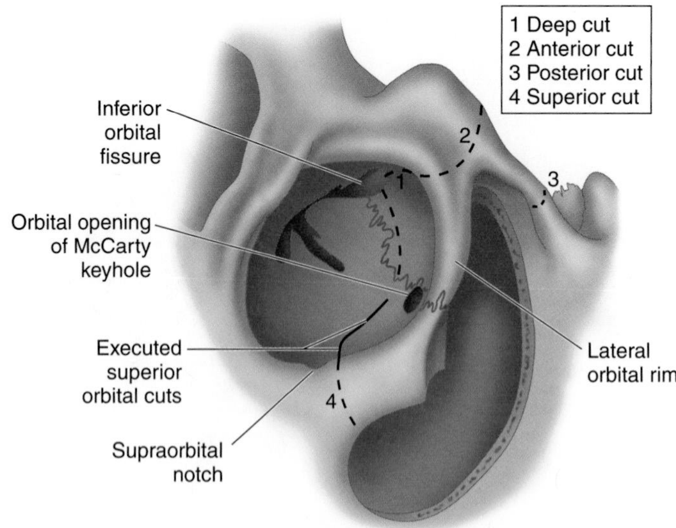

FIGURE 15-7

forehead come as anterior as possible. The footplate ideally should catch on the floor of the anterior fossa before turning laterally to the keyhole; this greatly simplifies the orbital cuts during the osteotomy.

- **Figure 15-7:** Orbitozygomatic osteotomy. The exact location of the cuts from this osteotomy can be a source of confusion, but this can be greatly simplified if the six cuts are thought of as achieving two primary goals: two cuts to remove the superior orbit and four cuts to disconnect the maxillary buttress at its points of attachment.

Removal of Superior Orbit

- Two cuts are made at right angles to each other through the roof of the orbit and superior orbital rim.
- The first is an anteroposteriorly directed cut through the superior orbital rim just lateral to the supraorbital notch. This cut is carried as far posteriorly as possible.
- A second cut is made perpendicular to this cut, proceeding laterally and exiting the orbit at the keyhole burr hole.

Disconnection of Maxillary Buttress

- The maxillary buttress is a complex structure but is essentially attached to the skull in four places: deep, anterior, posterior, and superior. Each of the remaining four cuts of the osteotomy is directed at one of these attachments.
  - *Deep cut*: The saw is placed into the lateral orbit and introduced into the inferior orbital fissure. The cut proceeds laterally until the lateral orbital rim is encountered.
  - *Anterior cut*: This cut enters the inferolateral orbital rim and maxilla from the lateral edge of the deep cut and proceeds inferolaterally across the maxilla just posterior to the zygomaticofacial nerve. It continues across the entire maxillary buttress until the buttress is disconnected from the facial skeleton anteriorly.
  - *Posterior cut*: This cut disconnects the zygomatic arch just anterior to its root. Repair is made easier by angling this cut and plating before disconnecting the osteotomy.
  - *Superior cut*: This is the disconnecting cut that enters the inferior orbital fissure from the temporalis side. This cut runs superiorly through the lateral orbit until joining with the keyhole burr hole. By uniting with the orbital cuts, this cut disconnects the superior attachment of the maxillary buttress and removes the superolateral orbital rim through a C-shaped orbitotomy.

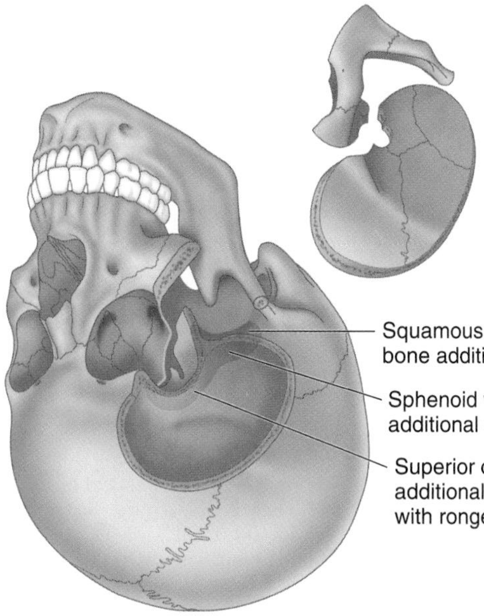

Squamous and temporal bone additional craniectomy

Sphenoid wing additional craniectomy

Superior orbit additional craniectomy with rongeur

FIGURE 15-8

- **Figure 15-7:** Additional craniotomy. To take advantage of the visualization provided by the orbitozygomatic osteotomy, it is wise to perform an additional craniectomy to eliminate bony obstruction to viewing angles. The superior orbit should be removed with a rongeur to as close to the orbital apex and sphenoid wing as possible. Additionally, after using the additional temporalis retraction made possible by the zygomatic arch removal, the squamous temporal bone should be removed down to the floor of the middle fossa. If necessary, the lesser sphenoid wing should be drilled until no bony elevation exists between the globe and the anterior clinoid process.
- **Figure 15-8:** The dura is opened in a C-shaped fashion across the sylvian fissure, with the ends of the "C" roughly bifurcating the exposed portion of the frontal and temporal lobes, and carried as anteriorly as possible. The dura is flapped anteriorly to retract the periorbita and eye out of the field and is sutured to the scalp, with the stitches into the dura placed as low as possible to retract the dura as flat and out of the working view as possible.

TIPS FROM THE MASTERS

- Placing the incision as close to the tragus as possible can complicate closure but is probably cosmetically superior.
- It is wise to attempt to spare the superficial temporal artery (STA) for several reasons. First, delayed bleeding from the STA is a frequent source of postoperative epidural hematomas requiring evacuation, and dealing with STA bleeding can often consume more time than it takes to spare the artery. Additionally, the STA is the principal blood supply to the scalp flap, and maintaining good scalp blood flow likely improves wound healing. Finally, the anterior branch of the STA runs roughly parallel and posterior to the frontalis branch of the facial nerve in the scalp and is a good indicator of how far the scalp can be separated from the temporalis fascia before the frontalis nerve needs to be separated from the temporalis muscle and protected.
- The STA typically lies in the subgaleal space above the temporalis fascia just anterior to the tragus. Metzenbaum scissors are used to dissect the galea away from the temporalis fascia to identify the STA before cutting it with the scissors.
- Care should be taken to preserve the periorbita because violation of this protective covering not only risks injury to the intraorbital contents, but also makes visualization of the reciprocating saw during the orbital osteotomy much more difficult.

PITFALLS

Care should be taken not to extend the inferior limb of the incision below the zygoma to avoid injuring the facial nerve branches that lie in the subcutaneous tissue of the subzygomatic face.

Dissection of the periorbita medial to the supraorbital nerve is unnecessary and risks injury to the trochlear attachment of the superior oblique muscle with resultant diplopia.

The lateral orbital wall should be preserved as much as possible to prevent the development of pulsatile enophthalmos postoperatively.

SUGGESTED READINGS

Chang CW, Wang LC, Lee JS, et al. Orbitozygomatic approach for excisions of orbital tumors with 1 piece of craniotomy bone flap: 2 case reports. Surg Neurol 2007;68(Suppl. 1):S56–9.

D'Ambrosio AL, Mocco J, Hankinson TC, et al. Quantification of the frontotemporal orbitozygomatic approach using a three-dimensional visualization and modeling application. Neurosurgery 2008;62:251–60.

Froelich S, Aziz KA, Levine NB, et al. Extension of the one-piece orbitozygomatic frontotemporal approach to the glenoid fossa: cadaveric study. Neurosurgery 2008;62:ONS312–6.

Martins C, Li X, Rhoton AL Jr. Role of the zygomaticofacial foramen in the orbitozygomatic craniotomy: anatomic report. Neurosurgery 2003;53:168–72.

Seckin H, Avci E, Uluc K, et al. The work horse of skull base surgery: orbitozygomatic approach: technique, modifications, and applications. Neurosurg Focus 2008;25:E4.

Shimizu S, Tanriover N, Rhoton AL Jr, et al. MacCarty keyhole and inferior orbital fissure in orbitozygomatic craniotomy. Neurosurgery 2005;57:152–9.

Tanriover N, Ulm AJ, Rhoton AL Jr, et al. One-piece versus two-piece orbitozygomatic craniotomy: quantitative and qualitative considerations. Neurosurgery 2006;58:ONS229–37.

Procedure 16

Subfrontal and Bifrontal Craniotomies with or without Orbital Osteotomy

Michael E. Sughrue, Andrew T. Parsa

INDICATIONS

- The unilateral and bilateral subfrontal approaches are the workhorse approaches for access to nearly the entire anterior cranial fossa floor; anterior midline parasellar structures such as the tuberculum sella, anterior communicating artery, and optic chiasm; posterior orbit; and orbital apex.
- A unilateral subfrontal approach is sufficient for most orbital lesions and midline lesions that are largely eccentric to one side.
- For large or purely midline lesions, the increased flexibility of view provided by a bifrontal approach is preferable.
- In smaller and more posterior lesions or lesions with significant superior extension, removal of the supraorbital bar may reduce retraction-related cortical injury and improves visualization.

CONTRAINDICATIONS

- Lesions in the middle fossa are difficult to access with this approach.
- Retrochiasmatic and subchiasmatic lesions are best accessed via a lateral approach.

PLANNING AND POSITIONING

- **Figure 16-1:** Positioning for bilateral subfrontal approach. The positioning for either approach is supine.

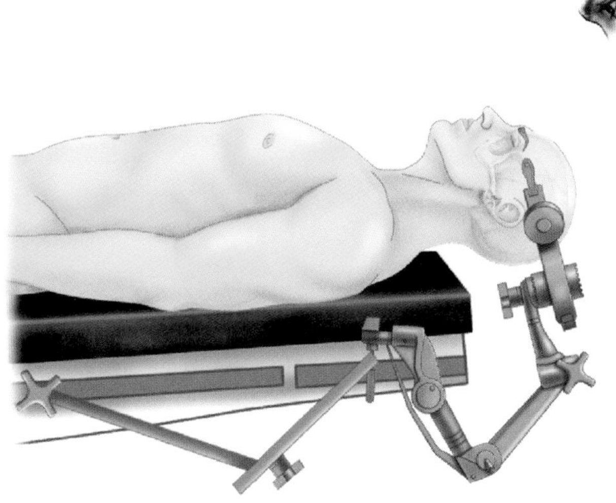

FIGURE 16-1

- For the unilateral approach, the inferior pins are placed above the mastoid process, and the single pin is placed in the forehead just behind the hairline. The head is rotated approximately 15 degrees toward the contralateral shoulder, the neck is slightly extended, and the head is elevated such that the ipsilateral orbital rim is the highest point of the head. The neck is slightly extended and elevated.

PROCEDURE

- **Figure 16-2:** Skin incision. The skin incision for either side of this approach begins at the posterior aspect slightly anterior to the tragus and reaches the zygomatic root at its inferiormost extent. Care should be taken to preserve the superficial temporal artery if possible. The incision extends superior and anterior in a curvilinear fashion to reach the hairline in the sagittal midline. If a bifrontal approach is planned, these incisions should meet in a gradual anteriorly directed peak.
- **Figure 16-3:** Soft tissue elevation. Forehead pericranium should be harvested with any subfrontal or bifrontal approach for repair of anterior fossa floor bony defects and for exclusion of the frontal sinus from the intracranial space. After the scalp has been

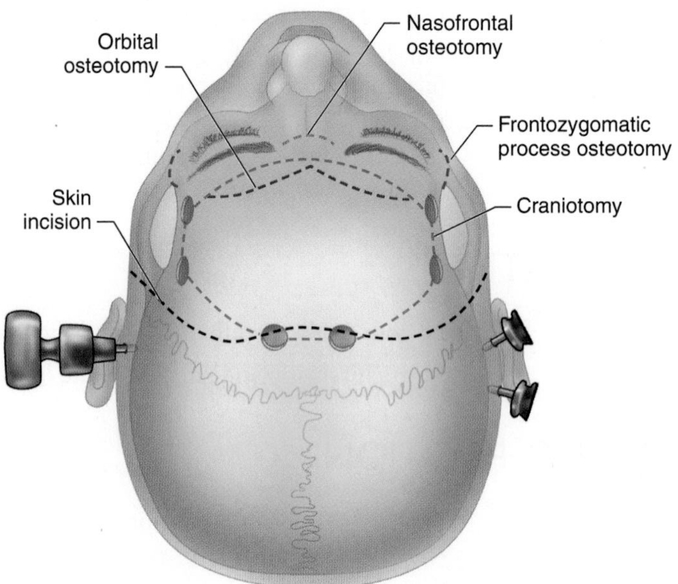

FIGURE 16-2

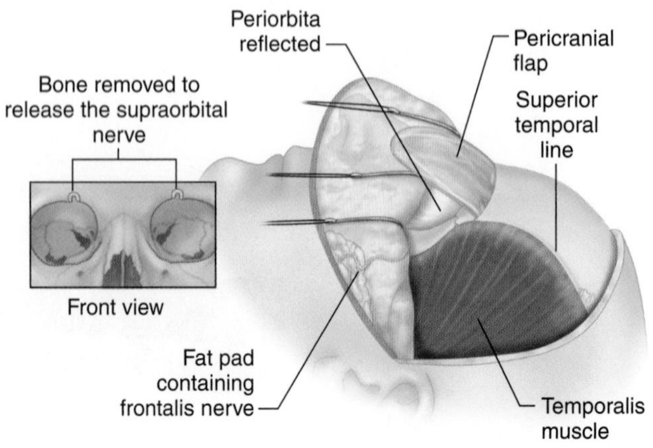

FIGURE 16-3

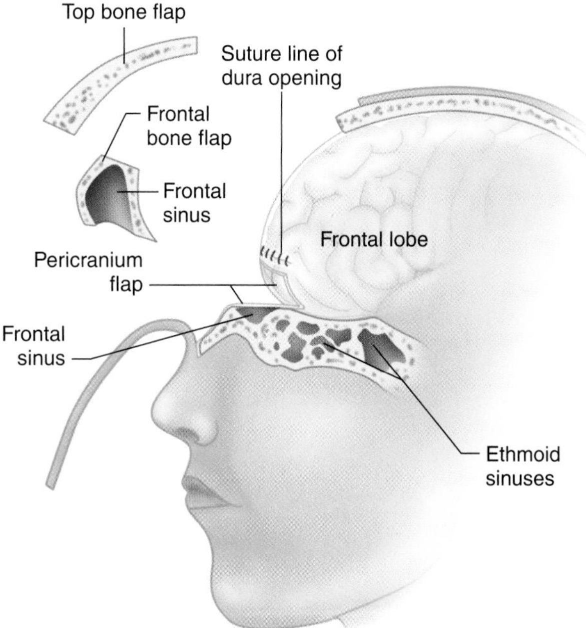

FIGURE 16-4

reflected forward over the superior orbital rim, a large rectangular piece of pericranium is cut with a monopolar cautery and reflected anteriorly over the forehead with its blood supply. The frontalis nerve is contained in a fat pad that lies superficial to the temporalis fascia. This fat pad should be reflected over the frontozygomatic process using either a suprafascial or a subfascial technique.

- **Figure 16-4:** Identification of landmarks. If orbital osteotomy is planned, it is important to dissect the periorbita away from the orbital bone using gentle dissection because tears in the periorbita, besides increasing the risk of orbital complications, cause the orbital fat to extrude outward, making the osteotomy much more difficult. For unilateral orbital osteotomies, the dissection should begin underneath the superior orbital rim slightly medial to the supraorbital foramen and notch and extend laterally underneath the lateral orbital rim down to the level of the frontozygomatic suture. The dissection should continue as far posteriorly into the orbit as is possible. If the supraorbital nerve is restrained by a bony foramen, this can be freed using an oblique cut with an osteotome to convert the foramen to a notch. The scalp dissection should continue down until the nasofrontal suture is visualized because the detaching cut of a bifrontal orbital osteotomy would run slightly superior to this suture.
- **Figure 16-5:** Unilateral or bifrontal craniotomy. Ideally, two burr holes—one placed at the McCarty keyhole and one placed directly posterior to this under the temporalis—should be enough to turn a frontal bone flap on one side. The bone flaps should extend laterally a few centimeters below the temporalis muscle cuff and as far anteriorly as allowed by the footplate.
- **Figure 16-6:** Orbital osteotomy (if needed). The cuts needed to remove the orbit in these approaches are more straightforward than the cuts needed for the orbitozygomatic approach. After dissecting the dura away from the orbital roof with a No. 1 Penfield, the orbit is entered first laterally with a reciprocating saw, and the lateral orbital rim is cut just above the frontozygomatic suture extending posteriorly into the burr hole at the keyhole. The roof is cut from lateral to medial in a plane just anterior to the crista galli. For the unilateral osteotomy, the cut is directed anteriorly slightly medial to the supraorbital foramen and proceeds anteriorly through the anterior face of the superior orbital rim, which detaches the orbital piece. In the bifrontal approach, the lateral orbital rim is cut bilaterally, and the orbital rim is cut

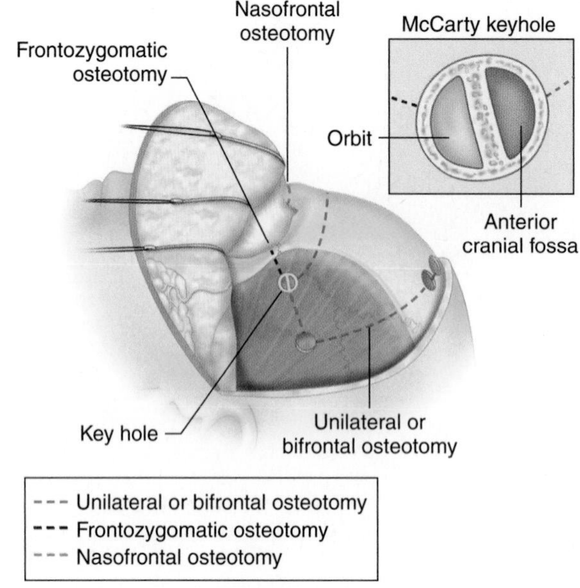

FIGURE 16-5

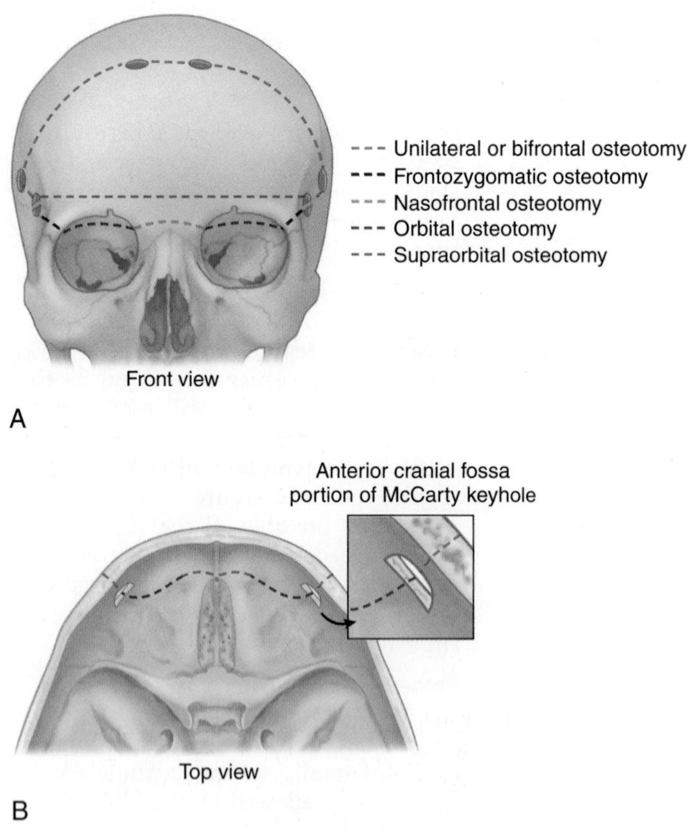

FIGURE 16-6

from keyhole to keyhole running just anterior to the crista galli. Finally, the supraorbital bar is disconnected with a horizontal cut across the nasofrontal process just above the nasofrontal suture.

- **Figure 16-7:** Dural incision. After the bone work is done, the dura is opened with each side opened horizontally and as close to the frontal floor as possible (steps *1* and *2*). The cut on each side should stop short of the superior sagittal sinus anteriorly. For a

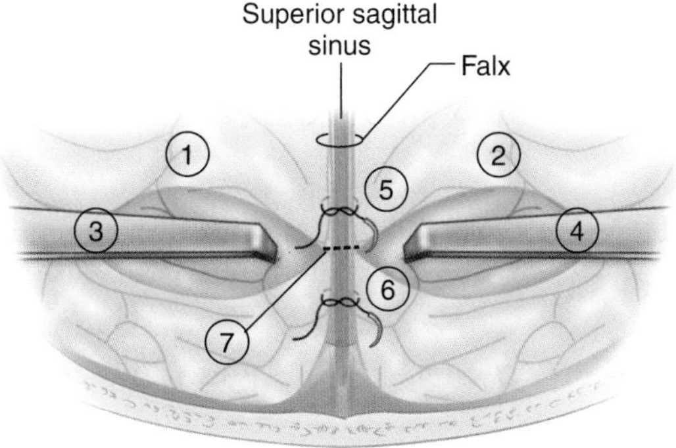

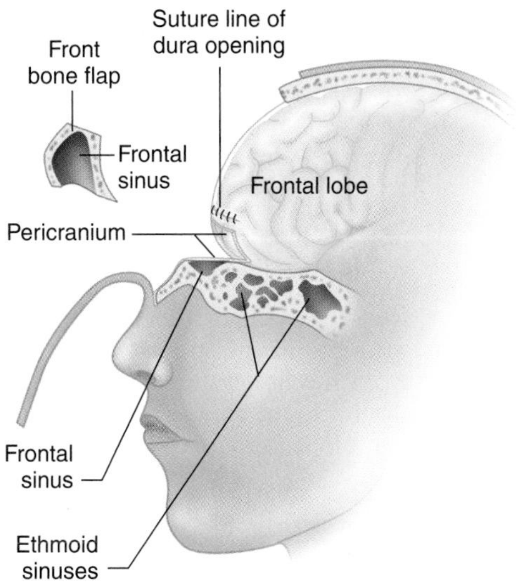

FIGURE 16-7

unilateral approach, this is all the dural opening required. Bifrontal approaches require that the sagittal sinus and falx be divided anteriorly. After a horizontal incision on both sides of the sinus, the frontal lobes are gently retracted away from the falx (steps *3* and *4*) so that two 2-0 silk sutures can be passed through the falx below the sinus (steps *5* and *6*). These sutures should ideally be placed as far anteriorly as possible. After tying these sutures over the top of the sinus, the sinus and falx are divided (step *7*), and the basal dura is put under mild tension so that it lays as flat as possible and does not obstruct vision.

Closure

- Proper closure of these cases can be complex but is important for achieving good outcomes. First, the frontal sinus should be excluded from the intracranial space to prevent infection or mucoceles. The frontal sinus mucosa on the bone flap or orbital osteotomy piece should be completely stripped and lightly débrided from the inner table with a diamond drill bit. The remnant mucosa on the frontal sinus can also be stripped and drilled, or it can merely be folded inward on itself because sinus drainage remains adequate in most cases. The pericranial patch can be used to cover the sinus and should be placed below the osteotomy piece. In many cases, tumor resection leaves a defect in the anterior fossa that should be repaired by laying the vascularized pericranial patch under the frontal lobe and lightly tacking it in place with sutures laterally.
- The horizontal dural opening is closed by circumferentially sewing the dura to the pericranial patch that has replaced the basal dura.
- It is important to consider the final cosmetic result of the bony repair and to consider additional cranioplasty with hydroxyapatite or methyl methacrylate in this region because it is a prominent part of the patient's face.

TIPS FROM THE MASTERS

- It is usually wise to place a lumbar drain in these cases if an anterior fossa floor defect is anticipated.
- It is important that the eye is prepared into the field and that the drapes are placed below the globe so that the drape does not impede the forward folding of the scalp over the supraorbital rim, particularly if removal of the supraorbital bar is planned.
- If a combined rhinologic approach is planned for either closure or tumor resection purposes, the entire upper face and midface should be included in the field, with the lower drape being placed over the upper lip.
- For removal of tumors arising from the anterior midline skull base, such as olfactory groove meningiomas, it is helpful to dissect along the medial orbit until the anterior ethmoid arteries are visualized exiting the orbit through the lamina papyracea. By cauterizing and dividing these arteries, the dural blood supply to these lesions can be eliminated.
- The frontal bone flap should be created taking into account the highly cosmetic nature of the forehead region.
- In elderly patients, it is sometimes wise to put a paramedian burr hole on one side to prevent dural tears near bridging veins near the superior sagittal sinus; these burr holes should ideally be placed behind the hair line.
- Regardless of whether a unilateral or bilateral approach is being performed, we prefer to turn a unilateral bone flap stopping short of midline first and to dissect the sinus away from the bone under direct vision before performing the contralateral flap needed for the bifrontal approach. We believe this reduces the risk of sinus injury and prolonged hemorrhage that could occur while turning this extensive bone flap.
- In cases in which significant frontal retraction is anticipated, it is often wise to remove the orbital bar.

PITFALLS

The eyes are protected against the preparation solution by either suture tarsorrhaphy or Tegaderm dressings and ophthalmic ointment.

Care should be taken to avoid severing the supraorbital nerve anteriorly as it exits the orbit and to avoid going too laterally over the frontozygomatic process until the supratemporal fat pad has been dissected over the frontozygomatic process to protect the facial nerve.

It is important with unilateral orbital osteotomies that the periorbita not be stripped from the medial portions of the orbital roof because it is unnecessary and risks detaching the trochlear pulley of the superior oblique muscle, causing diplopia.

Bilateral approaches differ in that the periorbita should be stripped from the orbital roof medially and laterally. In our experience, patients do not notice diplopia from bilateral superior oblique trochlear detachment.

Removal of the orbital roof or lateral orbital wall is unnecessary (unless the orbital contents need to be exposed), in contrast to in the orbitozygomatic approach. The principal purpose of this osteotomy is to facilitate a low and flat trajectory toward the back of the anterior cranial fossa and less to remove visual obstructions around the sphenoid wing, as with lateral approaches. By avoiding excessive orbital bone removal, the risk of pulsatile enophthalmos is decreased.

SUGGESTED READINGS

Chi JH, Parsa AT, Berger MS, et al. Extended bifrontal craniotomy for midline anterior fossa meningiomas: minimization of retraction-related edema and surgical outcomes. Neurosurgery 2006;59:ONS426–33.

Gazzeri R, Galarza M, Gazzeri G. Giant olfactory groove meningioma: ophthalmological and cognitive outcome after bifrontal microsurgical approach. Acta Neurochir (Wien) 2008;150:1117–25.

Kawakami K, Yamanouchi Y, Kawamura Y, et al. Operative approach to the frontal skull base: extensive transbasal approach. Neurosurgery 1991;28:720–24.

Kawakami K, Yamanouchi Y, Kubota C, et al. An extensive transbasal approach to frontal skull-base tumors: technical note. J Neurosurg 1991;74:1011–3.

Nakamura M, Struck M, Roser F, et al. Olfactory groove meningiomas: clinical outcome and recurrence rates after tumor removal through the frontolateral and bifrontal approach. Neurosurgery 2008;62:1224–32.

Park MC, Goldman MA, Donahue JE, et al. Endonasal ethmoidectomy and bifrontal craniotomy with craniofacial approach for resection of frontoethmoidal osteoma causing tension pneumocephalus. Skull Base 2008;18:67–72.

Procedure 17

Far-Lateral Suboccipital Approach

Michael E. Sughrue, Andrew T. Parsa

INDICATIONS

- The suboccipital approach with C1 laminectomy provides adequate visualization of approximately 270 degrees of the circumference around the medulla. This approach does not provide safe access to the 90 degrees anterior to the medulla, however, because the visual angle needed to see this region is obscured by the occipital condyle, which must be drilled in most cases to allow access along this visual trajectory.
- The muscular bulk in the midline approach performed in a conventional suboccipital craniectomy effectively limits the surgeon's ability to dissect safely laterally enough to visualize the extracranial vertebral artery and to drill away the posterior occipital condyle.

CONTRAINDICATIONS

- The limits of this approach are the ventral clivus and brainstem above the pontomedullary junction.

PLANNING AND POSITIONING

- Positioning for the far-lateral approach is perhaps the most complex of any common neurosurgical procedure.
- After turning the table at least 120 degrees away from the anesthesia team, the patient is placed in a three-quarter prone position on the operating table, with the contralateral shoulder down. The superior (ipsilateral) shoulder is in mild flexion on an arm rest in mild flexion. The contralateral arm is draped off the edge of the bed and placed in a shoulder sling, which is secured to the edge of the bed with towel clamps.
- The head is placed in a Mayfield head holder with two pins placed just behind the contralateral occiput. The single pin is placed in the ipsilateral frontal bone, above the superior temporal line. After pinning, the head is slightly flexed, rotated toward the contralateral shoulder, and elevated slightly. By positioning the patient three quarters prone, the appropriate head position is achieved.
- **Figure 17-1:** Positioning for far-lateral suboccipital approach.

PROCEDURE

- **Figure 17-2:** The skin incision is roughly hockey stick–shaped, consisting of three unequal-length limbs that are roughly perpendicular to each other. The long limb of the incision is midline and begins just below the spinous process of C3 and extends to just above the inion. The horizontal incision extends laterally from just above the inion to just above the mastoid tip. The short limb of the incision begins just below the mastoid tip and extends upward to meet the horizontal limb. This incision parallels the transverse and sigmoid sinuses and provides the ability to fold the myocutaneous flap laterally enough to expose the entire hemiocciput and the arch of C1 out to the tip of the transverse process.
- **Figure 17-3:** Soft tissue elevation and identification of landmarks. Soft tissue dissection is performed with a combination of periosteal dissectors and monopolar cautery to expose three key landmarks in their entirety. The hemiocciput should be cleared of soft tissue down to the foramen magnum. Also, the mastoid process should be

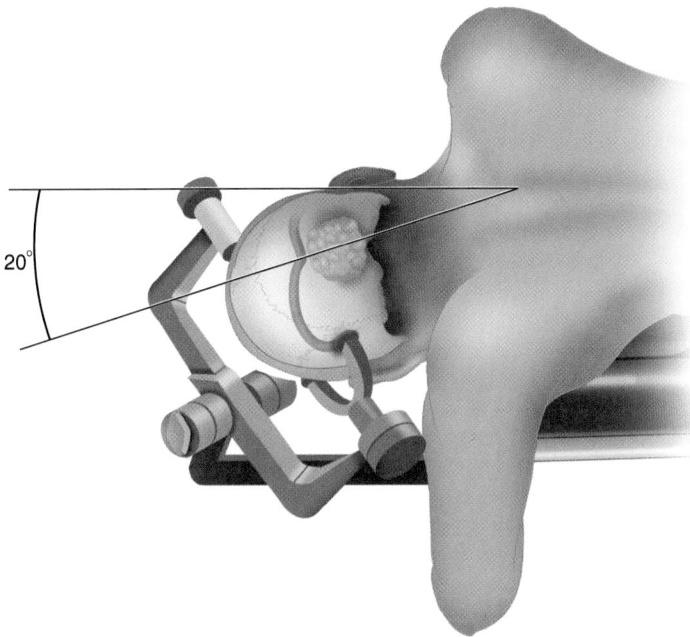

FIGURE 17-1

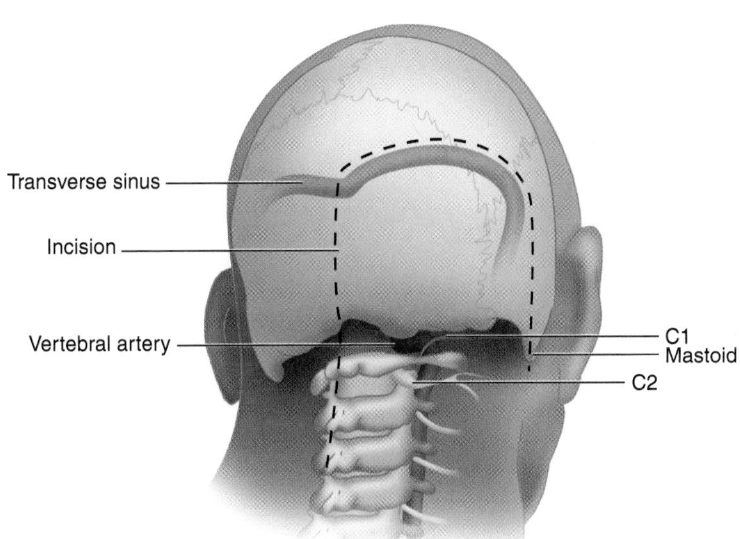

FIGURE 17-2

exposed down to the point where the mastoid tip begins to curve medially and anteriorly until the mastoid curves anteriorly. Finally, the lamina of C1 should be exposed laterally until the tip of the C1 transverse process can be palpated under the superior and inferior oblique muscles of the suboccipital triangle.

- **Figure 17-4:** Identification and mobilization of the vertebral artery. After reflecting the scalp flap with the inferior and superior oblique muscles laterally and posteriorly, the interlaminar and perivascular venous plexus is slowly controlled with bipolar cautery and direct pressure and divided with microscissors. Through this process, the course of the vertebral artery is delineated and prepared for mobilization. The posterior bony portion of the foramen transversarium is removed with a diamond bit drill to free the vertebral artery posteriorly. Multiple periosteal attachments that tether the vertebral artery into the foramen superiorly and inferiorly may be present; these should be sharply divided. The vertebral artery is mobilized away from the occipital condyle with a vessel loop and protected.

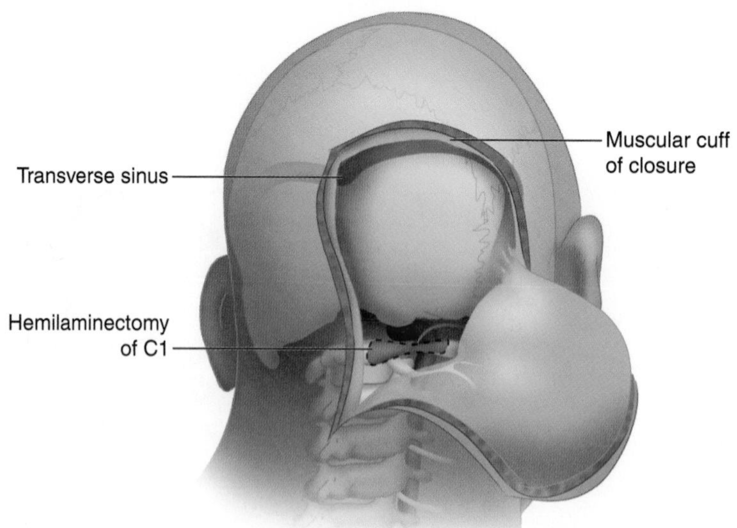

FIGURE 17-3

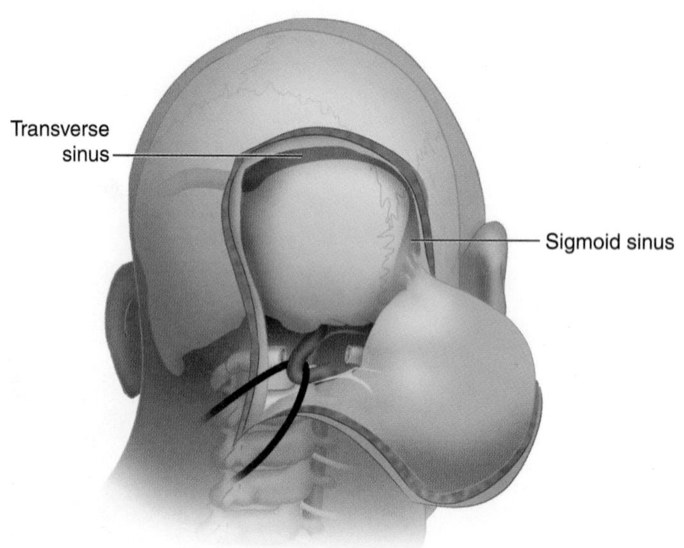

FIGURE 17-4

- **Figure 17-5:** Unilateral suboccipital craniotomy and C1 hemilaminectomy. The bone flap involves three bone cuts that viewed from above remove a J-shaped plate of hemioccipital bone. The medial vertical limb of the bone flap extends upward from the foramen magnum to just shy of the transverse sinus, which is just lateral to midline. The lateral vertical limb begins just inferomedial to the asterion and extends inferiorly and medially in a curvilinear fashion to reach the foramen magnum as lateral as possible. The horizontal limb connects the upper portions of each vertical limb at right angles and roughly parallels the transverse sinus. A C1 hemilaminectomy is necessary to lengthen the dural incision to achieve the desired exposure in this approach. The hemilaminectomy is performed either piecemeal or using a side-cutting bur with a footplate.
- **Figure 17-6:** Retrosigmoid mastoidectomy. In contrast to the transpetrosal approaches, the goal of mastoidectomy in the far-lateral approach is to expose the transverse and sigmoid sinuses from the torcular Herophili to the beginning of the jugular bulb,

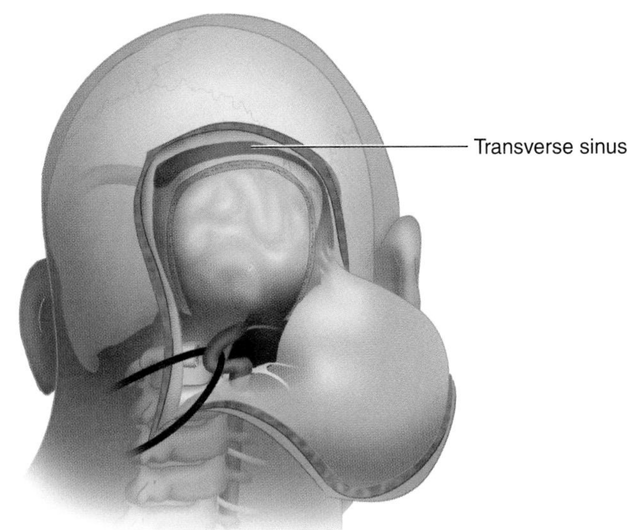

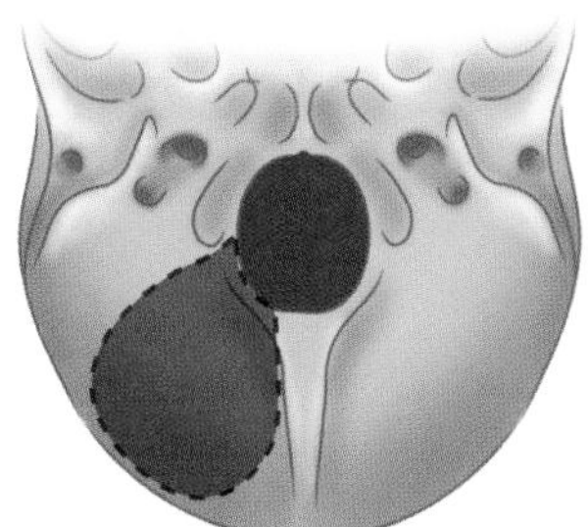

FIGURE 17-5

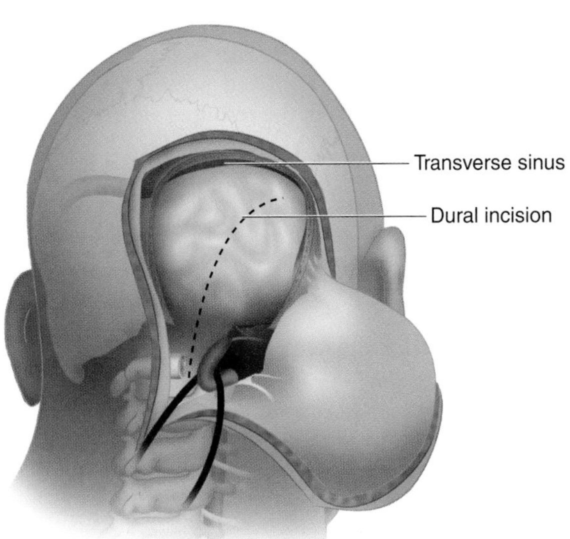

FIGURE 17-6

defining the superior and lateral extent of the dural incision. This is performed with a sequence of dural dissection away from the bone, bony thinning with the drill, and removal with a Kerrison punch.

- **Figure 17-7:** Drilling of occipital condyle. Removal of the occipital condyle and associated lip of foramen magnum allows the additional anterior visualization that this approach provides. Although the posterior half of the condyle can be removed with relatively

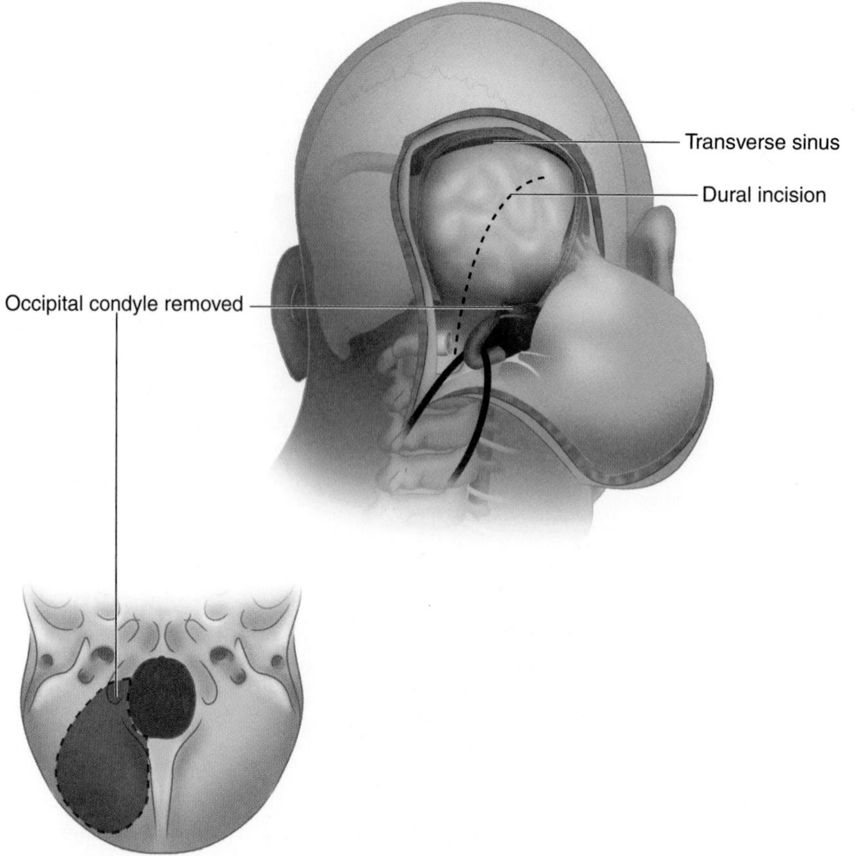

FIGURE 17-7

minimal adverse effects, additional condylar removal provides increased visualization at the cost of decreased stability of the atlantooccipital joint. Roughly 8 mm of condyle can be safely removed posteriorly before occipitocervical fusion should be considered. Before drilling, the rerouted vertebral artery should be protected well away from the site of drilling.

- **Figure 17-8:** Dural incision. The dura is opened in a lazy J-shaped fashion from the transverse sigmoid junction curving medial and inferiorly so that it crosses the foramen magnum just posteriorly to the intradural entry point of the vertebral artery.

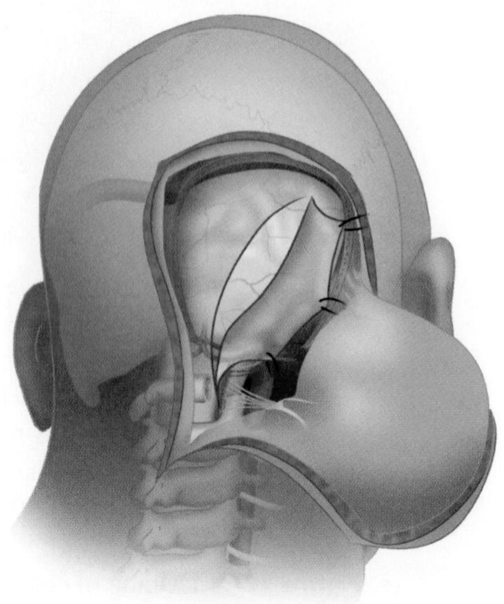

FIGURE 17-8

The cervical dura should be opened in a linear and paramedian fashion down to at least the upper edge of the C2 lamina. If a large circular sinus is encountered while crossing the foramen magnum, this should be controlled with Weck clips, divided, and oversewn with dural sutures. At least some dural cuff should be left around the vertebral artery so that the dura can be repaired safely in this region. The dura should be reflected anteriorly with sutures placed as deeply as possible to keep the dura flat against the bony surface of the drilled condyle.

TIPS FROM THE MASTERS

- The theoretical goal of head positioning is to place the posteromedial portion of the ipsilateral occipital condyle at the highest point in the room. By doing so, the corridor of attack just medial to the condyle is placed basically vertical, maximizing the retraction obtained by gravity.
- Ideally, as much of the bone removal as possible should be performed as part of a bone flap because replacement of bony surface is cosmetically superior and possibly prevents muscular adhesion to the dura and suboccipital pain.
- If necessary, hemilaminectomy of C2 and C3 can further improve visualization.
- Although it is possible to use the foramen magnum as the sole entry point for the side-cutting bur, we prefer to add two burr holes. One burr hole is placed inferolateral to the inion and torcular Herophili and one is placed inferomedial to the asterion to help dissect a clear epidural plane to turn the bone flap in, preventing injury to the venous sinuses.

PITFALLS

It is important to check motor and sensory evoked potentials before and after positioning and to adjust the positioning if there are adverse changes from baseline. We have done these cases with the patient awake in some instances when positioning without neuromonitoring changes was impossible while the patient was asleep.

It is important to remain oriented to the spinal midline; this can be confusing because of the degree of head rotation in this position, which is much greater than the typical suboccipital approach. A loss of one's sense of midline not only can increase blood loss owing to muscle dissection, but also can lead to inappropriate trajectories toward critical structures such as the vertebral artery. For this reason, we begin this approach by finding the intramuscular septum early and cautiously identifying the spinal midline and exposing the C1-3 hemilamina from medial to lateral until the C1 transverse process can be palpated.

During muscle dissection, it is possible to encounter large muscular branches of the vertebral artery.

It is important in either approach that the thick dural attachments at the foramen magnum are bluntly separated from the bony rim of the foramen magnum because dural tears in this region risk injuring the circular sinus.

After the sigmoid sinus is exposed, it is essential that the remaining mastoid air cells are aggressively obliterated with bone wax to prevent cerebrospinal fluid egress through the middle ear.

BAILOUT OPTIONS

- It is wise to have a set of permanent and temporary aneurysm clips on the field throughout the case if needed to address vertebral injury.

SUGGESTED READINGS

Dowd GC, Zeiller S, Awasthi D. Far lateral transcondylar approach: dimensional anatomy. Neurosurgery 1999;45:95–9.

Jiang T, Wang Z, Yu C. [Microsurgical anatomy of far-lateral transcondylar approach]. Zhonghua Yi Xue Za Zhi 1998;78:448–51.

Liu JK, Couldwell WT. Far-lateral transcondylar approach: surgical technique and its application in neurenteric cysts of the cervicomedullary junction: report of two cases. Neurosurg Focus 2005;19:E9.

Puzzilli F, Mastronardi L, Agrillo U, et al. Glossopharyngeal nerve schwannoma: report of a case operated on by the far-lateral transcondylar approach. Skull Base Surg 1999;9:57–63.

Rhoton AL Jr. The far-lateral approach and its transcondylar, supracondylar, and paracondylar extensions. Neurosurgery 2000;47:S195–209.

Seckin H, Ates O, Bauer AM, et al. Microsurgical anatomy of the posterior spinal artery via a far-lateral transcondylar approach. J Neurosurg Spine 2009;10:228–33.

Spektor S, Anderson GJ, McMenomey SO, et al. Quantitative description of the far-lateral transcondylar transtubercular approach to the foramen magnum and clivus. J Neurosurg 2000;92:824–31.

Zhang HZ, Lan Q. [Anatomic study on the design of far-lateral transcondylar transtubercular keyhole approach assisted by neuro-navigation]. Zhonghua Yi Xue Za Zhi 2006;86:736–9.

Procedure 18

Temporopolar (Half-and-Half) Approach to the Basilar Artery and the Retrosellar Space*

Michael E. Sughrue, Andrew T. Parsa

INDICATIONS

- Transsylvian approaches enter the parasellar cisterns on a superior-to-inferior trajectory, forcing the surgeon to work past the carotid artery through the opticocarotid or carotid-oculomotor triangles to access this region, making access of the mid-basilar and interpeduncular cisterns difficult.
- Although the subtemporal approach provides a good view of the basilar artery at the level of the tentorium, it is limited in its rostral visualization, which can be necessary for high-riding basilar apex aneurysms or tumors with significant superior extension. Also, the flat trajectory of this approach limits the ability to see the retrosellar space.
- The temporopolar approach combines these approaches largely through microsurgical mobilization of the temporal lobe, which is retracted posteriorly and laterally to add the exposure of the tentorial incisura to the visualization obtained with a transsylvian approach.

CONTRAINDICATIONS

- Laterally projecting posterior communicating artery or middle cerebral artery aneurysms because these might be attached to the temporal lobe and rupture with retraction.

PLANNING AND POSITIONING

- The patient is positioned supine.
- The head is pinned similar to the orbitozygomatic approach.
- The malar eminence needs to be the highest point in the field.
- **Figure 18-1:** Positioning for the temporopolar approach.

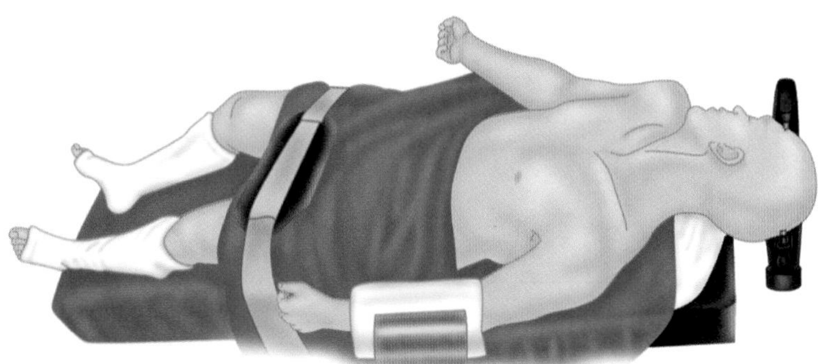

FIGURE 18-1

*See also Procedure 15.

PROCEDURE

- **Figure 18-2:** The skin incision is C-shaped from the zygomatic root up to the widow's peak similar to the incision used for the orbitozygomatic approach. The scalp flap is elevated, and pericranium is harvested for closure.
- **Figure 18-3:** Soft tissue elevation and identification of landmarks. The temporalis fat pad is mobilized similar to the orbitozygomatic approach to protect the frontalis branch of the facial nerve. The temporalis muscle is elevated down the root of the zygoma inferiorly and the inferior orbital fissure anteriorly. It is wise to attempt to preserve the superficial temporal artery if possible. If an orbitozygomatic osteotomy is planned, the attachment of the temporalis fascia to the zygomatic arch should be cut, and the soft tissue should be elevated off the zygoma over the maxillary buttress and frontozygomatic suture. The periorbita should also be freed from the orbital bone. These soft tissue dissection steps are described in more detail in Procedure 15.

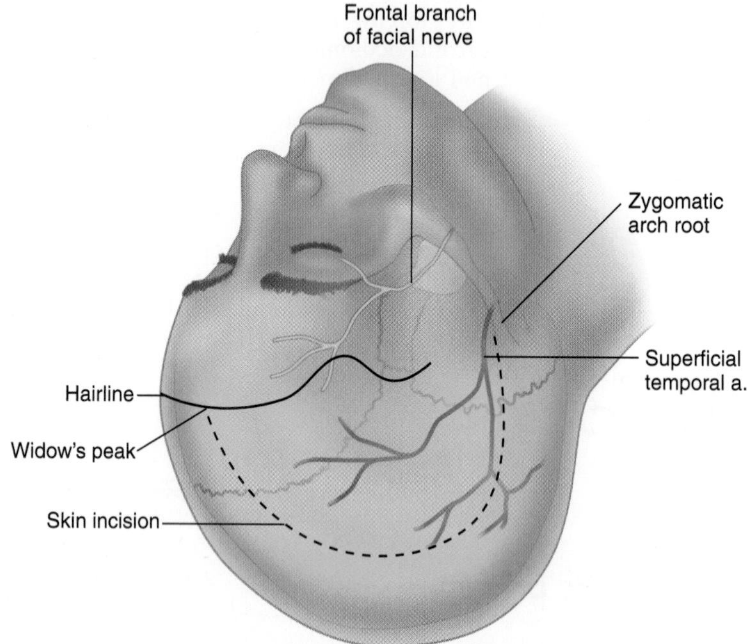

FIGURE 18-2

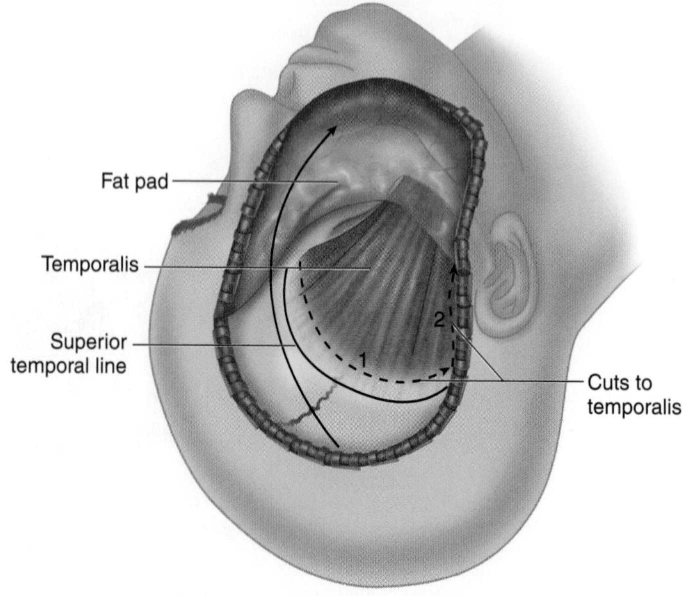

FIGURE 18-3

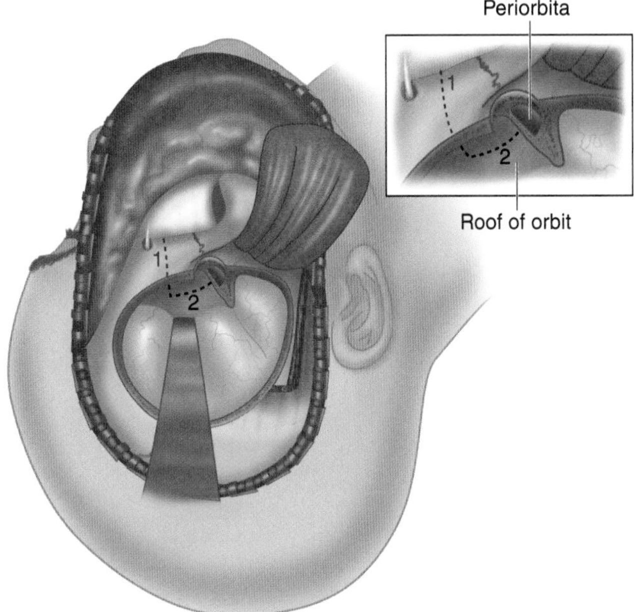

FIGURE 18-4

- **Figure 18-4:** Frontotemporal craniotomy. The craniotomy performed for the temporopolar approach is identical to the frontotemporal craniotomy performed for the pterional or orbitozygomatic approach. Aggressive craniectomy of the squamous temporal bone, from the temporal pole back to the root of the zygoma, until it is flush with the middle fossa floor is particularly important for this approach. This craniectomy is critical for safely mobilizing the temporal lobe posteriorly and working along the middle fossa floor.
- **Figure 18-5:** Zygomatic or orbitozygomatic osteotomy (if necessary). Although the temporopolar approach was initially described as an extension of a pterional craniotomy, we have found additional osteotomies indispensable in this approach. Removal of the zygomatic arch permits additional temporalis dissection and assists with temporal lobe mobilization. Removal of the superolateral orbital rim allows for a flatter, more anterior trajectory, which is invaluable in visualization of the basilar apex.

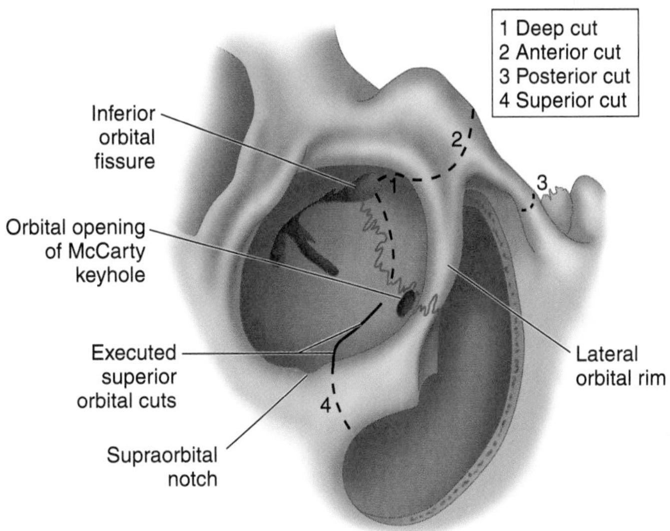

FIGURE 18-5

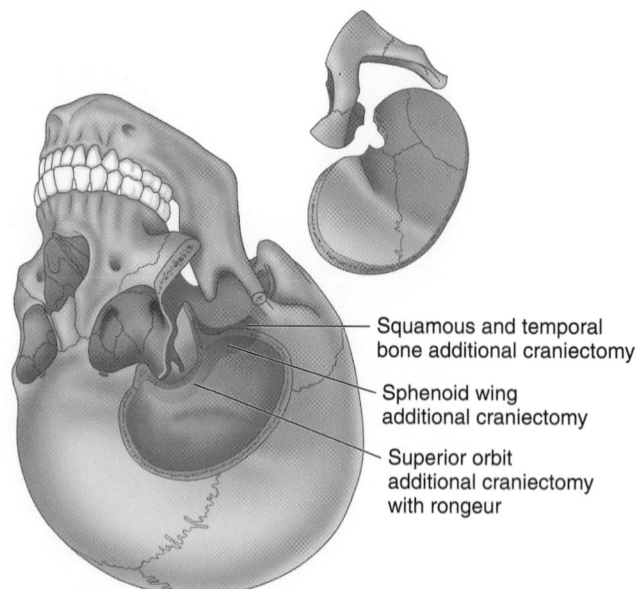

FIGURE 18-6

- **Figure 18-6:** Removal of lesser sphenoid wing. Regardless of whether or not an orbitozygomatic osteotomy is performed, it is necessary to drill the lesser sphenoid wing and orbital roof as flat as possible down to the anterior clinoid process. To perform this, the dura is first stripped from the orbit and sphenoid wing using a No. 1 Penfield dissector. The bony elevation of this region is achieved using a side-cutting drill that is held parallel to the orbital bone with the hand resting on the temporalis muscle. The drilling should avoid entering the orbit but should thin the bone in this region as close to this as possible. In deeper portions, thin spicules of bone need to be removed using a fine rongeur.
- **Figure 18-6:** The dural incision is a C-shaped incision that extends over the sylvian fissure and is convex posteriorly. The ends of the "C" should roughly bifurcate the frontal and temporal limbs of the frontotemporal bone flap. Dural sutures should be placed as low as possible and sutured tightly to the scalp.
- **Figure 18-7:** Sylvian dissection. After dural opening, the arachnoid bridging from frontal to temporal lobe over the anterior sylvian fissure should be meticulously divided using microscissors, No. 6 Rhoton dissector, and bipolar cautery, as necessary. By continuing laterally from the carotid, the middle cerebral artery or a middle cerebral vein can be identified and followed into the sylvian fissure. Arachnoid dissection continues until the frontal and temporal lobes are separated roughly back to the limen insulae. Brain retractors are placed on the frontal and temporal lobes to permit visualization of the basal cisterns.

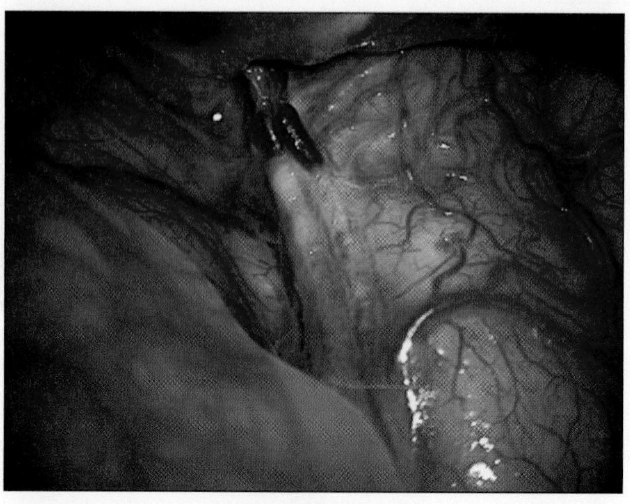

FIGURE 18-7

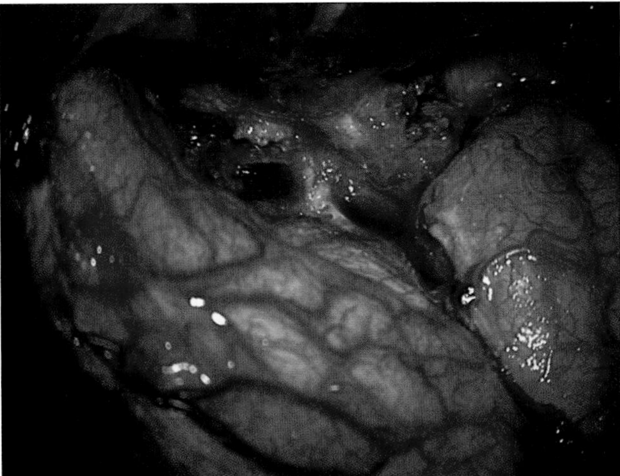

FIGURE 18-8

- **Figure 18-8:** Cisternal dissection. After completing the sylvian fissure dissection, the arachnoid surrounding all visible cisternal spaces should be opened sharply with microscissors. This dissection improves visualization and provides further brain relaxation. The posterior communicating artery should be identified exiting from the supraclinoid carotid artery, and the arachnoid of the opticocarotid and carotid-oculomotor triangle should be opened so that its course is clearly visualized and can be followed posteriorly.
- **Figure 18-9:** Temporal lobe mobilization. At this point, attention should be turned to the temporal pole and subtemporal region. With gentle posterior temporal retraction, any veins bridging from the temporal pole to the sphenoparietal sinus should be identified and divided. Additionally, the subtemporal space should be inspected for bridging veins, which should be divided. With the increased relaxation provided by opening the cisterns, the temporal lobe should be retracted slightly posterolaterally so that the arachnoid overlying the uncus can be identified. After mobilizing the temporal lobe, the posterior communicating artery should be followed posteriorly along the tentorial incisura. This can be followed to the membrane of Lillequist, which can be opened to expose the basilar apex and retrosellar space.

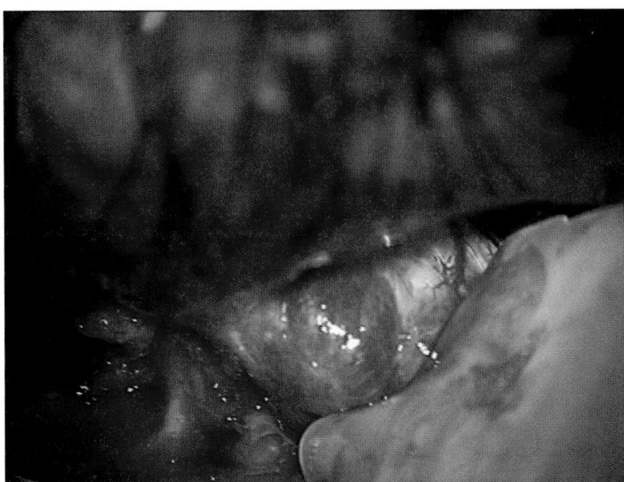

A

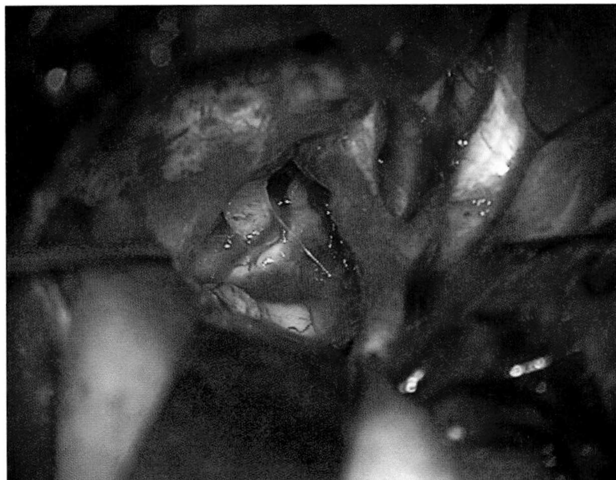

B

FIGURE 18-9

TIPS FROM THE MASTERS

- The dura needs to be tightly sutured flat against the bone so that it does not obscure visualization.
- Often the frontal and temporal operculum can overlap, making entering an arachnoid plane difficult. It is usually wise in these situations to elevate the frontal lobe gently, identify the opticocarotid cistern, and open this sharply to drain cerebrospinal fluid and identify the supraclinoid carotid artery.
- The cerebrum should be routinely protected at this point because these procedures can take some time. Brain retractors should be padded with Telfa.
- Additionally, it is a good idea to cover any cortical region that would be out of direct view of the microscope during the microdissection. Moistened rubber from powder-free gloves provides good protection and keeps the cortex moist.

PITFALLS

It should never be necessary to take a vein crossing the fissure because these can always be separated to one lobe or another through careful dissection.

BAILOUT OPTIONS

- If more posterior exposure of the ambient cistern is needed, the temporal lobe can be retracted upward, converting this approach to a subtemporal approach.

SUGGESTED READINGS

Chanda A, Nanda A. Anatomical study of the orbitozygomatic transsellar-transcavernous-transclinoidal approach to the basilar artery bifurcation. J Neurosurg 2002;97:151–60.

Ikeda K, Yamashita J, Hashimoto M, et al. Orbitozygomatic temporopolar approach for a high basilar tip aneurysm associated with a short intracranial internal carotid artery: a new surgical approach. Neurosurgery 1991;28:105–10.

Levy ML, Khoo LT, Day JD, et al. Optimization of the operative corridor for the resection of craniopharyngiomas in children: the combined frontoorbitozygomatic temporopolar approach: technical note. Neurosurg Focus 1997;3:e5.

Shiokawa Y, Saito I, Aoki N, et al. Zygomatic temporopolar approach for basilar artery aneurysms. Neurosurgery 1989;25:793–6.

Zada G, Day JD, Giannotta SL. The extradural temporopolar approach: a review of indications and operative technique. Neurosurg Focus 2008;25:E3.

Procedure 19 Middle Fossa Craniotomy and Approach to the Internal Auditory Canal or Petrous Apex

Michael E. Sughrue, Andrew T. Parsa

INDICATIONS

- The middle fossa approach is a largely extradural approach to the bony structures that make up the floor of the middle fossa.
- Although the convex floor of the middle fossa is the most straightforward region to access with this approach, this approach is commonly the starting point for anterior transpetrosal approaches to the internal auditory canal (IAC) or petroclival junction.

CONTRAINDICATIONS

- Tumors with significant posterior fossa extension
- Tumors caudal to the IAC

PLANNING AND POSITIONING

- The patient is placed in a semilateral position with the head turned toward the contralateral side until the zygomatic arch is roughly parallel to the floor.
- The pins of the Mayfield head holder are placed in the forehead and occiput, and the top of the head is lowered to help the temporal lobe fall away from the middle fossa floor.
- **Figure 19-1:** Positioning for middle fossa approach.

PROCEDURE

- **Figure 19-2: A,** Skin incision and soft tissue elevation (IAC approach). The skin incision in the middle fossa approach to the IAC is a horseshoe incision that begins just anterior to the tragus down to the inferior zygomatic root, extends upward, and curves

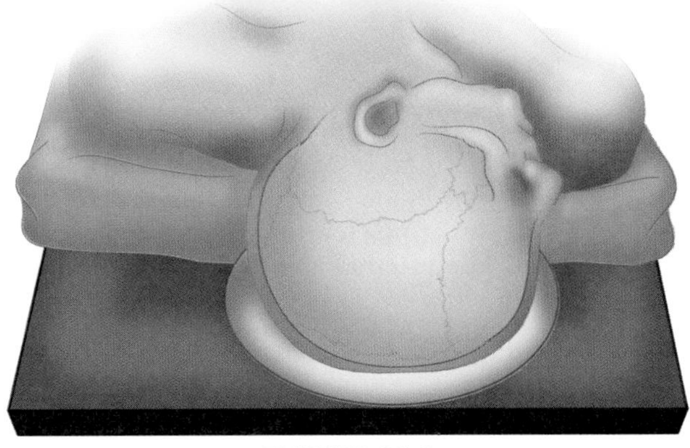

FIGURE 19-1

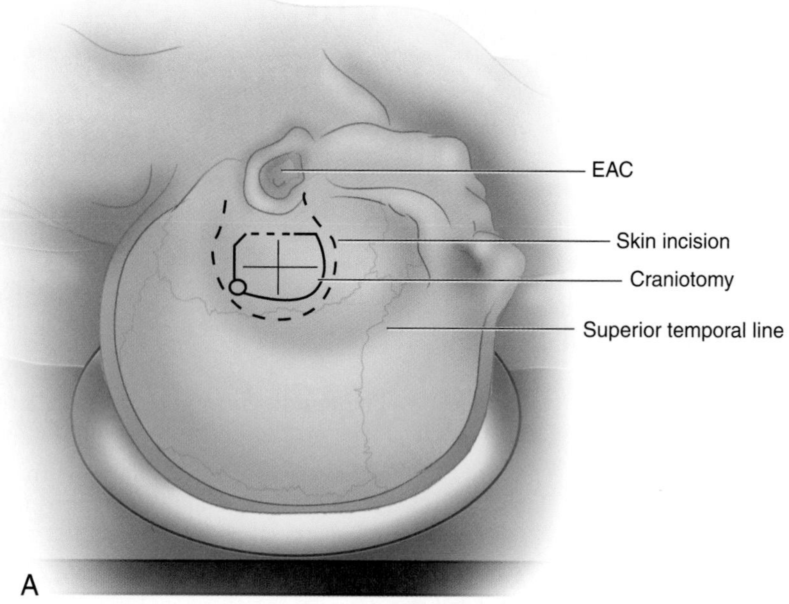

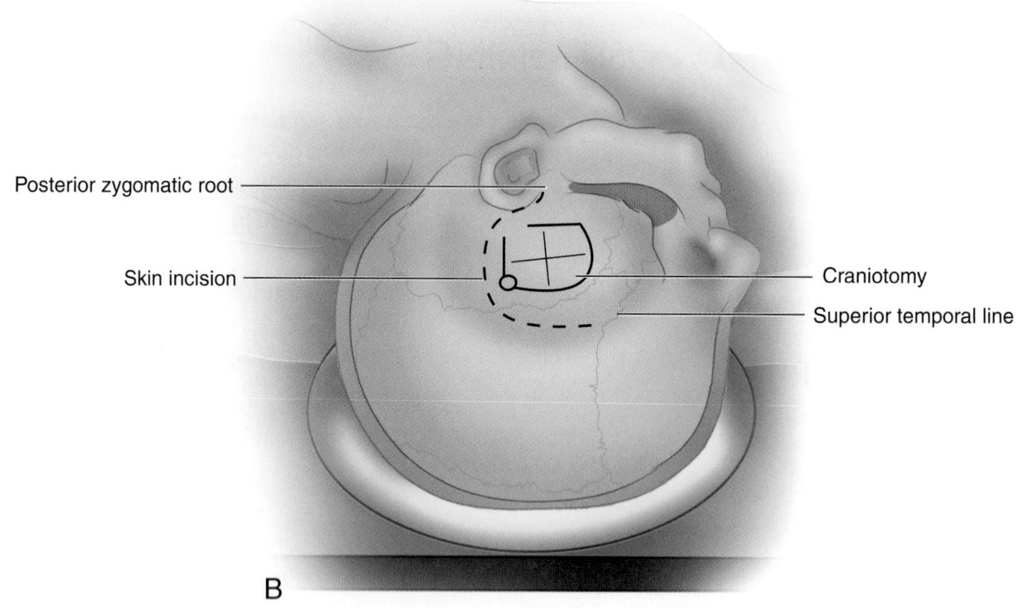

FIGURE 19-2

posteriorly around the pinna before curving inferiorly down to the mastoid tip. The horseshoe should be centered roughly over the IAC. It is wise to harvest pericranium with the elevation of the scalp flap. The soft tissue is elevated until the soft tissue of the external auditory canal (*EAC*) is palpable but not exposed. Temporalis muscle is elevated with the scalp flap as a myocutaneous flap. **B,** Soft tissue elevation and identification of landmarks (petrous apex approach). The skin incision in the middle fossa approach to the petrous apex is a small reverse question mark that begins just anterior to the tragus at the zygomatic root, extends upward to the top of the pinna root, and curves posteriorly for 1 cm before turning superiorly and anteriorly to run just above the superior temporal line. The temporalis muscle is divided in the plane

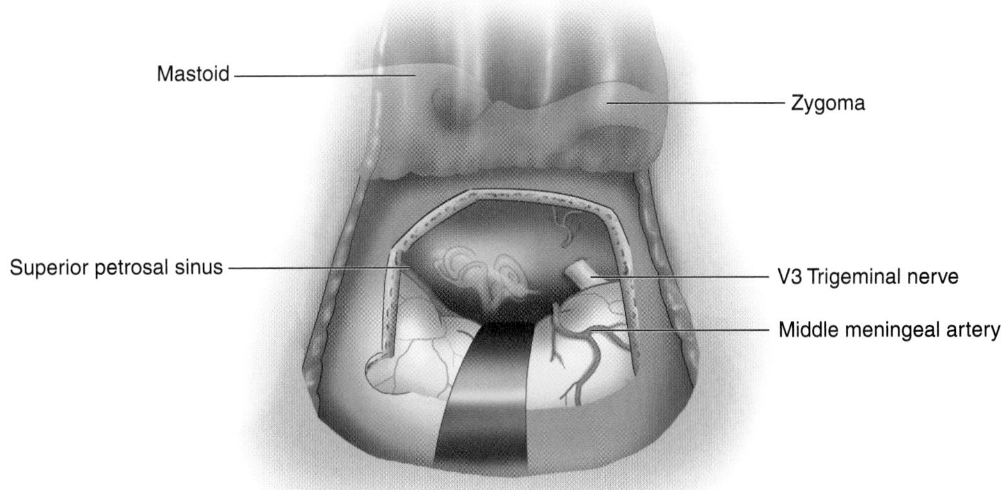

FIGURE 19-3

of its fibers and raised off the bone either as a myocutaneous flap or separated from the flap if a zygomatic arch osteotomy is planned. A limited posterior zygomatic arch osteotomy can allow for more temporalis retraction and a lower, flatter trajectory along the middle fossa floor.

- **Figure 19-3:** The temporal craniotomy is roughly rectangular. It is centered over the EAC for approaches to the IAC and over the posterior zygomatic root for approaches to the petrous apex. It is cosmetically superior to hide the burr holes below the temporalis muscle.
- **Figure 19-4:** Extradural approach. Following the craniotomy, the region of interest is approached extradurally by sequentially dissecting the dura away from the middle fossa floor. The first notable structure encountered in the extradural dissection is the foramen spinosum and middle meningeal artery. Although the middle meningeal artery can be sacrificed, a few centimeters should be spared because this can supply the facial nerve. Otherwise, the dural elevation continues to the edge of the superior petrosal sinus at the posterior edge of the petrous ridge.

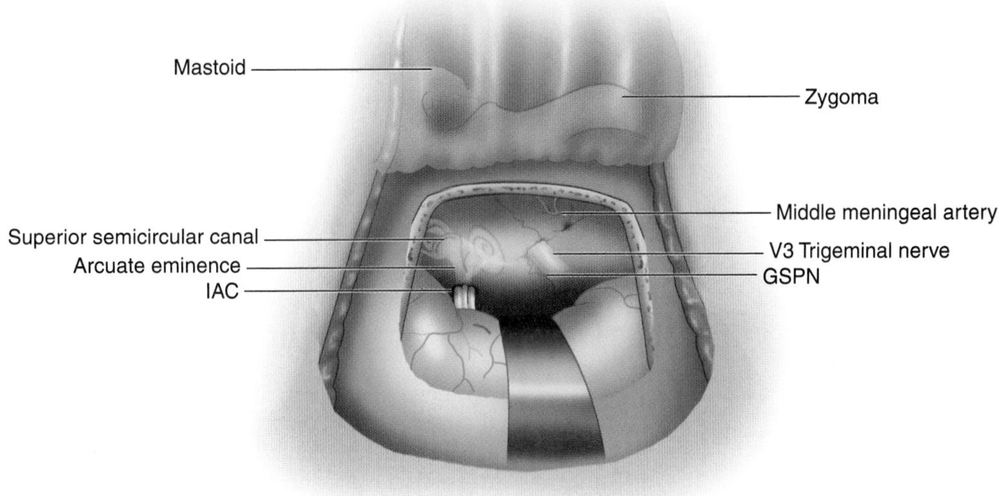

FIGURE 19-4

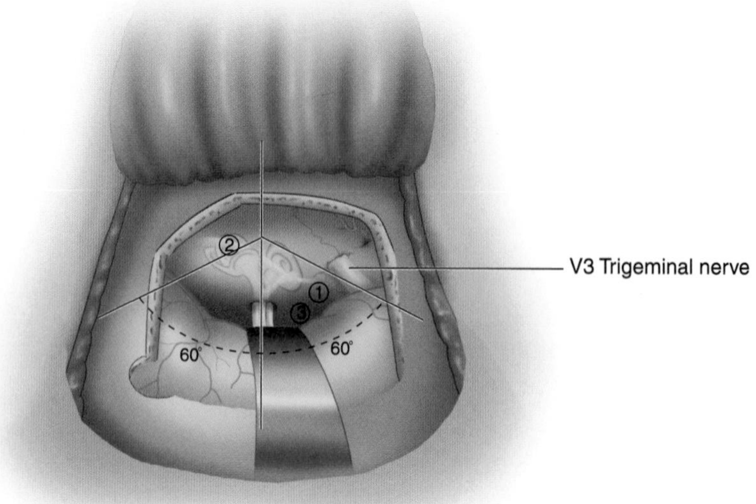

FIGURE 19-5

- Two important landmarks in anterior transpetrosal approaches are the greater superficial petrosal nerve (GSPN) and the arcuate eminence. The GSPN is an early branch of the facial nerve and not only defines the medial part of the cochlea (known as the Kawase triangle), but also meets the petrous carotid artery as it exits the carotid canal. The arcuate eminence is formed by the superior semicircular canal and can be used to identify the location of the IAC from above.
- **Figure 19-5:** Identification of IAC. Multiple methods for identifying the site to begin drilling to expose the IAC have been published. One approach is to identify the GSPN and follow it back to its exit point from the bone. The petrous bone is drilled at this point to follow the GPSN to the geniculate ganglion and subsequently to the ICA. Another approach involves gentle drilling over the arcuate eminence until the direction of blue line of the superior semicircular canal is appreciated. Care should be taken to avoid injury to the superior semicircular canal. The IAC can be identified by imagining a plane that bisects the angle between the superior canal and the GSPN. The plane of the IAC meets the plane of the GPSN or the superior canal at 60 degrees posteriorly. A final approach involves drilling the dorsal anterior petrous bone, well anterior to the hypothetical location of the IAC. Drilling is continued slowly until the facial nerve is encountered at the porus acusticus.
- **Figure 19-6:** Anterior petrosectomy (if indicated). Using the GSPN as a guide, the petrous bone is removed at the apex until the superior petrosal sinus (*SPS*) and tentorium are encountered and divided. It is important to avoid drilling too laterally because this risks injury to the cochlea or important to drill anterior to the petrous ridge because the carotid artery is located in this region. When this bone is removed extradurally, the dura is incised, the superior petrosal sinus is divided, and the tentorium is cut. This provides access to the petroclival junction.

TIPS FROM THE MASTERS

- The best skin incision and craniotomy for the middle fossa approach vary depending on the eventual target of the surgery. Surface landmarks can provide helpful information in planning these approaches. The EAC is roughly coplanar with the IAC. The ideal craniotomy for approaching the IAC is centered over the EAC. Similarly, the anterior petrous apex is roughly deep to the root of the zygoma in this position, and the skin incision and craniotomy are placed more anteriorly.

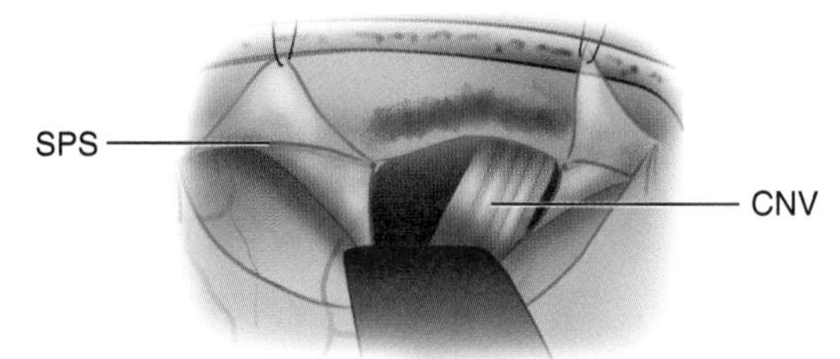

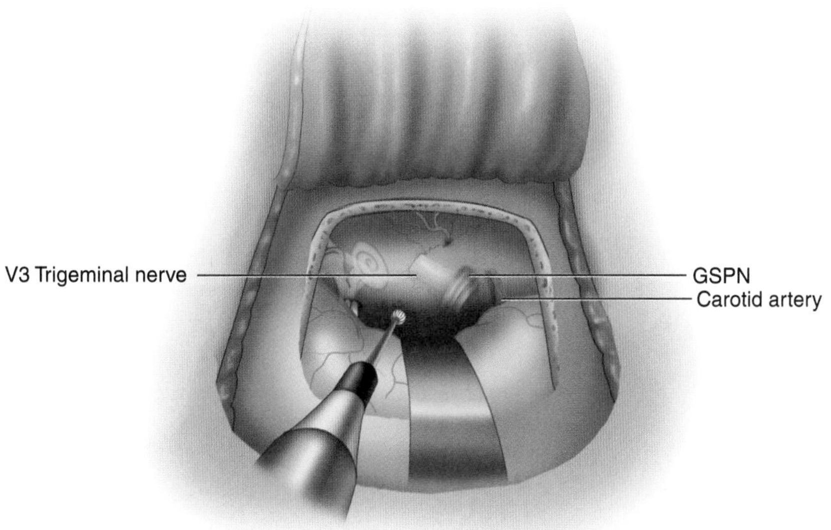

FIGURE 19-6

- Although the superior three limbs of the rectangular bone flap can be cut with the side-cutting foot plate, it is probably best to drill the inferior limb as a trough and to take the bone down with a Kerrison punch because the dura is easily torn in this location.
- Bleeding from the epidural veins during extradural dissection is typical, especially anteriorly.

PITFALLS

Drilling the petrous apex too laterally or too anteriorly risks entering the cochlea or the petrous carotid.

Traction on the GSPN should be avoided because this can injure the facial nerve.

SUGGESTED READINGS

Aristegui M, Cokkeser Y, Saleh E, et al. Surgical anatomy of the extended middle cranial fossa approach. Skull Base Surg 1994;4:181–8.

Kawase T, Shiobara R, Toya S. Middle fossa transpetrosal-transtentorial approaches for petroclival meningiomas: selective pyramid resection and radicality. Acta Neurochir (Wien) 1994;129:113–20.

Landolfi M, Arsistegui M, Taibah A, et al. [The extended middle cranial fossa approach: a morphometric analysis]. Acta Otorhinolaryngol Ital 1994;14:127–34.

Little KM, Friedman AH, Sampson JH, et al. Surgical management of petroclival meningiomas: defining resection goals based on risk of neurological morbidity and tumor recurrence rates in 137 patients. Neurosurgery 2005;56:546–59.

Silverstein H, Norrell H, Haberkamp T. A comparison of retrosigmoid IAC, retrolabyrinthine, and middle fossa vestibular neurectomy for treatment of vertigo. Laryngoscope 1987;97:165–73.

Procedure 20

Retrolabyrinthine Approach

Michael E. Sughrue, Andrew T. Parsa

INDICATIONS

- The retrolabyrinthine approach is a hearing-preserving presigmoid approach that uses a mastoidectomy and skeletonization of the sigmoid sinus to expose the presigmoid dura behind the semicircular canals.
- The principal appeal of this approach is its ability to expose widely the posterior petrous face and cisternal portions of cranial nerves VII and VIII with a minimal degree of cerebellar retraction.
- The retrolabyrinthine approach additionally is used to identify and expose the superior petrosal sinus, as a first step for division of the tentorium.

CONTRAINDICATIONS

- This approach is unable to access the internal auditory canal or petrous apex directly because of the interposition of the labyrinthine and cochlear structures between the surgeon and these regions.

PLANNING AND POSITIONING

- The patient generally is placed in a semilateral position on the operating table, with a bump under the ipsilateral shoulder.
- The head is placed in a Mayfield head holder with two pins placed in the occiput just off midline. The single pin is placed in the ipsilateral forehead, lateral to the mid-pupillary line ideally behind the hairline.
- After pinning, the head is usually positioned such that the region just behind the pinna just superior to the mastoid process is the highest point on the patient's head. With adequate ipsilateral shoulder elevation, this position is achieved by a slight amount of contralateral head rotation, minimal neck flexion, and head elevation.
- **Figure 20-1:** Positioning for retrolabyrinthine approach.

PROCEDURE

- **Figure 20-2:** The skin incision is C-shaped with the convex portion of the "C" pointing posteriorly. The upper limb of the incision begins just superior to the pinna. The height of this superior limb can estimated by drawing a line from the zygomatic arch to the inion and beginning the upper limb just above the external auditory canal along this line, which should overlie the linea temporalis. The incision terminates just inferior and anterior to the mastoid tip. The apex of the "C" should be far enough back to expose fully the asterion, which is roughly one third of the way from the pinna to the inion.
- **Figure 20-3:** Soft tissue elevation and identification of landmarks. Following incision, the scalp is separated from the underlying pericranium sharply and elevated anteriorly. A pericranial flap is also harvested and reflected anteriorly. The soft tissue dissection should proceed anteriorly until the external auditory canal can be palpated. When the mastoid process has been exposed, the attachments of the sternocleidomastoid and splenius capitus muscles are partially detached from the mastoid tip until the bone begins to curve medially.

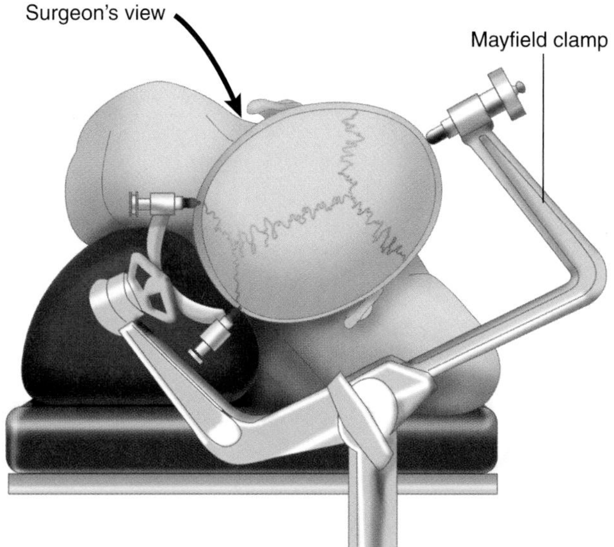

FIGURE 20-1

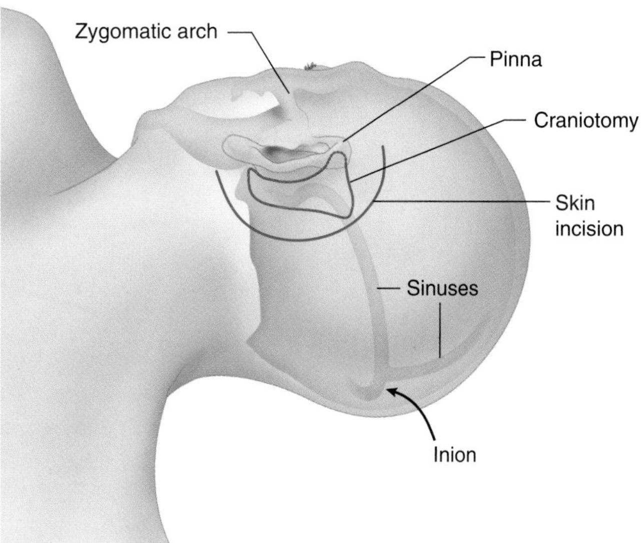

FIGURE 20-2

- **Figure 20-4:** The mastoidectomy is roughly a right triangle with the curvilinear hypotenuse just posterior to the external auditory canal. The superior limb of the triangle runs parallel and inferior to the linea temporalis from just posterior to the zygomatic root to just posterior to the asterion. The anterior limb of the triangle runs in from the anteriormost point of the superior limb inferiorly, following the curve dictated by the external auditory canal, terminating inferiorly at the mastoid tip. The posterior limb finishes the triangle, running from the asterion to the mastoid tip. An important landmark is the spine of Henle, just posterior and superior to the external meatus. This point roughly overlies the mastoid antrum where the semicircular canals and facial nerve are located.
- **Figure 20-5:** Delineation of the sinodural angle. After exposure of the sinuses and dura, the epitympanum is drilled open with a diamond bit. The bony labyrinth overlying the semicircular canals is skeletonized, with care taken not to violate this protective bone. When the boundaries of the labyrinths are well delineated, retrolabyrinthine bone removal can continue safely until the sinodural angle is defined and the adjacent middle and presigmoid dura are completely exposed up to the sinodural angle.

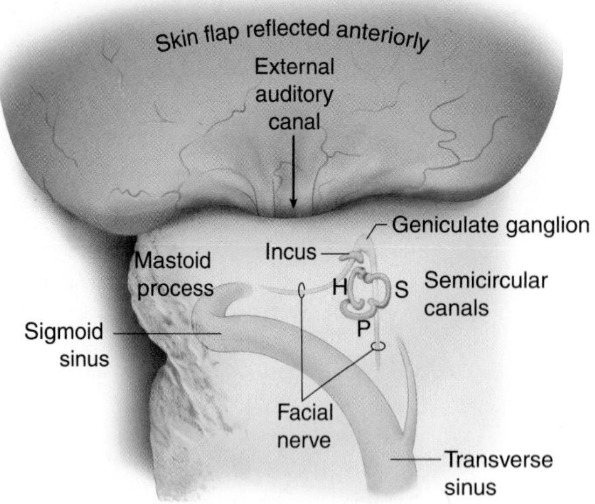

FIGURE 20-3

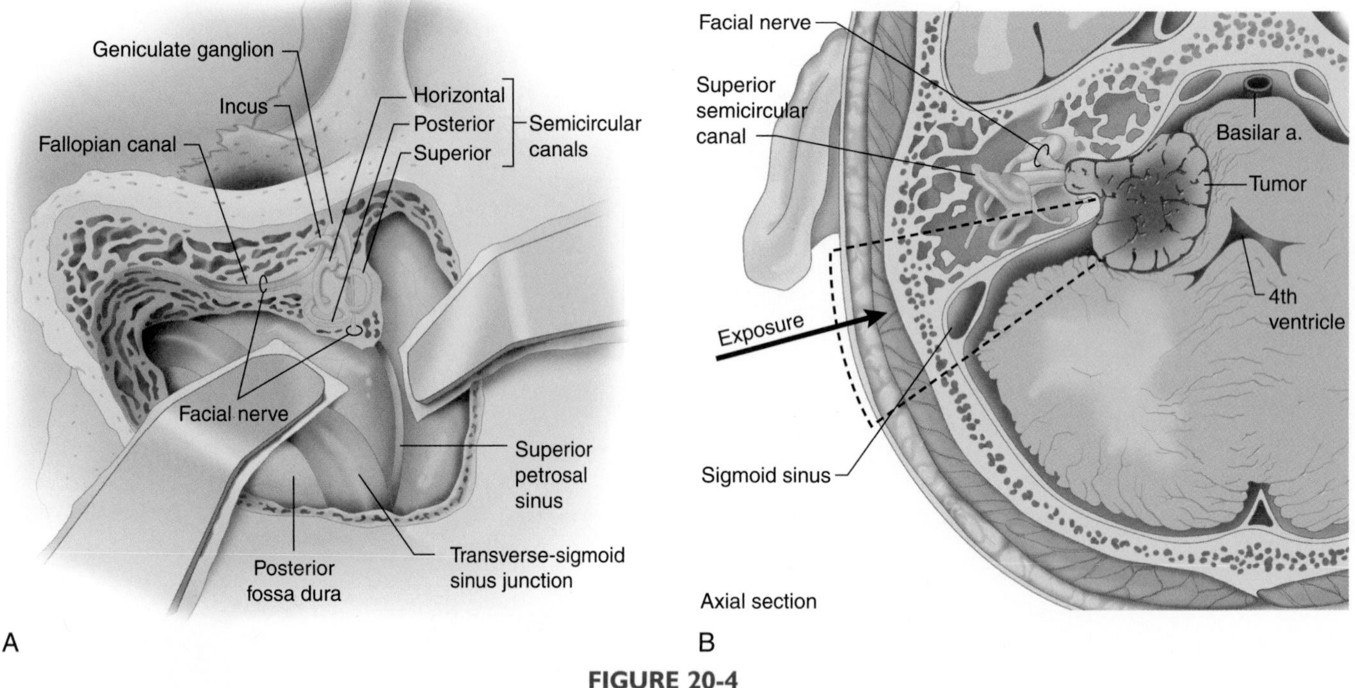

FIGURE 20-4

- **Figure 20-6:** Delineation of the fallopian canal. Adequate exposure in this approach requires that the presigmoid dura be exposed down to the jugular bulb. The vertical portion of the facial nerve overlies the jugular bulb and dura in this region. The fallopian canal is identified anterior and inferior to the bony labyrinths in the epitympanum. When identified, the canal is skeletonized with a diamond bit, particularly on its deep surface in a rostral-to-caudal direction, until its relationship to the jugular bulb is known. Bony removal can be continued as far anteroinferior as possible underneath the facial nerve.
- **Figure 20-7:** Dural incision. The dura is opened in a C-shaped fashion around the epitympanum with the base centered around the labyrinths. It is important that the endolymphatic sac is identified and included with the dural flap so that endolymphatic flow is not disrupted. Depending on the goals of surgery, the superior petrosal sinus can be sacrificed as part of a tentorial division, and the middle fossa dura can be opened to provide visualization of the petrous apex, tentorial incisura, or middle fossa floor.

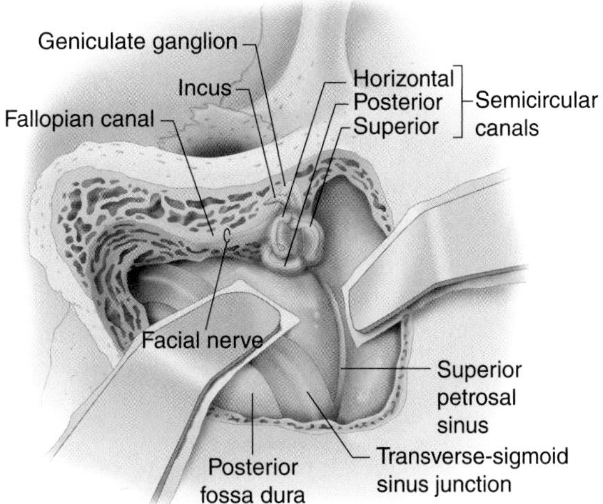

FIGURE 20-5

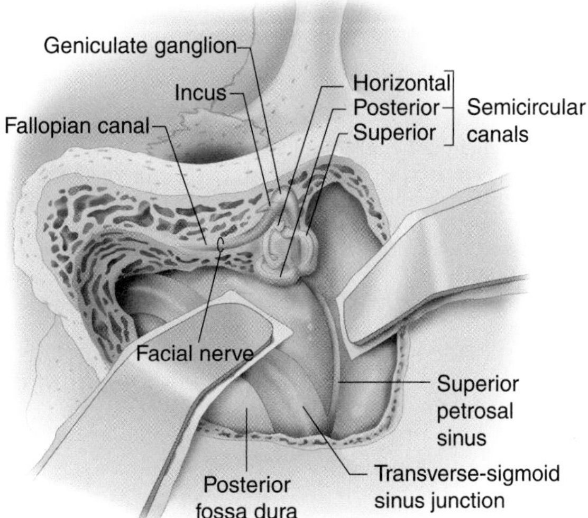

FIGURE 20-6

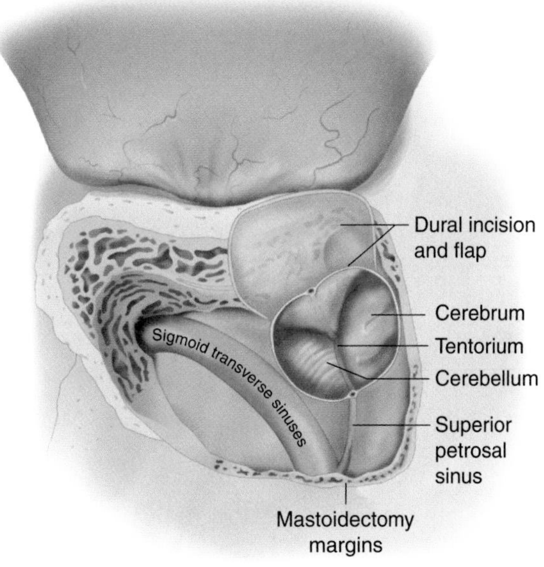

FIGURE 20-7

TIPS FROM THE MASTERS

- Numerous mastoid emissary veins can be encountered during this dissection, and when bleeding from one of these veins is encountered, it is best to continue dissection until well beyond these veins before attempting to control the bleeding with bone wax.
- The drilling should start with a large cutting bur and proceed to diamond burs as critical structures such as the facial nerve and sigmoid sinus are encountered.
- The largest burs possible for a given drilling task should be used because these are less likely to pierce a small hole in a vessel or nerve than a small bur.

PITFALLS

Care should be taken not to cause kinking of the contralateral jugular vein with the head position.

Care should be taken to avoid entering the external auditory canal during soft tissue dissection.

SUGGESTED READINGS

Alliez JR, Pellet W, Roche PH. [Value of retrolabyrinthine approach for surgical resection of meningiomas inserted around the lateral sinus between the transverse and sigmoid parts]. Neurochirurgie 2006;52:419–31.

Darrouzet V, Franco-Vidal V, Hilton M, et al. Surgery of cerebellopontine angle epidermoid cysts: role of the widened retrolabyrinthine approach combined with endoscopy. Otolaryngol Head Neck Surg 2004;131:120–5.

Goksu N, Yilmaz M, Bayramoglu I, et al. Combined retrosigmoid retrolabyrinthine vestibular nerve section: results of our experience over 10 years. Otol Neurotol 2005;26:481–3.

Lu H, Zhang X, Jiang G, et al. [A study of applied microanatomy by endoscope-assisted via retrolabyrinthine approach]. Lin Chung Er Bi Yan Hou Tou Jing Wai Ke Za Zhi 2007;21:724–6.

Russell SM, Roland JT Jr, Golfinos JG. Retrolabyrinthine craniectomy: the unsung hero of skull base surgery. Skull Base 2004;14:63–71.

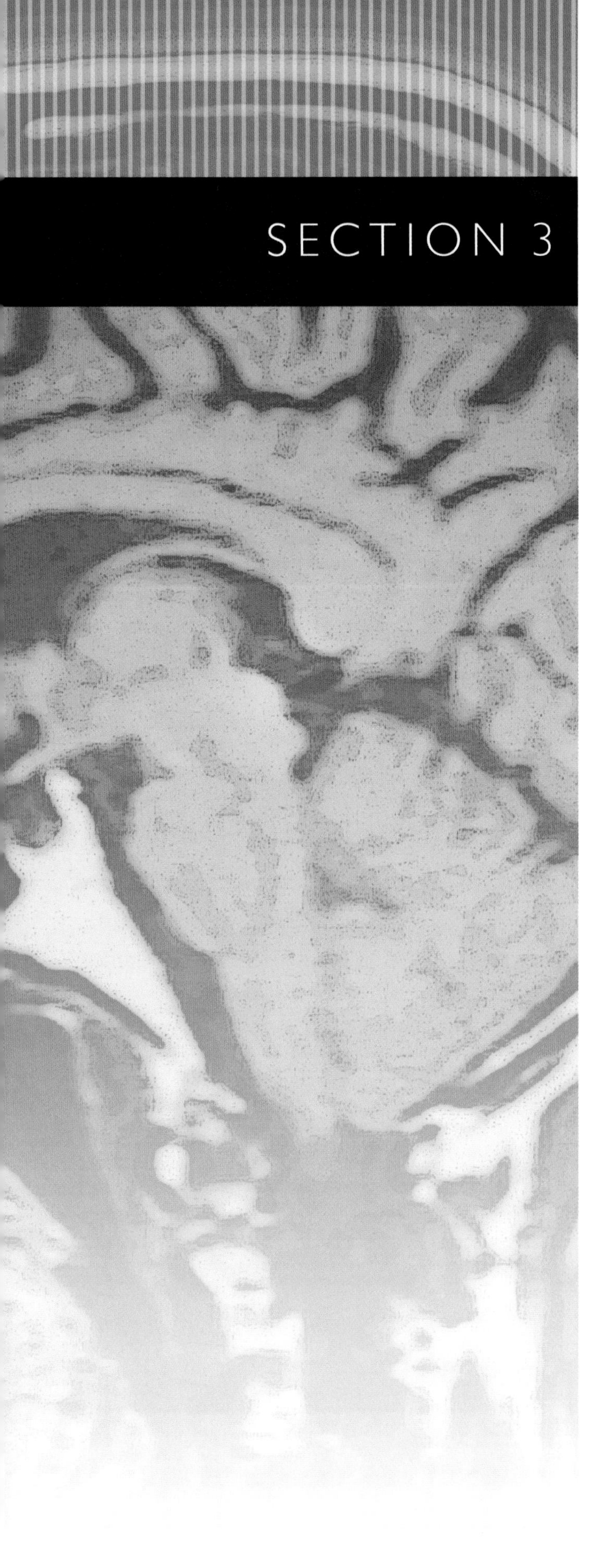

SECTION 3 Vascular

SECTION EDITORS — STEVEN GIANNOTTA, WITH AZADEH FARIN

Procedure 21

Pterional Craniotomy for Anterior Communicating Artery Aneurysm Clipping

Chad W. Washington, Ralph G. Dacey, Jr., Gregory J. Zipfel

INDICATIONS

Absolute

- Subarachnoid hemorrhage with intraparenchymal hemorrhage requiring emergent evacuation
- Subarachnoid hemorrhage with anterior communicating artery (Acomm) aneurysm not repairable by endovascular coiling

Strong

- Large aneurysm (≥10 mm)
- Unruptured aneurysm (≥7 mm) in a patient 50 years old or younger
- Aneurysm with intraluminal thrombus
- Anterior projecting aneurysm
- Hunt and Hess grade I, II, or III in a patient 50 years old or younger

CONTRAINDICATIONS

Strong

- Aneurysm with significant calcification or atheroma

Relative

- Hunt and Hess grade IV or V with aneurysm repairable by endovascular coiling
- Subarachnoid hemorrhage with aneurysm repairable by coiling in a patient older than 60 years
- Unruptured aneurysm less than 7 mm in a patient older than 70 years
- Posterior-projecting aneurysm

PLANNING AND POSITIONING

- It is generally preferred that the aneurysm be approached from the patient's nondominant side. Contraindications to this approach are the following:
  - The patient possesses a dominant-sided intraparenchymal hemorrhage requiring evacuation.
  - Early access to a dominant A1 branch would be difficult.
  - It is planned to clip multiple aneurysms during the same operation (e.g., left middle cerebral artery and anterior cerebral artery).
- Placement of an external ventricular drain or lumbar drain during the preoperative period for cerebrospinal fluid drainage is frequently advantageous.
- A radiolucent head holder should be used in case intraoperative angiography is performed.

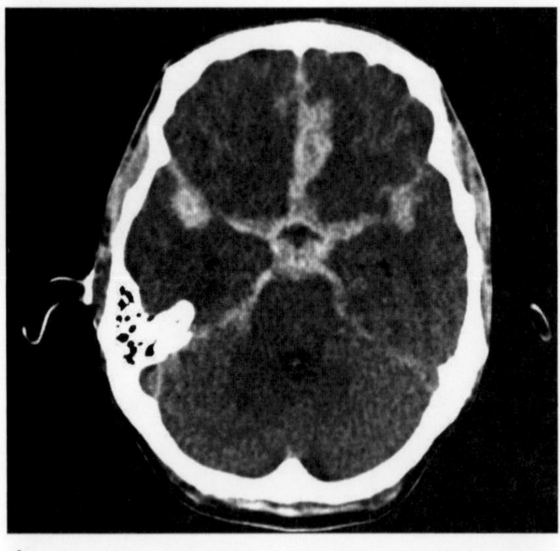

A

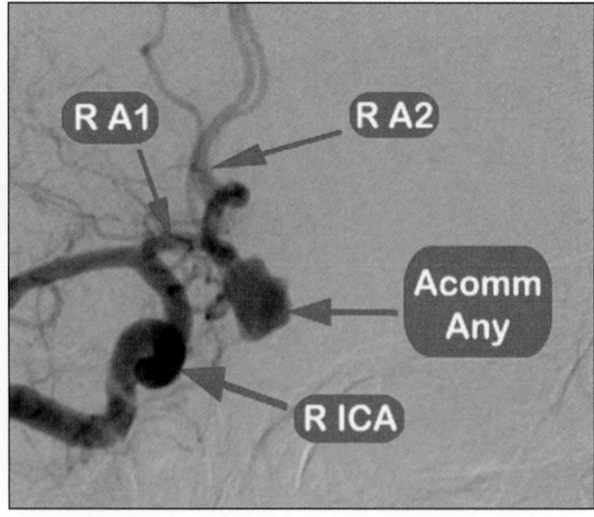

B

C

FIGURE 21-1

- Proper head positioning helps to minimize brain retraction.
- Antibiotic prophylaxis should be administered before skin incision.
- Mannitol given at the time of skin incision helps with brain relaxation.
- **Figure 21-1:** Preoperative imaging is essential in helping to define a patient's anatomy and may consist of a combination of modalities, including computed tomography (CT) scan, magnetic resonance imaging and magnetic resonance angiography, CT angiography, and four-vessel cerebral angiography. Examples of noncontrast head CT scan (**A**), cerebral angiography (**B**), and digital subtraction three-dimensional reconstruction (**C**) are shown. CT scan shows a common finding associated with ruptured Acomm aneurysms with intraparenchymal hemorrhage into the left gyrus rectus. Angiogram and three-dimensional reconstruction show a lobulated Acomm aneurysm being filled from right A1 segment with hypoplastic left A1.
- **Figure 21-2:** Pterional craniotomy is the standard approach for aneurysms arising from the Acomm complex. The patient's head is placed in a three-pin radiolucent head holder with the head rotated 30 to 60 degrees contralateral to the craniotomy site. The degree of rotation depends on the patient's anatomy. The goal is to provide a vertical corridor through which the Acomm complex may be accessed.

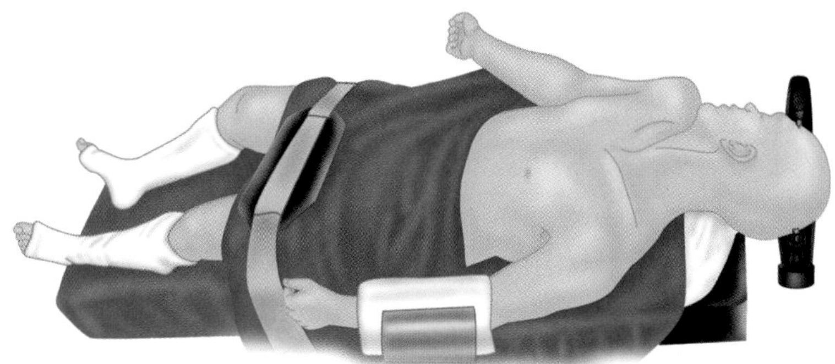

FIGURE 21-2

PROCEDURE

- **Figure 21-3:** Much of the complexity of Acomm aneurysm is related to the anatomic variation that can occur. **A,** Equal A1 arteries and recurrent arteries arising from proximal A2 arteries. **B,** Most common variation associated with aneurysms, with a dominant left A1 artery and hypoplastic right A1 artery. **C,** Bifid Acomm with left recurrent artery originating from distal A1 artery. **D,** Third A2 artery arising from Acomm complex.
- **Figure 21-4:** Incision for pterional craniotomy is curvilinear beginning within 1 cm anterior to the tragus at the level of the zygoma and traverses anteriorly. The incision ends approximately at the midline. Care should be taken to remain behind the patient's hairline if possible. An adequate exposure is obtained as well as an esthetic closure. Positioning has provided the vertical corridor needed for the approach.
- **Figure 21-5:** Generally, skin flap and temporalis muscle may be reflected together. By doing so, the frontalis branch of the facial nerve is protected from injury. There are occasions, however, in which an interfascial exposure is advantageous. Numerous burr hole configurations provide the exposure for the pterional craniotomy. Regardless of the number of burr holes used, it is important to extend the craniotomy 2 to 3 cm along the supraorbital rim to obtain the needed access to the floor of the anterior fossa.
- **Figure 21-6:** A key portion of the bony work is adequate removal of the sphenoid wing. This is accomplished with the use of a high-speed drill and dural protection (**A**). Sometimes access to the anterior portion of the planum sphenoidale is needed for larger aneurysms. For this, one may extend the craniotomy to include orbital osteotomies (**B**).
- **Figure 21-7:** The dural incision is made in a C-shaped fashion with the pedicle centered over the removed sphenoid wing. Dural tack-up sutures are used to help tamponade any epidural bleeding and to help provide adequate exposure (**A**). A key to the procedure is an extensive division of the sylvian fissure. This division is accomplished from lateral to medial using sharp and blunt dissection. The goal is to release the temporal lobe so that it may be retracted freely without placing stress on the Acomm complex (**B**).
- **Figure 21-8:** The rationale behind a significant portion of the procedure is to minimize brain retraction. An effective technique is resection of a portion of the gyrus rectus. This resection is accomplished through a corticectomy medial to the olfactory nerve, approximately 1 to 2 cm in length. By using blunt suction and electrocautery, the gyrus is resected in a subpial fashion. The aneurysm is protected from inadvertent injury by remaining subpial.
- **Figure 21-9:** After the gyrus rectus has been removed, a slow and deliberate dissection of the Acomm complex can be undertaken. Great care should be taken to prevent retraction on the aneurysm dome, particularly in previously ruptured aneurysms. The goal for dissection is to expose the neck of the aneurysm and the six major vessels of the complex (bilateral A1 arteries, A2 arteries, and recurrent arteries of Heubner).
- **Figure 21-10:** Although not an absolute, it is often beneficial to clip the A1 arteries temporarily (occasionally the A2 arteries as well) before placing the permanent clip on

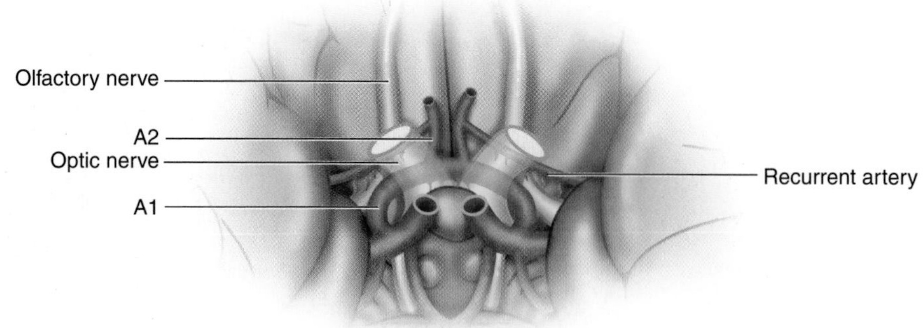
Olfactory nerve
A2
Optic nerve
A1
Recurrent artery

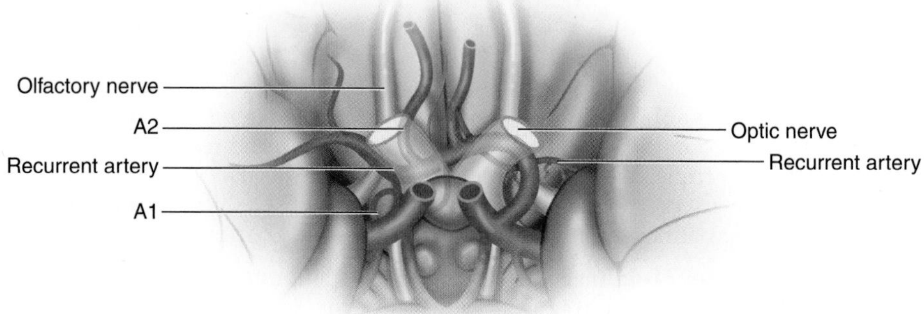
Olfactory nerve
A2
Recurrent artery
A1
Optic nerve
Recurrent artery

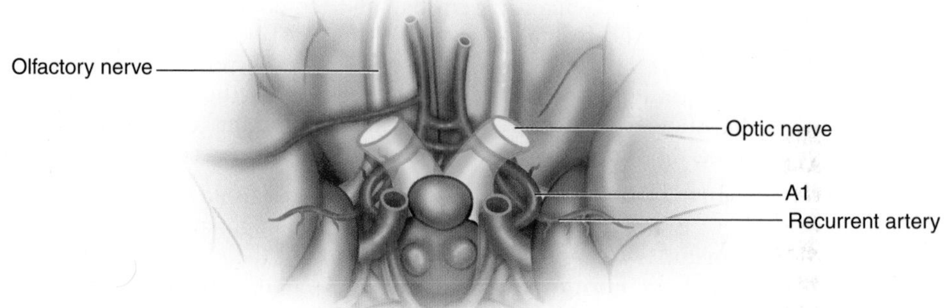
Olfactory nerve
Optic nerve
A1
Recurrent artery

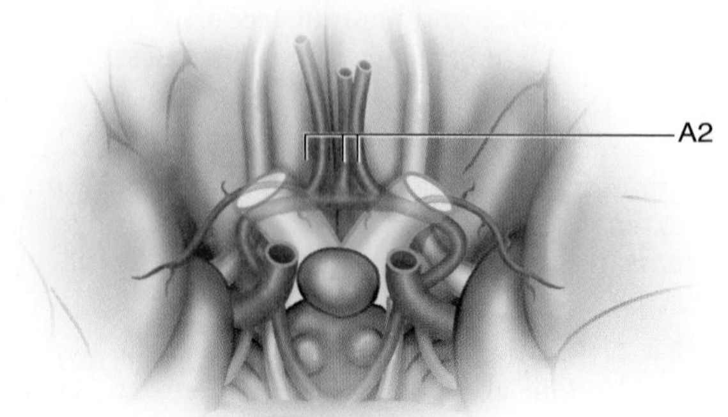
A2

FIGURE 21-3

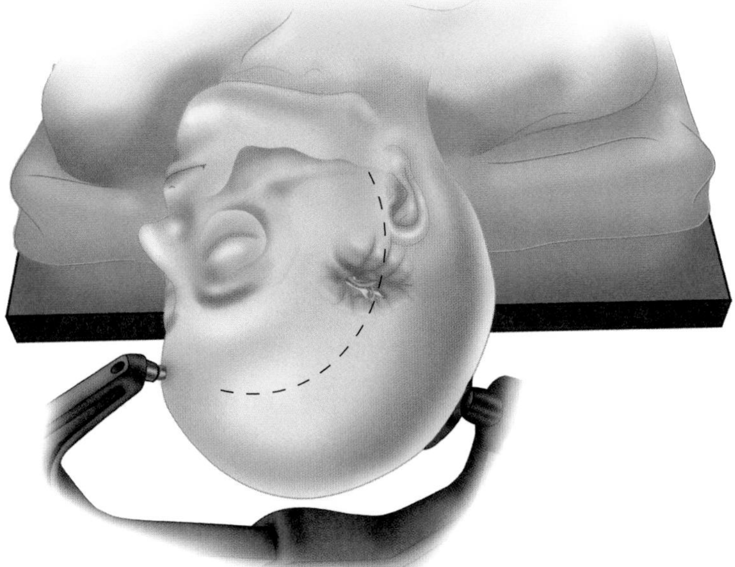

FIGURE 21-4

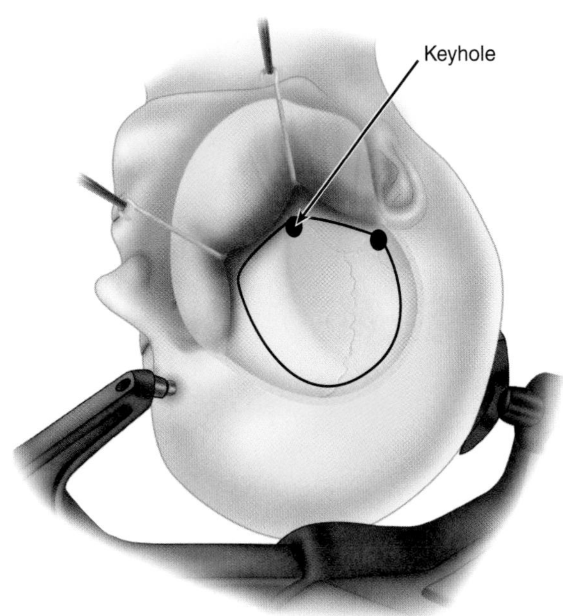

FIGURE 21-5

the aneurysm. This temporary clipping helps to decompress the aneurysm before permanent clipping and provides some protection against intraoperative rupture. Precautions should be taken not to occlude the recurrent arteries of Heubner.

- **Figure 21-11:** Clipping Acomm aneurysms is not always straightforward and often requires unique clip applications (**A**). After the permanent clip has been applied, it is essential that the surgeon determine that the surrounding vessels are still patent. Vessel patency can be

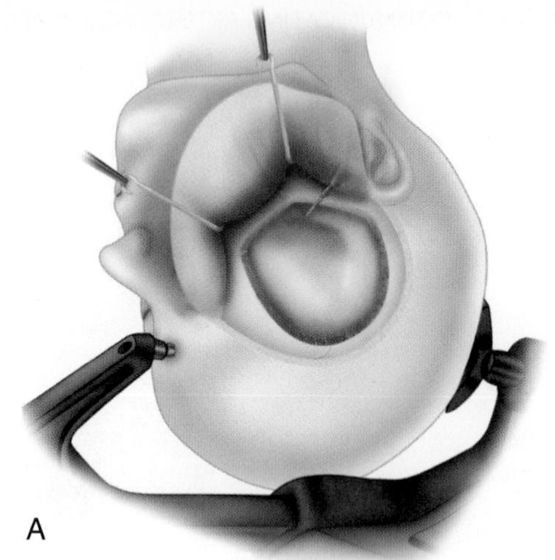

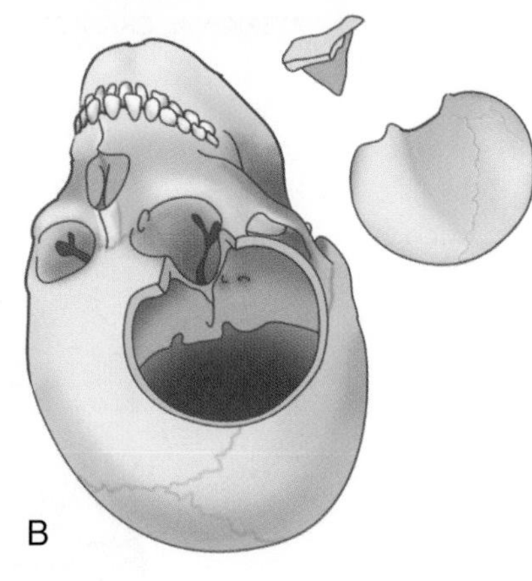

FIGURE 21-6

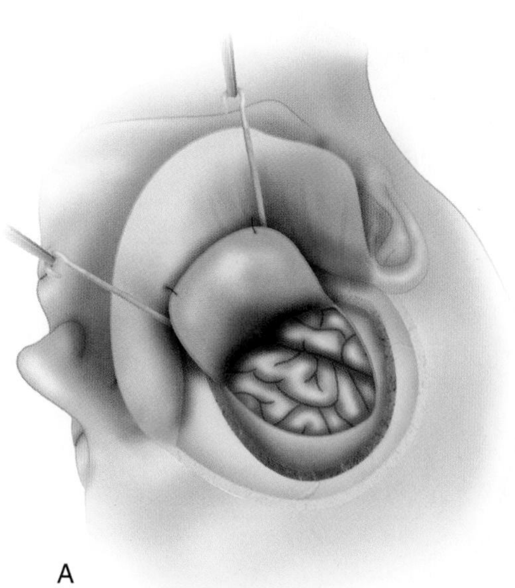

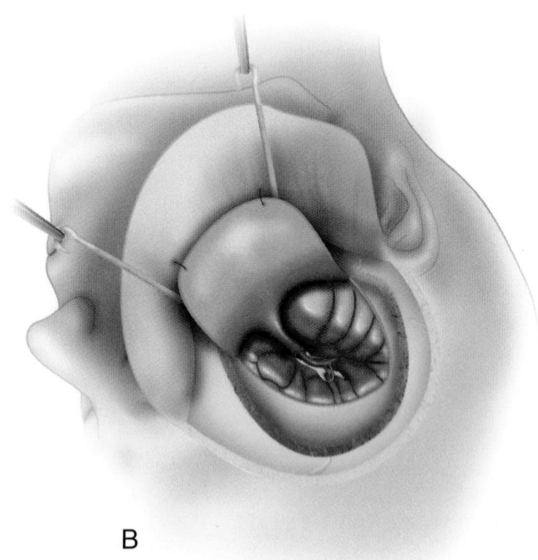

FIGURE 21-7

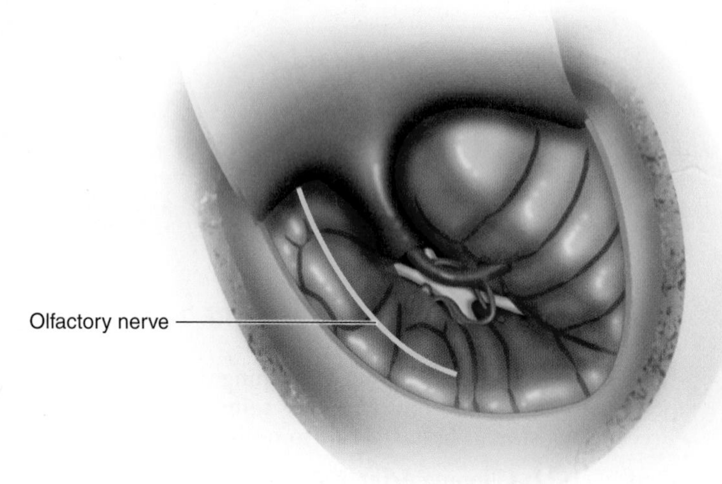

FIGURE 21-8

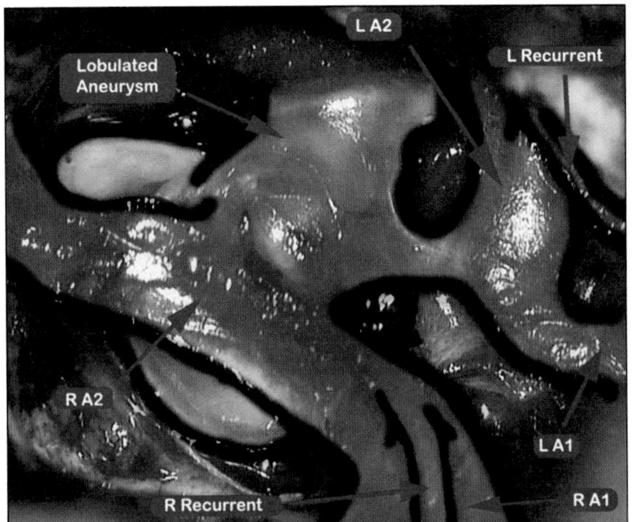

FIGURE 21-9

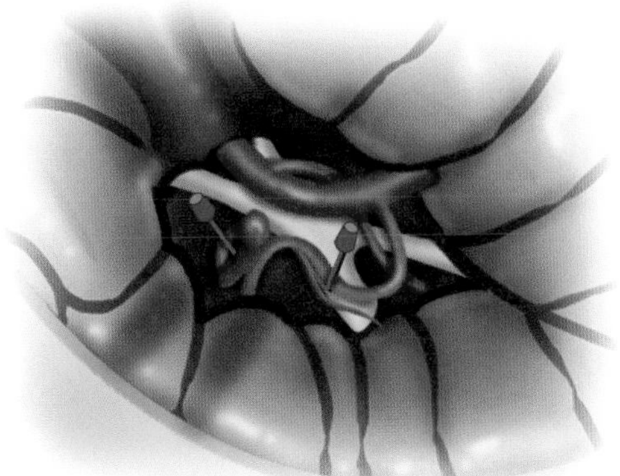

FIGURE 21-10

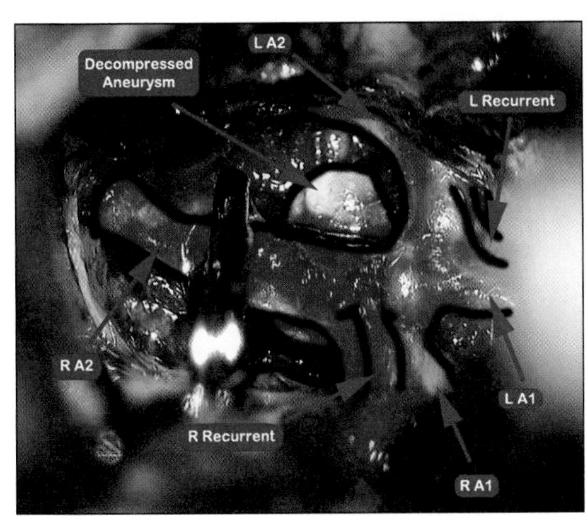

A

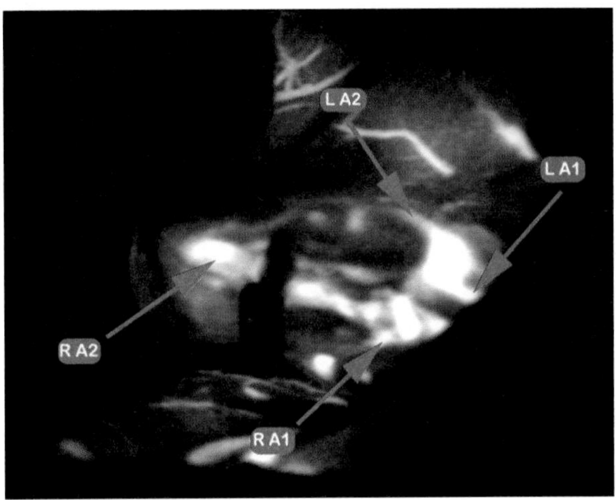

B

FIGURE 21-11

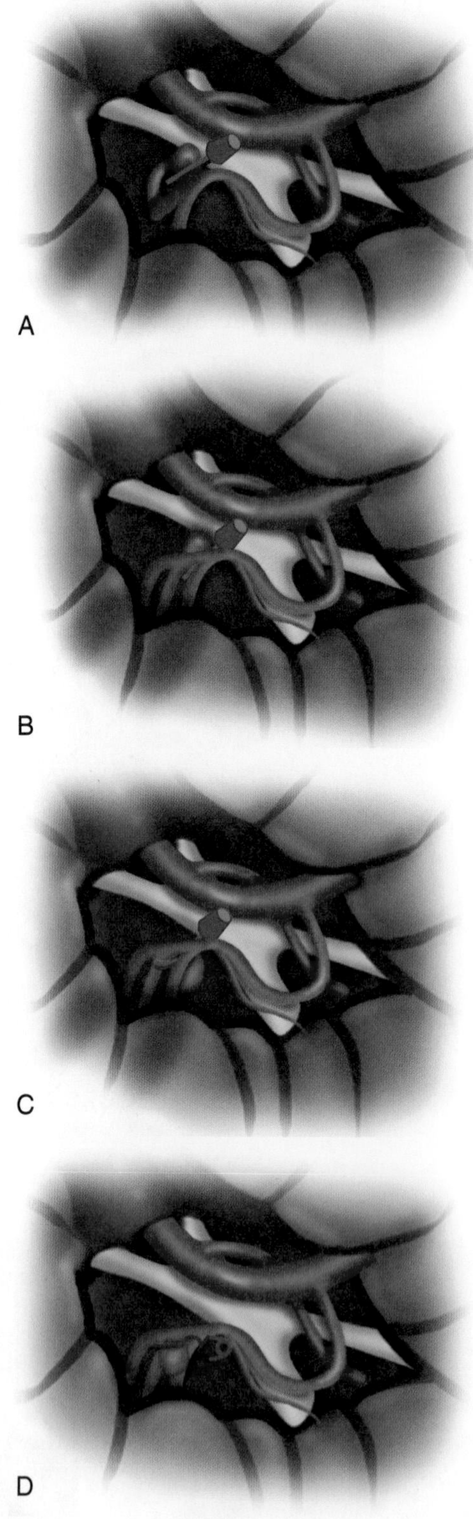

FIGURE 21-12

assessed with intraoperative indocyanine green (ICG) (**B**), intraoperative Doppler ultrasound, and intraoperative cerebral angiography (our preference).

- **Figure 21-12:** Aneurysms of the Acomm complex exhibit a wide range of variability. They may be categorized generally into anterior with a straight clip (**A**), inferior with a straight clip (**B**), posterior using a curved clip (**C**), and superiorly projecting with a fenestrated clip applied (**D**).

TIPS FROM THE MASTERS

- Unless contraindicated, approach the aneurysm from the patient's nondominant side.
- Use cerebrospinal fluid drainage, mannitol, and proper positioning to provide adequate brain relaxation.
- Wide opening of the sylvian fissure and arachnoid cisterns is essential in minimizing retraction.
- Use temporary clipping to assist during aneurysm dissection.
- Use a combination of tools (intraoperative Doppler, ICG, intraoperative angiography) to ensure patency of vessels.

PITFALLS

Overuse of a self-retaining retractor system is to be avoided. (At this institution, if possible, no retractor system is used.)

Early retraction of the frontal lobe with an inferior projecting aneurysm can lead to intraoperative rupture.

Sometimes there is an inability to define anatomy fully. It can be particularly difficult to find the proximal, contralateral A2 artery. It is essential that all of the arterial vessels be defined before clip application.

BAILOUT OPTIONS

- If adequate relaxation has not been obtained, opening the lamina terminalis may provide further cerebrospinal fluid release.
- The proximal, contralateral A2 may be found:
  - By dissecting toward the Acomm complex along the medial edge of the ipsilateral A2
  - By searching distally within the interhemispheric fissure
- Early temporary clipping of a hypoplastic, contralateral A1 artery can provide relaxation of the aneurysm and protection during dissection.

SUGGESTED READINGS

Hernesniemi J, Dashti R, Lehecka M, et al. Microneurosurgical management of anterior communicating artery aneurysms. Surg Neurol 2008;70:8–28.

Mira J, Costa F, Horta B, et al. Risk of rupture in unruptured anterior communicating artery aneurysms: meta-analysis of natural history studies. Surg Neurol 2006;66(S3):12–9.

Molyneux A, Kerr A, Stratton I, et al. International Subarachnoid Aneurysm Trial (ISAT) of neurosurgical clipping versus endovascular coiling in 2143 patients with ruptured intracranial aneurysms: a randomized trial. Lancet 2002;360:1267–74.

Rhoton AJ, Perlmutter D. Microsurgical anatomy of anterior communicating artery aneurysms. Neurol Res 1980;2:217–51.

Unruptured intracranial aneurysms—risk of rupture and risks of surgical intervention. International Study of Unruptured Intracranial Aneurysms Investigators. N Engl J Med 1998;339:1725–33.

Yasargil M. Microneurosurgery I. New York: Thieme Stratton; 1994.

Procedure 22

Pterional Craniotomy for Posterior Communicating Artery Aneurysm Clipping

Paul Gigante, Christopher P. Kellner, E. Sander Connolly, Jr.

INDICATIONS

Absolute

- Subarachnoid hemorrhage with intraparenchymal hemorrhage requiring emergent evacuation
- Subarachnoid hemorrhage with posterior communicating artery (Pcomm) aneurysm not repairable by endovascular coiling

Strong

- Large aneurysm (≥10 mm)
- Unruptured aneurysm (≥7 mm) in a patient 50 years old or younger
- Aneurysm with intraluminal thrombus
- Anterior projecting aneurysm
- Hunt and Hess grade I, II, or III in a patient 50 years old or younger
- Neurologic symptoms, classically manifesting as ophthalmoplegia owing to direct compression of the oculomotor nerve from the aneurysm

CONTRAINDICATIONS

Strong

- Aneurysm with significant calcification or atheroma

Relative

- Hunt and Hess grade IV or V with aneurysm repairable by endovascular coiling
- Subarachnoid hemorrhage with aneurysm repairable by coiling in a patient older than 60 years
- Unruptured aneurysm less than 7 mm in a patient older than 70 years

PLANNING AND POSITIONING

- The approach is chosen based on the location of the aneurysm.
- Placement of an external ventricular drain or lumbar drain during the preoperative period for cerebrospinal fluid drainage is frequently advantageous.
- A radiolucent head holder should be used in case intraoperative angiography is performed.
- Proper head positioning helps to minimize brain retraction.
- Antibiotic prophylaxis should be administered before skin incision.
- Mannitol given at the time of skin incision also helps with brain relaxation.

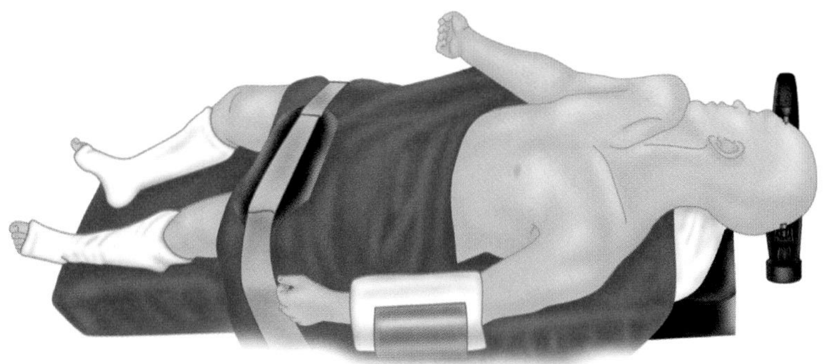

FIGURE 22-1

- **Figure 22-1:** The patient's head is placed in a three-pin radiolucent head holder with the head rotated 30 to 60 degrees contralateral to the craniotomy site. The degree of rotation depends on the patient's anatomy.

PROCEDURE

- **Figure 22-2:** The dissection is continued deeper in the direction of the optic chiasm. The right optic nerve and carotid artery are seen.
- **Figure 22-3:** With gentle retraction, the arachnoid is dissected, and cerebrospinal fluid is drained. The internal carotid artery (ICA) is carefully followed and dissected to visualize the posterior communicating artery (Pcomm) and aneurysm.
- **Figure 22-4:** A temporary aneurysm clip is applied to the ICA proximal to the Pcomm branch to acquire proximal control during exploration of the Pcomm aneurysm.
- **Figure 22-5:** With proximal control of the ICA, aneurysm clips are applied to the base of the aneurysm and readjusted while examining the aneurysm and its parent artery for perforators that may have been inadvertently occluded.
- **Figure 22-6:** Proximal ICA aneurysm clip is removed, and the aneurysm is examined for refilling and bleeding. Without proximal control, the aneurysm clips are not readjusted.

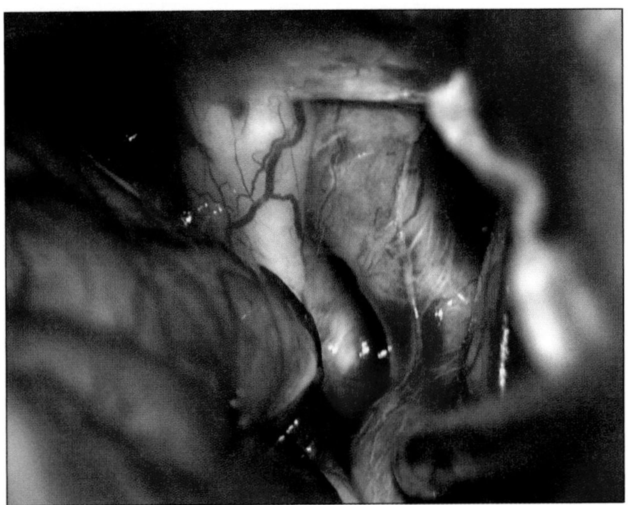

FIGURE 22-2

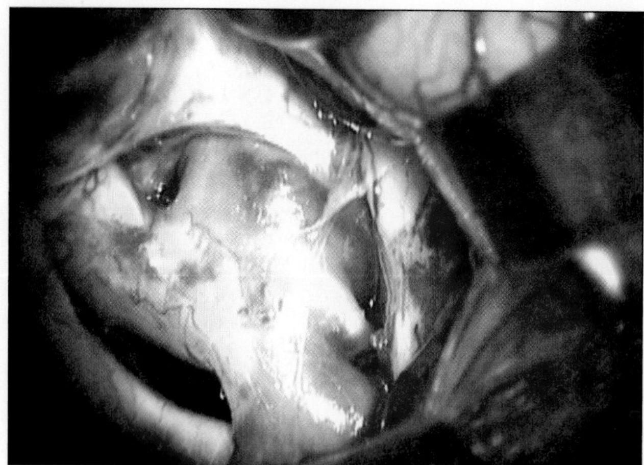

FIGURE 22-3

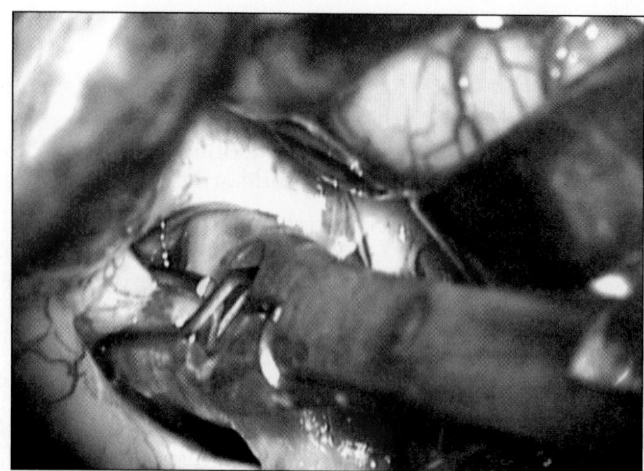

FIGURE 22-4

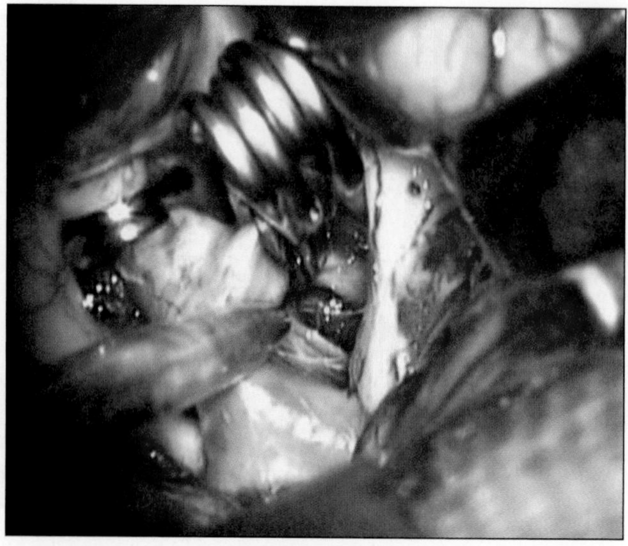

FIGURE 22-5

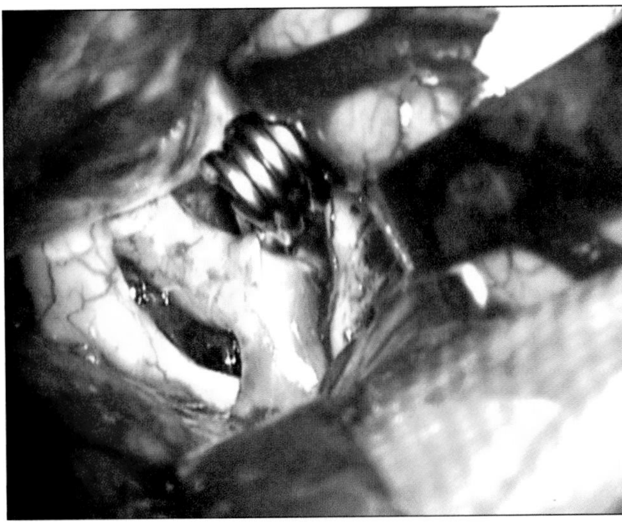

FIGURE 22-6

TIPS FROM THE MASTERS

- The aneurysm projection should be carefully analyzed on preoperative imaging. A lateral projection requires caution when retracting the temporal lobe to avoid unroofing of the aneurysm, whereas a posterior or medial projection would make the Pcomm origin more difficult to visualize.
- An excessively large neck of the aneurysm in the axis perpendicular to the long axis of the ICA that incorporates the Pcomm or posterior cerebral artery origin may require the use of a fenestrated clip.

PITFALLS

Check preoperative imaging for the presence of a fetal posterior cerebral artery, which would require increased care to preserve the Pcomm origin.

Be prepared for a very proximal Pcomm aneurysm, which requires clinoid process resection for proximal control.

BAILOUT OPTIONS

- In the case of premature rupture, temporary clipping of the ICA distal to the aneurysm and the Pcomm itself markedly improves visualization over proximal ICA occlusion alone.
- Before securing the proximal ICA in the case of premature rupture, compression of the ipsilateral neck may also facilitate control.

SUGGESTED READINGS

Bederson JB, Awad IA, Wiebers DO, et al. Recommendations for the management of patients with unruptured intracranial aneurysms: a statement for healthcare professionals from the Stroke Council of the American Heart Association. Stroke 2000;31:2742–50.

Lee KC, Lee KS, Shin YS, et al. Surgery for posterior communicating artery aneurysms. Surg Neurol 2003;59:107–13.

Unruptured intracranial aneurysms—risk of rupture and risks of surgical intervention. International Study of Unruptured Intracranial Aneurysms Investigators. N Engl J Med 1998;339:1725–33.

Wiebers DO. Unruptured intracranial aneurysms: natural history and clinical management. Update on the International Study of Unruptured Intracranial Aneurysms. Neuroimaging Clin N Am 2006;16:383–90.

Yasargil MG, Fox JL. The microsurgical approach to intracranial aneurysms. Surg Neurol 1975;3:7–14.

Procedure 23

Paraclinoid Carotid Artery Aneurysms

Anil Nanda, Vijayakumar Javalkar

INDICATIONS

Ruptured Aneurysm

- All ruptured paraclinoid aneurysms with subarachnoid hemorrhage as the presentation need to be treated. Multiple and bilateral aneurysms are more common among this group of aneurysms. In case of multiple aneurysms with subarachnoid hemorrhage, if the paraclinoid aneurysm is present ipsilateral to the ruptured aneurysm, occasionally it can be clipped at the same sitting.

Symptomatic Unruptured Aneurysm

- Generally, large or giant aneurysms are symptomatic from mass effect. Because of close proximity to anterior optic pathways, these aneurysms may cause visual disturbances as presenting symptoms. These cases need to be treated to prevent further visual loss or for improvement of vision.

Asymptomatic Unruptured Aneurysm

- The yearly risk of subarachnoid hemorrhage from an unruptured intracranial aneurysm is estimated to be around 1% for lesions 7 to 10 mm in diameter.
- For small incidental aneurysms less than 5 mm, conservative management is recommended.
- Patients younger than 60 years old with aneurysms larger than 5 mm should be offered treatment unless there is a significant contraindication.
- Large, incidental aneurysms greater than 10 mm should be treated in all healthy patients younger than 70 years.

CONTRAINDICATIONS

- Aneurysms that are large or giant, have calcified walls, are complex, or have ill-defined necks are difficult to clip and may require carotid occlusion and a bypass as a definitive treatment.
- Other relative contraindications for definitive surgical clipping are patient factors such as advanced age and serious comorbidities.

PLANNING AND POSITIONING

Preoperative Radiologic Evaluation

- Preoperative radiologic evaluation includes cerebral angiography to assess the size and shape of the aneurysm.
- In the case of thrombosed aneurysms, magnetic resonance imaging (MRI) is indicated to assess the true size of the aneurysm.
- MRI not only shows the relationship of the aneurysm with adjacent structures, but also shows calcification of the wall of the aneurysm.
- MRI source images may be useful in studying not only the neck and dome, but also the surrounding structures.

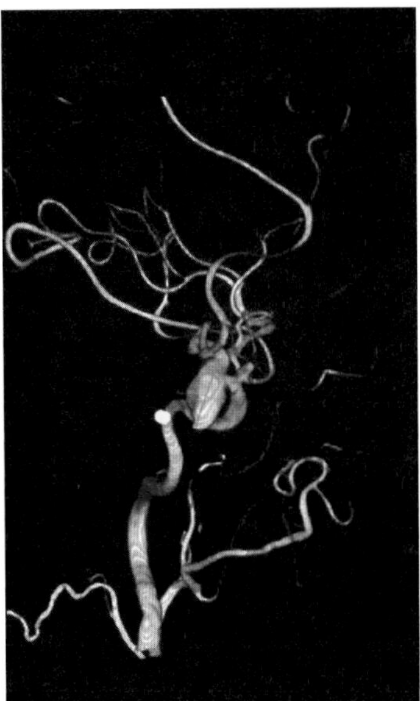

FIGURE 23-1

- Preoperative computed tomography (CT) angiography with three-dimensional reconstruction of the cranial base shows the relationship of the aneurysm to the bony anatomy. This information might help in cranial base drilling.
- **Figure 23-1:** Three-dimensional reconstruction of the aneurysm in complex cases is useful to study the morphology of the aneurysm.
- Thin CT sections through the region of the clinoid process may show calcification in the aneurysm wall and any erosion of the clinoid process.
- CT scans with 0.5-mm thickness with reconstructions through the clinoid process area are helpful in assessing the pneumatization of the anterior clinoid process (ACP). Preoperative evaluation for pneumatization of the ACP may help to avoid cerebrospinal fluid rhinorrhea.

Balloon Test Occlusion

- Aneurysms that are difficult to clip may require carotid occlusion as a bailout option or treatment alternative. In such cases, balloon test occlusion (BTO) is needed to assess the collateral circulation.
- Complete angiography with and without compression of the involved carotid artery to assess the collateral circulation is required when BTO is planned.
- Monitoring of cerebral perfusion with single photon emission computed tomography (SPECT) or xenon CT is also advised. If the patient tolerates the test clinically and without any perfusion defects on SPECT, permanent occlusion of the internal carotid artery (ICA) and trapping of the aneurysm can be performed safely. Patients who do not tolerate BTO either clinically or radiologically may require a bypass graft.
- According to the protocol developed by Sekhar et al, patients who tolerate BTO with cerebral blood flow greater than 35 mL/100 g/min need no revascularization. Patients who tolerate BTO with cerebral blood flow 15 to 35 mL/100 g/min have a moderate risk and typically require revascularization. Patients who develop neurologic deficits during BTO are at high risk and may require a revascularization.

Positioning

- **Figure 23-2:** The patient is positioned supine with the head turned by 30 to 35 degrees to the contralateral side fixed on a radiolucent Mayfield head holder, which facilitates intraoperative angiography. The vertex is tilted toward the floor until the zygoma is at the highest point.

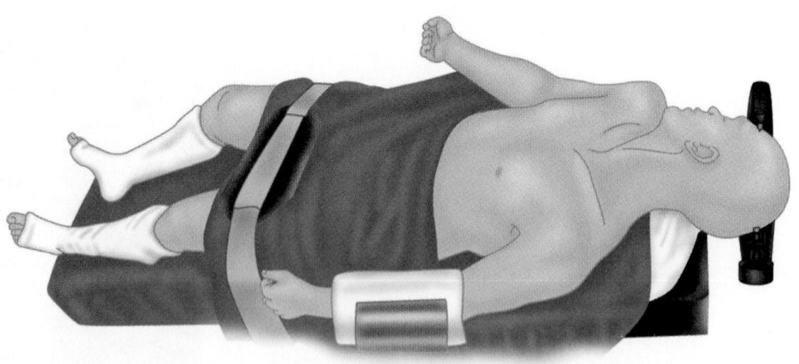

FIGURE 23-2

PROCEDURE

Proximal Control

- Traditionally, proximal control is achieved by exposing and clamping the carotid artery in the neck, before craniotomy. The aneurysm may be trapped by a temporary clip on the ICA proximal to the posterior communicating artery.
- Dolenc has advocated proximal control of the subclinoid ICA by a combined epidural and subdural approach.
- **Figure 23-3:** Batjer and Sampson in 1990 described retrograde suction decompression of giant paraclinoid aneurysms. A vascular clamp is placed across the cervical ICA, and a temporary clip is placed across the supraclinoid ICA immediately proximal to the posterior communicating artery. After temporary trapping, a No. 18 angiocatheter is inserted into the cervical ICA. An extension set and stopcock are connected, and a 7F surgical suction tube is inserted into the stopcock port. Through controlled digital manipulation of the suction, the collateral flow into the trapped arterial segment via the ophthalmic artery and cavernous branches can be removed.
- **Figure 23-4:** Endovascular retrograde suction decompression is achieved by placing a double lumen balloon catheter in the ICA by the transfemoral route. After balloon inflation and placement of a temporary clip distal to the aneurysm, the trapped segment and the aneurysm can be deflated.
- In large and more proximal aneurysms, we routinely establish proximal control by exposing the ICA in the neck before craniotomy.
- We have occasionally used retrograde suction decompression in selected cases.

Skin Incision and Craniotomy

- **Figure 23-5:** Curvilinear skin incision is made just behind the hairline starting 1 cm in front of the tragus. Branches of the superficial temporal artery are preserved. The skin flap is reflected anteriorly along with pericranium. The frontalis branch of the facial nerve is preserved by careful subfascial dissection of the temporalis muscle.

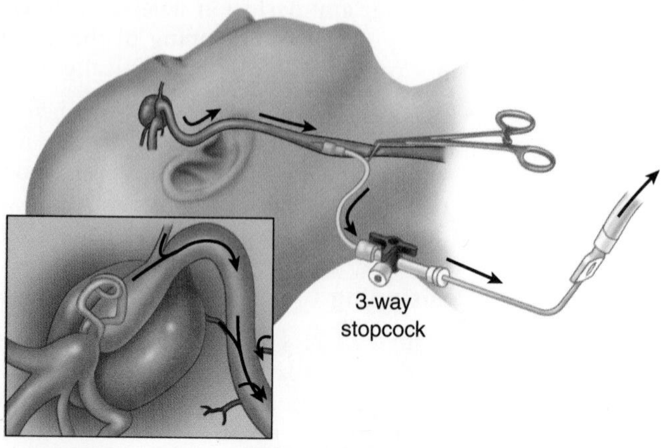

FIGURE 23-3

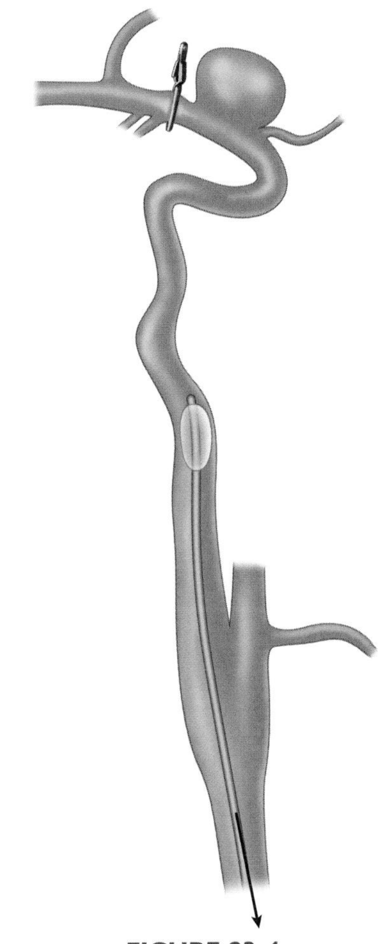

FIGURE 23-4

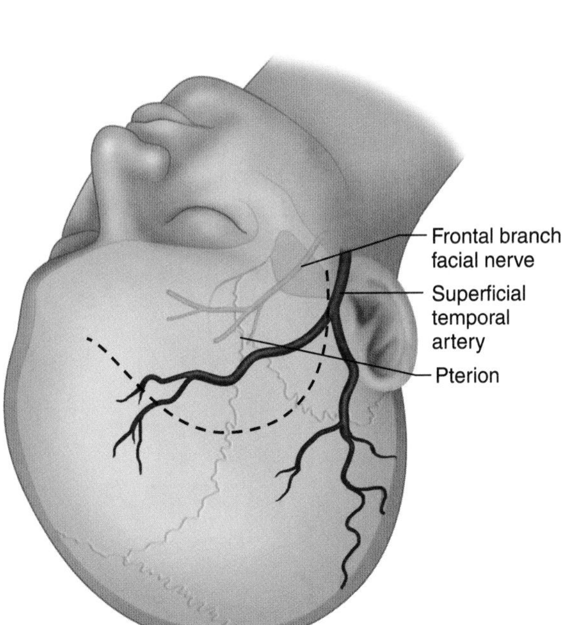

FIGURE 23-5

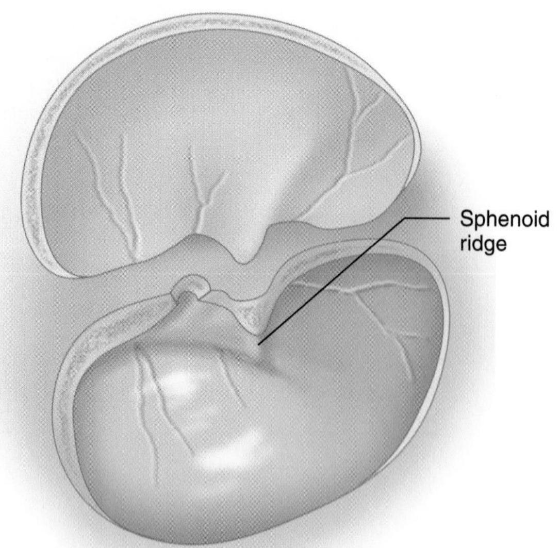

FIGURE 23-6

- There is no uniform agreement among neurosurgeons regarding approaches and surgical techniques. Some neurosurgeons advocate routine use of orbital osteotomy, and others believe that routine orbitozygomatic osteotomy is unnecessary in these cases. We believe that standard pterional craniotomy with flattening of the sphenoid ridge would be sufficient to tackle most of these aneurysms. In our series of 86 ophthalmic segment ICA aneurysms, standard pterional craniotomy was used in 66% of the operations.
- **Figure 23-6:** Ipsilateral standard pterional craniotomy with flattening of the sphenoid ridge is performed. In most cases, we have used pterional craniotomy without skull base modification.
- **Figure 23-7:** In selected cases, orbitozygomatic osteotomy is added. We generally use skull base modification in giant or large aneurysms. In our series of 86 ophthalmic segment ICA aneurysms, we used the frontotemporal orbitozygomatic approach in only 34% of our cases.

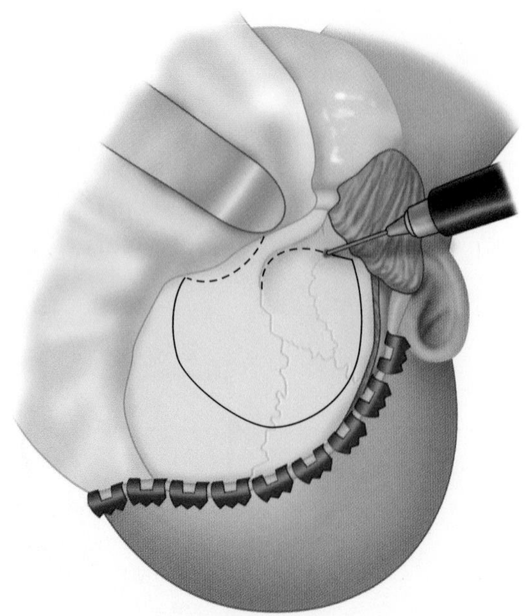

FIGURE 23-7

- There is no consensus on whether to perform clinoidectomy extradurally or intradurally. Advocates of extradural removal of the ACP maintain that the dura protects the aneurysm while drilling. Some neurosurgeons would argue that the dura does not remain a safe barrier with current high-speed drills, and this maneuver may invite untoward consequences, especially if the ACP is eroded by the aneurysm.
- We routinely use an intradural clinoidectomy in most cases when ACP excision is needed. Extradural clinoidectomy is performed occasionally in some patients.

Extradural Anterior Clinoidectomy

- **Figure 23-8:** The important key step in extradural anterior clinoidectomy is incision of the orbitotemporal periosteal fold (**A**), which facilitates exposure of the ACP (**B**).
- After craniotomy, the dura covering the middle and anterior cranial fossa is carefully elevated from the underlying bone. The sphenoid ridge is drilled out. After the superolateral bony edge of the superior orbital fissure is opened, the orbitotemporal periosteal fold is visualized. Some advocate incising the orbitofrontal dural fold at the level of the sphenoid ridge to avoid cranial nerve injury coursing through the superior orbital fissure.

Intradural Microdissection

- After the dural opening, the sylvian fissure is opened, and the aneurysm is inspected. The origin and projection of the aneurysm and its relationship to the optic nerve are carefully studied.
- **Figure 23-9:** Exposure of the sylvian fissure in this case showed the ICA, optic nerve, and ophthalmic segment ICA aneurysm. There is also a small supraclinoid ICA aneurysm.
- The need for further steps such as sectioning of the falciform ligament, optic nerve mobilization, ACP resection (if not already performed extradurally), and unroofing of the optic nerve canal depends on the visibility of the neck of the aneurysm and origin and projection of the aneurysm.

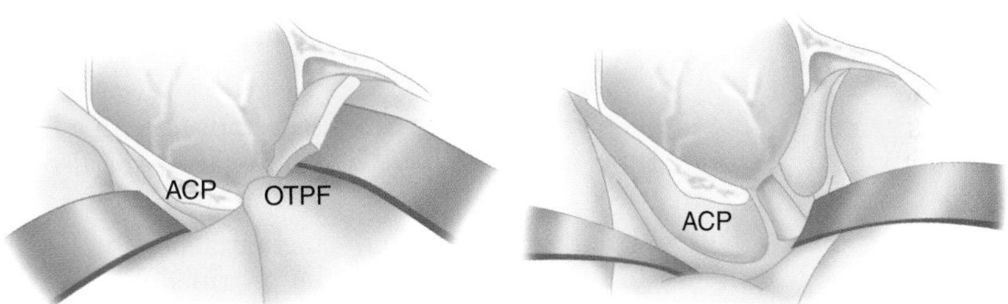

FIGURE 23-8

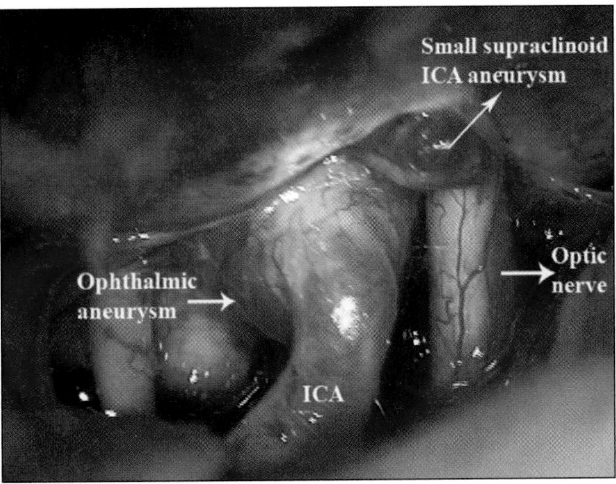

FIGURE 23-9

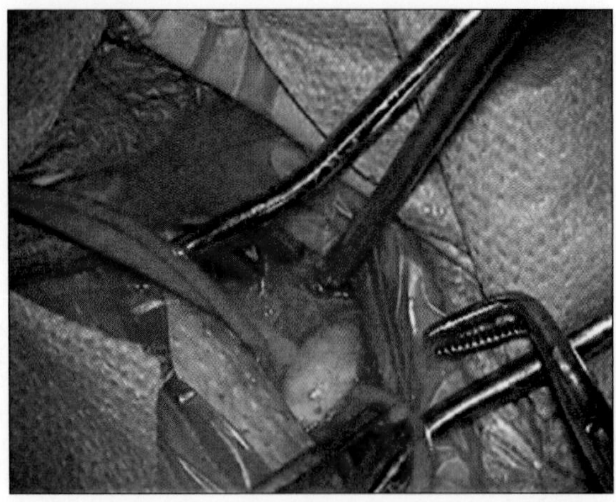
A

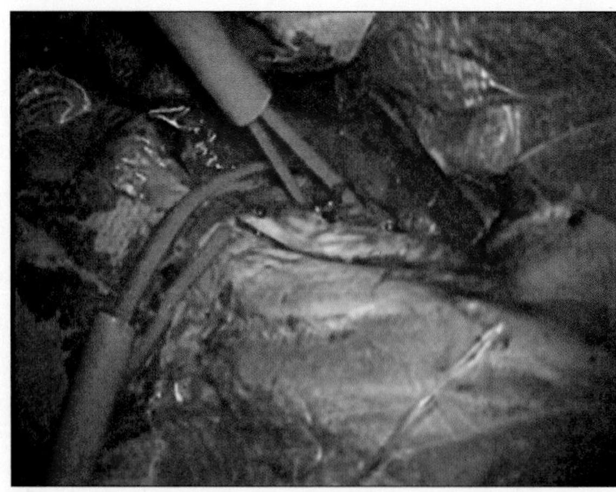
B

FIGURE 23-10

At this stage, proximal control as described in the previous section is needed for further dissection of the aneurysm.

- **Figure 23-10:** For large and more proximal aneurysms, we routinely expose the cervical ICA in the neck and pass loops around the common carotid artery and ICA for proximal control.
- We have occasionally used retrograde suction decompression technique to achieve proximal control.
- **Figure 23-11:** The falciform ligament is carefully incised. This step facilitates mobilization of the optic nerve. Sectioning of the falciform ligament usually yields exposure of the origin of the ophthalmic artery and proximal ICA. Extreme care needs to be taken to protect the pial vasculature of the optic nerve.
- **Figure 23-12:** For intradural drilling of the ACP, a small dural flap is created around the ACP. Gentle palpation of the clinoid process is done using a microinstrument to look for any bony erosion.
- **Figure 23-13:** The ACP is removed with a high-speed drill with a diamond bur (**A**) and fine rongeurs (**B**). The optic canal can also be unroofed. Initially, the central core is drilled out, and the peripheral shell can be removed with fine rongeurs.
- The distal dural ring, which attaches the ICA radially to the adjacent structures, needs to be incised to define the proximal neck of the aneurysm.
- **Figure 23-14:** Giant aneurysms may require multiple clips placed in tandem or in sequence.

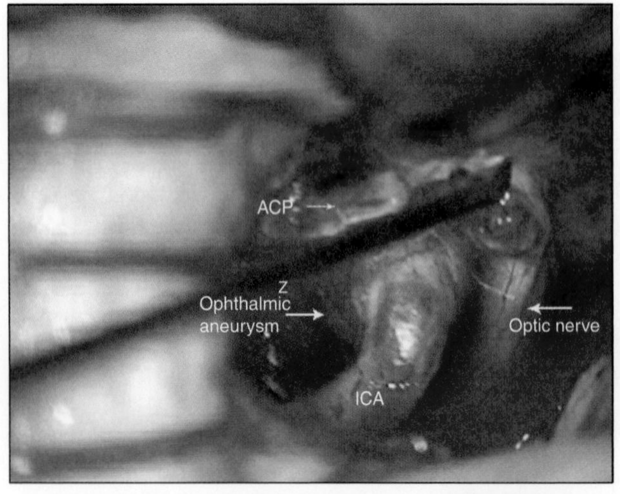

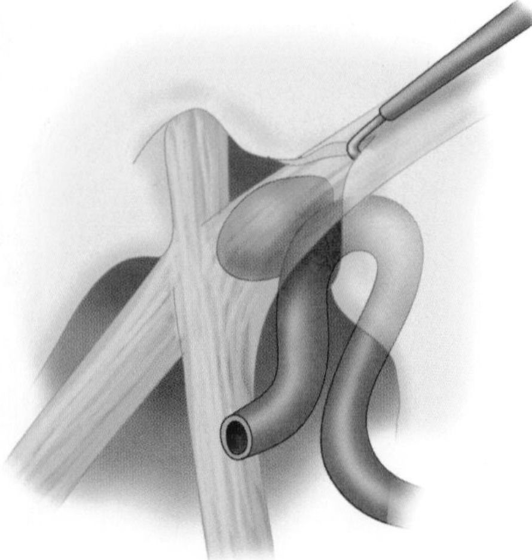

FIGURE 23-11

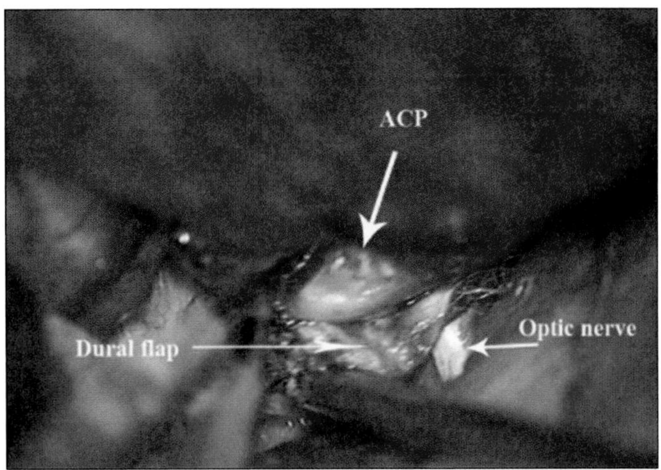

FIGURE 23-12

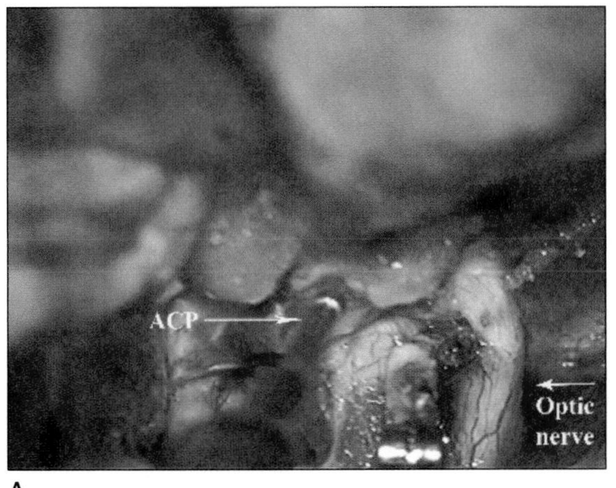

A

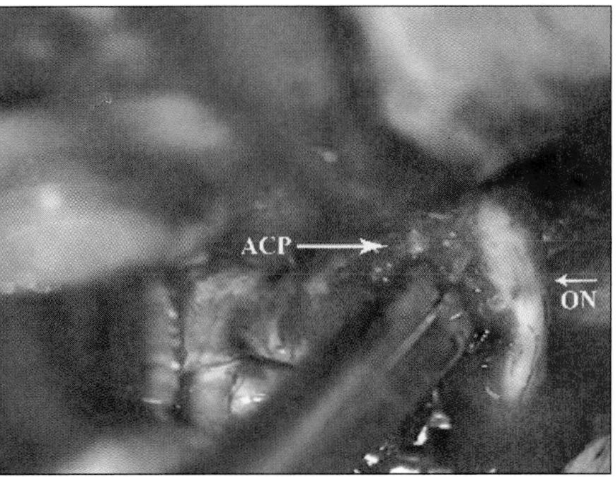

B

FIGURE 23-13

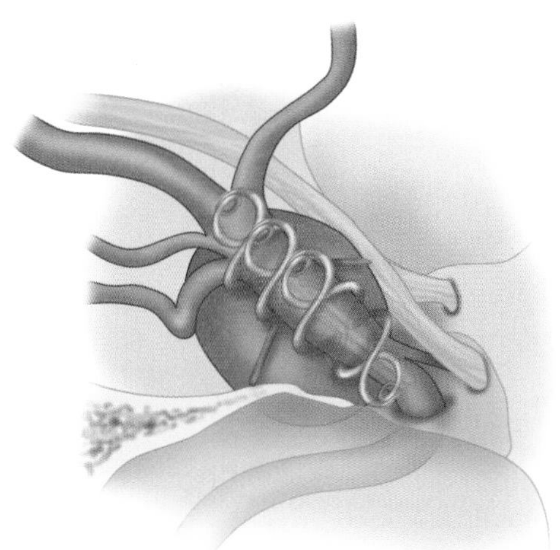

FIGURE 23-14

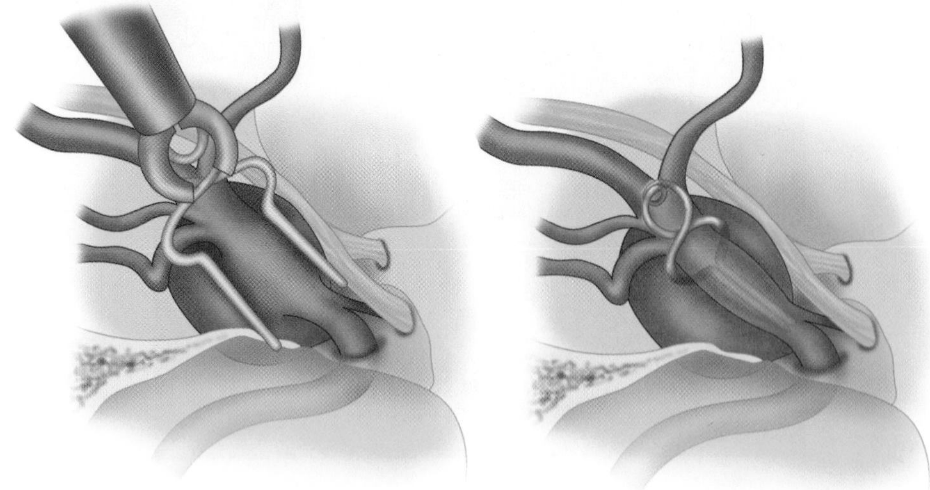

FIGURE 23-15

- **Figure 23-15:** Ventrally placed large or giant aneurysms may require a fenestrated clip. The fenestrated clip is applied parallel to the ICA.
- In addition, intraoperative microvascular Doppler ultrasonography can be performed during aneurysm clipping.
- Any defect in the ACP needs to be repaired especially in cases where sphenoid sinus extends into the ACP. The defect can be closed with fat graft reinforced with fibrin glue. This step is necessary to prevent cerebrospinal fluid rhinorrhea in cases in which anterior clinoidectomy is performed when the optic strut is pneumatized.

Intraoperative Angiogram and Indocyanine Green Angiogram

- **Figure 23-16:** For complex aneurysms, we routinely perform intraoperative angiography to look for obliteration of the aneurysm and parent vessel patency. In this case, there is total obliteration of the aneurysm with a patent ICA.
- **Figure 23-17:** We perform intraoperative indocyanine green angiography to look for obliteration of the aneurysm and to look for patency of the parent vessel. In this case, there is total obliteration of the aneurysm with patency of the ICA.

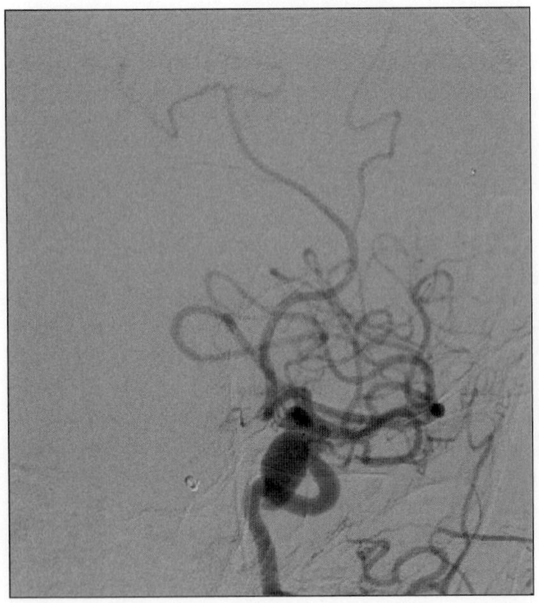

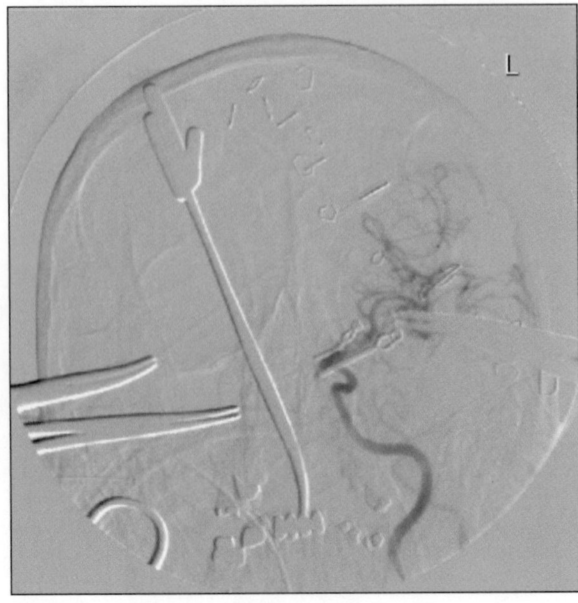

FIGURE 23-16

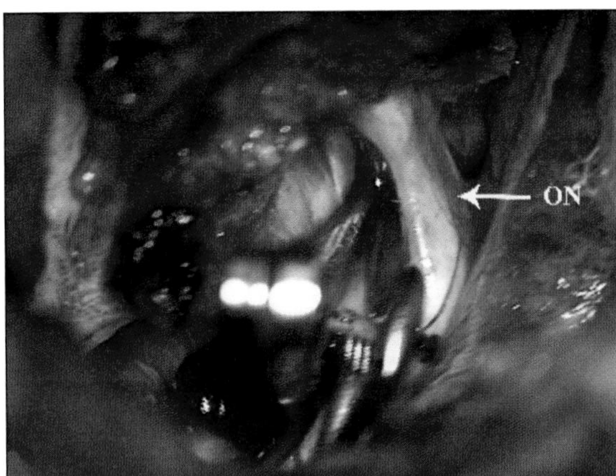

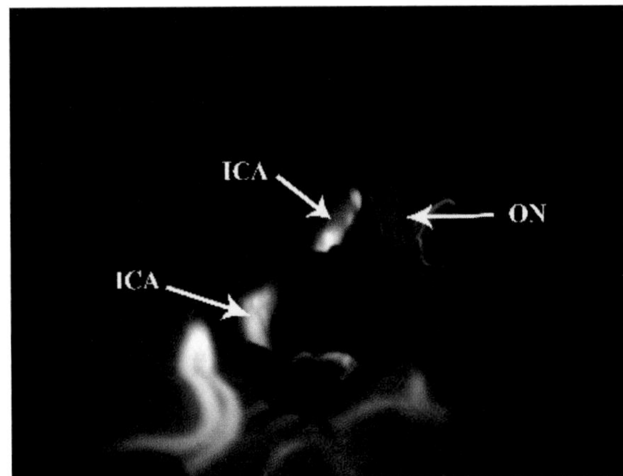

FIGURE 23-17

- If there is a compromise of the ICA after clip application, a bypass graft may need to be performed.

Contralateral Approach

- As many as 7% of ophthalmic aneurysms could be bilateral, and managing both lesions with a single approach should be considered whenever possible.
- The contralateral aneurysm preferably should be unruptured and reasonably small (<15 mm).
- Some authors do not advocate a contralateral approach in cases with prefixed chiasm or large or giant aneurysms. Other authors advocate drilling of planum sphenoidale in cases with prefixed chiasm.

TIPS FROM THE MASTERS

- Great caution needs to be exercised for aneurysms projecting anterosuperiorly. When trying to elevate the frontal lobe, such aneurysms may be densely adherent to the frontal lobe and may rupture.
- The falciform ligament needs to be sectioned before any aneurysm dissection is undertaken.
- The optic nerve should not be dissected circumferentially in all patients because it may result in devascularization of the nerve.
- Pial vessels of the optic nerve must not be disrupted while the dura is incised.
- Clinoid resection for the posterior carotid wall aneurysms is more lateral and posterior to the resection required for carotid-ophthalmic artery aneurysms.
- Superior hypophyseal artery aneurysms arising from the medial wall of the ICA and projecting inferomedially may not require bone removal and sectioning of the falciform ligament to yield an exposure to identify the origin of the ophthalmic artery and the proximal ICA.
- For aneurysms with broad necks, clip application should be parallel to the ICA. Clips placed perpendicular are ineffective in collapsing the aneurysm, and clip jaws occasionally open.

PITFALLS
Risk of optic nerve injury
Risk of third nerve injury
Risk of cerebrospinal fluid rhinorrhea from pneumatization of ACP
Risk of ischemic stroke

BAILOUT OPTIONS

- For complex aneurysms that cannot be clipped, one may have to consider carotid ligation or balloon occlusion as an alternative to clipping or coiling when combined with a revascularization procedure.
- If the aneurysm is heavily calcified, one may have to consider carotid ligation or balloon occlusion as an alternative to clipping or coiling when combined with a revascularization procedure.
- If there is a compromise of the ICA after clip application, it may be necessary to perform a bypass graft as a bailout maneuver if the clips cannot be adjusted.

SUGGESTED READINGS

Barami K, Hernandez VS, Diaz FG, et al. Paraclinoid carotid aneurysms: surgical management, complications, and outcome based on a new classification scheme. Skull Base 2003;13:31–41.

Batjer HH, Kopitnik TA, Giller CA, et al. Surgery for paraclinoidal carotid artery aneurysms. J Neurosurg 1994;80:650–8.

Batjer HH, Samson DS. Retrograde suction decompression of giant paraclinoidal aneurysms. Technical note. J Neurosurg 1990;73:305–6.

Beretta F, Andaluz N, Zuccarello M. Aneurysms of the ophthalmic (C6) segment of the internal carotid artery: treatment options and strategies based on a clinical series. J Neurosurg Sci 2004;48:149–56.

Day AL. Aneurysms of the ophthalmic segment: a clinical and anatomical analysis. J Neurosurg 1990;72:677–91.

De Jesus O, Sekhar LN, Riedel CJ. Clinoid and paraclinoid aneurysms: surgical anatomy, operative techniques, and outcome. Surg Neurol 1999;51:477–87.

Dolenc VV. A combined epi- and subdural direct approach to carotid-ophthalmic artery aneurysms. J Neurosurg 1985;62:667–72.

Froelich SC, Aziz KM, Levine NB, et al. Refinement of the extradural anterior clinoidectomy: surgical anatomy of the orbitotemporal periosteal fold. Neurosurgery 2007;61:179–85.

Giannotta SL. Ophthalmic segment aneurysm surgery. Neurosurgery 2002;50:558–62.

Heros RC, Nelson PB, Ojemann RG, et al. Large and giant paraclinoid aneurysms: surgical techniques, complications, and results. Neurosurgery 1983;12:153–63.

Hoh BL, Carter BS, Budzik RF, et al. Results after surgical and endovascular treatment of paraclinoid aneurysms by a combined neurovascular team. Neurosurgery 2001;48:78–89.

Kakizawa Y, Tanaka Y, Orz Y, et al. Parameters for contralateral approach to ophthalmic segment aneurysms of the internal carotid artery. Neurosurgery 2000;47:1130–6.

Komotar RJ, Mocco J, Solomon RA. Guidelines for the surgical treatment of unruptured intracranial aneurysms: the first annual J. Lawrence Pool Memorial Research Symposium—Controversies in the Management of Cerebral Aneurysms. Neurosurgery 2008;62:183–93.

Nagasawa S, Deguchi J, Arai M, et al. Topographic anatomy of paraclinoid carotid artery aneurysms: usefulness of MR angiographic source images. Neuroradiology 1997;39:341–3.

Nakao S, Kikuchi H, Takahashi N. Successful clipping of carotid-ophthalmic aneurysms through a contralateral pterional approach: report of two cases. J Neurosurg 1981;54:532–6.

Nanda A. Middle cerebral artery aneurysm. In: Rengachary S, editor. Neurosurgical Operative Color Atlas. Park Ridge, IL: AANS; 2000.

Parkinson RJ, Bendok BR, Getch CC, et al. Retrograde suction decompression of giant paraclinoid aneurysms using a No. 7 French balloon-containing guide catheter. Technical note. J Neurosurg 2006;105:479–81.

Sekhar LN, DeJesus O. Clinoid and paraclinoid aneurysms. In: Sekhar LN, DeOlivera E, editors. Cranial Microsurgery Approaches and Techniques. New York: Thieme; 1999, 151–75.

Sekhar LN, Sen CN, Jho HD. Saphenous vein graft bypass of the cavernous internal carotid artery. J Neurosurg 1990;72:35–41.

Procedure 24

Middle Cerebral Artery Aneurysms: Pterional (Frontotemporal) Craniotomy for Clipping

Mohamed Samy Elhammady, Roberto C. Heros

INDICATIONS

- We prefer surgical clipping of most ruptured and unruptured middle cerebral artery (MCA) aneurysms because of the accessibility of their location and the relatively low morbidity and durability of clipping compared with endovascular therapy. The exception is in patients in poor neurologic condition (Hunt and Hess grade III, IV, or V); for these patients, we generally prefer endovascular treatment if feasible.
- The decision to treat an unruptured MCA aneurysm is based on an understanding of the natural history and must be weighed against the risk of surgical intervention. Factors that must be considered include the patient's age, general health, clinical presentation (headaches, seizures), smoking history, family history of subarachnoid hemorrhage, and aneurysm size.

CONTRAINDICATIONS

- Relative contraindications include advanced age, the presence of serious medical comorbidities, and poor neurologic condition. If treatment is contemplated in patients with these relative contraindications, endovascular coiling may be a reasonable alternative.

PLANNING AND POSITIONING

- Preoperative evaluation includes assessment of the patient's cardiopulmonary status, laboratory values (complete blood count, basic metabolic profile, coagulation profile), chest x-ray, and electrocardiogram. The aneurysm configuration and associated vascular anatomy are defined by digital subtraction angiography with or without three-dimensional reconstruction, computed tomography angiography, or magnetic resonance angiography.
- The patient is given a dose of preoperative antibiotics before skin incision. Brain relaxation is achieved with intravenous mannitol and mild hyperventilation.
- **Figure 24-1:** The patient is positioned supine with the head elevated above the level of the heart. The head is placed in a three-pin fixation device and turned 30 degrees contralateral to the side of surgery with slight extension so that the malar eminence is highest in the surgical field. The scalp is shaved and sterilized in a standard fashion.
- **Figure 24-2:** The planned skin incision is marked starting at the level of the zygomatic arch just anterior to the tragus, to avoid injury to the frontalis branch of the facial nerve, and extended anterosuperiorly behind the hairline as a gentle curve to the midline.
- **Figure 24-3:** The skin is covered with self-adhesive transparent plastic. The incision line is infiltrated with a mixture of local anesthetic and epinephrine.

PROCEDURE

- **Figure 24-4:** The skin incision is made layer by layer starting anteriorly where the scalp overlies the bone. An attempt is made to identify and preserve the frontal branch of the superficial temporal artery, which may be used for a bypass graft if needed. Raney

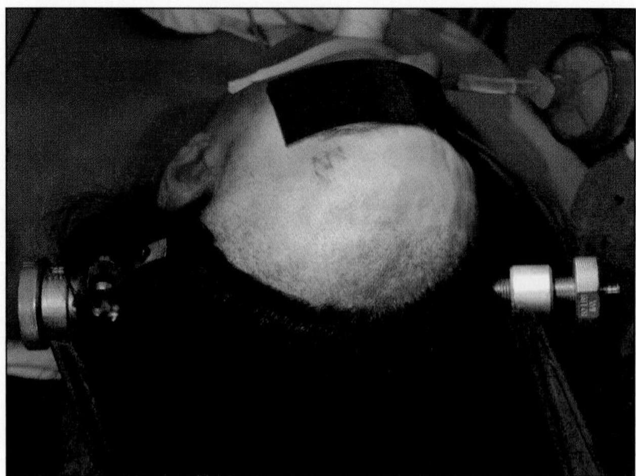

FIGURE 24-1

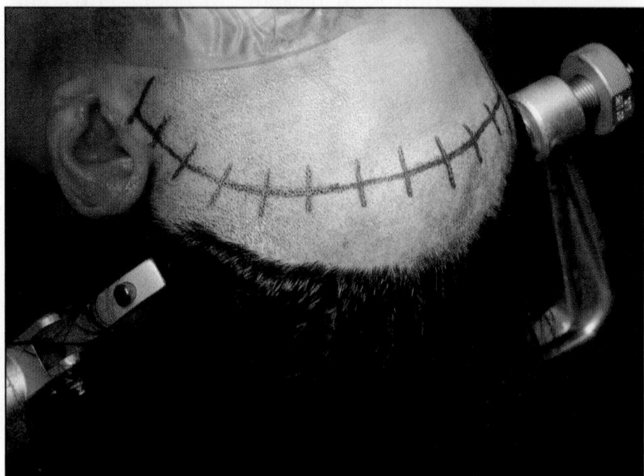

FIGURE 24-2

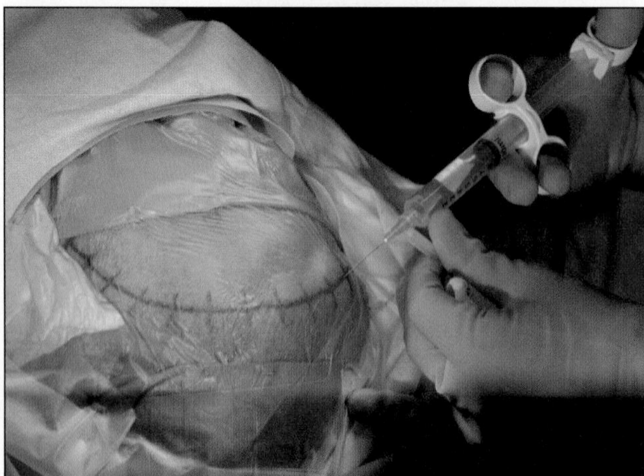

FIGURE 24-3

clips are applied to the full thickness of the scalp to control bleeding. The temporalis fascia and muscle are cut posteriorly along the same line of the skin incision.

- **Figure 24-5:** **A,** Muscle is detached from the bone by subperiosteal dissection and elevated along with the scalp flap as a single musculocutaneous unit until the orbital rim and frontozygomatic suture are exposed. **B,** The scalp flap is reflected anteriorly over a roll of gauze to prevent acute angulation, which may compromise the vascular

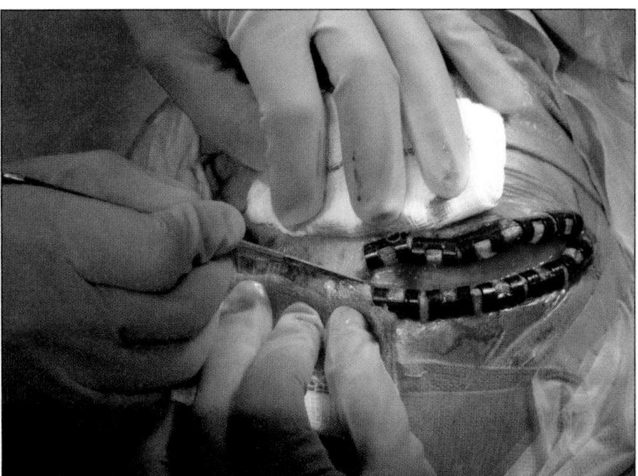

FIGURE 24-4

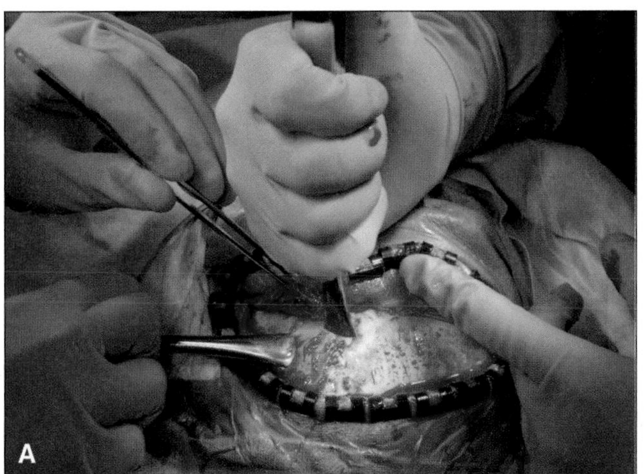

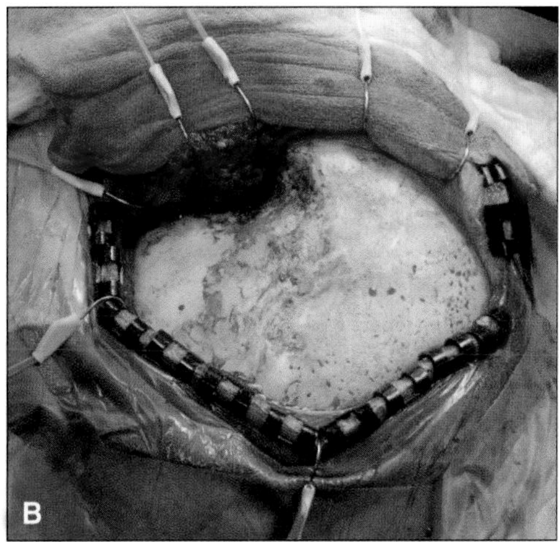

FIGURE 24-5

supply to the flap, and retracted with blunt fish hooks. Vigorous downward retraction of temporalis muscle toward the temporal fossa is important to avoid overhanging of muscle and obstruction of view. This retraction may be facilitated by cutting the anterior attachments of the muscle fibers and should be performed deep to the fat pad between the temporalis fascia and muscle to avoid injury of the frontalis branch. It is important to resuture the muscle anteriorly during closure to avoid a cosmetically unpleasant depression over the pterional region.

- **Figure 24-6:** **A,** Standard pterional (frontotemporal) craniotomy is performed to access the M1 artery and bifurcation aneurysms. Burr holes are placed at the key hole and in the temporal region and occasionally posteriorly along the superior temporal line if the dura is firmly adherent to the skull. Peripherally located aneurysms may require extension of the craniotomy posteriorly on to the temporal and parietal bones. **B,** After stripping the dura from the undersurface of the skull, a free bone flap is cut using a craniotome. The bone flap should extend at least 2 cm in the supraorbital area to allow adequate exposure of the proximal sylvian fissure. **C,** Dural tack-up sutures are placed along the bone edges.
- **Figure 24-7:** **A,** The pterion and lateral aspect of the lesser wing of the sphenoid bone are thoroughly drilled down to the frontodural fold to provide a low approach and avoid unnecessary brain retraction. Drilling also allows dissection of the aneurysm and clip application from an anterolateral direction and from a posterior direction. **B,** Dura is opened in a C-shaped fashion straddling the lateral sylvian fissure and sphenoid ridge. The dural flap is reflected anteriorly and tented with stay sutures.

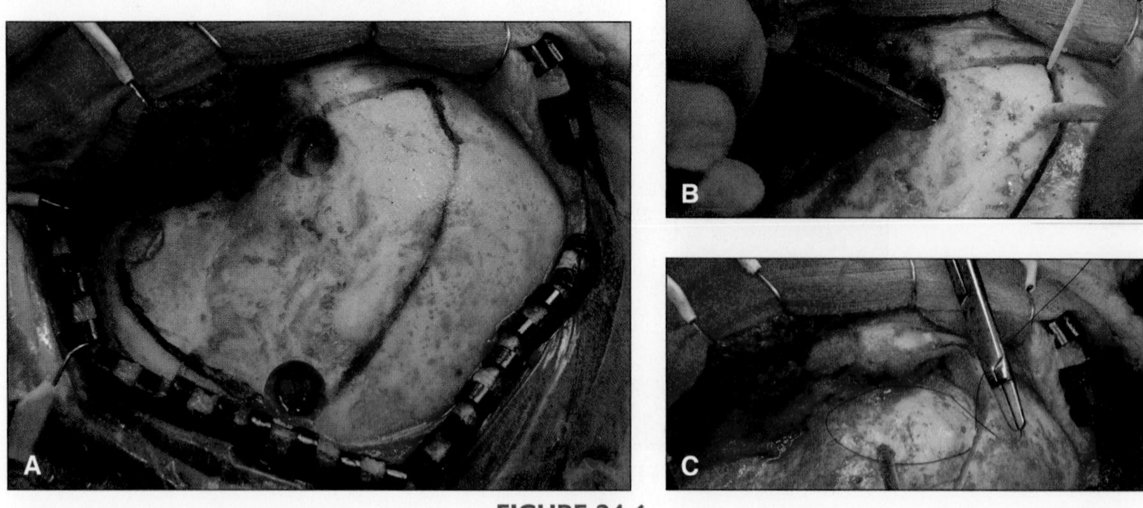

FIGURE 24-6

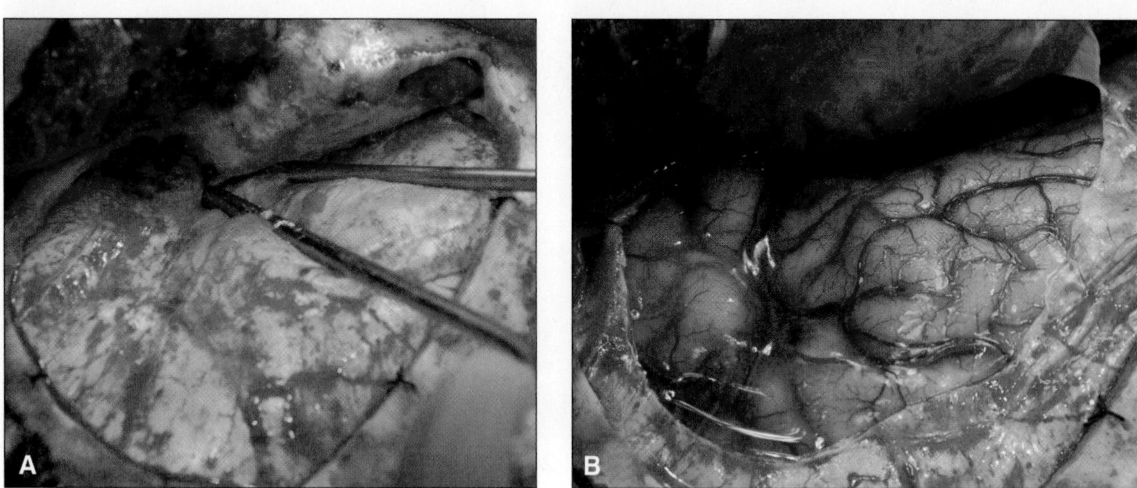

FIGURE 24-7

- The operating microscope is brought into the surgical field. There are three basic approaches to MCA aneurysms, described next.

Medial Transsylvian Approach

- Medial transsylvian approach is used sometimes for ruptured or complicated MCA aneurysms that arise from the M1 trunk or from an early temporal branch or bifurcation aneurysms in patients with a short M1 segment and early bifurcation. The approach allows early identification of the M1 trunk and proximal control, and it may be used when distal opening of the sylvian fissure is difficult because of the venous anatomy. Ordinarily, it is more difficult to open the sylvian fissure from proximal to distal, however, and that is why we generally prefer the lateral transsylvian approach, where the fissure is opened from distal to proximal.
- **Figure 24-8:** The laterobasal frontal lobe is gently retracted medially to expose the optic nerve and internal carotid artery. The optic and carotid cisterns are opened by sharp arachnoidal dissection to release cerebrospinal fluid and achieve adequate brain relaxation. If necessary, further cerebrospinal fluid drainage may be obtained by opening the lamina terminalis.
- **Figure 24-9: A,** Dissection is continued distally along the internal carotid artery toward the bifurcation. **B,** The sylvian cistern is opened medial to lateral by following the proximal MCA along its anteroinferior aspect, away from the perforating vessels. Dissection should

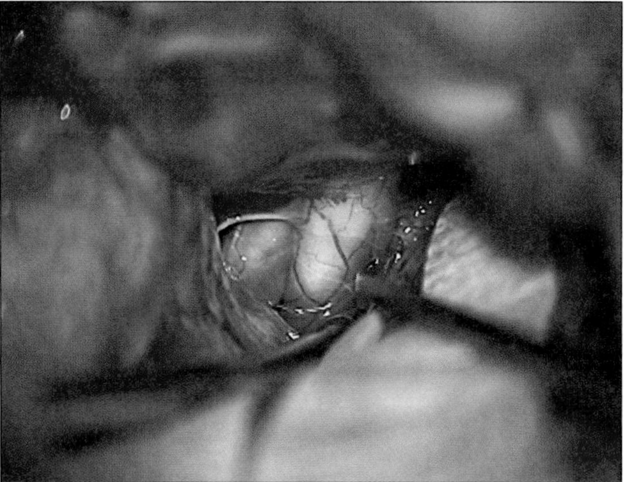

FIGURE 24-8

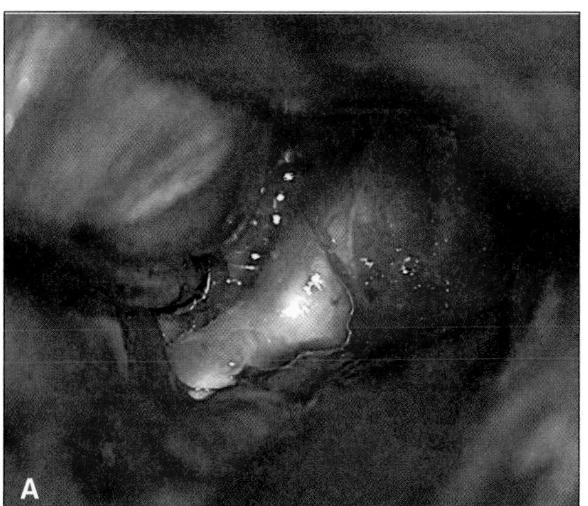

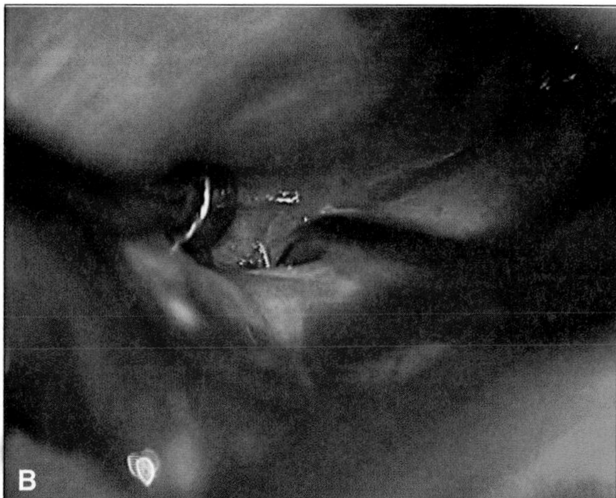

FIGURE 24-9

proceed on the frontal side of the superficial sylvian veins, which ultimately drain into the sphenoparietal or cavernous sinuses. Frequently, small crossing frontal veins are encountered and must be unavoidably sacrificed to facilitate complete separation of the frontal and temporal lobes; this can generally be performed without consequence.

Lateral Transsylvian Approach

- The lateral transsylvian approach is preferred for most MCA aneurysms. This approach facilitates exposure of the distal anatomy of the aneurysm complex, but it results in exposure of the aneurysm before achieving proximal control. This exposure is generally not a problem because as soon as the aneurysm base is identified, the surgeon can work behind or in front of the aneurysm following one division to the distal MCA trunk without dissecting the dome of the aneurysm. With large and giant aneurysms, this may be difficult.
- **Figure 24-10: A,** Opening of the sylvian fissure begins with sharp dissection along an area where the arachnoid is transparent on the frontal side of the superficial sylvian veins. **B,** Dissection proceeds by gently spreading the lips of the fissure until an M3 branch is identified. The artery is followed into the depth of the fissure toward an M2 branch. Subsequent dissection is carried from "inside out" by gently spreading the banks of the fissure and sharply cutting any superficial bridging arachnoidal bands.
- The M2 branches are followed proximally toward the M1 trunk along the side away from the aneurysm without disturbing the dome. Alternatively, the M1 vessel may be identified by opening the carotid cistern and following the artery from medial to lateral as described earlier.

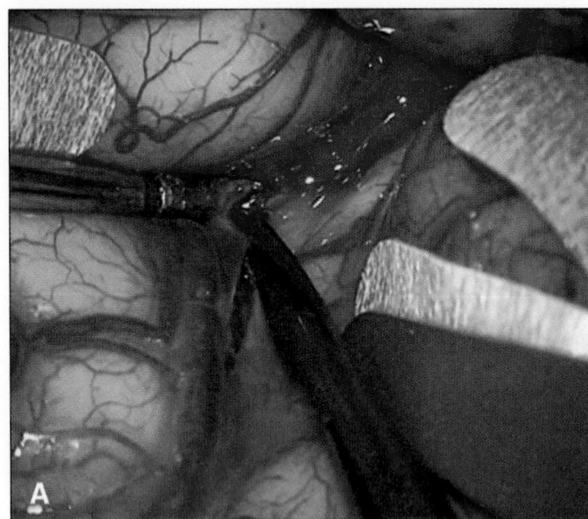

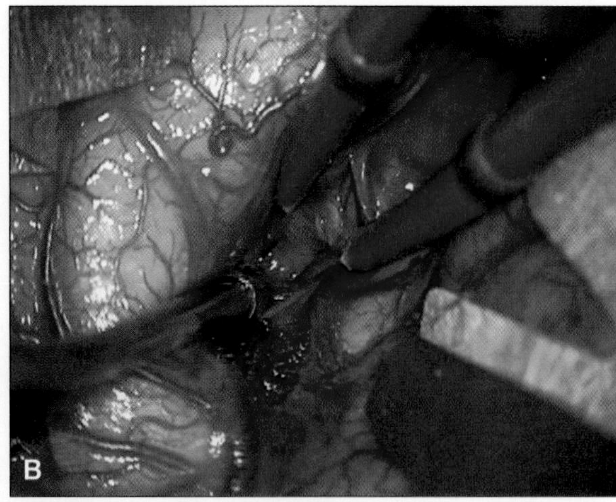

FIGURE 24-10

Superior Temporal Gyrus Approach

- The superior temporal gyrus approach is preferred for ruptured MCA bifurcation aneurysms associated with large temporal hematomas or in situations in which distal sylvian fissure splitting proves to be traumatic, which is usually due to complex venous anatomy.
- A 2- to 3-cm cortical incision is made in the anterior aspect of the superior temporal gyrus parallel to the sylvian fissure. Any associated hematoma is cautiously suctioned to achieve brain relaxation without disturbance of the aneurysm.
- Subpial resection is carried medially into the vertical segment of the fissure over the insula without disturbing the sylvian veins or frontal operculum.
- The MCA branches are followed proximally as described previously.
- The lenticulostriate, anterior temporal, and major distal arteries must be identified before aneurysm dissection and clipping. Enough room must be created along the M1 trunk, preferably distal to the lenticulostriate arteries, for placement of a temporary clip if required.
- **Figure 24-11:** Dissection of the aneurysm is carried out with a blunt dissector and should be initially limited to the neck until a space to pass the clip is developed. After the neck is defined, the rest of the aneurysm can be dissected with confidence. Adherent divisions or small branches at the neck must be separated with sharp dissection under high magnification. Any tethering arachnoidal bands must be cut sharply to avoid excessive traction on the aneurysm dome. Enough space must be created before any attempts at clip application to allow unhindered passage of the aneurysm clip.
- The permanent clip is applied across the neck of the aneurysm, while preserving M1 and M2 vessels.

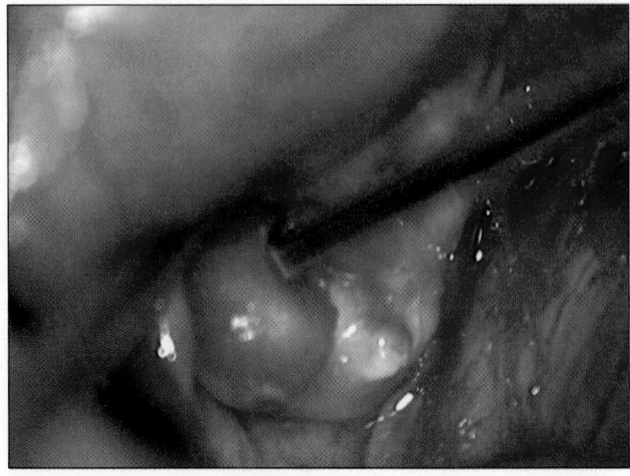

FIGURE 24-11

TIPS FROM THE MASTERS

- Broad-based, thick-necked aneurysms may require temporary clipping to deflate the aneurysm and facilitate proper permanent clip application.
- Fenestrated clips are useful in large or complex aneurysms. Incorporation of one or more of the MCA branches or lenticulostriate arteries within the clip fenestration may avoid unnecessary torque or compromise of these vessels. To ensure adequate closing force along the aneurysm neck, a fenestrated clip may be applied first to obliterate the distal neck followed by a second parallel clip to occlude the proximal neck.
- Large or giant, partially thrombosed or calcified aneurysms may require aneurysmorrhaphy and evacuation of the hematoma or atheroma to allow definitive clip application or suturing of the aneurysm base "cuff" after excision of the bulk of the aneurysm.
- Arterial reimplantation and extracranial-intracranial bypass (the description of which is beyond the scope of this chapter) may be necessary, particularly with a giant aneurysm, if complete clip placement is impossible without compromising a major MCA branch.

PITFALLS

Overrotating the head causes the temporal lobe to overlie the sylvian fissure, necessitating greater temporal lobe retraction and difficulty in aneurysm dissection.

Overextension of the head may result in obstruction of view by the orbital rim.

Care must be taken when opening the dura because the aneurysm may point superficially and be attached to the dura of the sphenoid wing.

Any visible stenosis, even if minimal, of either the M1 or the M2 arteries after clip placement should not be accepted because it is frequently associated with severe luminal constriction. Confirmation of vessel patency can be made by intraoperative angiography, indocyanine green videoangiography, or ultrasound flow probe measurements.

BAILOUT OPTIONS

- Intraoperative rupture before aneurysm dissection can be managed by several maneuvers. Temporary clip placement on the M1 trunk to reduce bleeding and use of large-bore suction usually clear enough blood to allow dissection and permanent clip placement. Another useful maneuver is to tamponade the bleeding point using suction over a cotton pad, while the surgeon completes the dissection with the other hand. If an experienced assistant is available, he or she can use the suction on the aneurysm to allow the surgeon to complete the dissection and place the clip using two hands. If bleeding is still too excessive to allow proper visualization, additional temporary clips may be placed on the M2 vessels. Occasionally, the tear in the aneurysm extends into the neck and may require several microsutures before final clip placement. Blind attempts at permanent clip placement in an incompletely dissected aneurysm may result in a tear at the neck that cannot be repaired or inadvertent injury to adjacent arteries and must be avoided.
- Intraoperative rupture during permanent aneurysm clip application may result from shearing the aneurysm wall, particularly if the neck has not been adequately dissected. A common mistake is reopening and then advancing the clip, which may lead to enlargement of the tear. In such circumstances, the clip should be quickly removed, and further dissection should be performed under temporary clipping. Occasionally, an aneurysm may rupture as the blades of the clip are closed owing to retraction of the dome away from adherent structures. If the surgeon is confident that the aneurysm is within the blades of the clip, advancing beyond the neck and closure of the clip usually stops the bleeding.
- Finally, the surgeon needs to be prepared and remain calm.

SUGGESTED READINGS

Heros R. Middle cerebral artery aneurysms. In: Wilkins R, Rengachary SS, editors. Neurosurgery. New York: McGraw-Hill; 1996. p. 2311–6.

Heros RC, Ojemann RG, Crowell RM. Superior temporal gyrus approach to middle cerebral artery aneurysms: technique and results. Neurosurgery 1982;10:308–13.

Yasargil MG. Microneurosurgery, vol. II, Stuttgart: Georg Thieme Verlag; 1984. p. 124–64.

Procedure 25 Paramedian Craniotomy and Unilateral Anterior Interhemispheric Approach for Clipping of Distal Anterior Cerebral Artery Aneurysm

Martin Lehecka, Mika Niemelä, Juha Hernesniemi

INDICATIONS

- Clipping of distal anterior cerebral artery (DACA) aneurysms has a long-lasting effect; rerupture of previously clipped aneurysm is very rare.
- DACA aneurysms are usually small, with a relatively broad base; are distally located; and have one or more branches originating from their base. These factors, together with the relatively small diameter of the parent artery, favor clipping over coiling.
- When DACA aneurysms rupture, about 50% manifest with frontal intracranial hemorrhage (ICH), which needs to be (at least partially) removed during clipping.
- DACA aneurysms rupture at a smaller size (mean 6 mm) than aneurysms in many other locations, so treatment of small (<7 mm), unruptured DACA aneurysms is reasonable in young, healthy patients.
- Multiple aneurysms are found in about 50% of patients with DACA aneurysms, and multiple DACA aneurysms are found in 10%. All DACA aneurysms can usually be accessed via the same interhemispheric approach and clipped during one operation.
- Even patients with poor Hunt and Hess grade with ruptured DACA aneurysm should be treated because mortality for this aneurysm location is lower than for other aneurysms.

CONTRAINDICATIONS

- In acute subarachnoid hemorrhage, only aneurysms that can be easily accessed through the same approach should be clipped. Extensive dissection and manipulation of cingulate gyri should be avoided to prevent neuropsychologic deficits.
- Patient with poor Hunt and Hess grade and subarachnoid hemorrhage with fixed dilated pupils and no proper reaction to pain would not benefit from active treatment.
- Old age, poor condition, and additional comorbidities are relative contraindications.

PLANNING AND POSITIONING

- Preoperative planning is based on computed tomography angiography or digital subtraction angiography images. Special attention is paid to (1) the vascular configuration of the anterior communicating artery region, (2) the number and course of the pericallosal arteries, (3) the actual originating artery, (4) aneurysm location with respect to the genu of corpus callosum, (5) dome projection, (6) possible ICH, (7) number and orientation of branches at the aneurysm base, (8) presence of vascular anomalies, and (9) additional aneurysms.
- Of DACA aneurysms, 85% originate from the A3 segment of the anterior cerebral artery (ACA), at the genu of corpus callosum.

- DACA aneurysms are generally approached via an anterior interhemispheric approach, the only exception being aneurysms located on the proximal A2 segment of the ACA and aneurysms located distally on the frontobasal branches of the ACA, the limit being 15 mm or less of vertical distance from the floor of the anterior fossa. These aneurysms are operated via a lateral supraorbital approach, a frontal modification of the pterional approach.
- For right-handed surgeons, the right-sided approach is more convenient because both pericallosal arteries can be reached under the lower margin of the falx for most of their course. Only very distal DACA aneurysms (A5 segment or distal callosomarginal artery) require an approach from the same side as the aneurysm. Left-sided ICH may require a left-sided approach.
- The location of the DACA aneurysm with respect to the genu of corpus callosum determines the exact location of the bone flap and the angle of approach. The more proximal the aneurysm, the more frontal the craniotomy to prevent the genu of the corpus callosum from obstructing the view toward the aneurysm base. Partial resection of the genu of corpus callosum is not recommended because it leads to cognitive impairment.
- Neuronavigation may be helpful in planning and executing the approach to the aneurysm.
- **Figure 25-1:** Positioning of the bone flap during interhemispheric approach for DACA aneurysms at different locations along the DACA.
- **Figure 25-2:** After minimal shaving, the skin is sterilized and infiltrated with a local anesthetic combined with epinephrine. An oblique skin incision is made just behind the hairline, with the base frontally and over the midline and extended more to the side of the planned bone flap.
- The patient is placed in the supine position with the head elevated about 20 cm above the heart level. The head should be in a neutral position with the nose pointing exactly upward. Tilting the head to either side risks the chance of placing the bone flap too lateral from the midline, making entry into the interhemispheric space difficult.
- The neck of the patient is slightly flexed or extended according to how proximal or distal the DACA aneurysm lies. In optimal position, the surgical trajectory is almost vertical.
- Anesthesia is maintained with propofol infusion, and mannitol is given.

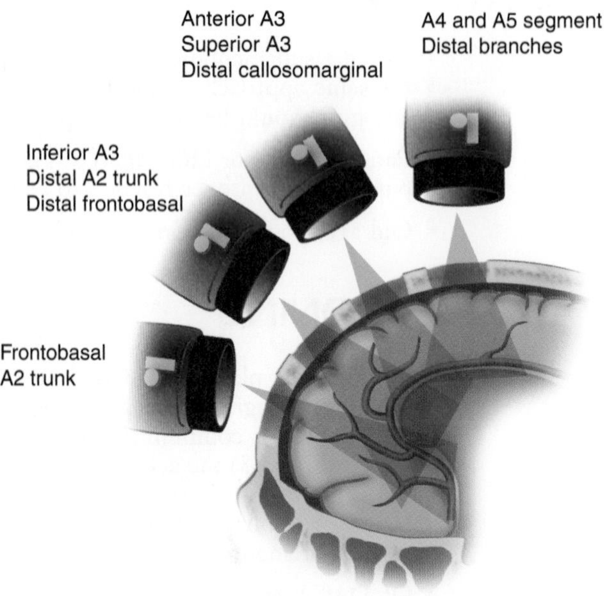

FIGURE 25-1

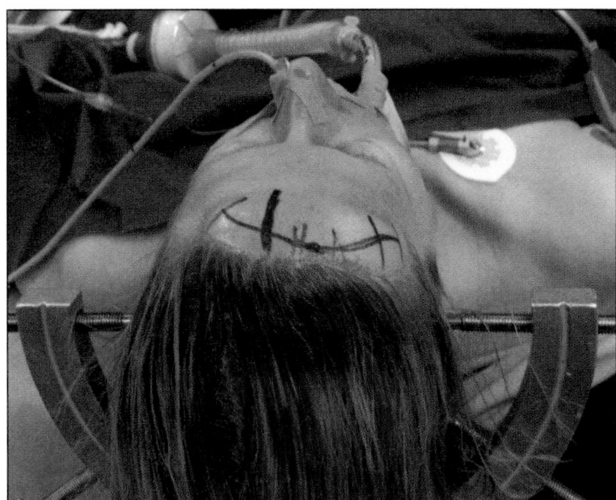

FIGURE 25-2

PROCEDURE

- **Figure 25-3:** One-layer skin flap is reflected frontally with spring hooks exposing the frontal bone. A 3- to 4-cm diameter bone flap is planned slightly over the midline to allow better retraction of the falx medially during dissection. A flap that is too small may provide insufficient space for working between the bridging veins.
- **Figure 25-4:** Only one burr hole in the midline over the superior sagittal sinus at the posterior border of the bone flap is needed. Bone is detached from the underlying dura with care using a curved dissector.
- **Figure 25-5:** The bone flap is removed using a side-cutting drill. Two cuts are made lateral to the sagittal sinus, avoiding cutting directly over the sinus. This remaining bony ridge is thinned down, and the bone flap is cracked. A high-speed drill can be used to smooth the edges or enlarge the craniotomy. Holes are drilled to be used with dural tack-up sutures.
- **Figure 25-6:** The dura is opened as a C-shaped flap with the base medially. The incision is made first laterally and then extended toward the midline in the anterior and posterior direction. The dural opening should be planned so that possible meningeal venous sinuses or lacunae remain intact. Bridging veins may be attached to the dura for several centimeters along the midline.
- **Figure 25-7:** Careful dissection and mobilization of the bridging veins is performed under the magnification of the operating microscope. Damage to the bridging veins

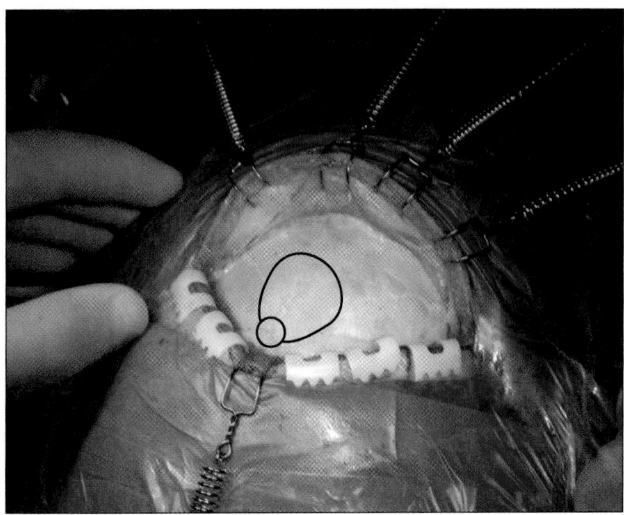

FIGURE 25-3

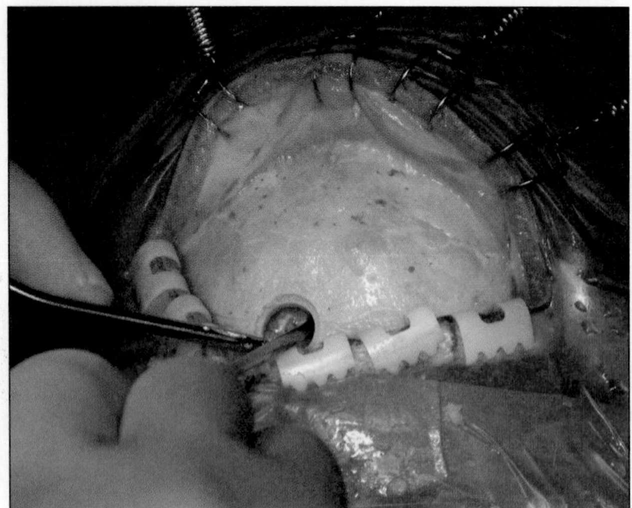

FIGURE 25-4

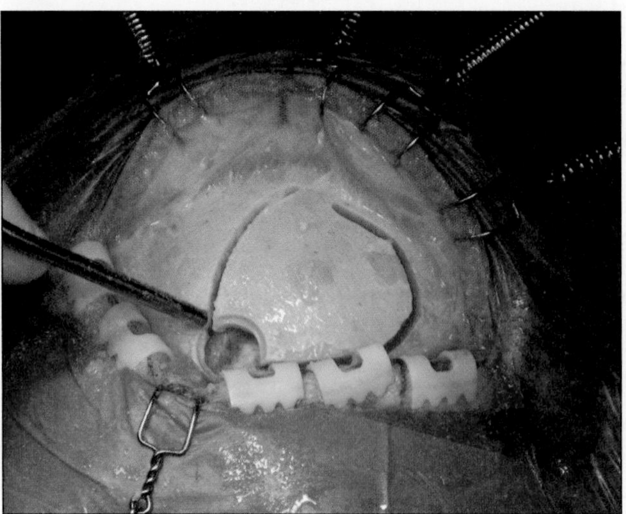

FIGURE 25-5

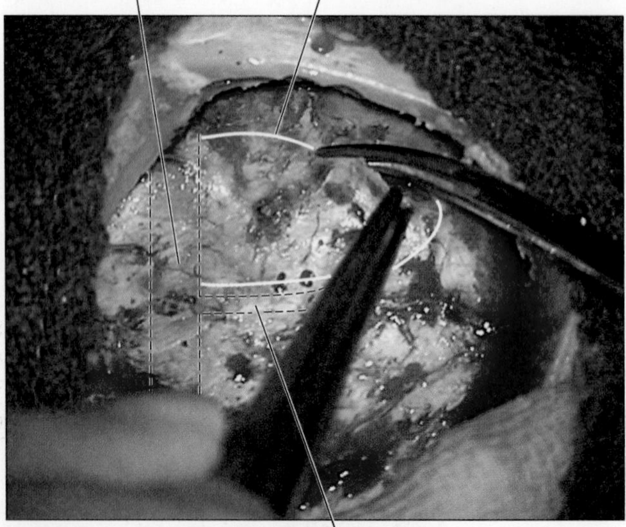

FIGURE 25-6

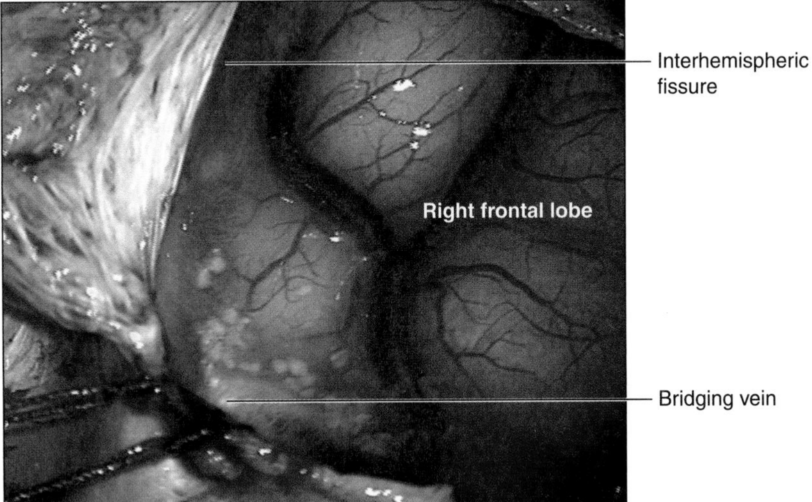

FIGURE 25-7

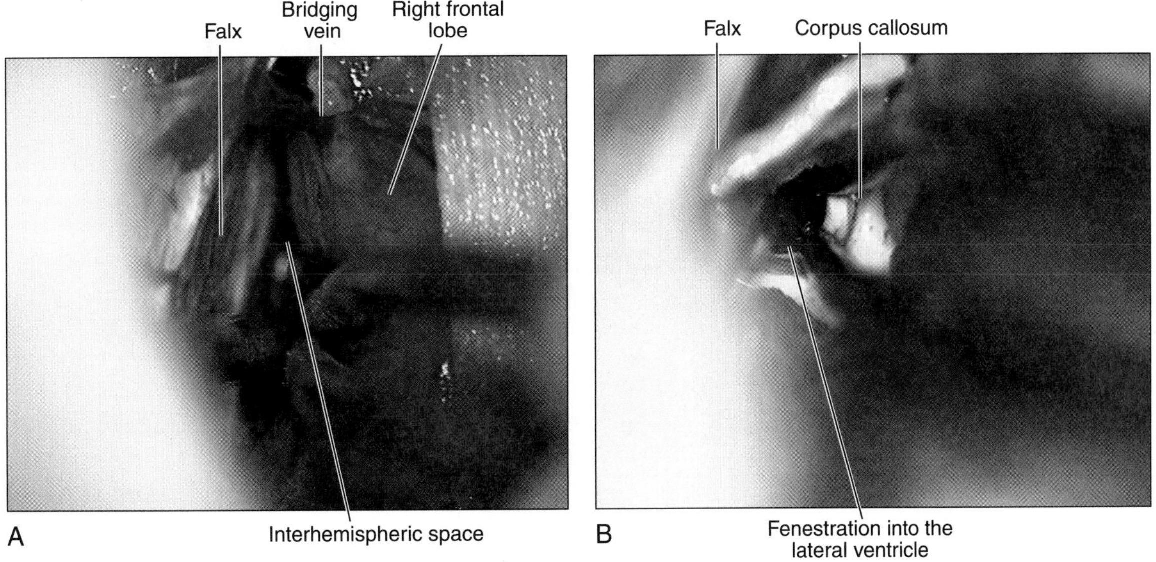

FIGURE 25-8

usually occurs during the opening of the dura. Dural edges are elevated over the craniotomy dressings to prevent epidural oozing into the surgical field.

- **Figure 25-8:** The interhemispheric fissure is entered in between the bridging veins, which should be left intact. The dissection is oriented deeper along the falx while removing cerebrospinal fluid with suction (**A**). The interhemispheric space and pericallosal cistern are narrow, so only a limited amount of cerebrospinal fluid can be released to gain space. In unruptured DACA aneurysms, this space is sufficient. In ruptured aneurysms, lumbar drainage or transcortical ventricular puncture at the lateral border of the craniotomy or a puncture with bipolar forceps through corpus callosum into the lateral ventricle later during the dissection may be used (**B**).
- **Figure 25-9:** Inside the interhemispheric fissure, the arachnoid adhesions are cleared by sharp dissection with microscissors. The interhemispheric fissure is opened, and the frontal lobe is mobilized. Injecting physiologic saline with syringe "water dissection" is used to expand the dissection planes, and suction and bipolar forceps and small cottonoids are used as microretractors.
- **Figure 25-10:** The first aim of the dissection is to identify the lower margin of the falx and the dissection plane in between the two tightly attached cingulate gyri. The depth

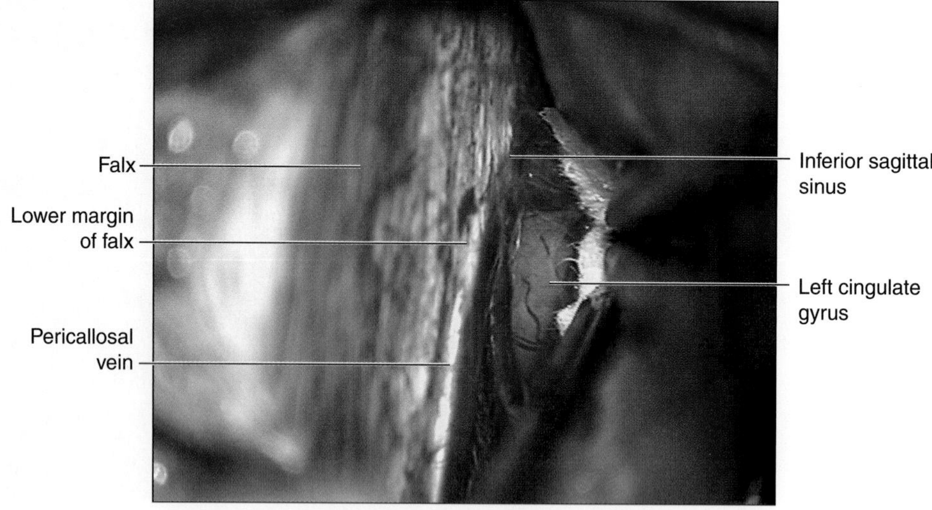

FIGURE 25-9

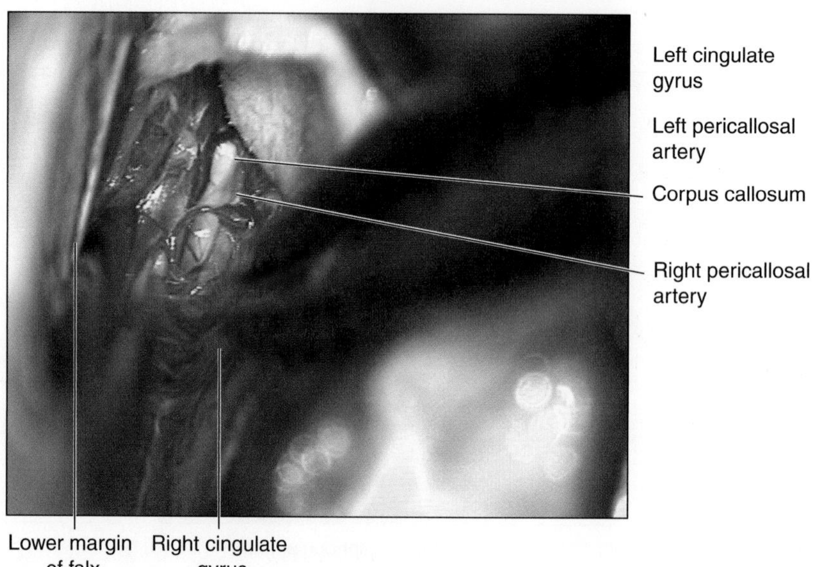

FIGURE 25-10

of the falx varies, and so does the course of the pericallosal artery. Sometimes the pericallosal artery can be found already in the cingulate sulcus, but usually it runs still deeper along the corpus callosum. The dissection continues deeper in between the cingulate gyri toward the corpus callosum.

- **Figure 25-11:** The corpus callosum is identified by its white color and parallel running transverse fibers. Both pericallosal arteries must be visualized, and the proper one is followed in a proximal direction toward the aneurysm. The aneurysm is often pointing lateral toward either side and can be embedded in the pial layer of the cingulate gyrus. Traversing along the opposite cingulate gyrus should provide visualization of the proximal parent artery, the possible site for temporary clipping.
- **Figure 25-12:** Obtaining proximal control is often the most difficult part of the interhemispheric approach for DACA aneurysms. The direction of the aneurysm may change owing to retraction, and blood may obscure the anatomy, making identification of the aneurysm difficult. Strong retraction of the frontal lobe is also likely to cause intraoperative rupture. For DACA aneurysms, only a proximal temporary clip is often sufficient; the distal one is seldom needed. If access to the proximal parent artery cannot be achieved, a pilot clip is the only choice.

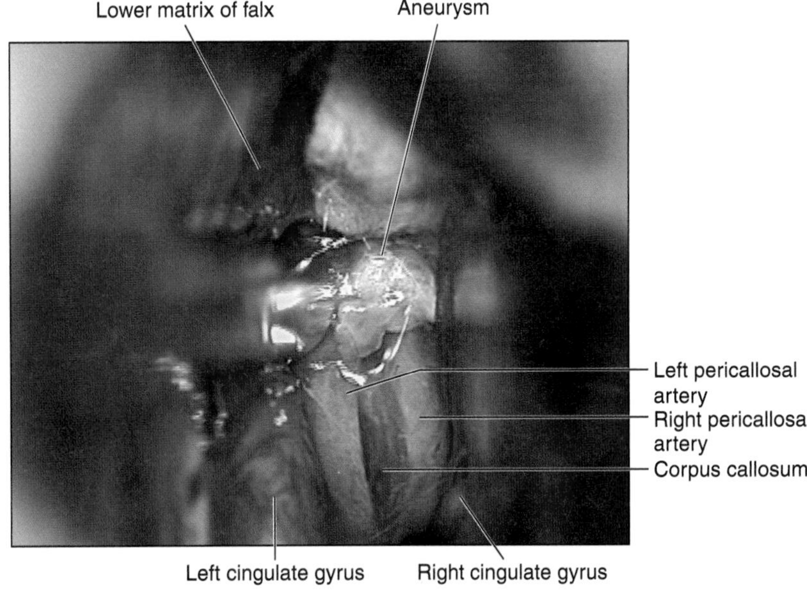

FIGURE 25-11

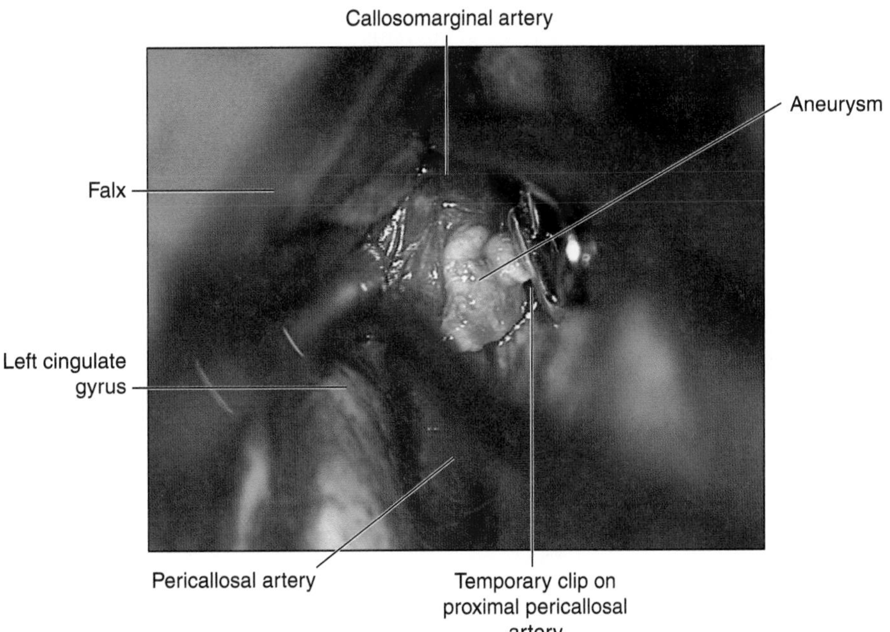

FIGURE 25-12

- **Figure 25-13:** Under the control of the temporary clip or possibly the pilot clip, the whole aneurysm dome is dissected free, all the surrounding branches are visualized, and the final clip is applied. The final clip should be as small and light as possible to prevent kinking, twisting, or occlusion of the parent artery or the surrounding branches. Papaverine is applied locally to prevent vasospasm.

TIPS FROM THE MASTERS

- The interhemispheric approach lacks good consistent anatomic landmarks, so intraoperative orientation is difficult. In acute subarachnoid hemorrhage, with blood clots and swelling obstructing the view, this approach is even more demanding. Careful

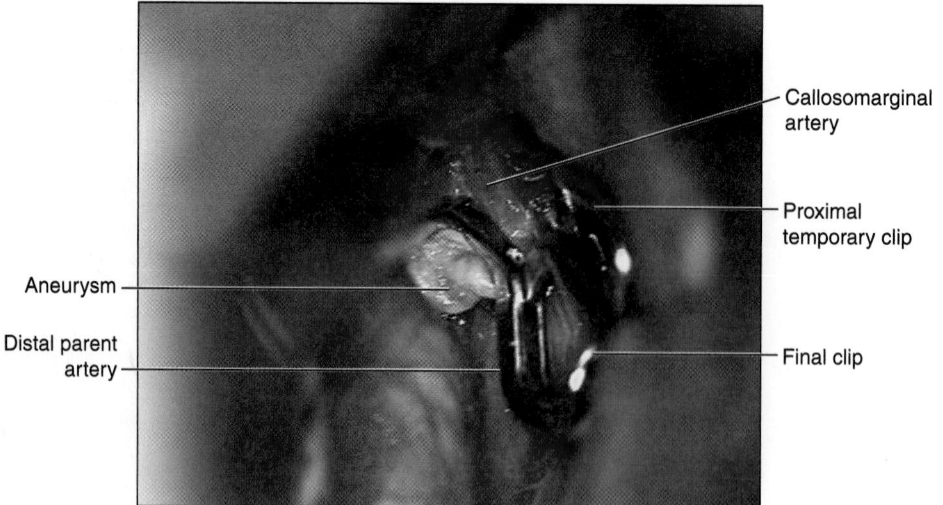

FIGURE 25-13

planning of the approach trajectory is crucial. Good landmarks for the entry point are the distance from the coronal suture or the nasion. In addition, distance from the cranium to the aneurysm at the entry point should be measured.

- DACA aneurysms with less than 15 mm vertical distance from the anterior skull base are better approached with a lateral supraorbital approach, which provides better proximal control and easier release of cerebrospinal fluid from the basal cisterns. To locate the aneurysm, the distance is measured from the optic chiasm to enter the interhemispheric space in the right place. A small frontobasal resection of the gyrus rectus is needed.
- Almost all DACA aneurysms except for the very distal ones can be reached below the lower margin of the falx. The depth of falx varies, but the inferior sagittal sinus can usually be seen on preoperative images.
- If the bone flap is too small, it might be difficult to find a proper working space in between the bridging veins. Dural opening can be tailored according to the veins. A working channel of 1.5 to 2 cm in diameter is often enough.
- The angle of the optics of the microscope should be checked to ensure that the approach trajectory is correct.
- When the angle of approach is wrong, the trajectory is usually too anterior.
- Corpus callosum is identified by its white color and parallel running transverse fibers, which distinguish it from the cingulate gyri.
- It may be difficult to decide from the preoperative images whether the aneurysm originates from the left or the right pericallosal artery.
- The pericallosal arteries may be running on either side of the midline. Both arteries should be visualized before continuing with the dissection toward the aneurysm.
- The aneurysm dome is often encountered before proximal control has been established. A too strong lateral retraction of the frontal lobe should be avoided to prevent intraoperative aneurysm rupture.
- Sometimes proximal control of the parent artery can be obtained better from below and behind the aneurysm dome than from above the aneurysm dome.
- In almost every case, there is at least one branch originating from the base. The whole base should be dissected free before final clipping of the aneurysm.
- During the final clipping, if the first clip slides, exposing some of the neck, another clip may be applied proximal to the first one (i.e., "double clipping").
- With aneurysm at the bifurcation of an azygos pericallosal artery, complications may lead to damage of both hemispheres.

PITFALLS

Craniotomy is placed too lateral from the midline, preventing easy access into the interhemispheric space.

The bridging veins are damaged or overstretched while opening the dura or later by excessive retraction of the frontal lobe.

Lack of working space in the interhemispheric space and pericallosal cistern is due to insufficient cerebrospinal fluid release or expansive ICH.

The cingulate gyri with dense adhesions are mistaken for the corpus callosum and other paired arteries for pericallosal arteries; this results in getting totally lost inside the interhemispheric fissure.

Intraoperative aneurysm rupture occurs before proximal control has been established.

DACA aneurysm has a sclerotic wall and broad base preventing proper final clipping.

A too large and too heavy final clip causes kinking of the parent artery.

BAILOUT OPTIONS

- If one gets lost inside the interhemispheric fissure, to prevent excessive dissection, a large aneurysm clip can be used as a mark, and a sagittal view of C-arm fluoroscopy is performed to help navigation.
- During intraoperative aneurysm rupture, control should be attempted first via suction and compressing the bleeding site with cottonoids while preparing the site for a temporary clip or pilot clip. Sudden and short hypotension by cardiac arrest, induced by intravenous adenosine (9 to 18 mg intravenous bolus), can be used to facilitate quick dissection and application of the pilot clip.
- If a small, thin aneurysm ruptures at the neck during dissection, under temporary clipping, reconstruction of the base involving a part of the parent artery in the clip should be attempted.

SUGGESTED READINGS

Hernesniemi J, Niemelä M, Karatas A, et al. Some collected principles of microneurosurgery: simple and fast, while preserving normal anatomy: a review. Surg Neurol 2005;64:195–200.

Lehecka M, Dashti R, Hernesniemi J, et al. Microneurosurgical management of aneurysms at A3 segment of anterior cerebral artery. Surg Neurol 2008;70:135–51.

Lehecka M, Lehto H, Niemelä M, et al. Distal anterior cerebral artery aneurysms: treatment and outcome analysis of 501 patients. Neurosurgery 2008;62:590–601.

Lehecka M, Porras M, Dashti R, et al. Anatomic features of distal anterior cerebral artery aneurysms: a detailed angiographic analysis of 101 patients. Neurosurgery 2008;63:219–28.

Yasargil MG. Distal anterior cerebral artery aneurysms. In: Yasargil MG, editor. Microneurosurgery, vol II. Stuttgart: Georg Thieme Verlag; 1984. p. 224–31.

Procedure 26

Vertebral Artery Aneurysms: Far-Lateral Suboccipital Approach for Clipping

Gavin P. Dunn, Christopher S. Ogilvy

INDICATIONS

- Ruptured or unruptured aneurysms of the vertebral artery, vertebrobasilar junction, and proximal posterior inferior cerebellar artery (PICA) have a particularly high rerupture rate and morbidity and mortality if left untreated. Unless the patient is tenuously unstable medically, treatment is indicated.
- In aneurysms deemed appropriate for surgical management, the far-lateral approach provides appropriate access to these lesions that are ventral or ventrolateral to the brainstem and below the mid-clival region.

CONTRAINDICATIONS

- As with all aneurysms, open and endovascular approaches should be considered. If aneurysms in these locations have anatomy favorable for embolization, this approach should be attempted before open surgery if possible.
- If PICA aneurysms are distal and involve the telovelotonsillar or cortical segments of the PICA, they may be more midline, and a far-lateral approach may be inappropriate. A midline suboccipital or combined lateral and medial suboccipital approach may provide requisite access to the aneurysm.
- Patients who are medically unstable may not tolerate open surgery.

PLANNING AND POSITIONING

- The three-dimensional anatomy of the aneurysm and its relationship to its parent vessel must be clearly delineated. We routinely employ high-resolution computed tomography (CT) angiography with three-dimensional reformatting in preoperative planning. The bony anatomy detail on CT angiography studies is particularly useful in planning the far-lateral suboccipital exposure. In some cases, conventional catheter-based cerebral angiography is necessary to clarify the aneurysm better. Using either approach, it is critical to determine the relevant vascular anatomy, including (1) whether the PICA is duplicated, (2) whether PICA territory is supplied by neighboring vessels, (3) the size of the posterior communicating artery, and (4) the orientation of the aneurysm dome relative to its neck.
- Antibiotics and dexamethasone (Decadron) are routinely administered before skin incision.
- **Figure 26-1:** High-resolution CT angiography studies are becoming increasingly important for preoperative planning. Thin-section source images (**A**) are reformatted into three-dimensional images that can be easily manipulated on a radiology workstation (**B**).
- **Figure 26-2:** There are multiple surgical approaches to the vertebral artery, PICA, and vertebrobasilar junction. The appropriate approach is dictated primarily by the specific location of the aneurysm in this region. This schematic diagram summarizes our surgical approach strategies.
- **Figure 26-3:** The patient is placed in a straight lateral position with a pad placed under the axilla. The ipsilateral arm rests on pillows. The ipsilateral shoulder is pulled down

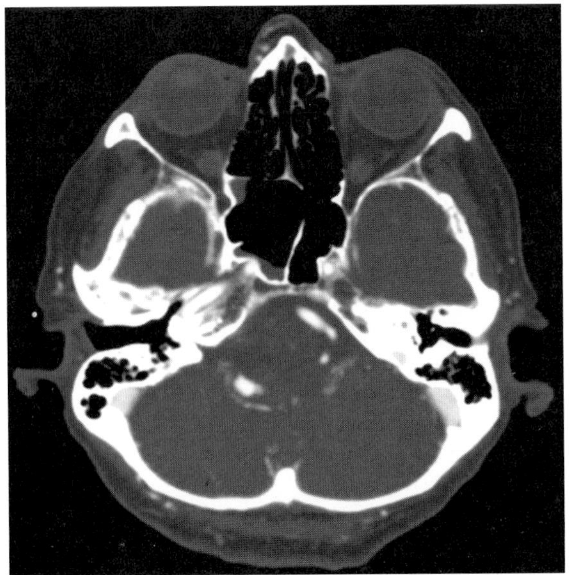

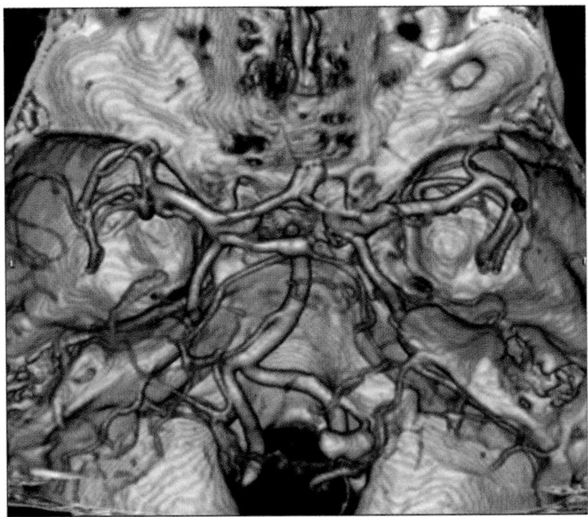

FIGURE 26-1

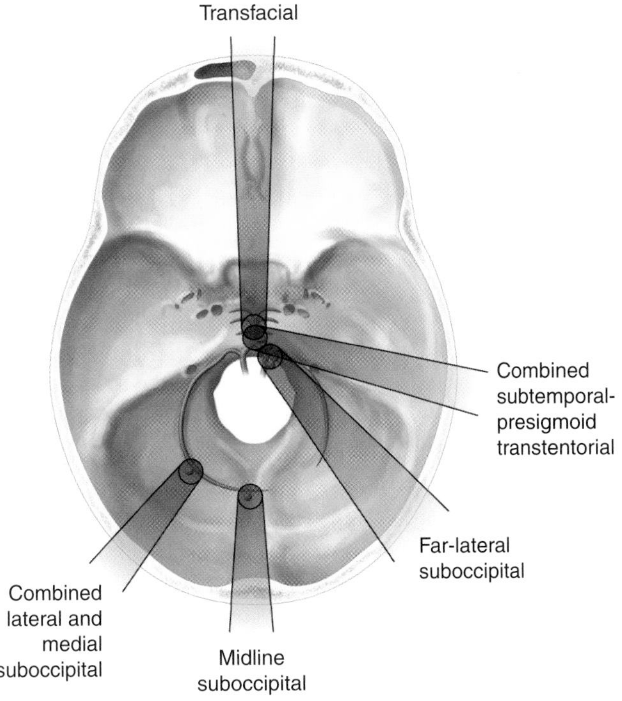

FIGURE 26-2

using thick adhesive tape to allow greater freedom of movement with the microscope, and the head is tilted approximately 30 degrees toward the ipsilateral shoulder to facilitate venous and cerebrospinal fluid drainage. When the final position is obtained, the head is secured in a Mayfield head holder, and the patient's body should be well secured with tape and blankets.

- **Figure 26-4:** We plan an S-shaped skin incision, which starts approximately 3 fingerbreadths medial to the mastoid at the level of the superior aspect of the pinna. The incision runs inferiorly before gently curving to the midline under the inion and terminating at the spinous process of C2. Translucent drapes are used to border the operative field before sterile preparation.

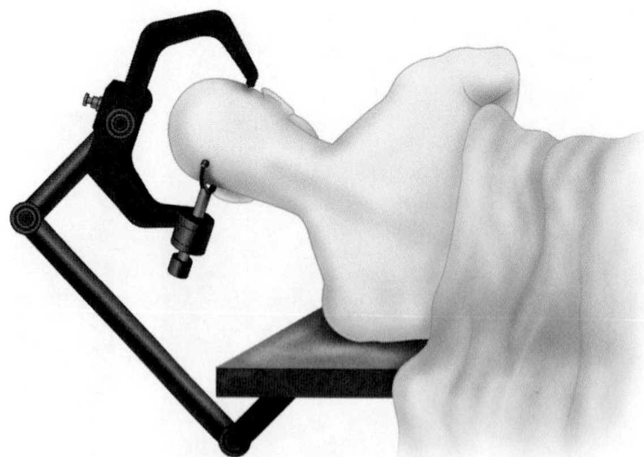

FIGURE 26-3

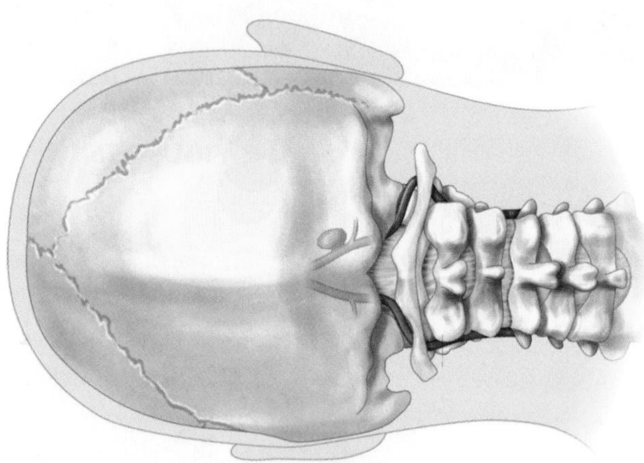

FIGURE 26-4

PROCEDURE

- **Figure 26-5:** We prepare early for the dural closure at the end of the procedure. To minimize the risk of infection, we prefer to use autologous pericranium for duraplasty in the event that primary dural closure is not feasible, which is often the case. **A,** The skin incision near the superior nuchal line at the level of the inion is carried to the galea. Sharp dissection with Metzenbaum scissors is used to develop a plane

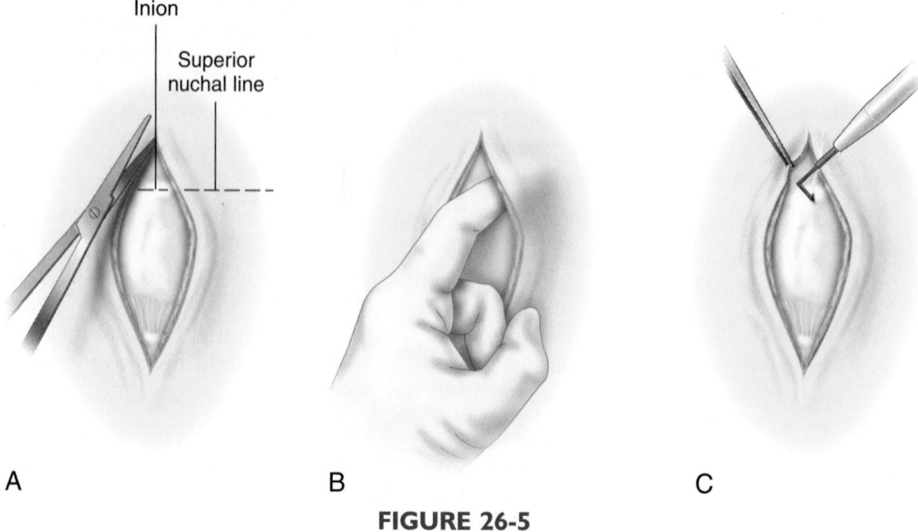

FIGURE 26-5

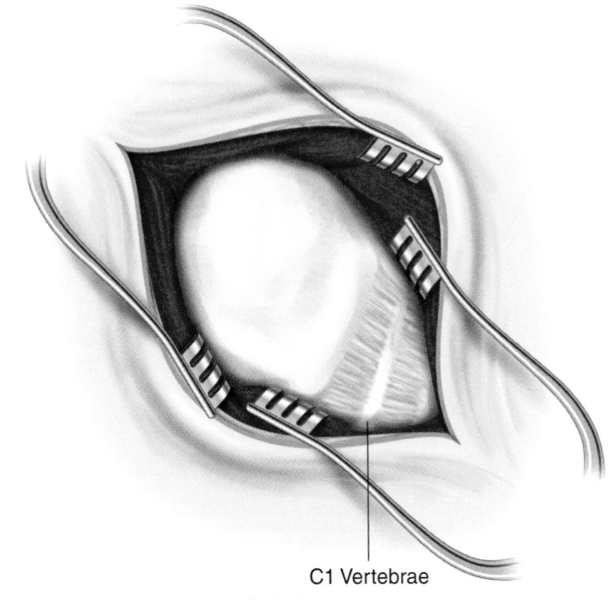

FIGURE 26-6

immediately underneath the galea to identify pericranium. **B,** When the pericranial layer has been identified, blunt finger dissection is used to develop the pericranial layer under retraction. **C,** Monopolar cautery with a 90-degree angled tip is used to define the extent of the graft, and meticulous harvest with a periosteal elevator brings the pericranium off the underlying bone into the field.

- **Figure 26-6:** After harvest of autologous pericranium, the incision is continued down to the bone using monopolar cautery. As dissection proceeds inferiorly below the superior nuchal line, it is imperative to remain in the midline avascular plane to avoid unnecessary muscle bleeding. C1 and the spinous process of C2 are exposed at the caudal end of the incision. A teardrop craniectomy is performed from the transverse-sigmoid sinus junction to just past the midline of the foramen magnum. We initiate the craniectomy with a perforator and turn a bone flap with the footplate of a high-speed drill; further bony removal is achieved using rongeurs and a cutting bur drill. Radical bone removal at this step is imperative to the effective use of this approach; the craniectomy should extend laterally to the occipital condyle, the medial aspect of which can be drilled further.
- The ipsilateral posterior arch of C1 is removed using a combination of a rongeur and high-speed drill. During this step, it is important to visualize the extradural portion of the vertebral artery, especially as it runs in the sulcus arteriosus. The dural opening starts superiorly at the junction of the transverse and sigmoid sinuses and curves gently to the midline just below the removed ipsilateral arch of C1. The operating microscope is brought into the field.
- **Figure 26-7:** The ipsilateral cerebellar tonsil and hemisphere are gently retracted to reveal the neurovascular landscape. The arachnoid is opened, and cerebrospinal fluid may be drained from the cisterna magna to improve brain relaxation. Two critical working corridors are identified that may provide access to the aneurysm, depending on its location. The caudal corridor (*dark arrow*) is accessed through the window bordered by cranial nerve XI inferiorly, cranial nerves IX and X superiorly, and the medulla medially. The cranial corridor (*white arrow*) is accessed through the window bordered by cranial nerves IX and X inferiorly, cranial nerves VII and VIII superiorly, and the medulla laterally.
- **Figure 26-8:** The aneurysm is secured by surgical clipping through the appropriate corridor. Blood flow through the distal parent vessel is confirmed via ultrasound using a micro-Doppler.

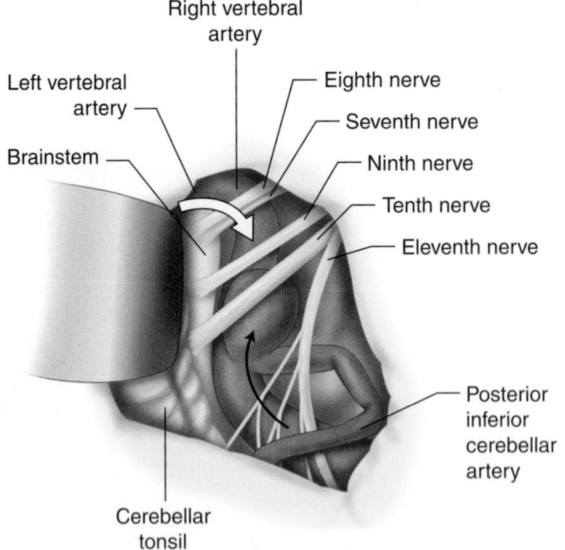

FIGURE 26-7

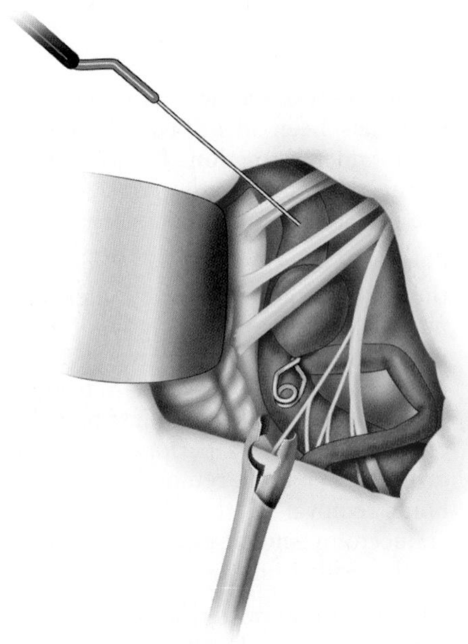

FIGURE 26-8

Closure

- **Figure 26-9:** The dura may be closed primarily but often requires graft placement. If duraplasty is required, previously harvested pericranium is sutured to native dura with a running 4-0 nylon on either side. Muscle and fascia are closed in layers with interrupted polyglactin 910 (Vicryl) suture, and the skin is closed with a running 3-0 nylon.

TIPS FROM THE MASTERS

- The key to this approach is the bony exposure. Specifically, the occipital condyle in the far-lateral approach is analogous to the sphenoid ridge in the pterional approach—there should be enough bone drilled away ventrally so that it does not obscure the surgeon's view after the dura is opened and reflected laterally. The medial and superior exposures should not be minimized to allow room for appropriate cerebellar retraction when needed.

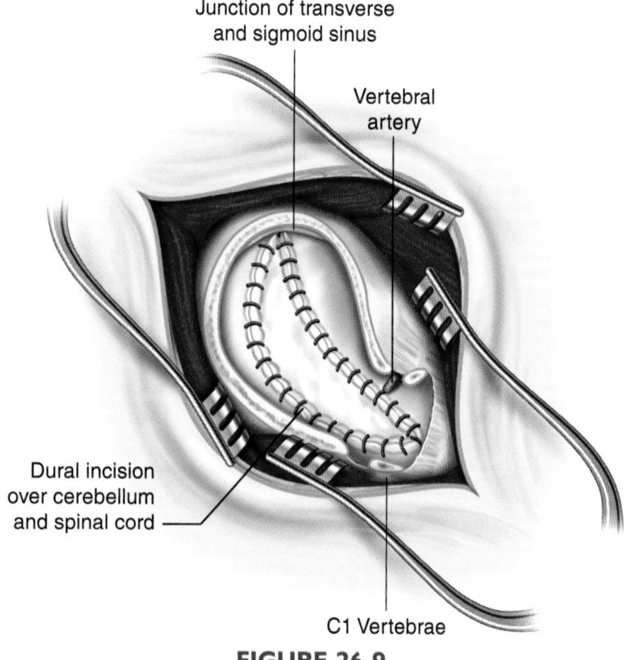

FIGURE 26-9

PITFALLS

Inadequate bony exposure before the dural opening necessitates excessive retraction.

The lower cranial nerves are enmeshed in the neurovascular landscape of this exposure. Even with gentle manipulation during surgery, patients may experience postoperative dysphagia, and care should exercised regarding diet advancement in this period.

A watertight dural closure, either primarily or with a dural graft, is pivotal in avoiding a cerebrospinal fluid leak.

BAILOUT OPTIONS

- Vertebral artery control proximal and distal to the aneurysm should be achieved early in the procedure. This control allows for temporary or permanent vessel occlusion should an inadvertent aneurysm or vessel tear occur.
- Consider PICA-PICA bypass with proximal occlusion for fusiform aneurysms or in situations in which the origin of the PICA vessel is injured or abnormal.
- Occipital artery–PICA bypass may be employed if the proximal PICA vessel is involved with the aneurysmal disease or is injured and not amenable to bypass.

SUGGESTED READINGS

D'Ambrosio AL, Kreiter KT, Bush CA, et al. Far lateral suboccipital approach for the treatment of proximal posteroinferior cerebellar artery aneurysms: surgical results and long-term outcome. Neurosurgery 2004;55:39–50.

Heros RC. Lateral suboccipital approach for vertebral and vertebrobasilar artery lesions. J Neurosurg 1986;64:559–62.

Ogilvy CS, Quinones-Hinojosa A. Surgical treatment of vertebral and posterior inferior cerebellar artery aneurysms. Neurosurg Clin N Am 1998;9:851–60.

Sanai N, Tarapore P, Lee AC, et al. The current role of microsurgery for posterior circulation aneurysms: a selective approach in the endovascular era. Neurosurgery 2008;62:1236–49.

Stevens EA, Powers AK, Sweasey TA, et al. Simplified harvest of autologous pericranium for duraplasty in Chiari malformation type I. Technical note. J Neurosurg Spine 2009;11:80–3.

Figure 26-4 is from Heros R. Lateral suboccipital approach for vertebral and vertebrobasilar artery lesions. J Neurosurg 1986;64:559–62.

Procedure 27

Basilar Artery Aneurysm: Orbitozygomatic Craniotomy for Clipping

Nader Sanai, Michael T. Lawton

INDICATIONS

- Basilar apex aneurysms include ruptured or unruptured basilar bifurcation aneurysms, superior cerebellar artery (SCA) aneurysms, and P1 posterior cerebral artery (PCA) aneurysms.
- Patients who are young and have good clinical grades (Hunt and Hess grades 1 to 3), with broad aneurysm neck, complex branching of the PCA or SCA, branches originating from side walls, intraluminal thrombus, or significant mass effect from the aneurysm should be considered for microsurgical clipping.

CONTRAINDICATIONS

- Patients who are elderly (≥70 years old) and have poor clinical grades (Hunt and Hess grades 4 and 5) and have calcified aneurysms or aneurysm anatomy that is favorable for coiling (narrow neck, acute-angle branches of the PCA, or posterior aneurysm projection) should be considered for endovascular therapy.

PLANNING AND POSITIONING

- Diagnostic imaging should include a computed tomography (CT) scan to evaluate for hydrocephalus and performance of ventriculostomy if ventricles are enlarged. Calcium or atherosclerotic changes in the aneurysm wall might preclude microsurgical clipping. Brain asymmetry (temporal lobe encephalomalacia, prior surgery, or sylvian anatomy) might affect the side of surgical approach. The relationship of the aneurysm neck to the posterior clinoid processes, dorsum sella, and clivus should be noted. The size of frontal sinuses is relevant. Intraluminal thrombus, which might be more apparent on CT angiography, should be noted and may be the inadvertent cause of distal emboli during manipulation of the aneurysm.
- Angiography details aneurysm size, neck size, morphology, laterality, aneurysm projection (anterior, posterior, superior, or lateral), and location of aneurysm neck relative to the posterior clinoid processes, dorsum sella, and clivus. Anatomy of branches at the aneurysm neck (P1 PCA, SCA, and perforating arteries) is evident, as is any discrepancy between intraluminal size on angiography and extraluminal size on CT or magnetic resonance imaging (MRI) to suggest intraluminal thrombus. The posterior communicating artery (PCoA) and P1 PCA are examined for fetal anatomy and anterior-to-posterior collateral circulation. Other aneurysms might influence the side of surgical approach. The location of perforating arteries relative to the neck should be assessed. Other angiographic abnormalities may also be evident, such as early vasospasm, arterial occlusions, associated arteriovenous malformations, and moyamoya disease.
- Special equipment may include a radiolucent head holder in the event an intraoperative angiogram is needed, reciprocating saw for orbitozygomatic osteotomies, diamond burr (1- or 2-mm-diameter ball tip) or ultrasonic aspirator with bone curettage tip for removal of the posterior clinoid process with low-lying basilar apex aneurysms, aneurysm clips (permanent and temporary), Rhoton dissectors, Doppler flow probe, and intraoperative angiography either with conventional catheter angiography or indocyanine green dye.

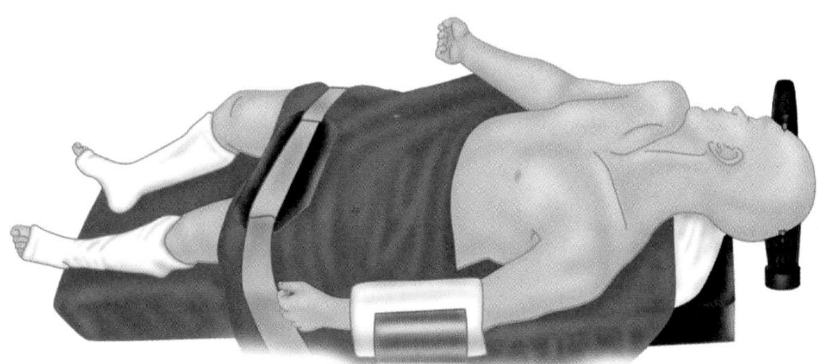

FIGURE 27-1

- The operating room setup may include bipolar cautery and Bovie cautery; operating microscope (foot pedal for focus and zoom, mouthpiece for fine adjustments); chair with arm rests and floor wheels; and neurophysiologic monitoring equipment with somatosensory evoked potentials, motor evoked potentials, and electroencephalography.
- Anesthetic issues include the following: On skin incision, 1 g of Ancef, 10 mg of dexamethasone (Decadron), and 1 g/kg of mannitol are administered. Cerebral perfusion pressure is maintained at greater than 70 mm Hg to prevent ischemia from brain retraction, temporary blood vessel occlusion, or vasospasm. Severe hypertension is treated aggressively with propofol, thiopental, or vasoactive drugs. Temperature is allowed to drift toward 34° C (93.2° F), and rewarming is started after aneurysm clipping. Relative hypervolemia and above-normal blood pressure are allowed after aneurysm clipping in patients with vasospasm.

Positioning for Orbitozygomatic Craniotomy

- **Figure 27-1:** The patient is supine with the head fixed in a Mayfield head holder.
- Head tilted 15 degrees from midline to contralateral side of approach, with moderate head extension and elevation
- Bilateral kidney rests to allow operating table to be laterally rotated
- Leyla bar holder attached to the operating table on the side opposite to the craniotomy

PROCEDURE

Orbitozygomatic Craniotomy

- Orbitozygomatic craniotomy is the preferred exposure for all basilar apex aneurysms because it allows for the full range of approaches to the basilar apex, from an anterior supraorbital trajectory to lateral subtemporal trajectories.
- In patients with large frontal sinuses likely to be entered with craniotomy or orbital osteotomy, pericranium is harvested after the scalp flap is reflected.
- Orbital rim and zygoma are exposed with a subfascial dissection, which is preferred over interfascial dissection, to preserve frontalis nerve function.
- Careful preservation of periorbital fascia facilitates later osteotomy cuts and reduces postoperative orbital edema.
- The orbitozygomatic piece is removed as a single unit after the craniotomy flap is removed, with notched cuts in the zygomatic root and maxillary bone for better seating of the unit on closure.
- Plating holes are drilled before the orbitozygomatic unit is removed for better cosmesis.
- The medial osteotomy lies just lateral to the supraorbital notch; the craniotomy should extend approximately 1 cm medial to this landmark.
- Orbital roof and lateral orbital wall are removed back to the orbital apex.
- Lateral temporal bone is drilled flush with the middle fossa floor to facilitate lateral temporal lobe retraction.

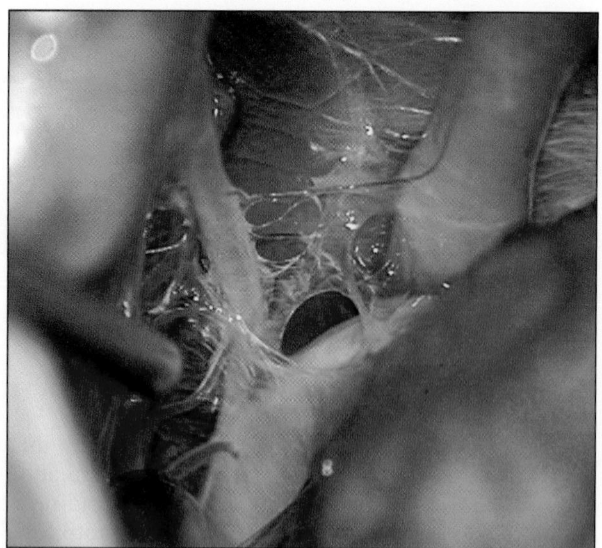

FIGURE 27-2

- Multiple tacking sutures in the reflected dura flap are needed to depress the eye and maximize the surgical corridor.
- Meticulous hemostasis is necessary to prevent blood from running down into the surgical corridor.

Dissection

- **Figure 27-2:** Wide splitting of the sylvian fissure is essential, exposing the middle cerebral artery trifurcation, M1 segment, and distal M2 middle cerebral artery branches.
- A frontal, self-retaining (Greenberg) retractor is placed on the frontal lobe at the junction of olfactory and optic nerves.
- The carotid cisterns are opened to drain cerebrospinal fluid, and the A1 anterior cerebral artery is followed out of the lamina terminalis for fenestration and additional cerebrospinal fluid drainage.
- The temporal lobe is mobilized by coagulating and cutting arachnoid adhesions between the inferior temporal lobe and middle fossa dura, then coagulating and cutting the temporal pole vein bridging to the sphenoparietal sinus.
- The arachnoid planes are opened along the tentorial edge, freeing the oculomotor nerve from its connections to the temporal lobe.
- The PCoA and anterior choroidal artery are identified. The PCoA leads to the membrane of Lillequist, which is carefully opened to enter the posterior fossa. The anterior choroidal artery leads to the choroidal fissure, and careful dissection of this artery separates the deep adhesions between frontal and temporal lobes to maximize temporal lobe mobilization.
- Temporal lobe is retracted posteriorly and laterally, with the retractor tip placed on the uncus.
- In patients with subarachnoid hemorrhage, clot obscures the vascular anatomy and should be removed carefully along normal anatomy as it is uncovered. The PCoA serves as the guiding landmark into thick clot, leading the dissection to the P1-P2 PCA junction and preventing inadvertent encounters with the aneurysm dome.
- The PCoA and its perforating arteries can be swept superiorly to open the surgical corridor to more medial structures. Occasionally, the PCoA may require sacrifice to widen the exposure, but this maneuver should be performed only when the PCoA is small and the ipsilateral P1 PCA can be preserved with microsurgical clipping. The PCoA should not be sacrificed when there is fetal anatomy or when clipping might compromise flow in the P1 PCA.

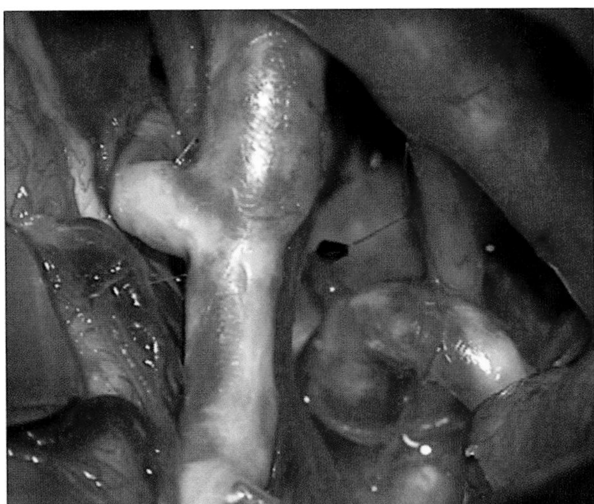

FIGURE 27-3

- **Figure 27-3:** The undersurface of the P1 PCA is followed medially to its intersection with the basilar artery, where the SCA is also identified.
- Aneurysm dissection is avoided until a segment of the basilar artery is secured below the SCA for proximal control.
- Identify the four vessels arising from the apex and decrease the patient's head rotation as needed to bring the basilar trunk and contralateral vessels into view.
- Identify and exclude posterior P1 perforating arteries by dissecting along the back wall of the basilar artery proximal to the ipsilateral P1 toward the base of the contralateral P1.
- For low-riding lesions, the posterior clinoid and upper portion of the clivus can be drilled off with a diamond burr or ultrasonic aspirator equipped with a bone curettage tip. Bleeding from the posteromedial cavernous sinus is controlled with bone wax or absorbable hemostat.

Temporary Clipping

- Temporary clipping should be considered when the aneurysm appears fragile or thin-walled and mobilization is required to visualize relevant anatomy. Temporary clipping softens the aneurysm to facilitate its manipulation and reduces the risk of intraoperative rupture.
- An area below the SCA relatively free of circumflex perforating arteries is identified for temporary clipping.
- Application of the temporary clip below the oculomotor nerve is preferred. Application of the temporary clip above the oculomotor nerve places the clip in the limited working space around the aneurysm and can crowd the field.
- Perforating arteries at the base of the aneurysm are dissected away from the neck, taking care to deflect the aneurysm rather than the perforating arteries. Dissection of these delicate perforating arteries is minimized because of their susceptibility to spasm. Perforating arteries do not need to be freed along their entire length, only enough to pass the posterior blade of the clip.
- **Figure 27-4:** The origin of the contralateral P1 PCA is carefully dissected and inspected because it determines the lie of the clip and can harbor the perforating arteries that are the most difficult to visualize.
- If the aneurysm remains tense with proximal temporary clipping, temporary clips may be needed on the PCoA.

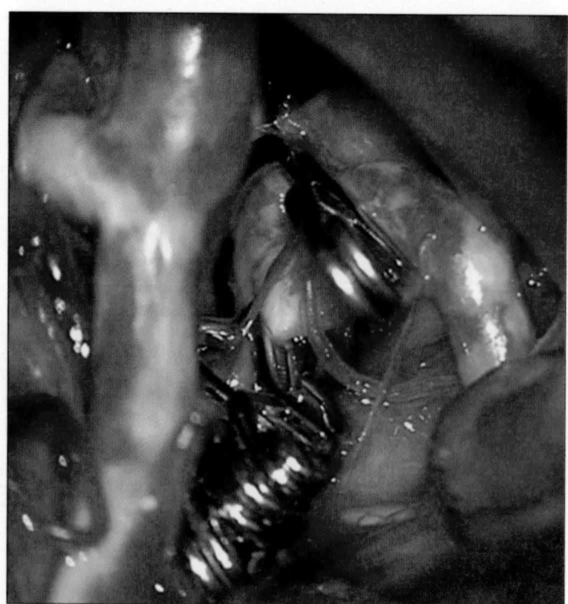

FIGURE 27-4

Permanent Clipping of the Aneurysm

- Permanent clip placement should be performed with the aneurysm, both sides of the neck, and perforating arteries under direct and complete visualization.
- Generally, long, straight clips are most useful to clip basilar aneurysms because the view is tangential along the clip, and long blades keep the shank of the clip from obstructing the view (see Figure 27-4).
- Small aneurysms with narrow necks often can be clipped with a single clip.
- Large aneurysms with wide necks often require clipping with multiple clips. Fenestrated clips are ideally suited for closing the distal neck, with the fenestration transmitting the proximal aneurysm neck and sometimes perforating arteries originating from the ipsilateral P1 PCA. A second nonfenestrated clip is used to close the fenestration and complete the clip reconstruction.
- Temporary clip time is minimized, and these clips should be used only during the final stages of the dissection and permanent clip application.

Reexamination of the Complex Aneurysm

- The aneurysm is palpated with a No. 6 Rhoton dissector, and if aneurysm pulsation indicates residual filling, the temporary clip should be replaced and the permanent clips should be inspected. The site of residual filling is usually at the distal neck, and the first clip can be advanced to address this problem. Visualization is often improved after this initial tentative clipping.
- If a perforating artery is caught in a clip, it must be freed.
- Sometimes a well-placed clip fails to close an aneurysm because of splaying of the tips of the blades. In these cases, an additional clip can be stacked above the initial clip to reinforce the closure.
- **Figure 27-5:** When the aneurysm looks well clipped, an intraoperative angiogram (catheter digital subtraction angiography or indocyanine green dye) is performed or the aneurysm is punctured for confirmation.
- Neurophysiologic monitoring data are carefully analyzed for changes as the clipping is inspected.

Postoperative Care

- Dexamethasone (Decadron) is given for 48 hours.
- Noncontrast brain CT scan is obtained on postoperative day 1.

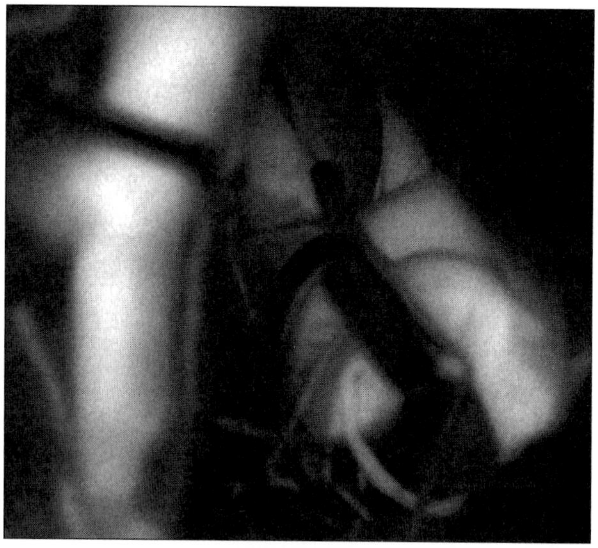

FIGURE 27-5

- Digital subtraction angiography is performed before hospital discharge to confirm exclusion of the aneurysm, absence of neck remnants, and preservation of parent and branch arteries.
- Patients with ruptured aneurysm require careful surveillance for vasospasm.

TIPS FROM THE MASTERS

- The secret to good results with basilar artery aneurysms is patient selection. In this endovascular era, it is important to identify aneurysms that are favorable for microsurgical clipping or, conversely, unfavorable for endovascular coiling. Factors that complicate microsurgical clipping include swollen brain with increased intracranial pressure and poor Hunt and Hess grade; posterior projection of the aneurysm; unusually high-lying or low-lying neck, relative to the posterior clinoid process; and calcified atherosclerotic tissue at the aneurysm neck. These patients should be considered for endovascular coiling. Factors that complicate microsurgical clipping but still make it preferable over coiling include large or giant size, broad neck, complex branching of the PCA or SCA or both, and intraluminal thrombus.
- Temporary clipping is important because it softens the aneurysm and enables aggressive mobilization of the aneurysm. In such a tight space with limited viewing room, it is crucial to be able to move the aneurysm safely to free perforating arteries or visualize contralateral anatomy.
- Morbidity results from the perforating arteries, particularly the adherent ones that are poorly visualized on the far side of the neck. These perforating arteries must be anticipated and dissected painstakingly until free. After clipping, this blind side should be checked and double-checked for perforating arteries not seen before clipping.
- The problem with poorly clipped aneurysms usually lies at the distal neck, which is the deepest spot, hardest to visualize, and the first to be clipped. Aneurysms that still fill after permanent clipping often need to be redone by removing the second and third clips and carefully readjusting the initial clip. Fenestrated clips are useful in completely shutting this particular spot on the neck.
- Basilar artery aneurysms have a difficult learning curve, and poor outcomes should be studied thoroughly to advance one's technical abilities and avoid repeating past mistakes.

PITFALLS

Premature Rupture of Aneurysm before Control of Basilar Artery

- *Avoidance*: Careful placement of initial retractor; brain relaxation with release of cerebrospinal fluid from carotid cisterns and third ventricle via lamina terminalis fenestration; avoidance of hypertension; judicious removal of clot in the interpeduncular cistern, leaving thrombus over the dome and removing thrombus only at the neck
- *Intervention*: Hypotension and pack basilar cisterns with cotton; continue dissection when bleeding abates

Rupture of Aneurysm during Clipping

- *Avoidance*: Gentle dissection under temporary occlusion; stay away from dome where the walls are thinnest; focus dissection on the aneurysm base where the blades need to lie; save the riskiest maneuvers until the final steps
- *Intervention*: Prepare for rupture before it happens (administer cerebroprotective agents, preselect temporary and permanent clips, plan the clip configurations); do not panic; apply a cottonoid to the rupture site to clear the field; switch to a larger suction if necessary; apply a temporary clip to the proximal basilar artery; apply permanent clips; maintain normal blood pressure or increase blood pressure if neurophysiologic signals change

Injury to Brainstem Perforating Arteries

- *Avoidance*: Delicate handling of perforating arteries; under temporary clipping, mobilize aneurysm wall instead of already stretched perforating artery; dissect only enough artery to pass the clip blade; do not apply the permanent clip until the entire posterior wall is dissected and perforating arteries are identified; do not use cautery to control bleeding around perforating arteries
- *Intervention*: If a perforating artery is included in the permanent clip, reposition the clip; if perforating artery is in spasm, apply papaverine; if artery cannot be dissected off the aneurysm base, use fenestrated clips to clip around it

Injury to Oculomotor Nerve

- *Avoidance*: Minimize direct contact with the nerve, dissecting its arachnoidal layers and handling only these supporting tissues; separate its arachnoidal connections to the temporal lobe; carefully preserve its vascular supply; do not use cautery around the nerve
- *Intervention*: Steroids; counsel patient that the deficit is usually transient

SUGGESTED READINGS

Hsu FP, Clatterbuck RE, Spetzler RF. Orbitozygomatic approach to basilar apex aneurysms. Neurosurgery 2005;56(1 Suppl):172–7; discussion 172–7.

Lawton MT, Daspit CP, Spetzler RF. Technical aspects and recent trends in the management of large and giant midbasilar artery aneurysms. Neurosurgery 1997;41(3):513–20; discussion 520–1.

Sanai N, Zador Z, Lawton MT. Bypass surgery for complex brain aneurysms: an assessment of intracranial-intracranial bypass. Neurosurgery 2009;65(4):670–83; discussion 683.

Procedure 28

Craniotomy for Resection of Intracranial Cortical Arteriovenous Malformation

Christopher S. Eddleman, Christopher C. Getch, Bernard R. Bendok, H. Hunt Batjer

INDICATIONS

- Eloquently located ruptured arteriovenous malformation (AVM) with significant hematoma and neurologic deficit
- Angioarchitectural features that deem the cortical AVM at higher risk of hemorrhage (e.g., deep venous drainage, intranidal aneurysms, venous stenosis, venous hypertension, previous hemorrhage)
- Worsening neurologic deficits or seizures despite optimal nonsurgical therapy
- Safely treatable cortical AVM in a young patient with lifelong exposure to natural history risks of an AVM
- Psychological burden or personal limitations of activities of living with knowledge of the lesion and its natural history risks of an AVM

CONTRAINDICATIONS

- Premorbid conditions increasing surgical risks beyond natural history risks, including coagulopathies or cardiopulmonary compromise
- Asymptomatic AVM within functionally eloquent cortex as defined by location and functional magnetic resonance imaging (MRI)
- Angioarchitectural features that present a high surgical risk, such as a diffuse nidus near or within eloquent cortex in unruptured AVM
- Personal, religious and nonreligious, wishes of patient or family
- Older age or limited life expectancy in asymptomatic patient with fewer years of natural history risk

PLANNING AND POSITIONING

- Preoperative planning includes a detailed study of the location and angioarchitectural features of the AVM, including any angiomatous change, location of the feeding arteries, draining veins, and extent of the nidus. Preoperative imaging should include MRI and catheter-based angiography. Computed tomography (CT) angiography and magnetic resonance angiography may also be performed. Functional and diffusion tensor MRI may be used to assess the functional status and pathway of white matter tracts of the surrounding brain parenchyma.
- Intraoperative mapping may be used in cases in which the AVM is located in or near functionally eloquent cortex.
- **Figure 28-1:** The patient is placed in a Mayfield head clamp. Shoulder rolls may be used for patients with limited neck mobility. For frontal, temporal, and sylvian AVMs, the head is turned so that the craniotomy flap is at the highest point of the head. For lesions in the posterior parietal, occipital, and posterior fossa, patients can be positioned in the lateral prone position or, rarely, in the sitting position.

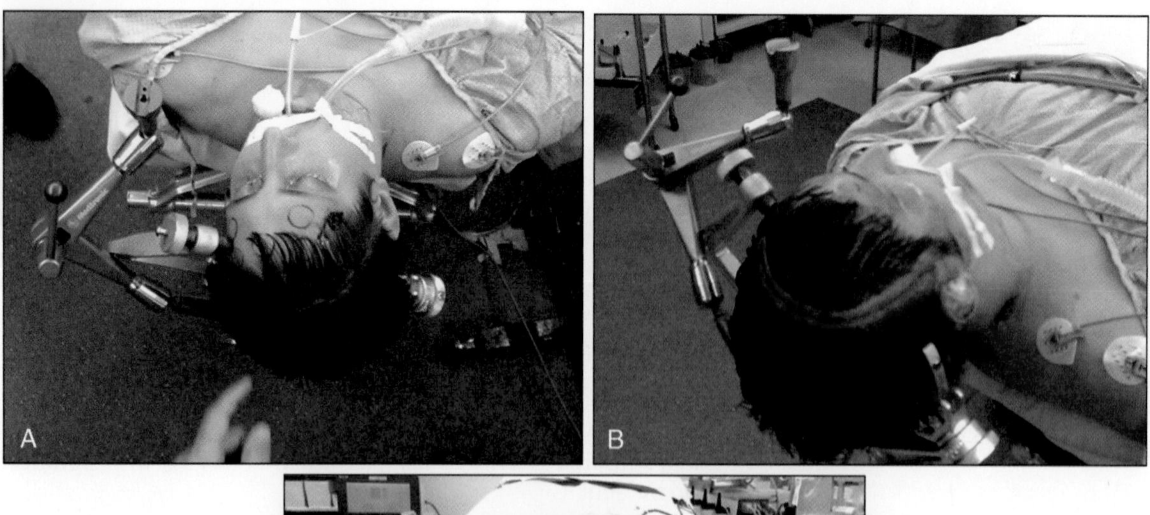

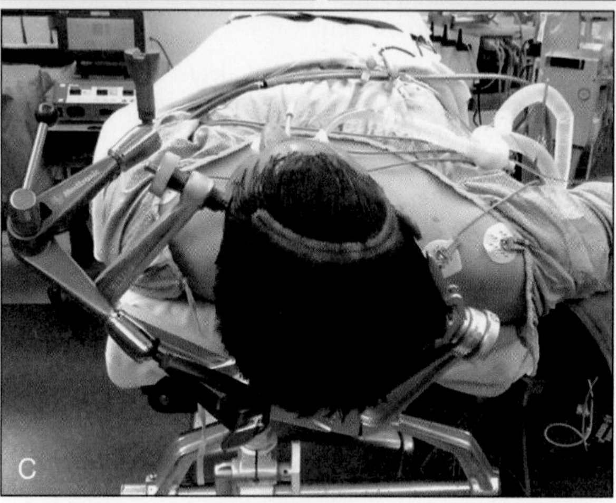

FIGURE 28-1

- **Figure 28-2:** After positioning, AVM architecture is mapped out using neuronavigation so that the skin incision is adequate for the bone flap to encompass the brain parenchyma beyond the AVM nidus and all of the cortical arterial feeders and draining veins.

PROCEDURE

- **Figure 28-3:** Skin is incised in the standard fashion. Extra precaution should be taken if arterial feeders emanating from the external carotid arteries feed the AVM nidus because this can lead to significant bleeding. When the skull is exposed, the AVM is mapped out again using a neuronavigation system for bone flap planning. Burr holes should be placed beyond the borders of the AVM nidus so that adequate exposure can be accomplished, and potential nidal rupture with plunging of the perforating drill can be avoided. Care should be exercised when crossing locations of draining veins with a craniotome to avoid unnecessary bleeding.
- **Figure 28-4:** When the bone flap has been removed, the dura should be tacked up to the surrounding bone, taking care not to penetrate vessels underlying the dura. The dural opening should be adequate enough to expose entire AVM nidus, feeding arteries, and draining veins on the cortical surface. The dura can be opened using a knife along with a dural guide or scissors. The dura should be reflected very gently because vessels associated with the AVM can be adherent to the dura, and tearing could result in AVM bleeding.
- **Figure 28-5:** When the dura is opened, the cortical angioarchitecture of the AVM, arachnoid planes associated with the feeding arteries and draining veins, and sulci

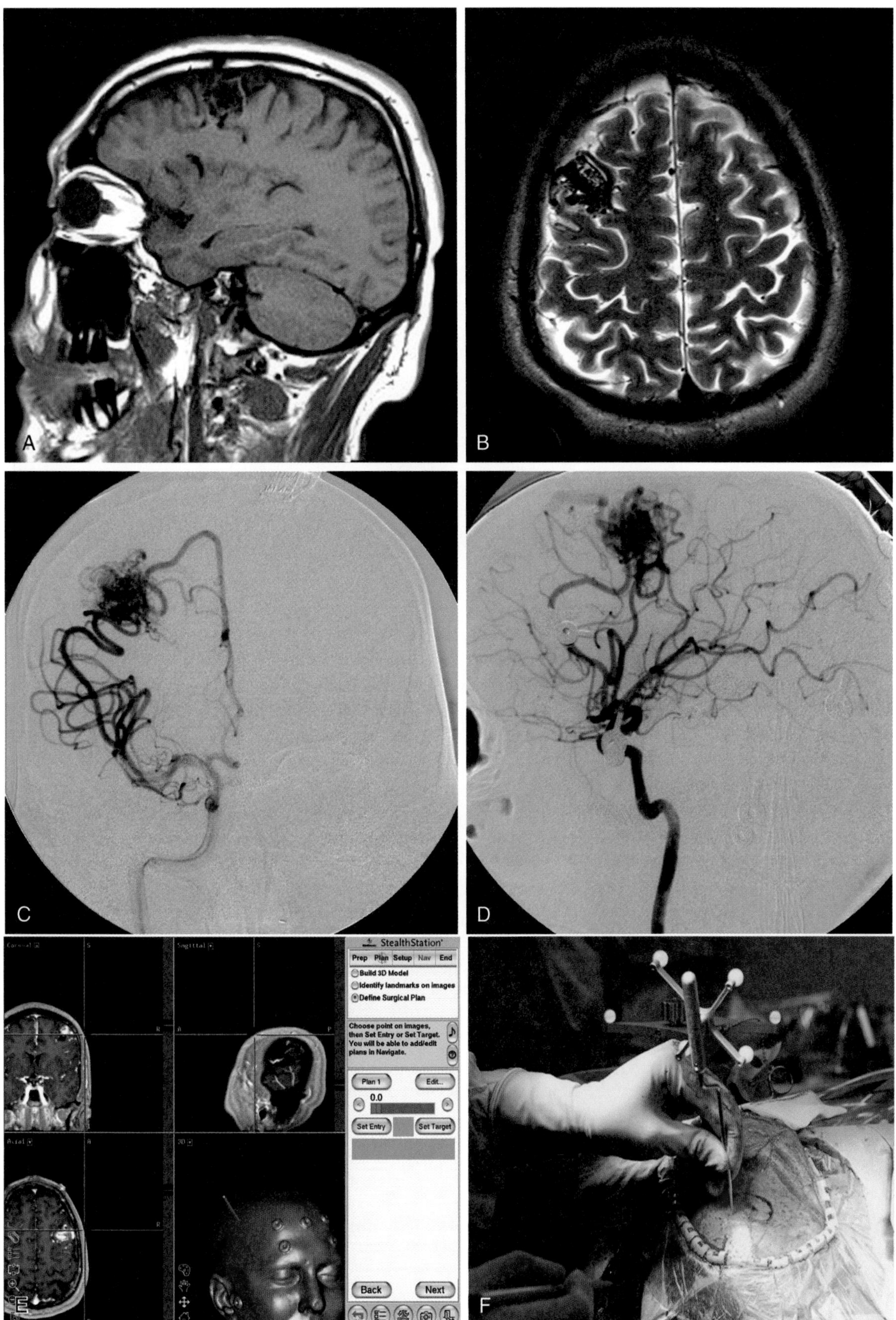
A
B
C
D
StealthStation
Prep Plan Setup Nav End
Build 3D Model
Identify landmarks on images
Define Surgical Plan
Choose point on images, then Set Entry or Set Target. You will be able to add/edit plans in Navigate.
Plan 1
Edit...
0.0
Set Entry
Set Target
Back
Next
E
F

FIGURE 28-2

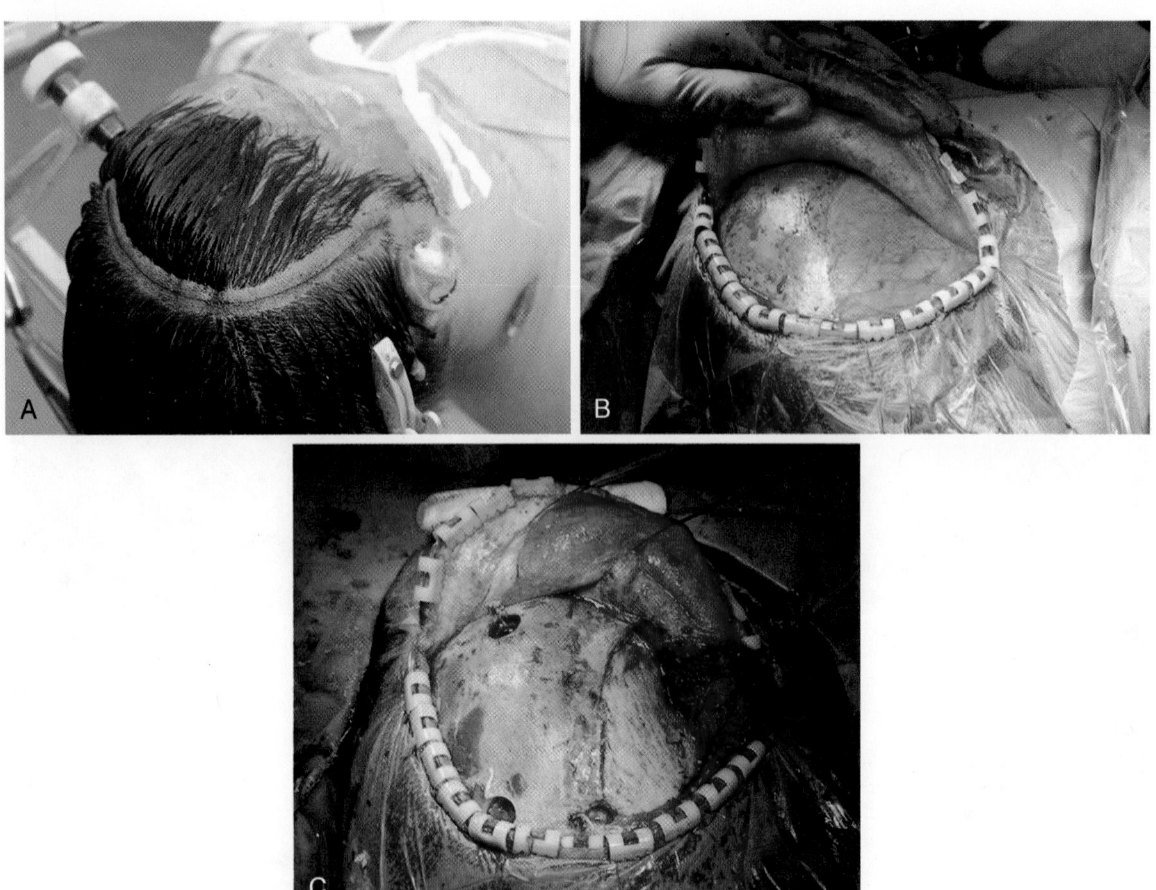

FIGURE 28-3

should be identified. The arachnoidal phase of the dissection can begin by dissecting out all of the associated vessels with the cortical AVM. This dissection allows improved mobilization and identification of associated vessels and en passage vessels. The AVM can be initially devascularized by clipping of the cortical feeding arteries.

- **Figure 28-6:** When all components of the AVM are identified on the cortical surface, the parenchymal phase of the dissection can begin, dissecting around the AVM in a spiral fashion. A gliotic tissue plane frequently exists because of chronic ischemic changes that facilitate identification of such a plane. Each plane of the dissection can be delineated with Telfa or cotton pledgets so that the plane can be more easily identified later. Retraction during dissection should always be on the AVM nidus and not on the surrounding brain parenchyma.
- **Figure 28-7:** Draining veins should always be maintained until the end of the dissection. Inadvertent sacrifice might cause congestion of the AVM nidus leading to rupture. Arterial feeders should be sacrificed throughout the parenchymal dissection. Although bipolar cautery can be used for numerous feeders, small AVM clips may be used on larger arterial feeders with or without subsequent electrocautery. Careful attention should be paid to loops of vessels and potential en passage vessels because these could be important for distal blood supply and merely incidentally associated with the nidus, making their sacrifice unnecessary and a potential cause of morbidity.
- **Figure 28-8:** When the dissection plane has led to the apex of the nidus, special attention must be paid to the deep arterial supply. Often these arterial feeders are small and high flow, making their control difficult with electrocautery. Small AVM clips are useful. If the bleeding cannot be controlled, it may be necessary to remove the bulk of the AVM nidus so that the remaining AVM deep in the resection bed can be better controlled.

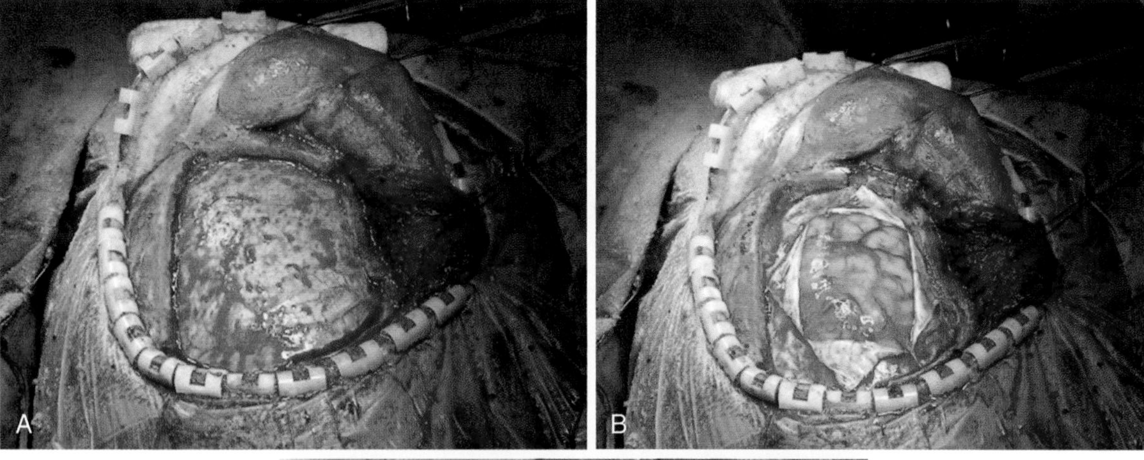

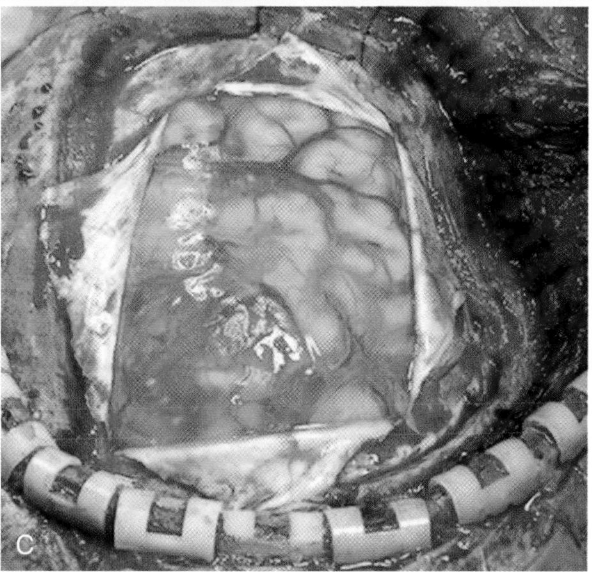

FIGURE 28-4

- **Figure 28-9:** After the AVM nidus has been removed, the resection bed must be examined for residual nidus and areas of bleeding. Continuous bleeding often means residual nidus and should be examined closely. Intraoperative imaging may consist of digital subtraction angiography with or without supplementary indocyanine green dye videoangiography. The resection bed must be completely dry because increases in systolic blood pressure can easily lead to rebleeding necessitating evacuation. Systolic blood pressure can be increased temporarily to high-normal levels to check for areas of potential bleeding.
- **Figure 28-10:** The bone flap and incision are closed in the standard fashion. Definitive postoperative imaging (catheter-based angiography) should be performed when possible to ensure complete resection of the AVM nidus.

TIPS FROM THE MASTERS

- Three-dimensional knowledge of the AVM and its associated vessels is key for planning an effective and efficient strategy for removal. High-resolution vascular imaging and intraoperative neuronavigation are extremely helpful.
- Adequate surgical exposure is important to avoid the risks of working through a narrow surgical corridor. Wide bony exposure allows improved visualization and the room required if an assistant is needed to help clear the field from blood. In a parasagittal AVM that may not have pial representation in the interhemispheric fissure,

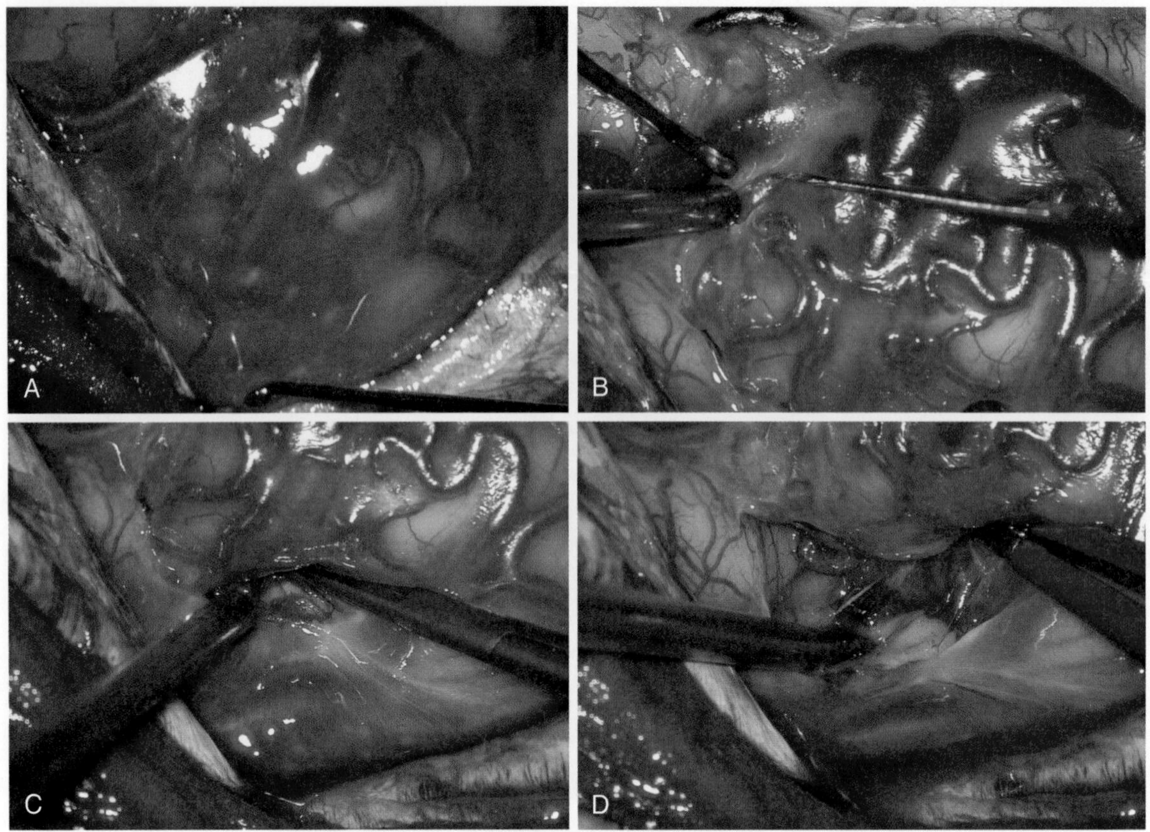

FIGURE 28-5

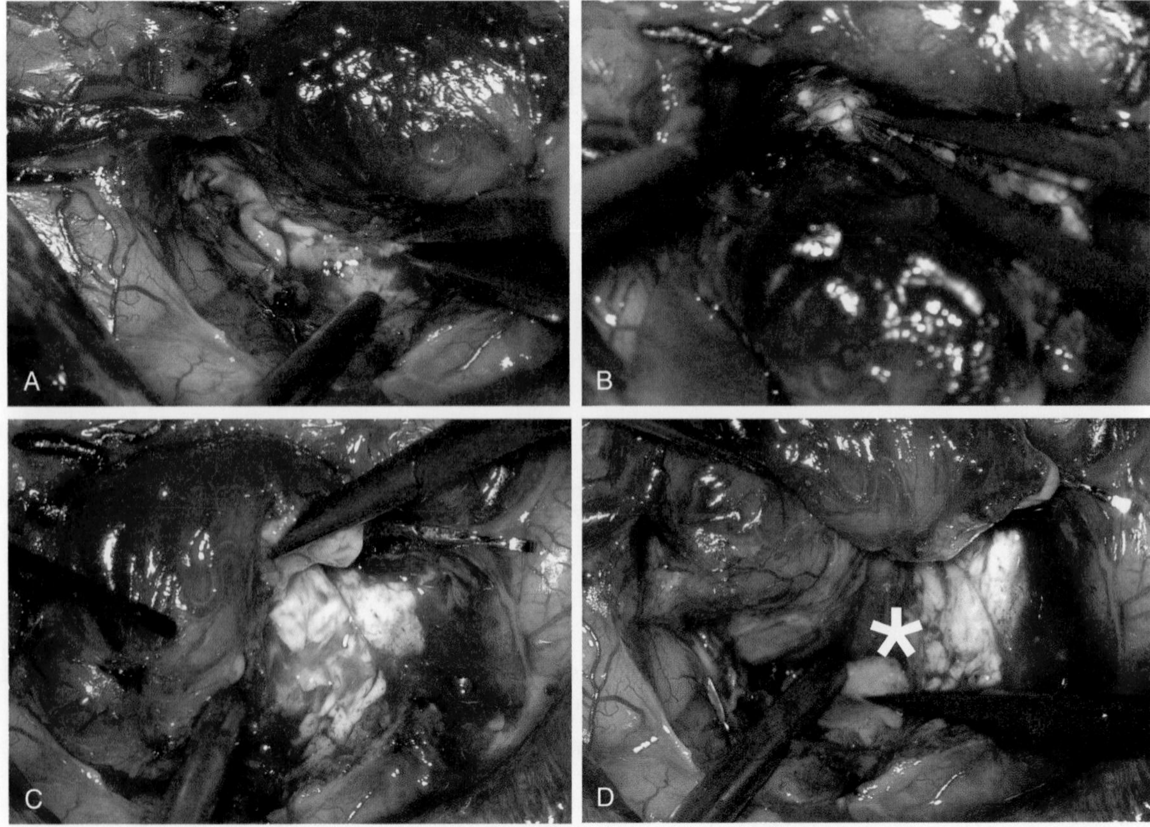

FIGURE 28-6

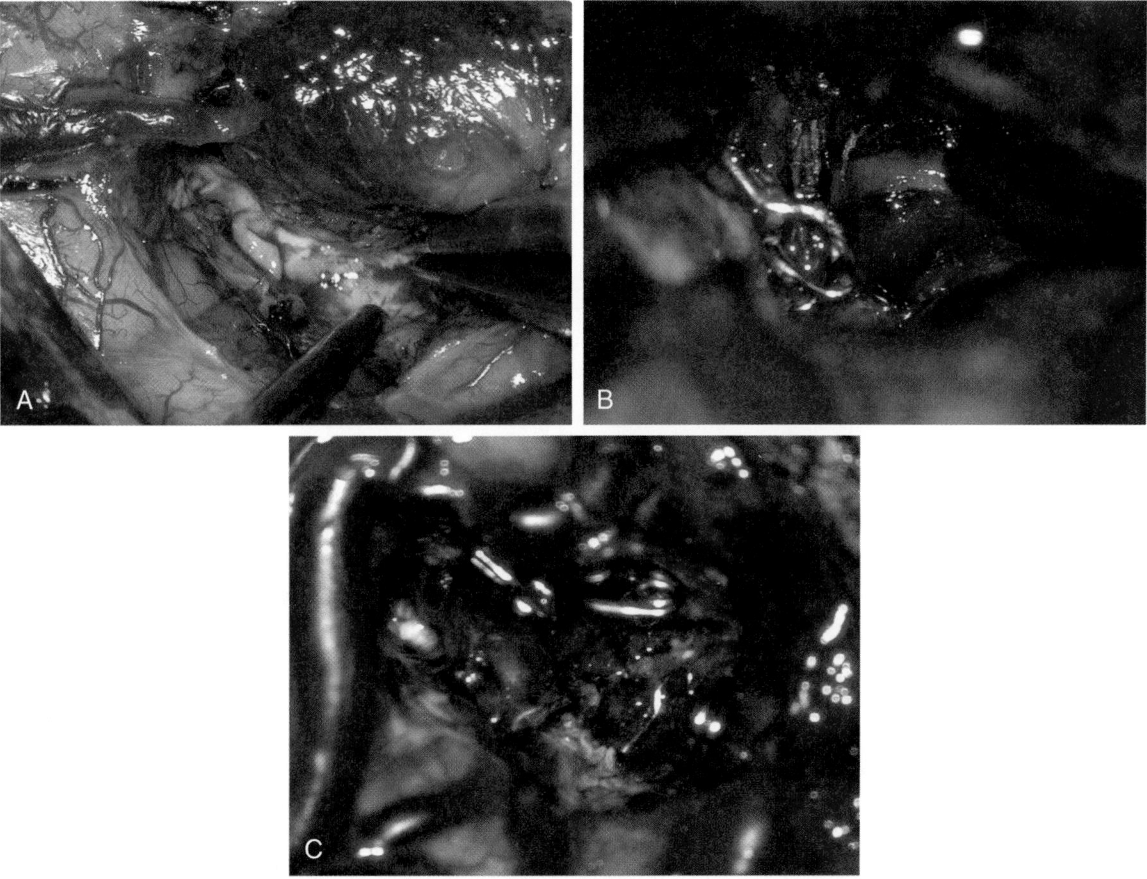

FIGURE 28-7

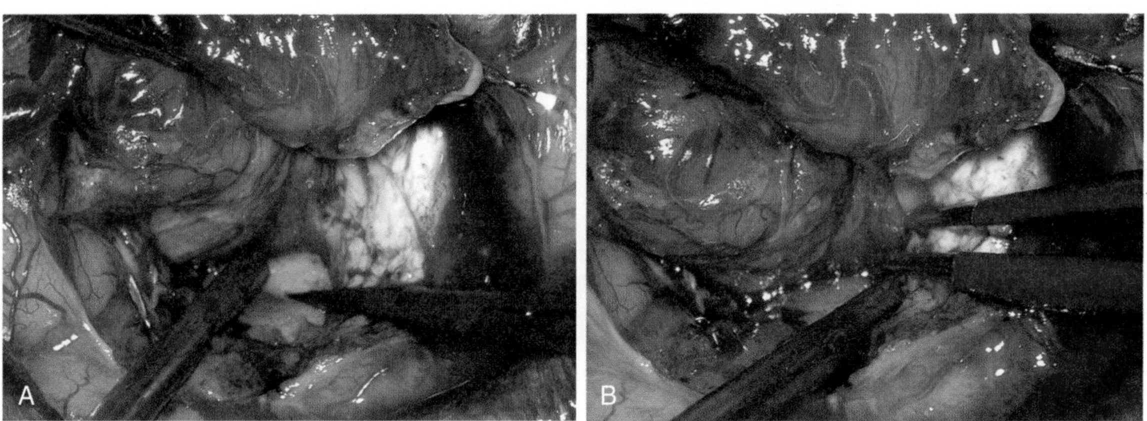

FIGURE 28-8

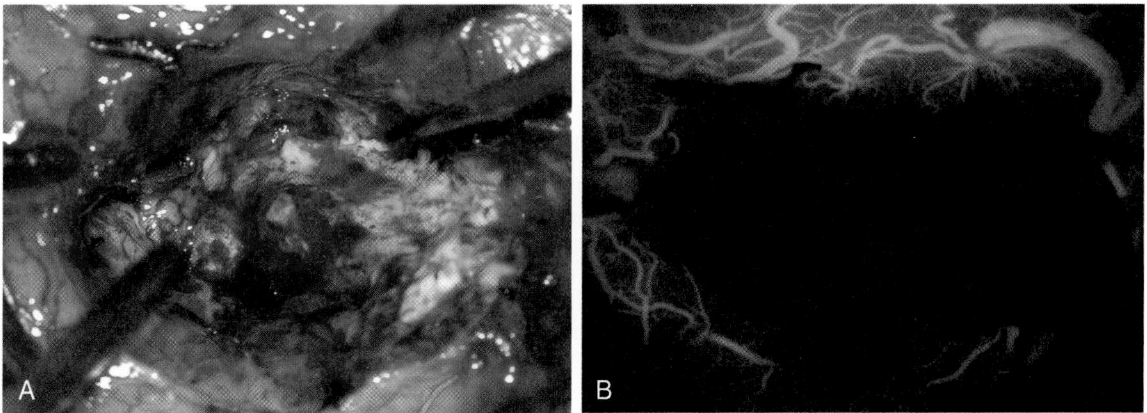

FIGURE 28-9

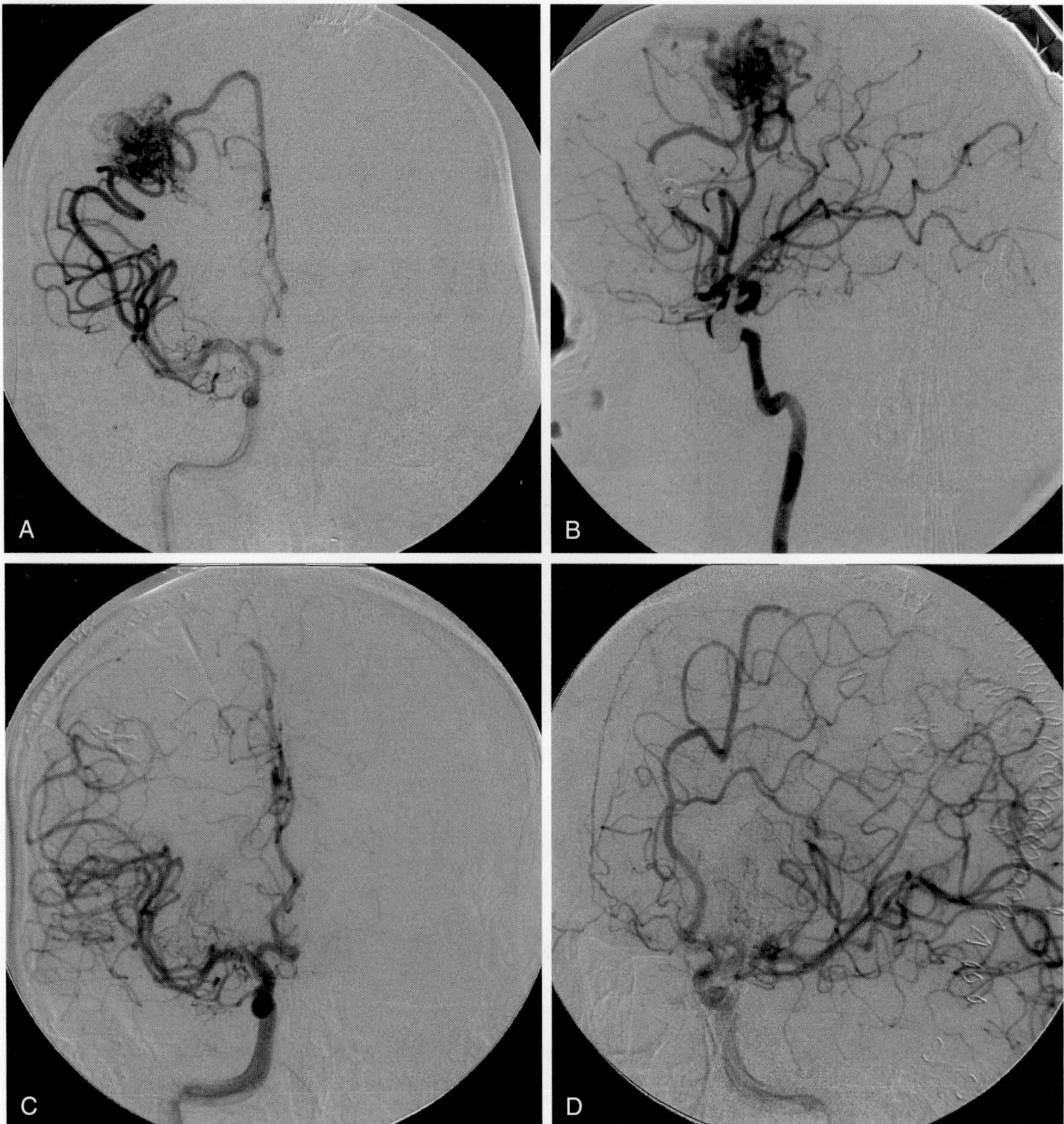

FIGURE 28-10

if substantial anterior cerebral feeding is present, it may be helpful to perform the craniotomy crossing the midline to facilitate access to the interhemispheric fissure for proximal control.

- Preoperative embolization can be helpful for staged flow reduction in larger AVMs in cases of inaccessible deep feeding vessels and in perisylvian lesions in which Onyx landmark can help facilitate rapid identification of vessels en passant in distinction to vessels heading for the malformation.
- During the parenchymal phase of dissection, persistent bleeding can be controlled either by using small cotton balls to tamponade the bleeding site gently and decrease arterial flow to facilitate coagulation or by moving the focus of dissection slightly so that the bleeding area on the malformation can be actively retracted. Packing the area of hemorrhage with cotton and other hemostatic agents can be problematic because hemorrhage can be diverted into the brain parenchyma and ventricles with catastrophic results. If nidal penetration is suspected, the surgeon must withdraw to a more superficial location and reenter a dissection plane outside the nidus. It is futile to continue attempts at coagulation when a malformation has been violated early in the course of the procedure.

PITFALLS

Arteriolar feeding vessels, particularly near the ventricle, can be difficult to manage. The flow through these vessels is so rapid that the bipolar coagulation device simply cannot heat the vessels adequately to facilitate coagulation. If this technique is applied too aggressively, the vessels rupture and retract into deeper tissue, increasing the morbidity of the procedure. A much more desirable technique includes the early use of small AVM clips followed by successful coagulation, division of the vessel, and removal of the clips.

Sacrifice of the dominant draining vein early in the procedure leads to nidal congestion and increases the turgor of the AVM during dissection and poses an increased risk of deep bleeding into the parenchyma or ventricular system.

Persistence and strategy regarding hemostasis are critical. In difficult situations, when the dissection planes are becoming increasingly difficult because of congestion and ongoing bleeding, it may be necessary to deliver the AVM nidus quickly. Clipping feeding vessels before cutting them is helpful, as is the use of two functioning surgeons working in tandem. Small cotton balls applied with gentle pressure can control aggressive bleeding. The cotton ball can be rolled around to facilitate precise exposure of the bleeding site.

After resection, meticulous hemostasis in the resection cavity is crucial because the hemodynamic impact of the resection is significant, and postoperative hematomas are a risk. Careful blood pressure control during closure, awakening, and in the first 24 to 36 hours is also critical. Extended periods of normal blood pressure to hypotension may be necessary depending on the size or complexity of the AVM.

SUGGESTED READINGS

Batjer HH. Treatment decisions in brain AVMs: the case for and against surgery. Clin Neurosurg 2000;46:319–25.

Getch CC, Eddleman CS, Swope MK, et al. Surgical principles. In: Intracranial Arteriovenous Malformations. London: Informa Healthcare; 2006.

McCarthy DP, Bendok BR, Getch CC, et al. Surgical approaches. In: Intracranial Arteriovenous Malformations. London: Informa Healthcare; 2006.

Nussbaum ES, Heros RC, Camarata PJ. Surgical treatment of intracranial arteriovenous malformations with an analysis of cost-effectiveness. Clin Neurosurg 1995;42:348–69.

Starke RM, Komotar RJ, Hwang BY, et al. Treatment guidelines for cerebral arteriovenous malformation microsurgery. Br J Neurosurg 2009;23:376–86.

Procedure 29

Subcortical Arteriovenous Malformations: Corpus Callosum, Lateral Ventricle, Thalamus, and Basal Ganglia

Marco Lee, Gary K. Steinberg

INDICATIONS

- Surgery is indicated for patients with arteriovenous malformations (AVMs) that have ruptured or are causing intractable seizures, progressive neurologic deficits, or intractable debilitating headaches. Often, failure of alternative therapies—embolization and stereotactic radiosurgery in symptomatic patients—is an indication for microsurgical intervention.
- It is mandatory to consider embolization and stereotactic radiosurgery for subcortical AVMs because of their location in eloquent structures. Multimodality approaches are usual, and staged resection of large AVMs is sometimes necessary.
- We favor resection of the AVM when the patient is stable and over the immediate acute period; this often means 3 to 4 weeks after the hemorrhage when the patient has had some recovery and the blood is liquefied. We also favor emergent evacuation of a hematoma that is producing significant mass effect and resecting the AVM at a later stage if possible.

CONTRAINDICATIONS

- Surgery is contraindicated in patients who are in a poor clinical condition; patients with medical conditions that preclude surgery; very elderly patients; and patients with AVMs that are located within eloquent areas without safe surgical corridors for approach, such as the intact motor, language, or visual cortices.

PLANNING AND POSITIONING

- Close study of a four-vessel cerebral angiogram is necessary to evaluate the arterial, capillary, and venous phases of the vessels; presence of aneurysms; size and configuration of the nidus; and the relationship of the nidus to feeding arteries and venous drainages. Magnetic resonance imaging (MRI) details the relationship of the AVM with the surrounding neuroanatomic structures, which helps in selecting the most appropriate surgical approach. Operative or endovascular treatment of ruptured proximal aneurysms should proceed before resection of the AVM.
- Brain relaxation techniques, such as the use of mannitol and lumbar cerebrospinal fluid drainage, should be considered, especially if the ventricles are not being entered. For patients with seizures, anticonvulsants and cortical mapping to locate the epileptic foci are indicated. Localization of language dominance with amobarbital (Amytal) studies or functional MRI may be helpful.
- We routinely administer prophylactic antibiotics, employ mild hypothermia, use electrophysiologic monitoring, insert a femoral catheter sheath for intraoperative angiography, and induce hypotension during the resection. Routine equipment includes a radiolucent three-point head fixation device, neuronavigation system, microscope, microsurgical instruments, self-retaining retractor system, nonadhering bipolar forceps, aneurysm microclips, and AVM miniclips.

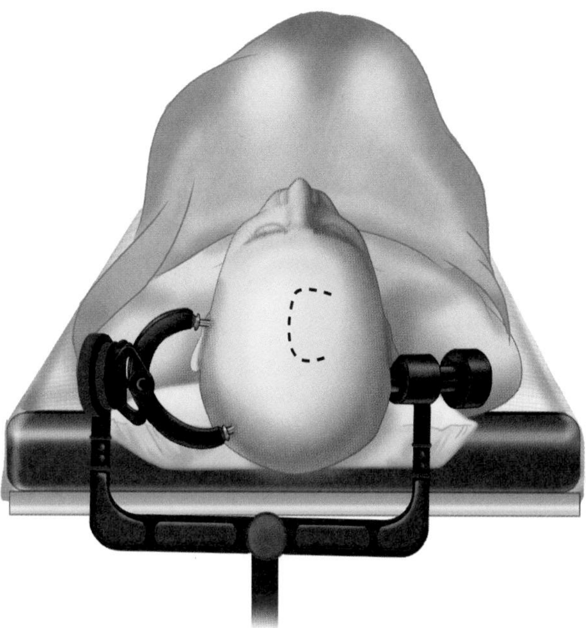

FIGURE 29-1

- **Figure 29-1:** Positioning of patients with callosal AVMs depends on the rostral-caudal location of the AVM. For frontal and parietal callosal AVMs, we prefer to have the patient supine, with the thorax raised 15 degrees and the head neutral and slightly flexed. The U-shaped skin flap is optimally centered over the nidus as guided by the neuronavigation system, based laterally and crossing the midline. A large enough scalp flap is fashioned to avoid compromise to the bridging veins from the medial cortex to the sagittal sinus.
- **Figure 29-2:** For occipital (splenial) callosal AVMs, we prefer to have the patient in a lateral position with the lesion side down and the thorax slightly elevated. A U-shaped incision centered over the AVM and large enough to incorporate the draining veins is marked, based over the superior nuchal line with the medial edge crossing the midline. This posterior interhemispheric approach is also suitable for intraventricular AVMs in the medial trigonal area.
- **Figure 29-3:** A transcallosal approach is favored for medial caudothalamic AVMs with the head turned so that the lesion side is down. The flap is similarly fashioned as in

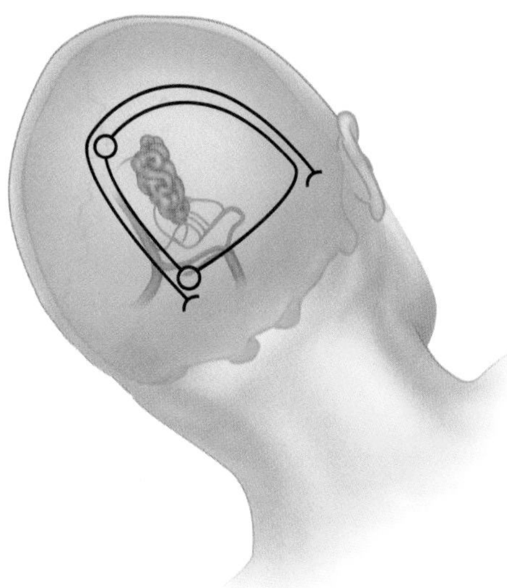

FIGURE 29-2

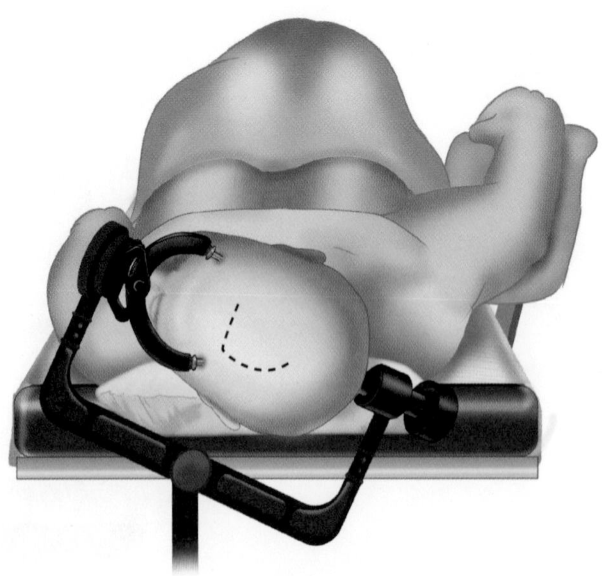

FIGURE 29-3

Figure 29-1, guided by the neuronavigation system. For more lateral and dorsally placed pulvinar AVMs, a transcortical approach is used, with the head turned, the lesion uppermost, and an inferiorly based parietooccipital skin flap fashioned.

PROCEDURE

- **Figure 29-4:** For frontal or parietal callosal AVM, the superior sagittal sinus should be exposed and the dura opened in a U shape based along the sagittal sinus. The medial cortical surface is dissected and gently retracted away from the falx with a self-retaining retractor. The dissection gradually deepens until the callosal marginal and pericallosal vessels are identified. A medial retractor may be used sometimes to retract the contralateral cingulate gyrus and improve exposure to the corpus callosum, although this additional retractor can decrease the working space.
- **Figure 29-5:** Anterior callosal AVMs are usually fed by branches of the ipsilateral callosal marginal and pericallosal arteries and venous drainage to the superior and inferior sagittal sinuses superficially and the subependymal veins deep within the ventricles. Care is taken to avoid damaging the draining veins when exposing the ipsilateral cingulate gyrus where dissection of the AVM begins, and the feeders from both arteries are gradually coagulated and cut.

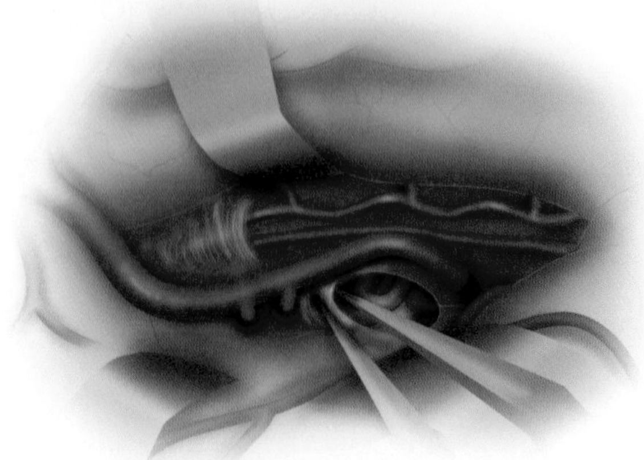

FIGURE 29-4

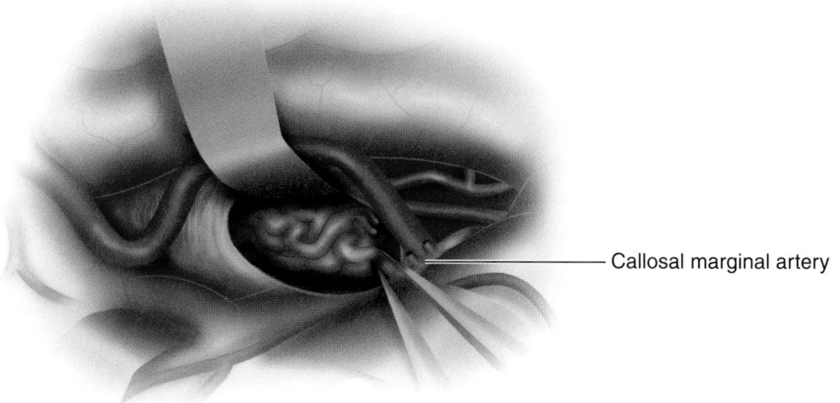

FIGURE 29-5

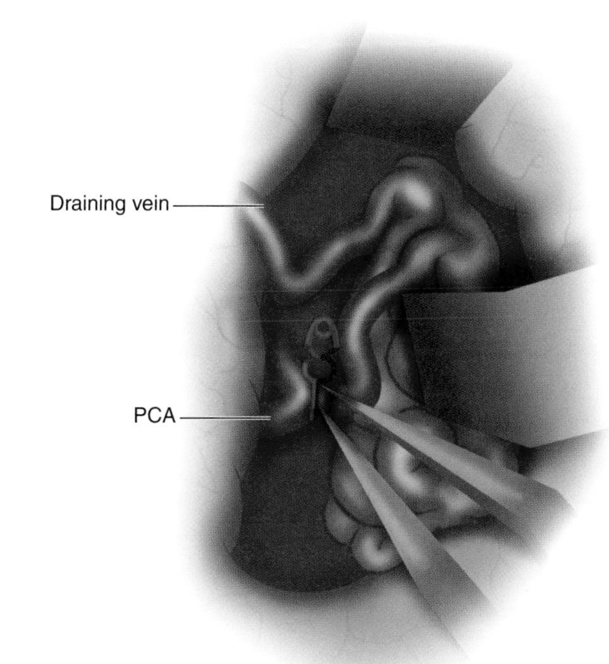

FIGURE 29-6

- **Figure 29-6:** In addition to pericallosal arteries, splenial AVMs are also fed by posterior choroidal arteries and other branches of the posterior cerebral artery. Venous drainage is usually to the internal cerebral veins and Galen veins. The parietal and occipital lobes are dissected away from the falx, and the dissection is similarly performed as in Figure 29-5. This approach is also suitable for AVMs located medial to the trigone, but the deep venous drainage is usually encountered before the arterial feeders.
- **Figure 29-7:** Medial caudothalamic lesions may be approached via the transcallosal-transventricular route. The lesions are most often fed by the anterior and posterior choroidal arteries with venous drainage to the thalamostriate and internal cerebral veins. The dissection begins as described in Figure 29-4 with the lesion side down. The retractors are deepened to aid separation of the two pericallosal arteries, and a 2- to 3-cm incision is made on the exposed corpus callosum.
- **Figure 29-8:** The ipsilateral ventricle is entered, and the AVM nidus is visualized. Most of the feeders are deep to the AVM, and dissection of the nidus alternately along the

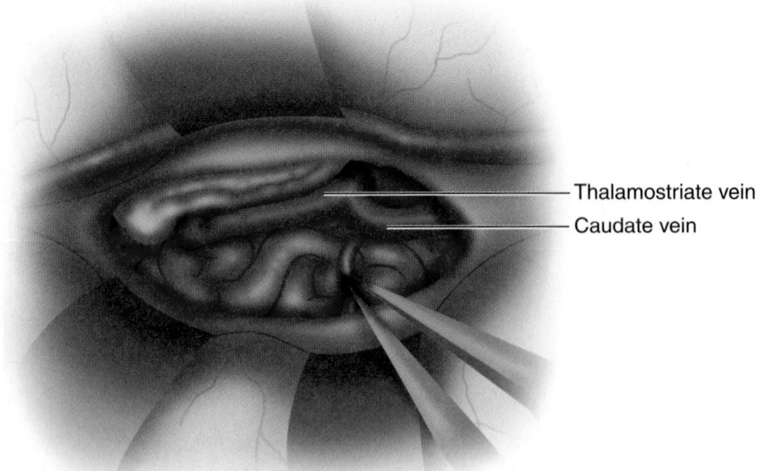

FIGURE 29-7

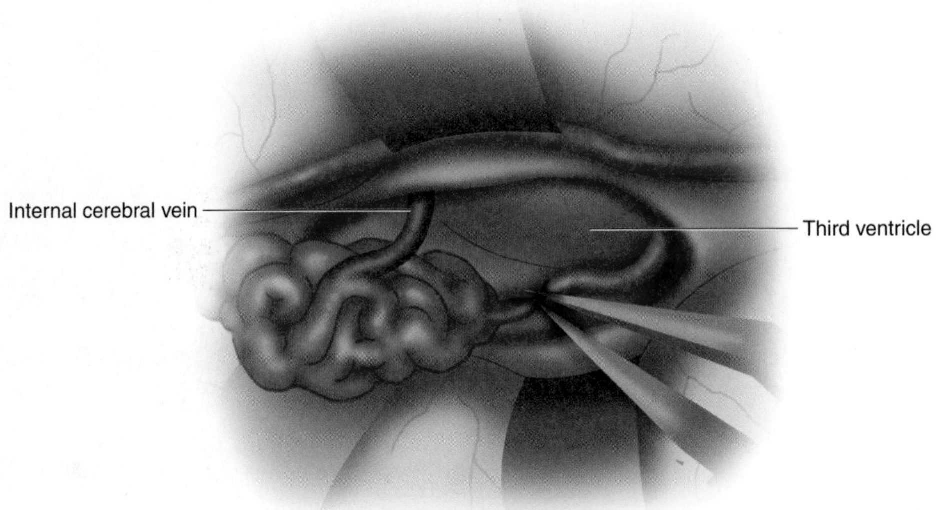

FIGURE 29-8

lateral and medial border is carried out progressively with coagulation or clipping of the feeders. The posterior thalamostriate and ependymal veins together with the distal choroid plexus are coagulated until the nidus is free and attached only to the internal cerebral vein, which is clipped and cut at the end.

- **Figure 29-9:** AVMs in the lateral dorsal pulvinar or posterior atrial regions may be approached via a transcortical parietooccipital route with the lesion uppermost. The dura is opened and based inferiorly. The trigone of the ipsilateral ventricle is entered by a cannula, which is passed through the parietooccipital fissure or using stereotactic guidance and brain retraction. The fissure is incised, deepened, and retracted until the ventricle is entered, and the pulvinar and choroid plexus are identified.
- **Figure 29-10:** The main feeders arise from branches of the posterior cerebral and posterior choroidal arteries, with the venous drainage mainly flowing to the internal cerebral vein and Galen veins. The arterial feeders are coagulated along the base of the AVM along with the choroid plexus, and the posterior choroidal fissure is opened laterally.

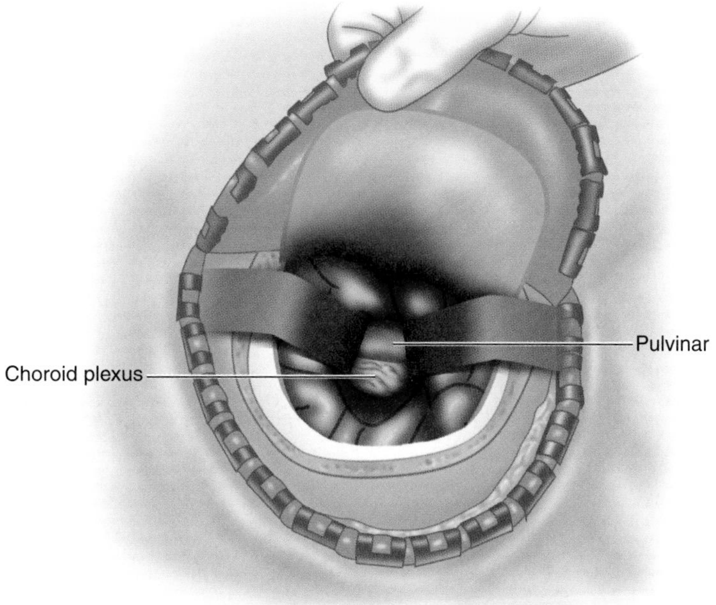

FIGURE 29-9

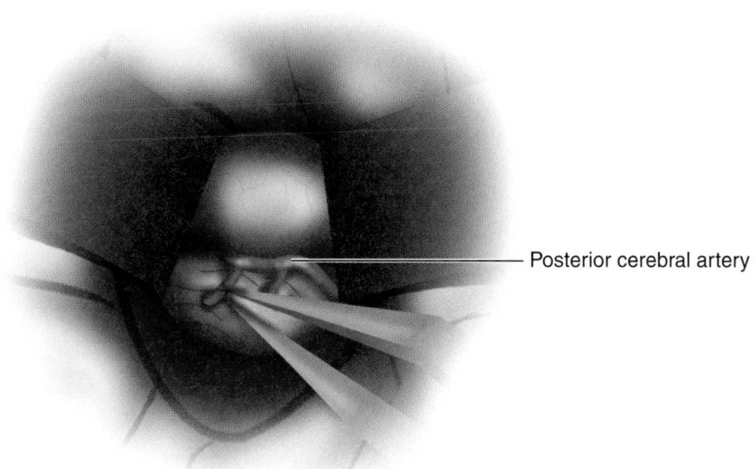

FIGURE 29-10

- **Figure 29-11:** As the dissection proceeds medial and lateral to the nidus, the septum pellucidum is opened medially, and the internal cerebral and Galen veins are exposed. After the bulk of the nidus is freed, the internal cerebral vein is coagulated and cut.

TIPS FROM THE MASTERS

- Generous craniotomy flaps should be used in deep AVM surgery.
- If the AVM is not visible at the cortical surface, the nidus may be located by following the draining vein or hematoma. Intraoperative stereotactic surgical navigation is essential.
- Gentle traction of the nidus with a moist cottonoid can aid visualization of the feeders.
- Arterial feeders are often difficult to coagulate but can be occluded using AVM microclips.

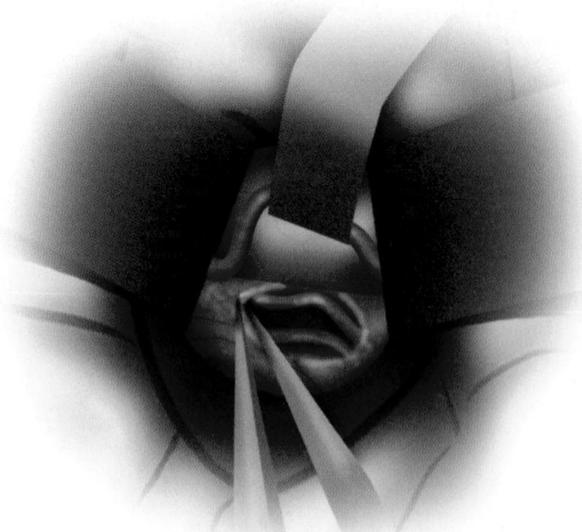

FIGURE 29-11

- The draining vein should be temporarily occluded before cutting it, and the nidus should be observed to ensure that all significant feeders are cut and the nidus does not swell or bleed.

PITFALLS

A stroke may occur when arteries en passant to supply normal brain are coagulated because they are mistakenly thought to be feeding the nidus.

Residual AVM is unrecognized with resultant postoperative hemorrhage. The resection bed always should be thoroughly inspected under the microscope and at normal blood pressure.

Straying outside the gliotic plane close to the nidus can damage the surrounding brain parenchyma, and veering inside this plane can cause the nidus to hemorrhage.

Packing in an attempt to stop bleeding from deep feeding arteries that retract should be avoided.

BAILOUT OPTIONS

- If bleeding from fragile retracted deep perforating arteries occurs from the depth of the dissection, packing should be avoided, and the perforating arteries should be pursued with AVM microclips.
- Sometimes excessive bleeding from residual AVM toward the end of the resection can be controlled only by quickly removing the remaining nidus and then obtaining hemostasis.

SUGGESTED READINGS

Chang SD, Marcellus ML, Marks MP, et al. Multimodality treatment of giant intracranial arteriovenous malformations. Neurosurgery 2007;61(1 Suppl.):432–42.

Drake CG. Cerebral arteriovenous malformations: considerations for and experience with surgical treatment in 166 cases. Clin Neurosurg 1979;26:145–208.

Fleetwood IG, Marcellus ML, Levy RP, et al. Deep arteriovenous malformations of the basal ganglia and thalamus: natural history. J Neurosurg 2003;98:747–50.

Heros RC. Brain resection for exposure of deep extracerebral and paraventricular lesions. Surg Neurol 1990;34:188–95.

Spetzler RF, Martin NA. A proposed grading system for arteriovenous malformations. J Neurosurg 1986;65:476–83.

Procedure 30

Cranial Dural Arteriovenous Fistula Disconnection

Ivan Radovanovic, M. Christopher Wallace

INDICATIONS

General Indications for Treatment of Dural Arteriovenous Fistulas

- The indication for treatment of cranial dural arteriovenous malformations (DAVFs) is dictated by their natural history. Because the risk of hemorrhage and neurologic deficit is directly correlated to the presence of cortical venous reflux (CVR), a general principle is that only these lesions should be treated.
- Two accepted classifications, the Borden and the Cognard classification, relate the different hemodynamic patterns of DAVFs and stratify their risk of aggressive progression by considering CVR and the involvement of major venous sinus drainage. These classification systems are important to determine the indication for treatment and to direct the treatment strategy. For simplicity, only the Borden classification is used in this chapter.

Borden I Dural Arteriovenous Fistula: Sinus Drainage without Cortical Venous Reflux

- Because the risk of hemorrhage is very low in these lesions, they should be treated only in patients with intolerable symptoms, such as tinnitus, ophthalmologic symptoms, or pain. These benign lesions should be observed clinically and radiologically, however, because a small percentage (2% to 3%) eventually develop CVR.

Borden II Dural Arteriovenous Fistula: Sinus Drainage with Cortical Venous Reflux

- Patients with these lesions should be treated because they have CVR. In patients with neurologic deficits, most often secondary to venous congestion, the sinus cannot be sacrificed, generally precluding a total obliteration of the fistula by surgery or endovascular therapy. The treatment is limited to disconnecting the arterial feeders and skeletonization of the involved sinus. In patients without neurologic deficits, CVR can be disconnected; the fistula can be totally excised with sacrifice of the sinus only if the brain does not use the draining sinus.

Borden III Dural Arteriovenous Fistula: Direct Cortical Venous Reflux without Sinus Drainage

- Patients with these lesions have the highest risk of bleeding and neurologic deficit. In patients without neurologic deficits, the treatment strategy depends on whether the functional brain uses the veins with cortical reflux from the DAVF. This can be assessed on the venous phase of angiography. In the event the brain uses cortical reflux veins for drainage (especially if there is reflux in the vein of Labbé), only arterial feeder disconnection should be done without disturbing the venous aspect of the lesion. If there is no evidence of brain dependence on cortical reflux veins, a classic CVR disconnection can be done. In patients with neurologic deficits that may be due to venous congestion, only arterial feeders are disconnected.

Location of Dural Arteriovenous Fistulas

- The classic locations of cranial DAVFs are (1) transverse and sigmoid sinus (40%), (2) cavernous sinus (30%), (3) deep venous and tentorial incisura (10%), (4) superior sagittal sinus and convexity (5%), (5) foramen magnum (5%), (6) anterior cranial fossa (4%), (7) temporal fossa (2%), and (8) superior petrosal sinus (1%). Treatment is determined by the criteria discussed earlier and not the location of the DAVF. Some DVAFs, such as anterior cranial fossa lesions, always have a CVR, however, and are always treated because there is no venous sinus in the proximity of the fistula to route the venous drainage away from cortical veins.

Treatment Options

- When the indication and the goals of treatment are established, the different management options generally include endovascular embolization through transarterial or transvenous routes and surgery. Although radiosurgery is described for the treatment of DVAFs, it is rarely used. Endovascular treatment should be the first choice whenever it is possible to achieve the goals of the treatment with low risk, and surgery is recommended whenever endovascular therapy fails or is technically not feasible.

Endovascular Therapy

- Transarterial endovascular treatment involves superselective catheterization of arterial feeding vessels that can be occluded, but the fistula itself is rarely obliterated. Most of the time, treatment through a transarterial route reduces the flow in the fistula by eliminating major feeder arteries, but it is not curative because many smaller feeders cannot be embolized. If residual flow is present in the fistula, further feeders are likely to be recruited leading to recurrence. Some arteries are too microscopic to be occluded, and because of small arterioles in the dura and wall of sinus, these lesions often are hard to cure. Arterial embolization is a very effective adjunct before surgical treatment of DAVF because it can significantly reduce procedural blood loss. Transvenous embolization using a retrograde venous route to access the venous compartment of the fistula is a well-established treatment of DAVFs. It usually involves the occlusion and sacrifice of the DAVF draining sinus. Transvenous embolization is feasible only if venous phase angiography has documented the absence of venous drainage of normal brain by the involved sinus. Most of the time, venous access is impossible in Borden III lesions, which do not drain through a venous sinus but directly in cortical veins.

Surgery

- When endovascular therapy fails or is not possible, three main surgical strategies exist to treat cranial DAVFs.
- The first option is direct surgical exposure, catheterization, and packing of the involved sinus with coils or other thrombogenic material (e.g., Gelfoam, silk sutures).
- Another option, which is the traditional surgical treatment of DAVFs, is a complete excision of the fistula and the surrounding dura. This approach involves the disconnection of all feeding arteries and arterialized leptomeningeal veins and excision of the draining sinus, when not used by brain, together with pathologic dura. If the brain uses the sinus, the sinus is skeletonized and left patent.
- The third option is a selective disconnection of the arterialized leptomeningeal veins with CVR, which is the procedure described here. The rationale of this simpler, less invasive, and less morbid option is based on our understanding of the natural history and physiopathology of DAVFs. Because CVR is the major risk factor for aggressive behavior of DVAFs, it seems plausible that selectively eliminating CVR would convert DVAFs into benign lesions and eliminate the risk of bleeding and neurologic deficit. Based on our positive experience and several reports in the literature, we currently prefer this strategy to complete excision to treat most aggressive DAVFs. As discussed previously, disconnection of CVR is safe only when the brain does not use the reflux veins for its own drainage.

Radiosurgery

- Although there are a few reports on radiosurgical treatment of DAVFs, its current role is unclear. The long interval between treatment and the expected obliteration of DAVFs may be unacceptable for lesions having a CVR and a bleeding or neurologic deterioration risk of about 15% per year.

CONTRAINDICATIONS

- In DAVFs with no CVR (Borden I) without signs or symptoms or with minor tolerable symptoms, no treatment is justified because the risk of hemorrhage is very low.
- In Borden type II DAVFs, a neurologic deficit owing to venous engorgement from the DAVF is a contraindication for disconnection of the CVR. Only disconnection of arterial feeders should be done, with meticulous preservation of veins.
- Another contraindication for CVR disconnection is use of draining vein by normal brain shown on angiography. A disconnection of arterial feeders is preferred.
- Use of draining sinus by normal brain shown on angiography is a contraindication for the sacrifice of the sinus.
- The procedure is also contraindicated in patients with medical conditions that prohibit general anesthesia.

PLANNING AND POSITIONING

- **Figure 30-1:** Different locations and approaches for cranial DAVFs. The approaches shown are in bold.
- **Figure 30-2:** Angiography and magnetic resonance imaging (MRI) of Borden type II DAVF of the tentorium, torcular Herophili, and transverse sinus. **A,** Magnetic resonance angiography showing dilated vessels in the region of the torcular Herophili suggestive of DAVF. **B,** Injection of the right external carotid artery (RECA) showing a large occipital artery (*black arrowheads*) and its branches feeding the fistula (*asterisk*). The enlarged draining veins and venous pouches that participate in CVR and the filling of the transverse and sigmoid sinus make this lesion a Borden type II DAVF. **C,** Injection of the left external carotid artery showing participation of the left occipital artery (*arrowheads*) to the DAVF. **D,** Injection of the right vertebral artery showing leptomeningeal branches of the vertebral artery feeding the fistula.
- DAVF type is carefully identified based on angiography.
- The exact anatomic location of fistulous point should be determined.
- All arterial feeders, draining veins, and sinuses and cortical veins with reflux should be identified on preoperative angiography.
- The approach is chosen based on the location of the fistula.
- **Figure 30-3:** A patient with Borden type II fistula of the torcular Herophili is placed in the prone position.
- **Figure 30-4:** The head is fixed in a three-pin or four-pin head rest and slightly flexed for maximal exposure of suboccipital bone.
- A straight or S-shaped incision is planned on the midline from the inion to the mid-cervical spine or laterally approximately two fingerbreadths from the ear depending on lesion location.
- The craniotomy is planned with surgical guidance to expose the transverse sinus, the torcular Herophili, the suboccipital dura below the sinus, and the temporooccipital dura above the sinus.

PROCEDURE

- **Figure 30-5:** Suboccipital and occipital craniotomy has been performed, exposing the whole breadth of the transverse sinus. The dura has been opened in a Y fashion over the posterior fossa, and the cisterna magna has been opened. The arachnoid over the vermis has been sharply dissected. Dilated arterialized red draining vein is visualized.
- **Figure 30-6:** The large draining vein is dissected and followed toward the transverse sinus. The vein takes a supracerebellar infratentorial course and is adherent to the transverse sinus and the tent.

DAVF location	Approach	Surgical view
Transverse/sigmoid sinus	Temporal, occipital and/or **suboccipital**	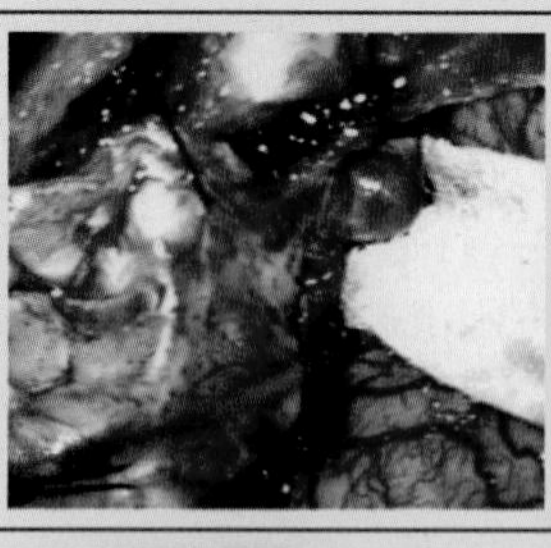 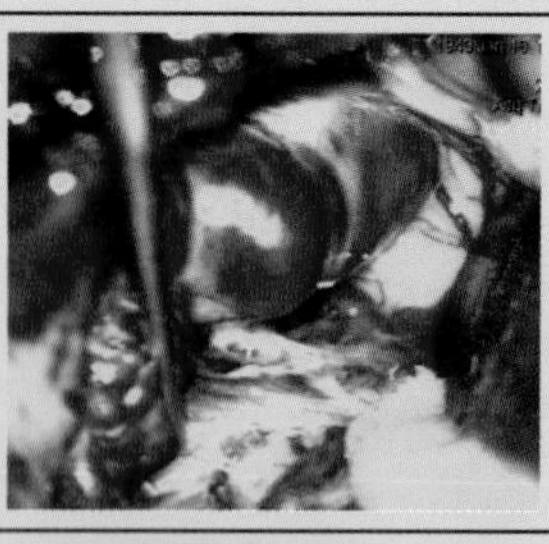
Anterior cranial fossa/ethmoidal	**Supraorbital subfrontal**	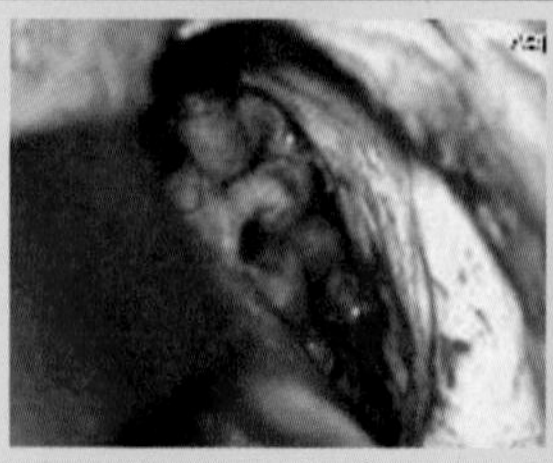 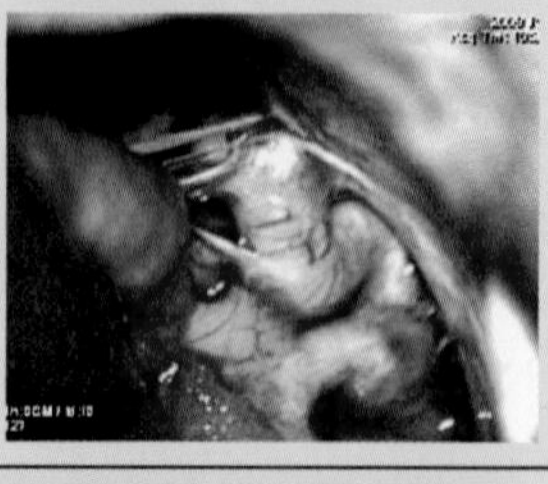
Superior sagittal sinus/ convexity	**Median and paramedian**	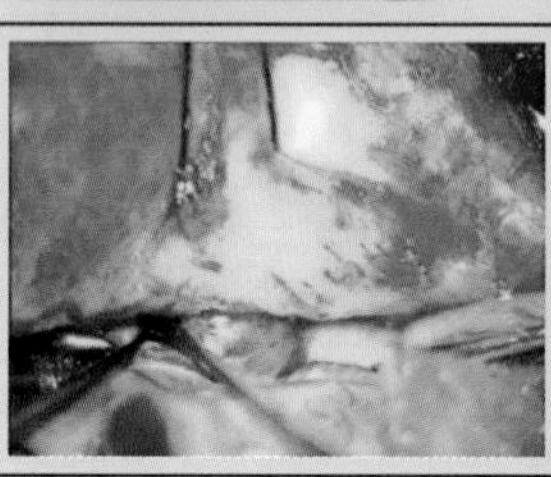 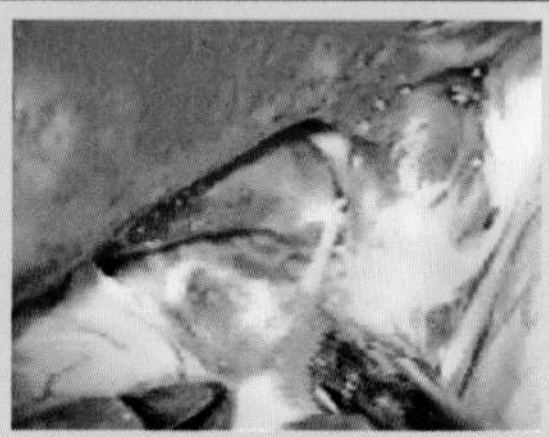
Temporal fossa	**Pterional transsylvian**, subtemporal, pretemporal	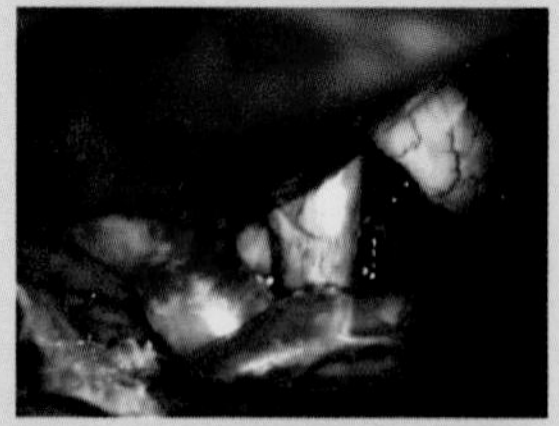
Foramen magnum	**Suboccipital**, far lateral	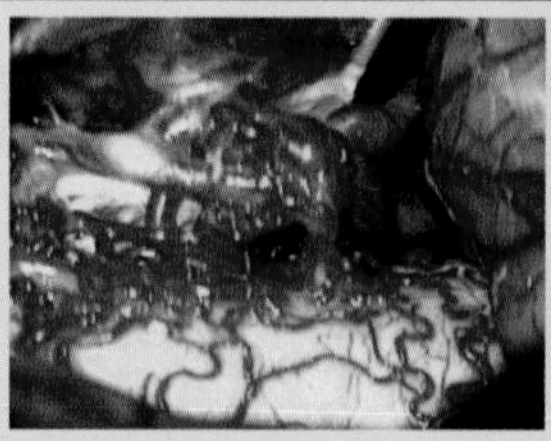 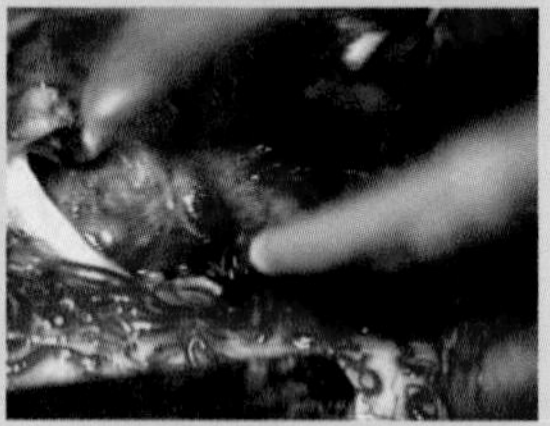
Superior petrosal sinus	**Lateral suboccipital**	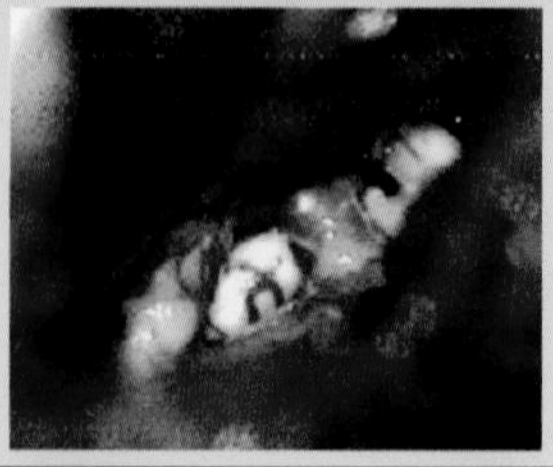
Cavernous	Pterional transsylvian, **subtemporal**	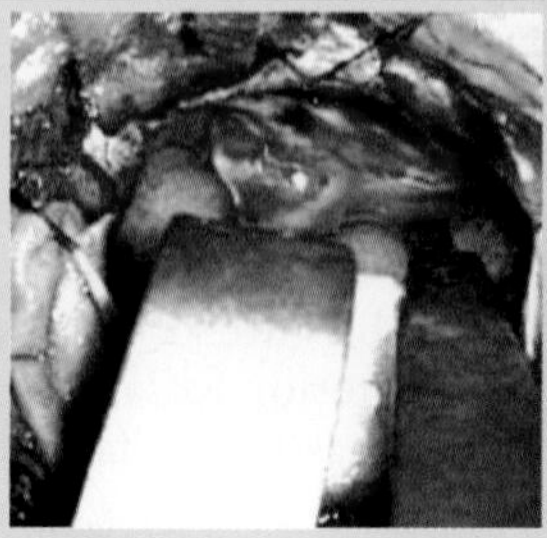 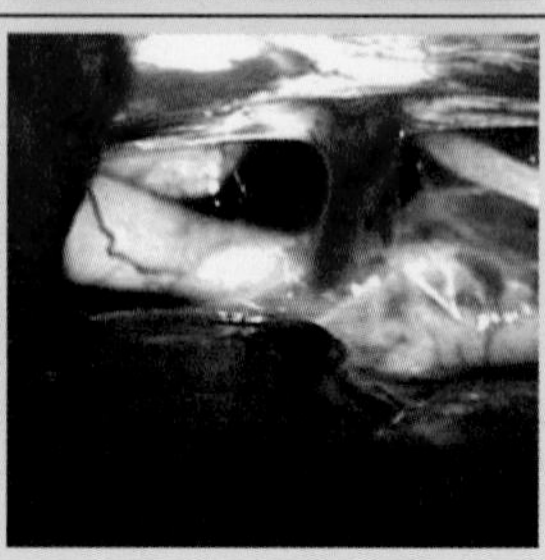

FIGURE 30-1

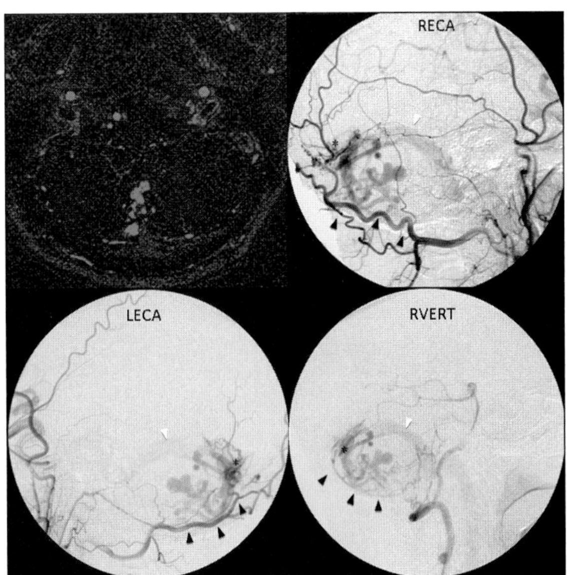

FIGURE 30-2

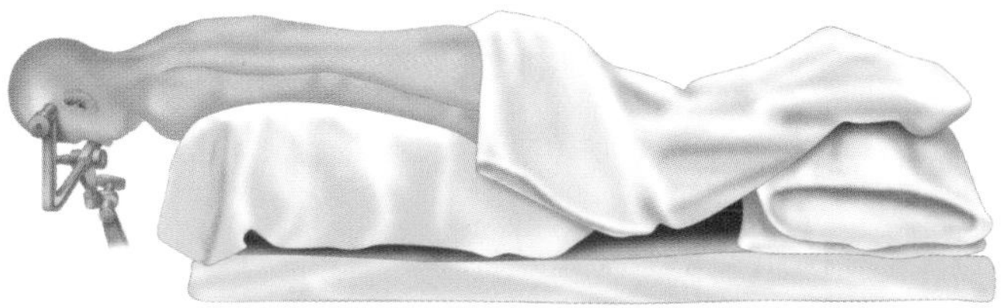

FIGURE 30-3

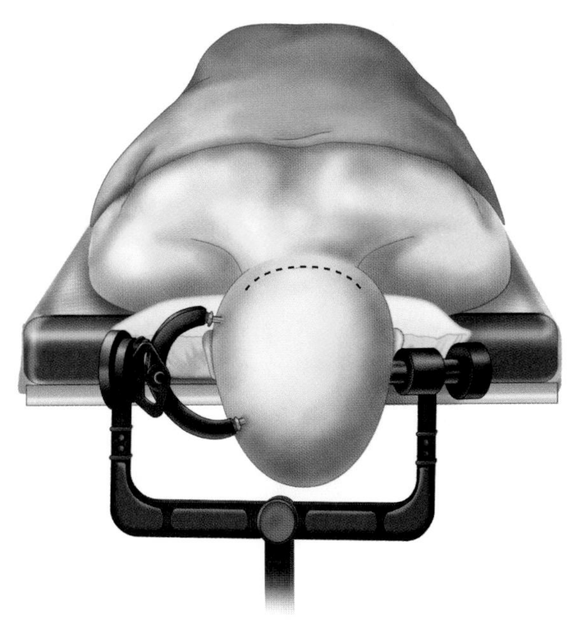

FIGURE 30-4

- **Figure 30-7:** Further dissection is carried out, and a more proximal portion of the vein is visualized curving back where it takes its origin on the transverse sinus.
- **Figure 30-8:** The bridging portion of the vein connecting to the transverse sinus is completely dissected.

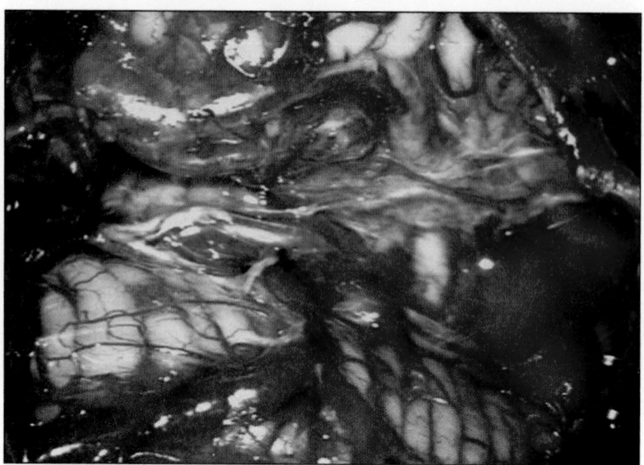

FIGURE 30-5

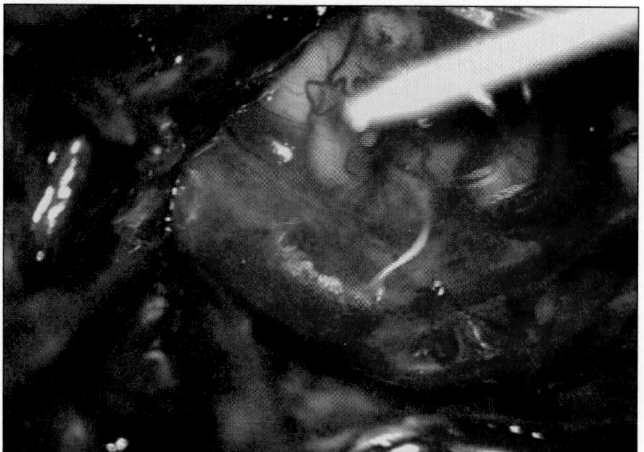

FIGURE 30-6

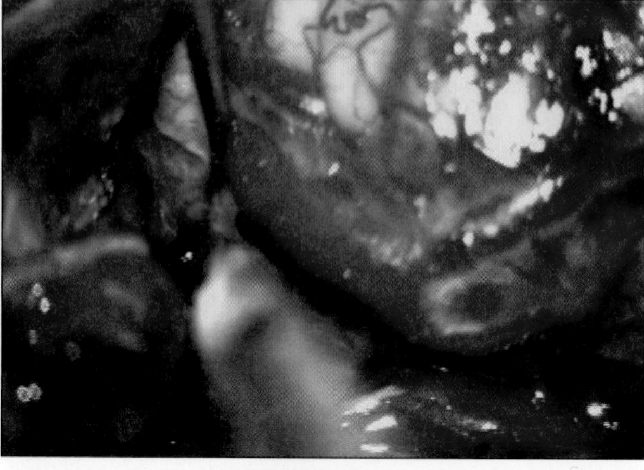

FIGURE 30-7

- **Figure 30-9:** The vein is mobilized medially clearing a view along the lateral aspect of the tent. No other draining veins are identified in this area. Small collateral dilated vessels are seen around the exit of the main draining vein from the sinus.
- **Figure 30-10:** The medial aspect of the draining vein is inspected. No other major dilated draining veins are identified.
- **Figure 30-11:** The aneurysm clip is applied on the main draining vein.

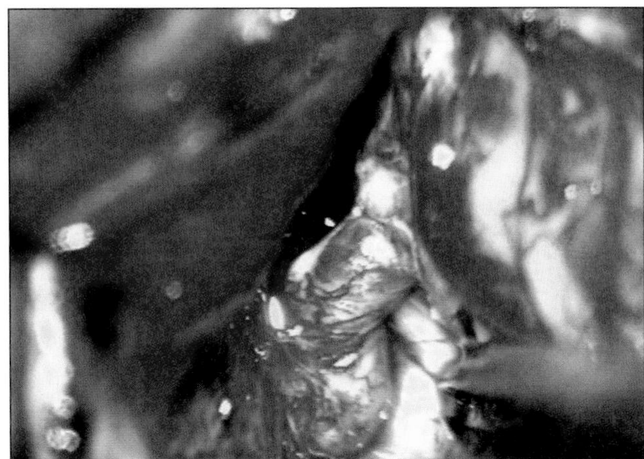

FIGURE 30-8

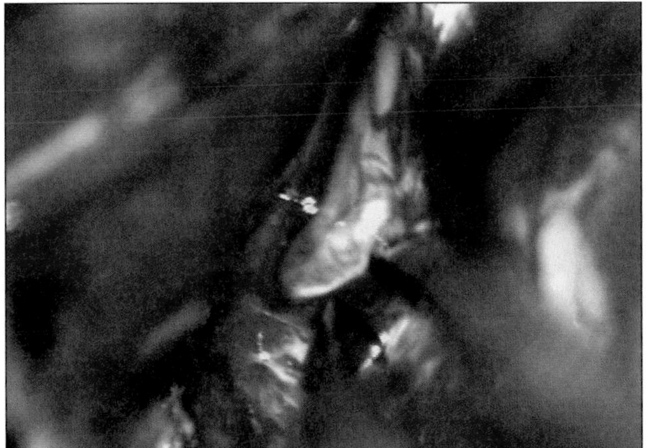

FIGURE 30-9

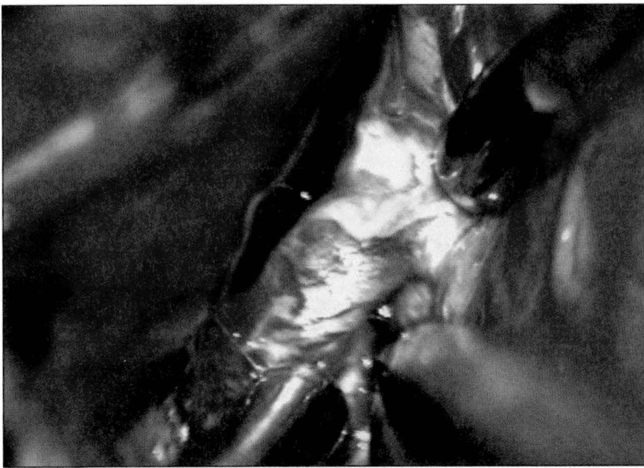

FIGURE 30-10

- **Figure 30-12:** The large draining vein is coagulated and divided.
- **Figure 30-13:** The final view of the operative site. Distal course of the divided draining vein is seen over the cerebellum. The vein is now filling with venous blood and has a blue color (compare with Figure 30-5).

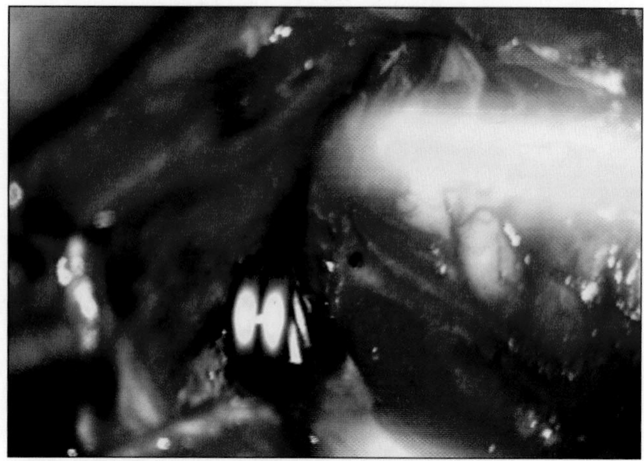

FIGURE 30-11

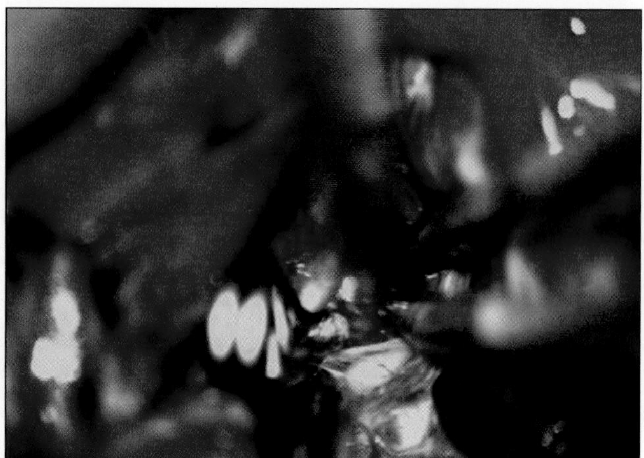

FIGURE 30-12

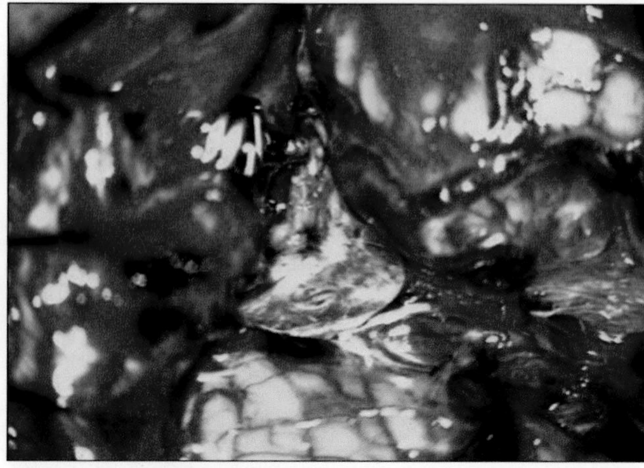

FIGURE 30-13

TIPS FROM THE MASTERS

- The occipital and posterior auricular arteries, which are usually enlarged, should be doubly ligated and divided as they are encountered during the approach because this sometimes interrupts the main arterial supply to the DAVF and significantly reduces intraoperative bleeding.
- Transosseous veins can be prominent and torrentially bleed when bone is exposed or during craniotomy. It is important to take care during bone exposure to recognize these vessels early and occlude them in a controlled way with bone wax.
- In transverse and sigmoid sinus DAVF, venous drainage can be through the ipsilateral transverse and sigmoid sinuses or through the contralateral side if the ipsilateral side is occluded. Occasionally, these lesions drain into the diploic veins, which may lead to significant hemorrhage during craniotomy. CVR may occur through temporal, occipital, or cerebellar veins. Careful identification of this pattern is important.
- Even if it is judged from angiography that CVR veins do not drain normal brain, it is safer to apply a clip on major draining veins before disconnecting them. The brain should be observed for any swelling resulting from impaired venous drainage for a few minutes before coagulating and anatomically dividing the vein.
- Because several veins can contribute to the fistula, some of them being smaller and more difficult to identify than the major draining vein, it cannot be stressed enough how important it is to ensure all arterialized veins are identified and disconnected.

PITFALLS

A catastrophic hemorrhage can occur during craniotomy and after bone flap elevation from nonembolized fistulas. Preoperative embolization and reduction of arterial feeders is a useful adjunct to surgery. Great care should be taken when drilling burr holes and craniotomy sections and handling the dura.

We stress the importance of preoperative identification of all the vessels contributing to the DAVF and understanding of DAVF anatomy, architecture, and flow pattern because unrecognized feeders, such as an artery of the falx cerebelli feeding a transverse sinus fistula, might be missed during surgery.

BAILOUT OPTIONS

- If a profuse venous bleeding is encountered from a tear at the junction of a vein and its draining sinus, compression and holding patiently until the bleeding stops generally works well.

SUGGESTED READINGS

Borden JA, Wu JK, Shucart WA. A proposed classification for spinal and cranial dural arteriovenous fistulous malformations and implications for treatment. J Neurosurg 1995;82:166–79.

Cognard C, Gobin YP, Pierot L, et al. Cerebral dural arteriovenous fistulas: clinical and angiographic correlation with a revised classification of venous drainage. Radiology 1995;194:671–80.

Collice M, D'Aliberti G, Talamonti G, et al. Surgical interruption of leptomeningeal drainage as treatment for intracranial dural arteriovenous fistulas without dural sinus drainage. J Neurosurg 1996;84:810–7.

da Costa LB, Terbrugge K, Farb R, et al. Surgical disconnection of cortical venous reflux as a treatment for Borden type II dural arteriovenous fistulae. Acta Neurochir (Wien) 2007;149:1103–8.

Satomi J, van Dijk JM, Terbrugge KG, et al. Benign cranial dural arteriovenous fistulas: outcome of conservative management based on the natural history of the lesion. J Neurosurg 2002;97:767–70.

van Dijk JM, TerBrugge KG, Willinsky RA, et al. Clinical course of cranial dural arteriovenous fistulas with long-term persistent cortical venous reflux. Stroke 2002;33:1233–6.

van Dijk JM, TerBrugge KG, Willinsky RA, et al. Selective disconnection of cortical venous reflux as treatment for cranial dural arteriovenous fistulas. J Neurosurg 2004;101:31–5.

Procedure 31 Cavernous Malformations

Giuliano Giliberto, Giuseppe Lanzino

INDICATIONS

- Cavernous malformations are "low-pressure" vascular malformations that typically come to clinical attention because of seizures or acute hemorrhage. With widespread use of noninvasive axial imaging, many cavernous malformations are now being diagnosed incidentally.
- Surgery is recommended in symptomatic patients with seizures or after at least one symptomatic bleed. In patients with symptomatic brainstem and thalamic cavernous malformations, surgery is usually recommended if the lesion comes to a pial or ependymal surface.

CONTRAINDICATIONS

- Asymptomatic incidental cavernous malformations
- Patients with significant medical systemic comorbidities or with short life expectancy

PLANNING AND POSITIONING

- In planning surgery for a cavernous malformation, the main factors crucial to the success of the operation are the location of the lesion and its relationship to surrounding eloquent structures. Positioning and approaches for supratentorial cortical and subcortical cavernous malformations do not differ from basic craniotomies for other neoplastic or vascular supratentorial lesions. We discuss only the basic surgical techniques for the resection of supratentorial cavernous malformations. Resection of brainstem and thalamic cavernous malformations poses specific problems and technical pitfalls that are discussed in more detail.
- In preparing patients for resection of brainstem and thalamic cavernous malformations, proper counseling is important to alert them to the possibility of transient worsening of symptoms that mimic prior bleeding episodes. If the operation is conducted correctly, most patients return to their preoperative baseline after a possible transient postoperative worsening.
- Planning of the correct approach depends on the location of the cavernous malformation itself; the pattern of bleeding, which may have opened a "surgical corridor"; and the location at which the cavernous malformation approaches the pial or ependymal surface. Location of associated developmental venous anomalies is also a very important aspect in the planning of the correct approach. We believe strongly, as do other authors, that every attempt must be made to preserve the associated developmental venous anomaly (which is present in virtually all brainstem cavernous malformations even when not shown on preoperative magnetic resonance imaging [MRI]). Damage of the developmental venous anomaly invariably results in a venous infarct and poor outcome.
- Ideally, we prefer to operate 2 to 3 weeks after a symptomatic bleed. Operation within this time frame allows for partial liquefaction of the hematoma, limiting the mechanical trauma related to the surgery. In such cases, the liquefied hematoma allows for easy internal decompression with minimal trauma. We try to avoid surgery months after a symptomatic bleed because organization of the hematoma leads to more adhesions with the surrounding hemosiderin-stained brainstem parenchyma and increases trauma related to resection. Despite the brainstem location, immediate clinical improvement can be observed after resection of some large "hemorrhagic" cavernous malformations in which the symptoms are partially related to mechanical displacement and compression of the surrounding parenchyma rather than destruction.

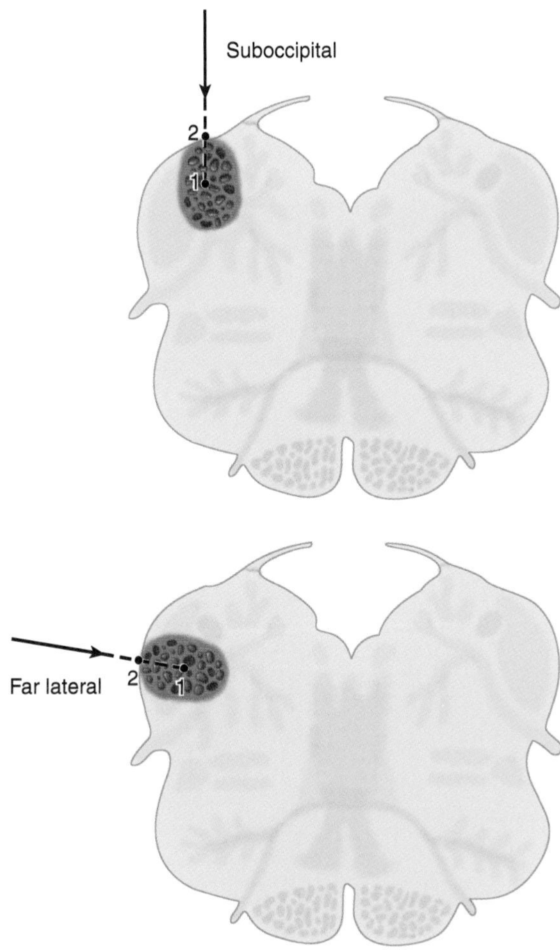

FIGURE 31-1

- **Figure 31-1:** A simple principle to follow in deciding which approach to choose is the two-point method. In deciding the most superficial location of the cavernous malformation, T1-weighted images must be used instead of T2-weighted images. On T2 images, a "blooming" artifact gives the false impression of a larger extension and superficiality of the cavernous malformation.
- Frameless stereotaxy registered to the focus of the surgical microscope is very helpful to provide real-time feedback during surgery. It is particularly useful, in combination with intraoperative monitoring and mapping, to identify the point of entry and initial incision in cases in which, despite suggestion on MRI of a superficial extension, exploration of the outer surface of the brainstem or thalamus does not provide direct or indirect clues regarding the exact location of the cavernous malformation.
- Many thalamic and caudate cavernous malformations are adjacent to the ventricular surface. For these lesions, we prefer a contralateral transcallosal approach with the head parallel to the floor and the symptomatic side up. In such a manner, the surgeon takes advantage of gravity, which drops the ipsilateral (to the approach) hemisphere away from the falx. Having the head parallel to the floor allows for the surgeon's hands to be side by side in a more physiologic working position. The contralateral approach also affords a more direct trajectory to the lesion.
- **Figure 31-2:** In the contralateral transcallosal approach, the ipsilateral (to the approach) hemisphere "falls" away from the falx by gravity and allows the surgeon to work without any additional brain retraction (**C** and **D**). In addition, the contralateral approach with the head positioned as in **A** and **B** provides a more direct and optimal (trajectory *B* in **D**) trajectory to the lesion than an ipsilateral (to the target lesion) approach (trajectory *A* in **D**).

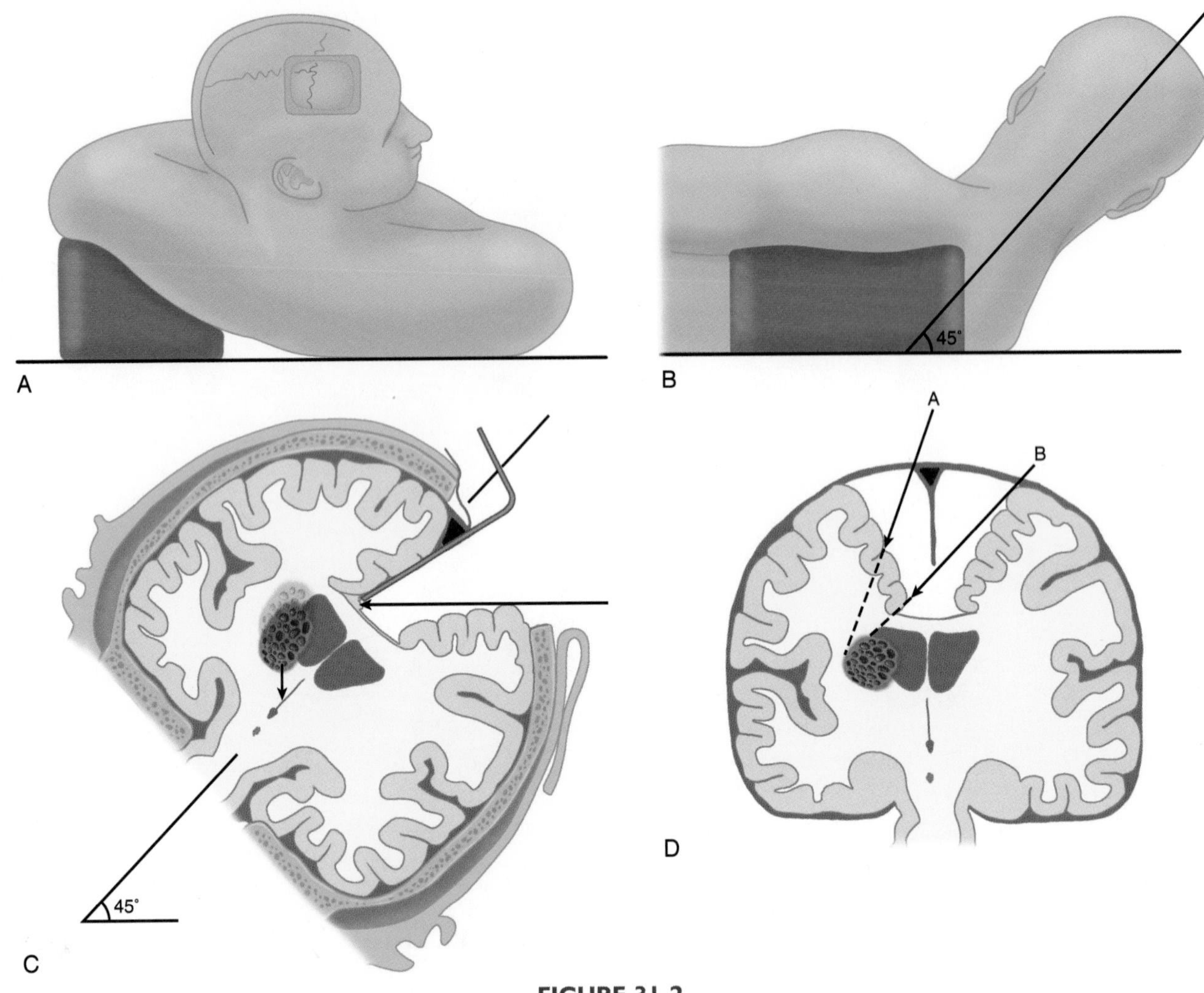

FIGURE 31-2

- **Figure 31-3:** Various approaches are available when treating cavernous malformations of the brainstem. The choice of the approach depends on the location and superficiality of portions of the cavernous malformation, the patient's preoperative deficits, the location of associated venous developmental anomalies, and the surgeon's preference and level of comfort with one approach over the other.
- **Figure 31-4:** Various safe entry zones in the brainstem have been described. We prefer whenever possible to enter through areas of frank hemorrhage or portions of the cavernous malformations directly evident on the brainstem surface because every attempt must be made to preserve intact parenchyma.

PROCEDURE

- **Figure 31-5:** To avoid damage to eloquent parenchyma, a longitudinal incision is made following the direction of the tracts and nuclei present at that specific level. Most tracts and nuclei in the brainstem are organized in a vertical orientation. A longitudinal vertical incision minimizes the chances of direct damage from the incision itself. Similarly, to avoid thermal damage, no cautery is used, and the incision is made sharply with a blade or gently with a blunt dissector.
- **Figure 31-6:** Brainstem cavernous malformations are often removed through a parenchymal incision much smaller than the malformation itself. In contrast to many supratentorial cavernous malformations, the principles of piecemeal resection are applied here. After incision, the lesion is emptied internally targeting cavities with liquefied old blood.

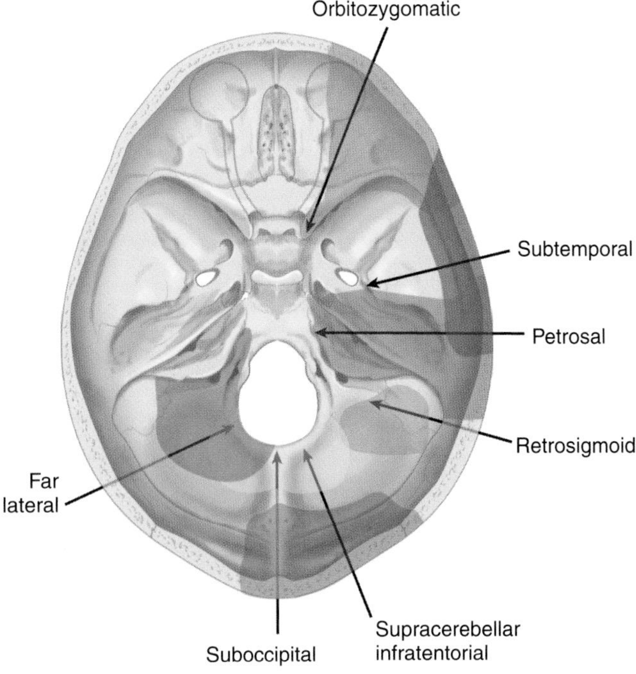

FIGURE 31-3

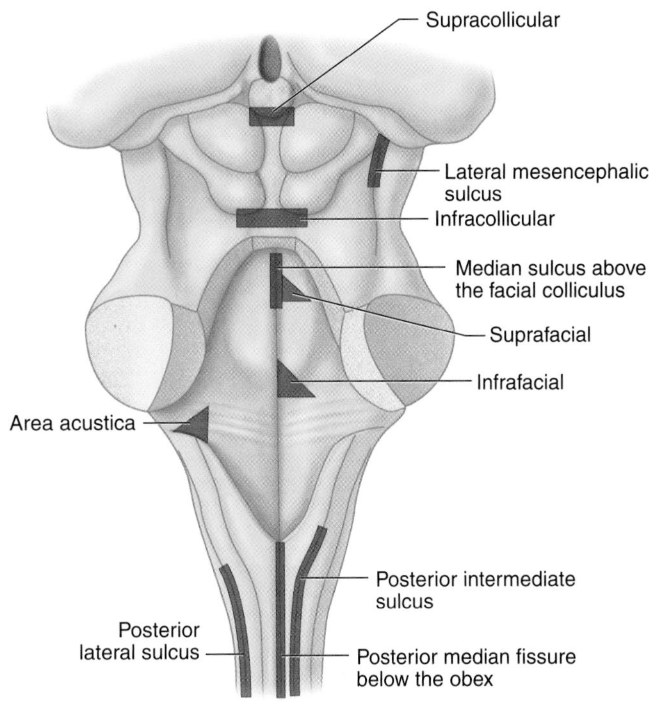

FIGURE 31-4

- **Figure 31-7:** When the malformation has been partially internally decompressed, a cleavage plane between the lesion and the surrounding gliotic hemosiderin-stained parenchyma is developed beginning in the portion of the capsule and surface of the malformation closest to the entry point. Specifically designed round dissectors (**A**) or gentle spread of the bipolar forceps (**B**) can be used for this maneuver. During this maneuver, gentle traction can be applied to the cavernous malformation with the suction in the surgeon's left hand, minimizing the mechanical trauma to the surrounding parenchyma.
- **Figure 31-8:** Principles of separation of the cavernous malformation from the brainstem parenchyma. The separation between the surface of the cavernous malformation and the

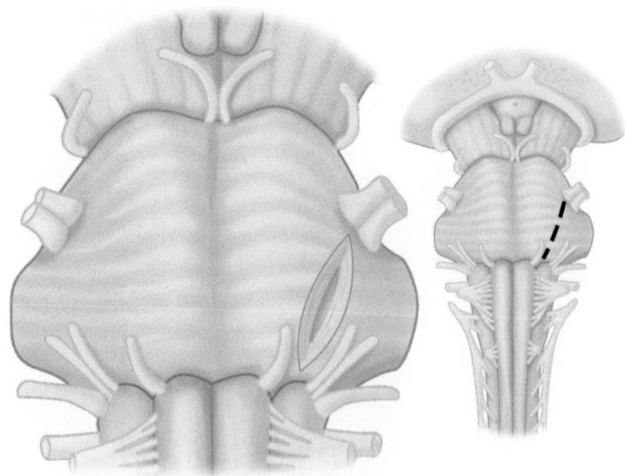

FIGURE 31-5

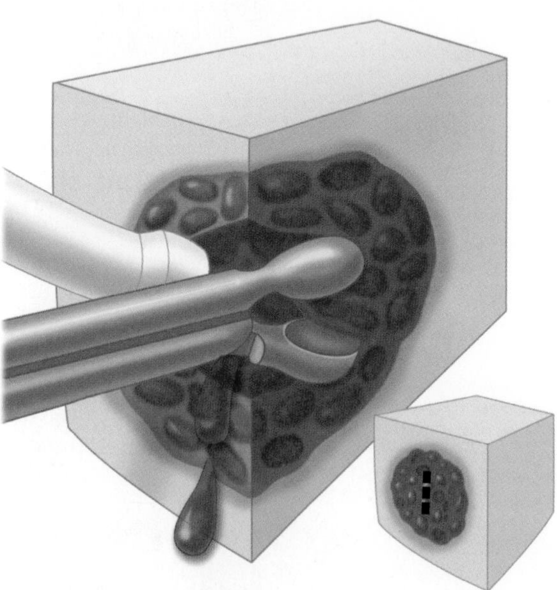

FIGURE 31-6

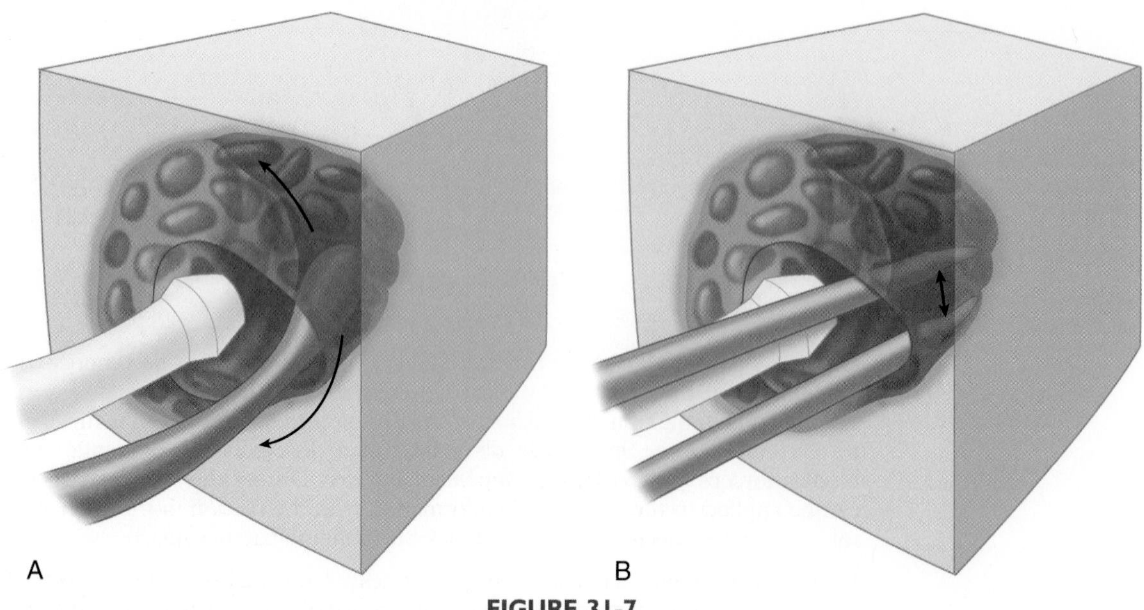

FIGURE 31-7

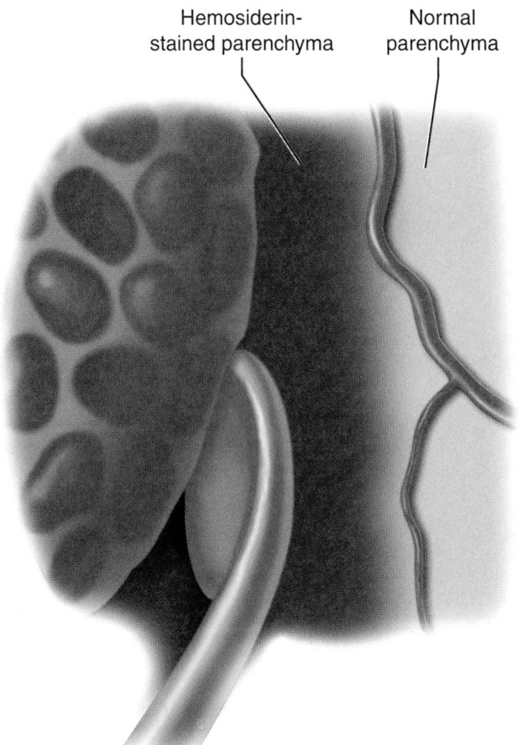

FIGURE 31-8

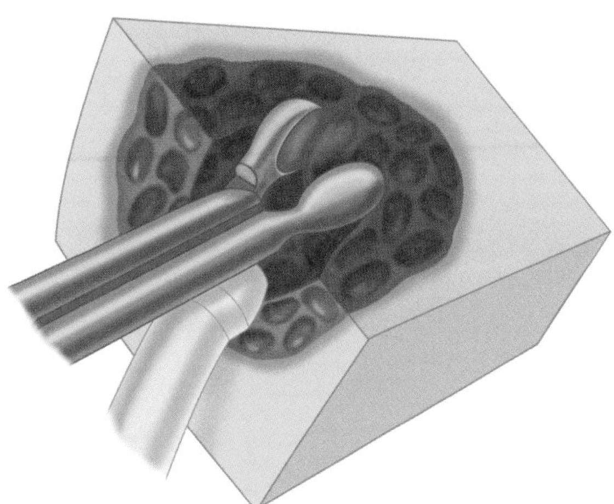

FIGURE 31-9

surrounding hemosiderin-stained parenchyma is obvious in some areas but becomes less evident in others. In such instances, the separation should be halted as soon as any transition from brownish yellow to yellowish white is noted because this indicates transition into normal parenchyma.

- **Figure 31-9:** As the plane is developed and the capsule starts collapsing further, internal emptying by gentle removal of cavernous malformation fragments with pituitary microforceps is carried out.
- **Figure 31-10:** After further internal emptying of the malformation, the cleavage plane is dissected further with a round dissector. Because of the depth of the field and the limited size of the entry incision, this portion of the operation is done more by "feel" than by direct vision. Extreme caution and gentle touch must be exercised to avoid any damage to portions of parenchyma not under direct vision.
- **Figure 31-11:** After the bulk of the cavernous malformation has been released from the surrounding parenchyma, gentle traction with pituitary forceps is applied to the edges of

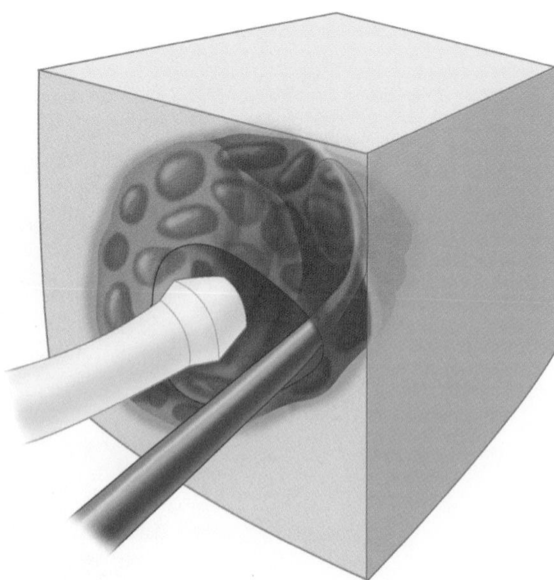

FIGURE 31-10

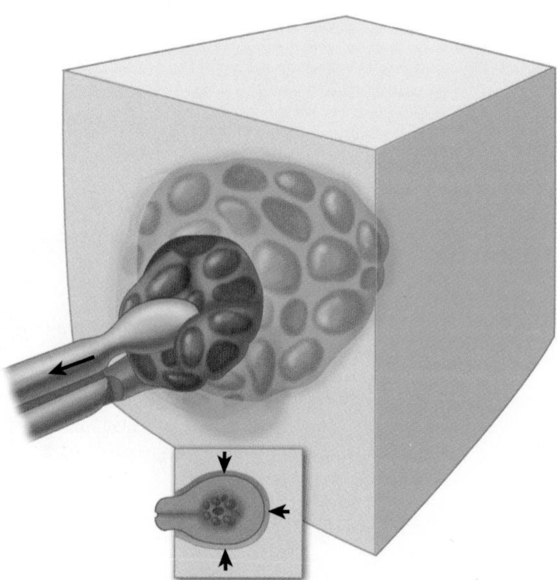

FIGURE 31-11

the most superficial portion of the lesion. If the cavernous malformation has been properly separated, very gentle but steady traction at this point often leads to the malformation eventually "giving in."

- **Figure 31-12:** When the cavernous malformation starts delivering itself through the opening, gentle traction with the pituitary forceps is continued (**A**), and as the malformation starts delivering, the forceps are advanced to the base (**B**) of the partially delivered cavernous malformation. If any undue resistance is felt in this phase, the process of further partial internal debulking and further separation is restarted.
- **Figure 31-13:** Eventually, the malformation delivers itself through the hole, and because of the internal emptying and the soft rubbery consistency, a large portion of cavernous malformation, often larger than the original incision, "transiently deforms" as it exits the incision into the brainstem. This maneuver is facilitated further by the natural tendency of the compressed brainstem parenchyma to regain its normal shape after decompression. After delivery of the malformation, it is not unusual that the cavity left is much smaller than the original cavernous malformation as the compressed brain parenchyma regains its original shape.

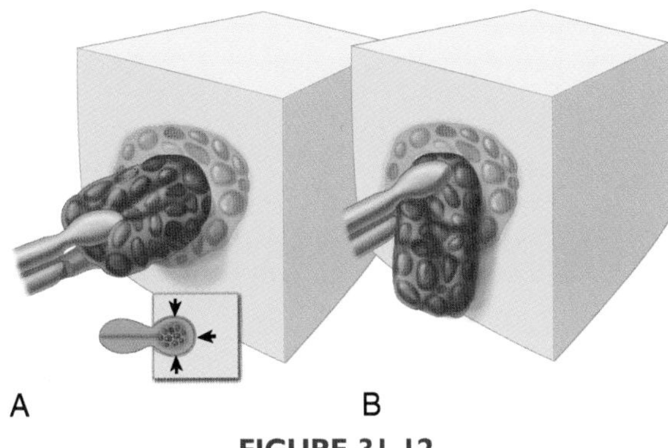

FIGURE 31-12

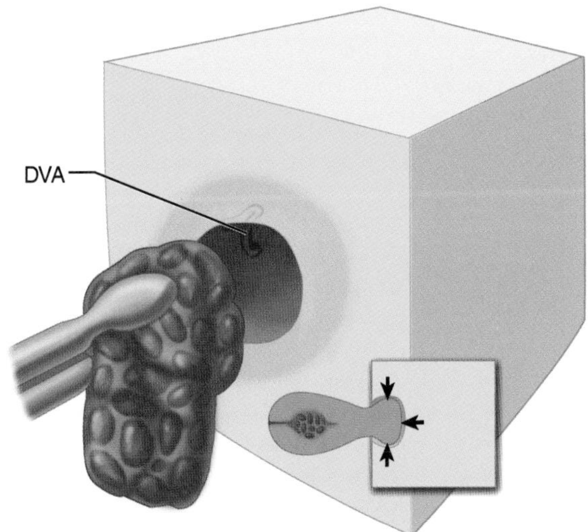

FIGURE 31-13

- **Figure 31-14:** After delivery of the malformation, it is not unusual to have some bleeding from the limits of the cavity, often from radicles of the associated developmental venous anomaly. This bleeding is not brisk, but instead is a low-pressure venous ooze. It is important to avoid using bipolar cautery to control this bleeding; irrigation with warm saline and gentle pressure with hemostatic agent is sufficient to control this bleeding successfully.
- **Figure 31-15:** After bleeding is controlled and hemostasis achieved, the cavity is inspected under high magnification. We often use a small mirror to inspect the cavity

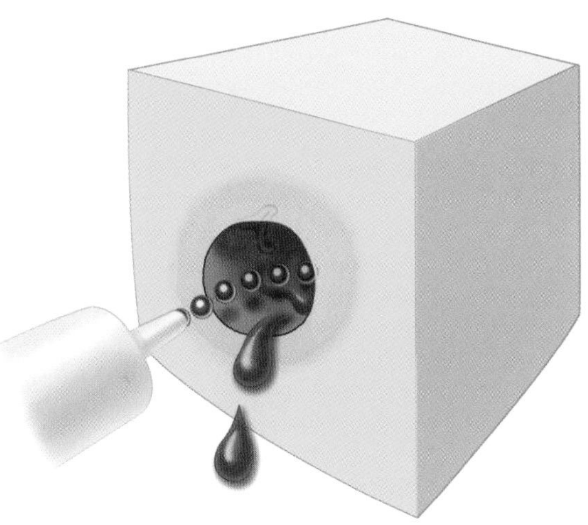
FIGURE 31-14

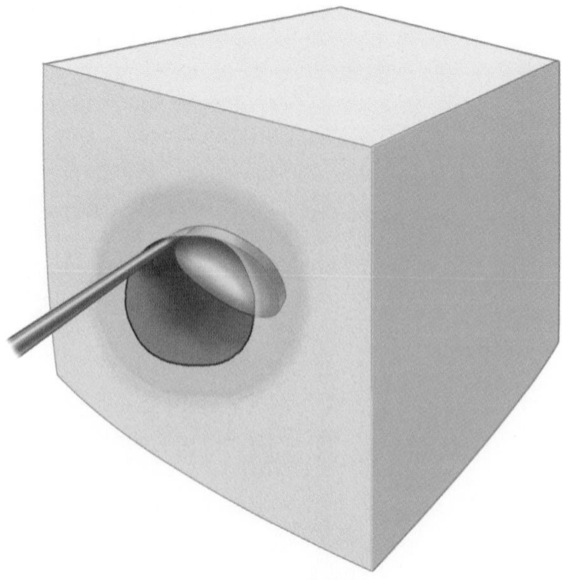

FIGURE 31-15

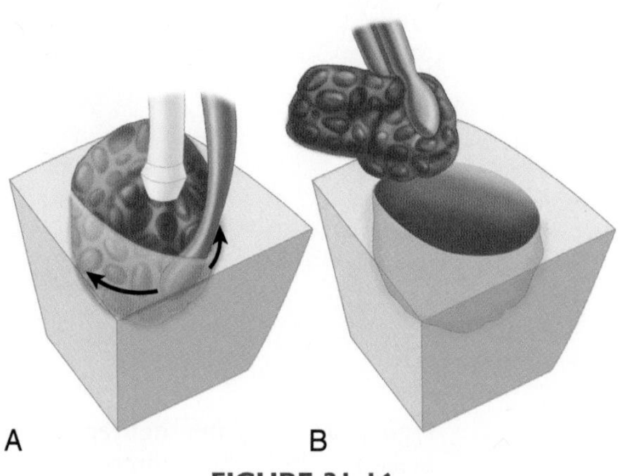

FIGURE 31-16

in angles hidden behind the opening through the brainstem. No attempt should be made to resect the surrounding hemosiderin-stained brainstem parenchyma.

- **Figure 31-16:** Superficial supratentorial cavernous malformations can often be exposed circumferentially. In such cases, the plane of dissection is progressively developed around the cavernous malformation (**A**), and the lesion is removed in a single piece (**B**). If the lesion is not in an eloquent area, every attempt is made to remove the surrounding hemosiderin-stained brain, especially if the indication for surgery is treatment of associated seizures.

TIPS FROM THE MASTERS

- Surgery done 2 to 4 weeks after a symptomatic brainstem bleed allows for partial liquefaction of the hematoma, facilitating internal decompression and delivery of the cavernous malformation.
- During resection of a brainstem cavernous malformation, a change in tissue color from yellowish brown to yellowish white indicates the cavernous malformation–brainstem interface, and extreme caution must be exercised in this stage of the dissection.
- There is often bleeding from the cavity after resection of a cavernous malformation in eloquent parenchyma. This bleeding is usually related to a low-pressure venous ooze and can be controlled with irrigation and gentle pressure with hemostatic agent. Cautery should be avoided as much as possible.

PITFALLS

Distinguishing the interface between the cavernous malformation and the surrounding hemosiderin-stained parenchyma can be challenging, especially in a deep, poorly illuminated field.

Resection of brainstem and thalamic cavernous malformations is often performed through an incision much smaller than the malformation itself. Separation of the cavernous malformation from the surrounding parenchyma deep in the cavity or around corners is often done by "feel," rather than under direct vision. Patience and a "gentle touch" are critical in these phases.

Postoperative imaging is often difficult to interpret because of the residual hemosiderin-stained parenchyma in eloquent areas. We prefer to obtain MRI the day after the procedure to use as a baseline against which we compare later follow-up studies.

BAILOUT OPTIONS

- Radical removal of cavernous malformations is the goal of any surgery for these lesions. Partial removal can result in higher risk of rebleeding as shown by anecdotal cases. Immediate reexploration should be considered for any obvious residual cavernous malformation.

SUGGESTED READINGS

Bricolo A. Surgical management of intrinsic brain stem gliomas. Oper Tech Neurosurg 2000;3:137–54.
Gross BA, Bajer HH, Awad AA, et al. Brainstem cavernous malformations. Neurosurgery 2009;64:805–18.
Lanzino G, Spetzler RF. Cavernous Malformations of the Brain and Spinal Cord. New York: Thieme; 2008.
Porter RW, Detwiler PW, Spetzler RF. Surgical approaches to the brain stem. Oper Tech Neurosurg 2000;3:114–23.
Recalde RJ, Figueiredo EG, De Oliveira E. Microsurgical anatomy of the safe entry zones on the anterolateral brainstem related to surgical approaches to cavernous malformations. Neurosurgery 2008;62(Suppl. 1):9–17.

Procedure 32 Superficial Temporal Artery–Middle Cerebral Artery Bypass

Matthew R. Reynolds, Gregory J. Zipfel

INDICATIONS

- *Atherosclerotic carotid artery occlusion with hemodynamic insufficiency*. In nonselected patient populations, a multicenter randomized controlled trial showed no benefit of superficial temporal artery–middle cerebral artery (STA-MCA) bypass for patients with symptomatic carotid occlusive disease. Two more recent natural history studies suggest, however, that a discrete subpopulation of patients with symptomatic carotid occlusion—patients with "misery perfusion," defined as increased oxygen extraction fraction on positron emission tomography (PET)—are at very high risk for future ischemic events and that this patient population may benefit from surgical revascularization. The Carotid Occlusion Surgery Study was designed to examine the effect of STA-MCA bypass (vs. best medical therapy) on the incidence of recurrent ischemic stroke in patients with symptomatic carotid occlusion and "misery perfusion" on PET. Results from this ongoing clinical trial are likely to provide a definitive answer to this important question.
- *Moyamoya disease with ischemic symptoms*. Although not validated by a large randomized controlled trial, it is generally accepted that surgical revascularization for patients with moyamoya disease with ischemic symptoms is beneficial. This conclusion is based on multiple case series indicating that STA-MCA bypass provides long-term reduction in ischemic symptoms in adult patients with moyamoya disease. Whether adult patients with moyamoya disease with hemorrhagic symptoms also benefit from STA-MCA bypass is unknown.
- *Complex intracranial aneurysms and skull base tumors*. Surgical revascularization is frequently performed during complex intracranial procedures to prevent ischemic complications after planned sacrifice of a major intracerebral artery. STA-MCA bypass is often the procedure of choice when the amount of flow augmentation required is modest (e.g., sacrifice of an M2 branch of the MCA, occlusion of the internal carotid artery in a patient with mild hemodynamic compromise by temporary balloon occlusion testing).

CONTRAINDICATIONS

- *Atherosclerotic carotid artery occlusion without hemodynamic insufficiency*. These patients have a documented benign natural history that does not justify surgical revascularization.
- *Atherosclerotic intracranial artery stenosis*. These patients were at high risk for ischemic complications after STA-MCA bypass in the aforementioned randomized controlled trial.
- *Cerebral vasospasm*. Emergent STA-MCA bypass for the treatment of cerebral vasospasm has been reported in a few small case series to date; however, its efficacy in these patients remains unproven.
- *Planned sacrifice of a major intracerebral artery in patients with marked hemodynamic compromise by temporary balloon occlusion testing*. These patients require a high-flow bypass procedure using a radial artery or saphenous venous graft.

PLANNING AND POSITIONING

- All patients should undergo the following: (1) Detailed history and physical examination with particular attention paid to cardiovascular risk factors; (2) computed tomography (CT) or magnetic resonance imaging (MRI) study of the brain (or both); and (3) catheter cerebral angiogram, including select injections of the external carotid arteries to assess adequacy of the STA for bypass. For patients with chronic ischemia, radiographic assessment of cerebrovascular reserve should be considered (e.g., PET, transcranial Doppler ultrasonography, single photon emission computed tomography, xenon CT, perfusion CT). For patients in whom sacrifice of a major intracerebral artery is being contemplated, temporary balloon occlusion testing should be considered to assess adequacy of the collateral circulation and to help determine the extent of revascularization required.

- For patients undergoing STA-MCA bypass for chronic ischemia (e.g., patients with carotid occlusion or moyamoya disease), special anesthetic considerations must be adhered to throughout the procedure. Specifically, normal-to-high mean arterial pressures and normal arterial carbon dioxide levels (38 to 42 mm Hg) must be strictly maintained to avoid ischemic complications related to the vulnerable hypoperfused cerebral hemispheres.
- **Figure 32-1:** Preoperative catheter angiogram showing select injection of the right internal carotid artery (ICA) in a patient with moyamoya disease. The supraclinoid portion of the ICA cannot be visualized because of stenoocclusion. The anterior (frontal) and posterior (parietal) branches of the STA are easily distinguishable. The middle meningeal artery (MMA) may also be delineated given its location just proximal to the STA.
- **Figure 32-2:** The patient is administered general endotracheal anesthesia with a combination of inhaled and intravenous agents. The patient is placed in the supine position with the head immobilized in three-point fixation pins and a bump underneath the ipsilateral shoulder. The presumed site of arterial anastomosis should be positioned at the apex to avoid pooling of cerebrospinal fluid in the operative field. The head is elevated 10 to 15 degrees to promote venous drainage.

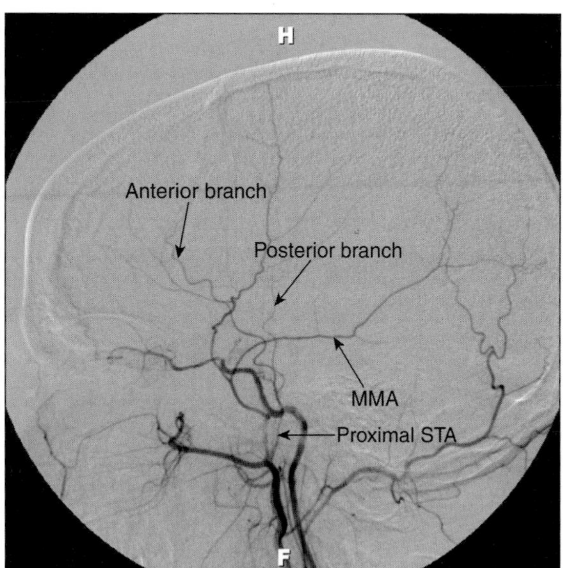

FIGURE 32-1

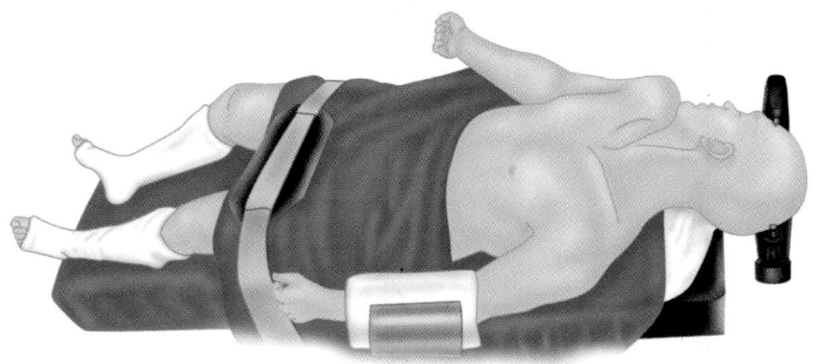

FIGURE 32-2

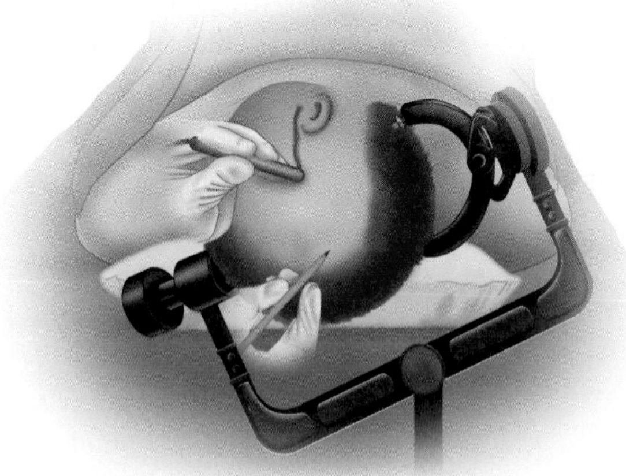

FIGURE 32-3

PROCEDURE

- **Figure 32-3:** The location of both branches of the STA is determined via Doppler ultrasonography and outlined with a marking pen. Based on the preoperative angiogram, the surgeon decides whether the anterior (frontal) or posterior (parietal) branch is more suitable for anastomosis.
- **Figure 32-4:** Local anesthetic is *not* used to avoid needle-induced injury or spasm of the STA. Most commonly, the posterior branch of the STA is selected because of its proximity to the posterior aspect of the sylvian fissure (located approximately 6 cm above the external acoustic meatus) where M4 vessels sufficient for bypass are commonly located. The anterior branch of the STA is selected when the posterior branch is of insufficient size or has been occluded during a prior craniotomy. When the posterior branch is used, a linear skin incision is made directly over the artery from above the superior temporal line to the zygoma (**A**; *solid line* depicts skin incision site). When the anterior branch is used, two options for the skin incision exist: (1) a linear incision directly over the artery (**A**), or (2) a curvilinear incision behind the hairline with separate dissection of the underlying STA from the skin flap (**B**). We prefer the latter because it provides better bony exposure to the posterior aspect of the sylvian fissure and avoids a skin incision that often extends anterior to the patient's hairline.
- **Figure 32-5:** Loupe magnification is encouraged to assist in visualization of the dissection field. We advocate starting the dissection along the distal aspect of the STA to avoid proximal vessel injury that would prematurely end the bypass procedure. The skin is first opened sharply with a scalpel, and the subcuticular tissue is dissected with small, blunt-tip scissors or hemostats until the STA is identified. A plane above the STA is developed, permitting safe and efficient continuation of the skin incision until the entire vessel is exposed. Two-point bipolar cautery is used intermittently to assist in hemostasis, taking care to avoid thermal injury to the STA.
- **Figure 32-6:** When the STA branch is exposed, it is mobilized along with a 5- to 10-mm cuff of soft tissue surrounding the artery. In so doing, unnecessary manipulation of the STA is avoided, which helps protect the vessel from thermal and mechanical injury. The authors advocate preservation of the STA until the time of anastomosis, as opposed to early ligation. Preservation of the STA permits conversion to an indirect revascularization procedure, such as an encephaloduroarteriosynangiosis, in the case where an appropriate recipient M4 vessel is not found after craniotomy.
- **Figure 32-7:** The temporalis muscle is incised and reflected to either side using fish hooks. During this time, the STA is safely positioned outside the operative field to protect against inadvertent damage. A craniotomy flap is fashioned with its center approximately 6 cm above the external acoustic meatus (Chaters point) by placing burr holes at the root of the zygoma and superior temporal line. This location is where large M4 branches of the MCA typically emanate from the distal sylvian fissure.

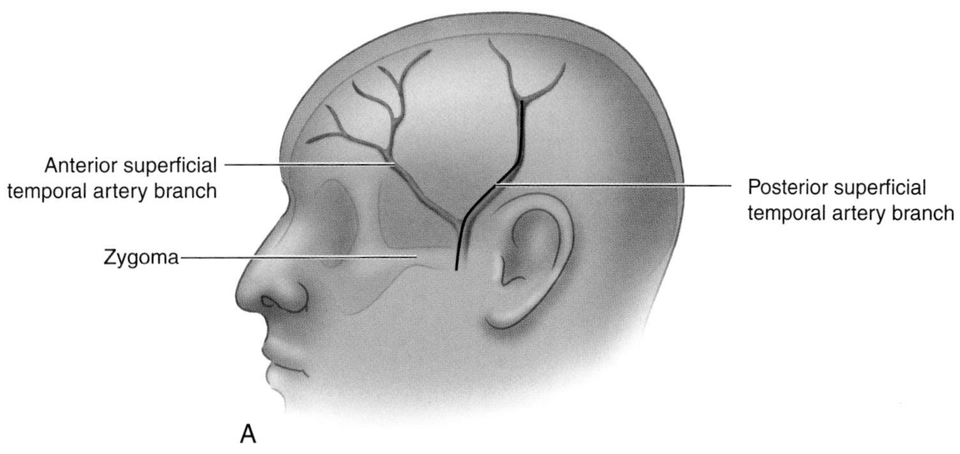

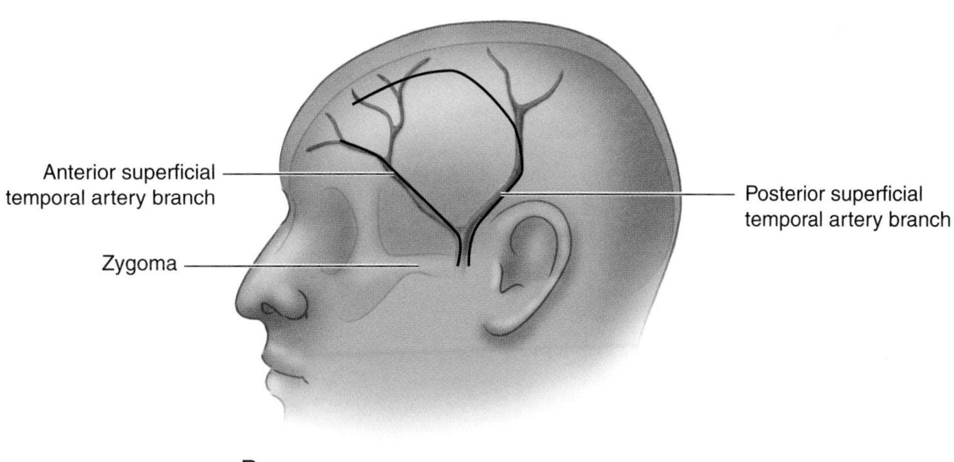

FIGURE 32-4

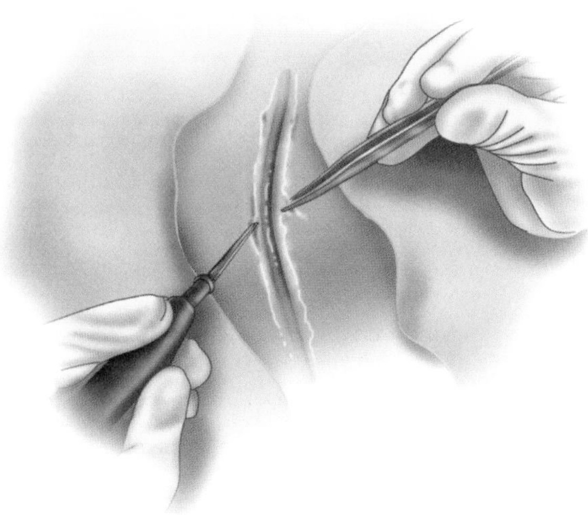

FIGURE 32-5

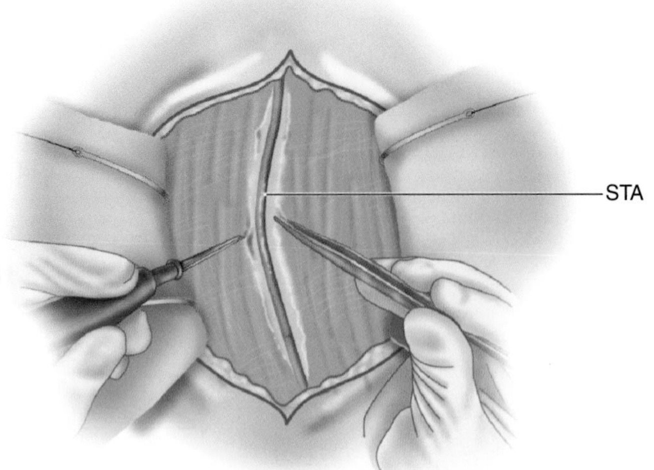

FIGURE 32-6

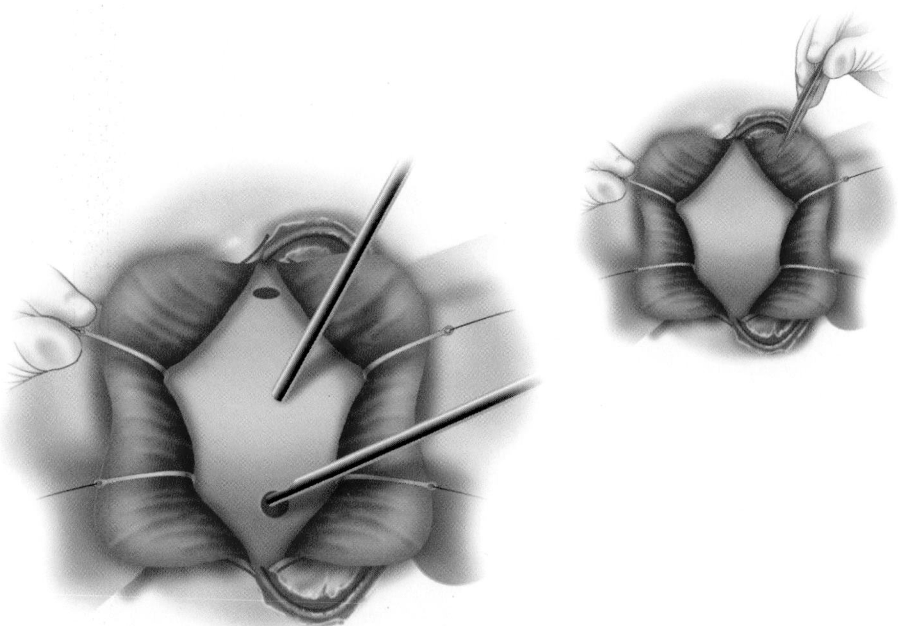

FIGURE 32-7

- **Figure 32-8:** The dura is sharply incised in a cruciate fashion, taking care not to injure the main middle meningeal branches that can provide essential collateral branches to the brain. The operative microscope is brought into the field to assist in the identification and dissection of the M4 branches that are selected as a recipient vessel. Generally, the largest M4 branch is chosen. Some consideration to the presenting ischemic territory should be given (e.g., a presenting temporal lobe infarction suggests that a temporal M4 may be preferable, whereas a frontoparietal infarction suggests that a frontoparietal M4 may be preferable). Recipient vessels of 1 mm or greater are generally considered sufficient for bypass, although some authors have reported success with vessels 0.7 to 0.9 mm in diameter.
- **Figure 32-9:** Under microscopic visualization, the arachnoid is opened sharply, and the recipient M4 vessel is dissected free for at least 1 cm. Small perforators emanating from the vessel segment are cauterized and divided with microscissors—a critical step toward maintaining a blood-free field during arteriotomy and anastomosis. A small rubber dam is cut to size and placed beneath the recipient vessel in preparation for anastomosis. A dilute papaverine-soaked pledget may be placed on the artery at any time during the operation to address mechanical vasospasm if it develops.

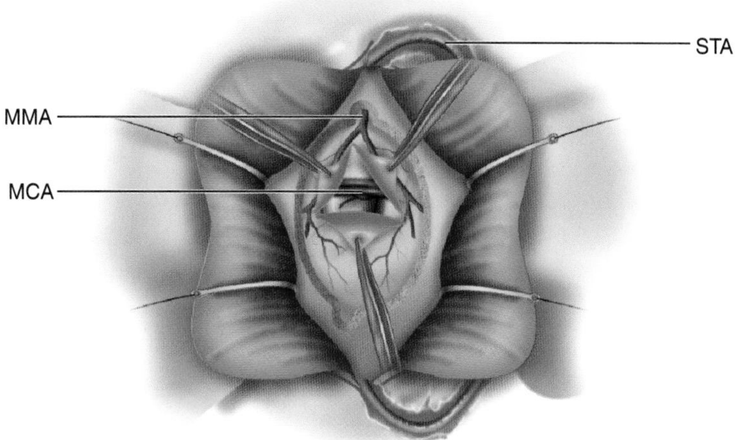

FIGURE 32-8

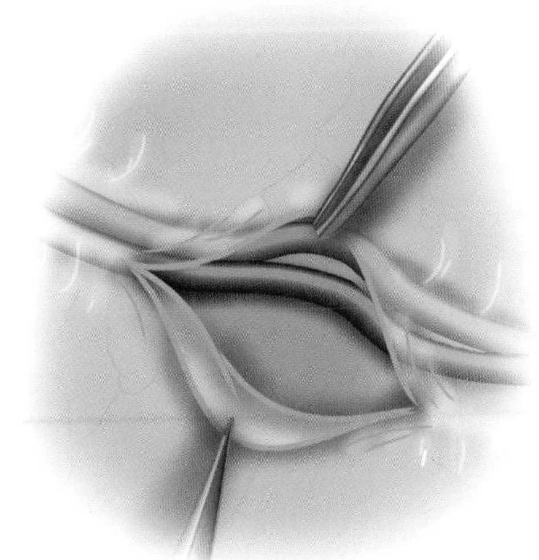

FIGURE 32-9

- **Figure 32-10:** The donor STA branch is brought into the operative field and occluded proximally with a temporary aneurysm clip and distally with ligated suture. The STA is cut obliquely at a point along the vessel whereby some redundancy is maintained to avoid tension at the planned site of anastomosis. The artery is flushed retrogradely with a heparinized saline solution. Great care is given to removing all adventitial tissue for several millimeters along the cut end of the STA. "Pinching" maneuvers of the STA with microforceps are strictly avoided. The donor vessel is spatulated with microscissors to create a "fish mouth" opening (the diameter of the opening should be approximately 2 to 2.5 times the diameter of the recipient vessel). At this time, the free flow from the cut end of the STA, or "cut flow," may be quantified using an ultrasonic flow probe (Charbel Micro-Flowprobe; Transonics Systems, Inc, Ithaca, NY). The cut flow index (bypass flow [mL/min]/cut flow [mL/min]) has been identified as a predictor of bypass patency.
- **Figure 32-11:** The recipient MCA branch is isolated using two temporary low-tension microvascular clips. A linear arteriotomy is made in the recipient vessel approximately 2 to 2.5 times the diameter of the artery. The authors advocate use of a sickle-shaped arachnoid knife to open the vessel initially. Microscissors can be used to complete the arteriotomy. The artery is flushed with a heparinized saline solution and is now ready for anastomosis. The cut edge of the MCA is marked with a blue marking pen to delineate the graft edges more precisely during anastomosis. Two suturing methods have been described: continuous and interrupted. We prefer the continuous method,

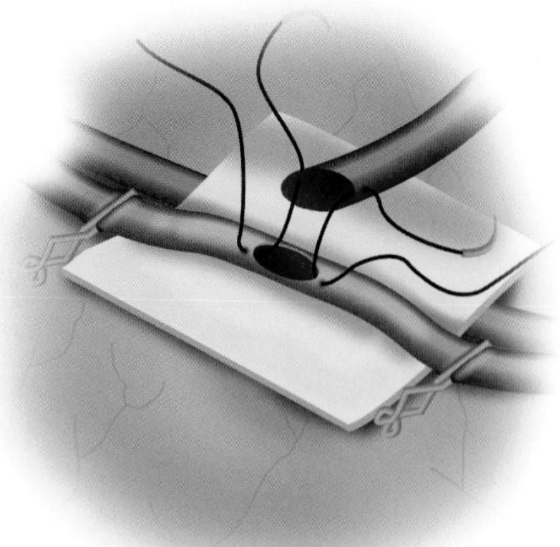

FIGURE 32-10

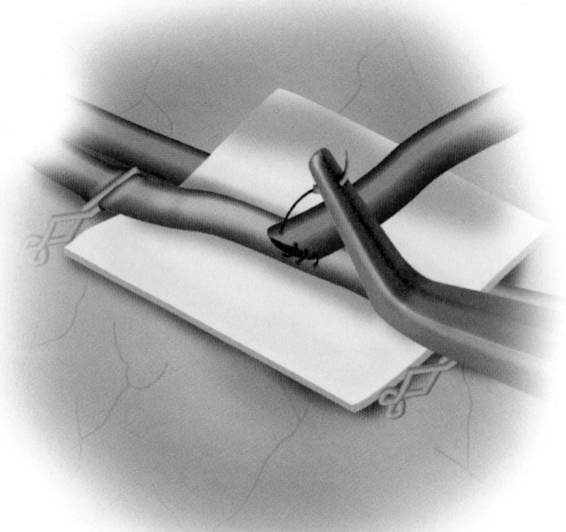

FIGURE 32-11

which is briefly described. First, the heel and foot of the STA graft are anchored to the recipient vessel using 10-0 monofilament microsuture with a tapered needle. The anchoring sutures are used to complete the anastomosis. Generally, the more anatomically difficult suture line is completed first so that the lumen can be inspected to ensure that the suture line is adequate and that the back wall has not been entrapped. Thereafter, the second, more straightforward suture line is completed. When using a running suture method, the suture needs to be "cinched" before tying to ensure the anastomosis remains watertight.

- **Figure 32-12:** Arterial blood flow is restored by removing the distal MCA temporary clip followed by the proximal MCA clip. Hemostasis along the suture line can usually be achieved with application of oxidized regenerated cellulose (Surgicel). If not, additional interrupted sutures may be necessary. When hemostasis is achieved, the temporary STA clip is removed, and graft patency is assessed. Multiple techniques may be used to verify arterial flow, including Doppler ultrasonography, cut flow indices (Charbel Micro-Flowprobe), indocyanine green angiography, and catheter angiography.

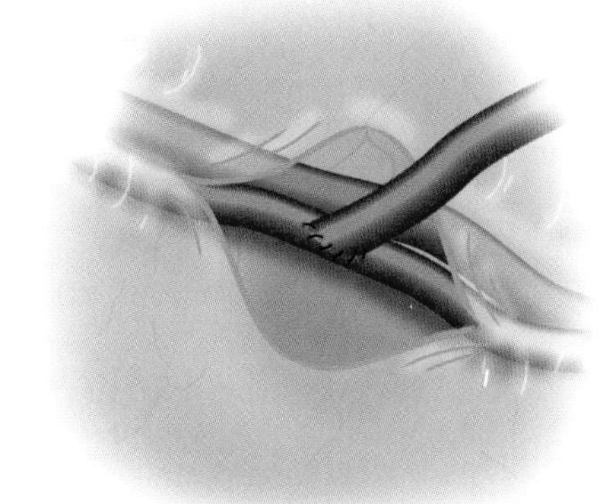

FIGURE 32-12

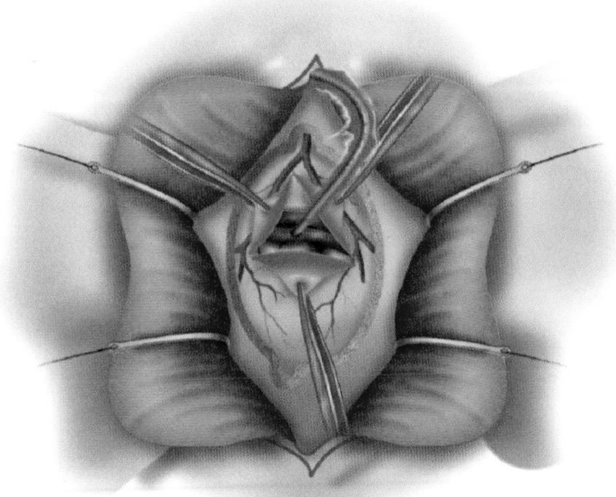

FIGURE 32-13

- **Figure 32-13:** The dura is carefully closed leaving a large durotomy window for the bypass. The bone flap is secured into place after sufficient bone has been removed with rongeurs allowing unhindered passage of the bypass. The temporalis muscle is reapproximated, taking care to avoid tethering or kinking the bypass. The scalp is closed using 3-0 Vicryl sutures and staples.

TIPS FROM THE MASTERS

- *Preoperative antiplatelet therapy*. We initiate aspirin therapy the day before surgery (e.g., 325 mg orally daily) to help minimize risk of intraoperative bypass thrombosis.
- *Neuroprotection*. We advocate use of several neuroprotective measures during STA-MCA bypass to help minimize the risk of ischemic complications caused by temporary MCA occlusion. First, mild hypothermia (33° C to 35° C) is achieved to suppress cerebral metabolism. Second, barbiturate-induced burst suppression, as verified by intraoperative electroencephalography, is performed. Third, mild hypertension is induced to maximize collateral cerebral blood flow. Finally, reagents or maneuvers that reduce intracranial pressure, such as mannitol or hyperventilation, are generally avoided to ensure that the cerebral cortex remains in close approximation with the dural edges and that undue tension is not placed on the anastomotic site.
- *Strict adherence to surgical technique*. Most bypass failures are due to lapses in surgical technique. We emphasize the following: (1) Maintain a clear, blood-free surgical field during anastomosis (e.g., use a silicone suction tube with multiple holes placed beneath

the rubber dam to remove cerebrospinal fluid continuously from the field). (2) Meticulously prepare the cut end of the STA including complete removal of the perivascular soft tissues. (3) Create an arteriotomy that is appropriately long (e.g., approximately 2 to 2.5 times the recipient vessel diameter). (4) Avoid "pinching" of the donor and recipient vessels, which may cause endothelial damage and promote graft thrombosis. (5) Perform the more difficult suture line first, and then check the lumen to ensure that the suture did not stenose or occlude the recipient vessel. (6) Primarily use tamponade with Surgicel to address postreperfusion bleeding because frequent and repeated use of interrupted sutures to achieve hemostasis risks causing stenosis and potentially occlusion of the bypass.

- *Postoperative care.* We advocate the following maneuvers to minimize risk of bypass occlusion in the postoperative period. Aspirin therapy is continued in the postoperative period (325 mg orally daily). Permissive hypertension is allowed in the immediate postoperative period, with mean arterial pressure goals of 100 to 120 mm Hg to facilitate collateral cerebral blood flow. Head wraps are avoided to prevent undue pressure on the graft, and the patient is encouraged to wear loose-fitting eyeglasses or to remove temporarily the ipsilateral eyeglass stem to ensure graft patency.

PITFALLS

Small reductions in mean arterial pressure or arterial carbon dioxide, or both, can lead to ischemic complications in patients undergoing STA-MCA bypass for chronic ischemia. A close working relationship between the neurosurgeon and the anesthesiologist is essential.

Lack of absolute hemostasis before performing anastomosis can lengthen the period of temporary circulatory arrest.

An arteriotomy that is too short (<2 times the diameter of the recipient vessel) predisposes the bypass to failure.

Poorly placed sutures, typically at the foot or heel of the anastomotic site, can lead to MCA stenosis or occlusion and, ultimately, bypass failure.

Discontinuation of aspirin therapy (especially in the early postoperative period) can lead to bypass thrombosis.

BAILOUT OPTIONS

- *Indirect revascularization.* If the recipient or donor vessels are deemed unsuitable for STA-MCA bypass, or if the bypass is attempted and fails, conversion to an indirect revascularization procedure where the STA is sewn to the pial surface (e.g., encephaloduroarteriosynangiosis) is a useful bailout option. Although an indirect procedure does not provide immediate revascularization, it can produce substantial pial collaterals and improve cerebral blood flow over time (typically months).

SUGGESTED READINGS

Adams HP Jr, Powers WJ, Grubb RL, et al. Preview of a new trial of extracranial-to-intracranial arterial anastomosis: the Carotid Occlusion Surgery Study. Neurosurg Clin N Am 2001;12:613–24.

Derdeyn CP, Yundt KD, Videen TO, et al. Increased oxygen extraction fraction is associated with prior ischemic events in patients with carotid occlusion. Stroke 1998;29:754–8.

Failure of extracranial-intracranial arterial bypass to reduce the risk of ischemic stroke: results of an international randomized trial. The EC/IC bypass study group. N Engl J Med 1985;313:1191–200.

Grubb RL Jr, Derdeyn CP, Fritsch SM, et al. Importance of hemodynamic factors in the prognosis of symptomatic carotid occlusion. JAMA 1998;280:1055–60.

Grubb RL Jr, Powers WJ, Derdeyn CP, et al. The carotid occlusion surgery study. Neurosurg Focus 2003;14:e9.

Zipfel GJ, Fox DJ, Rived DJ. Moyamoya disease in adults: the role of cerebral revascularization. Skull Base 2005;15:27–41.

Procedure 33

Extracranial-Intracranial High-Flow Bypass

Takanori Fukushima

INDICATIONS

- Despite advances in endovascular neurosurgery, cerebral bypass operations remain essential components in the management of giant aneurysms and some skull base tumors involving the carotid artery. Sacrifice of the internal carotid artery (ICA), either inadvertently or in a planned fashion, can be associated with substantial mortality (5%) and morbidity (15%).
- For the management of intracavernous or proximal carotid aneurysms and carotid-cavernous fistulas and radical resection of cavernous tumors and infratemporal fossa lesions, maintenance of the ICA flow is crucial.
- For cavernous sinus lesions, C6 petrous carotid to paraophthalmic C2 segment interposition saphenous vein graft or external carotid to submandibular subzygomatic pterygoid subtemporal saphenous vein bypass to the M2 inferior branch anastomosis is indicated. For an infratemporal vascular or neoplastic lesion, submandibular external carotid to subtemporal petrous carotid saphenous bypass can be performed, eliminating the infratemporal process or pathology.

CONTRAINDICATIONS

- This procedure is relatively contraindicated in elderly patients, patients with serious medical comorbidities, and patients in poor neurologic condition.

PLANNING AND POSITIONING

Types of High-Flow Carotid Bypass

- **Figure 33-1:** Fukushima bypass type 1. Petrous carotid C6 to paraophthalmic C2 saphenous interposition graft.
- Type 1 bypass is indicated for the management of intracavernous giant aneurysms and cavernous carotid stenosis and for radical resection of invasive meningioma or malignant tumors in this location.
- **Figure 33-2:** Fukushima bypass type 2. External carotid to petrous C6 infratemporal saphenous graft.
- Type 2 bypass is indicated for the repair of infratemporal or high cervical aneurysms, dissecting aneurysms, and stenosis and radical resection of infratemporal meningiomas or glomus tumors.
- **Figure 33-3:** Fukushima bypass type 3. External carotid to M2 saphenous vein graft.
- Type 3 bypass is used for management of proximal carotid aneurysms and intracavernous aneurysms.
- **Figure 33-4:** Fukushima bypass type 4. External carotid to P2 segment saphenous graft.

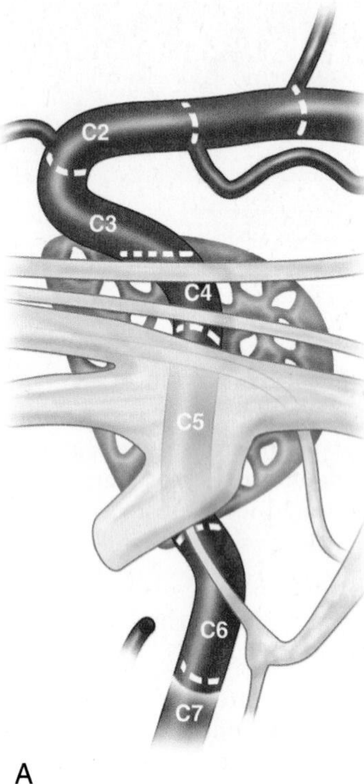

A

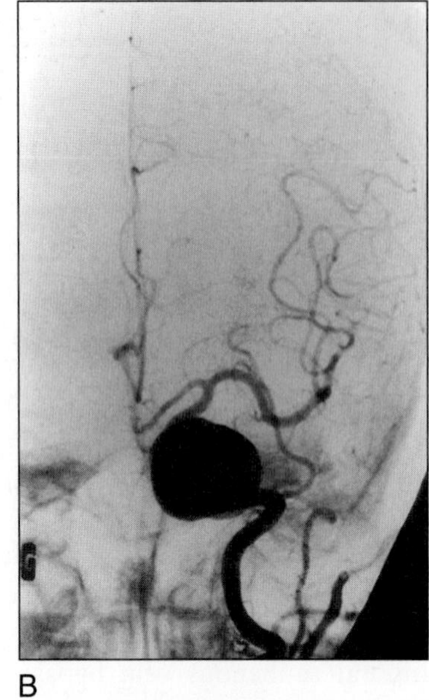

B

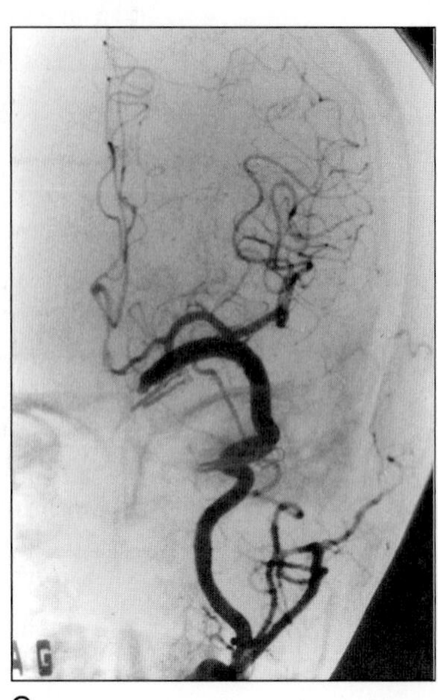

C

FIGURE 33-1

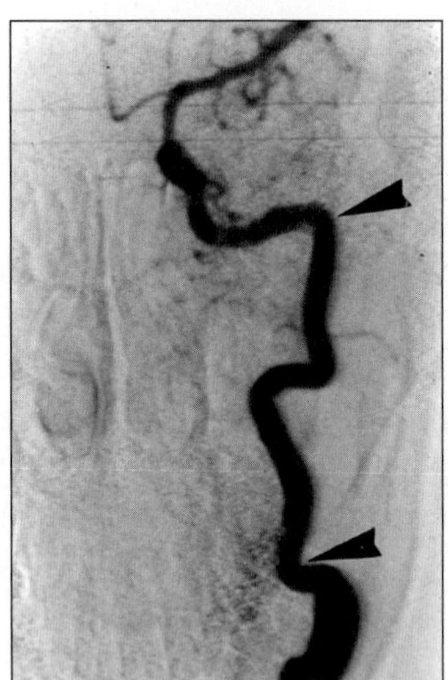

FIGURE 33-2

- Type 4 bypass is used for the management of basilar artery giant aneurysms.
- Preoperative evaluation includes a complete neurologic examination and assessments for visual function, respiratory status, cardiovascular status, diabetes mellitus, and gastrointestinal function. Preoperative routine laboratory values (complete blood count, coagulation profile, electrolytes, chemistry, and basic metabolic profile), chest x-ray, and electrocardiogram are essential.
- In addition to the standard neurologic examinations of computed tomography (CT), magnetic resonance imaging (MRI), or magnetic resonance angiography, a four-vessel catheter angiogram is essential for neuroradiologic evaluation of the vascular process.

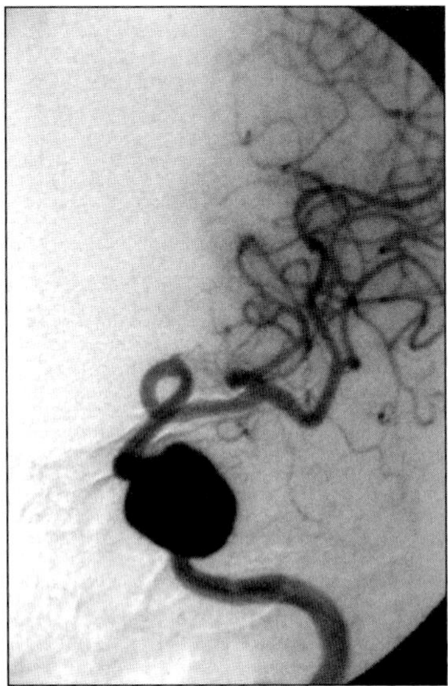
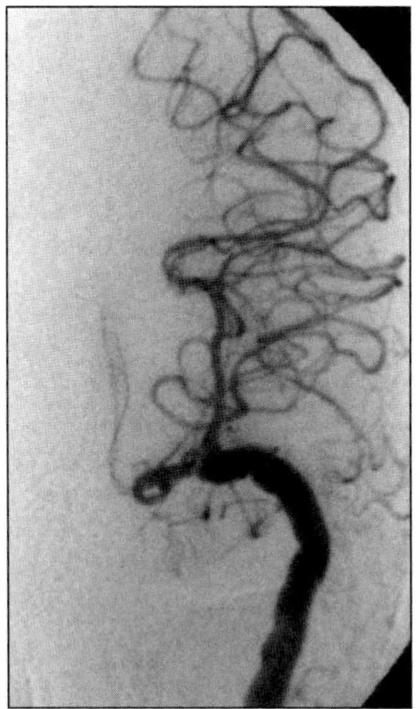

FIGURE 33-3

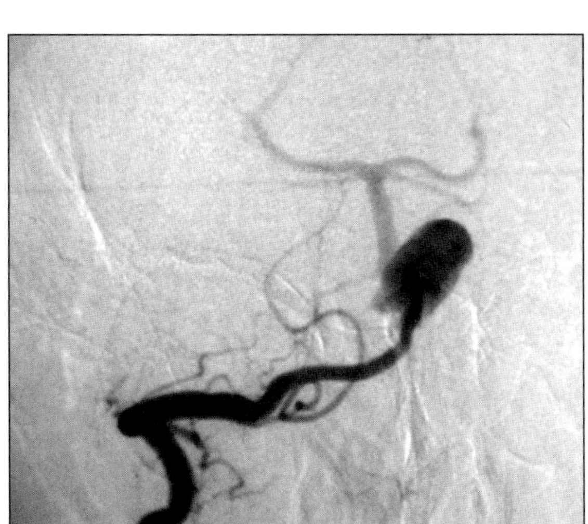
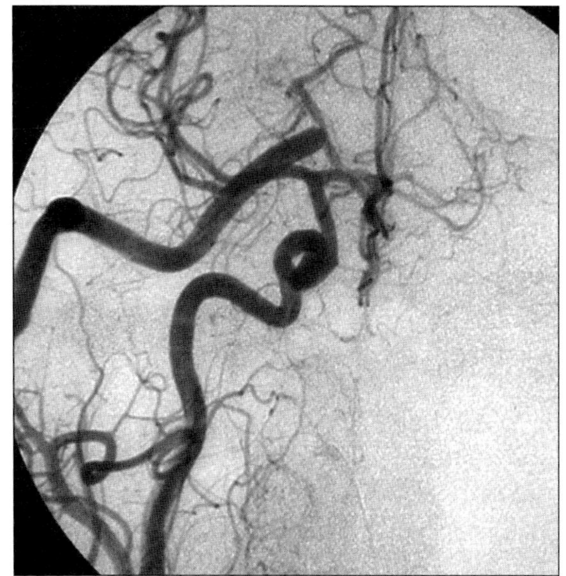

FIGURE 33-4

Frequently, a balloon occlusion test is indicated for assessment of cross flow or collateral circulation capacity.

- The patient is given a dose of preoperative antibiotics and dexamethasone (10 to 20 mg intravenously) before the skin incision. Brain relaxation is achieved with mannitol (25 to 50 g intravenously), furosemide (Lasix; 20 to 40 mg intravenously), and hyperventilation. When a tight brain is expected, a lumbar catheter may be inserted for continuous cerebrospinal fluid drainage intraoperatively and postoperatively. For temporary arterial occlusion during a difficult anastomosis procedure, a moderate dose of intravenous heparin (2000 to 4000 U), moderate hypothermia (33° C to 35° C), and barbiturate burst suppression pharmacologic brain protection may be used.

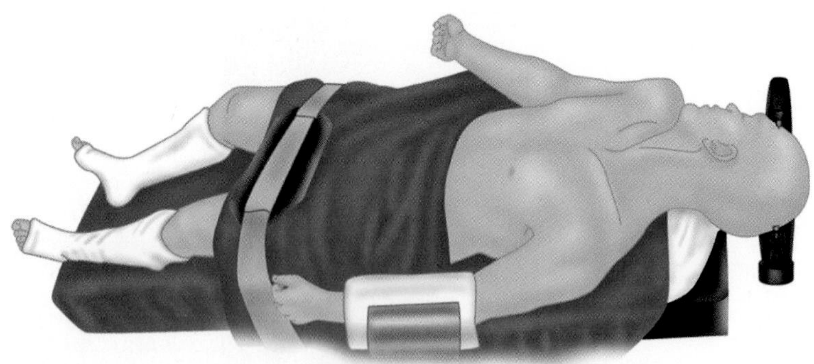

FIGURE 33-5

Positioning

- **Figure 33-5:** The patient is placed in the supine position with the head supported on an ear, nose, and throat (ENT) silicone pillow. The head is rotated to the other side for easy access to the frontotemporal craniotomy and to the submandibular cervical region. Most of the time, a three-pin skull clamp is avoided to facilitate opening of the cervical carotid artery and saphenous vein passage through submandibular, pterygoid, and subzygomatic areas to the subtemporal area. After the scalp and muscle layer are elevated, the head can be fixated securely with multiple blunt scalp hooks and blue silicone rubber bands anteriorly and posteriorly.
- Generally, the patient's upper torso is elevated 15 degrees, and the operating table is positioned at 15 degrees reverse Trendelenburg position to maintain the head above the level of the heart.

PROCEDURE

Skin Incision

- **Figure 33-6:** Skin incision starts usually from the preauricular zygomatic point 10 mm anterior to the tragus of the ear to avoid injury to the zygomatic and frontalis branches of the peripheral facial nerve and is extended anterosuperiorly behind the

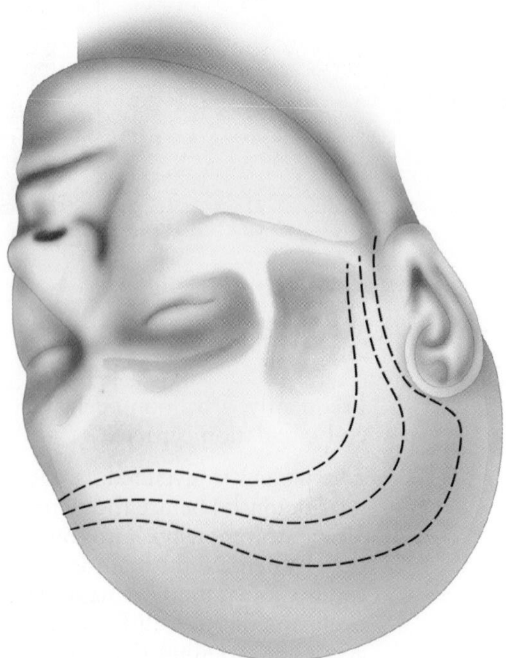

FIGURE 33-6

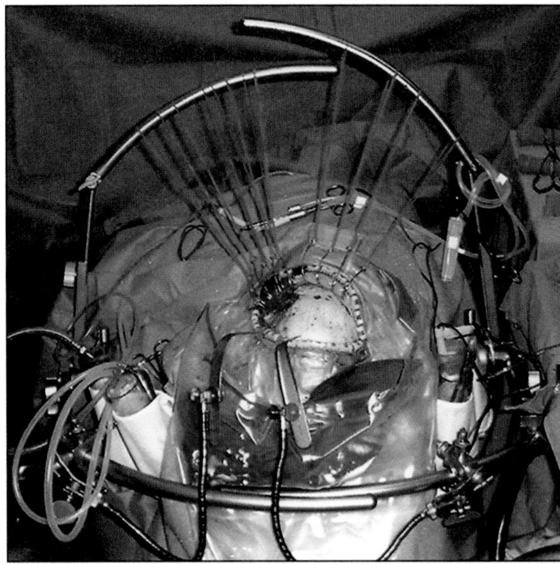

FIGURE 33-7

hairline as a gentle curve, crossing the midline a few centimeters to the other side. This incision is mostly done as a simple one-layer scalp elevation including the skin, galea, and temporal muscle together in a single unit.

Skin Flap Reflection

- **Figure 33-7:** The reflected skin is covered and protected with moist Telfa to prevent the skin drying up and then retracted anterosuperiorly with multiple blunt scalp hooks and rubber bands hooked to the front bar of the retraction system. The temporalis fascia and muscle are cut posteriorly along the same line of the scalp incision using monopolar cautery. Usually, we keep 1.5 cm of muscle from the root of zygoma to prevent devascularization and denervation of the posterior portion of the temporalis muscle. The temporal muscle and the periosteum are detached from the bone by monopolar or periosteal elevators (Adson Joker and Langebeck periosteal elevators). The scalp and muscle flap are reflected using multiple blunt hooks (5 to 10 hooks—sizes small, medium, and large). It is important to elevate the scalp and temporal muscle 45 degrees anteriorly to avoid any compression to the eyes. The orbital ridge, lateral orbital rim, and frontozygomatic suture are identified. A regular standard frontotemporal pterional craniotomy is then made.
- As mentioned before, for high-flow saphenous vein bypass, the head is supported on an ENT pillow without three-pin fixation so that the surgeon can adjust the head positioning. Generally, the head is rotated 45 degrees to the other side in moderate extension to facilitate access to the submandibular cervical carotid artery and to the frontotemporal, subtemporal, and infratemporal regions.

Craniotomy

- **Figure 33-8:** A small burr hole is made posteriorly around the temporal squama. We never use a conventional 14-mm large perforator. A 5-mm extra-coarse diamond drill is used to make a 6-mm burr hole opening with just enough space to pass the craniotome footplate. The outer table and diploic cancellous bone are removed, and the inner table is shaved, leaving a thin shell of bone over the dura. After the eggshelling procedure, the remaining thin inner cortical table is removed with a curet or dissector. After the small bone opening is made, the dura is dissected with a 90-degree Fukushima burr hole dural elevator. Next, the triangular construct of the sphenoid wing is drilled away, exposing the frontal and temporal dura. Triangular pterional drilling is continued downward to the orbitotemporal junction detachment, and then subtemporal groove drilling is performed in a golf club shape. In patients older than 60 years, usually the frontal dura is very thin and adherent to the inner cortical plate, so a small frontal burr hole is made near the orbital ridge near the supraorbital rim. This second burr hole

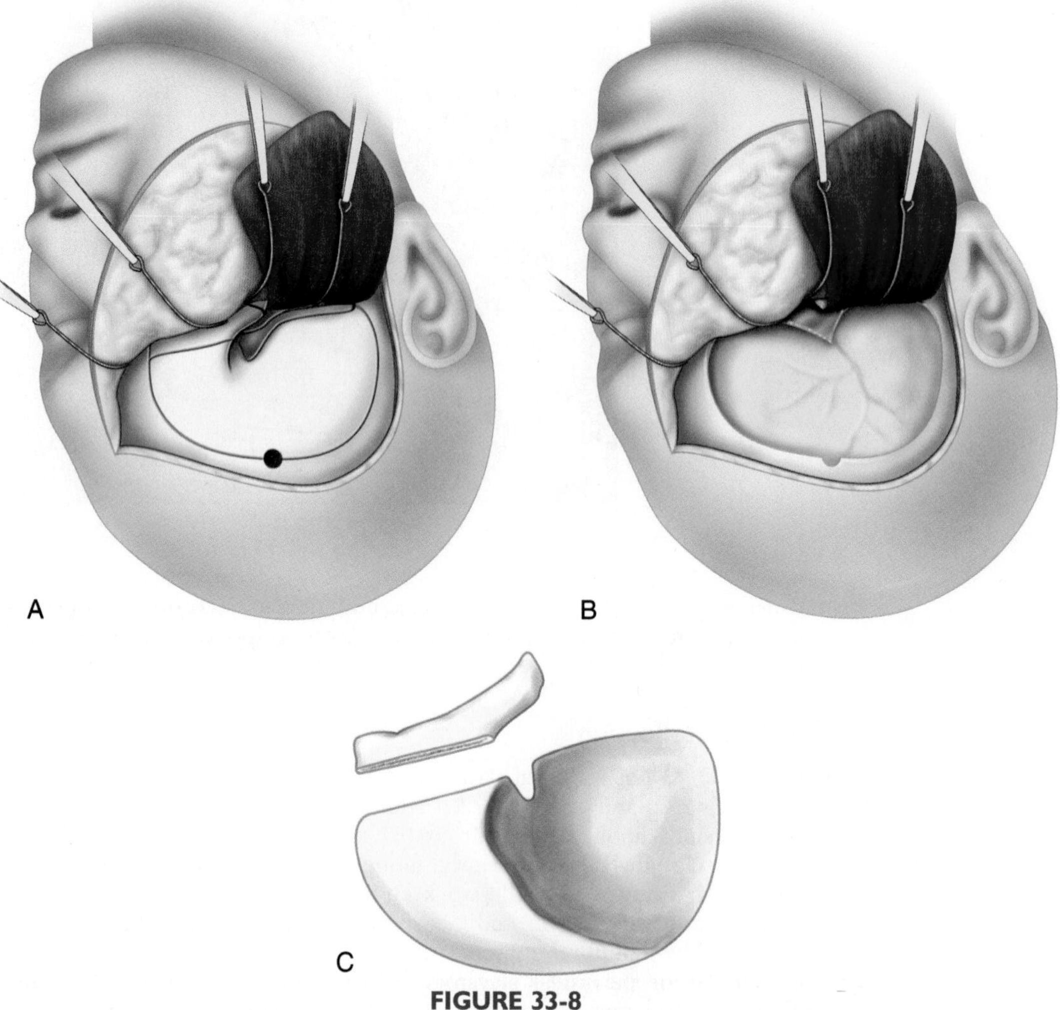

FIGURE 33-8

prevents damage and disruption of the anteromedial frontal dura. A small craniotome is used to achieve minimum bone loss in a cosmetic fashion. When the kidney-shaped frontotemporal bone flap is turned, the dural tack-up stitches are made posteriorly with multiple bone holes. The epidural dissection is advanced to the frontal base, pterion, sphenoid ridge, and subtemporal area.

- For type 1 bypass, exposure of the C6 petrous carotid and C2–3 clinoid and paraophthalmic carotid segments is necessary; a Dolenc-type anteromedial and Fukushima-type anterolateral extradural elevation of the dura and anterior clinoidectomy and optic canal unroofing should be performed.
- Dural elevation begins from the anterior skull base to the sphenoid ridge and to the anterior middle fossa. The frontal dura is elevated with a Joker dissector or skull base sharp A dissector to confirm the olfactory dural line, ethmoid band, and planum sphenoidale. First, the entire sphenoid ridge is drilled off to the meningoorbital band, and then the orbital roof is shaved flat to the eggshell. The anterior clinoid process starts from the meningoorbital band, and this triangular shark tooth–like bone is firmly attached to the sphenoid bone by the optic strut.

Anterior Clinoidectomy

- **Figure 33-9:** Removal of the anterior clinoid process is the most important and the most frequently used technique in cavernous sinus surgery. There are some risks from drill bur slippage or thermal injury to the optic nerve; extreme care and attention needs to be focused on the proper technique of the drill procedure. We start with a 4-mm or

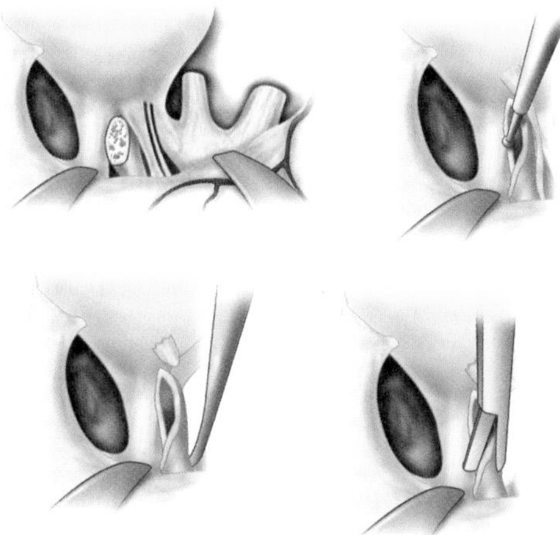

FIGURE 33-9

3-mm coarse diamond bur to make the anterior clinoid process inside hollow and empty. Using a 2-mm or 3-mm diamond bur, the medial half of the anterior clinoid process is removed from the optic strut anteriorly and posteriorly, avoiding damage to the optic nerve dura. When the medial half of the anterior clinoid process is removed, the lateral half can be elevated with a sharp A or D dissector and then twisted and removed with alligator forceps.

Optic Canal Unroofing

- **Figure 33-10:** Optic canal unroofing is started from the orbital side to the falciform ligament. Most of the time, medially the sphenoid bone is not drilled to avoid sphenoid sinus opening. The drilling of the anterior clinoid process and the optic canal should be performed very gently with cooling irrigation. There is some risk of visual compromise during this step in the procedure.
- It is incumbent on the surgeon to have practiced this technique in the anatomy laboratory. Next, dural elevation is continued in the anterolateral direction to the temporal base to elevate the dura while achieving meticulous hemostasis with bone wax, monopolar and bipolar cautery, and Surgicel. Care must be taken when using the monopolar cautery not to propagate the electric current and heat to any neurovascular structures. Typically, the dura propria is elevated from the V2 and V3 foramen rotundum and foramen ovale, and then the dura is elevated posteriorly, and the middle meningeal artery is coagulated and divided. In most cases, the midpoint of the root of zygoma indicates the foramen spinosum and middle meningeal artery. The surgeon starts the posterior cavernous dissection.

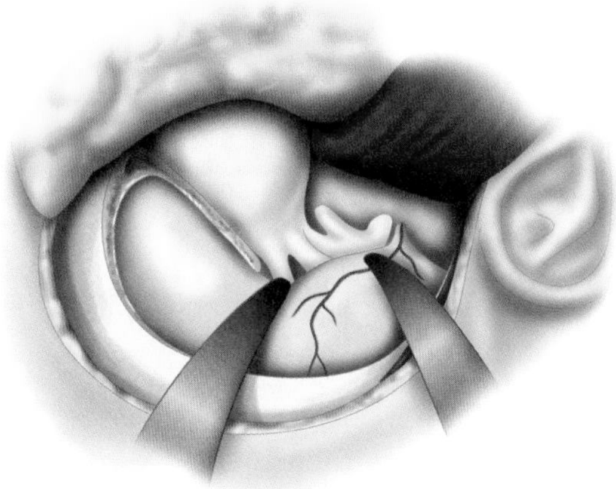

FIGURE 33-10

Identification of Greater Superficial Petrosal Nerve and Internal Carotid Artery C6 Portion

- **Figure 33-11:** After detachment of the middle meningeal artery, the dura and the dura propria are elevated continuously from the trigeminal third branch. Just medial to the foramen spinosum, the lesser petrosal nerve and then the greater superficial petrosal nerve (GSPN) and the facial hiatus can be confirmed. After the identification of the GSPN, further dural elevation to the petrous ridge is performed while holding the dura with 2-mm rigid extradural tapered retractors. The posterior border of the trigeminal third branch can be retracted anteriorly to expose the longer C6 petrous carotid artery. To obtain sufficient length of the C6 petrous carotid, often the GSPN needs to be incised at the facial hiatus, and posteriorly the geniculate ganglion can be located with a facial nerve stimulator. Using a 3-mm or 4-mm diamond drill, the surgeon now uncovers the petrous C6 segment of the carotid artery at the Glasscock cavernous sinus triangle. The petrous carotid artery is located just under the GSPN and can be exposed about 10 mm. The C6 petrous carotid genu in the carotid canal resides only 1 or 2 mm from the cochlea; extreme care must be taken when drilling. Most of the time, with gentle retraction of the trigeminal third branch, about 12 mm of the C6 petrous carotid can be exposed, which is sufficient to perform the end-to-side or end-to-end saphenous vein microanastomosis.

Opening of the Fibrous Ring

- **Figure 33-12:** For exposure of the C2–3 paraophthalmic carotid artery, the dura needs to be incised at the frontotemporal base and then longitudinally along the lateral margin of the optic nerve. The optic dural sheath is incised, and removal of the carotid fibrous ring is accomplished with rigid curved microscissors.

Bypass Type 1 (C6 to C3)

- **Figure 33-13:** In my 70 cases of C6 to C3 saphenous bypass, 7% of patients have experienced a visual deficit owing to the temporary occlusion of the ophthalmic artery for 30 to 50 minutes. Before anastomosis to the paraophthalmic segment, preoperative balloon occlusion testing is necessary to determine ophthalmic artery ischemic tolerance. If the ophthalmic artery temporary occlusion is not tolerated, M2 inferior trunk microanastomosis can be considered.

Bypass Type 3

- **Figure 33-14:** When high-flow carotid bypass or carotid replacement is necessary to treat intracavernous giant aneurysms or proximal carotid vascular lesions, the submandibular cervical external carotid to M2 saphenous bypass can be employed. To accomplish this, the cervical ICA and the external carotid artery is exposed at the submandibular region with a transverse incision. Usually, the saphenous vein is anastomosed to the external carotid artery end-to-side with 8-0 monofilament nylon

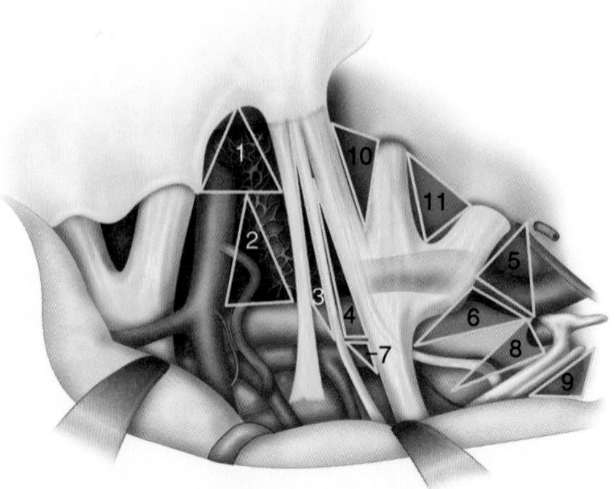

FIGURE 33-11

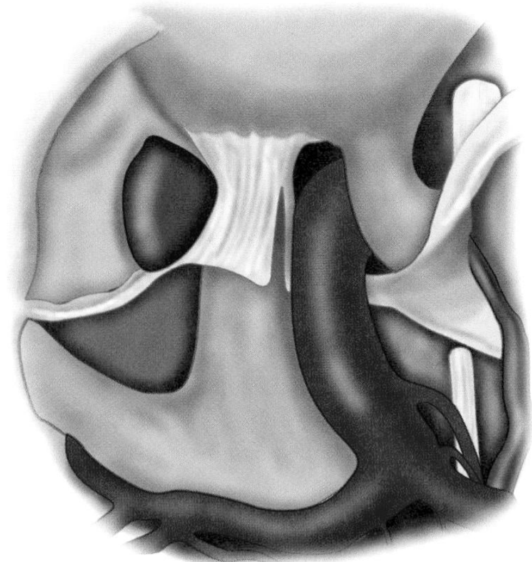

FIGURE 33-12

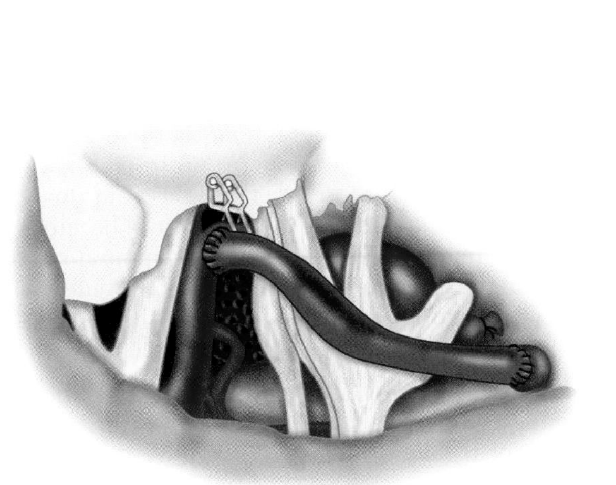

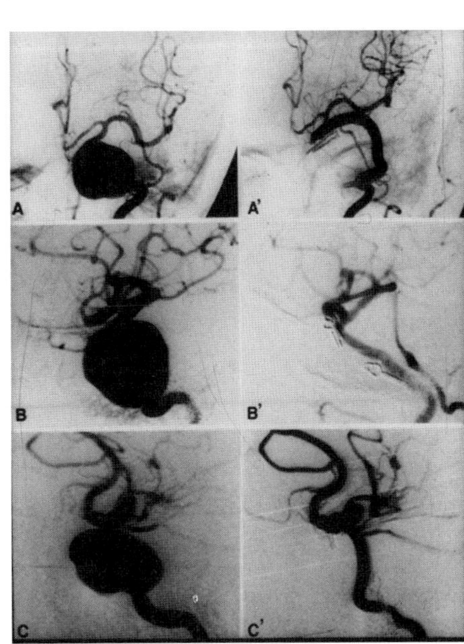

FIGURE 33-13

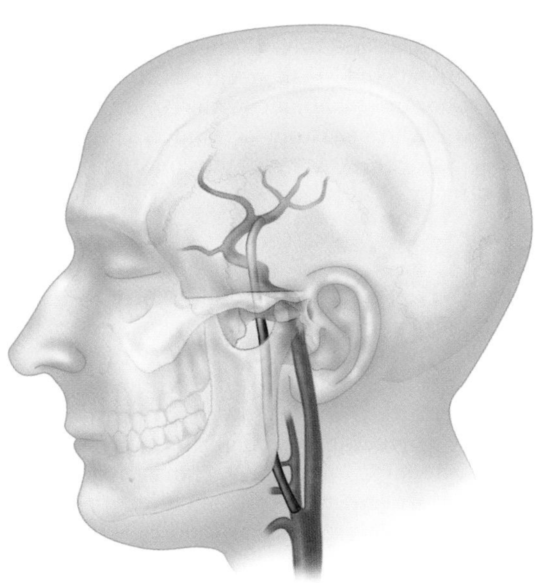

FIGURE 33-14

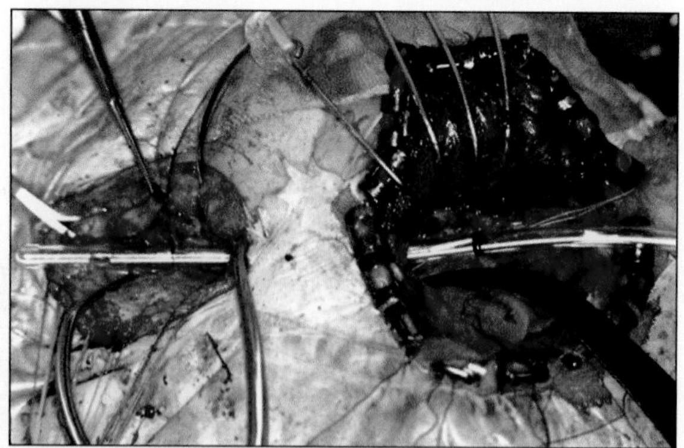

FIGURE 33-15

sutures. The external carotid artery is temporarily ligated with vascular tourniquet or a large Mizuho clip proximally and distally. Most of the time, after the incision to the external carotid artery, I use a 3-mm or 4-mm vascular punch to make an oval aperture for easy anastomosis with the saphenous vein. Microanastomosis is performed with 1-mm deep, full-thickness stitches and with strict intima-to-intima approximation with interrupted sutures 1 mm apart from each other.

Chest Tube Technique

- **Figure 33-15:** The saphenous vein can be passed from the submandibular to the subzygomatic infratemporal area by the subtemporal and infratemporal drill procedure to expose the infratemporal fascia. A small hole around the lateral pterygoid muscle is made. Blunt dissection through this infratemporal hole via the posterior pterygoid fossa connects to the submandibular external carotid area. Also, the surgeon can bluntly dissect from the submandibular space toward the pterygoid fossa and from the infratemporal region down, creating a corridor for the graft. The surgeon then passes a large Kelly clamp from the subtemporal area to the infratemporal region, grasping the No. 28 chest tube and passing the tube through this pterygoid route. A 1-0 silk suture is pulled into the chest tube with suction irrigation. This 1-0 silk suture is tied to the end of the saphenous vein graft. The saphenous vein graft is passed through the chest tube.
- The saphenous vein distally is anastomosed to the external carotid, and the proximal saphenous end is anastomosed to the M2 segment. Usually after transsylvian exposure, we prefer the posterior inferior trunk of the M2. This M2 vessel is elevated with a rubber dam resting on Gelfoam.
- **Figure 33-16:** Under barbiturate, mannitol, and phenytoin (Dilantin) pharmacologic protection, a temporary clip is applied to the M2. Within 30 minutes, the saphenous vein is microanastomosed to the M2 segment end-to-side. A 9-0 monofilament nylon stitch with tapered small needle is used. To avoid any postanastomosis leak, 1-mm intima-to-intima technique with 1-mm increments of interrupted sutures should be used. To secure anastomosis and to prevent leakage, a small piece of Surgicel is applied. Sometimes I wrap the anastomotic site with shredded Teflon tape and a small amount of fibrin glue.

Bypass Type 2

- **Figure 33-17:** For infratemporal lesions, to remove glomus vagale tumors or to repair high cervical infratemporal aneurysms, external carotid-to-petrous C6 anastomosis is performed. Most of the time, after the passage of the saphenous vein graft, the saphenous vein is anastomosed to the petrous C6 carotid end-to-end, which provides direct carotid flow to the cavernous carotid artery to replace the infratemporal ICA. To secure patency of the high-flow bypass, the surgeon's skill of microanastomosis suture is the most important technical issue. A smaller, thinner curved tapered needle with monofilament nylon of 2-inch length suture is used. Usually four or five sutures are needed for one microanastomosis. The key element of the anastomosis technique is intima-to-intima precise approximation for each stitch.

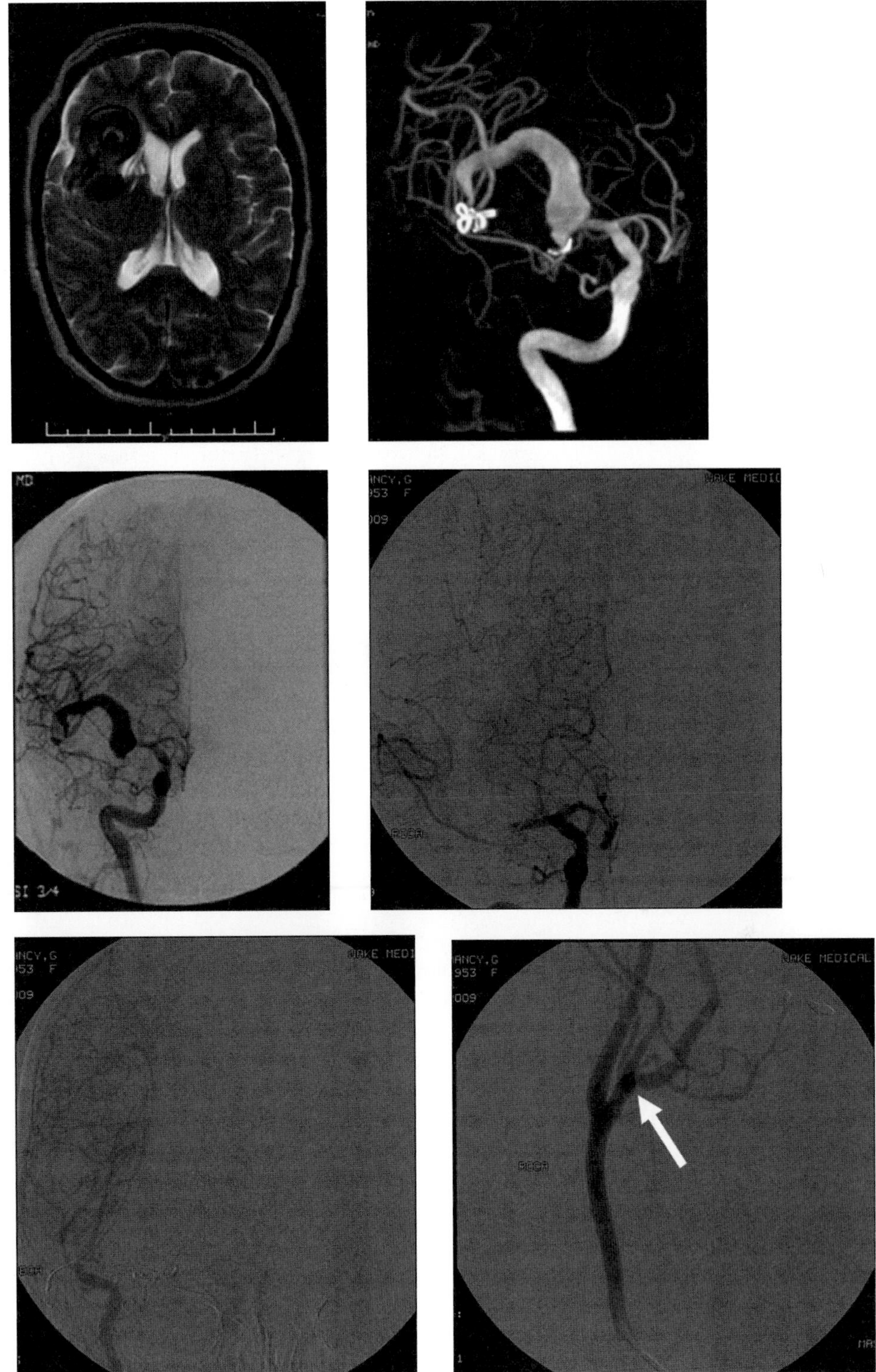

FIGURE 33-16

TIPS FROM THE MASTERS

- Maintain a bloodless clean operative field by meticulous hemostasis and sharp dissection technique from the skin incision until closure.
- Use accurate, efficient, and speedy microanastomosis to minimize temporary occlusion time, possibly one microanastomosis within 30 minutes.
- Perform intima-to-intima full layer 1 × 1 mm microsuture technique.

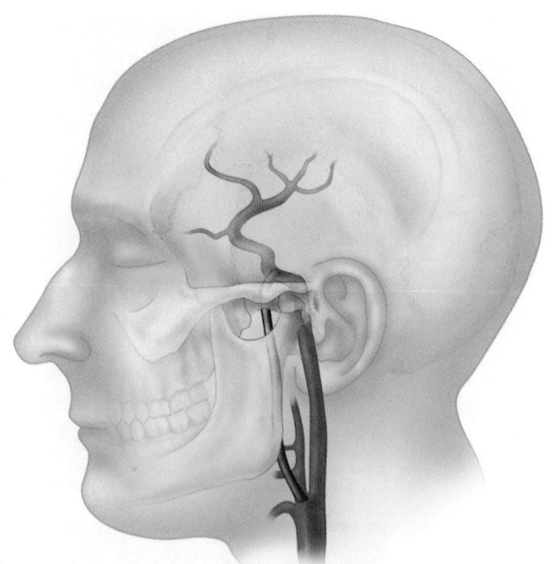

FIGURE 33-17

PITFALLS

Avoid involvement of the opposite side vessel wall when suturing because it would cause postoperative occlusion.

Avoid blood leakage after microanastomosis.

Avoid visual deficit by using extremely careful drilling and dissection around the optic canal and the anterior clinoid process. Temporary clipping of the ophthalmic artery may cause 7% incidence of visual deficit.

Temporary clips may cause low flow, poor collateral circulation, and ischemic complications. Pay attention and use all possible brain protection measures and monitoring methods such as electroencephalogram or cerebral blood flow.

BAILOUT OPTIONS

- If any vessel—external carotid, paraophthalmic carotid, or middle cerebral artery—is calcified or has thick atherosclerosis, choose other locations of the vessel to prevent anastomosis occlusion.
- If the recipient vessel caliber is too small—less than one third of the saphenous vein—congestion of the high-flow bypass occurs, and this may lead to postoperative occlusion or thrombosis. It is best for the recipient vessel to be at least half the size of the saphenous vein.

SUGGESTED READINGS

Bulsara KR, Patel T, Fukushima T. Cerebral bypass surgery for skull base lesions: technical notes incorporating lessons learned over two decades. Neurosurg Focus 2008;24:E11.

Spetzler RF, Fukushima T, Martin N, et al. Petrous carotid-to-intradural carotid saphenous vein graft for intracavernous giant aneurysm, tumor, and occlusive cerebrovascular disease. J Neurosurg 1990;73:496–501.

Procedure 34

Open Evacuation of Intracerebral Hematoma

Issam Awad, Mahua Dey, Jennifer Jaffe

INDICATIONS

- Symptomatic intracerebral hemorrhage (ICH) causing progressive neurologic symptoms or impending cerebral herniation syndromes is best managed with open evacuation, especially in younger patients, in whom there is less atrophy and cerebral compliance to accommodate mass effect.
- ICH that is associated with suspected underlying structural etiology (vascular malformation, tumor, aneurysm) is best managed with open surgical evacuation, allowing evacuation of hematoma and addressing the underlying structural lesion as appropriate. Lobar hemorrhage, especially in younger patients, is more likely associated with underlying structural abnormalities compared with deep ICH, which is more commonly associated with hypertension.
- ICH associated with more diffuse cerebral edema (e.g., in the setting of trauma or hemorrhagic conversion of arterial or venous infarction) is best evacuated by an open approach, which also allows decompression craniectomy and expansive duraplasty if necessary.
- Infratentorial hematomas causing mass effect on the brainstem and hydrocephalus from compression of the fourth ventricle (or extension of bleed to the ventricular system) are best managed by prompt open surgical evacuation.

CONTRAINDICATIONS

- Hemorrhages involving deep nuclei are best managed with stereotactic aspiration rather than open surgery.
- Lobar hemorrhages in older patients, without rapid deterioration in neurologic condition or suspected structural lesion, may be managed expectantly or by stereotactic catheter aspiration.
- Surgical evacuation of ICH should not be attempted in the setting of uncorrected coagulopathy or platelet dysfunction.

PLANNING AND POSITIONING

- Initial evaluation of a patient with ICH should involve evaluation with an imaging modality such as computed tomography (CT). In almost all cases, a few additional minutes are taken to obtain computed tomography angiography (CTA) to rule out underlying vascular etiology.
- In stable patients, a more complete diagnostic evaluation is done if CTA provides insufficient information to allow appropriate management of the underlying structural lesion (magnetic resonance imaging [MRI] or formal angiography if tumor [MRI] or aneurysm [angiography] is suspected). In stable patients, fiducial scalp markers or other preparations are undertaken for image-guided planning and execution of the surgery.
- In the presence of a large ICH with associated shift, mannitol (0.5 to 1 g/kg) is administered intravenously, and judicious hyperventilation is instituted after induction of general anesthesia. Prophylactic anticonvulsant is administered in all cases but infratentorial ICH.

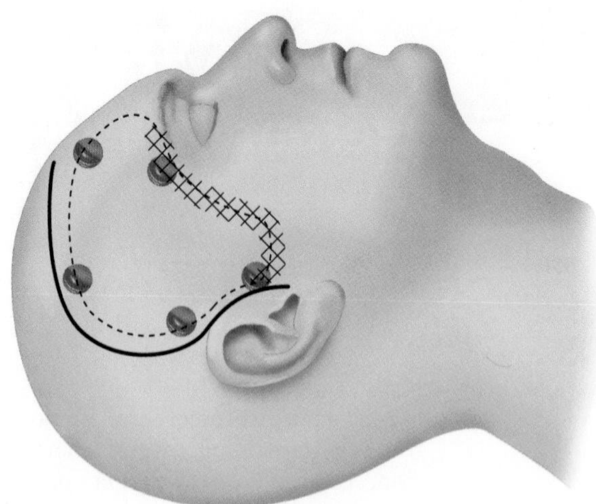

FIGURE 34-1

- Normotension is instituted and insured especially if underlying aneurysm or vascular malformation is suspected. Blood pressure control should be particularly insured during placement of skull fixation pins and on skin incision.
- **Figure 34-1:** In the case of a supratentorial hematoma involving the frontoparietal region, the patient is positioned in supine position with the head turned opposite to the side of operation and the neck slightly extended, making the zygoma the highest point of the face. Position is fixed using a three-point Mayfield headrest set. This incision is used for all cases of frontotemporal ICH. Bony exposure at the skull base is indicated to accommodate potential temporal lobe edema, and frontobasal resection of the lesser wing of the sphenoid (*hatched areas*) is indicated to address associated aneurysms. Aneurysms are secured at the same time as ICH evacuation to prevent rebleeding. Resection of associated arteriovenous malformation (AVM) or other vascular anomaly should be planned unless the AVM is complex and requires preparatory embolization. In such cases, bony exposure should be wide enough to accommodate AVM resection at the same or a subsequent procedure.
- **Figure 34-2:** In the case of hematoma involving the posterior temporal, parietal, or occipital regions, a more posterior flap is planned as shown, with the patient positioned supine, the ipsilateral shoulder elevated on a roll, and the head turned into the lateral position and fixed in a three-point Mayfield headrest. The flap should be generous to accommodate potential brain swelling and to address associated vascular or tumor pathology.

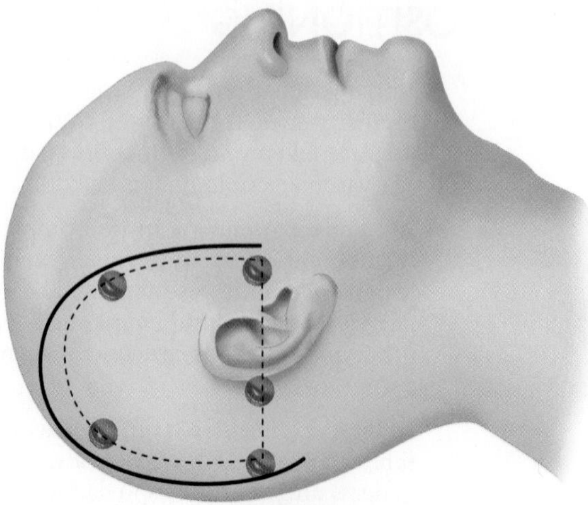

FIGURE 34-2

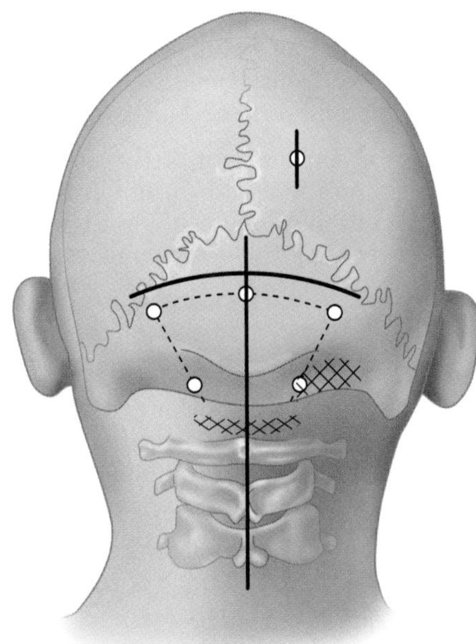

FIGURE 34-3

- **Figure 34-3:** In the case of infratentorial hematoma, the patient is first intubated in the supine position and then turned to the prone position with the neck slightly flexed. The position is fixed using a three-point Mayfield headrest set. Bony exposure should be generous, extending more on the side of the ICH and typically including the rim of the foramen magnum, allowing for potential cerebellar edema. The arch of the atlas (C1 vertebra) should be resected in cases of large cerebellar hematomas or in the setting of associated vascular anomaly, and resection of the ipsilateral condyle should be planned for cases associated with posterior inferior cerebellar aneurysms (*hatched areas*). A point above the lambdoid suture (6 cm above the inion and 2 to 3 cm lateral to the midline) should be marked and prepared in the surgical field to allow ventricular drainage if needed (see Tips from the Masters section).

PROCEDURE

- The flap and bony exposure should be generous, extending well beyond the area of the hematoma.
- With the dura tight in most cases, a small cruciate opening is made over the area of the hematoma, and a small corticectomy is performed with gentle suction of enough hematoma to decompress some of the mass effect. At this stage, neither radical evacuation of the ICH nor resection of associated tumor or vascular anomaly should be attempted.
- The surface of the cortex right above the hematoma is gently coagulated with a bipolar cautery, and a small cortical incision is made. Gently using a bipolar cautery and suction, the incision is widened to approach the hematoma. Image guidance is used, if available, in more stable patients to optimize location of the initial durotomy and corticectomy.
- After initial decompression of mass effect, the durotomy is widened in a cruciate fashion. The operating microscope is used in all but the most emergent situations to evacuate the rest of the ICH, while watching for active bleeding sources and securing hemostasis with irrigating bipolar cautery. The hematoma is resected under direct visualization, until the brain border is reached; this is covered with cottonoid patties to assist with hemostasis and to reach deeper portions of the ICH.
- In cases of suspected tumor or vascular anomalies, these are looked for carefully and addressed in all but large complex AVMs. In cases of primary ICH, the brain surface is carefully explored for active bleeding points, which are sequentially secured using irrigating bipolar cautery. Active bleeding should not be simply covered by hemostatic materials.

- In cases of large complex AVMs that have not been treated with embolization, enough ICH is resected to accomplish decompression, but the AVM is carefully avoided to avoid uncontrolled bleeding. Bleeding from the AVM nidus can be controlled using Avitene Hemostat or gentle pressure on a thrombin-soaked Gelfoam patty.
- Hemostasis of the brain surface and within the AVM nidus is attained by careful compression with thrombin-soaked Gelfoam. Aneurysms and tumors are addressed definitively along with evacuation of the ICH to prevent rebleeding or tumor swelling during the postoperative period.
- The ICH cavity is irrigated with cool saline to enhance hemostasis, and when the irrigant is crystal clear, the cavity is lined by a thin layer of Surgicel (http://www.ethicon360.com/products/surgicel-family-absorbable-hemostats).
- In cases of documented or anticipated brain swelling, a wide durotomy is created; the brain surface is covered by two layers of DuraGen (one beneath and one above the dural leaflets), and the bone craniotomy bone is freeze-stored for later cranioplasty (http://www.medcompare.com/details/1611/Duragen-Dural-Graft-Matrix.html).
- In cases in which the brain is fully relaxed (sunken), primary dural closure is accomplished, and bone is returned and the wound closed in layers as per routine technique.

TIPS FROM THE MASTERS

- If the hematoma does not extend to the cortical surface, the corticectomy site to access the ICH should be chosen anterior or posterior to eloquent motor or language cortex, as close as possible to the surface extension of the hematoma.
- The corticectomy should be widened to allow cottonoid patties to be placed in the ICH cavity for optimal visualization and hemostasis.
- In large supratentorial ICH in which the cerebral ventricle is entered, a ventricular catheter may be placed in the ventricular system under direct microsurgical visualization to exit through the corticectomy and a burr hole, tunneled through an exit site adjacent to the main incision for postoperative external ventricular drainage.
- In infratentorial hemorrhages, opening of the cisterna magna allows significant cerebellar relaxation, which enhances exposure and the ability to resect the hematoma and explore the cavity for hemostasis. In comatose patients without an external ventricular drain, the previously marked supratentorial burr hole site should be used to tap the lateral ventricle and place a ventricular catheter. Imaging guidance and a passive catheter introducer should be used when available for safer and more accurate placement of the ventricular catheter.

PITFALLS

Operating in a patient with a coagulopathy typically is counterproductive, with frequent recurrence of larger ICH postoperatively. In cases of emergent surgery, correction of a coagulopathy should be performed concurrently, including the use of recombinant factor VIIa (NovoSeven) and platelet transfusions.

Do not simply suck the ICH and plug the cavity with hemostatic agents, because this is ineffective. Always think of visualization and hemostasis.

Always plan a wider craniotomy than the ICH and to accommodate potential decompression craniectomy for edema.

In most instances, aneurysms and most tumors are addressed at the same time as ICH evacuation. For difficult aneurysms, a conservative lifesaving ICH evacuation is performed with immediate postoperative endovascular treatment of the aneurysm. Do not delay securing the aneurysm.

Do not dig into an AVM while evacuating associated ICH ("do not disturb the tiger unless you are prepared to tackle it").

BAILOUT OPTIONS

- External ventricular drainage
- Decompressive craniectomy
- NovoSeven and platelet transfusion for uncontrolled bleeding

SUGGESTED READINGS

Mendelow AD. Investigators and the Steering Committee. The International Surgical Trial in Intracerebral Hemorrhage (ISTICH). Acta Neurochir Suppl 2003;86:441–53.

Mendelow AD, Gregson BA, Fernandes HM, et al. Early surgery versus initial conservative treatment in patient with spontaneous supratentorial intracerebral hematoma in the International Surgical Trial in Intracerebral Hemorrhage (STICH): a randomised trial. Lancet 2005;365:387–97.

Mitchell P, Gregson BA, Vindlacheruvu RR, et al. Surgical options in ICH including decompressive craniectomy. J Neurol Sci 2007;261:89–98.

Prasad K, Mendelow AD, Gregson B. Surgery for primary supratentorial intracerebral hemorrhage. Cochrane Database Syst Rev 2008;4.

Rabinstein AA, Wijdicks EF. Surgery for intracerebral hematoma: the search for the elusive right candidate. Rev Neurol Dis 2006;3:163–72.

Procedure 35

Image-Guided Catheter Evacuation and Thrombolysis for Intracerebral Hematoma

Issam Awad, Mahua Dey, Jennifer Jaffe

INDICATIONS

- Spontaneous intracerebral hemorrhage (ICH)
- Deep-seated and lobar hematomas with suspected underlying hypertension or cerebral amyloid angiopathy
- Moderate-sized and large hematomas (>20 mL)
- Normal coagulation parameters (international normalized ratio [INR] < 1.3, prothrombin time < 14, and partial thromboplastin time < 30 to 32 seconds or local normal range), platelet counts greater than 100,000/μL, and no evidence of platelet dysfunction other than aspirin effect (i.e., known use of clopidogrel [Plavix])
- Stable clot volume (as evidenced by radiographic imaging 6 hours later)
- Stable or slowly declining neurologic condition

CONTRAINDICATIONS

- The procedure is contraindicated in patients with poor functional status or multiple medical comorbidities that put them at a high surgical risk or preclude meaningful recovery or rehabilitation.
- Glasgow Coma Scale score 4 or less or extension of ICH into the brainstem typically precludes meaningful recovery.
- Infratentorial hemorrhage (including cerebellum) requiring surgery is better approached with open suboccipital craniotomy.
- Patients with rapidly deteriorating neurologic condition or signs of impending herniation, or both, are better treated with open surgical evacuation of ICH and other decompressive techniques.
- Secondary hematomas resulting from vascular malformation, tumor, or ruptured aneurysm are inappropriate for image-guided surgery and are better suited for an open procedure that can address the primary process causing the bleed.
- Small (<20 mL) or asymptomatic lesions should be managed expectantly because risk of intervention may not be justified.
- Progressively enlarging ICH should not be treated with catheter evacuation and may require open surgery to address an active bleeding source.
- Coagulopathy and abnormal platelet counts or function should be corrected, and clot stability should be established. Elevated INR and prothrombin time are often found in patients on warfarin and can be reversed with vitamin K, fresh frozen plasma, and recombinant factor VIIa (NovoSeven). Heparin-induced coagulopathy can be reversed with protamine sulfate. Patients with platelet counts less than 100,000/μL and known platelet dysfunction (other than aspirin effect) should be treated with platelet transfusions.

PLANNING AND POSITIONING

- Initial imaging of a patient with ICH-like symptoms is typically with a computed tomography (CT) scan because it quickly establishes diagnosis and assesses ICH volume. To ensure that the hematoma is not expanding, follow-up CT scan should be performed about 6 hours later. If the volume of the hematoma is significantly enlarged (>5 mL growth), catheter placement should be postponed until the clot has stopped expanding, or open surgical evacuation should be considered if the patient is rapidly deteriorating. Correction of coagulopathy is essential to allow stabilization of ICH before catheter placement.
- A search for the etiology should be performed, particularly in younger patients and patients without a history of uncontrolled hypertension, to exclude an underlying vascular malformation, tumor, or aneurysm. This evaluation can best be accomplished using contrast-enhanced CT and CT angiography (CTA). Magnetic resonance imaging (MRI) without and with gadolinium contrast agent is preferred if tumor or hemorrhagic conversion of ischemic stroke is suspected. Often the image guidance planning test (CTA or MRI) can also serve as the stabilization scan, so one should plan accordingly with placement of scalp fiducial markers if needed for the image guidance system. A catheter cerebral angiogram is required if CTA is negative but aneurysm is still strongly suspected (significant associated subarachnoid hemorrhage or ICH distribution adjacent to sylvian or interhemispheric cisterns).
- Entry point should be selected from the imaging studies so as to allow the least intrusive access to the ICH and a catheter trajectory along the long axis of the clot. For most deep ganglionic bleeds, a frontal or parietooccipital burr hole is most appropriate. For lobar hemorrhages, a burr hole is selected overlying the closest extension of the ICH to the cortical surface.
- Correction of coagulopathy should be verified (verify normal INR and partial thromboplastin time) before starting the procedure, and platelet transfusion may be initiated before and completed during the procedure.
- **Figure 35-1:** After induction of anesthesia, the patient's head is fixed in a three-point Mayfield head rest, and the frameless navigation base station is secured to the head clamp. Skull fixation is unnecessary if electromagnetic guidance is used. Fiducial markers (or surface anatomic landmarks) are registered with the treatment planning platform.
- **Figure 35-2:** Navigation is established and verified, aiming for 1- to 2-mm precision at the catheter trajectory. The surgical plan is selected, with desired catheter entry and target points and trajectory depth allowing catheter perforations within the depth of the clot.
- **Figure 35-3:** The entry point is marked, and the surgical field is shaved, prepared, and draped with full sterile technique. The entry point and catheter trajectory are verified using a passive catheter introducer (PCI) or an equivalent navigation probe.

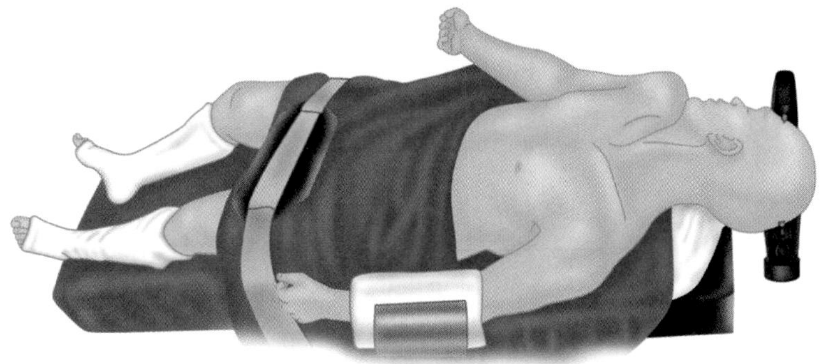

FIGURE 35-1

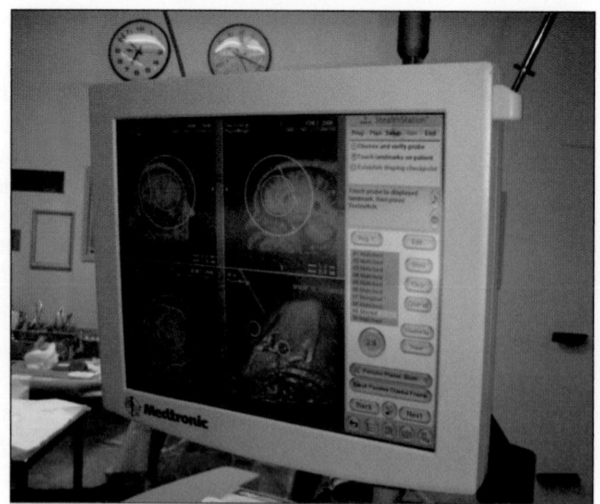

FIGURE 35-2

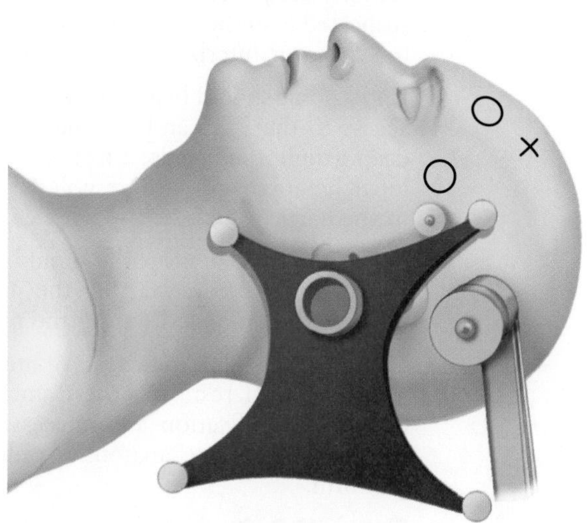

FIGURE 35-3

PROCEDURE

- **Figure 35-4:** The skin incision (2 to 3 cm) is made down to the pericranium, and scalp hemostasis is insured before the retractor is placed. The catheter entry point is again verified on the skull surface using the PCI or navigation wand.
- **Figure 35-5:** A standard burr hole is made using a power drill or Hudson brace. The hole is curetted to expose the dura, and perfect hemostasis is established with bone wax and bipolar coagulation as necessary.
- **Figure 35-6:** The dura is coagulated and slit using a No. 11 or No. 15 blade, and the dural edges are coagulated. The pial surface is coagulated and slit, making sure to avoid cortical arteries and veins.
- **Figure 35-7:** The cannula with a peel-away sheath (Codman 83-1326, Codeman and Shurtleff, Inc., Raynham, MA). The catheter introducer (cannula) is marked to the desired depth, and the PCI is used as a stylet. The PCI is used to guide the introducer along the treatment plan. It is placed with a single pass into and through two thirds of the overall hematoma diameter.
- **Figure 35-8:** The inner portion of the cannula is carefully removed while allowing the cannula to remain in the clot. Using a 10-mL syringe, manual aspiration is performed until resistance is met.

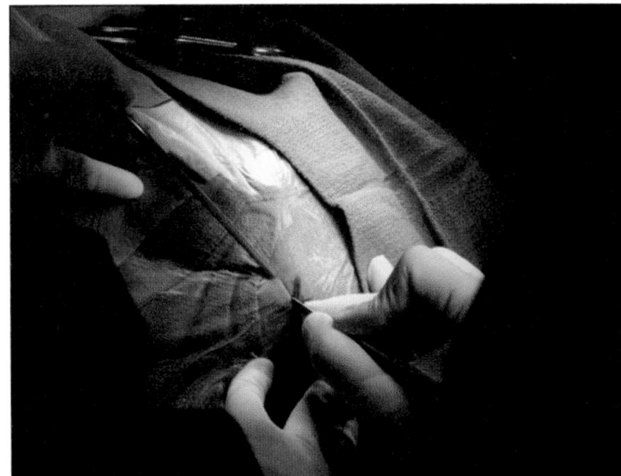

FIGURE 35-4

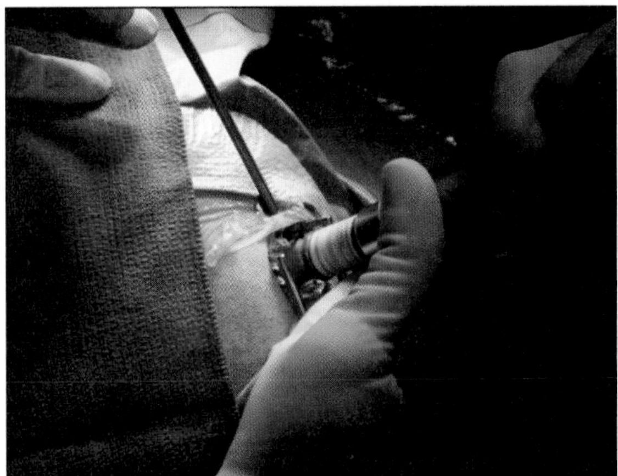

FIGURE 35-5

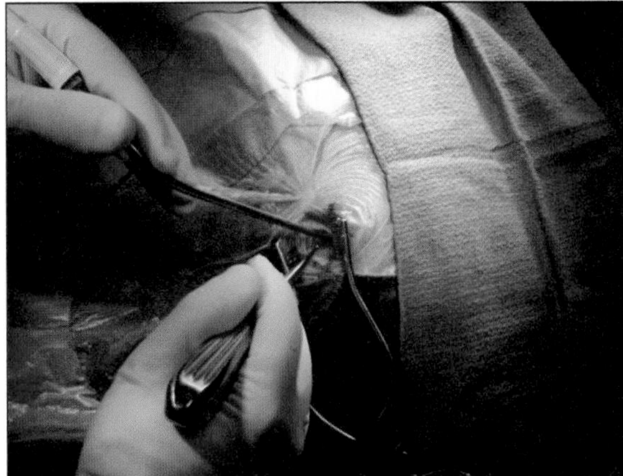

FIGURE 35-6

- **Figure 35-9:** A soft catheter is passed through the cannula into the residual hematoma.
- **Figure 35-10:** The cannula is peeled away, ensuring that the soft catheter remains in the hematoma core. While firmly clasping the catheter to prevent dislocation, the catheter is tunneled under the galea and exited using a trocar or hemostat forceps by a separate stab beyond the main incision. The principal incision is closed using a nylon suture through the full thickness of the scalp. The catheter is secured to the skin at its exit site using a second nylon suture, insuring that the catheter is not kinked or obstructed.

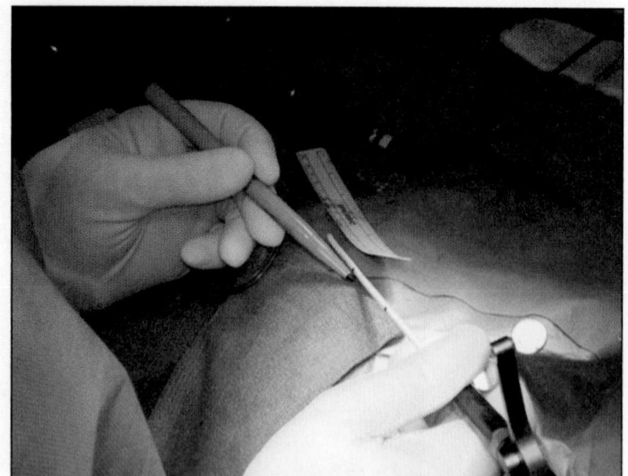

FIGURE 35-7

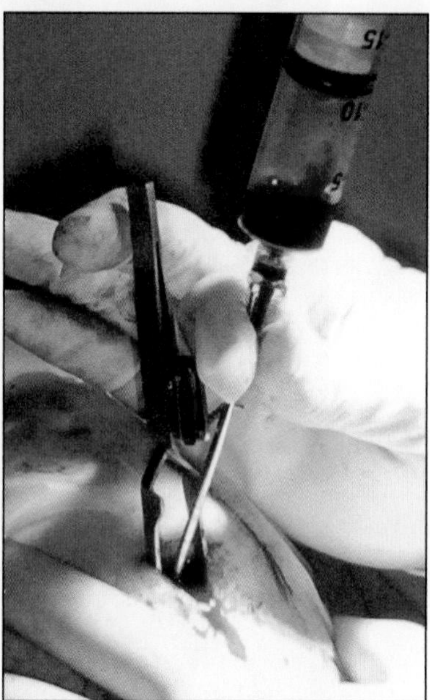

FIGURE 35-8

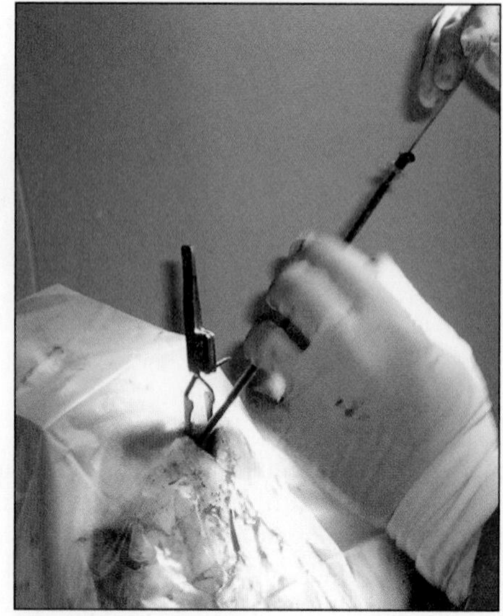

FIGURE 35-9

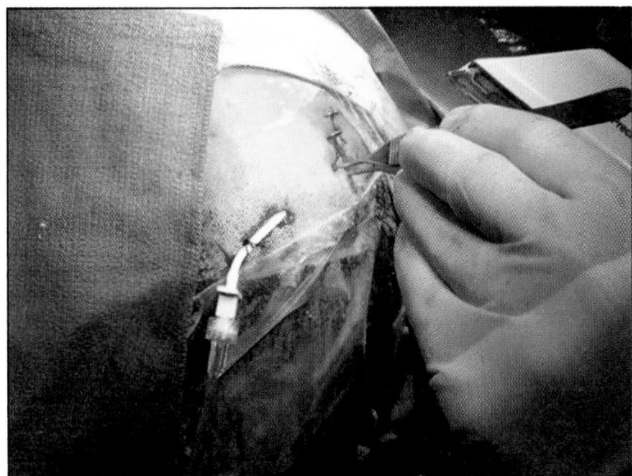

FIGURE 35-10

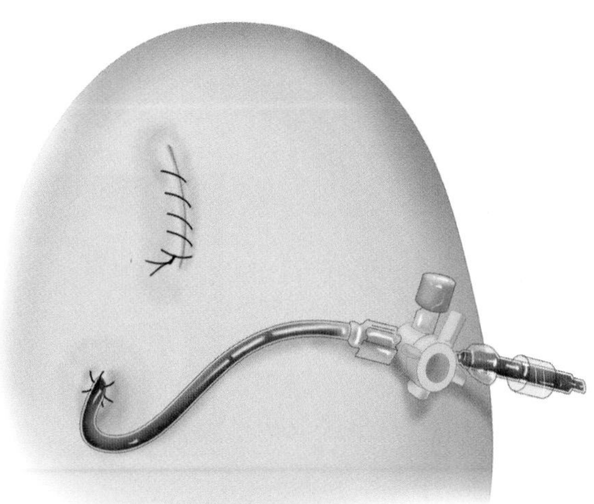

FIGURE 35-11

- **Figure 35-11:** The soft catheter is connected to the closed bag drainage system incorporating a three-way stopcock, with the collection chamber at head level.
- **Figure 35-12:** The catheter is used for closed bag drainage of ICH, enhanced by intermittent thrombolytic administration through the catheter. A dose of 1 to 2 mg (1 mg/mL) of recombinant tissue plasminogen activator (rTPA) is administered through a proximal three-way stopcock port into the ICH catheter every 8 to 12 hours, followed by flushing with sterile saline under full aseptic techniques. The catheter is closed for 30 to 60 minutes after rTPA administration and reopened to resume ICH drainage.
- **Figure 35-13:** CT scan is checked at least daily (more frequently if any neurologic change), and rTPA administration is stopped when ICH volume reaches less than 15 to 20 mL. The ICH catheter is left in place (open to bag drainage) for 12 to 24 hours after the last rTPA administration, before catheter removal.

TIPS FROM THE MASTERS

- NovoSeven is used when rapid reversal of coagulopathy is needed to prevent ICH growth and to allow quicker intervention for ICH evacuation. Its compassionate use should be carefully individualized, depending on the size of the ICH, required urgency of evacuation, and severity of coagulopathy. At the same time, the risks of prothrombotic complications should be considered when administering NovoSeven (e.g., hypercoagulable states, mechanical heart valves, multiple coronary stents). Considering risks and benefits,

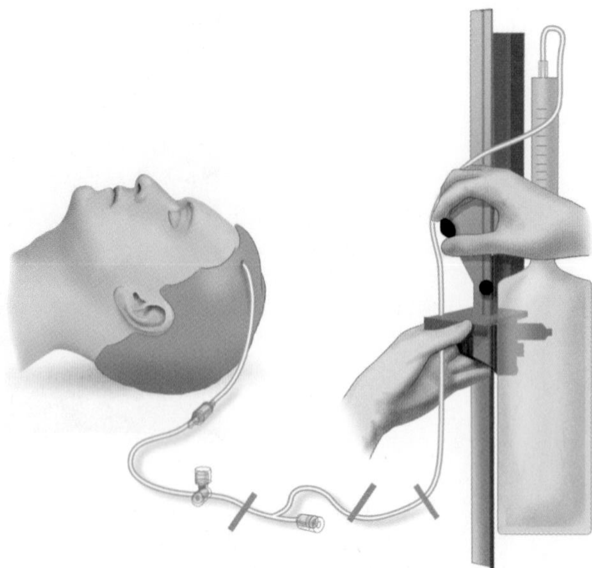

FIGURE 35-12

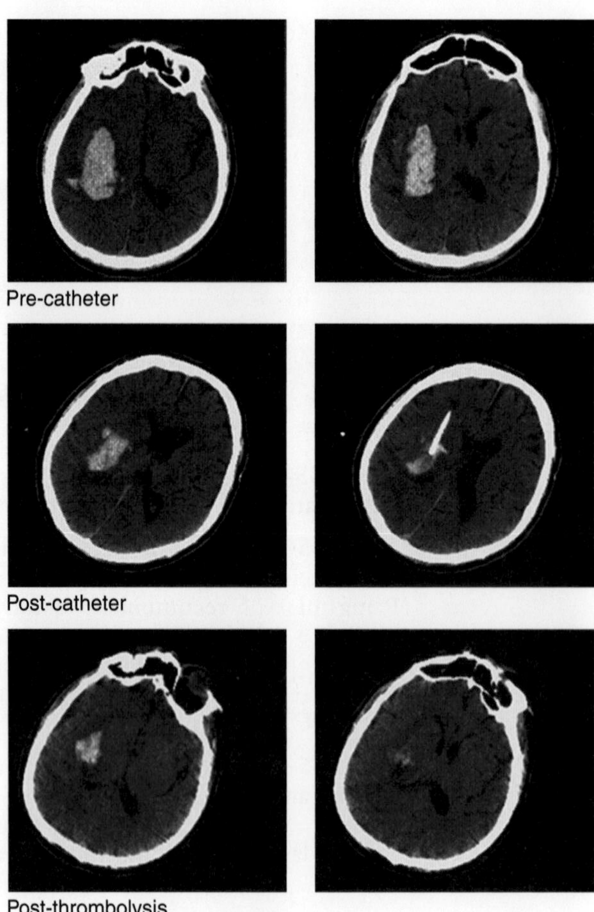

FIGURE 35-13

the dose of NovoSeven can be individualized, with low doses (20 to 50 μg/kg) used in milder coagulopathy or greater concern about prothrombotic complications and higher doses (50 to 80 μg/kg) used in expanding ICH with severe coagulopathy. This agent should not be used if coagulopathy is mild enough and the hematoma and clinical condition are stable enough to permit the reversal with fresh frozen plasma and vitamin K alone, which is typically much slower. Given the shorter half-life of NovoSeven compared with warfarin, coagulation parameters should continue to be monitored closely in the hours and days after initial reversal, and additional fresh frozen plasma and vitamin K administered as needed. Repeat administration of NovoSeven is rarely needed.

- After draping the head, the entry point and trajectory should be reregistered, and this should be repeated again at the bony surface and after placement of the burr hole.
- As an alternative to the catheter–cannula–peel-away sheath procedure described earlier, the surgeon may perform initial ICH aspiration using a Dandy blunt-tipped metal brain needle with a side port and the PCI used as stylet. The catheter is placed as a separate pass with the PCI after removing the brain needle. This procedure may allow more efficient initial manual aspiration and the placement of a larger brain catheter, which is less prone to clog.
- When significant ICH is evacuated by initial aspiration, the catheter tip should be revised to a slightly more shallow target than initially planned, allowing for smaller ICH residual volume.
- The optimal dosage of thrombolytic is currently under investigation in an ongoing phase II clinical trial (http://mistietrial.com). Until a standard dosage is determined, the lower dosage frequency (1 mg every 8 to 12 hours) should be used for smaller residual ICH.
- Coagulation parameters should continue to be monitored closely and corrected if necessary as long as the catheter is in place.
- Thrombolysis should be terminated if CT scan reveals catheter perforations without contact with residual ICH.
- Some ICHs communicate with the ventricular system, so blood-tinged cerebrospinal fluid may sometimes drain through the ICH catheter. This drainage may enhance the clearance of ICH.
- Catheter manipulations for each injection of thrombolytic and any revision of catheter placement must be performed under full aseptic technique. Intravenous antibiotics are used for the duration of catheter implantation.
- An external ventricular drain may be placed in addition to the ICH catheter in cases with associated intraventricular hemorrhage or hydrocephalus or to monitor intracranial pressure in comatose patients.

PITFALLS

The catheter is often placed deeper in the ICH than planned because the residual ICH is more shallow than before initial aspiration.

Thrombolysis should not be administered if the catheter perforations are no longer in contact with residual ICH.

The catheter should not be revised, withdrawn, or removed within 12 hours of thrombolytic administration.

BAILOUT OPTIONS

- If the catheter position is suboptimal initially or at any time during thrombolytic evacuation, the surgeon must decide whether to replace the catheter in more optimal placement, depending on the volume of residual ICH (>20 mL); this requires a repeat procedure as outlined earlier or alternative catheter repositioning in the CT scanner.
- **Figure 35-14:** Catheter replacement may be performed in real time under sterile technique in the CT scanner for real-time optimization of catheter placement. This may also be performed for initial ICH aspiration and catheter placement, as an alternative to frameless stereotactic image guidance.

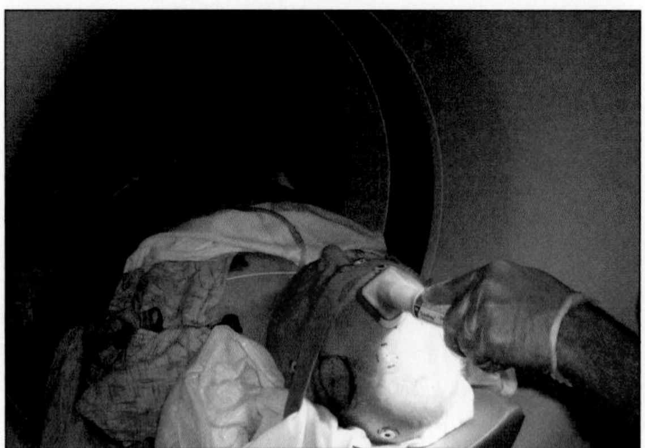

FIGURE 35-14

SUGGESTED READINGS

Miller DW, Barnett GH, Kormos DW, et al. Stereotactically guided thrombolysis of deep cerebral hemorrhage: preliminary results. Cleve Clin J Med 1993;60:321–4.

Montes J, Gunel M, Wong J, et al. Stereotactic computed tomographic guided aspiration and thrombolysis of intracerebral hematoma: protocol and preliminary experience. Stroke 2000;31:834–40.

Morgan T, Zuccarello M, Narayan R, et al. Preliminary findings of the minimally-invasive surgery plus rtPA for intracerebral hemorrhage evacuation (MISTIE) clinical trial. Acta Neurochir Suppl 2008;105:147–51.

Park P, Fewel ME, Garton HJ, et al. Recombinant activated factor VII for the rapid correction of coagulopathy in nonhemophilic neurosurgical patients. Neurosurgery 2003;53:34–8.

Schaller C, Rohde V, Meyer B, et al. Stereotactic puncture and lysis of spontaneous intracerebral hemorrhage using recombinant tissue-plasminogen activator. Neurosurgery 1995;36:328–35.

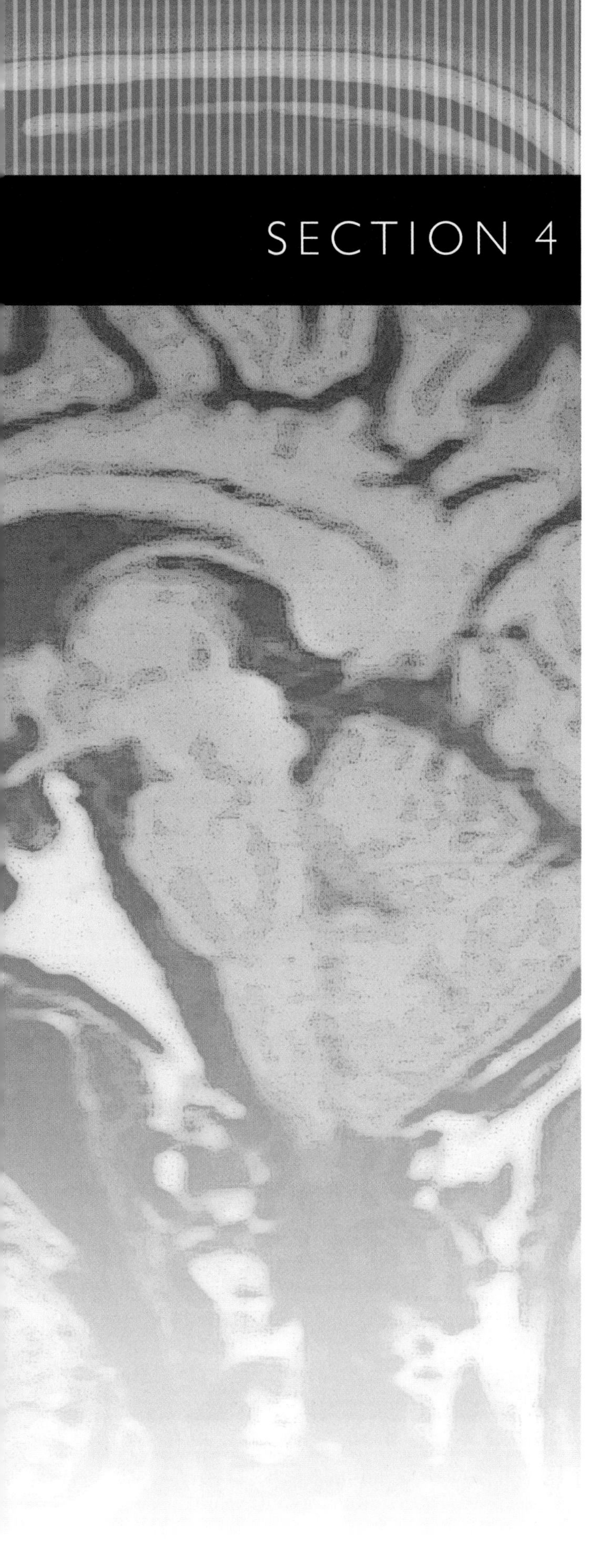

SECTION 4 Functional

SECTION EDITOR — KIM BURCHIEL, WITH SAMUEL A. HUGHES

Procedure 36

Anteromedial Temporal Lobe Resection

Alexander M. Papanastassiou, Kenneth P. Vives, Dennis D. Spencer

INDICATIONS

- Medial temporal lobe epilepsy associated with mesial temporal sclerosis pathology consisting of neuronal cell loss, gliosis, and synaptic reorganization
    - Presumed mesial temporal sclerosis can be determined preoperatively as hippocampal atrophy or increased hippocampal fluid attenuated inversion recovery (FLAIR) signal on magnetic resonance imaging (MRI).
- Lesion-related temporal lobe epilepsy
    - Common lesions include vascular cavernous angiomas, focal developmental abnormalities, and low-grade neoplasms.
    - Lesions may be associated with hippocampal atrophy, in which case dual pathology exists. In such cases, it is uncertain whether the atrophic hippocampus is nonfunctional and epileptogenic and should be removed, or whether it is capable of normal function and resection would result in cognitive deficits. Neuropsychologic evaluation and the intracarotid amobarbital procedure are performed to address this uncertainty.
- Cryptogenic temporal lobe epilepsy, in which there is no imaged lesion or atrophy and the temporal lobe is identified as the putative epileptogenic region primarily based on intracranial electrophysiology

CONTRAINDICATIONS

- Localization of epileptogenesis in the dominant temporal lobe with preserved memory on neuropsychologic testing
    - If there is support for memory function on the nondominant side as tested by the intracarotid amobarbital procedure, anteromedial temporal lobe resection (AMTR) still leads to a decline in verbal memory function that is noticeable to the patient.
    - If memory function is lacking on the nondominant side as tested by the intracarotid amobarbital procedure, AMTR has the theoretical risk of causing global amnesia.
- Localization of epileptogenesis in the dominant temporal lobe with poor memory on neuropsychologic testing and no or little support for verbal memory on the nondominant side as tested by the intracarotid amobarbital procedure
    - In this group, AMTR has the theoretical risk of causing global amnesia.
- Nonepileptic seizures
    - All patients should undergo noninvasive continuous audiovisual electroencephalography monitoring even in the presence of seemingly appropriate clinical and radiologic findings to rule out nonepileptic seizures.

PLANNING AND POSITIONING

- Valproate may lead to bleeding complications. At our institution, we routinely measure prothrombin time, partial thromboplastin time, fibrinogen level, platelet count, and bleeding time. If values are abnormal, we decrease or discontinue valproate and recheck values before surgery.
- Neuronavigation may be used when available.

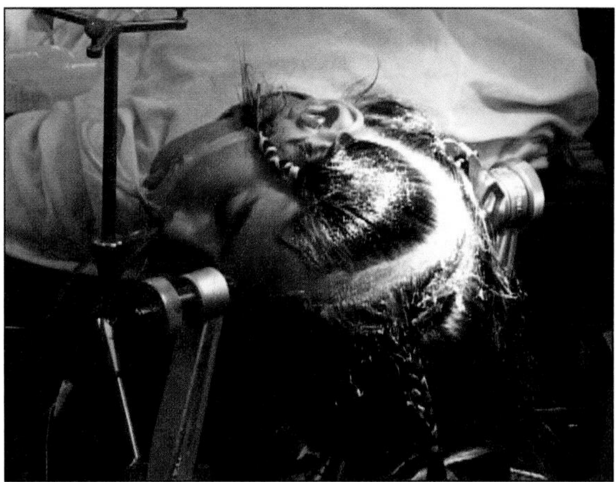

FIGURE 36-1

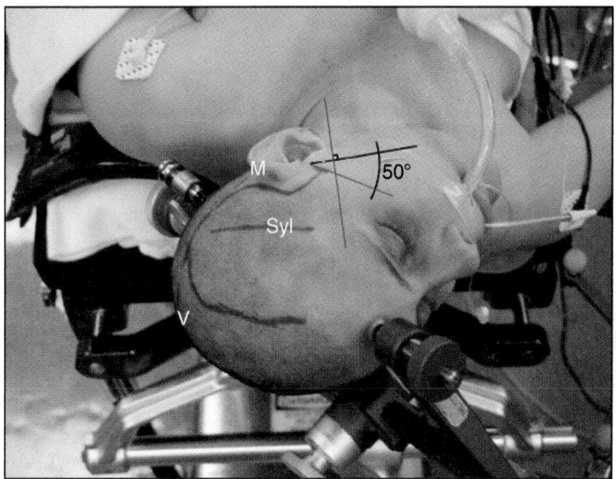

FIGURE 36-2

- Antiepileptic drugs should be taken on the morning of surgery with a small sip of water.
- The patient is positioned supine with a foam wedge or shoulder roll ipsilateral to the side of surgery.
- The head is fixed in a Mayfield head holder, turned to the contralateral side, and extended 50 degrees. The vertex of the head is lowered 10 degrees. Head extension allows the surgeon to view the long axis of the hippocampus with the microscope.
- **Figure 36-1:** Example of patient position with hair clipped along the planned incision for right AMTR, which is our routine. The position of the frameless stereotactic system's reference star (Brainlab, Inc., Westchester, IL) for neuronavigation is also shown.
- **Figure 36-2:** Second example of patient position, this time for left AMTR, with all hair clipped. The head is extended 50 degrees. The skin incision starts at the zygoma anterior to the tragus and curves superiorly and posteriorly. The posterior margin of the incision is a line drawn from the mastoid tip (*M*) to the vertex (*V*). The incision must expose enough of the cranium to remove a bone flap that allows for retraction of the superior temporal gyrus and frontal lobe without compressing brain against the skull edge. The approximate position of the Sylvian fissure (*Syl*) is shown. The superior extent of incision varies based on the patient's hairline.

PROCEDURE

- **Figure 36-3:** The skin is incised, and the scalp and temporalis muscle are reflected anteriorly and retracted with perforating towel clips attached to a Leyla bar with rubber bands. A cuff of temporalis muscle is preserved along the superior temporal line for reattaching the temporalis muscle during closure.

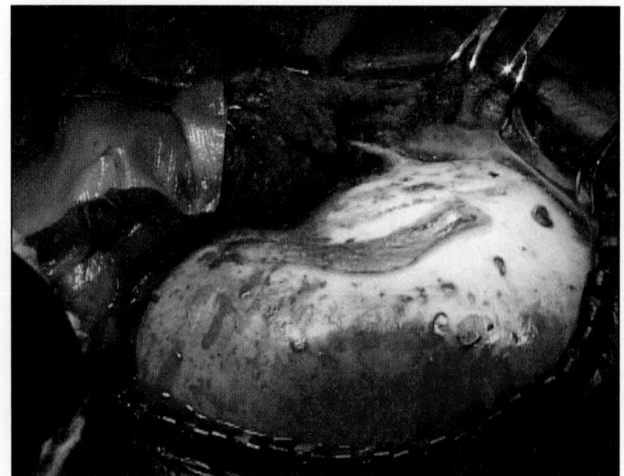

FIGURE 36-3

- **Figure 36-4:** Three to four burr holes are created, and the dura is stripped from the bone. Bone flap is completed with a craniotome and elevated to expose the dura. Entry into mastoid air cells is avoided, and any opening into mastoid air cells is sealed closed with bone wax. Epidural tack-up stitches are placed.
- **Figure 36-5:** The dura is opened in the shape of a C and reflected anteriorly. To plan the posterior margin of the lateral cortical resection of the middle and inferior temporal gyri, a No. 4 Penfield and a mosquito clamp are used to measure from the temporal tip to a prominent cortical vein approximately 3 to 3.5 cm from the temporal tip.

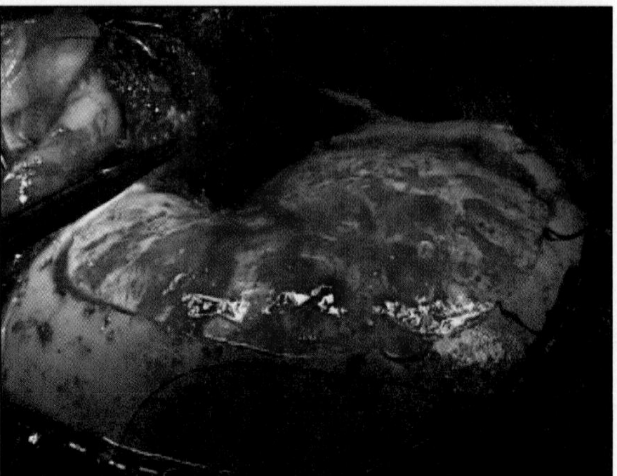

FIGURE 36-4

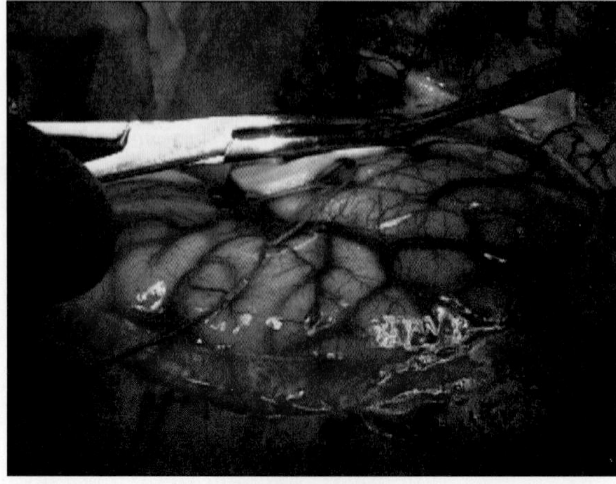

FIGURE 36-5

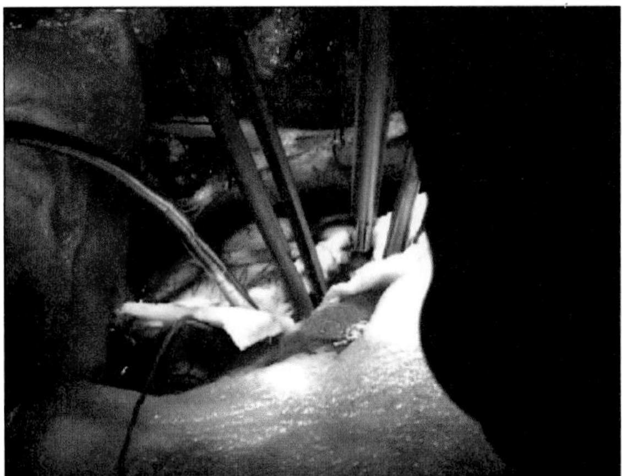

FIGURE 36-6

- **Figure 36-6:** The pia is coagulated and then incised sharply in front of the vein to preserve it, extending from the inferior temporal gyrus along the middle temporal gyrus superiorly to the superior temporal sulcus (STS). The superior temporal gyrus is preserved on the dominant side to protect language and on the nondominant side for uniformity. The cortical incision is extended anteriorly along the STS, dissecting inferior to the STS in the subpial plane. The cortical incision is deepened with ultrasonic aspiration.
- **Figure 36-7:** As the cortical incision is deepened, the temporal horn (*TH*) is identified by following the arachnoid of the fusiform gyrus from inferior to superior. The TH is

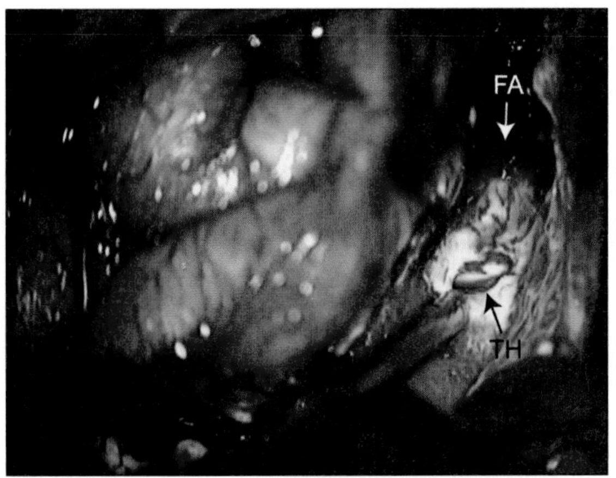

A

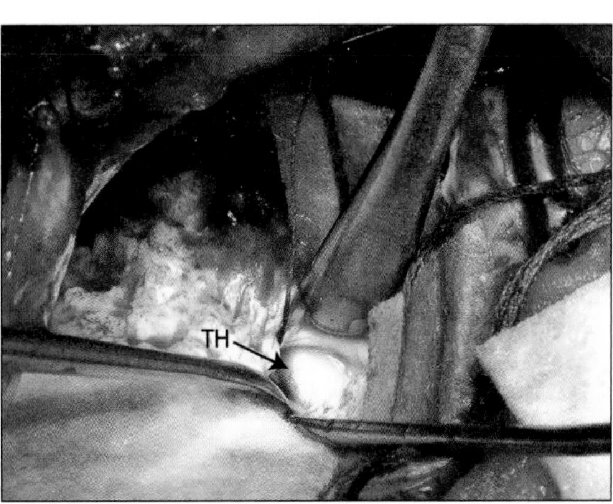

B

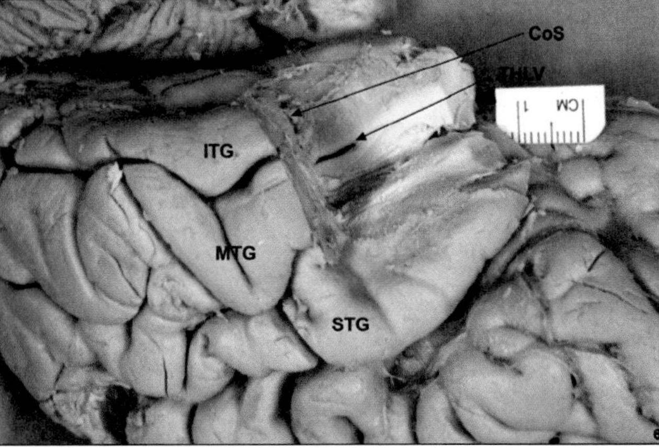

C

FIGURE 36-7

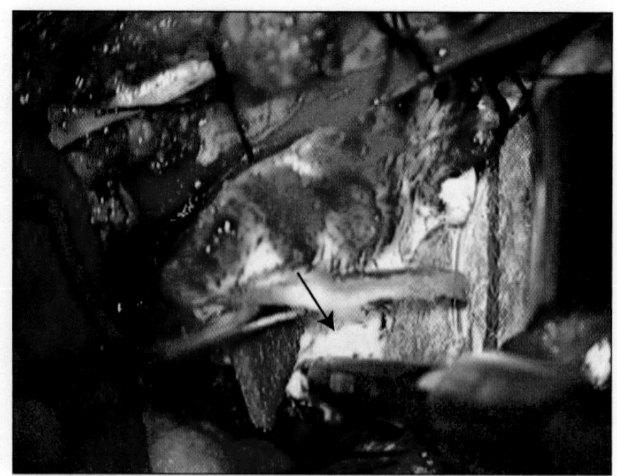

FIGURE 36-8

perpendicular to the cortical surface at the inferior temporal sulcus. Care is taken not to dissect superiorly into the temporal stem. Superior to the TH, there is no intervening arachnoid plane if one were to dissect medially from the anterior temporal lobe white matter through the temporal stem and basal ganglia/amygdala complex into the crus cerebri. **A,** TH. Approximate location of the fusiform arachnoid (*FA*) is also indicated. **B,** TH is shown after resection of lateral neocortex and is opened more widely. **C,** TH in anatomic specimen. *CoS* = collateral sulcus; *ITG* = inferior temporal gyrus; *MTG* = middle temporal gyrus; *STG* = superior temporal gyrus; *THLV* = temporal horn of lateral ventricle.

- **Figure 36-8:** The temporal pole is undermined anteriorly along the white matter and removed. The *arrow* indicates temporal pole medial white matter.
- **Figure 36-9:** The medial temporal pole is resected subpially from its anterior aspect until the middle cerebral artery (MCA) is exposed, then the remainder of the amygdala is resected inferior to a line between the velum terminale and the genu of the MCA at the junction between the M1 and M2 segments. The velum terminale is the union of the taeniae of the fimbria fornicis and the stria terminalis at the origin of the choroid plexus. Resecting inferior to this line prevents injuring the basal ganglia and crus cerebri. **A,** A patty string has been laid along this line before resection of the amygdala. **B,** After resection of the amygdala, the genu at the M1-M2 junction and the velum terminale are more easily seen. **C,** Illustration of this line. **D,** This line on a parasagittal MRI slice that includes the amygdala and hippocampus.
- As shown in Figure 36-9B and C, two retractors are placed. Care must be taken not to injure the vein of Labbé during placement of retractors. The superior retractor gently holds the superior temporal gyrus, and the choroid plexus is protected underneath a patty and retracted medially toward the thalamus. The choroid plexus should not be coagulated because this may lead to injury of the anterior choroidal artery and subsequent ischemia of the internal capsule and lateral thalamus. Manipulation of the choroid plexus should be minimized to prevent it from bleeding. The posterior retractor is curved under the lateral temporal cortex to elevate it gently laterally and posteriorly. This elevation of the lateral temporal cortex allows the lateral temporal neocortex to be gradually elevated, exposing the entire hippocampus.
- **Figure 36-10:** **A,** The medial occipitotemporal fasciculus is transected longitudinally from the anterior hippocampus to the hippocampal tail. **B,** Cadaveric dissection.
- **Figure 36-11:** The next step is resection of the anterior parahippocampus including the entorhinal cortex, ambient gyrus, semilunar gyrus, uncinate gyrus, and intralimbic gyrus using ultrasonic aspiration or a round dissector. The intralimbic gyrus of the parahippocampus lies lateral to the peduncle of the midbrain. This is a photograph of an anatomic specimen showing the medial surface of the temporal lobe: *14* and *15* are the posterior uncus; *16* is the parahippocampal gyrus; *13* is the uncal sulcus, which is the arachnoid plane in the uncus where the uncus folds back on itself; and 7 is the velum terminale.

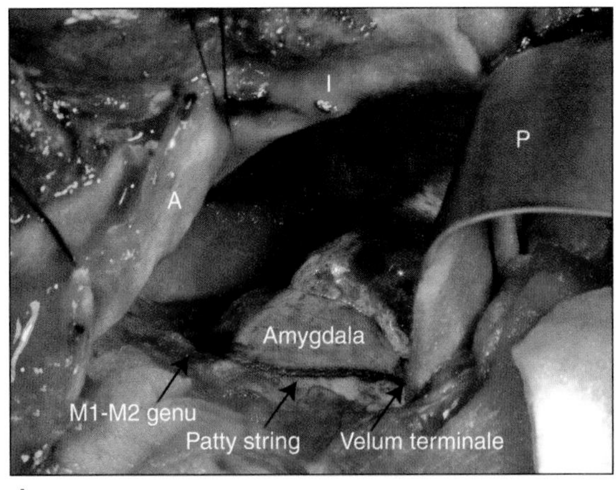

A

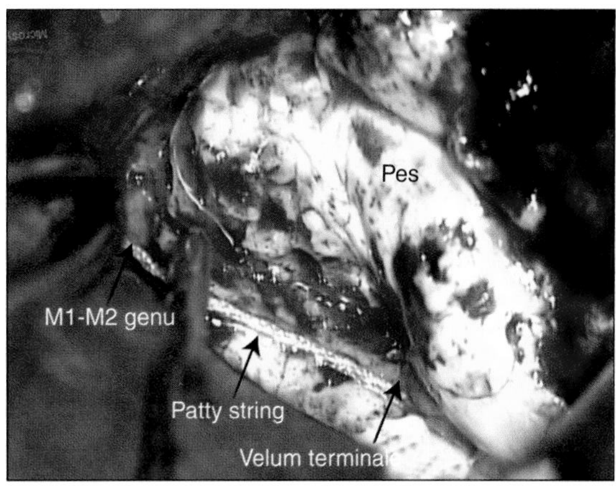

B

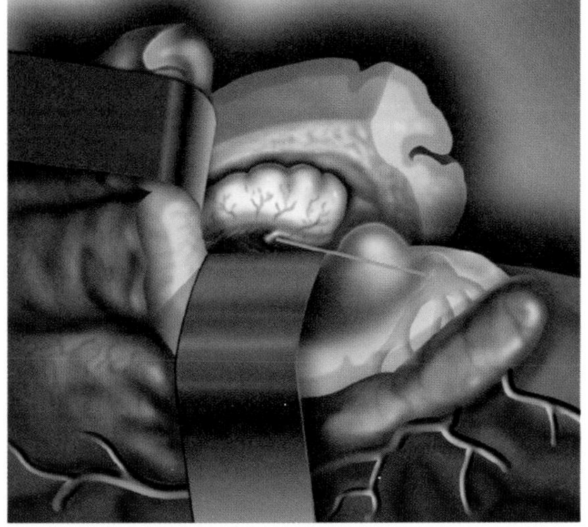

C

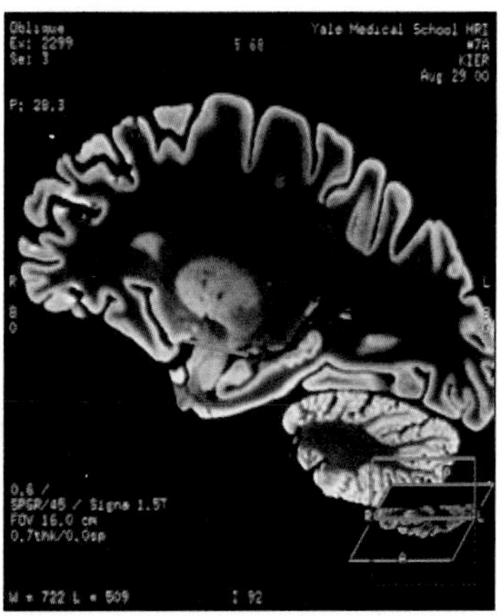

D

FIGURE 36-9

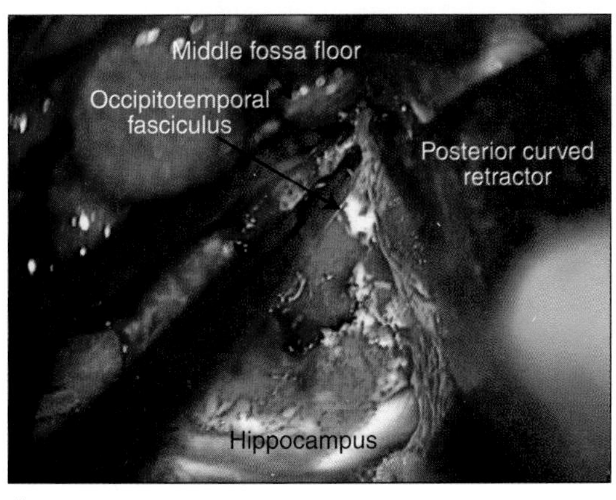

A

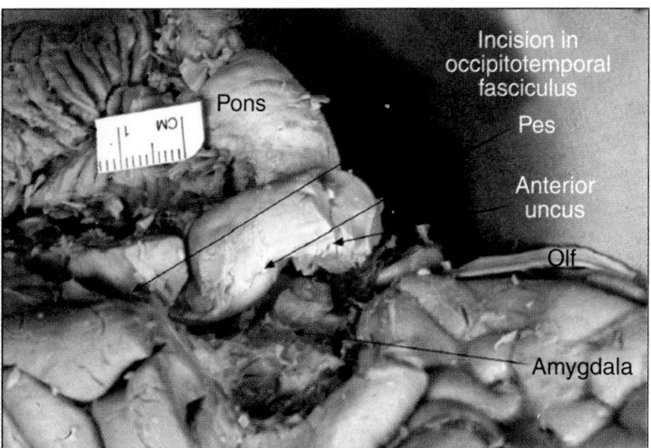

B

FIGURE 36-10

- **Figure 36-12:** As dissection proceeds, numerous small vessels emanating from the posterior cerebral artery (*PCA*) lie in the arachnoid plane of the uncal sulcus (*arrows*). PCA branches in the uncal sulcus may return and supply the thalamus. Complete dissection of the uncal sulcus is crucial for distinguishing perforators that supply the hippocampus from perforators that travel superiorly to the thalamus. The uncal sulcus

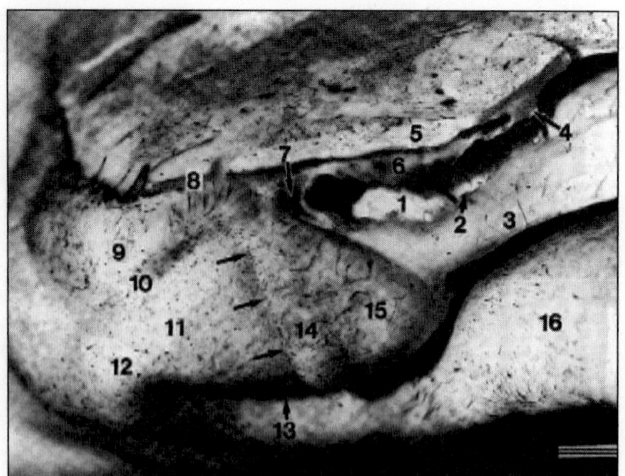

FIGURE 36-11

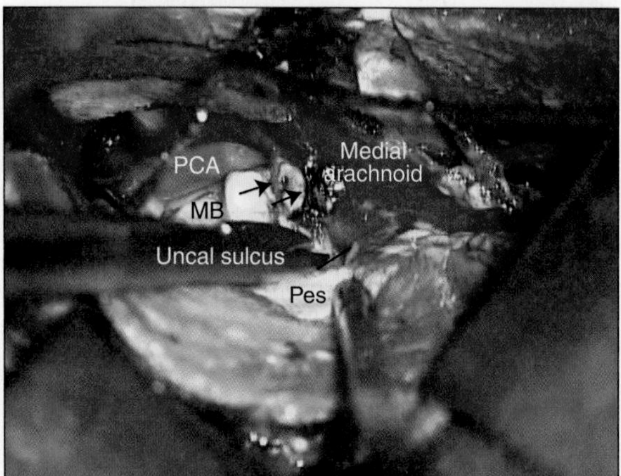

FIGURE 36-12

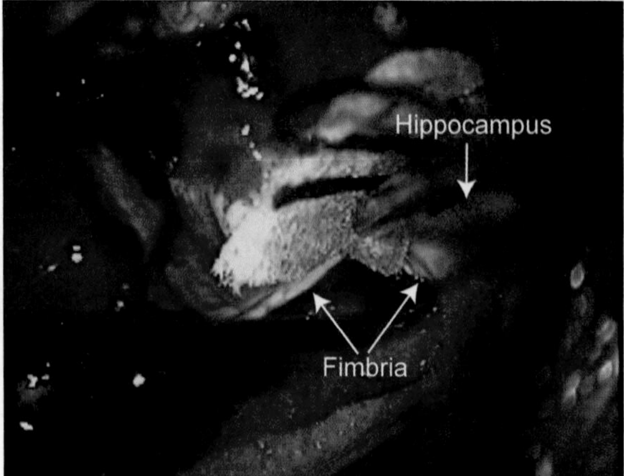

FIGURE 36-13

is indicated by the *black line*. The midbrain (*MB*) lies just medial to the PCA. When the fold of arachnoid is well dissected, it is sometimes easier to divide the *pes* from the body of the hippocampus.

- **Figure 36-13:** When the anterior hippocampus and pes hippocampi have been removed, the medial dissection of the hippocampus is started by separating the fimbria of the fornix from the medial arachnoid and reflecting it back onto the surface of the hippocampus. The anterior body of the hippocampus then can be gently retracted laterally, exposing the arachnoid that covers the superior surface of the parahippocampal gyrus. Care is taken to

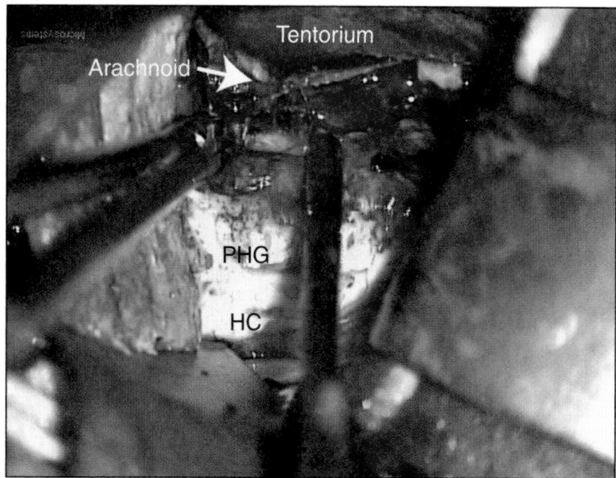

FIGURE 36-14

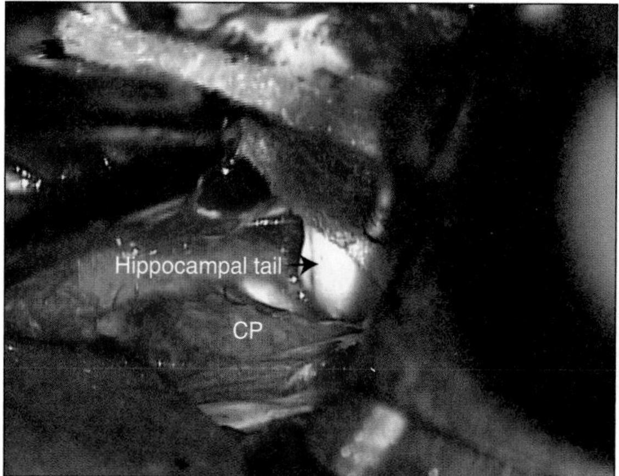

FIGURE 36-15

avoid dividing any vessels that are not clearly going into the hippocampus because occasionally thalamic perforators can be seen in this area as well.

- **Figure 36-14:** The parahippocampal gyrus (*PHG*) can be entered with a bipolar cautery and suction or ultrasonic aspirator and dissected in a longitudinal plane from anterior to posterior. This dissection is carried out from medial and inferolateral approaches to the PHG, with the inferolateral trajectory shown here. The inferior arachnoid of the parahippocampal gyrus is seen superior to the tentorium, and the hippocampus (*HC*) is at the superior margin of the parahippocampal gyrus.
- **Figure 36-15:** The hippocampus is gently retracted laterally, showing the tail as it curves medially. The choroid plexus (*CP*) lies over the lateral geniculate nucleus. The PCA temporal branch is protected as the hippocampal tail is divided.
- **Figure 36-16:** The specimen is removed, photographed, and sent for histologic and laboratory analysis. Closure is performed in typical fashion, reattaching the reflected temporalis muscle to the cuff of muscle that was preserved on the bone flap.

TIPS FROM THE MASTERS

- The most important part of positioning is extension of the head to facilitate hippocampal resection.
- Bony exposure must extend inferiorly to the root of the zygoma and anteriorly as close to the temporal tip as possible.
- On opening dura, identify and protect the vein of Labbé. Attention to the vein of Labbé is particularly important during retractor placement.

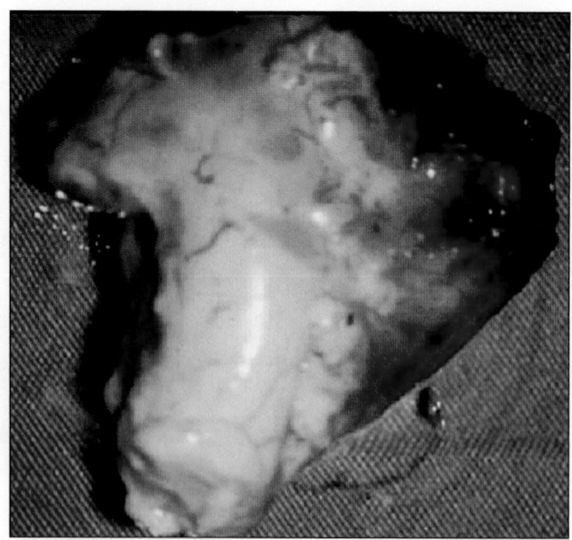

FIGURE 36-16

- Search for the temporal horn by following the arachnoid of the fusiform gyrus from inferior to superior. The temporal horn is perpendicular to the cortical surface at the inferior temporal sulcus. Neuronavigation may be helpful for locating the temporal horn.
- The lateral temporal cortex should be elevated laterally more than retracted posteriorly.
- Determine the superior extent of amygdalar resection by imagining a line between the velum terminale and the genu of the MCA at the junction between the M1 and M2 segments.
- Retract the choroid plexus toward the thalamus. Do not coagulate it.
- Dissect the uncal sulcus to distinguish PCA perforators to the hippocampus from recurrent thalamic branches.
- Identify and protect the posterior temporal branch of the PCA as the hippocampal tail is divided.

PITFALLS

Injury to the vein of Labbé must be avoided.

While searching for the temporal horn, if one misses it and dissects too far superiorly, the temporal stem, basal ganglia/amygdala complex, and then the crus cerebri may be entered. Superior to the temporal horn, there is no arachnoid plane along this medial trajectory.

If the surgeon resects tissue above the line between the M1 MCA branch and the velum terminale, the temporal stem, basal ganglia/amygdala complex, and crus cerebri also may be injured.

Coagulation of the choroid plexus in the temporal horn may lead to injury of the anterior choroidal artery.

Injury of recurrent thalamic perforators from the PCA in the uncal sulcus can occur.

Injury of the posterior temporal branch of the PCA as the hippocampal tail is divided can occur.

BAILOUT OPTIONS

- If you do not find the temporal horn, use neuronavigation or resect further posteriorly and inferiorly along the middle and inferior temporal gyri to identify the hippocampus.

SUGGESTED READINGS

Duvernoy H. The Human Hippocampus. Munich: JF Bergmann Verlag; 1988.

Helmstaedter C, Richter S, Roske S, et al. Differential effects of temporal pole resection with amygdalohippocampectomy versus selective amygdalohippocampectomy on material-specific memory in patients with mesial temporal lobe epilepsy. Epilepsia 2008;49:88–97.

Spencer DD, Spencer SS, Mattson RH, et al. Access to the posterior medial temporal lobe structures in the surgical treatment of temporal lobe epilepsy. Neurosurgery 1984;15:667–71.

Spencer SS, Berg AT, Vickrey BG, et al. Predicting long-term seizure outcome after resective epilepsy surgery. The Multicenter Study. Neurology 2005;65:912–8.

Wiebe S, Blume WT, Girvin JP, et al. A randomized controlled trial of surgery for temporal-lobe epilepsy. N Engl J Med 2001;345:311–8.

Wyler AR, Hermann BP, Somes G. Extent of medial temporal resection on outcome from anterior temporal lobectomy: a randomized prospective study. Neurosurgery 1995;37:982–90.

Figure 36-11 from Duvernoy H. The Human Hippocampus. Munich: JF Bergmann Verlag; 1988, p. 36.

Procedure 37

Selective Amygdalohippocampectomy

Ahmed Raslan, Samuel A. Hughes, Kim Burchiel

INDICATIONS

- Mesial temporal lobe epilepsy without evidence of neocortical involvement is an indication for selective amygdalohippocampectomy.
- The decision to proceed with surgery is usually made after medical intractability of epilepsy is established. In many institutions, a paradigm shift toward early consideration of surgery in mesial temporal lobe epilepsy has occurred because of the cognitive side effects of antiepileptic medications and the demonstration of superiority of resection over medical treatment.
- Invasive monitoring is often required to determine surgical candidacy and can include (1) foramen ovale electrodes (i.e., to localize the side of the epileptogenic focus), (2) depth electrodes, or (3) subdural grid electrodes.
- In many cases, bilateral medial temporal discharges are encountered on electroencephalogram (EEG). Accurate determination of the side of the epileptogenic focus is critical because bilateral amygdalohippocampectomy can be associated with severe and devastating short-term memory deficits.

CONTRAINDICATIONS

- Relatively speaking, neocortical foci in the temporal lobe require resection, and selective amygdalohippocampectomy would be inappropriate.
- Prior contralateral temporal lobectomy or amygdalohippocampectomy portends severe sequelae.

PLANNING AND POSITIONING

- In addition to routine evaluations (patient's cardiopulmonary status, laboratory values [complete blood count, basic metabolic profile, coagulation profile], chest x-ray, and electrocardiogram), preoperative evaluation includes video EEG, sphenoid or foramen ovale electrodes, and ictal single photon emission computed tomography (SPECT). In the strict sense of selective amygdalohippocampectomy, a Wada test (i.e., intracarotid sodium amobarbital procedure) may be unnecessary, given the absence of significant neocortical resection.
- At our institution, frameless stereotactic navigation is used to guide the approach. The most commonly used route—which is the one described here—is the trans–middle temporal gyrus–transventricular route. Other routes include the transsylvian and the subtemporal approaches, with modifications.
- The initial target in planning the transcortical dissection should be the temporal horn; registration of the entry point into the sulcus with confirmation of a distance less than 3 cm from the temporal tip is especially important in surgery in the dominant hemisphere.
- Whether the patient is placed in a supine or a lateral position, the key element in the positioning chosen is a full and straight lateral position of the patient's head in the region where the temple is flattest; this positioning is crucial for visualization of the posterior part of the hippocampus while maintaining a safe and adequate trajectory to the rest of the approach.

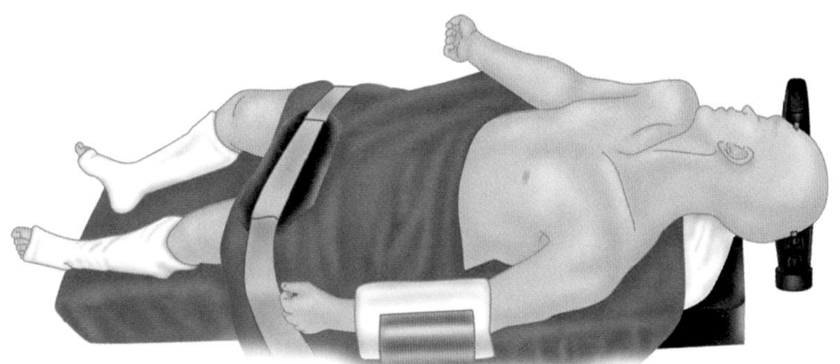

FIGURE 37-1

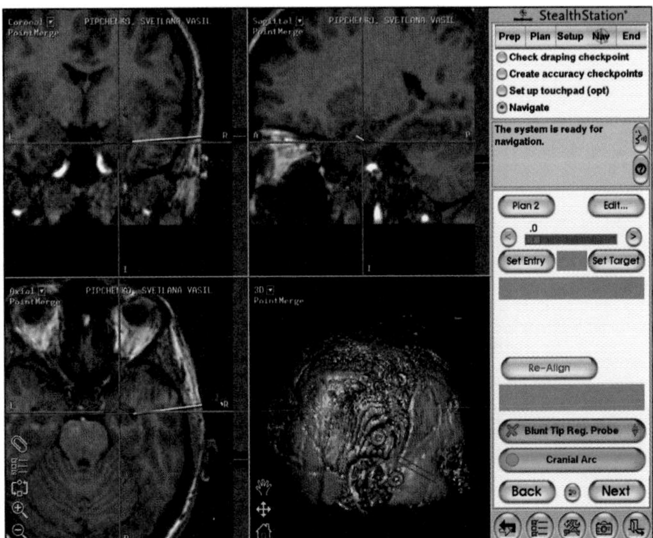

FIGURE 37-2

- **Figure 37-1:** The patient is placed supine or lateral, if neck rotation would not allow for appropriate head position. The objective is a flat and complete lateral position of the head. A shoulder roll can be helpful in achieving ideal positioning when the patient is supine.
- **Figure 37-2:** Planning the surgical trajectory from the skin surface down to the temporal horn, which is the cornerstone of the surgical trajectory.

PROCEDURE

- **Figure 37-3:** Skin incision planning. It is critical to extend the incision inferior enough to achieve adequate lower exposure. The incision does not need to extend above the superior temporal line.
- **Figure 37-4:** Craniotomy and incision into the middle temporal gyrus. Craniotomy should extend inferiorly as close to the root of the zygoma as possible. The cortical surface of middle temporal gyrus is exposed and confirmed with navigation.
- **Figure 37-5: A,** Line drawing showing the planned incision on the crus of the middle temporal gyrus (*T2*). **B,** Superimposition of the cortical incision on sagittal magnetic resonance imaging (MRI).
- **Figure 37-6:** Access into the ventricle. Identification of critical landmarks at the onset of surgical approach is crucial. *A* = amygdala; *CP* = choroid plexus; *H* = hippocampus; *LVS* = lateral ventricular sulcus or collateral sulcus; *PHG* = parahippocampal gyrus.

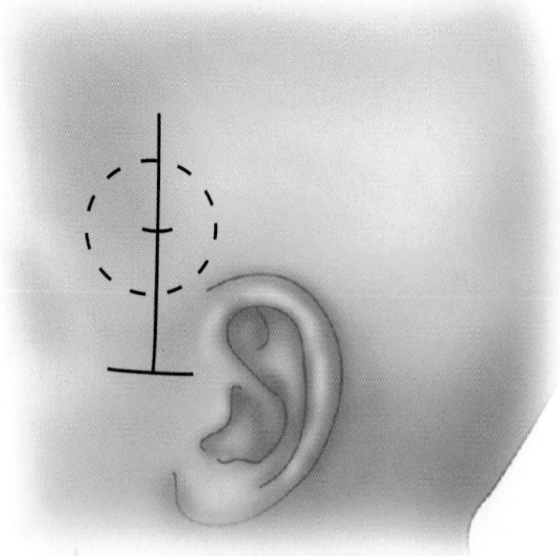

FIGURE 37-3

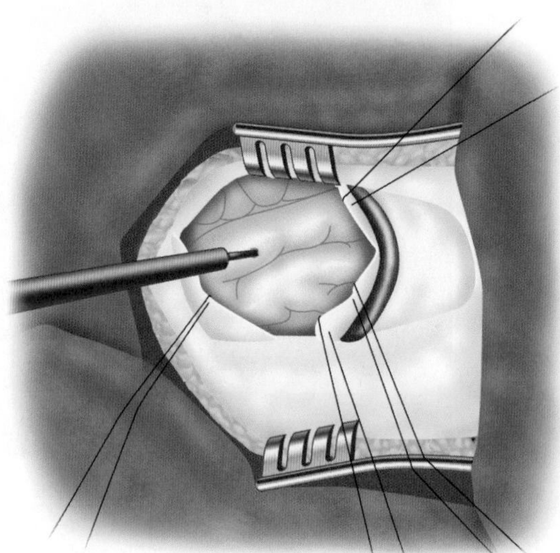

FIGURE 37-4

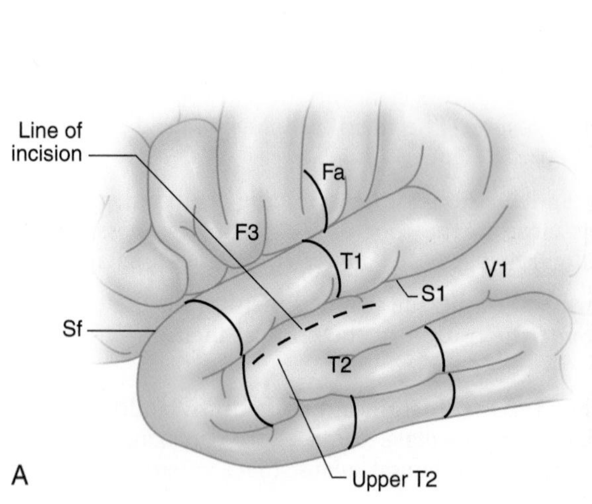

B

FIGURE 37-5

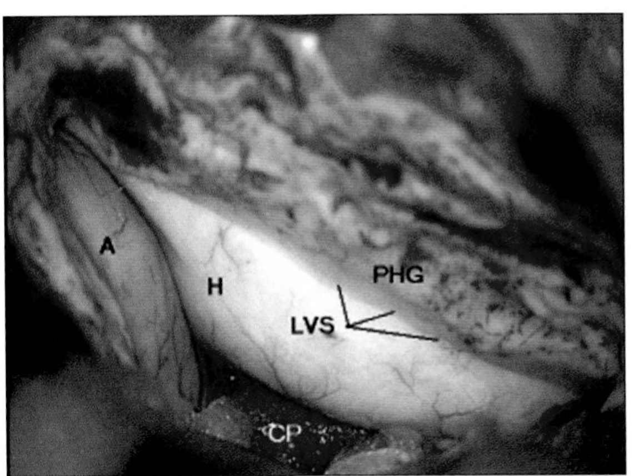

A

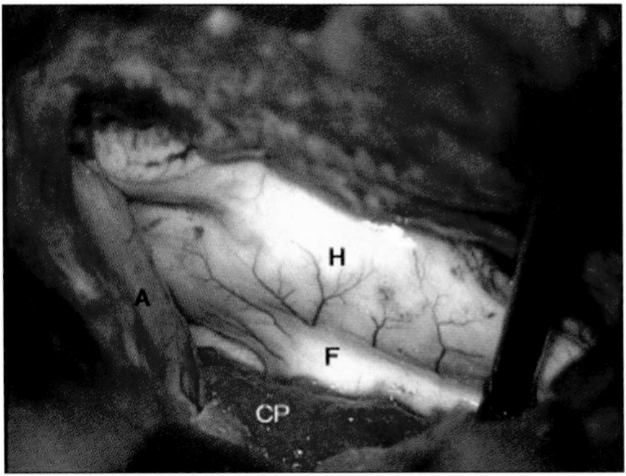

B

FIGURE 37-6

- **Figure 37-7:** Resection of the amygdala. The tip of the suction handpiece overlies the amygdala.
- **Figure 37-8:** **A,** Subpial-endopial approach and completion of amygdala and uncal resection. **B,** Navigation confirms resection.
- **Figure 37-9:** Hippocampal resection. Resection remains below the level of the choroidal fissure.

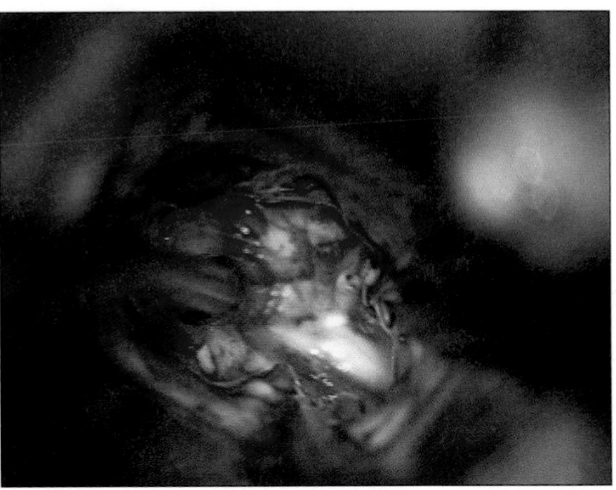

FIGURE 37-7

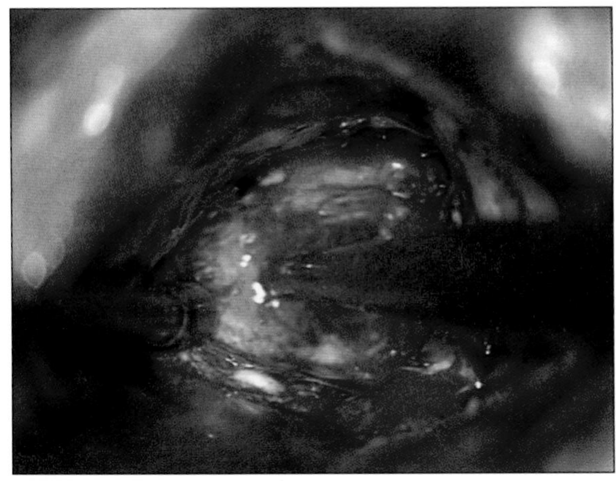

A

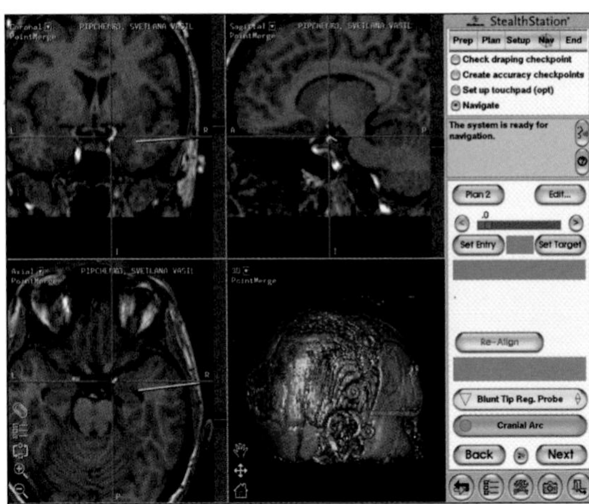

B

FIGURE 37-8

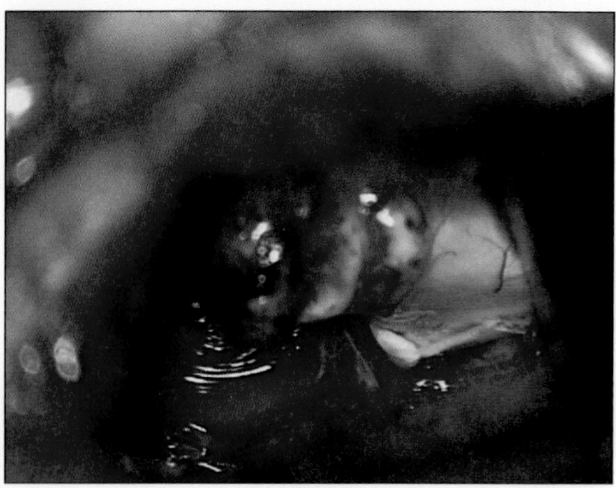

FIGURE 37-9

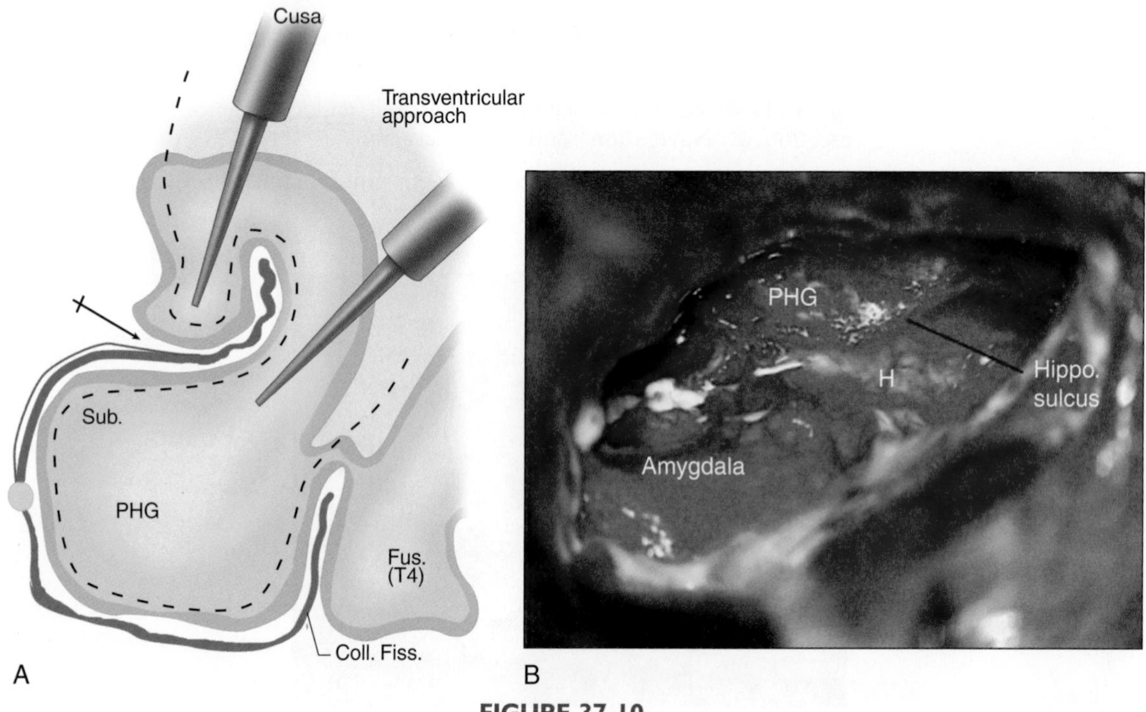

FIGURE 37-10

- **Figure 37-10: A,** Line drawing showing resection along both sides of the hippocampal sulcus. **B,** Hippocampal sulcus after hippocampal resection.
- **Figure 37-11:** Confirmation of posterior extent of resection. Frameless stereotactic neuronavigation screen capture depicting intraoperative confirmation of the extent of the resection cavity compared with preoperative imaging.
- **Figure 37-12:** Hemostasis. Intraoperative photograph showing the resection cavity and applied hemostatic agents at the conclusion of resection before closure of the dura.

TIPS FROM THE MASTERS

- Flat lateral positioning of the temporal region of the head is essential for the best possible intraoperative visualization.
- Also for optimal intraoperative visualization, efforts should be made to extend the craniotomy as inferior toward the root of the zygoma as possible.
- Remaining in the endopial surface during amygdala resection decreases the risk of inadvertent migration into the medial structures.

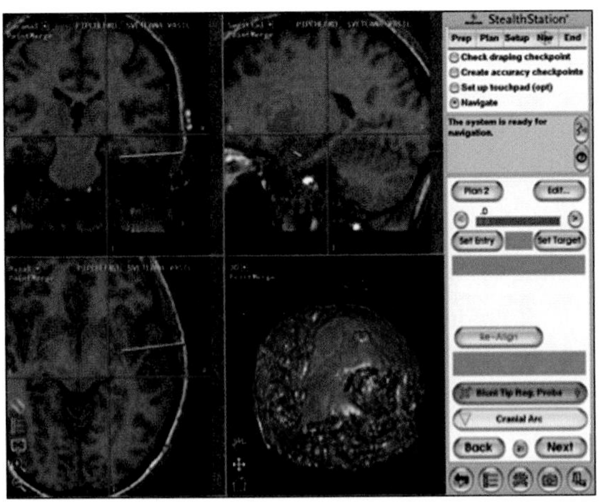

A

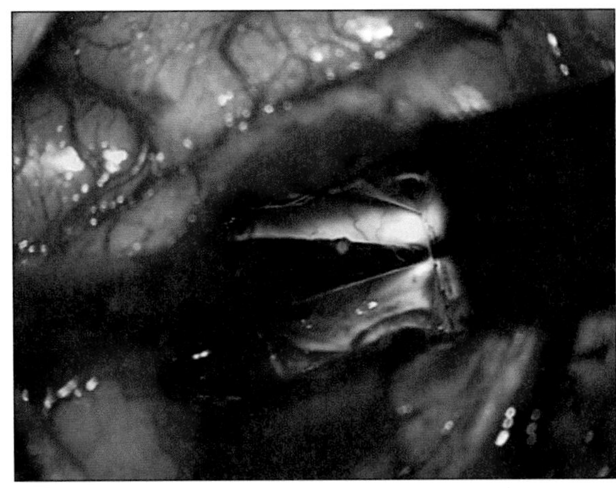

B

FIGURE 37-11

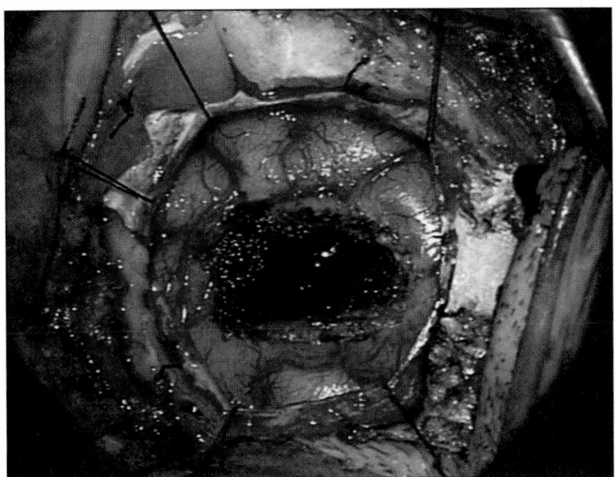

FIGURE 37-12

- It is best to err anteriorly and inferiorly for a safe starting point; resection lateral to the tentorial notch generally is safe.
- Piecemeal resection around both sides of the hippocampal sulcus is preferred to attempted en bloc resection.
- Resection of the amygdala should remain below the horizontal plane of the choroidal fissure.

PITFALLS

Inadequate exposure, especially anteriorly and inferiorly, hampers appropriate, safe visualization. It is critical to avoid shifting the trajectory posterior and superior to avoid unnecessary exposure and potential injury to the Sylvian fissure, language areas, or optic radiation.

The most common issue with selective hippocampectomy is incomplete resection; we consider the coronal plane of the collicular plate as the posterior extent of hippocampal resection.

Injury or spasm of the anterior choroidal artery can lead to temporary neurologic deficit, permanent neurologic deficit, or no sequelae. Avoiding injury of the vessels is facilitated by remaining in the endopial surface at all times.

Frequent confirmation with neuronavigation is crucial to avoid catastrophic injury to the cerebral peduncle.

BAILOUT OPTIONS

- The temporal horn is the cornerstone of the mental map of this approach. Whenever in doubt, return to the temporal horn. If the frameless stereotactic navigation appears not to correlate, the temporal horn is usually 3 cm deep to the surface of the middle temporal gyrus.
- When the approach is tight and the degree of freedom is limited, small corticectomy of the inferior temporal gyrus might ease the initial part of the approach.
- The choroid plexus is a very useful landmark to maintain the orientation of the exposure; the resection should remain inferior to the plane of the choroid plexus at all times. The free edge of the tentorium is another useful landmark for bailout.

SUGGESTED READINGS

Olivier A. Transcortical selective amygdalohippocampectomy in temporal lobe surgery. Can J Neurol Sci 2000; 27(Suppl. 1):S68–S76.

Tanriverdi T, Olivier A, Poulin N, et al. Long-term seizure outcome after mesial temporal lobe epilepsy surgery: corticalamygdalohippocampectomy versus selective amygdalohippocampectomy. J Neurosurg 2008;108:517–24.

Tellez-Zenteno J, Dhar R, Wiebe S. Long-term seizure outcomes following epilepsy surgery: a systematic review and meta-analysis. Brain 2005;128:1188–98.

Weibe S, Blume W, Girvin J, et al. A randomized controlled trial of surgery for temporal lobe epilepsy. N Engl J Med 2001;345:311–8.

Yasargil MG, Teddy PG, Roth P. Selective amygdalo-hippocampectomy: operative anatomy and surgical technique. Adv Tech Stand Neurosurg 1985;12:93–123.

Procedure 38

Seizure Focus Monitor Placement

Tsulee Chen, Jorge Alvaro Gonzalez-Martinez, William E. Bingaman

This procedure describes subdural and depth electrode implantation for long-term invasive recording of electroencephalography (EEG).

INDICATIONS

- Invasive monitoring of EEG in patients with medically refractory, focal-onset epilepsy can provide valuable information regarding an epileptogenic zone that is not clearly correlated with seizure symptoms and noninvasive studies, including scalp EEG, magnetic resonance imaging (MRI) of the brain, nuclear medicine studies, and magnetoencephalography (MEG).
- Invasive monitoring is indicated for the more precise identification of the epileptogenic zone in cases of "nonlesional" epilepsy, dual pathology, or discordant noninvasive data.
- Invasive electrodes can also provide important functional information about the underlying cortex and its relationship to the surrounding epileptogenic zone.
- Depth electrode recordings can provide valuable information regarding electrical activity in regions that are not easily or safely covered by subdural grid electrodes, including amygdala, various portions of the hippocampus, cingulate gyrus and mesial frontoparietal regions, and insula.
- Depth electrode recordings are indicated for the evaluation of temporal lobe epilepsy to identify a unilateral ictal onset within a mesial temporal lobe region.

CONTRAINDICATIONS

- Patients with extensive dural scarring, prior cranial infections, increased intracranial pressure, or other space-occupying lesions generally are not considered for implantation of subdural electrodes.
- Patients with significant medical or psychiatric comorbidities that would prevent them from safely undergoing surgery are ineligible for invasive monitoring.
- Invasive recordings are best avoided in young patients, less mature patients, and patients with violent seizure activity who are at risk for cranial injury during the monitoring period.

PLANNING AND POSITIONING

- All patients who are offered subdural grid electrode (SDE) implantation for monitoring have previously undergone the standard preoperative evaluation, which includes not only imaging studies but also neuropsychiatric testing. The decision regarding invasive monitoring is made during a multidisciplinary meeting including neurologists, neurosurgeons, neuroradiologists, and behavioral health specialists.
- Areas of coverage are determined based on preoperative noninvasive studies and seizure symptoms. Preoperative noninvasive studies include video scalp EEG monitoring, subtraction difference single photon emission computed tomography (SPECT) blood flow studies, interictal positron emission tomography (PET) using 18-FDG radionuclide, and MEG. All patients receive neuropsychologic testing, and some receive functional MRI or amobarbital sodium (Amytal Sodium) intracarotid testing for identification of language and memory function.

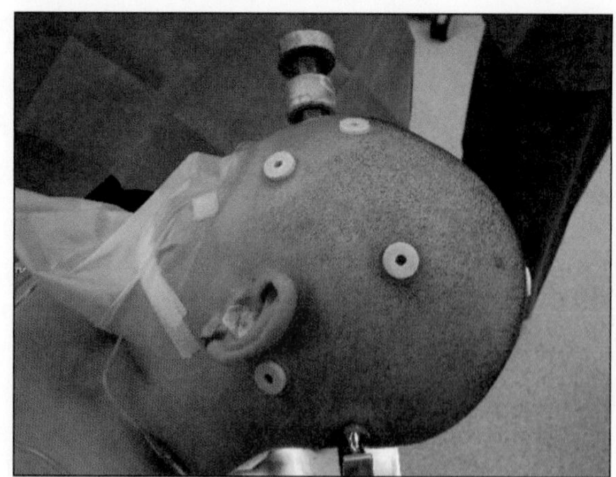

FIGURE 38-1

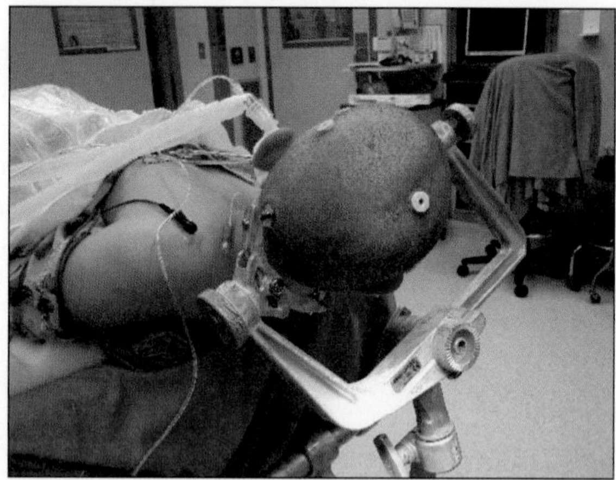

FIGURE 38-2

- Incision and craniotomy are individualized to provide the desired coverage according to the preoperative hypothesis. The exposure should allow for placement of electrodes in addition to access to the anticipated area of resection.
- Positioning of the patient should allow for stereotactic guidance in the event that depth electrodes are to be placed during the same operation.
- **Figure 38-1:** All patients have the hair fully clipped, with care taken not to disturb the fiducial markers for stereotactic guidance. Pinning of the patient's head within the head holder clamp is done such that a large incision and craniotomy can be turned; this usually involves fixing a single pin in the forehead, skewed to the contralateral side, and two pins in the occiput.
- **Figure 38-2:** The patient is placed in the supine position, with a shoulder roll positioned under the ipsilateral shoulder and the head turned 30 to 45 degrees toward the contralateral side, depending on the amount of parietal and occipital coverage needed. If mesial coverage is desired, the vertex is tipped superiorly. The frame is locked into place.
- **Figure 38-3:** When the patient is secured, the reference arm for the stereotactic guidance system is affixed to the head holder. Registration of the patient is completed and checked for accuracy. Planning of targets is performed to allow placement of depth electrodes and subdural electrodes during the same procedure.

PROCEDURE

- **Figure 38-4:** The incision should be large enough to allow for an adequate craniotomy. Usually a T-shaped or large question mark incision is used. If basitemporal coverage is needed, the incision should extend down to the zygoma. Orbitofrontal coverage can be

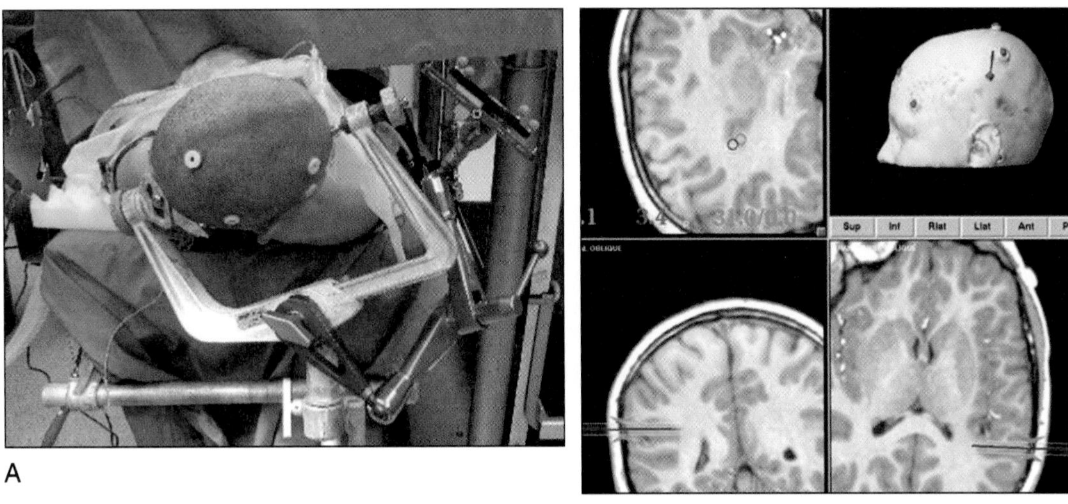

FIGURE 38-3

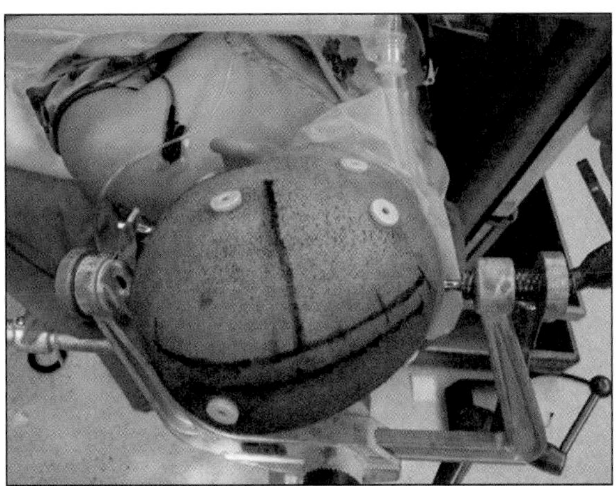

FIGURE 38-4

achieved easily as long as the incision allows for visualizing the keyhole region. Mesial hemispheric coverage necessitates an incision all the way to midline.

- **Figure 38-5:** When the scalp is opened, and the temporalis muscle is dissected from the bone, the craniotomy is made by placing burr holes that allow turning the flap and for exit of the electrode cables. When the bone flap is removed, tack-up holes are made

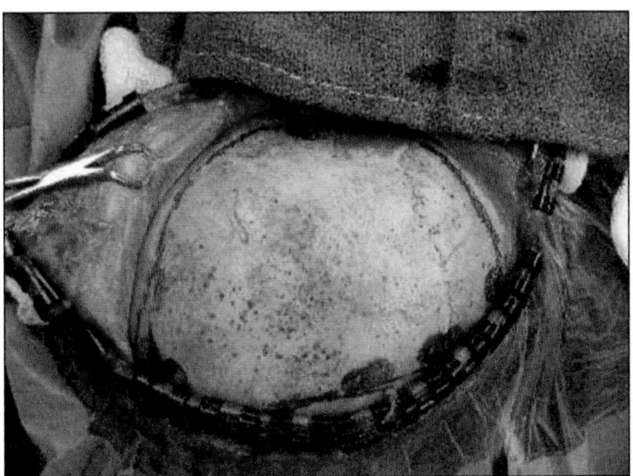

FIGURE 38-5

along the edges of the craniotomy, and tack-up sutures (3-0 or 4-0 braided monofilament) are placed to reduce the risk of postoperative epidural hematoma.

- **Figure 38-6:** Dural opening should allow for visualization of the necessary cortex and should provide a sufficient cuff for securing the electrode wires and a "watertight" closure. Attention to the presence of dural sinuses and draining veins is important to prevent injury.
- **Figure 38-7:** To facilitate placement of electrodes, the basal and mesial surfaces should be carefully inspected for cortical draining veins that could impede them. Using bayoneted forceps, the grid electrodes can be slid into place under a constant stream of irrigation. Any resistance may indicate the presence of a draining vein or cortical scarring, and the trajectory of the grid should be adjusted.
- **Figure 38-8:** Before covering the lateral cortex, any desired depth electrodes are inserted using stereotactic guidance. The entry point should be planned to avoid cortical sulci and blood vessels. Using stereotactic guidance, the trajectory from the entry point is identified, the pial surface is incised, and the electrode is inserted. Generally, targets chosen are regions of cortex, and submillimeter accuracy is unnecessary. The most important goal is to avoid vascular injury.
- **Figure 38-9:** When the depth electrodes are in place, the grids for lateral coverage can be placed. Again using bayoneted forceps, the larger grid electrodes are laid over the cortical surface, tucking the edges under the borders of the dural flap. The grid electrodes can be cut if necessary to allow exit of the depth electrodes. When in place, each electrode wire is secured to the nearest dural edge with a stitch to prevent movement during the monitoring period. After final electrode positioning, photographs can be taken to allow for postoperative planning and registration of the grid position to the preoperative MRI surface reconstruction.
- **Figure 38-10:** The dura is closed using 3-0 or 4-0 braided monofilament in either a running fashion or a simple interrupted fashion, trying to achieve a "watertight" closure to reduce the chances of postoperative cerebrospinal fluid (CSF) leak at the

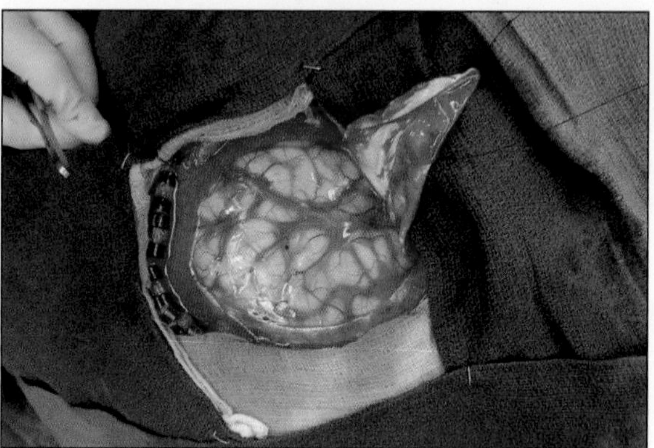

FIGURE 38-6

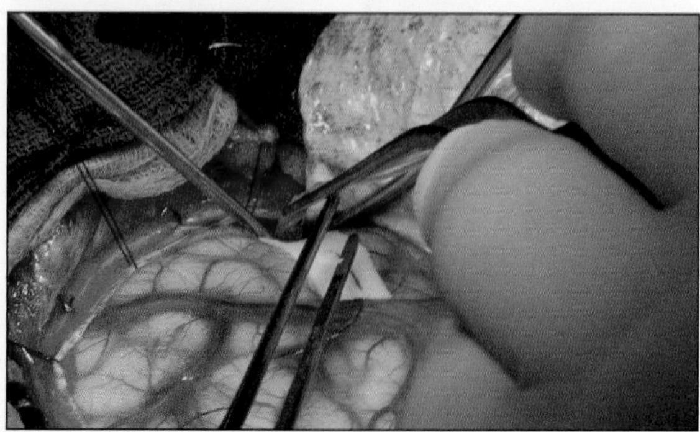

FIGURE 38-7

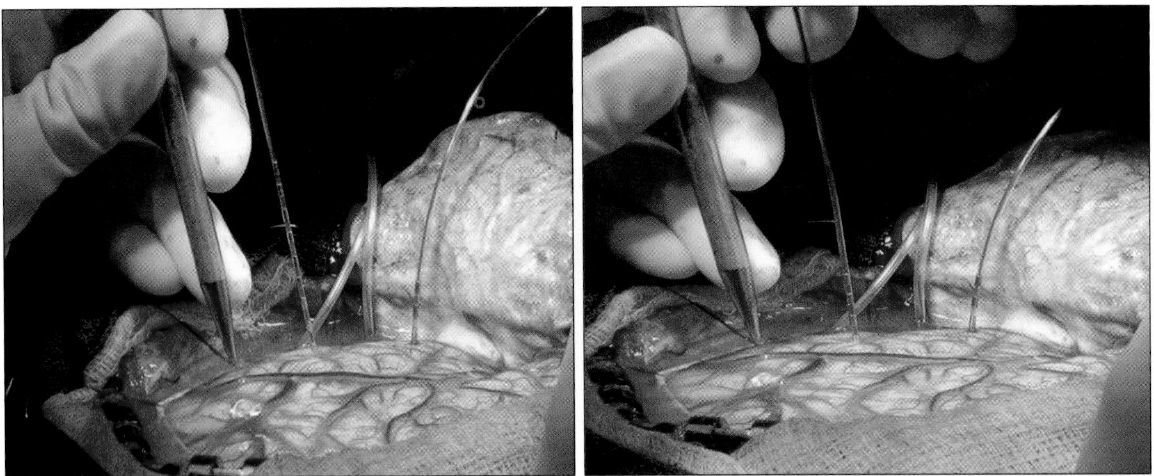

FIGURE 38-8

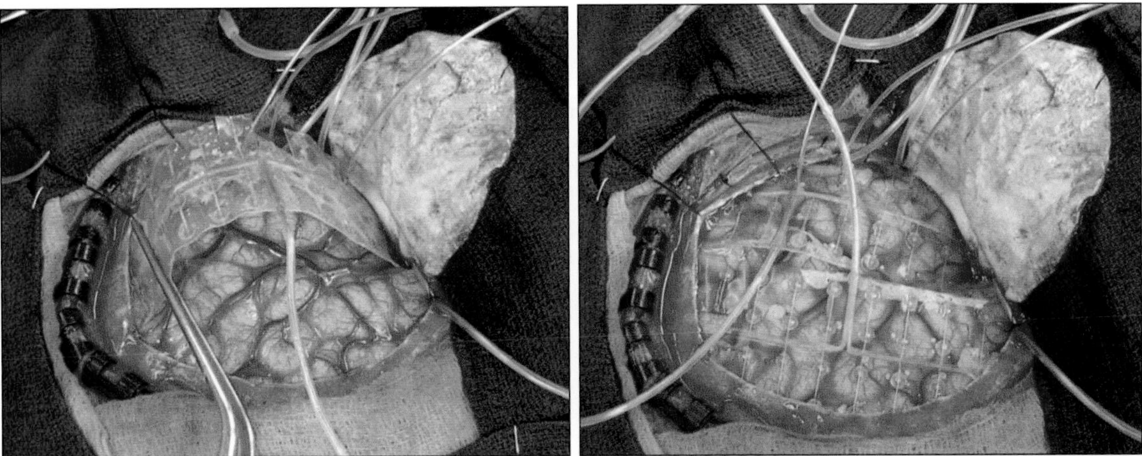

FIGURE 38-9

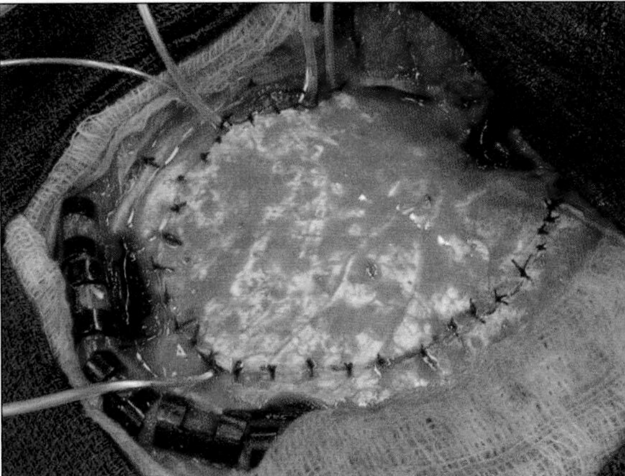

FIGURE 38-10

electrode exit site on the scalp. Revision craniotomies in patients can be particularly challenging and usually result in an incomplete closure of the dura because of compromised dural integrity. If adequate closure cannot be achieved, a dural substitute can be laid over the open areas. When the dura is closed and excess moisture is dried with a sponge, the dural opening is covered with a dural sealant.

- **Figure 38-11:** The bone flap is secured with titanium cranial fixation plates. Burr hole covers are not used because the electrode wires exit the craniotomy at these sites.

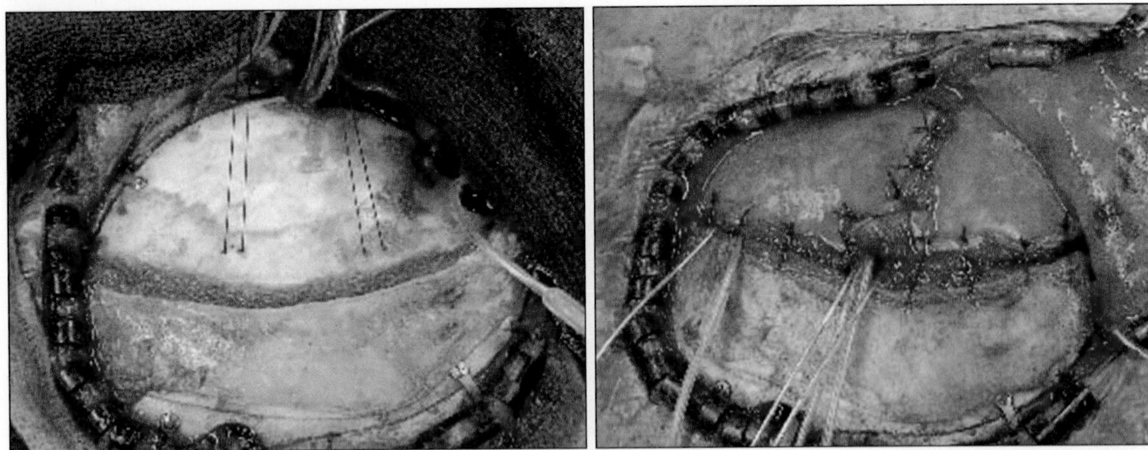

FIGURE 38-11

Dural tack-up sutures are pulled through tack-up holes in the middle of the bone flap and tied down after the plates are secured. The temporalis muscle is reapproximated when appropriate.

- **Figure 38-12:** A small 1-cm incision is made remote to the incision to serve as the exit site for the wires. The exit site should be planned as near to the top of the head as possible to help reduce the chances of postoperative CSF leak. Before tunneling the wires, a U-stitch is placed to close the exit site after tunneling in an effort to reduce the occurrence of CSF leak. Using a hemostat, the wires are carefully pulled through the separate incision from the inside out. The stitch is cinched, and the exit site is closed. The electrode cables are secured to the skin.

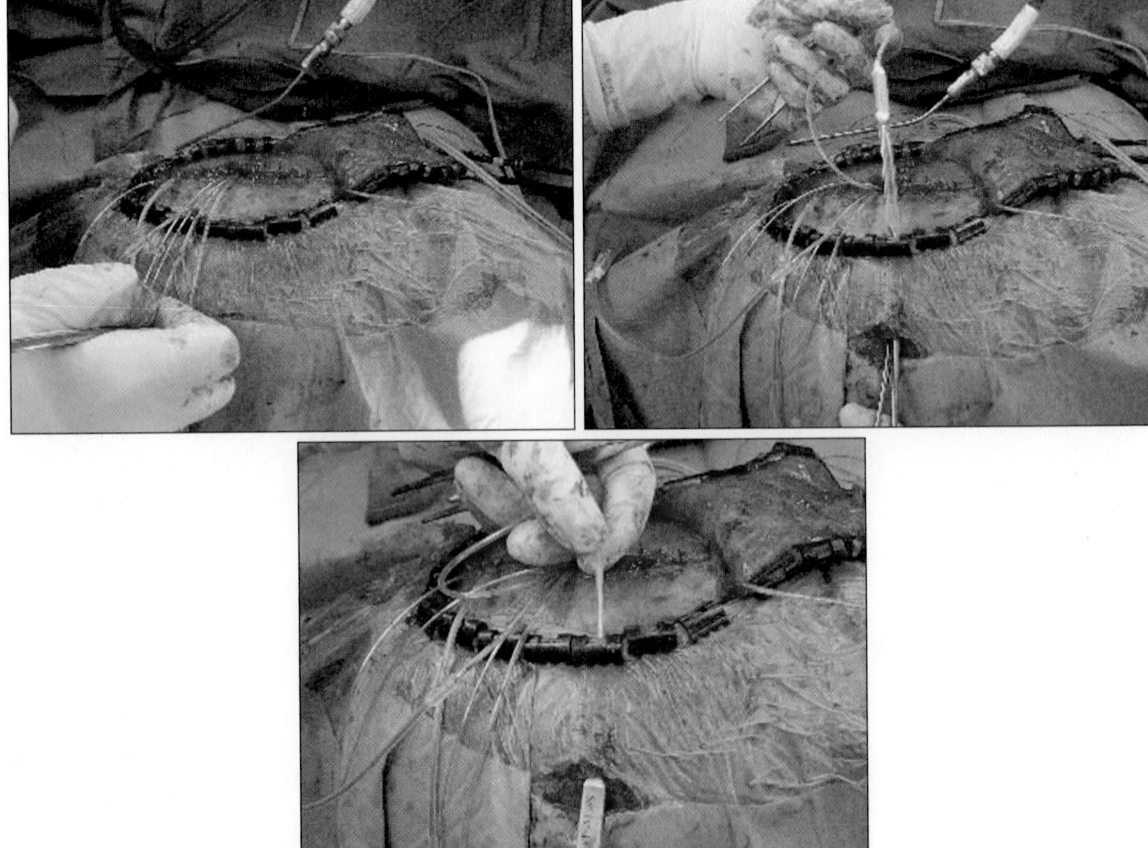

FIGURE 38-12

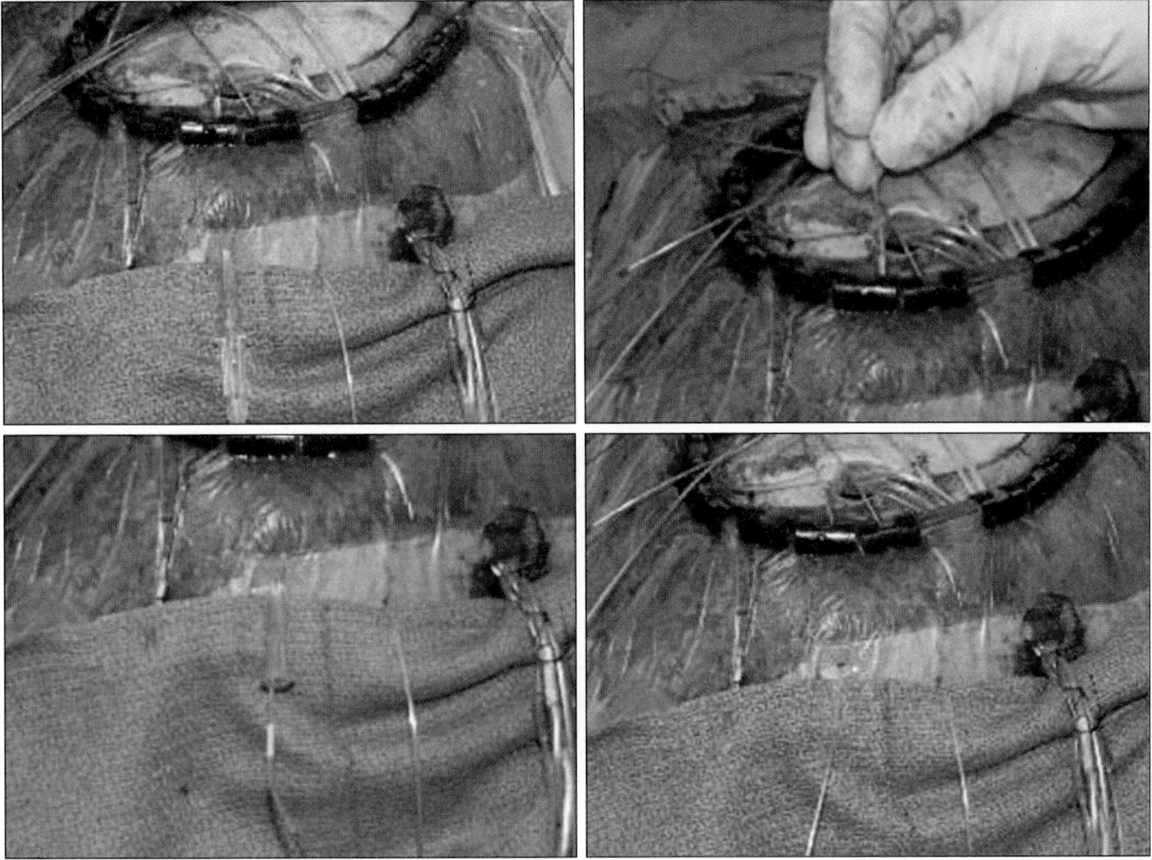

FIGURE 38-13

- **Figure 38-13:** Depth electrodes are tunneled away from the incision in a similar fashion with the aid of a 14-gauge intravenous catheter. The needle is inserted from a starting point approximately 2 to 3 cm away from the incision, to just inside the incision. The wire is fed through the catheter, which is removed when the electrode end is out of the skin. Each wire is secured to the scalp with a 3-0 monofilament. A subgaleal drain may be used to reduce postoperative swelling and may help to reduce the chances of postoperative CSF leak. All patients are maintained on intravenous antibiotics while the electrodes are in place.

TIPS FROM THE MASTERS

- Basitemporal coverage can be easily achieved with a few strip electrodes. In our institution, they can vary in size but are generally 1 × 6 or 2 × 6 strips. These electrodes record from the parahippocampal gyrus and may not accurately reflect ictal activity within the hippocampus and amygdala.
- Interhemispheric coverage is difficult because of the presence of draining cortical veins to the sagittal sinus. Pick an entry point close to the midline that is away from eloquent cortex and draining veins whenever possible. If bleeding occurs, elevate the head and irrigate the area. The bleeding often stops on its own. Use of bipolar coagulation in the interhemispheric region should be avoided to minimize the risk of venous injury.
- If the grid or strip electrode does not slide easily, do not force it. Bridging veins and adhesions can limit the ease or even the ability to slide an electrode in that area. Minor adjustments can be made to compensate; sometimes a suboptimal coverage is safer for the patient, however.
- Longer subcutaneous tunnels may help to reduce infection and CSF leaks after surgery. Also, the U-stitch in the exit site needs to be tied tightly enough to prevent CSF leak without causing skin edge necrosis.

- Postoperative skull x-rays can immediately show the relative placement of the electrodes and determine mass effect, pneumocephalus, and midline shift.
- Larger grids and strip electrodes can be cut to the desirable size. Take care not to cut the communication of the electrode contact with the exiting wire.
- Although areas of encephalomalacia can be covered, grids should be placed so that minimal contacts are located over a cyst or prior resection cavity.
- Careful attention while tunneling the cables is mandatory to prevent injury to the cables already in the tunnel and to prevent displacement of the electrodes on the cerebral surface.
- Dressing of the head is done in a standard fashion. Careful attention to how the electrode cables are placed in the dressing is necessary to prevent injury to the cables when the head wrap dressing is changed.

PITFALLS

Placement of invasive electrodes adds mass effect to the brain, and careful attention to hemostasis, electrolytes, and fluid status is necessary to reduce the risk of injury.

Invasive recordings necessitate two surgeries with all the inherent risks of craniotomy.

Obtaining coverage of deep gray matter structures, of the mesial frontal lobe, and of the basitemporal lobe can be challenging, and supplementation with depth electrodes should be considered.

The number of available channels for recording depends on the institution. A plan for placement of electrodes should be finalized with the epileptologist before the operation.

Placement of invasive recordings does not guarantee localization of the epileptogenic zone. The number of electrodes that can be safely placed is limited, and the region of cortex sampled is limited as well. The patient should be counseled regarding the possibility of not localizing the epileptogenic zone or the necessity of having to move the electrodes further based on the initial recordings.

Involvement of functional cortex is easily identified by cortical stimulation of electrodes overlying it. This trial of stimulation in no way means that surgical resection in eloquent cortex is better tolerated. Risks to cortical function during epilepsy resective surgery depend on many variables and may be better predicted with the use of invasive recordings.

BAILOUT OPTIONS

- If bleeding occurs, hemostasis should be obtained with irrigation and hemostatic agents, no electrocautery. This reduces the risk of venous infaret.

SUGGESTED READINGS

Fausser S, Sisodiya SM, Martinian L, et al. Multi-focal occurrence of cortical dysplasia in epilepsy patients. Brain 2009;132:2079–90.

Fountas KN, Smith JR. Subdural electrode-associated complications: a 20-year experience. Stereotact Funct Neurosurg 2007;85:264–72.

Koubeissi MZ, Puwanant A, Jehi L, et al. In-hospital complications of epilepsy surgery: a six-year nationwide experience. Br J Neurosurg 2009;23:524–9.

Musleh W, Yassari R, Hecox K, et al. Low incidence of subdural grid-related complications in prolonged pediatric EEG monitoring. Pediatr Neurosurg 2006;42:284–7.

Widdess-Walsh P, Jeha L, Nair D, et al. Subdural electrode analysis in focal cortical dysplasia: predictors of surgical outcome. Neurology 2007;69:660–7.

Procedure 39

Awake Craniotomy

Daniel L. Silbergeld, Adam O. Hebb

INDICATIONS

- When the planned resection site of a tumor is near essential language cortex, intraoperative language mapping is necessary.
- Occasionally, tumors in or near motor cortex are best removed with intraoperative testing of motor ability during surgery.

CONTRAINDICATIONS

- Patients who are unable to cooperate because of psychosocial issues or young age.
- Patients with airway concerns, including sleep apnea and obesity.
- Patients whose preoperative language baseline is less than 80% of objects named correctly at 4-second intervals. Because stimulation language mapping relies on the ability to block object naming, language cannot be localized when baseline errors are too high. Although some object slides can be discarded from the specific patient's slide set, the final set should have at least 50 slides. When the patient has normal naming ability (i.e., 100% of slides named correctly), slides are presented at 3-second intervals. This allows quicker mapping with a higher current because of less temporal current summation.

PLANNING AND POSITIONING

- All local anesthetics used comprise 1% lidocaine and 0.25% bupivacaine with 1:200,000 epinephrine. Typically, 80 to 110 mL of this mixture is administered.
- The patient's head must always be lateral or angled slightly above the horizon so that the airway is well protected and the patient can see the computer screen. Attention is directed toward positioning the head to optimize the patient's airway during sedation. Although we prefer to use the pin headrest, the procedure can be done with a horseshoe headrest or even a foam donut. Pins provide the greatest degree of head stability, however.
- A Foley catheter is always placed.
- Patients should have therapeutic serum levels of antiepileptic medication preoperatively.
- **Figure 39-1:** Applying a pin headrest after instillation of local anesthesia.

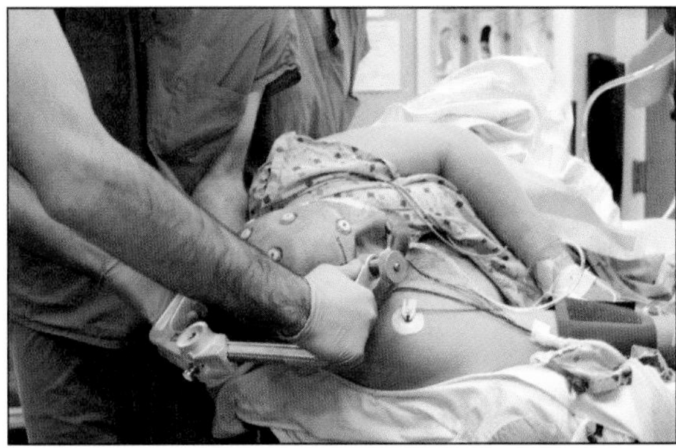

FIGURE 39-1

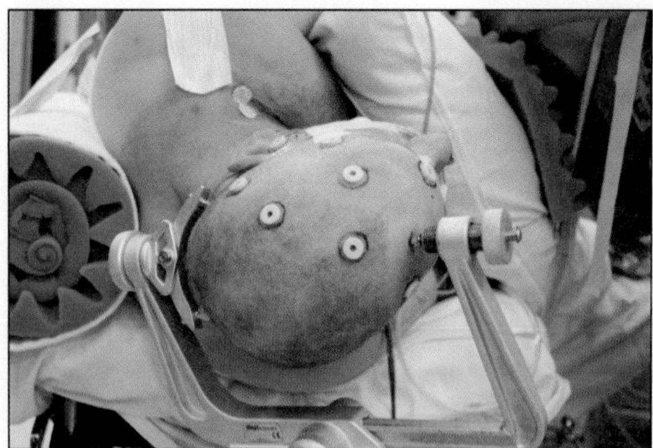

FIGURE 39-2

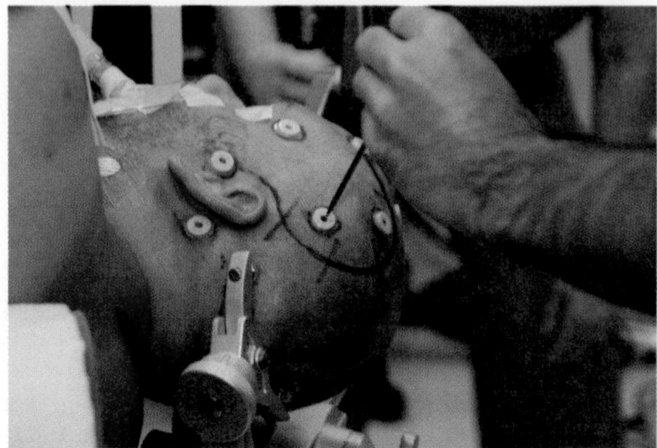

FIGURE 39-3

- **Figure 39-2:** The patient is turned to a 45- to 60-degree lateral position with the bed in 15 to 25 degrees of reverse Trendelenburg. All pressure points are carefully padded with the neck slightly extended to improve airway patency during propofol (Diprivan) anesthesia.
- **Figure 39-3:** Scalp fiducial markers are registered to preoperative magnetic resonance imaging (MRI) using the frameless neuronavigation system.

PROCEDURE

- **Figure 39-4:** After induction of neuroleptic propofol anesthesia, without intubation, the local anesthetic field block is placed, beginning in the regions of the preauricular, postauricular, and supraorbital nerves. By starting at these points, placement of the remainder of the block is less painful. Although some centers use a laryngeal airway throughout the "asleep" aspects of the procedure, we prefer to do this only when necessary to maintain airway control.

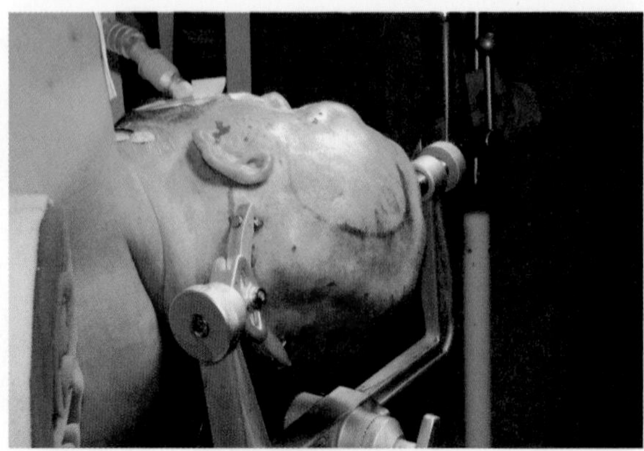

FIGURE 39-4

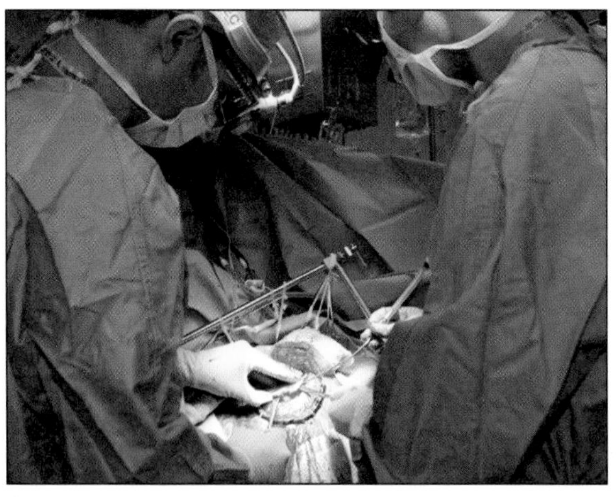

A

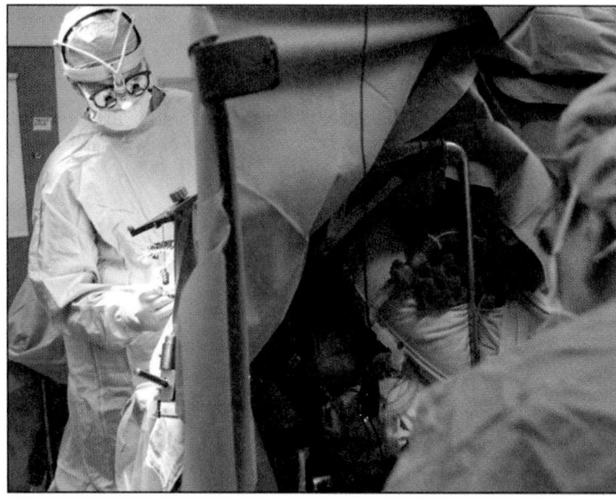

B

FIGURE 39-5

- **Figure 39-5:** Draping must be done so that the patient can see the stimulus presentation screen and the anesthesia team has access to the airway. **A,** Surgeons' view. **B,** Anesthesiologists' view.
- **Figure 39-6:** Because some patients awaken confused or slightly combative, the dura is not opened until the patient is completely awake and calm. To hold the electrode, two options are available: an epidural post, which clamps to the skull, or a post that screws into the bone. We prefer the post that screws into the skull (shown) because it is more stable and avoids potential epidural bleeding.
- **Figure 39-7:** After the brain is exposed, cortical electrodes are placed on the brain surface, followed by small numbers that identify which area has been stimulated.

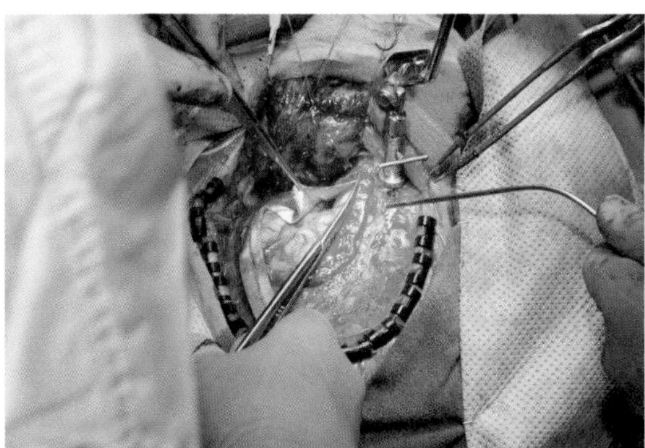

FIGURE 39-6

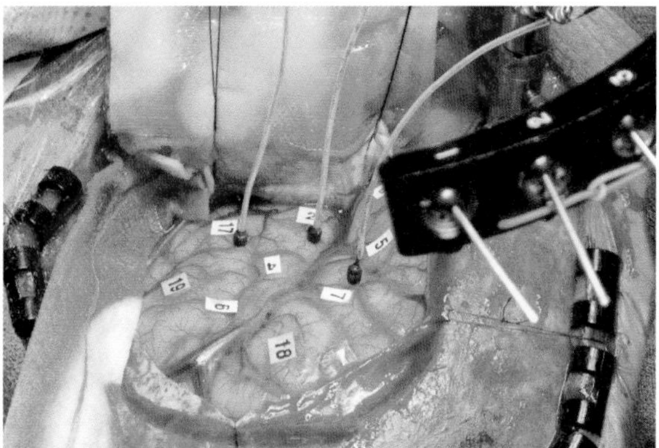

FIGURE 39-7

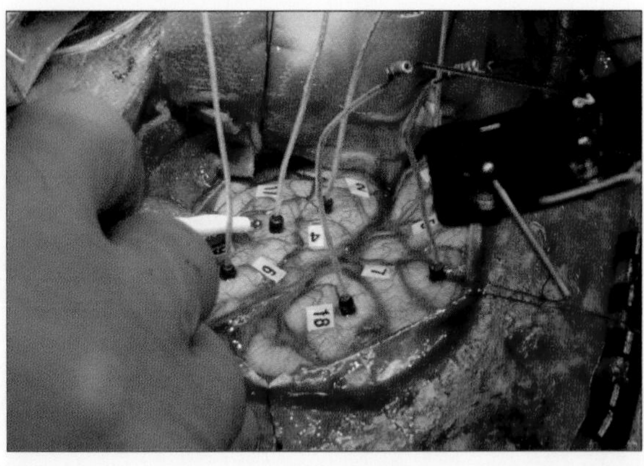

A

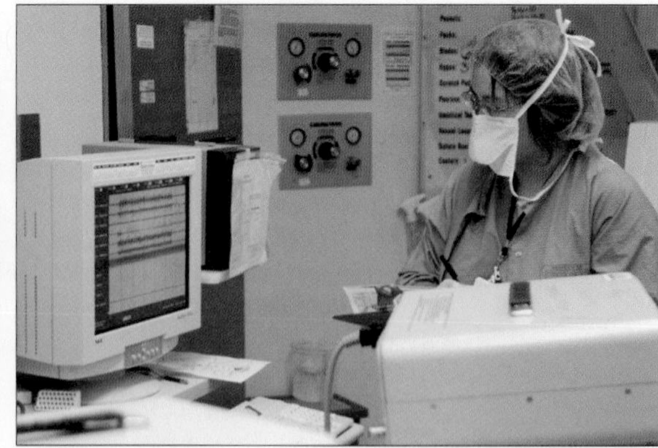

B

FIGURE 39-8

There are also many electrode options available, including carbon-tip electrodes (as shown), cotton-tip electrodes, and strip/grid electrodes. We prefer carbon-tip electrodes because they maintain good contact with the cortex while permitting the surgeon excellent access for cortical stimulation.

- **Figure 39-8:** The after-discharge (AD) threshold is determined next. Determining the AD threshold helps to prevent evoking clinical seizure activity and false localization. **A,** The cortex is stimulated while electrocorticography is performed. Beginning with 2-mA current, several spots on the cortex are stimulated for the same duration as the planned object image presentation epoch (3 or 4 seconds). Current is increased by 2 mA after several areas are tested without evoking ADs. This sequence is repeated until ADs are seen, then mapping is performed with current 1 to 2 mA below the AD threshold. The surgeon stimulates the brain as the patient names the object slides. After each stimulation, the surgeon calls out the number on the nearest ticket. **B,** The neurologist monitors electroencephalogram for ADs and seizures. If either ADs or a frank clinical seizure occurs, the brain is irrigated with iced irrigation fluid. If a seizure persists, midazolam (Versed) is administered in 1- to 2-mg increments until clinical seizure activity ceases. It is very rare to evoke seizures that persist or become problematic for continued mapping.
- **Figure 39-9:** **A,** After mapping is complete, borders of the surgical resection are identified based on the operative goal and location of eloquent cortex. The surgical resection border is identified here with silk suture. **B,** Resection proceeds with the patient again placed under propofol anesthesia for the remainder of the procedure. An exception is when the resection is very close to the language areas. In these instances, the patient continues naming during the portion of the resection that is closest to the language area and then goes back to sleep. Brain outside of the resection boundary is protected with BICOL Collagen Sponge (Codman & Shurtleff, Raynham, MA).

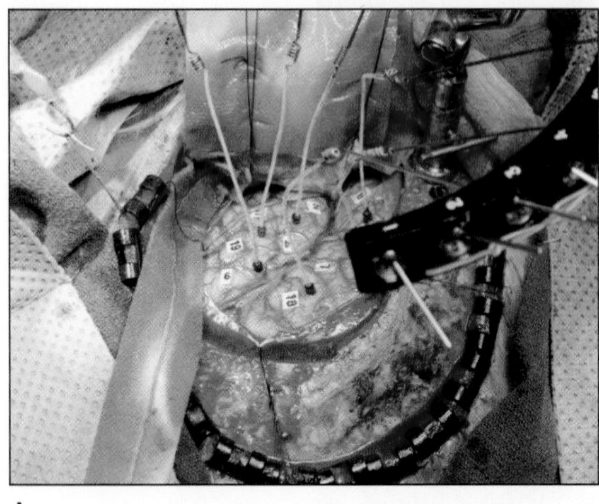

A

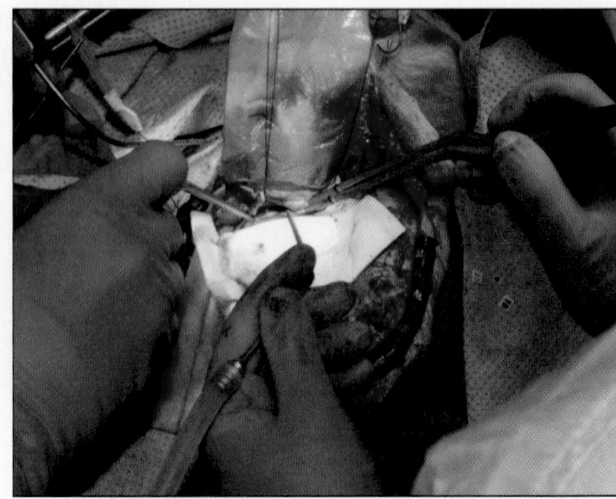

B

FIGURE 39-9

TIPS FROM THE MASTERS

- It is important to choose patients who can cooperate and who have adequate language ability.
- When undertaking awake cranial surgery in patients with significant intracranial masses, 0.5 g/kg of mannitol is administered. Using higher doses often causes significant nausea. The bed should be in reverse Trendelenburg, and the neck should be in neutral, anatomic position.
- Although it is critical for the neurosurgeon to have experience with awake craniotomies, it is of equal importance to have experienced anesthesiology and electroencephalography teams.

PITFALLS

Many people have multiple language areas. Finding one language area in either the temporal lobe or the frontal lobe does not mean that mapping is complete. The entire area at risk should be mapped. Similarly, in multilingual patients, each language must be mapped. Injury to the native tongue would disrupt all language function. Injury to secondary languages would not affect the native language.

Mapping is only the first step. During resection, the surgeon must avoid injuring subcortical connections and vascular structures. When in doubt, the patient should be kept awake and continue the object-naming task until the risk period is over.

BAILOUT OPTIONS

- A laryngeal airway should be available to prevent losing airway control.
- If the surgeon cannot find the language area, the patient should continue object naming throughout the resection.
- If a seizure persists, despite reasonable doses of midazolam and irrigation of the brain with cold fluid, an airway should be placed and the seizures stopped with other drugs as needed.

SUGGESTED READINGS

Lucas T, Silbergeld DL. Review of language mapping procedures for temporal resections. In: Silbergeld DL, Miller JW, editors. Epilepsy Surgery: Principles and Controversies. New York: Marcel Dekker; 2005.

Ojemann G, Ojemann J, Lettich E, et al. Cortical language localization in left, dominant hemisphere: an electrical stimulation mapping investigation in 117 patients. J Neurosurg 1989;71:316–26.

Ojemann GA. Cortical organization of language. J Neurosci 1991;11:2281–7.

Penfield W, Jasper H. Epilepsy and the Functional Anatomy of the Human Brain. Boston: Little, Brown; 1954.

Silbergeld DL. Cortical mapping. In: Luders HO, Comair YG, editors. Epilepsy Surgery. Philadelphia: Lippincott Williams & Wilkins; 2002, p. 633–5.

Silbergeld DL, Ojemann GA. The tailored temporal lobectomy. Neurosurg Clin N Am 1993;4:273–81.

Tozer K, Silbergeld DL. Neocortical resections and lesionectomies. In: Silbergeld DL, Miller JW, editors. Epilepsy Surgery: Principles and Controversies. New York: Marcel Dekker; 2005.

Procedure 40 Corpus Callosotomy (Anterior and Complete)

James M. Johnston, Jr., Matthew D. Smyth

INDICATIONS

- Medically intractable, generalized atonic seizures
- Secondarily generalized seizures without identifiable focus
- Medically intractable, Lennox-Gastaut syndrome with multiple seizure types
- Severe myoclonic absence seizures

CONTRAINDICATIONS

- Identifiable seizure focus
- Bleeding disorder
- Agenesis of corpus callosum

PLANNING AND POSITIONING

- Supine position with the head in neutral position; chin flexed; torso elevated 10 degrees above horizontal
- Transverse, sigmoid incision at coronal suture extending across midline
- Neuronavigation optional but helpful in planning craniotomy flap that ensures access to anterior and posterior callosum, while avoiding large, bridging cortical veins
- **Figure 40-1:** The patient is positioned supine, with the head flexed in a Mayfield head holder and the torso elevated approximately 10 to 20 degrees above the horizontal. Early use of mannitol and mild hyperventilation minimize frontal lobe retraction during the operation.

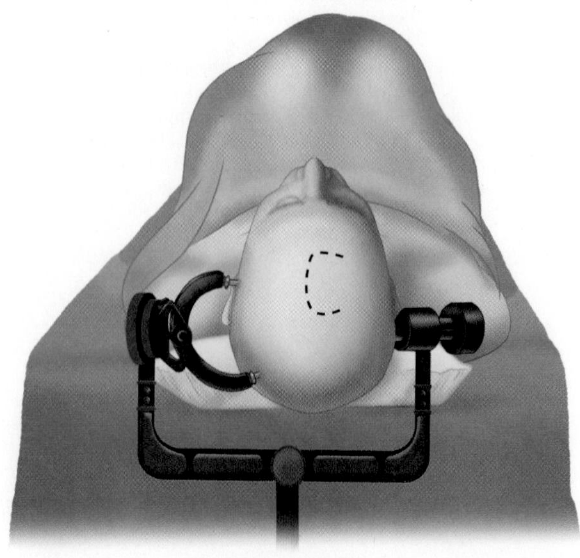

FIGURE 40-1

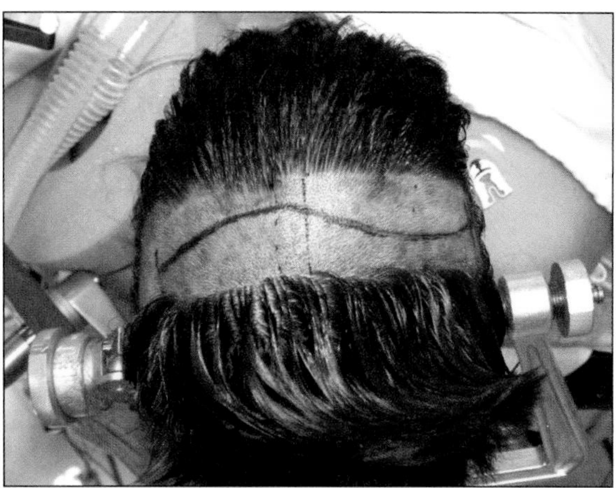

FIGURE 40-2

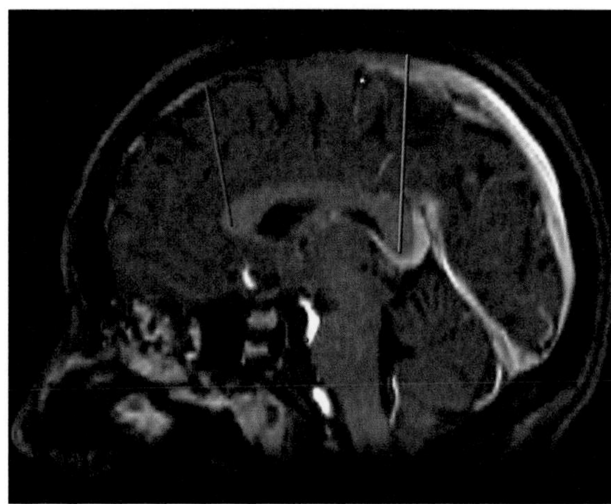

FIGURE 40-3

- **Figure 40-2:** After minimal clipping of the hair, a sigmoid incision located over the coronal suture is used.
- **Figure 40-3:** Frameless navigation may be used to optimize the craniotomy location to avoid cortical veins and plan trajectories to the anterior and posterior aspects of the corpus callosum.

PROCEDURE

- **Figure 40-4:** Craniotomy 4 cm × 8 cm is fashioned across the midline after placement of three to six burr holes for dural stripping. Bleeding from the dura overlying the superior sagittal sinus may be controlled with Surgicel, Gelfoam, and cottonoids. The craniotomy site should straddle the coronal suture to allow access to the splenium in cases of complete callosotomy.
- **Figure 40-5:** A careful dural opening is made and reflected toward the superior sagittal sinus until interhemispheric fissure is visualized. All cortical veins at or posterior to the coronal suture should be carefully preserved.
- **Figure 40-6:** Cotton strips or Telfa patties may be placed on the mesial frontal lobe to minimize injury over the course of the dissection.
- **Figure 40-7:** Interhemispheric fissure is visualized, and arachnoid bands are carefully dissected while retractor blades deepen the exposure. Pericallosal arteries are identified and should be carefully separated to find the avascular midline. In cases of an azygous anterior cerebral artery, the artery should be retracted to the side to minimize injury to bilateral perforators.

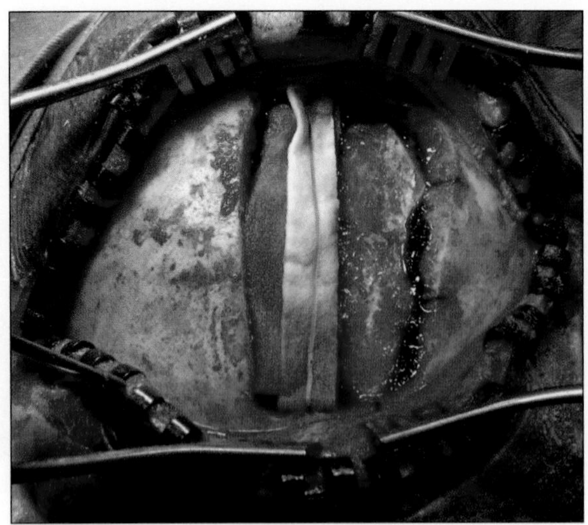

FIGURE 40-4

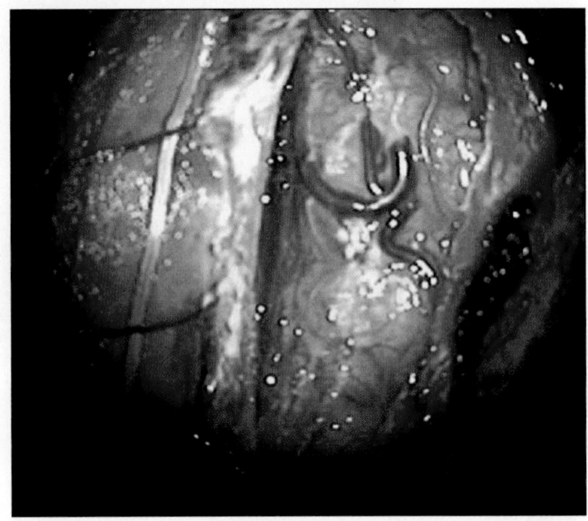

FIGURE 40-5

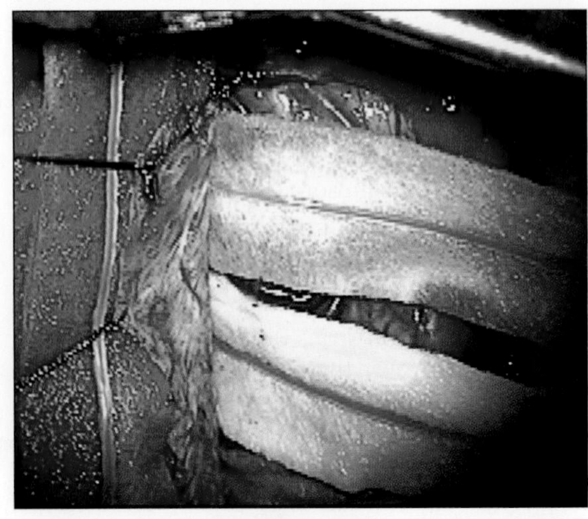

FIGURE 40-6

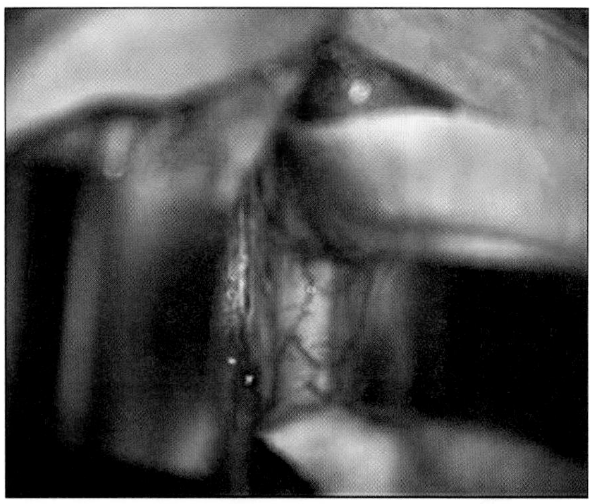

FIGURE 40-7

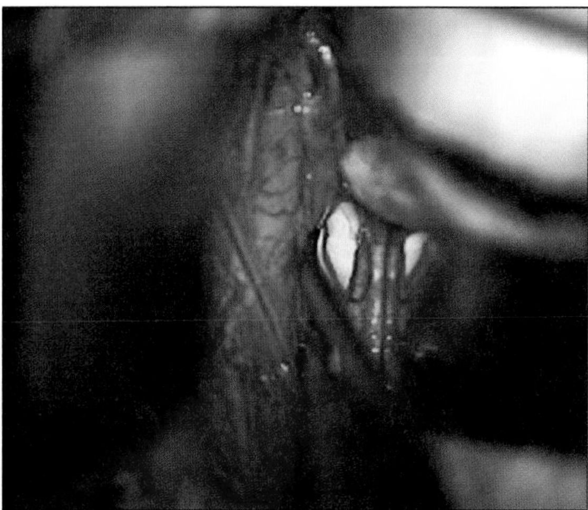

FIGURE 40-8

- **Figure 40-8:** The characteristic white appearance of the corpus callosum is visualized between the pericallosal arteries after sharp dissection of adherent arachnoid bands. It is helpful to expose the length of the intended disconnection completely before beginning the callosotomy.
- **Figure 40-9:** Callosotomy may be performed with a combination of low-power bipolar cautery and suction or ultrasonic aspiration. It can be helpful to confirm the midline with the use of frameless stereotactic neuronavigation before beginning the resection. It is important to stay between the midline leaves of the septum and preserve the ependymal lining of the ventricles to minimize postoperative cerebrospinal fluid accumulation.
- **Figure 40-10:** In cases of complete callosotomy, it is crucial to preserve the pial membrane protecting the internal cerebral vein and vein of Galen that lie just anterior to the splenial reflection of the callosum.
- **Figure 40-11:** Posterior callosotomy may be challenging because the angle of the splenium falls away from the operator.

TIPS FROM THE MASTERS

- Use mannitol and mild hyperventilation to minimize frontal lobe retraction.
- Preserve all bridging cortical veins posterior to coronal suture.

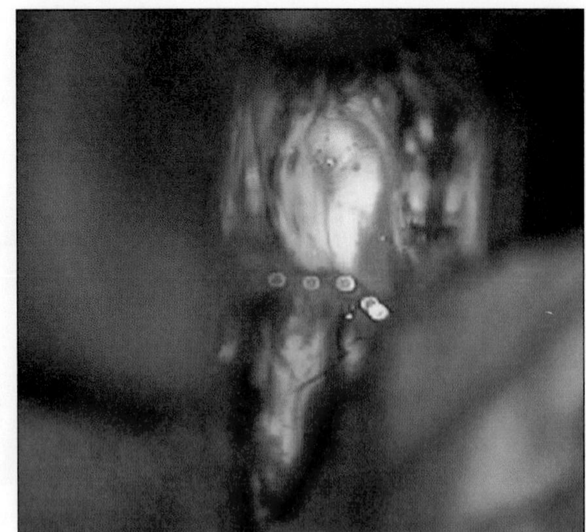

FIGURE 40-9

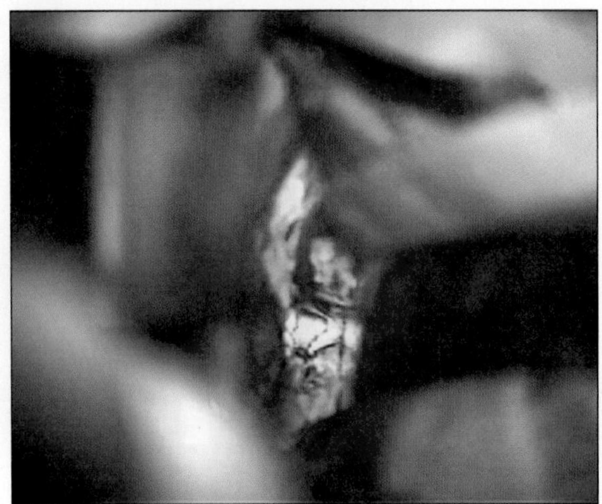

FIGURE 40-10

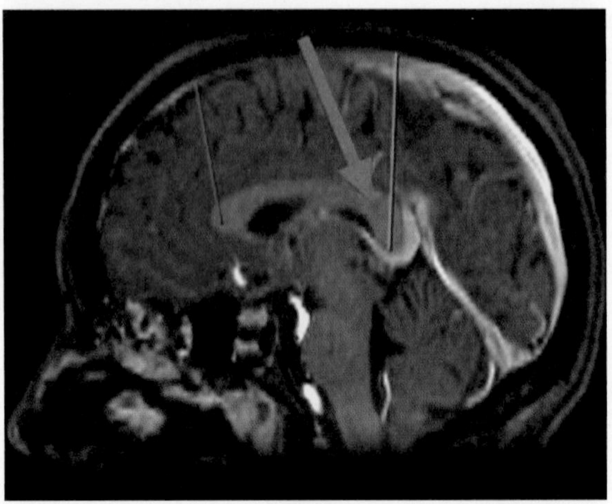

FIGURE 40-11

- Place cottonoids or Telfa patties along the mesial frontal lobe to minimize retraction injury.
- Completely expose the length of corpus callosum before beginning the callosotomy.
- Verify that the callosotomy is in the midline to avoid entry into the ventricle and minimize cerebrospinal fluid leakage.
- Perform intracallosal section of the posterior callosum and splenium when performing single-stage complete callosotomy with preservation of midline pia.

PITFALLS
Injury to crossing cortical veins, venous infarction
Retraction injury on mesial frontal lobes
Injury to anterior cerebral arteries
Entry into the ventricular system, cerebrospinal fluid fistula
Incomplete callosotomy

BAILOUT OPTIONS

- If the intended callosotomy is incomplete, a second-stage posterior approach through a separate posterior incision allows more direct access to the splenium.

SUGGESTED READINGS

Fuiks KS, Wyler AR, Hermann BP, et al. Seizure outcome from anterior and complete corpus callosotomy. J Neurosurg 1991;74:573–81.

Maehara T, Shimizu H. Surgical outcome of corpus callosotomy in patients with drop attacks. Epilepsia 2001;42:67–71.

Nei M, O'Connor M, Liporace J, et al. Refractory generalized seizures: response to corpus callosotomy and vagal nerve stimulation. Epilepsia 2006;47:115–22.

Sunaga S, Shimizu H, Sugano H. Long-term follow-up of seizure outcomes after corpus callosotomy. Seizure 2009;18:124–8.

Taniverdi T, Olivier A, Poulin N, et al. Long term seizure outcome after corpus callosotomy: a retrospective analysis of 95 patients. J Neurosurg 2009;110:332–42.

Procedure 41

Thalamotomy and Pallidotomy 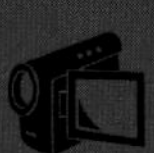

Jaliya R. Lokuketagoda, Robert E. Gross

INDICATIONS

- Pallidotomy
  - *Parkinson disease*: Complications of advancing disease and medical therapy including tremor, wearing off, motor fluctuations, and dyskinesia, in patients with a good response to levodopa therapy. Pallidotomy is performed unilaterally only in patients with Parkinson disease.
  - *Dystonia*: Disabling symptoms nonresponsive to medical therapy, including anticholinergics, benzodiazepines, and botulinum toxin. In certain cases, pallidotomy may be performed bilaterally in dystonic patients.
- Thalamotomy
  - *Essential tremor*: Disabling, predominantly upper extremity, unilateral kinetic tremor despite medical therapy, including beta blockers, primidone, and benzodiazepines
  - *Parkinson disease*: Unilateral rest tremor resistant to medical therapy in tremor-dominant disease
  - *Cerebellar outflow tremor*: Medically intractable unilateral kinetic, postural, or rest tremor secondary to multiple sclerosis or traumatic brain injury
- Contralateral to deep brain stimulation (DBS) system
  - In patients requiring bilateral surgery (e.g., patients with Parkinson disease, essential tremor), pallidotomy and thalamotomy may be performed contralateral to a DBS system.
  - Dystonia may be treated with bilateral pallidotomy or unilateral pallidotomy contralateral to a globus pallidus internus (GPi) DBS system.
- In place of DBS system
  - In patients who have undergone DBS (GPi, ventralis intermedius [Vim], possibly subthalamic nucleus), but in whom there have been hardware-related complications, such as chronic infection, the DBS may be removed and radiofrequency lesioning performed.

CONTRAINDICATIONS

- Unstable medical condition precluding awake stereotactic surgery
- Neuropsychiatric conditions, including untreated depression, psychotic symptoms (unless resulting from medical therapy such as dopamine agonists), and cognitive decline
- Multisystem atrophy in parkinsonian patients
- Poor response to levodopa therapy in Parkinson disease (except tremor)
- Contralateral homotopic lesion (except for dystonia)
- Need for general anesthesia during surgery
  - With rare exception, radiofrequency lesions should be created with constant neurologic evaluation, necessitating an awake patient.
  - General anesthesia can be used and the patient reversed for the lesioning part of the procedure, if necessary.

PLANNING AND POSITIONING

Frame Application

- The stereotactic frame is usually affixed under local anesthesia with or without conscious sedation on the morning of surgery.
- Because of severe movement disorder (e.g., dystonia, tremor) or anxiety, some patients may need the frame affixed or imaging obtained under general anesthesia for comfort or to obtain adequate imaging.
- The use of frameless systems developed after the era during which most pallidotomies and thalamotomies were performed, but these systems are adaptable for use with these procedures.

Imaging

- Volumetric imaging is obtained with the stereotactic frame and fiducial marker in place.
- T1-weighted magnetic resonance imaging (MRI) (with contrast agent to visualize venous anatomy) is sufficient.
- Stereotactic computed tomography (CT) scan also may be obtained and coregistered to MRI; in this case, MRI may be performed before frame application.
- In patients with contraindications to MRI (e.g., pacemaker), stereotactic CT alone may be used.

Target and Entry Planning

- Preplanning
  - The scan is loaded into a neuronavigation workstation; multiple scans, if obtained, are coregistered and checked for alignment.
  - Fiducial markers are indicated and checked for rectilinearity.
  - The locations of the anterior and posterior commissures (AC, PC) and midline points are marked, and the image sets are reformatted (automatically) orthogonal to the intercommissural line (ICL).
- Target planning
  - *Pallidotomy*: The target in the posteroventral GPi is selected using consensus coordinates for indirect targeting (e.g., 20 mm lateral, 2 mm anterior to mid-commissural point, 4 mm ventral to ICL). Alternatively, the target may be selected or refined by direct visualization of the GPi, facilitated by inversion recovery imaging.
  - *Thalamotomy*: The target in the Vim nucleus is selected using consensus coordinates for indirect targeting (e.g., 11.5 mm lateral to ventricle wall, 6 mm anterior to PC, at vertical level of AC-PC line.) No direct visualization of Vim is currently routinely possible.
- Entry planning
  - A precoronal entry point is selected that avoids venous, sulcal, or ventricular penetration, which may necessitate a double-oblique trajectory.

Stereotactic Frame Adjustment

- The stereotactic frame coordinates are adjusted to the target selected and checked.
- If available, a phantom is similarly adjusted, and the accuracy of the delivery of a test mandrel to the target is checked.

Patient Positioning

- The patient is positioned supine with slight neck flexion and counterflexion at the knees to prevent slipping down (and resultant airway compromise) during the procedure.
- Transparent drapes are used to increase visibility of and by the patient.
- The C-arm is aligned transversely at the patient's head.
- **Figure 41-1:** Target and entry planning. **A,** Volumetric T1 and inversion recovery images are imported into a neuronavigational functional neurosurgery platform (in this

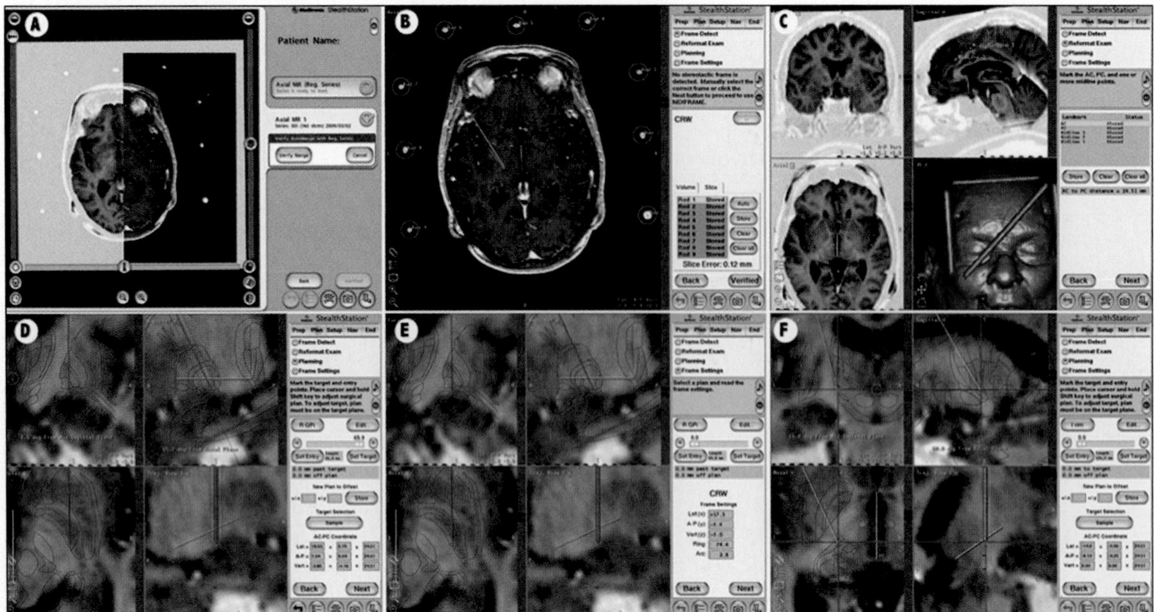

FIGURE 41-1

case, Stealth Station with Framelink software [Medtronic, Minneapolis, MN]) and merged (coregistered). **B,** The frame fiducial markers are indicated, and rectilinearity of the frame is checked. **C,** Internal landmarks are marked (AC, PC, and midline points) for reformatting of the examination along the plane of the ICL. **D-F,** Identification of the initial target in the GPi or Vim nucleus of thalamus can be done automatically using the software containing preloaded targeting formulas. **D,** GPi 20 mm lateral, 4 mm anterior to the mid-commissural point (MCP), 4 mm below the ICL. **F,** Vim 11.5 mm lateral to the third ventricle wall, 0.25 × ICL length anterior to the PC, at the level of the ICL. These targets can be modified as needed, which is facilitated by overlaying of the Schaltenbrand and Wahren stereotactic atlas. Entry point is selected at the appropriate angle of approach to the GPi or Vim (approximately 30 degrees from the vertical in the sagittal plane, lateral to the vertical in the coronal plane so as to miss penetrating the ventricle), modified to avoid prominent cerebral veins and sulci. The final stereotactic coordinates and angles are generated by the software **(E).**

- **Figure 41-2:** Adjustment of the stereotactic frame. The planned target coordinates are used to adjust the stereotactic frame (*X*, *Y*, and *Z*—lateral, anteroposterior, and vertical). Ideally, a phantom base is available, as with the Cosman-Robert-Wells (CRW) frame (Integra, Plainsboro, NJ), to check the accuracy of the physical setting of the frame coordinates and the stereotactic accuracy of the frame, which must be carefully maintained and calibrated.
- **Figure 41-3:** Patient positioning and room arrangement. The patient is positioned supine with neck flexion of 45 degrees or less, and the frame is affixed to the table through the Mayfield adapter. Knees are slightly flexed to provide comfort and countertraction to prevent the patient's torso from slipping toward the feet, which may lead to head extension and airway compromise. The C-arm is positioned before draping the patient so that it can be draped out of the sterile field.

PROCEDURE

- **Figure 41-4:** Stereotactic-guided skin incision and burr hole. After frame adjustment, skin preparation, and draping, the frame arc is mounted to the frame base and used to mark the skin incision site. A straight skin incision—in the coronal or sagittal plane—is made sufficient for a burr hole, or a twist drill craniostomy with smaller incision is possible to use. The burr hole (or twist drill) craniostomy is made after stereotactically marking the skull, and the dura and pia and arachnoid are opened (to avoid subdural hematoma from traction by the cannula). A curvilinear incision, as used in placement of a DBS system, is unnecessary with the absence of implanted hardware.

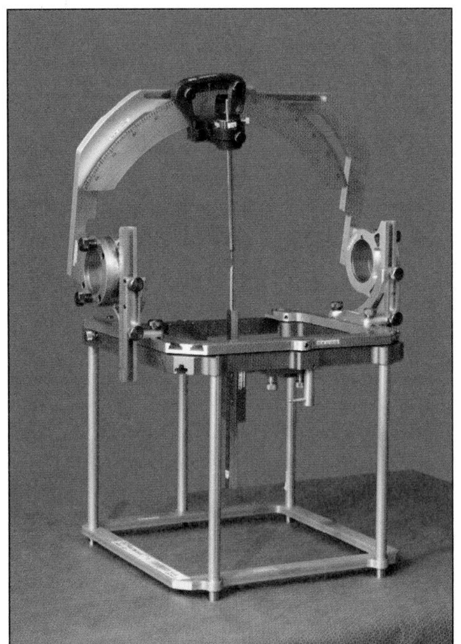

FIGURE 41-2

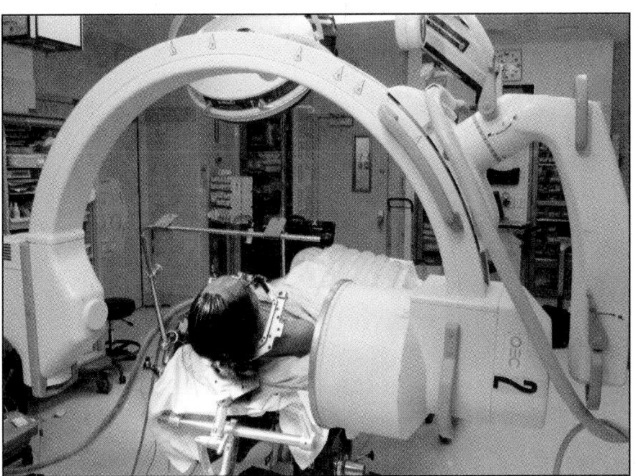

FIGURE 41-3

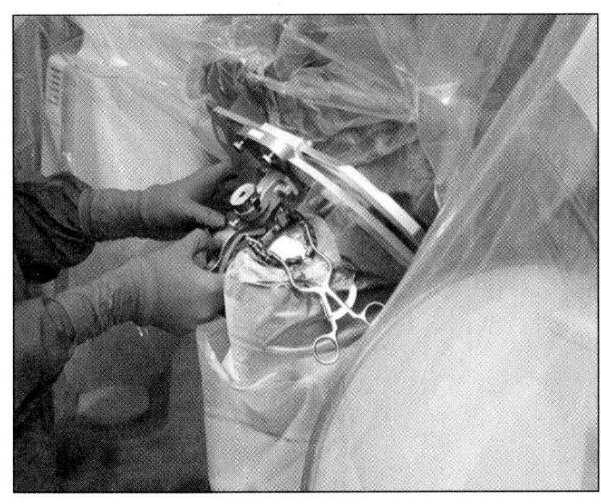

A

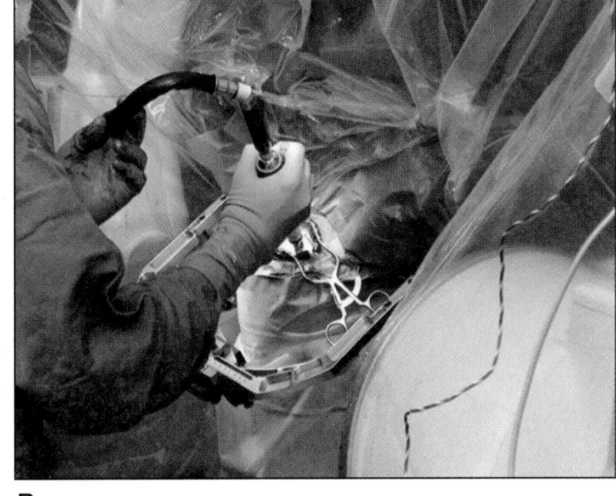

B

FIGURE 41-4

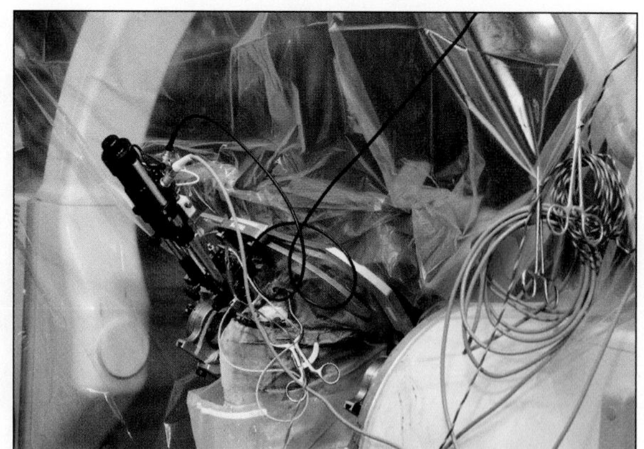

FIGURE 41-5

- **Figure 41-5:** The microelectrode platform and drive are mounted and microelectrode recording is initiated. The microdrive platform is mounted to the frame arc, and the microelectrode guide cannula and stylet are advanced slowly, followed by insertion of the microelectrode (details vary depending on the microdrive system. Pictured is the Guideline 3000 system [Fred Haer Corporation, Bowden, ME].)
- **Figure 41-6:** Stereotactic position of the microelectrode (or macroelectrode) is confirmed by C-arm fluoroscopy. After insertion of the microelectrode or macroelectrode (e.g., the stimulating or lesioning electrode) to the stereotactic target, the accuracy of the insertion is confirmed fluoroscopically after careful alignment of the C-arm. If there is an offset, this may be considered in interpretation of the data and in planning subsequent tracks, as needed.
- **Figure 41-7:** Neurophysiologic (e.g., microelectrode) mapping for pallidotomy. The first microelectrode track is run recording single units through the striatum, globus pallidus externus (GPe), GPi, and internal capsule (IC) or optic tract (OT), each characterized by stereotypic activity as shown. Light-evoked responses (via strobe or flashlight) can be recorded to confirm the location of the OT. The microelectrode can be used to perform electrical stimulation in the IC to elicit motor responses (typically in the mouth, face, or arm) or in the OT to elicit phosphenes. The microelectrode may be retracted, and macrostimulation can be performed from the end of the microelectrode guide cannula in some systems. Alternatively, the microelectrode may be removed and replaced by a stimulating electrode—typically the lesioning electrode itself—for macrostimulation results. Effects on clinical symptoms can be observed from macroelectrode stimulation as well. A second track is run in the same sagittal plane and sometimes additional ones to establish the location of the posterior border of the GPi with the IC; another one or two tracks are run laterally to establish the lateral border of the GPi with the GPe.

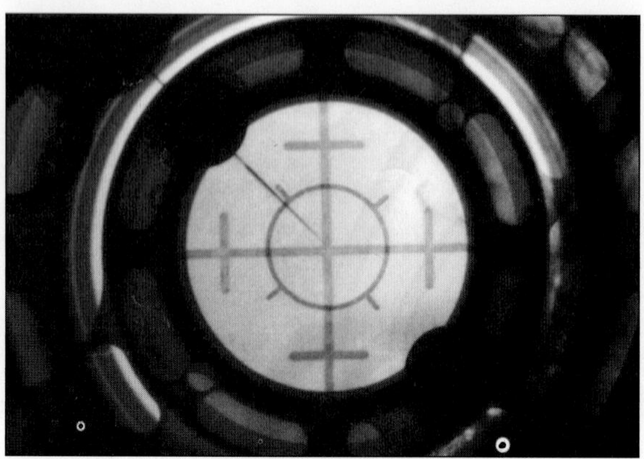

FIGURE 41-6

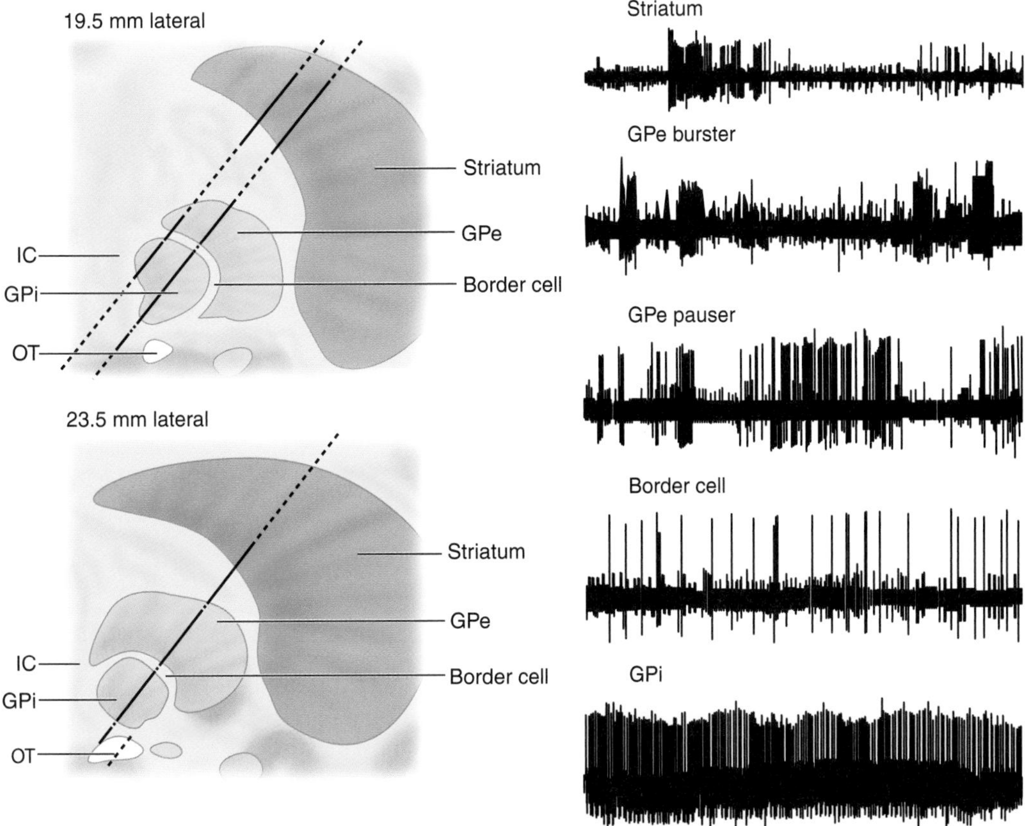

FIGURE 41-7

- **Figure 41-8:** Radiofrequency ablation of the GPi (pallidotomy). After mapping is completed, the lesioning electrode (approximately 1.1-mm-diameter, 3-mm-long exposed tip) is inserted into the chosen location and confirmed with fluoroscopy. It is positioned to lie approximately 2 to 3 mm anterior to the IC (lesion will have a radius of approximately 1.5 mm) (see Table 41-1). Test stimulation is performed, followed by temporary lesioning at 42° C, and if no adverse effects are observed, the permanent lesions are created with a radiofrequency generator at 60° C to 85° C, accompanied by neurologic testing of speech, motor strength, and visual fields. The electrode is retracted after cooling to less than 42° C.
- *Performing a complete pallidotomy* (Table 41-1): The lesioning electrode is repositioned in up to three tracks for complete controlled lesioning of the posteroventrolateral GPi with careful neurologic monitoring as noted. After the electrode has cooled, it is

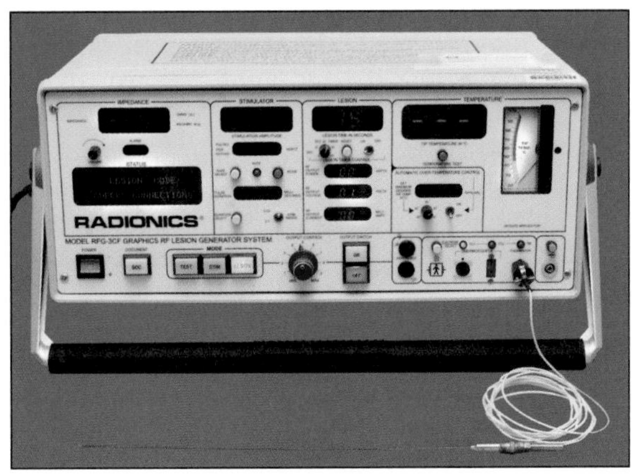

FIGURE 41-8

TABLE 41-1 Performing a Complete Pallidotomy

Track	Location	Step	Action*	Parameters	Duration	Comment
1	2.5 mm medial to lateral border with GPe 2.5-3 mm anterior to IC	1	Test stimulation: Advance from 2 mm above IC/OT by 0.5-mm steps until thresholds obtained	300 Hz; 100 μsec	1 sec trains	Thresholds: motor >0.5 mA; visual >1.0 mA
1		2	Test lesion at target above threshold	42° C	60 sec	Monitor for strength (facial-limb), visual, and speech changes. If deficits observed, retract electrode 2 mm
1		3	Temporary lesion	60° C	60 sec	
1		4	Lesion	75-80° C	60 sec	
1		5	Retract electrode 2 mm and repeat lesion	75-80° C	60 sec	
1		6	Retract electrode 2 mm if more GPI present based on mapping and repeat lesion	70-75° C	60 sec	
2	2 mm anterior to track 1	1-6	Repeat steps 1-6			
3	2-3 mm medial to track 1 and 2.5-3 mm anterior to IC	1-6	Repeat steps 1-6			
4	2-3 mm anterior to track 3	1-6	Repeat steps 1-6			

*Using 3-mm exposed tip; 1.1 mm diameter; lesion parameters are variable from group to group ranging from 70-90° C.
GPe = globus pallidus externus; IC = internal capsule; OT = optic tract.

removed, and the skin is closed in standard fashion in layers. The patient is observed in the postanesthesia care unit and then on a regular neurosurgical unit overnight. Parkinson medications are restarted in the postanesthesia care unit or on the regular ward as soon as the patient tolerates oral liquids.

- **Figure 41-9:** Postoperative imaging and reconstruction. Postoperative imaging is performed, typically by MRI (*left*); the timing is not critical so long as the patient is neurologically intact after the procedure. Depicted is a bilateral pallidotomy performed for generalized dystonia, with patient-specific deformation of the Schaltenbrand and Wahren atlas overlaid. A coronal reconstruction (*center*) shows the completeness of the lesioning of the posteroventral GPi, when the multiple overlapping–lesioning method is performed, as shown in two separate tracks in the 20.0-mm and 21.5-mm lateral planes (*right*). The microelectrode tracks performed in the 23.0-mm lateral plane verified the location of the lateral border of GPi.
- **Figure 41-10:** Neurophysiologic (e.g., microelectrode) mapping of the thalamus. Similar to the pallidum, with the thalamus, microelectrode recording tracks are run recording single-unit receptive fields in the thalamic nuclei, from rostral to caudal: ventralis oralis anterior (Voa), ventralis oralis posterior (Vop), Vim, and ventralis caudalis (Vc) (Hassler terminology). Microelectrode stimulation eliciting somatotopic organized projected fields (i.e., paresthesias) at low thresholds (1 to 5 μA) from Vc aids further in identifying the posterior border of Vim with Vc or, at higher thresholds, the medial lemniscus below the thalamus (in *black* in the figure). Macrostimulation through the microelectrode guide cannula tip or through the lesioning electrode definitively identifies correct location of the lesioning electrode. A second and possibly additional tracks are run as needed until the posterior border of Vim with Vc is mapped and until receptive and projected fields consistent with wrist or medial digits somatotopy are obtained.
- *Radiofrequency ablation of Vim thalamus* (Table 41-2): Under continuous neurologic monitoring, the thalamotomy is completed, 2 mm anterior to the Vim and Vc border (the lesion radius is approximately 1.5 mm) and at the ventralmost location within the thalamus. Usually, tremor is immediately relieved. A second lesion track may be performed more dorsally—in a more posterior track but rostrally within that track (as in Figure 41-11) for lesioning of the regions pertaining to more proximal tremor, for more complete tremor relief in some patients.
- **Figure 41-11:** Postoperative thalamotomy imaging. Overlap of thalamotomy with microelectrode recording tracks is shown. The hemorrhagic portion of the lesion measures approximately 7 mm high and approximately 3 mm wide, as expected. This portion corresponds to the destructive portion of the lesion on long-term follow-up imaging.

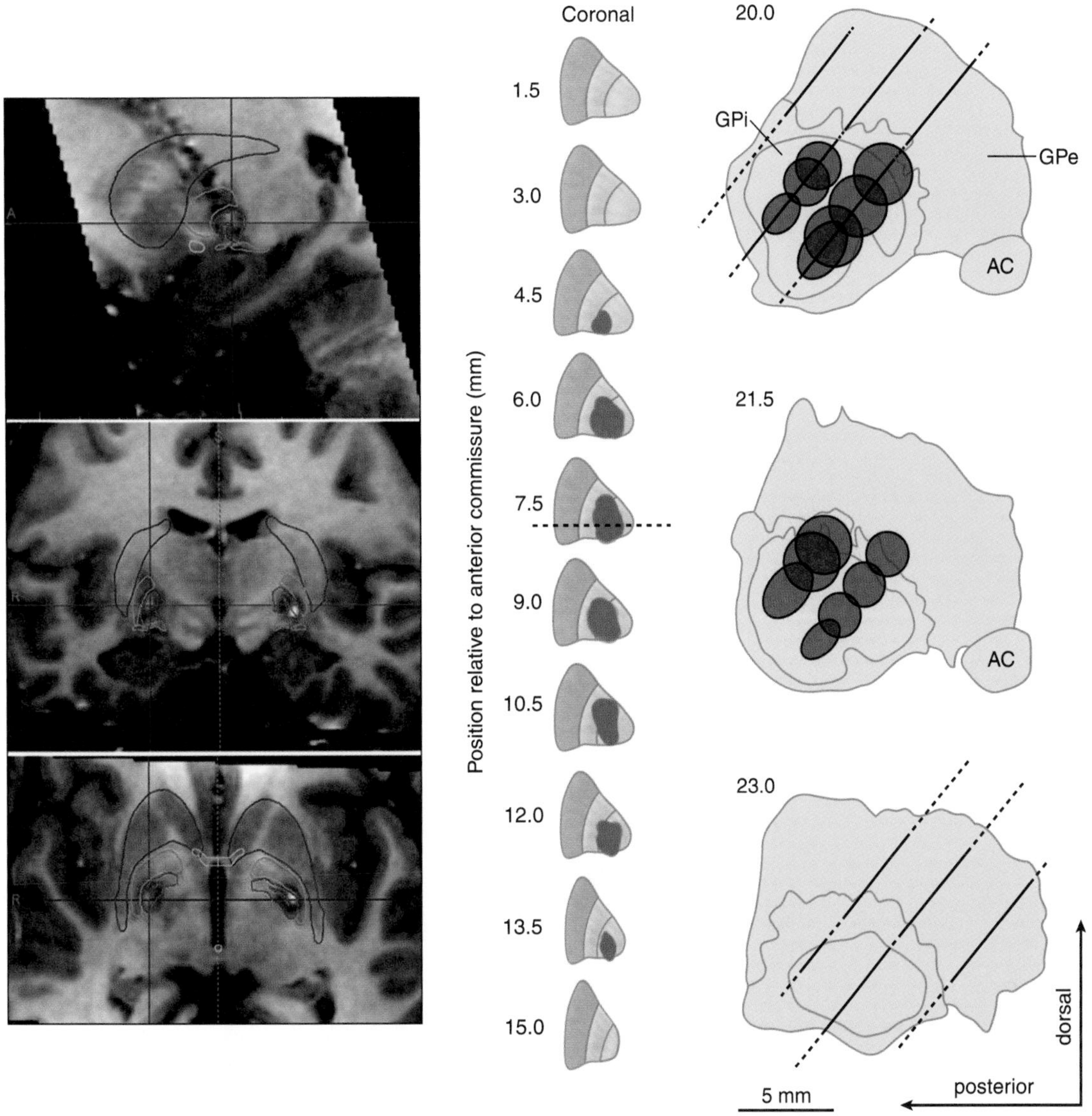

FIGURE 41-9

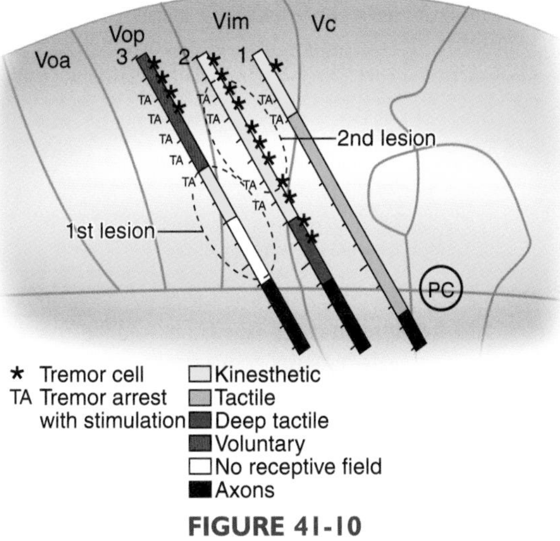

FIGURE 41-10

TABLE 41-2 Radiofrequency Ablation of Ventralis Intermedius Thalamus

Track	Location	Step	Action*	Parameters	Duration	Comment
1	2-3 mm anterior to Vim/Vc border in parasagittal plane of wrist receptive fields	1	Test stimulation: advance to ventral border of thalamus; if thresholds too low, reposition electrode 1 mm anterior	300 Hz; 100 μsec	1 sec trains	Thresholds: motor and sensory, >0.5 mA
		2	Test lesion ~3 mm rostral to ventral border	42° C	60 sec	Monitor for paresthesia, motor weakness, dysarthria, tremor arrest
		3	Temporary lesion	60° C	60 sec	
		4	Lesion	70-75° C	60 sec	
		5	Retract electrode 2 mm and repeat lesion	75-80° C	60 sec	
2	~2 mm posterior to track 1 but located dorsal to previous lesion	6	Repeat steps 1-4 (optional, depending on type and severity of tremor)			

*Using 3-mm exposed tip; 1.1 mm diameter; lesion parameters are variable from group to group ranging from 70-90° C.
Vim/Vc = ventralis intermedius/ventralis caudalis.

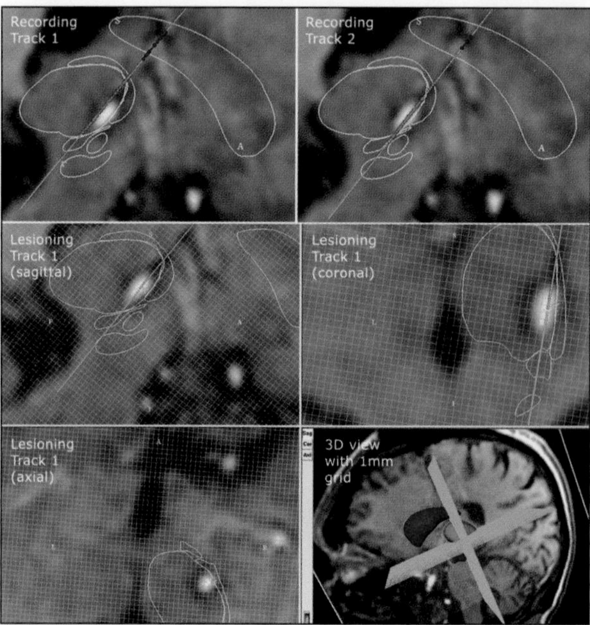

FIGURE 41-11

TIPS FROM THE MASTERS

- The initial key to pallidotomy is appropriate patient selection, in particular, avoiding patients with "Parkinson-plus" syndromes and with cognitive decline; the best response to pallidotomy is in drug-induced dyskinesia.
- Only rarely is thalamotomy an appropriate choice these days for parkinsonian tremor, given the benefits on all cardinal symptoms of either pallidotomy or GPi and subthalamic nucleus DBS.
- Occasionally, imaging must be performed with heavy sedation or general anesthesia to avoid movement artifacts that affect targeting accuracy, increasing the length and risks of the surgery.
- Frames and fiducial marker boxes should be sent frequently (e.g., twice yearly) for periodic maintenance to ensure accuracy (rectilinearity), especially frames that have adjustable calibration bars (e.g., CRW frame).
- Placing the patient in too much of a sitting position, with the idea of minimizing cerebrospinal fluid loss and "brain shift," should be avoided; this leads to increased pneumocephalus from inspiratory negative pressure, leading to further brain shift and occasionally seizures.

- Sedation can be used judiciously during creation of the burr hole craniostomy. Either propofol or dexmedetomidine (Precedex) can be used and then stopped after creating the burr hole and still allow for intraoperative mapping. Although mapping can be performed under general anesthesia (e.g., sevoflurane), lesioning must be performed with the patient awake to evaluate the neurologic examination.
- Blood pressure must be strictly controlled during surgery, especially before introducing the sharp microelectrode. We routinely insist that systolic blood pressure be 140 mm Hg or less throughout the case to limit the incidence of hemorrhage.
- After craniotomy, we wax the bone edges liberally to avoid venous air embolism, which may result from unappreciated venous lakes in the bone (or dura), especially when they are collapsed if the head is too high above the heart. In the event of hemodynamic changes during surgery, often heralded by coughing, the head should be lowered and the bone edges waxed further because this may be indicative of air embolism (confirmed with decreased end-tidal carbon dioxide readings).
- When venous bleeding is encountered while opening the dura or pia and arachnoid, the surgeon should avoid cauterizing for hemostasis, which can lead to venous infarction; rather, venous bleeding can almost always be stopped with Gelfoam and cottonoid patties, working around the site (rarely by extending the burr hole and dural opening) to implant the electrode.
- A completely dry surgical field is mandatory. Persistent bleeding, even in small amounts, can lead to acute subdural hematoma.
- We use fibrin glue in the burr hole to minimize cerebrospinal fluid drainage and the resultant brain shift.
- System accuracy should be checked with the microdrive in place using intraoperative fluoroscopy. The weight of the microdrive in some systems leads to anterior displacement of the tip of the cannula, for which the surgeon may need to compensate.
- Complete lesions of the posteroventral pallidum result in sustained long-term benefits. Failure to create a complete lesion, as in lesioning GPi in only one sagittal plane, can conversely lead to temporary benefits only and the need for repeat lesioning. The best way to avoid optic tract injury is not to lesion only the lateral GPi beyond the OT, but rather to map out the GPi completely as needed.
- In some cases, long-term tremor suppression is not obtained after thalamotomy, requiring repeat surgery for improved results.

PITFALLS

Hemodynamic or respiratory changes may be due to air embolism or airway compromise, the former resulting from inadequate waxing of the bone or coagulation of the dura in the setting of head elevation, and the latter resulting from the patient shifting down during the procedure. Both of these problems are increased by having the patient in too much of a sitting position.

In the event of neurologic compromise during the procedure (before the radiofrequency lesioning stage), beware that the differential diagnosis, in addition to "deep" hemorrhage, may include subdural hematoma. Subdural hematoma can occur from traction on the brain (i.e., by inadequately opening the pia and arachnoid), and, given the location of the burr hole on the top of the head, the blood can slowly run down toward the temporal lobe and not be appreciated until a precipitous decline in the neurologic examination.

If mapping is extended, brain shift—accentuated by brain atrophy in some patients—may lead to difficulties acquiring a consistent brain map, resulting in decreased certainty as to the location for the lesions. Final thresholds with electrical stimulation are critical to avoiding inadvertent capsular or optic tract injury.

Continued

PITFALLS—cont'd

During pallidotomy, mapping exclusively in the initially chosen sagittal plane cannot tell you how medial or lateral this plane is; whichever plane is chosen has a posterior border of the GPi with the IC. Moving medial brings you closer to the IC, which is anteromedially to posterolaterally inclined, and this too does not provide information about the laterality of that particular sagittal plane. Rather, defining the lateral border with the GPe by exploring *laterally* provides information about which sagittal planes need lesioning and allows more complete lesioning with improved long-term results on tremor, rigidity, akinesia, and dyskinesia. If lesions are solely placed in the initial sagittal plane explored, suboptimal long-term results may be obtained.

It is easy to avoid the ventricle during GPi surgery in most cases, whereas in the thalamus transventricular approaches can occasionally be difficult to avoid in patients with enlarged ventricles, as may often be encountered especially in elderly patients with essential tremor. Transventricular trajectories are prone to medial deflection of the lesioning electrode, which is blunt, at the ependymal border. This deflection can lead to a discrepancy between the map acquired with the *sharp* microelectrode, which may not be as prone to this deflection by the ependyma. It is recommended to avoid these transventricular routes; if this is impossible, always transgress the ependyma with the microelectrode, before inserting the lesioning electrode.

BAILOUT OPTIONS

- In the event of acute neurologic decline during surgery, check first for airway compromise, and rule out venous air embolism in cases with hemodynamic and ventilatory changes (e.g., decreased end-tidal carbon dioxide). If these reversible causes are ruled out, the surgery should be aborted, and a CT scan should be obtained immediately to evaluate for intraparenchymal hemorrhage.
- If a seizure occurs, midazolam is administered, and in some cases the surgery can resume when the postictal state resolves, *if the neurologic examination remains nonfocal*. If the postictal state does not resolve in several minutes, intraparenchymal hemorrhage must be suspected, and the case must be aborted.
- In the event of conflicting data from microelectrode mapping tracts, check to ensure that there has been no shift of the stereotactic frame; if there is suspicion for such shift, the surgery needs to be aborted.

SUGGESTED READINGS

de Bie RM, de Haan RJ, Nijssen PC, et al. Unilateral pallidotomy in Parkinson's disease: a randomised, single-blind, multicentre trial. Lancet 1999;354:1665–9.

Fine J, Duff J, Chen R, et al. Long-term follow-up of unilateral pallidotomy in advanced Parkinson's disease. N Engl J Med 2000;342:1708–14.

Gross RE, Lombardi WJ, Lang AE, et al. Relationship of lesion location to clinical outcome following microelectrode-guided pallidotomy for Parkinson's disease. Brain 1999;122:405–16.

Schuurman PR, Bosch DA, Bossuyt PM, et al. A comparison of continuous thalamic stimulation and thalamotomy for suppression of severe tremor. N Engl J Med 2000;342:461–8.

Vitek JL, Bakay RA, Freeman A, et al. Randomized trial of pallidotomy versus medical therapy for Parkinson's disease. Ann Neurol 2003;53:558–69.

Figure 41-7 redrawn from Gross RE, Krack P, Rodriguez-Oroz MC, et al. Electrophysiological mapping for the implantation of deep brain stimulators for Parkinson's disease and tremor. Mov Disord 2006;21(Suppl 14):S259–83.

Figure 41-9 center and right images redrawn from Vitek JL, Bakay RA, Hashimoto T, et al. Microelectrode-guided pallidotomy: technical approach and its application in medically intractable Parkinson's disease. J Neurosurg 1998;88:1027–43.

Figure 41-10 redrawn from original illustration provided courtesy of Dr. William Hutchison, University of Toronto.

Procedure 42 Deep Brain Stimulation

Ahmed Raslan, Kim Burchiel

INDICATIONS

- Medically refractory, dopamine-responsive Parkinson disease
- Medically refractory essential tremors
- Medically refractory dystonia
- Rare, off-label uses include treatment of chronic pain and of epilepsy

CONTRAINDICATIONS

- *Absolute contraindications*: Uncorrected bleeding tendencies and unstable cardiopulmonary status
- *Relative contraindications*: "Parkinson-plus" syndromes and dopamine-resistant Parkinson disease

PLANNING AND POSITIONING

- Under most circumstances, deep brain stimulation (DBS) is performed under local anesthesia. The exception is a rare situation in which an intractable movement disorder precludes stable positioning; general anesthesia might then be used.
- The most frequent targets are (1) subthalamic nucleus (STN), (2) globus pallidus internus (GPi), and (3) ventralis intermedius (Vim) nucleus of the thalamus. STN and GPi stimulation are used for Parkinson disease that involves all three cardinal manifestations (i.e., bradykinesia, rigidity, and tremors); GPi is preferred to STN when there is a question about the patient's mood status, given the potential depressive effect of STN stimulation. GPi stimulation is currently used for surgical treatment of dystonia. Vim stimulation is used for symptomatic treatment of tremors of Parkinson disease and essential tremors.
- Worldwide, some form of digital atlas is used for operative planning. Memorization of the coordinates of each target from the anterior commissure (AC), the posterior commissure (PC), and the mid-commissural point (the reference point) in stereotactic functional neurosurgery is unnecessary. The Schaltenbrand and Bailey atlas can be used to extract coordinates, if needed (Table 42-1). All coordinates constitute a range and can change with head size, age, degree of brain atrophy, and possible anatomic brain asymmetry.
- If a manual method of calculation is contemplated, accurate knowledge of the mathematical/trigonometric principle of the frame used is necessary for calculation (contact the manufacturer of the particular frame used).
- Surgery is undertaken in two stages: The first involves the placement of one or more DBS electrodes, and the second consists of the placement of a DBS generator and connection to the electrodes.
- Placement of one DBS electrode on one side is shown in the following figures; in the case of bilateral electrode placement, the same steps are repeated on the other side.
- **Figure 42-1:** Accurate positioning of the patient in the frame that is attached to the table using a special Mayfield adapter. The C-arm is placed around the patient at the beginning of the procedure.
- **Figure 42-2:** Magnetic resonance imaging (MRI) and data acquisition. T1-weighted (spoiled gradient echo) and T2-weighted (fast spin echo–inversion recovery) images

TABLE 42-1 Schaltenbrand and Bailey Atlas

Target Nucleus	Coordinates*	Corresponding Target
STN	Vertical = −4 Lateral = 12 AP = −3/−4	Center of motor territory of STN
GPi	Vertical = −5 Lateral = 18 from lateral ventricular wall AP = +2	Inferior border of motor territory of GPi, immediately superior to optic tract
Vim	Vertical = 0 or −1 Lateral = 50% of AC-PC distance but should be <12 mm of lateral ventricular wall AP = 25%-30% of AC-PC distance anterior to posterior commissure	Labial commissure of Vim

*Negative value in vertical axis = inferior; negative value in AP axis = posterior.
AC-PC = anterior commissure–posterior commissure; AP = anteroposterior; GPi = globus pallidus internus; STN = subthalamic nucleus; Vim = ventralis intermedius.

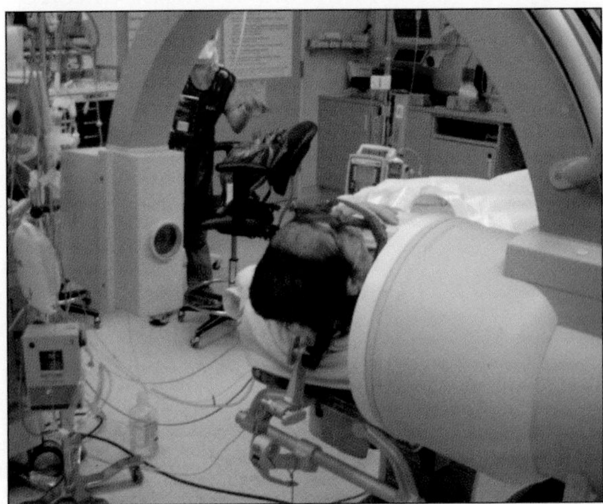

FIGURE 42-1

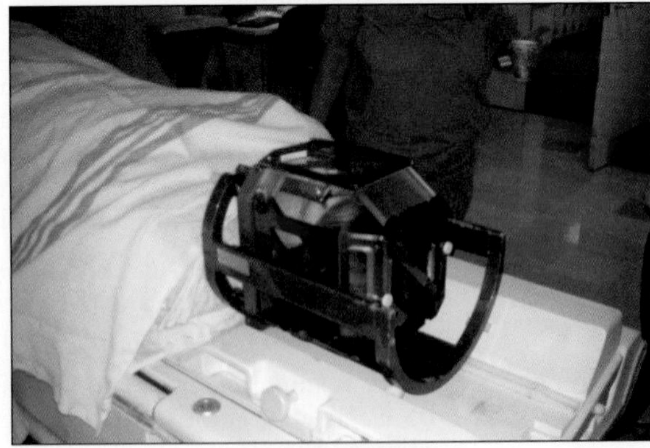

FIGURE 42-2

are the two most used sequences. T2 sequences are particularly important in GPi and STN targeting. The frame is fitted to the MRI table using a special adapter.

- **Figure 42-3:** Operative planning using a workstation. Identification of midline points: posterior edge of AC (**A**); anterior edge of PC (**B**); aqueduct of Sylvius (**C**); junction of septum pellucidum with splenium of corpus callosum (**D**); interpeduncular point (**E**); and final target, left Vim nucleus (**F**).

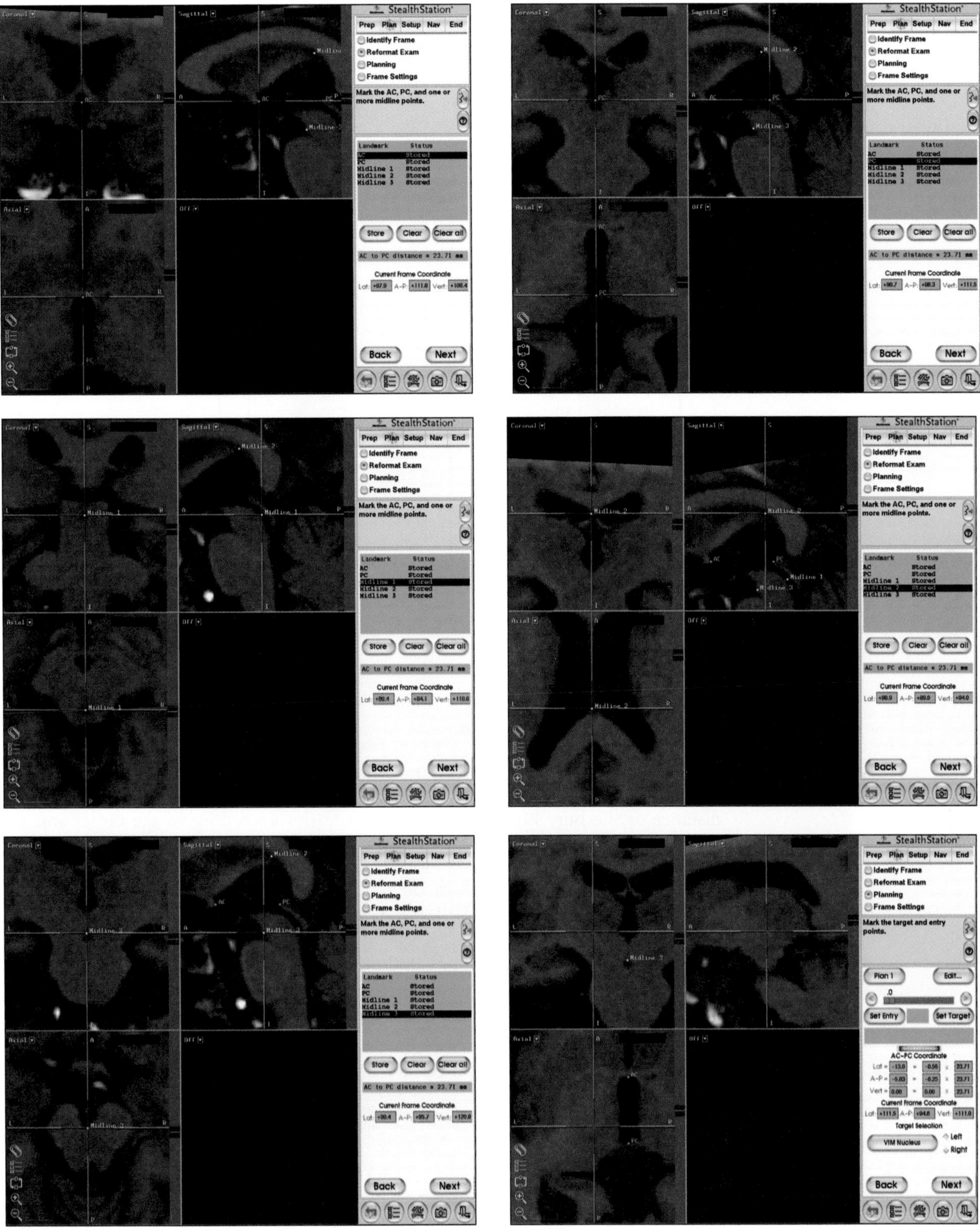

FIGURE 42-3

PROCEDURE

- **Figure 42-4:** Frame placement. **A,** Accurate frame placement under local anesthesia. **B,** Line drawing showing frame orientation on the patient's head. Accurate placement is parallel to the AC-PC line, with minimal roll and yaw; this can be aided by the use of ear bars.

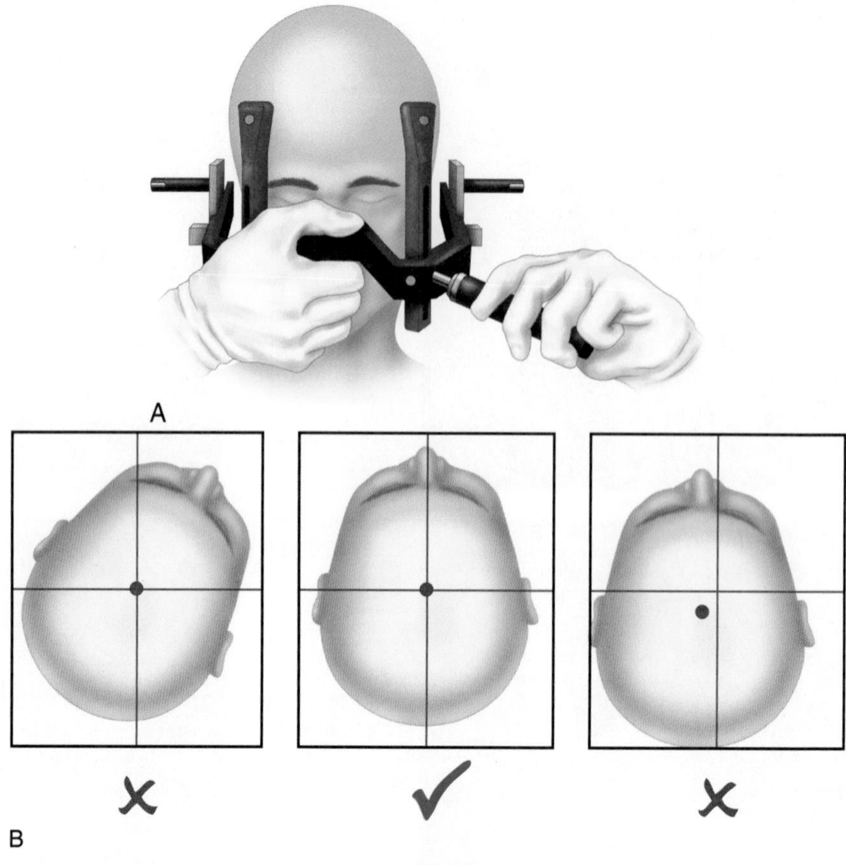

FIGURE 42-4

- **Figure 42-5:** Skin incision after attachment of the arc. Incisions should be placed to allow for bilateral burr hole placement 1 cm in front of the coronal suture. The distance of the burr hole from the midline varies according to the target and the size of the ventricle. The goal is to avoid entry into the ventricle and ensure more or less parallel electrode trajectories. Notice the transparent drapes used to allow interaction between the patient and the surgeon and other personnel.
- **Figure 42-6:** Burr hole placement. **A,** Burr holes should be placed just anterior to the coronal suture and on either side of midline. Improper frame placement, if extreme, can distort burr hole placement onto the midline, which, if not detected, can lead to inadvertent entry into the superior sagittal sinus. **B,** Intraoperative picture of the Stimloc (Medtronic, Minneapolis, MN) lead anchoring the burr hole system in place.

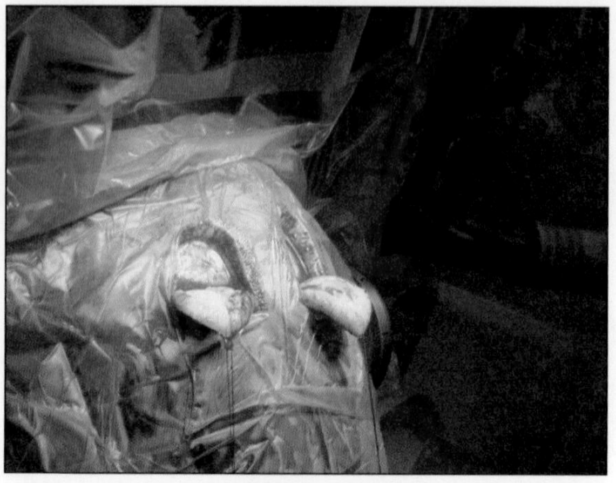

FIGURE 42-5

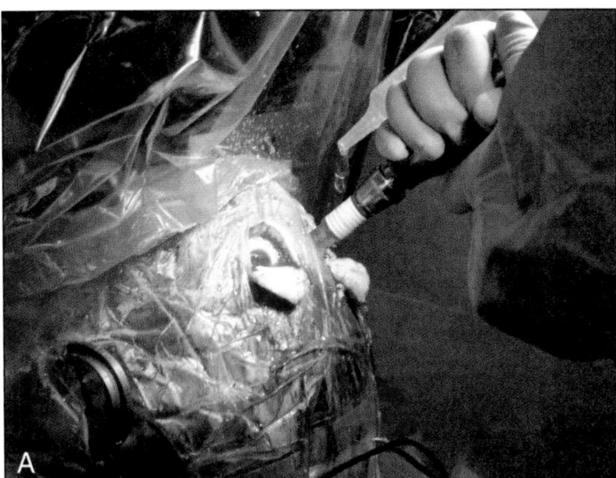

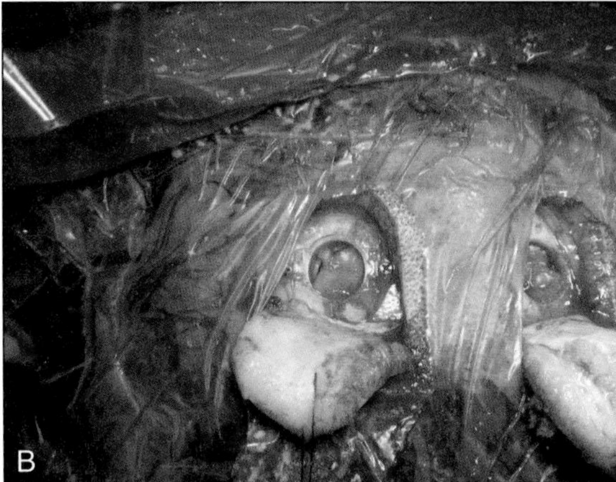

FIGURE 42-6

- **Figure 42-7:** Microelectrode recording unit assembly and attachment. **A,** Insertion of microelectrodes. A special cannula (guide tube) is inserted into the brain to harbor the microelectrode and DBS electrode. Institutions differ on the number of microelectrodes used. At our institution, we routinely record using two electrodes simultaneously; five electrodes can be used simultaneously. **B,** Pattern of microelectrode recording in GPi. Different patterns of neural activity occur during recording in GPi surgery.
- **Figure 42-8:** Electrode deployment, locking in position, and verification. **A,** The DBS electrode is placed and ready for macrostimulation. **B,** The DBS electrode is secured using Stimloc. **C,** X-ray verification of the electrode after being locked in place to verify nonmigration.

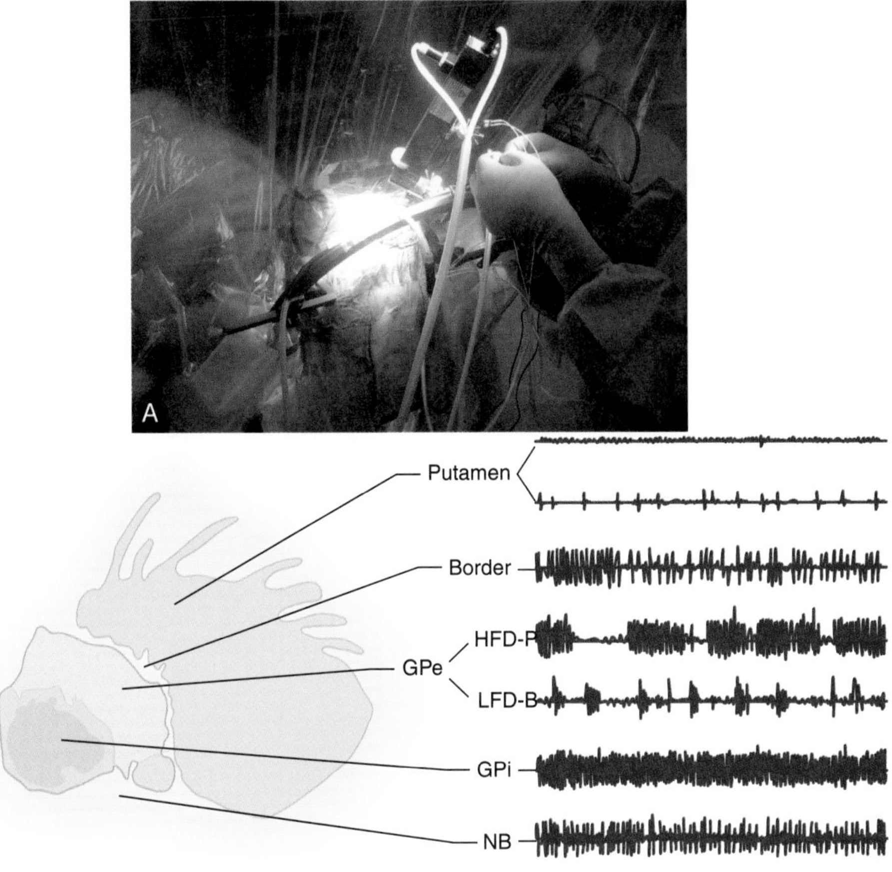

FIGURE 42-7

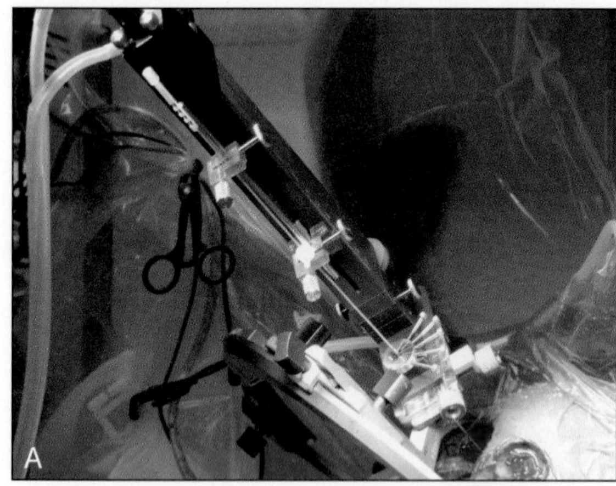

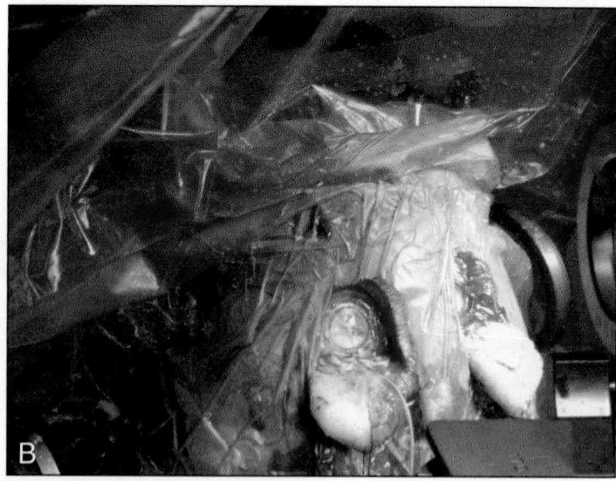

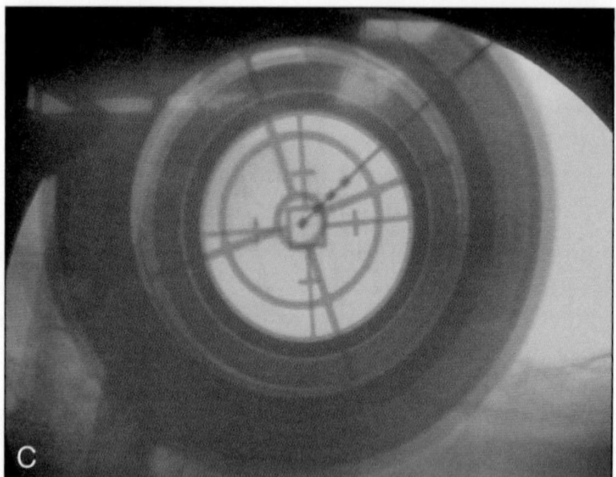

FIGURE 42-8

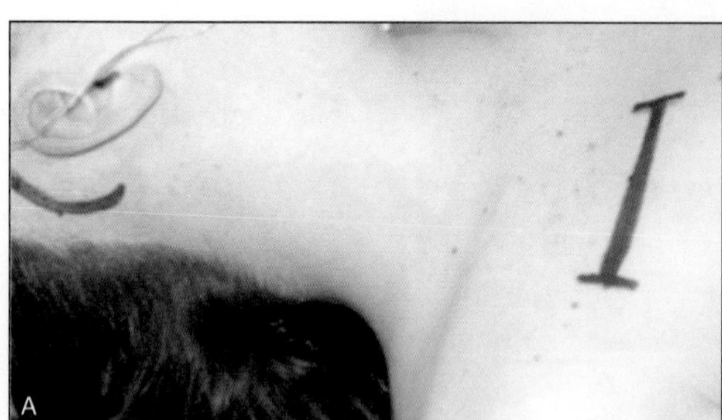

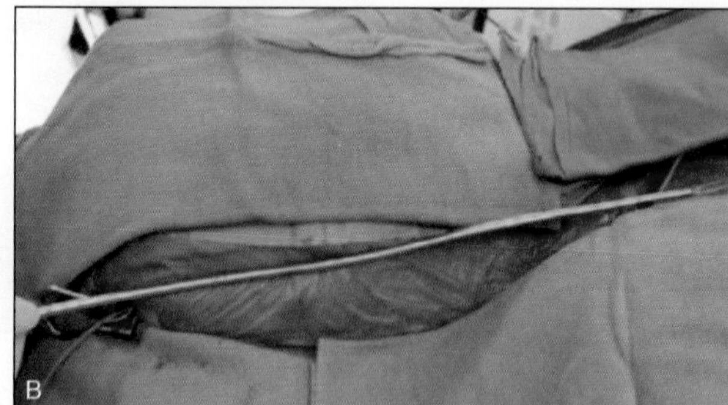

FIGURE 42-9

- **Figure 42-9:** Second stage of DBS surgery, which involves placement of the generator. We prefer the left infraclavicular area for right-handed patients. **A,** Approximate location of the incision. **B,** The area is prepared, and the tunneler is used for passing the extension cable that connects the electrodes to the battery.

TIPS FROM THE MASTERS

- Adequate frame placement is crucial and minimizes the risk of inaccurate burr hole placement.
- Double- and triple-check coordinates between the workstation and frame. Checks by multiple persons and at multiple times are paramount.

- If anything seems amiss, stop and retrace your steps. This retracing can substantially lessen the likelihood of methodologic flaws. Successful safe stereotactic surgery is based on optimal execution of numerous small steps.
- Avoid the loss of large amounts of cerebrospinal fluid during surgery to minimize brain shift.
- Frequent repeated fluoroscopic imaging can identify electrode migration before completion of the closure, allowing restoration before departure from the operating room.

PITFALLS

The most serious side effect of DBS surgery is intraparenchymal hemorrhage. This risk can be minimized by (1) cessation of antiplatelet medications at least 1 week before surgery; (2) control of blood pressure to less than 160 mm Hg systolic pressure before insertion of cannulas, microelectrodes, and DBS electrodes into the brain; and (3) limitation of the microelectrode passes to the minimum number necessary for proper placement.

Every effort should be made to minimize the risk of infection. Infection, if it occurs, requires removal of the entire system. Antibiotic treatment for 2 to 6 months is required before reimplantation.

Electrode migration during surgery can be a minor problem or a major problem if migration occurs after the frame is removed (i.e., at stage 2). Surgery needs to be reperformed if migration occurs at stage 2; confirmation of proper locking of the Stimloc is paramount, as is careful manipulation of the electrode.

BAILOUT OPTIONS

- Manual calculation can save the day if a digital atlas is dysfunctional.
- Having a digital copy of the MRI on a CD or optical drive can also save the day in case of lost digital imaging and communications in medicine (DICOM) connections.
- Do not hesitate to replace a burr hole if it appears too medial.
- If the cannula (i.e., electrode guide tube) passes through the ventricle on its approach to the target, keep the stylet inside the cannula as long as possible to avoid cerebrospinal fluid drainage that could distort brain morphology.

SUGGESTED READINGS

Deep-Brain Stimulation for Parkinson's Disease Study Group. Deep-brain stimulation of the subthalamic nucleus of the pars interna of the globus pallidus in Parkinson's disease. N Engl J Med 2001;345:956–63.

Deuschl G, Schade-Brittinger C, Krack P, et al. A randomized trial of deep brain stimulation for Parkinson disease. N Engl J Med 2006;355:896–908.

Kringelbach ML, Jenkinson N, Owen SLF, Aziz TZ. Translational principles of deep brain stimulation. Nat Rev Neurosci 2007;8:623–35.

Kupsch A, Benecke R, Muller J, et al. Pallidal deep brain stimulation in primary generalized or segmental dystonia. N Engl J Med 2006;355:1978–90.

Weaver F, Follett K, Stern M, et al. Bilateral deep brain stimulation vs best medical therapy for patients with advanced Parkinson disease: a randomized controlled trial. JAMA 2009;301:63–73.

Procedure 43 Motor Cortex Stimulator Placement

Louis Anthony Whitworth, Erika Anne Petersen

INDICATIONS

- Motor cortex stimulation (MCS) may be considered for patients with medically refractory deafferentation or neuropathic pain, including central pain syndromes related to stroke or, rarely, trauma or multiple sclerosis; trigeminal neuropathic pain (anesthesia dolorosa and postherpetic neuralgia); glossopharyngeal neuralgia; spinal cord injury; brachial plexus avulsion; and phantom limb or stump pain.
- Overall, efficacy is 40% to 70% for patients with refractory neuropathic pain, but identifying which patients would benefit from MCS is difficult because there is no definitive predictive factor. Likelihood of response to MCS may depend on the pain syndrome being treated or the anatomic location of the pain. Outcomes are better when patients present with no more than mild motor weakness in the region of pain. Patients with trigeminal neuropathic pain, phantom limb pain, and spinal cord injury have shown the most benefit, although at 1 year of follow-up, more than half of all patients, regardless of pain syndrome, responded to MCS.
- A proposed mechanism is that MCS activates descending axons, rather than apical dendrites or cell bodies, which is suggested by blood flow studies showing that the somatosensory cortex is not activated during stimulation. Cerebral blood flow studies show increased regional cerebral blood flow in the ipsilateral ventrolateral thalamus (the site where corticothalamic connections from the stimulated motor and premotor areas predominate) and in the medial thalamus, insula, subgenual cingulate, and brainstem as part of a cascading effect on a series of pain-related structures.
- Preliminary trials of limited duration MCS for poststroke recovery of motor function showed promise for improvement over rehabilitation alone. A phase III study sponsored by Northstar Neuroscience showed no advantage for the combination of concurrent invasive cortical stimulation and rehabilitation over rehabilitation alone. Initial investigations of MCS in patients with Parkinson disease showed promise for improvement in Unified Parkinson Disease Rating Scale–III scores at 6 months, but most initial benefits were lost by the end of 12 months, and tremor was poorly controlled by MCS.

CONTRAINDICATIONS

- Patients with severe motor weakness in the affected region, because it is believed that an intact corticospinal tract originating from the motor cortex is necessary for effective pain relief.
- Patients with neuropsychologic limitations to being able to participate fully in the evaluation and treatment process (including adequately communicating with health care workers about the effectiveness of alterations in their stimulation parameters) and patients with affective disorders, including severely depressive or neurotic tendencies.
- Patients with preexisting epilepsy or seizure disorders.
- The implantation of the MCS system is an elective surgical procedure that should be undertaken only when the patient's health status is stable; any active infection or uncontrolled comorbidities that would increase anesthesia risks (e.g., thrombocytopenia, leukopenia; renal, hepatic, and cardiac failure) should be addressed before considering surgery.

PLANNING AND POSITIONING

- McGill Pain Questionnaire and Visual Analogue Scale scores should be documented preoperatively to provide a baseline for tracking a patient's postoperative progress.
- Preoperative computed tomography (CT) and magnetic resonance imaging (MRI) of the brain facilitate identification of the central sulcus, sylvian fissure, and inferior and superior frontal sulci. Functional MRI studies may identify the motor cortex area. Frequently after a stroke there is a reorganization of motor areas that does not follow the usual somatotopic organization.
- Routine preoperative laboratory work should be performed, including prothrombin time, partial thromboplastin time, and platelet counts.
- **Figure 43-1:** The patient is positioned supine or in a lateral position with the side contralateral to the pain upward, with an axillary roll under the same shoulder to prevent venous congestion.
- **Figure 43-2:** Linear incision is planned to overlie the central sulcus using standard anatomic landmarks on the side contralateral to the patient's pain. A neuronavigation system is used for planning the incision and to map out the craniotomy to overlie the

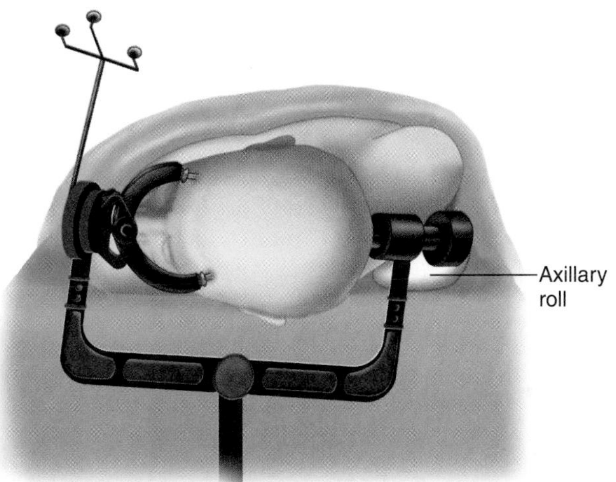

FIGURE 43-1

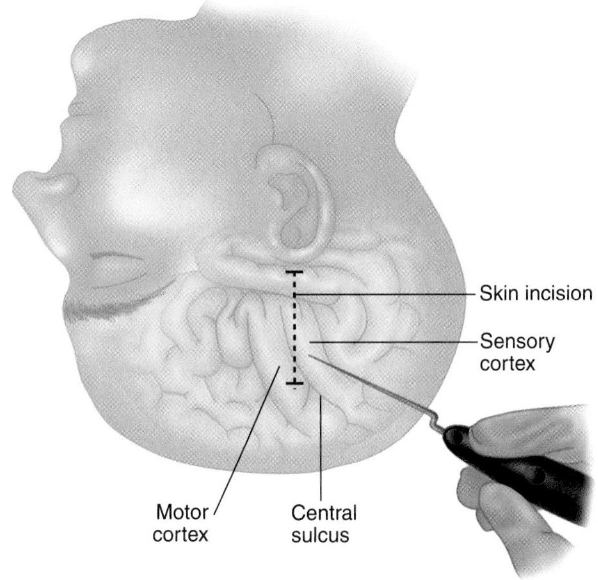

FIGURE 43-2

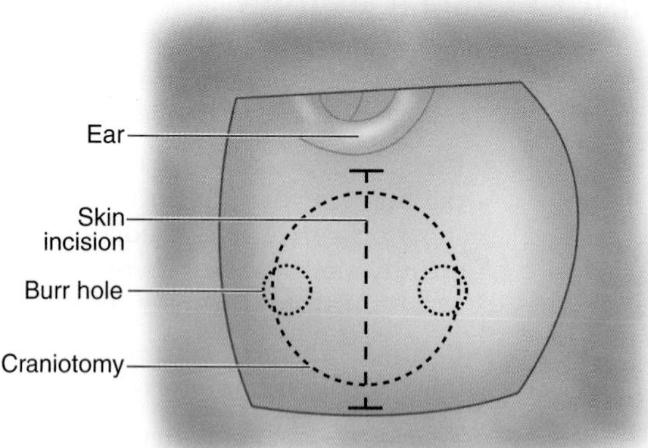

FIGURE 43-3

motor cortex. The incision should be long enough to allow for a circular craniotomy opening with an approximate diameter of at least 5 cm.

- **Figure 43-3:** Draping allows enough scalp exposure so that the electrode extensions can be externalized behind the ear. The draping may be modified to allow for observation of facial movement during intraoperative cortical stimulation if facial pain is to be treated.

PROCEDURE

- **Figure 43-4:** Burr hole placement of the electrode. Several disadvantages are associated with the limited exposure provided by this approach, including the possibility of inaccurate electrode placement. It is difficult to perform thorough electrophysiologic localization (i.e., somatosensory evoked potentials, motor stimulation) to confirm accurate electrode placement. Finally, the risk of developing an epidural hematoma may be increased with this approach, owing to the stripping of the dura from the skull without direct visualization before insertion of the electrode.
- **Figure 43-5:** A small (4 to 5 cm) craniotomy is favored over a burr hole because the larger exposure facilitates intraoperative somatosensory evoked potential recording and high-intensity, low-frequency stimulation to map the motor cortex in detail.
- **Figure 43-6:** Central sulcus is localized by the phase reversal of the N20/P20 wave (*at arrow*). Additional mapping of the motor cortex can be performed with cortical stimulation inducing contralateral motor responses.
- **Figure 43-7:** One or two quadripolar electrodes are placed either parallel or perpendicular to the central sulcus. There is no definite consensus on optimal electrode orientation.

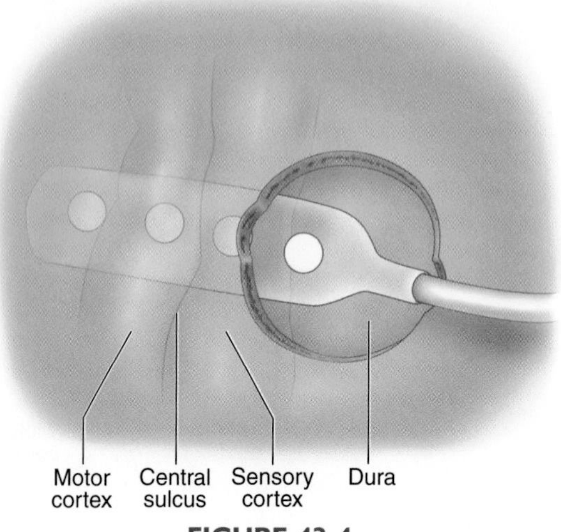

FIGURE 43-4

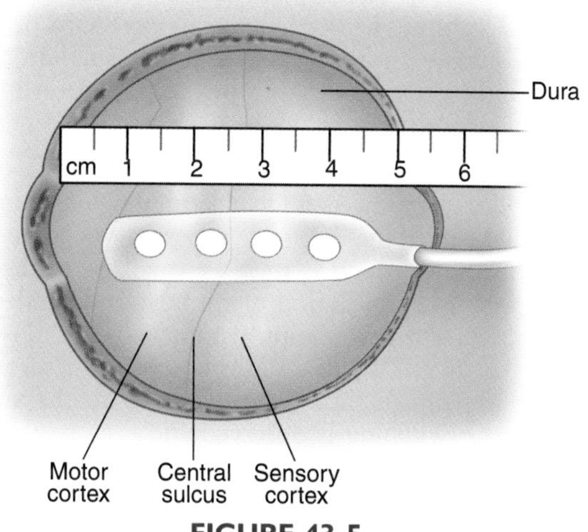

FIGURE 43-5

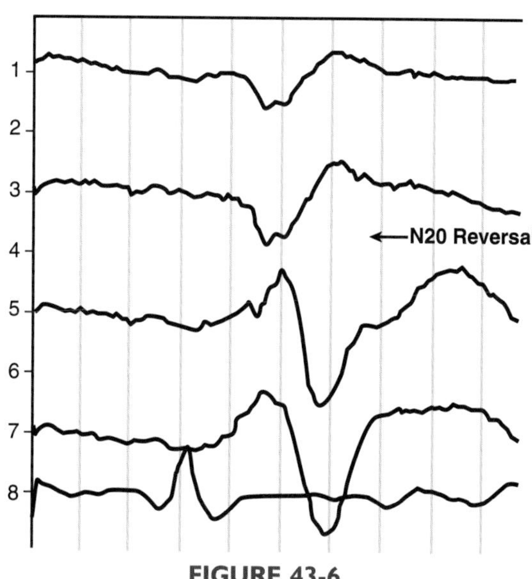

FIGURE 43-6

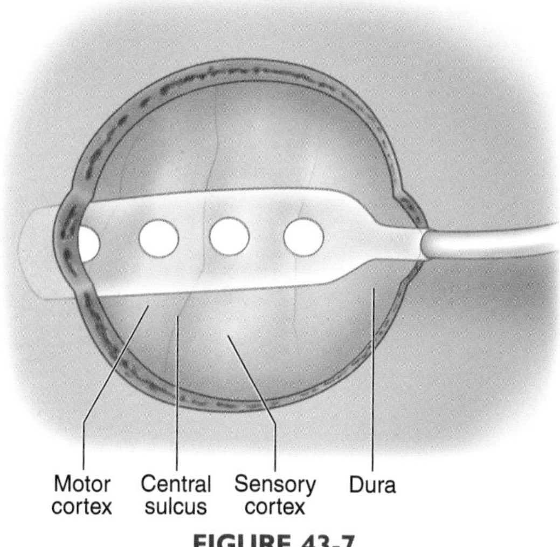

FIGURE 43-7

Some surgeons prefer a longitudinal orientation along the gyrus to maximize coverage of the gyrus, although more surgeons prefer to orient the electrode perpendicular to the central sulcus. In this case, a much smaller area of the postcentral gyrus can be stimulated, and the somatotopic organization must be well mapped to ensure proper electrode placement.

- **Figure 43-8:** The electrode is secured to the dura with 4-0 Nurolon (Ethicon, Inc., Somerville, NJ) sutures. Each electrode is sutured to the outer, periosteal layer of the dura. The distal end of the electrode is passed out of one of the burr holes and connected to the extension cable, which is then externalized in the retroauricular area through a separate stab incision. A trial period of stimulation is undertaken during an inpatient admission to test efficacy. For stimulation parameters, the most commonly used settings are 2 to 3 V (range 0.5 to 9.5 V), 25 to 50 Hz (range 15 to 130 Hz), and 200 μsec (range 60 to 450 μsec). The voltage should be increased to the submotor threshold; we increase voltage until motor twitching is observed and then reduce the voltage slightly until motor effects abate. Bipolar stimulation is used with the negative pole overlying the motor cortex and positive pole over the sensory cortex. Pain relief may last for hours after electrical stimulation is discontinued. For this reason, a pattern of a short interval of stimulation alternating with longer "off" periods can be programmed.
- **Figure 43-9:** Assuming a successful trial, the patient returns to the operating room for connection of new, permanent extension cables. These extensions are tunneled subcutaneously to a subcutaneous, infraclavicular pocket where the intermittent pulse generator (IPG) is implanted. The IPG should be no deeper than 2 cm below the skin to permit communication between the control unit and the battery. There are three incision points on the head and torso: (1) the site of the craniotomy, (2) a

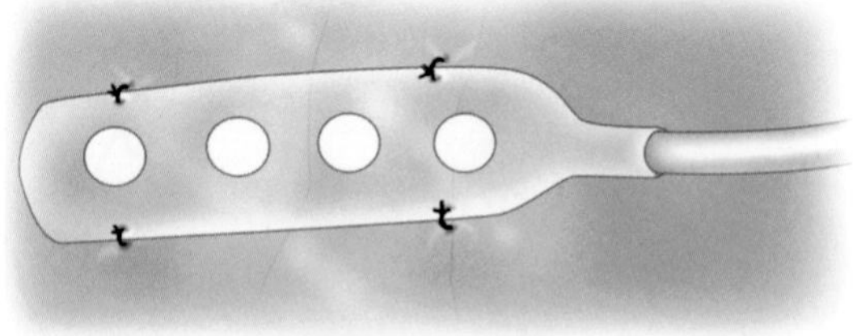

FIGURE 43-8

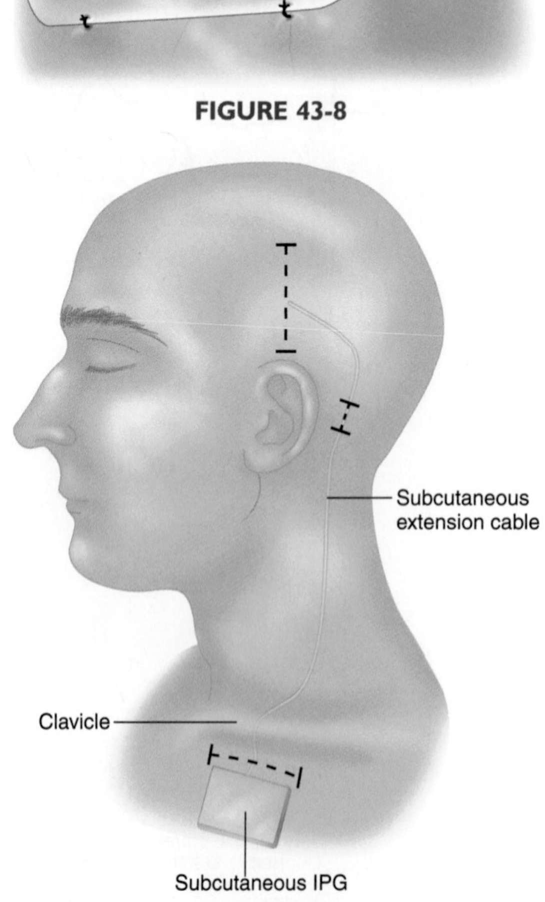

FIGURE 43-9

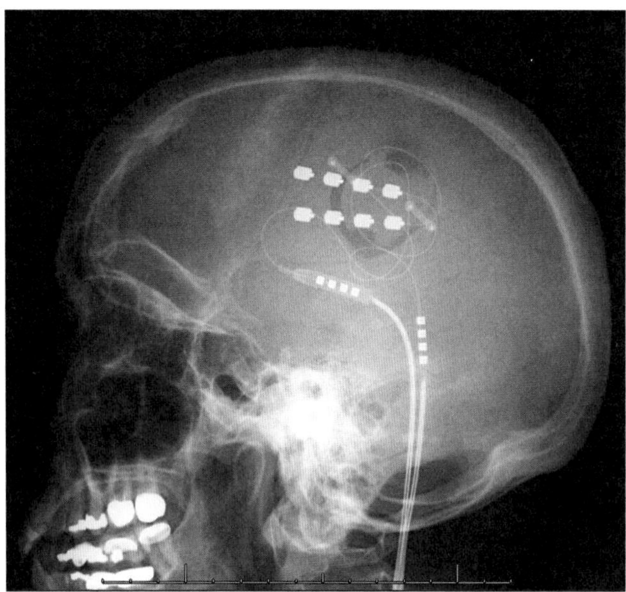

FIGURE 43-10

retroauricular site used as a "release" point for tunneling, and (3) the infraclavicular site of the IPG.

- **Figure 43-10:** Postoperative skull x-ray illustrates the position of two quadripolar electrodes, the extension connector points, and the cables continuing down toward the IPG.

TIPS FROM THE MASTERS

- Correct localization of the motor cortex is crucial. It is essential to position the electrode along the appropriate portion of the gyrus. This positioning can be accomplished by combining preoperative imaging studies including functional MRI with intraoperative phase reversals and cortical mapping. Use of a neuronavigation system can facilitate perioperative localization of the cortical gyri.
- To cover multiple areas of pain (e.g., a patient with central pain affecting the face and the hand), two separate electrodes may be placed over a wide cortical area. Current implantable generators can accommodate 16 electrode contacts.

PITFALLS

Epidural placement of electrodes may be less invasive than subdural placement, but relatively high voltage may be required for pain relief when the stimulated cerebral hemisphere is atrophic.

Hardware-related failure is a concern. There is a 5% risk of lead fractures, migration, and insulation fractures. Shifted epidural electrode position or development of granulation tissue may decrease the ability to deliver charge from the electrode to the cortex.

Subdural electrodes within the interhemispheric fissure (to address lower extremity pain) may migrate or lose their coverage.

The risk of subdural or epidural hematoma is 1% to 2%. Other reported complications include stimulation-induced seizures, dysphasia, upper extremity fatigue, burning sensations or pain in the area of stimulation, and gradual decline in degree of pain relief.

The risk of wound infection is 4% to 7%.

Patients with multiple pain sites may not gain relief at all sites, and improving coverage at one site may worsen it at another.

BAILOUT OPTIONS

- If the MCS trial is unsuccessful (decrease in Visual Analogue Scale score <50%), the patient returns to the operating room for removal of leads.

SUGGESTED READINGS

Brown JA, Pilitsis JG. Motor cortex stimulation for central and neuropathic facial pain: a prospective study of 10 patients and observations of enhanced sensory and motor function during stimulation. Neurosurgery 2005;56:290–7.

Fontaine D, Hamani C, Lozano A. Efficacy and safety of motor cortex stimulation for chronic neuropathic pain: critical review of the literature. J Neurosurg 2009;110:251–6.

Garcia-Larrea L, Peyron R. Motor cortex stimulation for neuropathic pain: from phenomenology to mechanisms. Neuroimage 2007;37(Suppl 1):S71–9.

Lefaucheur JP, Drouot X, Cunin P, et al. Motor cortex stimulation for the treatment of refractory peripheral neuropathic pain. Brain 2009;132(Pt 6):1463–71.

Plow EB, Carey JR, Nudo RJ, et al. Invasive cortical stimulation to promote recovery of function after stroke: a critical appraisal. Stroke 2009;40:1926–31.

Tsubokawa T, Katayama Y, Yamamoto T, et al. Chronic motor cortex stimulation in patients with thalamic pain. J Neurosurg 1993;78:393–401.

Velasco F, Arguelles C, Carrillo-Ruiz JD, et al. Efficacy of motor cortex stimulation in the treatment of neuropathic pain: a randomised double-blind trial. J Neurosurg 2008;108:698–706.

Procedure 44

Occipital and Supraorbital Nerve Stimulator Placement

Konstantin V. Slavin, Sebastian R. Herrera, Prasad Vannemreddy, Zilvinas Zakarevicius

INDICATIONS

- Peripheral nerve stimulation (PNS) is indicated for patients with chronic, medically refractory, severe neuropathic pain that involves distribution of the nerve to be stimulated.
- Occipital nerve stimulation (ONS) is indicated primarily for treatment of occipital neuralgia, including posttraumatic and postsurgical pain in the occipital nerve distribution.
- Supraorbital nerve stimulation (SNS) is indicated for patients with trigeminal neuropathic pain, mainly secondary to posttraumatic or postsurgical supraorbital neuralgia or neuropathy (e.g., after operations on frontal sinuses, after frontal craniotomies).
- ONS and SNS have been used for treatment of migraines and cluster headaches in research studies.

CONTRAINDICATIONS

- PNS is contraindicated in patients with complete sensory loss (e.g., in cases of anesthesia dolorosa).
- Patients with unfavorable psychological evaluation results.
- Patients with anticoagulation or who are receiving antiplatelet therapy.
- Patients with active infection.
- Failed trial of stimulation.

PLANNING AND POSITIONING

- Patients are positioned supine, with attention given to the electrode insertion point, the entire area where the electrode will be located, an anchoring incision, and the generator pocket (for internalization procedures). The entire area is shaved and prepared, and the planned location of electrodes is drawn on the skin with fluoroscopic assistance (i.e., with the C-arm positioned around the patient's head).
- For ONS implants, a gel roll is placed under the patient's ipsilateral shoulder, and the patient's head is turned into the lateral position. The insertion point for the ipsilateral electrode is placed behind the mastoid process, with the goal of reaching the midline with the needle along the radiographic level of the arch of C1. The contralateral electrode is inserted through a small incision at the midline aiming at the contralateral mastoid process; this electrode is tunneled backward so that both electrodes, in case of bilateral insertion, exit behind same ear.
- For supraorbital electrode insertion, the patient may be positioned supine, but the shoulder roll and head turning are needed for the second stage of surgery so that the electrodes may be anchored in the retromastoid region and then tunneled toward the generator pocket.
- A generator pocket for craniofacial PNS is planned in the infraclavicular region with an incision drawn 1 to 2 cm below the clavicle.
- **Figure 44-1:** Line of incision for anchoring the bilateral ONS electrodes with electrode direction drawn. Note the "X" mark through which temporary electrodes exit the skin during the trial period; it is placed a few centimeters away from the incisions for permanent implantation.

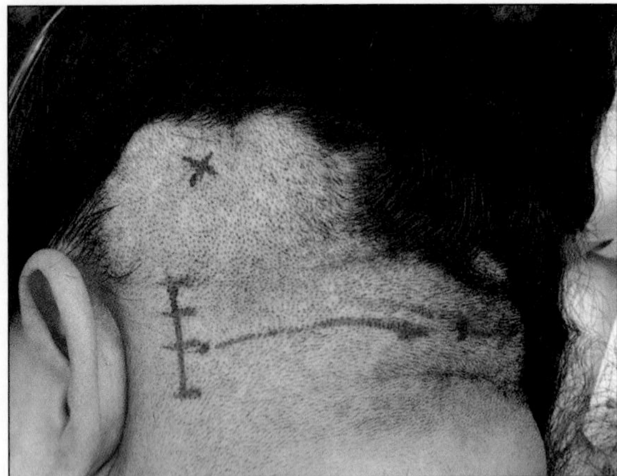

FIGURE 44-1

- **Figure 44-2: A,** Direction for insertion of the right supraorbital nerve stimulation electrode and the right auriculotemporal nerve stimulation electrode. Direction for insertion is from lateral to medial. **B,** Location of anchoring incision behind the ipsilateral ear. "X" marks indicate exit sites for temporary (trial) electrodes.
- **Figure 44-3:** Patient positioning within the aperture of the C-arm used for intraoperative fluoroscopy.

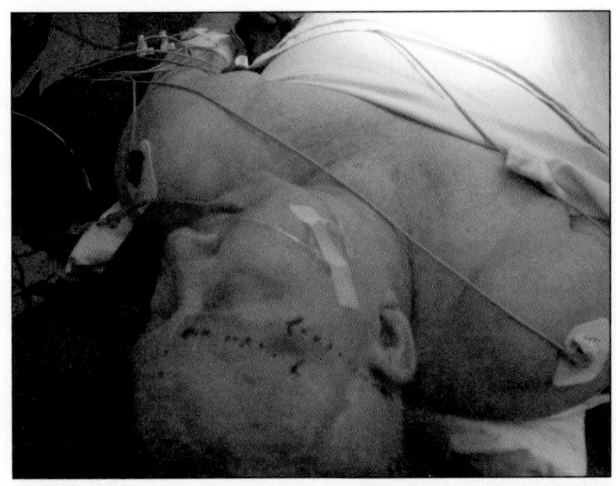

A

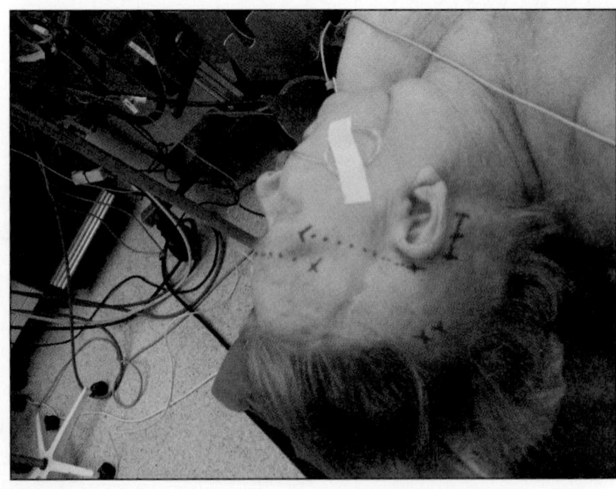

B

FIGURE 44-2

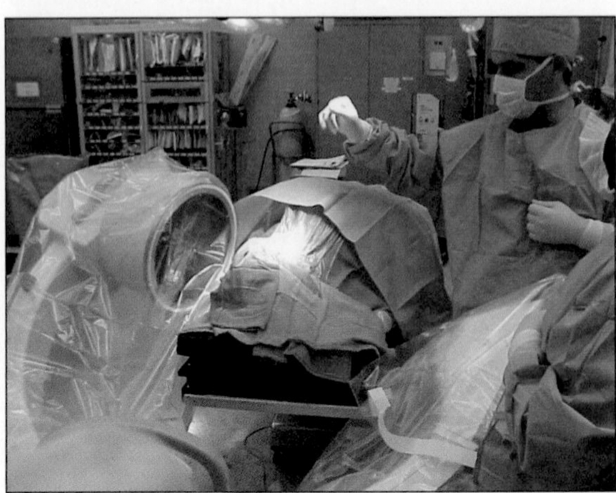

FIGURE 44-3

PROCEDURE

- **Figure 44-4:** The needle from the standard electrode kit is bent to conform with the curvature of the occipital or supraorbital region.
- **Figure 44-5:** The direction is chosen in such a way that the electrode contacts are positioned perpendicular to the course of the nerves selected for stimulation.
- **Figure 44-6:** The needle is inserted into the epifascial plane in the desired direction. This is the plane that offers the least resistance. Encountered resistance indicates that

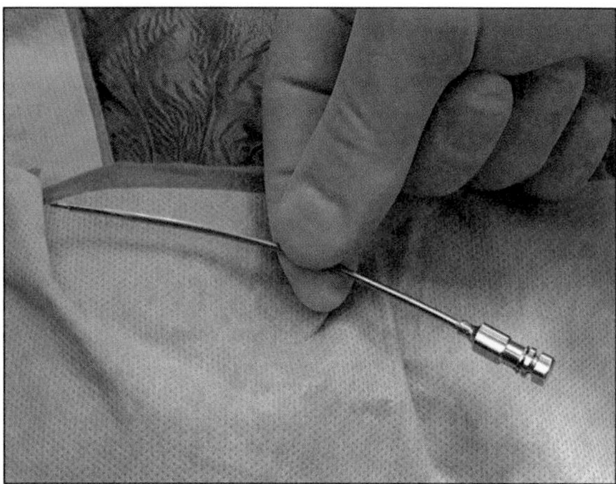

FIGURE 44-4

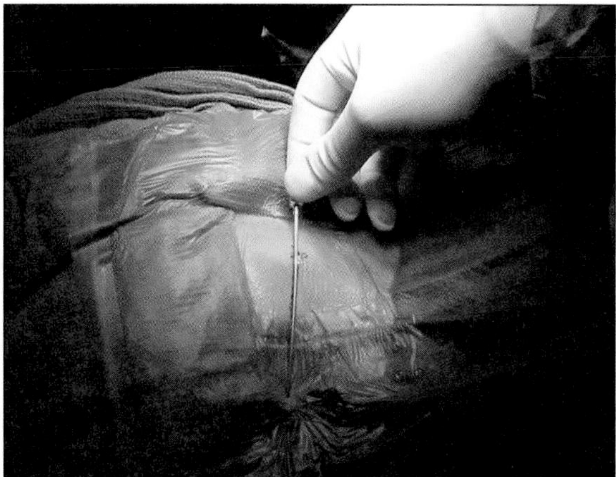

FIGURE 44-5

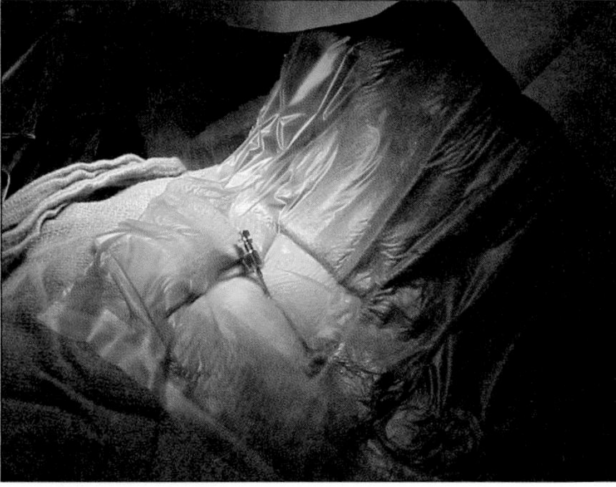

FIGURE 44-6

the needle is either traveling through the skin (too superficial) or penetrating the underlying fascia (too deep).

- **Figure 44-7:** A standard electrode (four-contact or eight-contact) is inserted through the needle after the stylet is removed.
- **Figure 44-8:** When the electrode reaches the desired location, the needle is removed.
- **Figure 44-9:** A temporary electrode may be sutured in place directly at the exit site.

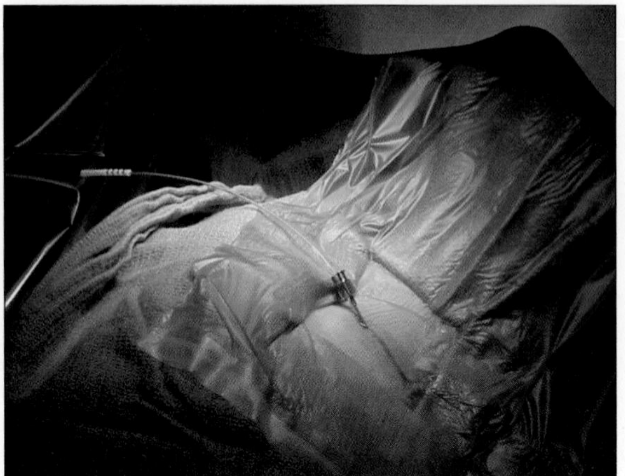

FIGURE 44-7

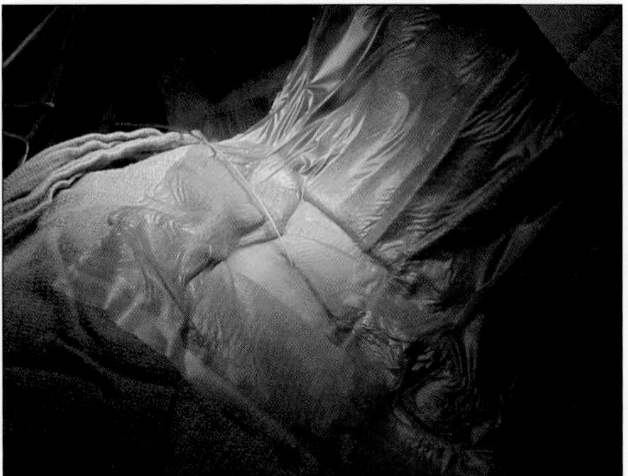

FIGURE 44-8

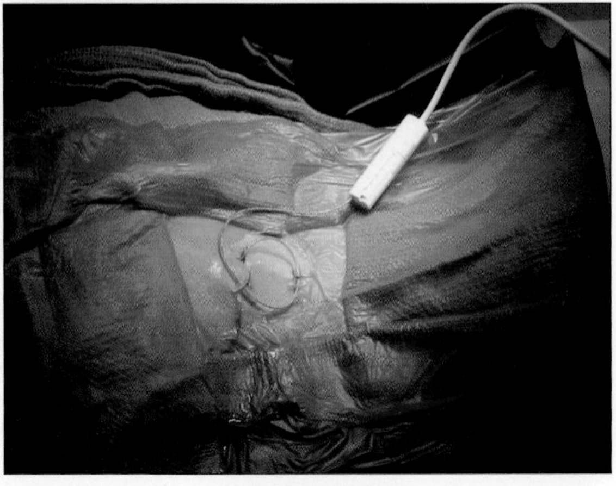

FIGURE 44-9

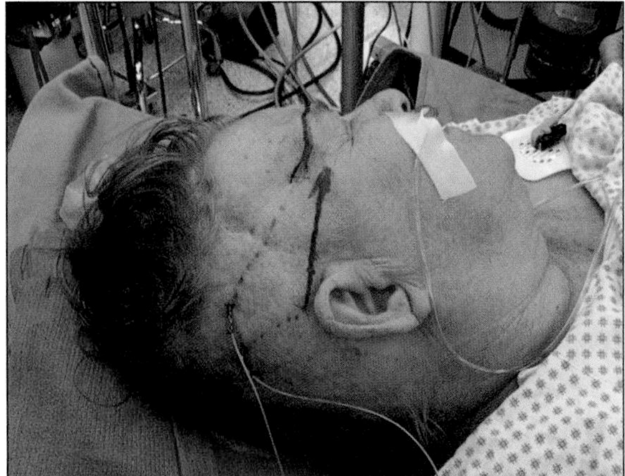

FIGURE 44-10

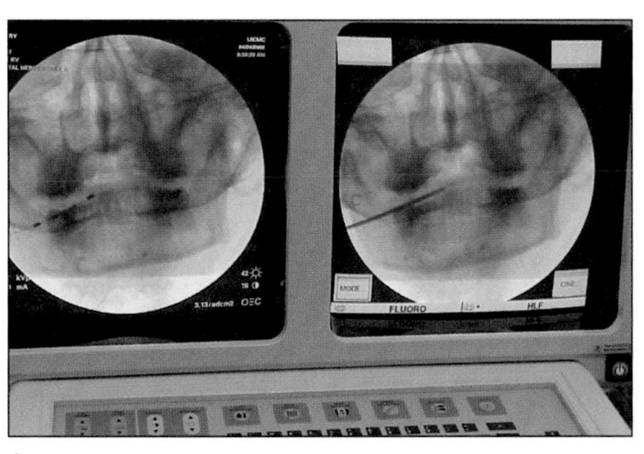

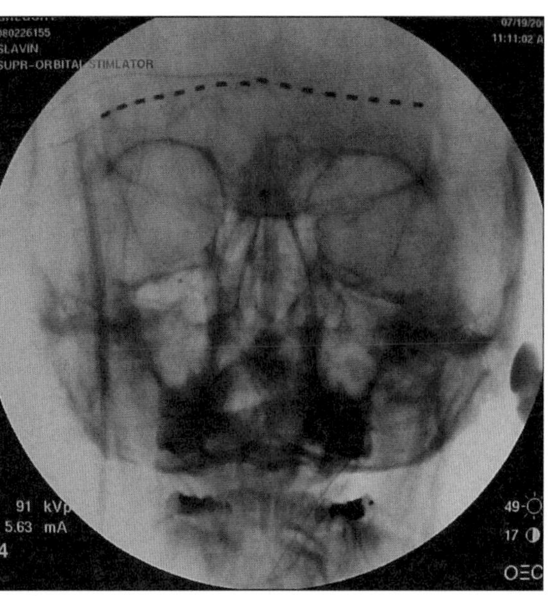

A B

FIGURE 44-11

- **Figure 44-10:** Alternatively, the electrode may be tunneled under the skin a few centimeters away from the insertion site so that the exit site does not interfere with any subsequent internalization path.
- **Figure 44-11:** **A,** Intraoperative fluoroscopic images of the needle and electrode during ONS implantation procedure. **B,** Fluoroscopic image of bilateral supraorbital electrode positioning.
- **Figure 44-12:** The generator is usually placed in the infraclavicular region with the incision made 1 to 2 cm below the clavicle.

TIPS FROM THE MASTERS

- The stimulatory electrodes should be anchored to the stiffest and least mobile tissue available. We suggest anchoring occipital and supraorbital electrodes to the retromastoid fascia. This is an immobile region with stiff tissue that is able to withstand the stress associated with head and neck movements. Loose anchoring may result in electrode migration, and attaching the anchor to a mobile part of the body may lead to metal fatigue and subsequent electrode fracture.

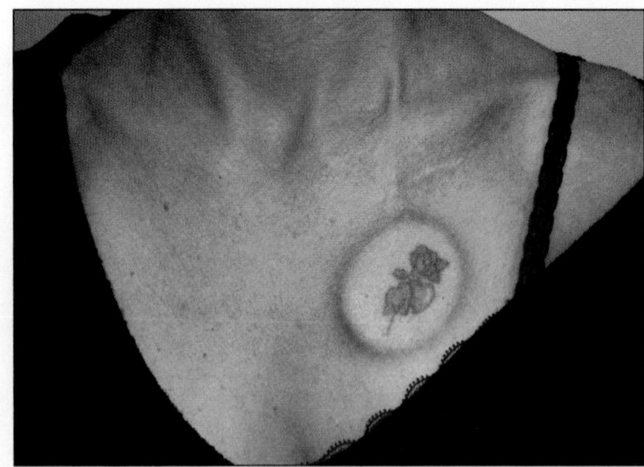

FIGURE 44-12

- We recommend placing electrodes perpendicular to the course of the nerves to be stimulated. Ideally, the middle contacts of the electrode should be in closest proximity to the nerve. This way, minor migration of an electrode may be dealt with by simple reprogramming instead of electrode revision.
- Any strain relief loop that is placed in the same tissue pocket as the anchor should be arranged to be between the anchor and the generator rather than between the anchor and stimulating contacts. This placement decreases the chance of migration and disconnection.

PITFALLS

Placing electrodes too superficial in the tissue may result in electrode erosion.

Placing electrodes too deep may result in uncomfortable stimulation that requires electrode removal or revision.

If the length of the electrodes does not compensate for natural stretch owing to change in body position, the tethering of hardware results in electrode migration or fracture depending on the tensile strength of the anchoring system.

BAILOUT OPTIONS

- In cases of electrode migration, fracture, or disconnection, revision surgery should include replacement of the affected component—with preparation of the entire field including the locations of electrodes and generator—in case troubleshooting requires examination or modification (or both) of the rest of the implanted system.
- In cases of erosion, one option is to remove the eroded electrode. Another option is to remove the most distal part of the electrode, leaving some of the contacts inside. This approach sometimes allows one to maintain positive effects of stimulation with few remaining contacts.
- In cases of infection, we recommend removal of the entire system followed by reimplantation 2 to 3 months later.

SUGGESTED READINGS

Slavin KV. Peripheral nerve stimulation for neuropathic pain. Neurotherapeutics 2008;5:100–6.

Slavin KV, Nersesyan H, Wess C. Peripheral neurostimulation for treatment of intractable occipital neuralgia. Neurosurgery 2006;58:112–9.

Slavin KV, Wess C. Trigeminal branch stimulation for intractable neuropathic pain: technical note. Neuromodulation 2005;8:9–15.

Trentman TL, Slavin KV, Freeman JA, et al. Occipital nerve stimulator placement via a retromastoid to infraclavicular approach: a technical report. Stereotact Funct Neurosurg 2010;88:121–5.

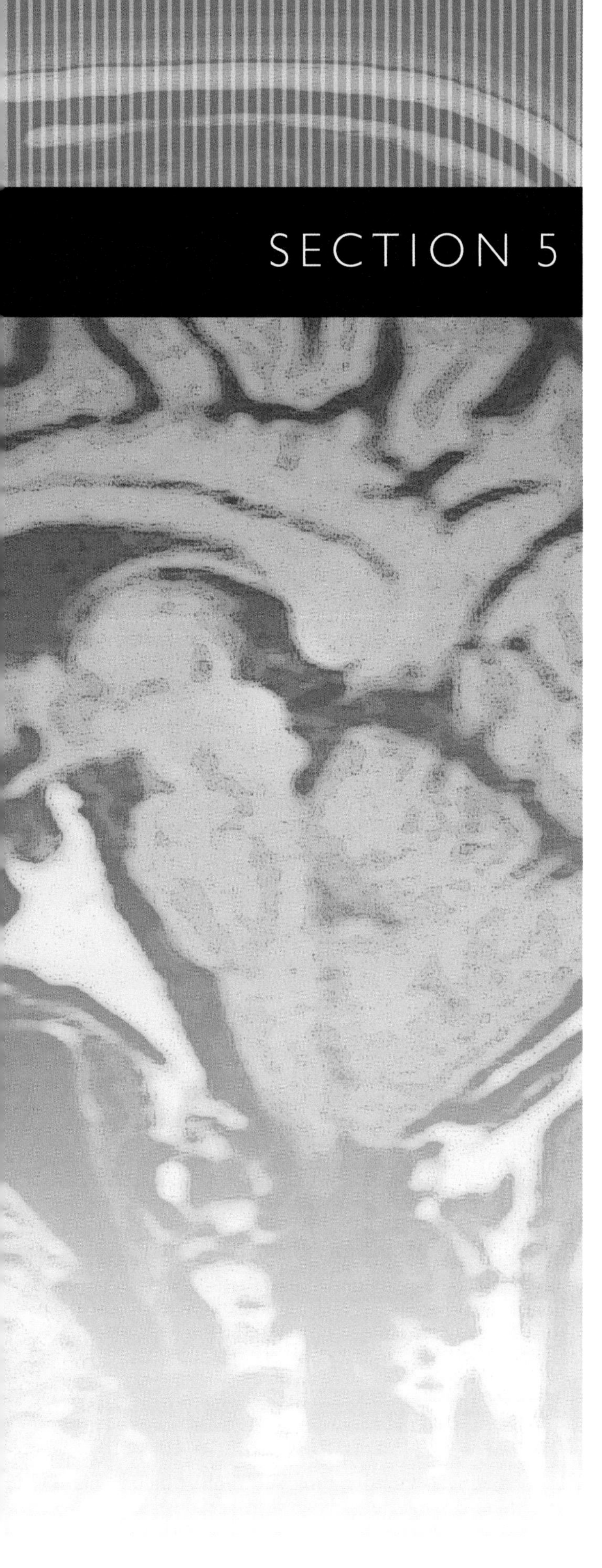

SECTION 5

Other

SECTION EDITOR — MICHAEL L. LEVY, WITH LISSA C. BAIRD

Procedure 45 Cranioplasty (Autogenous, Cadaveric, and Alloplastic)

Ryan C. Frank, Steven R. Cohen, Hal Meltzer

INDICATIONS

- We prefer to use autologous calvarial bone grafts as the primary material for cranioplasty and skull reconstruction. Autogenous graft has a lower incidence of infection, grows with the child, and heals the best of all other alternatives. It is generally close to the operative site, and resorption tends to be minimal. We prefer autologous calvarial bone when the defect size is not larger than the amount of remaining diploic bone available for harvest.
- We use split rib or iliac crest grafts in patients with large defects who are opposed to alloplastic reconstruction or in whom a prior infection has occurred. Autogenous bone is our first choice in patients with a history of scalp irradiation, provided that the scalp blood supply is intact. In patients with compromised soft tissue coverage, free tissue transfer may be necessary for coverage of autogenous or alloplastic calvarial reconstruction.
- In large defects in which an inadequate amount of bone is available, we prefer to use alloplastic reconstruction over split rib or iliac crest bone grafts to avoid donor site issues. Occasionally, patients may prefer autogenous reconstruction, however, or in heavily scarred tissue in which infection or dehiscence may occur, autogenous grafting with split rib or split iliac bone may still be preferable.
- When the defect is larger than the amount of remaining diploic bone available for harvest, we prefer to use prefabricated implants made of various synthetic materials, such as methyl methacrylate and porous, linear high-density polyethylene (MEDPOR, Porex Surgical, Inc., Newnan, GA). These implants are constructed using three-dimensional reconstructed images derived from "fine-cut" computed tomography (CT) scans.
- We prefer to use a calcium phosphate bone void filler when smaller gaps in bone are present (<2 to 3 cm) or when contour abnormalities require augmentation. Cadaveric bone and demineralized bone paste are viable options for filling in small bony gaps. In children younger than 5 years old, in whom the diploic space is not fully formed, demineralized bone grafts are also useful to fill moderately large defects. In using calcium phosphate bone cements or similar products, dural pulsations may be disruptive to the material before it hardens. In smaller defects, resorbable mesh may be used to cover the dura, dampening pulsations, and the bone cement is then overlaid on the mesh to fill the defect.

CONTRAINDICATIONS

- We do not use autologous calvarial bone when the defect is larger than the bone available. In smaller children with large defects, we avoid using rib and iliac crest grafts.
- Cranioplasty should not be performed if there is questionable soft tissue coverage present over the calvaria, or if there is active infection present in any of the layers of the scalp. Free tissue coverage should be considered in cases of questionable scalp viability or in the presence of irradiated tissue.

PLANNING AND POSITIONING

- Preoperative evaluation includes obtaining laboratory values (complete blood count) and crossmatching for packed red blood cells. A three-dimensional reconstruction of a CT scan of the head is obtained preoperatively in all patients.
- Patients are given a dose of preoperative antibiotics immediately before skin incision.

- Neuroanesthesia techniques are used in most patients, especially patients with larger defects.
- **Figure 45-1:** The patient is positioned so that easy, complete access to the defect site is obtainable.
- **Figure 45-2:** A bicoronal incision is planned.
- **Figure 45-3:** The planned incision is injected with a mixture of 0.25% bupivacaine (Marcaine) and 1:200,000 epinephrine.

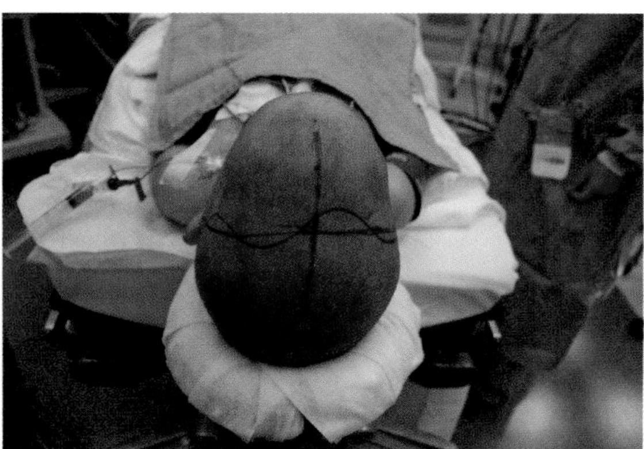

FIGURE 45-1

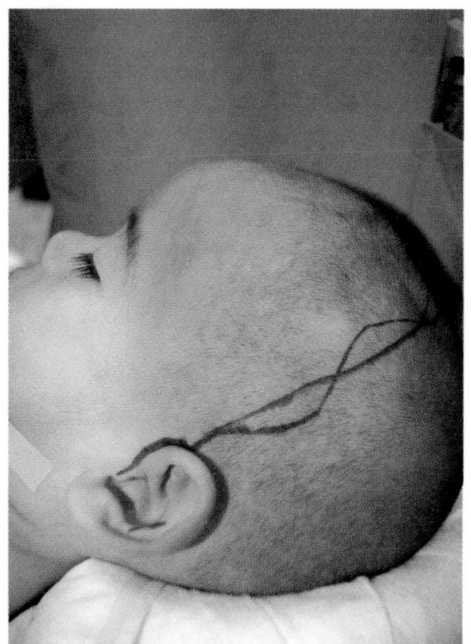

FIGURE 45-2

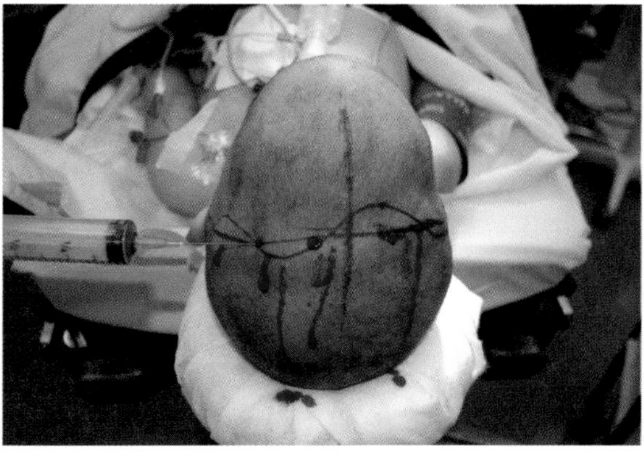

FIGURE 45-3

PROCEDURE

- **Figure 45-4:** The scalp incision is made with cutting frequency on monopolar, needle-tip cautery. Whenever possible, dissection is carried out in a subgaleal plane over the defect and surrounding calvaria. This dissection optimizes hemostasis and preserves the pericranium and frontogaleal muscle flap in the event these are needed for skull base or dural reconstruction.
- **Figure 45-5:** Dissection is performed in the subpericranial plane directly around the defect.
- **Figure 45-6:** When a preconstructed alloplastic implant is employed, the position of the implant is planned on a CT-developed mode.

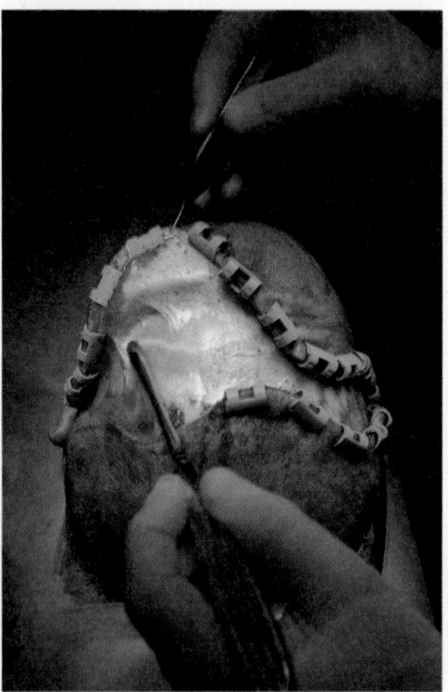

FIGURE 45-4

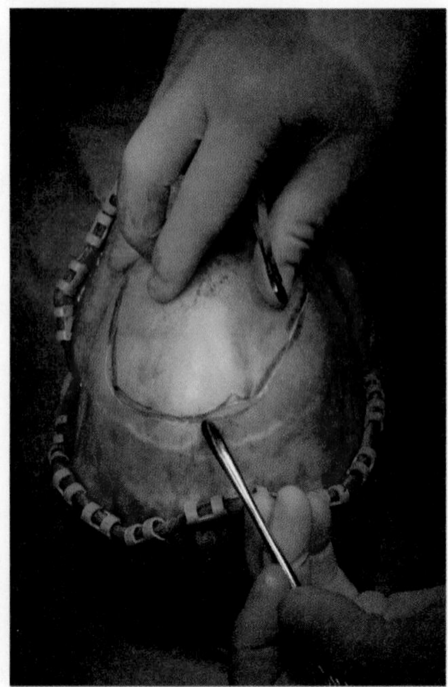

FIGURE 45-5

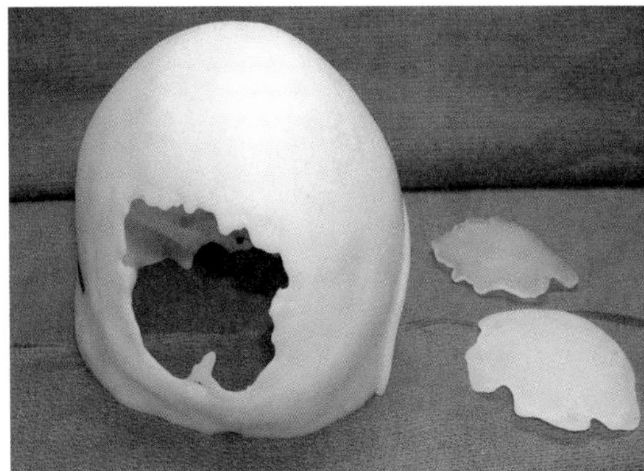

FIGURE 45-6

- **Figure 45-7:** Split calvarial grafts are obtained by two techniques. One technique is to harvest a full-thickness calvarial bone graft and on a side table, using a saw and fine osteotomes, separate the inner and outer tables cutting through the diploic space. When complete, the outer table is rigidly fixed into the donor site with either resorbable or metal plates and screws or mesh and screws, while the inner table is placed in the defect site, or vice versa.
- **Figure 45-8:** Iliac crest grafts can be used for autologous reconstruction.
- **Figure 45-9:** Split rib grafts can be used for autologous reconstruction.

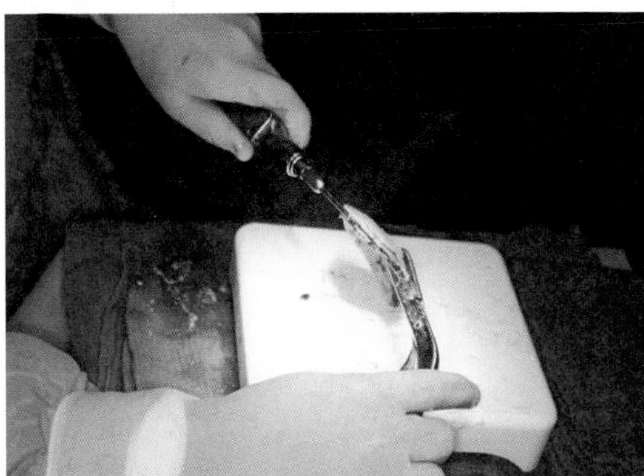

FIGURE 45-7

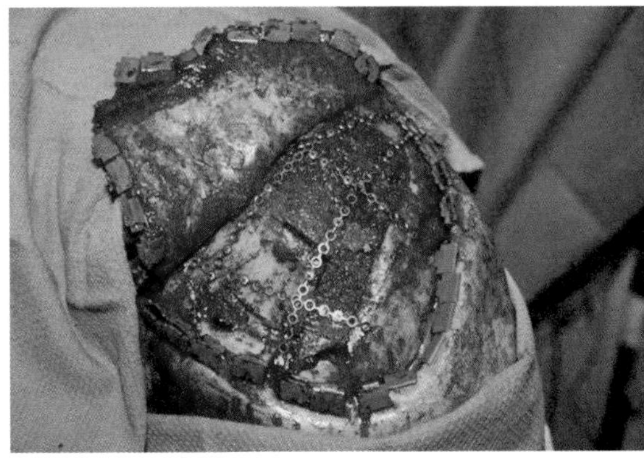

FIGURE 45-8

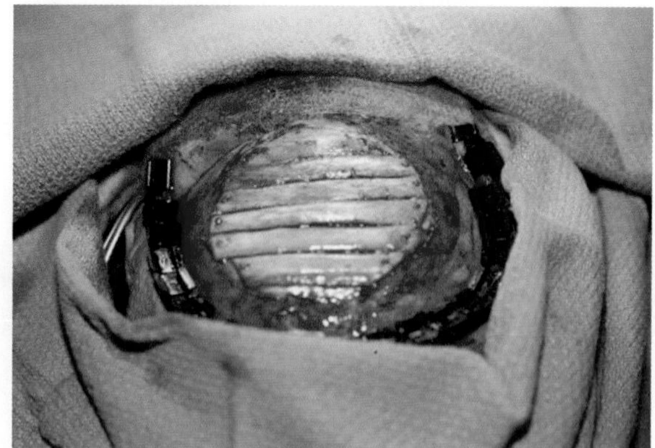

FIGURE 45-9

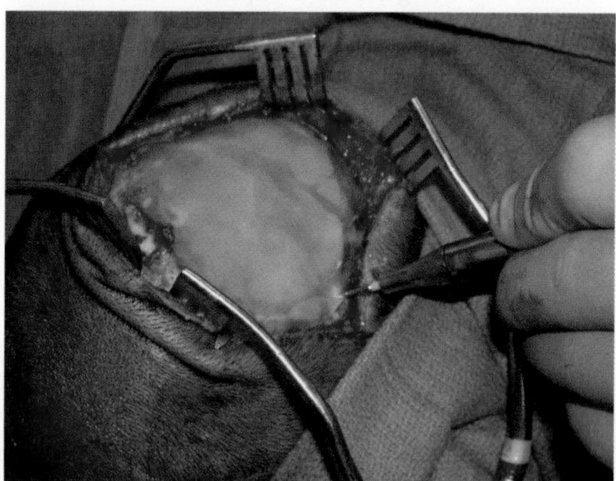

FIGURE 45-10

- **Figure 45-10:** A drill is used to create points of fixation of the implant to the surrounding margin of calvaria. Titanium screws are secured into the drill holes to stabilize the implant. If there is insufficient overlap of the implant with the calvarial margin, titanium plates can be used to secure the implant.
- The wound is thoroughly irrigated with antibiotic saline. Suture closure of the galea aponeurotica and scalp skin is performed.

TIPS FROM THE MASTERS

- Preoperative imaging and planning is essential to the success of this procedure. With preconstructed implants, the procedure is simplified immensely. Minor adjustments to the implant intraoperatively can be performed easily to ensure proper stabilization is achieved.

PITFALLS

This procedure cannot be performed if there is poor soft tissue coverage over the defect. Similarly, active infection of the scalp is an absolute contraindication to performing cranioplasty.

BAILOUT OPTIONS

- In the unlikely event that the preconstructed implant does not fit properly into the defect, other methods to reconstruct the defect can be employed. Autogenous split calvarial, split rib, or iliac crest grafts can be placed in remaining gaps and secured with screws and plates. Smaller remaining gaps can be filled with calcium phosphate cement or cadaveric bone paste.
- The use of postoperative hyperbaric oxygen treatments may salvage a failing cranioplasty wound, especially in the setting of a previously irradiated scalp.

SUGGESTED READINGS

Blum KS, Schneider SJ, Rosenthal AD. Methyl methacrylate cranioplasty in children: long-term results. Pediatr Neurosurg 1997;26:33–5.

Rish BL, Dillon DJ, Meirowsky AM, et al. Cranioplasty: a review of 1030 cases of penetrating head injury. Neurosurgery 1979;4:381–5.

Procedure 46

Endoscopic Transsphenoidal Approach

Justin F. Fraser, Vijay K. Anand, Theodore H. Schwartz

INDICATIONS

- Indications for the transsphenoidal approach have significantly increased with the addition of the endoscope. Using a team approach with a skilled endoscopic rhinologist has rendered the endoscopic transsphenoidal approach a valid minimal access method for exposing various midline skull base pathologies involving the planum sphenoidale, tuberculum sellae, medial cavernous sinus, pterygoid bone, and infrasellar clivus.
- The most common indication for the endoscopic transsphenoidal approach is a sellar mass. These lesions include pituitary adenomas, Rathke cleft cysts, and craniopharyngiomas. Although microadenomas and small macroadenomas do not require extended approaches, lesions with suprasellar, cavernous sinus and clival extension can be resected with the extended endoscopic transsphenoidal approaches.
- Extradural and intradural chordomas can be resected using an endoscopic transsphenoidal approach with transclival extension.
- Meningiomas of the planum sphenoidale, meningiomas of the tuberculum sellae, and some small olfactory groove meningiomas are amenable to endoscopic, endonasal resection.
- Juvenile nasal angiofibromas arising from the pterygopalatine fossa can be removed through an endoscopic endonasal approach, even with extension into the infratemporal fossa and Meckel cave.
- Malignant tumors such as esthesioneuroblastoma, squamous cell carcinoma, and adenocarcinoma can be resected through an endoscopic transsphenoidal approach if the surgeon is confident that negative margins can be achieved.
- Encephaloceles, meningoencephaloceles, and other midline skull base defects prone to cerebrospinal fluid (CSF) leakage can be repaired through endonasal endoscopic approaches, avoiding a craniotomy.
- Large tumors that cannot be completely removed with an endoscope are not always contraindications to this approach. Depending on the age of the patient and the surgical goals, an endoscopic approach may augment a secondary cranial approach with internal decompression or a staged resection.

CONTRAINDICATIONS

- Careful case selection is crucial to the success of this minimal access approach. Pathology extending laterally over the orbits or lateral and posterior to the carotid arteries is difficult to access, even when using extended endonasal approaches.
- Lesions extending into or posterior to the frontal sinus can be difficult to reach even with angled scopes. Additionally, the nasoseptal flap may not reach this far anteriorly, and skull base closure may be challenging.
- Invasion of the cavernous sinus is not an absolute contraindication but requires careful preoperative evaluation of surgical goals. The risk to surrounding neurovascular contents should be carefully assessed in the event the surgeon elects to enter the cavernous sinus to resect the tumor through a medial approach. Alternatively, an intentional subtotal resection or biopsy may be performed and augmented with planned postoperative stereotactic radiotherapy. Availability of an interventional neuroradiologist is crucial in preparation for endoscopic surgery around the carotid artery.

- The differential diagnosis of large sellar and suprasellar masses includes hypothalamic hamartomas, large intracranial aneurysms, and germ cell tumors. These lesions require a very different work-up and approach, and meticulous evaluation should be undertaken in appropriate patients to rule out such diagnoses preoperatively.

PLANNING AND POSITIONING

- Appropriate instrumentation for the endoscopic transsphenoidal approach differs from the instrumentation used for standard transcranial microsurgical approaches. Long, straight instruments with pistol grips are best for endoscopic approaches; specially designed bayoneted instruments can also be used. Monopolar cautery is favored for mucosal bleeding; bipolar coagulation is used with dural and intracranial structures. A tissue shaver or microdébrider is useful for resection of intranasal pathology; intracranial lesions require gentle bimanual suction, an ultrasonic aspirator, or a radiofrequency device. A micro-Doppler probe can be useful for identifying vascular structures. It is important to ensure that all endoscopic visualization equipment is working before starting the surgery. A range of endoscopes including 18-cm and 30-cm scopes with 0-degree, 30-degree, and 45-degree lenses should be available. High-definition cameras and widescreen displays allow the surgeon to visualize normal and abnormal structures. A sheath around the scope can be used to irrigate and clean the lens during the operation to minimize the need for repeated removal and introduction of the scope. Finally, a scope holder is often useful to maintain a fixed, steady field of view during aspects of the case in which mobile visualization is not required.
- After induction of general anesthesia, intravenous antibiotics (2 g of cefazolin or 1 g of vancomycin) and steroids (except in the setting of Cushing disease) are given. For large extended cases, we administer triple antibiotics. Injection of intrathecal fluorescein is an optional procedure that can help to identify CSF leaks during the surgery. After pretreating with antihistamines, 10 mL of CSF is removed via lumbar puncture, mixed with 0.2 mL of 10% fluorescein, and reinjected into the thecal sac. Alternatively, a lumbar drain may be placed for postoperative drainage if the risk of CSF leak is high. The head is placed in three-point pin fixation, elevated above the heart, and extended 10 to 15 degrees. If a fixed position is unnecessary, a horseshoe head holder may be used.
- Neuronavigation is not required but is highly recommended in endoscopic endonasal surgery. Navigation provides real-time information about the angle of approach and localization. Additionally, navigation allows the surgeon to tailor the approach for maximal visualization of pathology with minimal exposure and manipulation of vital neurovascular structures.
- The abdomen should be prepared for harvesting of a fat graft in case of CSF leak after resection of an intrasellar lesion. For extended approaches in which a large skull base defect is anticipated, the thigh should be prepared for harvesting fascia lata. A nasoseptal flap may also be harvested for large skull base defects.
- **Figure 46-1:** Operating room organization. Ergonomic placement of equipment is essential because endoscopic procedures require nondirect tools for visualization (i.e., viewing screens, neuronavigation). The patient's head is positioned in the center of the operating room, angled slightly away from the anesthesia team. Two projection screens are used to allow easy visualization for the main operator and the assistant. A primary surgeon who is right-handed should stand on the patient's right side.
- **Figure 46-2:** After positioning of the patient, the nose should be prepared and draped in a triangular fashion, exposing both nares. Cottonoids saturated with 4 mL of 4% cocaine are placed in the nares to vasoconstrict the nasal mucosa. Additional preparation and draping of the abdomen and lateral thigh should be done as necessary for harvest of fat and fascia lata.
- **Figure 46-3:** Neuronavigation through the nasal cavity assists in directing the approach to the sphenoid sinus. Navigation is also useful in determining the amount of bone that must be removed in the extended approach to expose the entire tumor. In this example, an extended approach with removal of the tuberculum sellae and planum sphenoidale is required to reach above the tumor and ensure a complete resection.

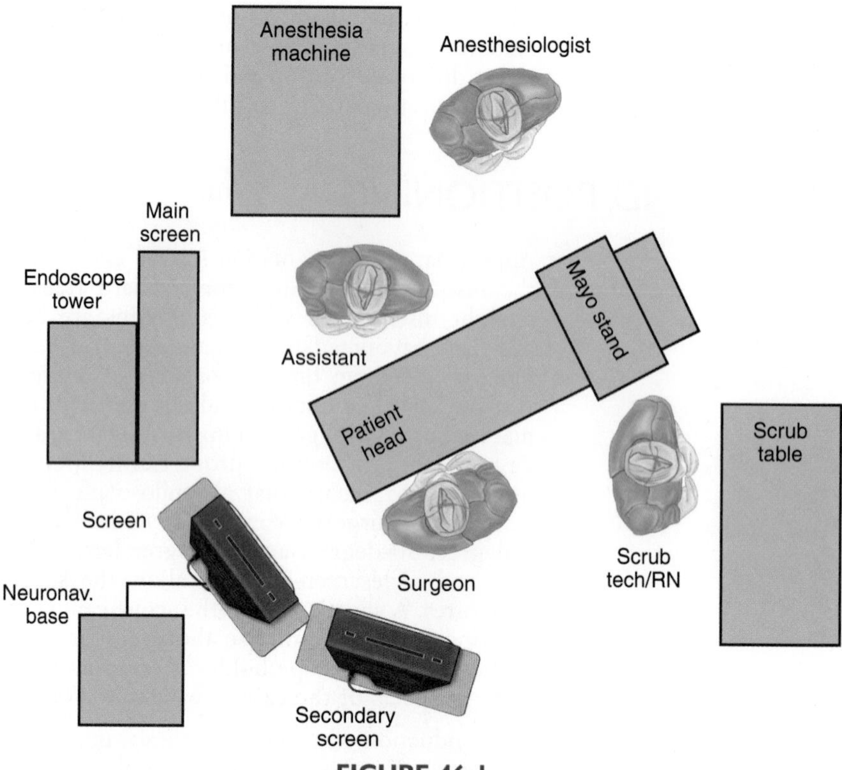

FIGURE 46-1

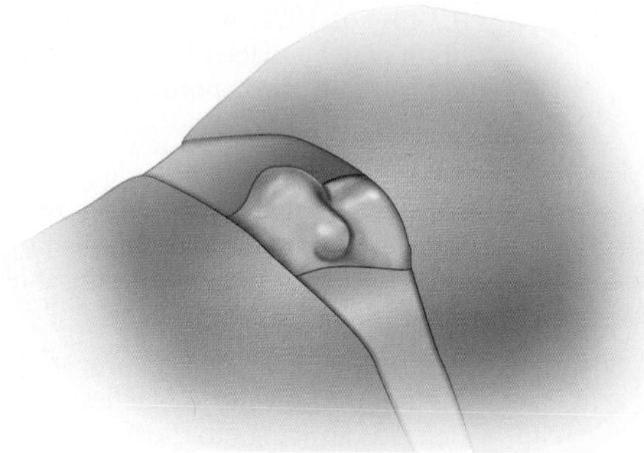

FIGURE 46-2

PROCEDURE

- **Figure 46-4:** A rigid 0-degree 4-mm endoscope is used for the nasal and sinus portion of the exposure. A one-handed technique, in which the endoscope is held and manipulated in one hand (usually the left) and the dissection is performed with the other hand, is used. Alternatively, an assistant may manipulate the endoscope. The middle turbinates (MT) and sphenopalatine artery are injected with 1% lidocaine and epinephrine (1:100,000).
- **Figure 46-5:** Harvesting of a nasoseptal flap should be performed at the beginning of the case through a hemitransfixation incision. After submucosal detachment or resection of the septum (or both), the middle and superior turbinates are retracted bilaterally, creating a larger working space. Vomer is removed.
- **Figure 46-6:** The sphenoid ostium is identified. The mucosa around the ostium is cauterized, and the opening is enlarged with rongeurs. The mucosa of the sphenoid sinus may be stripped or simply incised. If an intersinus sphenoid septum is present, it is removed with rongeurs.

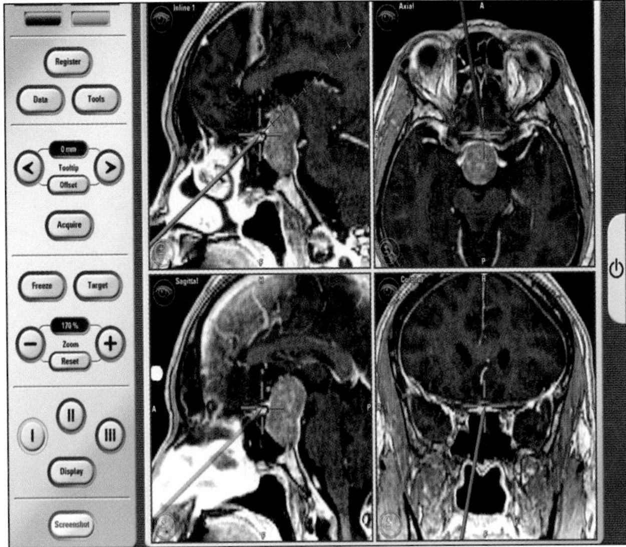

FIGURE 46-3

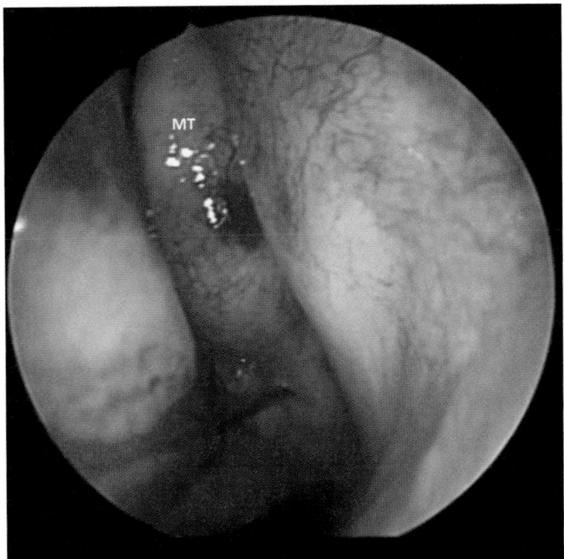

FIGURE 46-4

- **Figure 46-7:** A view of the posterior sphenoid sinus is obtained. Important anatomy to identify at this point includes the carotid prominences, the opticocarotid recesses (OCR), and the floor of the sella (S). At this point, we fix the endoscope in position with a flexible scope holder.
- **Figure 46-8:** The floor of the sella is opened with a high-speed drill, curets, and Kerrison rongeurs. The margins of the opening are the cavernous sinuses laterally and the tuberculum sella superiorly. Doppler ultrasound and neuronavigation should be used to verify the path of the carotid arteries.
- **Figure 46-9: A,** The dura is opened using a sickle knife in a cruciate fashion, and the leaflets are cauterized with a bipolar cautery. Care is taken to stay below the anterior intercavernous sinus to avoid unnecessary bleeding. A straight dissector is used to probe the sella and determine if a plane exists around the pathology. **B,** For hormone-producing adenomas, en bloc resection is the most complete method to ensure gross total resection. Visualization of yellow-green fluorescein demonstrates CSF. Venous bleeding often occurs when the sella is decompressed after tumor removal; gentle pressure with hemostatic agents such as thrombin-soaked Gelfoam should be applied.

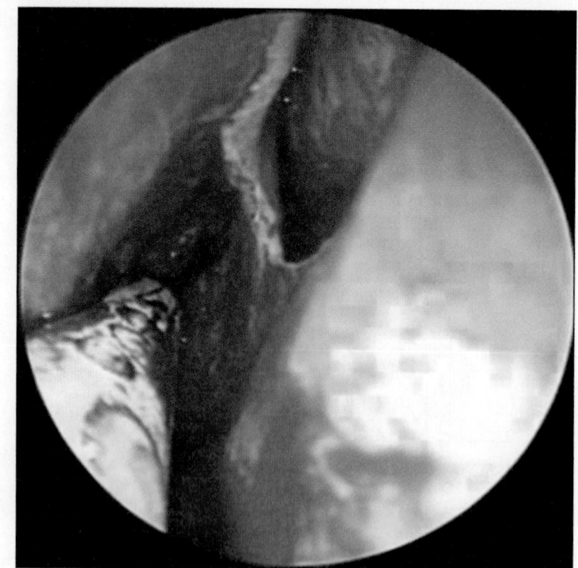

FIGURE 46-5

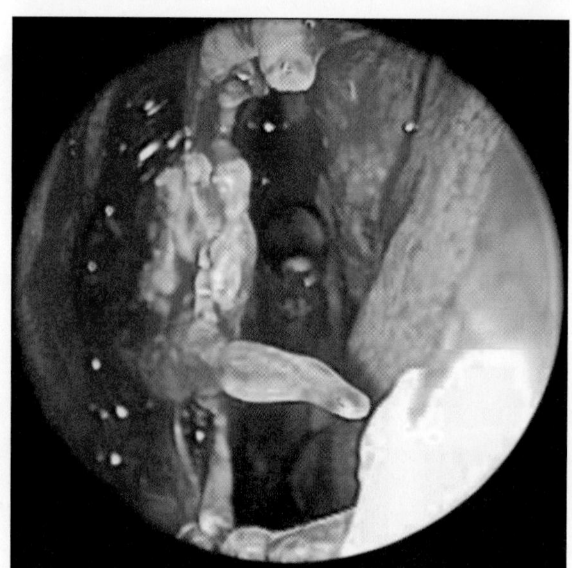

FIGURE 46-6

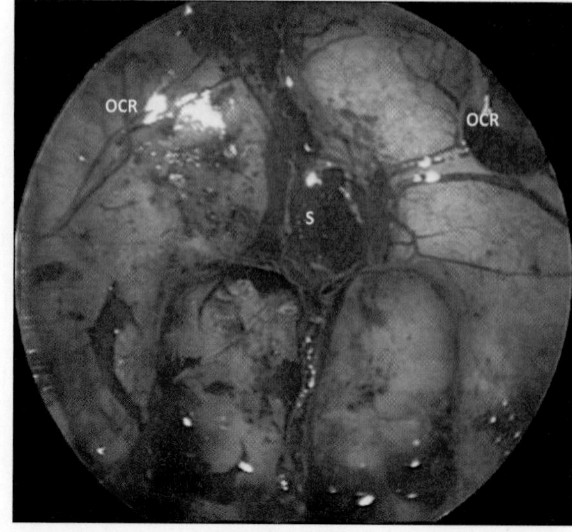

FIGURE 46-7

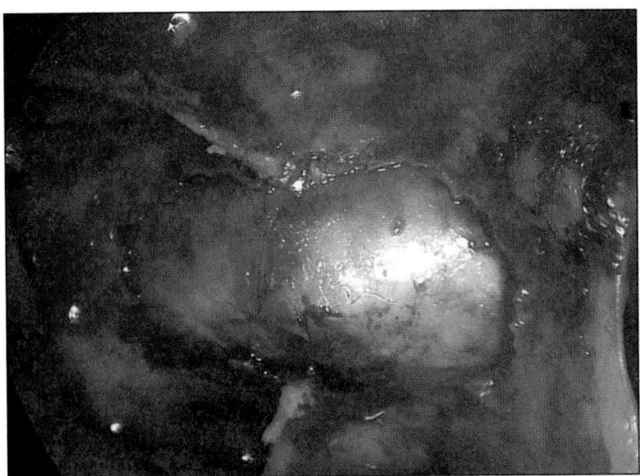

FIGURE 46-8

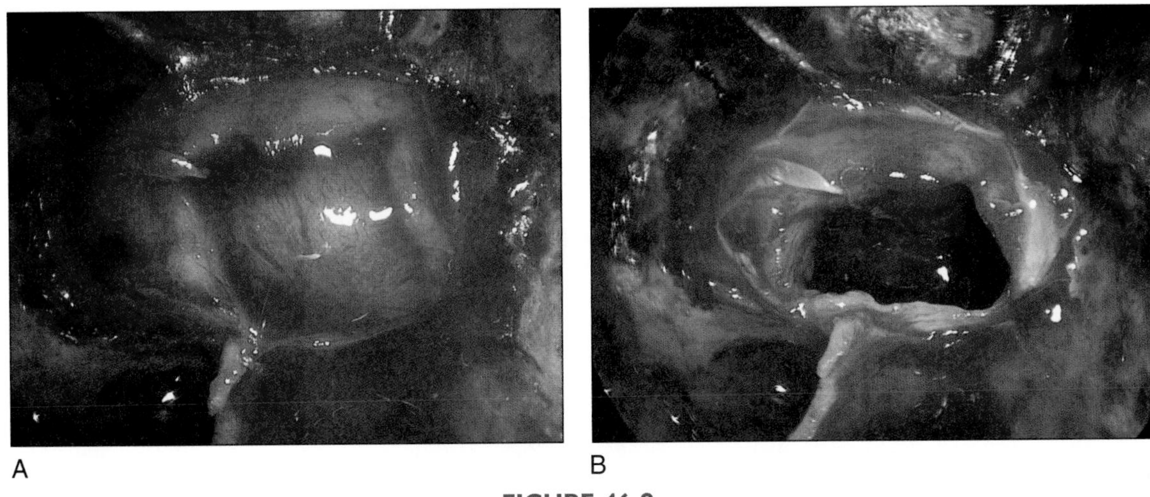

A B

FIGURE 46-9

- **Figure 46-10:** In the absence of en bloc resection, a repeating cycle of ring curets and micropituitary rongeurs is used to remove the tumor sequentially. Different angled ring curets may be used to elicit tumor from different corners of the sella.
- **Figure 46-11:** The superior margin of the tumor should be removed last because manipulation and dissection may cause the arachnoid membrane *(AM)* of the sella

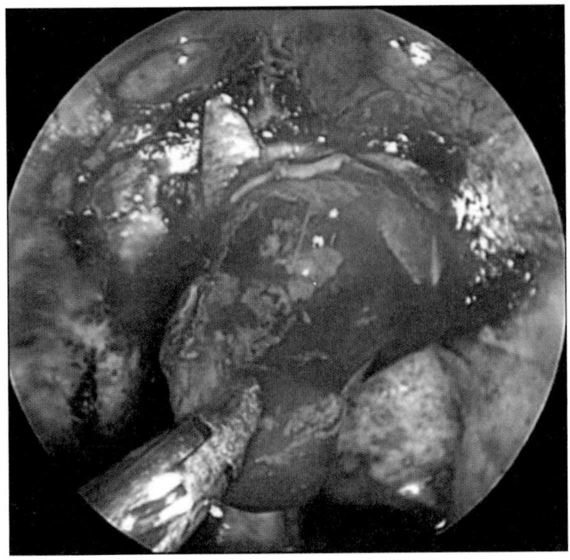

FIGURE 46-10

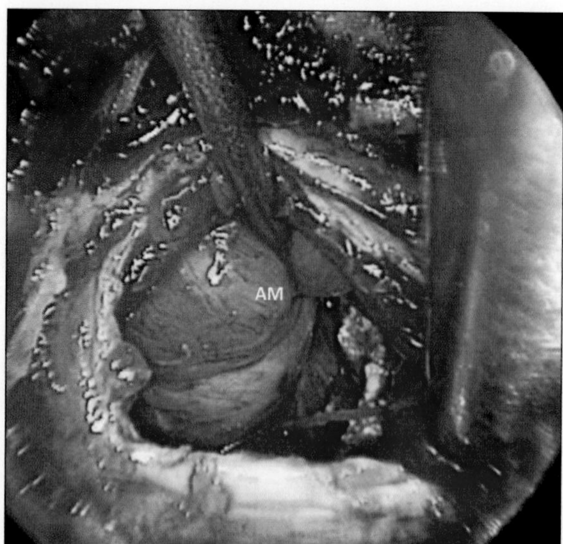

FIGURE 46-11

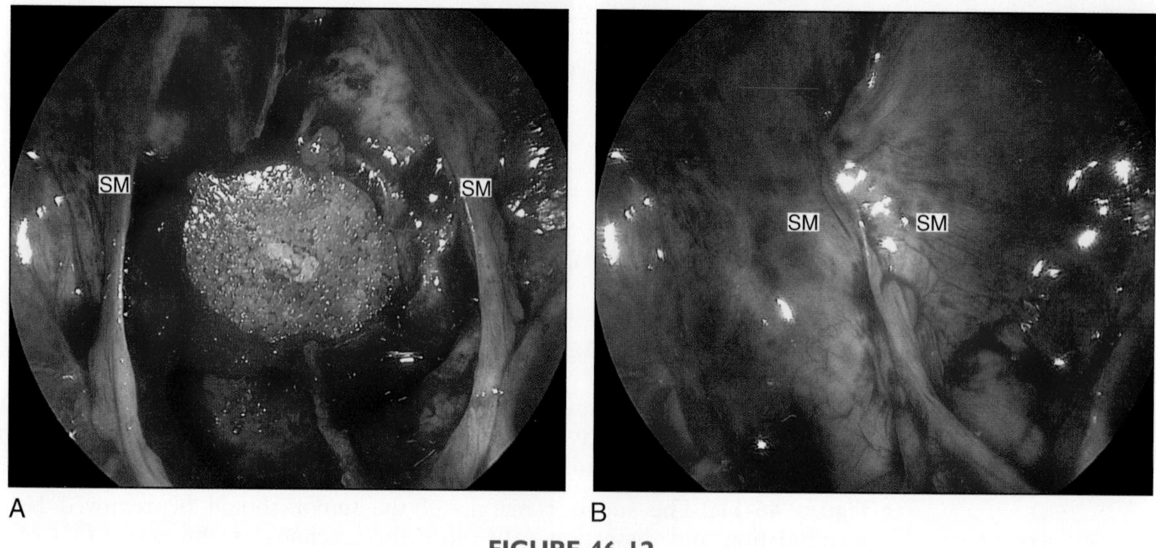

FIGURE 46-12

roof to drop into the operative field. It is important to maintain the integrity of this arachnoid if possible to reduce the risk of CSF leak. This arachnoid along with the pituitary should be retracted, and the superolateral corners of the sella should be investigated with angled endoscopes to ensure that no residual tumor is present.

- **Figure 46-12:** For closure of the standard transsphenoidal approach, the sella is investigated for CSF leak. If no leak is present, thrombin-soaked Gelfoam is placed in the sella for hemostasis. In the presence of CSF leak, we prefer abdominal fat. **A,** Harvested vomer or bone substitute is used to reconstruct the sella floor. A dural sealant is placed over the construct. **B,** If possible, intact sphenoid sinus mucosa *(SM)* (saved by opening it in a vertical linear fashion) may be closed over the posterior wall of the sella by bringing its edges together. Finally, the sphenoid sinus is filled with thrombin-infused gelatin, and Telfa packing is placed in each nostril overnight.
- **Figure 46-13:** **A,** For extended approaches to the midline anterior cranial fossa or in cases in which superior exposure of the tumor into the floor of the third ventricle is required, anterior extension of the transsphenoidal approach is necessary. **B,** Further anterior trajectories and targets in or around the orbital apex require a transethmoidal approach. **C,** The transplanum approach requires careful drilling of the planum and sella, followed by dural opening above and below the intercavernous sinus; these steps

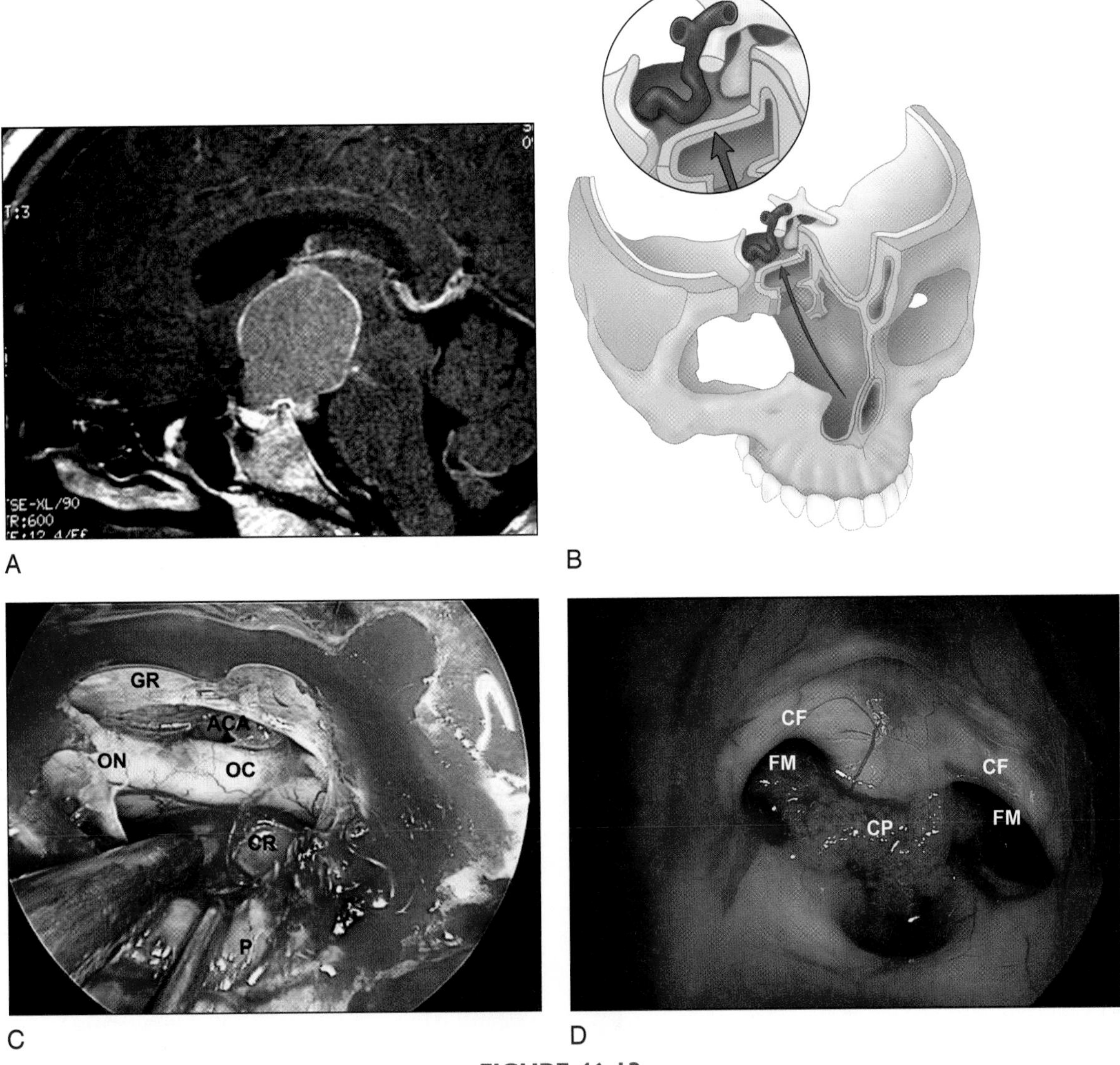

FIGURE 46-13

allow for control of bleeding because the intercavernous sinus can then be cauterized and cut. This approach provides clear visualization of the optic chiasm. *ACA* = anterior cerebral artery; *CR* = carotid recess; *GR* = gyrus rectus; *OC* = optic chiasm; *ON* = optic nerve; *P* = pituitary. **D,** The transplanum approach can be used to reach lesions that extend into the third ventricle. *CF* = column of the fornix; *CP* = choroid plexus; *FM* = foramen of Monro.

- **Figure 46-14: A,** For extended approaches to lesions of the clivus, inferior extension is required. For lesions in the inferior two thirds of the clivus, an inverted U-shaped incision is made in the basopharyngeal fascia and prevertebral musculature and flapped inferiorly. Drilling of the clivus extends from the sella, with the eustachian tubes representing the lateral border, although care must be taken when drilling over the carotid arteries. **B,** Dural opening, when necessary, is performed from medial to lateral in the shape of a capital I to avoid damaging the sixth cranial nerves. *A* = anterior inferior cerebellar artery; *B* = basilar artery; *ET* = eustachian tube; *ICA* = internal carotid artery; *M* = medulla; *P* = pons; *S* = sella; *VI* = abducens nerve.
- **Figure 46-15: A,** The transpterygoid approach uses a transmaxillary corridor extension of the transsphenoidal approach to obtain access from the petrous apex to the infratemporal fossa. The medial border of the maxillary sinus is marked by the sphenopalatine artery. After cauterization, drilling of bone posteriorly provides access

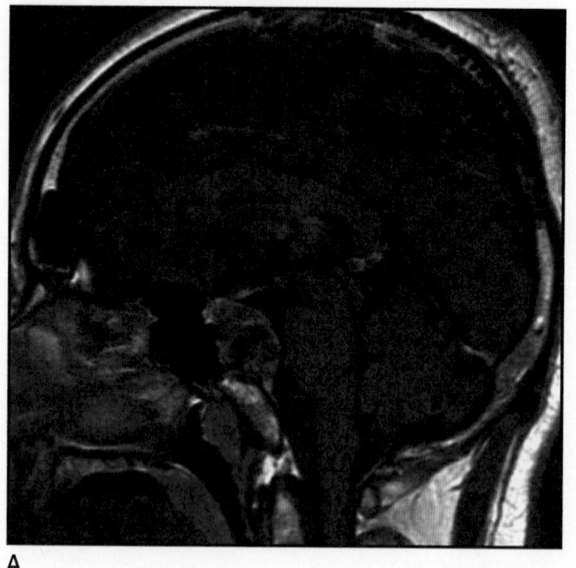
A

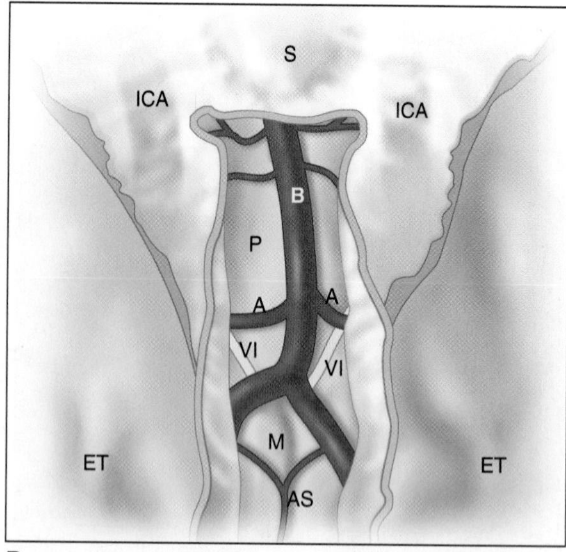

B

FIGURE 46-14

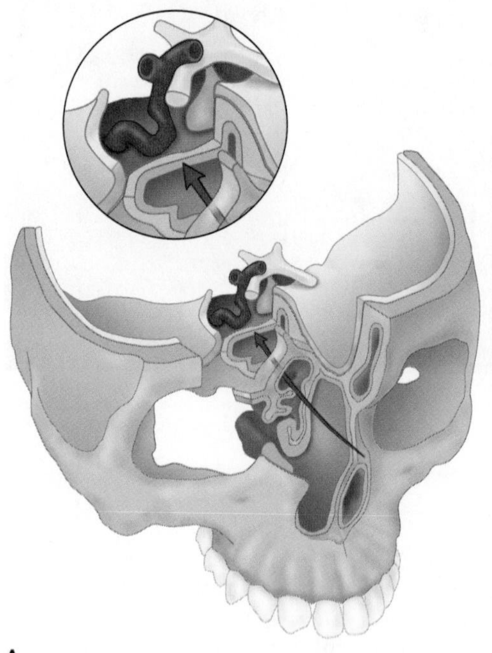
A

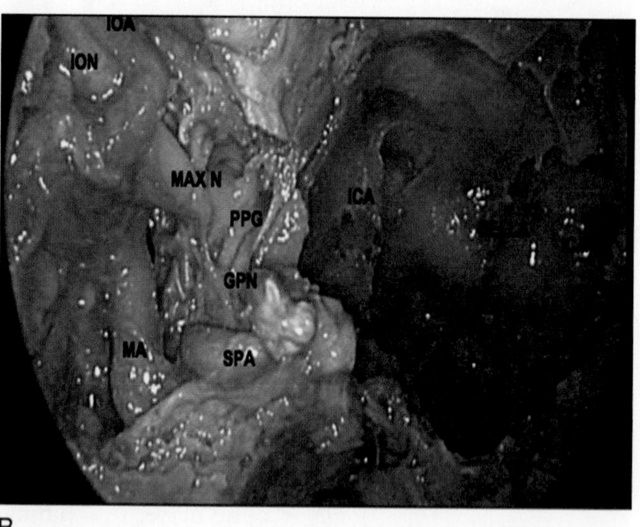

B

FIGURE 46-15

to the pterygopalatine fossa and maxillary nerve (V2), which can be followed to the foramen rotundum. **B,** Lateral drilling provides access to the infratemporal fossa. *GPN* = greater petrosal nerve; *ICA* = internal carotid artery; *IOA* = infraorbital artery; *ION* = infraorbital nerve; *MA* = maxillary artery; *MAX N* = maxillary nerve (V2); *PPG* = pterygopalatine ganglion; *SPA* = sphenopalatine artery.

- **Figure 46-16:** For extended skull base approaches, a gasket-seal closure with nasoseptal flap is favored to minimize CSF leak. **A,** A piece of fascia lata larger than the skull defect is shaped, and vomer or bone substitute buttress is wedged in place with redundant fascia creating a water-tight seal as it is draped around the bone. **B** and **C,** The nasoseptal flap *(NSF)* may be rotated to cover the defect; *dotted line* outlines the skull defect. Sealants such as DuraSeal (Covidien, Mansfield, MA) or fibrin glue are used to support the closure.

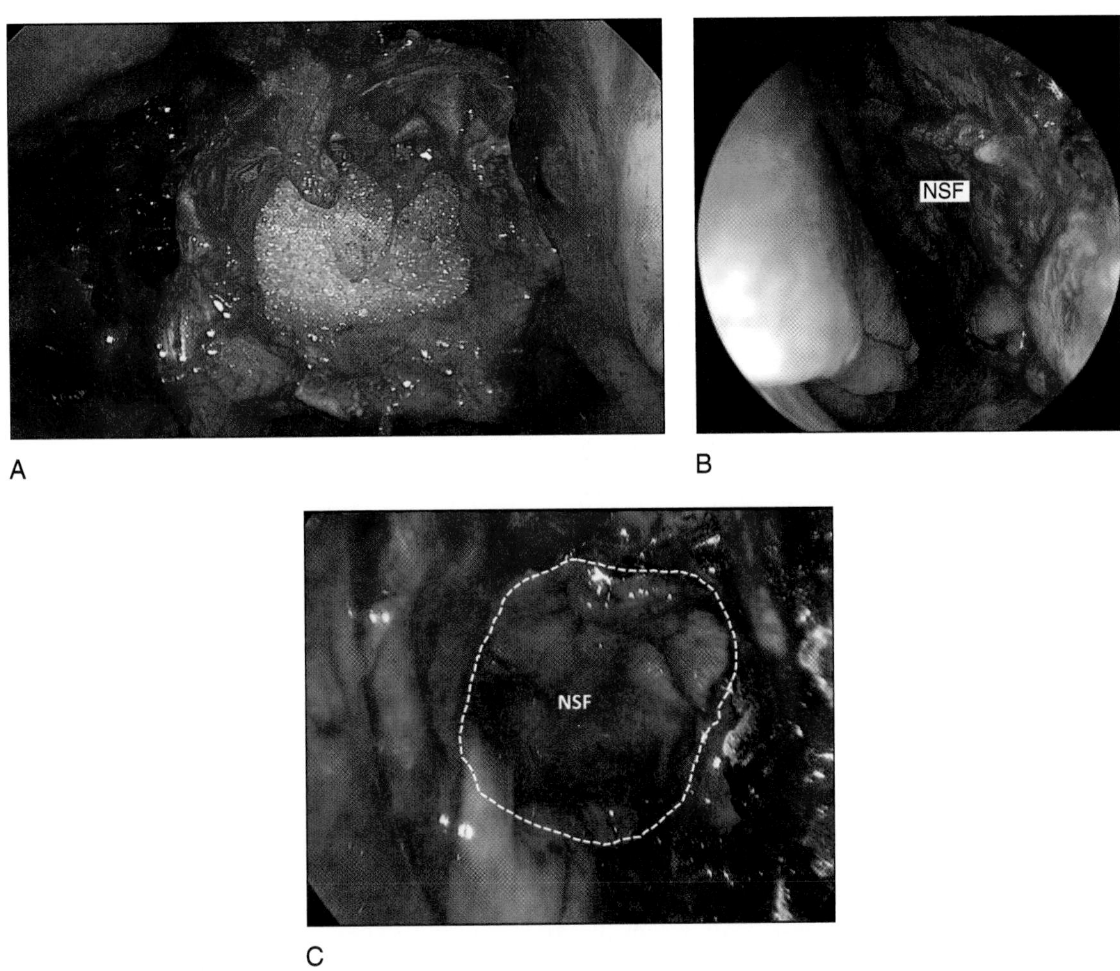

FIGURE 46-16

TIPS FROM THE MASTERS

- When opening the sphenoid ostium, avoid straying inferolaterally because this may result in injury to the sphenopalatine artery.
- For very large tumors and for extended approaches, the middle turbinate may be removed to provide additional visualization.
- The micro-Doppler should be used to identify the location of the carotid artery before opening the dura.
- For patients with Cushing disease with normal magnetic resonance imaging (MRI), exploration of the pituitary gland must be performed. Several small vertical incisions at 2- to 3-mm intervals are made in the pituitary gland. En bloc resection using the pseudocapsule should be attempted. If no tumor is identified, petrosal sinus sampling can be used to lateralize the tumor, in which case half the gland can be removed. Adrenalectomy may be preferable to complete resection of the gland.
- Carefully examine preoperative computed tomography (CT), CT angiography, or MRI to understand the relationship between the septations in the sphenoid sinus and the carotid artery. CT angiography navigation can be useful intraoperatively.
- Use a diamond rather than a cutting bur to remove bone over the dura and carotid artery.
- For extended approaches, it is important not to make the bone opening too small. Navigation is useful to plan the size of opening needed for adequate exposure of the tumor.

- Internal decompression and extracapsular dissection permits the surgeon to avoid blindly pulling the tumor into the surgical field.
- For extended transsphenoidal approaches in which there is significant risk of CSF leak, more elaborate methods of closure are necessary. We recommend either the "gasket-seal" closure using a fascia lata and vomer reconstruction or a MEDPOR (Porex Surgical, Inc., Newnan, GA) buttress with a vascularized nasoseptal flap. Intradural fat can decrease the dead space but can make postoperative imaging of residual tumor challenging.

PITFALLS

If the bone opening is too small, the surgeon is forced to pull the pathology into the field of view, which risks injury to vessels attached to the back of the tumor.

The venous plexus in the clival dura can be extensive. Slow, meticulous opening with careful hemostasis is imperative to ensure the success of this approach.

Visual identification of the pituitary and stalk is important because accidental injury to these structures must be avoided. The superior hypophyseal arteries should be identified and preserved because devascularization of the stalk can cause hypopituitarism.

Drilling over the carotid artery with a cutting bur should be avoided.

BAILOUT OPTIONS

- If carotid injury occurs, the sphenoid should be packed quickly, and a Foley catheter should be inserted and inflated to maintain pressure. The patient should be taken for emergent endovascular assessment and treatment.
- Hemostasis of venous bleeding is most effectively accomplished with hemostatic agents and gentle pressure.
- If reoperation is undertaken to close a CSF leak, it is useful to identify the source of the leak before surgery. The source of CSF leak can be identified with intrathecal iohexol injection before CT scan or intraoperatively with intrathecal fluorescein.

SUGGESTED READINGS

Cappabianca P, Cavallo LM, de Divitiis E, et al. Endoscopic endonasal transsphenoidal surgery. Neurosurgery 2004;55:933–40.

Fraser JF, Nyquist GG, Moore N, et al. Endoscopic endonasal transclival resection of chordomas: operative technique, clinical outcome, and review of the literature. J Neurosurg 2010;112:1061–9.

Jho HD. Endoscopic transsphenoidal surgery. J Neuro-oncol 2001;54:187–95.

Schwartz TH, Fraser JF, Brown S, et al. Endoscopic cranial base surgery: classification of operative approaches. Neurosurgery 2008;62:991–1002.

Tabaee A, Anand VK, Barron Y, et al. Endoscopic pituitary surgery: a systematic review and meta-analysis. J Neurosurg 2009;111:545–54.

Procedure 47

Endoscopic Colloid Cyst Removal 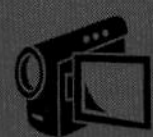

Charles Teo

INDICATIONS

- Symptomatic cysts
  - Symptoms may range from visual obscurations and loss of consciousness to positional headache, sensory disturbance, and short-term memory decline.
  - Symptoms of hydrocephalus, such as urinary incontinence, dementia, and ataxia, may also be present.
- Secondary hydrocephalus or unilateral ventriculomegaly
  - Treatment is indicated whether or not symptoms are present.
- Incidental colloid cysts without secondary hydrocephalus
  - Incidental cysts are a controversial indication for surgical intervention.
  - The patient's wishes, informed consent from the patient, and the surgeon's level of comfort all are key factors when determining treatment.

CONTRAINDICATIONS

- A patient with an incidental colloid cyst and small ventricles presents a relative contraindication to surgery.
- Size of the cyst is another relative contraindication to the endoscopic approach. Given the limitations of current endoscopic instrumentation, large cysts containing tenacious material may take significantly longer to remove than by an open approach.

PLANNING AND POSITIONING

- It is prudent to have all patients assessed by a neurologist to ascertain absolutely that headaches are related to the cyst.
- Preoperative imaging should include data acquisition for frameless stereotactic intraoperative guidance, especially in the setting of small ventricles.
- The video monitor needs to be directly across from the surgeon, and it should be ensured that all components of the video chain are fully functional before making the skin incision.
- The patient is placed supine on the table with the head in three-point pin fixation. The head is flexed approximately 45 degrees to the horizontal plane without lateral flexion or rotation. The burr hole is placed 8 cm behind the nasion and 5 to 7 cm from the midline. We recommend approaching the cyst from the nondominant side, although if the ventricle of the dominant hemisphere is significantly more dilated, it is reasonable to approach the cyst from the side of the larger ventricle.
- **Figures 47-1: A,** The patient is placed supine on the table with the head in three-point pin fixation. The head is flexed approximately 45 degrees to the horizontal plane without lateral flexion or rotation. **B,** The burr hole is placed 8 cm behind the nasion and 5 to 7 cm from the midline.

PROCEDURE

- **Figure 47-2:** A standard 11-mm burr hole gives ample room to maneuver the endoscope. The ventricle should be tapped with a brain needle and *not* the endoscope sheath. This is preferably done with stereotactic guidance. It is imperative to "target"

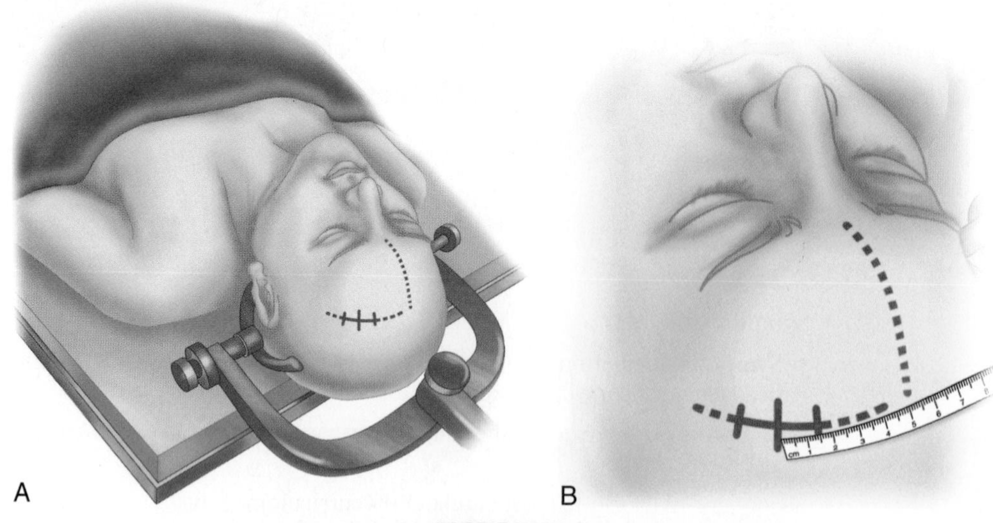

FIGURE 47-1

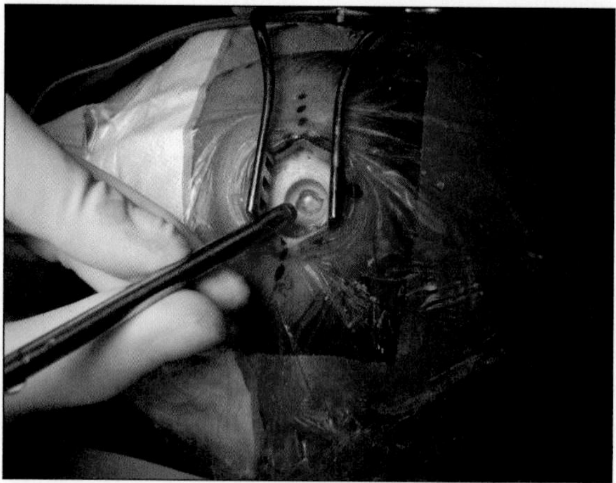

FIGURE 47-2

the frontal horn of the lateral ventricle and *not* the colloid cyst. If the cyst is the target, a trajectory from the burr hole necessarily traverses the head of the caudate nucleus.

- **Figure 47-3:** To avoid disorientation in the lateral ventricle, we recommend using a 0-degree scope initially rather than a 30-degree scope. Landmarks that assist in finding the foramen of Monro are the septal and thalamostriate veins and the choroid plexus. When the cyst can be seen through the foramen, we recommend changing to a 30-degree scope.

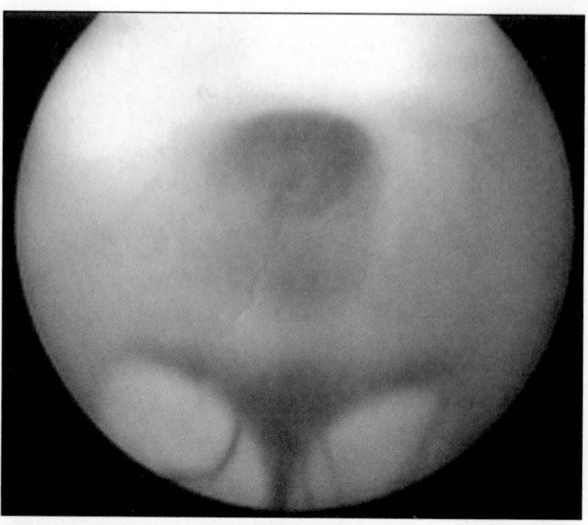

FIGURE 47-3

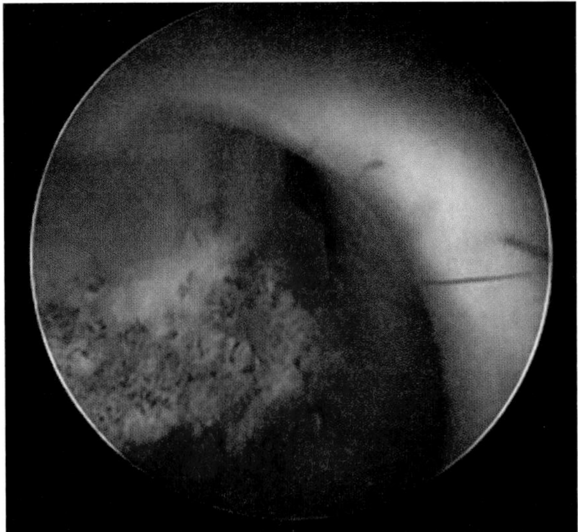

FIGURE 47-4

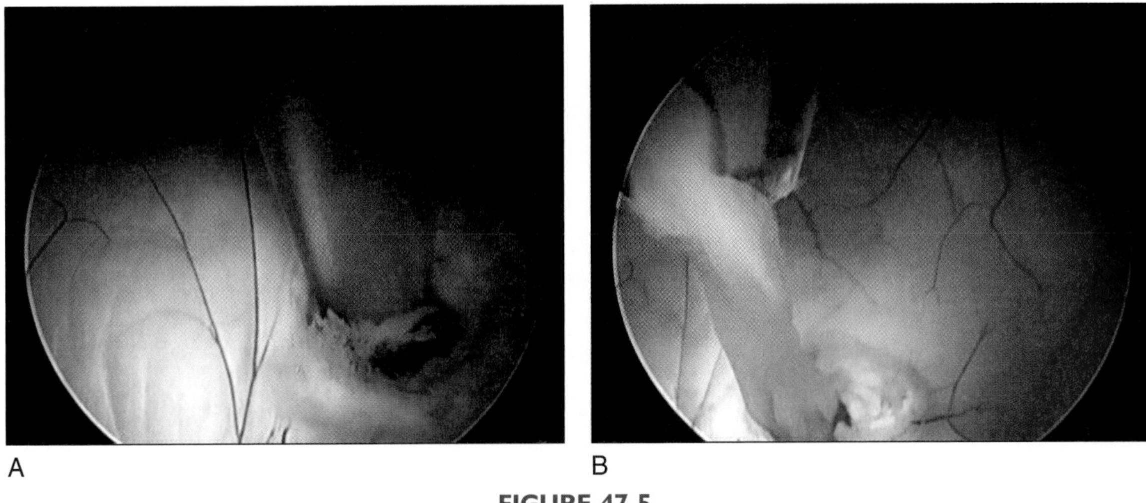

A B

FIGURE 47-5

- **Figure 47-4:** Small cysts can be removed by initially coagulating and cutting the overlying choroid plexus before grabbing the cyst to remove it en bloc. It is preferable to coagulate the contralateral choroid plexus before placing the cyst under traction, although this is a difficult maneuver when the foramen is minimally expanded.
- **Figure 47-5:** Large cysts should be initially decompressed either through a small opening in the tenuous ipsilateral fornix and septum pellucidum or through the foramen. Any access to the third ventricle through the fornix and septum should be performed with caution because this may leave the patient totally dependent on the contralateral fornix for memory.
- **Figure 47-6:** When the cyst has been decompressed, the cyst wall should be coagulated and removed. Most bleeding, even from a large vein such as the thalamostriate, is readily controlled with irrigation. If the vessel can be identified, other techniques to control hemorrhage include tamponade with the endoscope itself; coagulation with monopolar or bipolar probes; and, in extreme circumstances, draining CSF from the ventricles and coagulating in an air environment.

TIPS FROM THE MASTERS

- An anterolateral approach gives the best exposure.
- The incision is straight and preferably behind the hairline. A coronal incision is cosmetically preferable to a sagittal incision, which may be visible on the forehead. In a patient

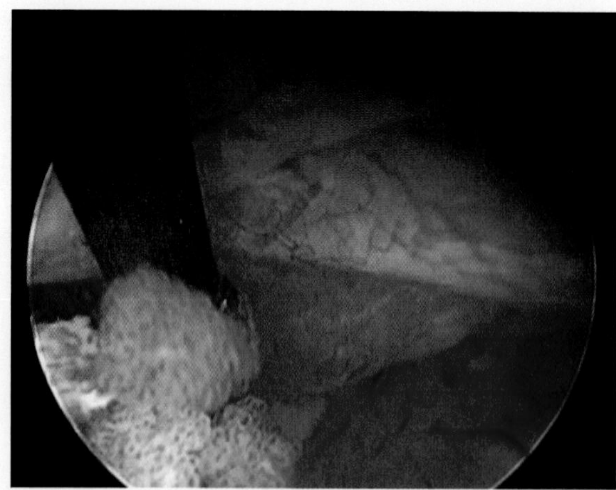

FIGURE 47-6

with frontal baldness, the incision would be exposed regardless, however, and a sagittal incision may limit damage to the plexus of sensory nerves coursing toward the supraorbital foramen. A sagittal incision would minimize postoperative scalp numbness.

- Keep the ventricle full with irrigation, avoiding ventricular collapse.

PITFALLS

Targeting cyst with stereotactic guidance damages caudate and causes problematic bleeding.
Tapping ventricle with scope or sheath instead of brain needle is dangerous.
Faulty instrumentation.

BAILOUT OPTIONS

- One should always be prepared for uncontrollable hemorrhage. In this situation, the burr hole is extended to a small craniotomy, and the operation is converted to a standard microsurgical transcortical, transventricular approach.

SUGGESTED READINGS

Greenlee JD, Teo C, Ghahreman A, et al. Purely endoscopic resection of colloid cysts. Neurosurgery 2008;62(3 Suppl 1):51–5.

Grondin RT, Hader W, MacRae ME, et al. Endoscopic versus microsurgical resection of third ventricle colloid cysts. Can J Neurol Sci 2007;34:197–207.

Hellwig D, Bauer BL, Schulte M, et al. Neuroendoscopic treatment for colloid cysts of the third ventricle: the experience of a decade. Neurosurgery 2008;62(6 Suppl 3):1101–9.

Horn EM, Feiz-Erfan I, Bristol RE, et al. Treatment options for third ventricular colloid cysts: comparison of open microsurgical versus endoscopic resection. Neurosurgery 2007;60:613–8.

Lewis AI, Crone KR, Taha J, et al. Surgical resection of third ventricle colloid cysts: preliminary results comparing transcallosal microsurgery with endoscopy. J Neurosurg 1994;81:174–8.

Procedure 48 Encephalocele Repair

David Gonda, Lissa C. Baird, Michael L. Levy

INDICATIONS

- The presence of an encephalocele is an indication for surgical repair. Encephaloceles are typically diagnosed at birth, although many are now identified in utero by ultrasound.
- Indications for the immediate repair of an encephalocele include open exposure to any meninges or brain, a ruptured encephalocele sac, and leakage of cerebrospinal fluid. Expeditious repair of the encephalocele in these circumstances minimizes the risk of a central nervous system infection.
- If the skin overlying the encephalocele is intact, surgical repair can be done on an elective basis.

CONTRAINDICATIONS

- There are few contraindications for repair of a congenital encephalocele because lethal meningitis eventually occurs if the encephalocele is left untreated. Surgical treatment is recommended unless the amount of herniated brain tissue exceeds the remaining intracranial brain tissue.
- Severe encephaloceles with other coexisting systemic or central nervous system abnormalities may be considered incompatible with long-term survival. Corrective or palliative surgery in these patients may have limited benefit.

PLANNING AND POSITIONING

- Of children with encephaloceles, 20% may have other congenital neurologic deformities that can affect the success of surgical treatment and long-term prognosis. Many of these children also have abnormalities of other organ systems that can affect treatment decisions. A complete multisystemic assessment of the patient is critical before surgical planning.
- **Figure 48-1:** Preoperative work-up should include magnetic resonance imaging (MRI) and magnetic resonance venography to determine the exact nature of the encephalocele and its contents. The extent of neural tissue herniation is the most important prognostic indicator and should be carefully assessed. The location of relevant vascular structures should be studied, especially venous sinus drainage.
- **Figure 48-2:** Positioning and surgical treatment of encephaloceles vary depending on the location of the lesion. In North America, approximately 80% of encephaloceles are found in the occipital region. These patients should be positioned prone on a horseshoe headrest after induction of anesthesia.

PROCEDURE

- **Figure 48-3:** After positioning of the patient, intravenous antibiotics are given. For occipital encephaloceles, the occipital and cervical areas are prepared with iodine solution and sterile drapes. For large encephalocele sacs, forceps can be used to elevate the sac gently to allow for complete skin preparation.
- **Figure 48-4:** Scalpel or monopolar cautery is used to divide the normal skin from the epithelialized skin circumferentially. A transverse incision can be extended to expose the underlying bone to elucidate the extent of the bony defect. The plane between the

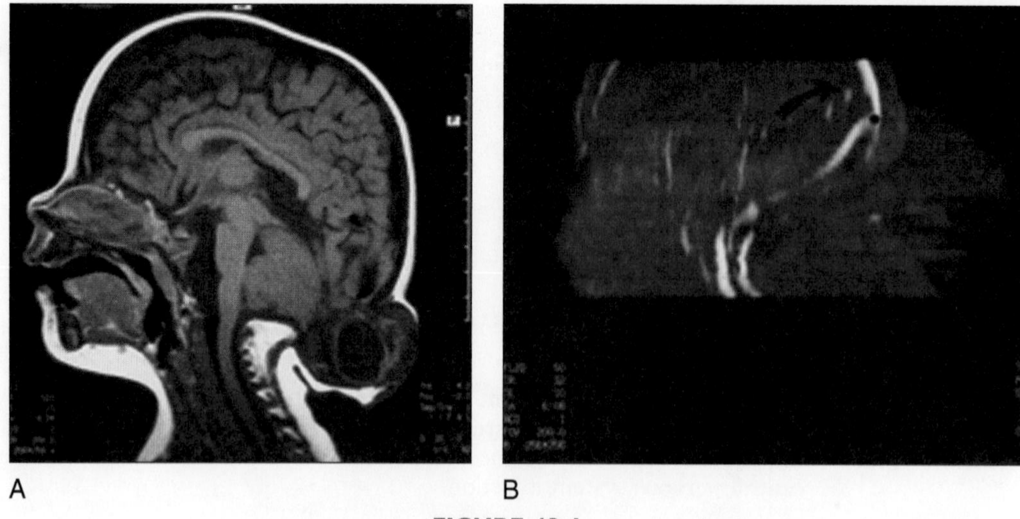

FIGURE 48-1

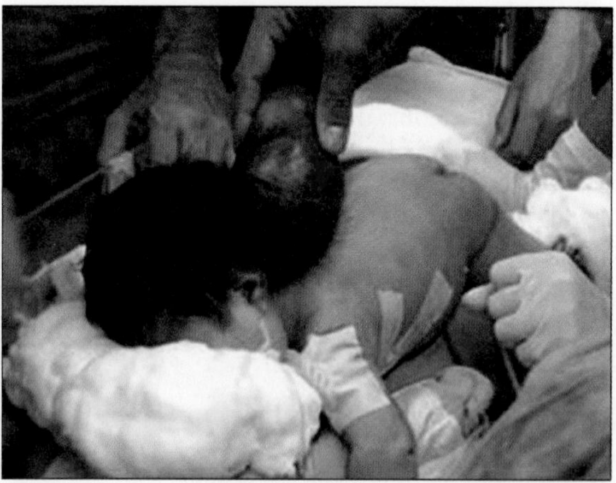

FIGURE 48-2

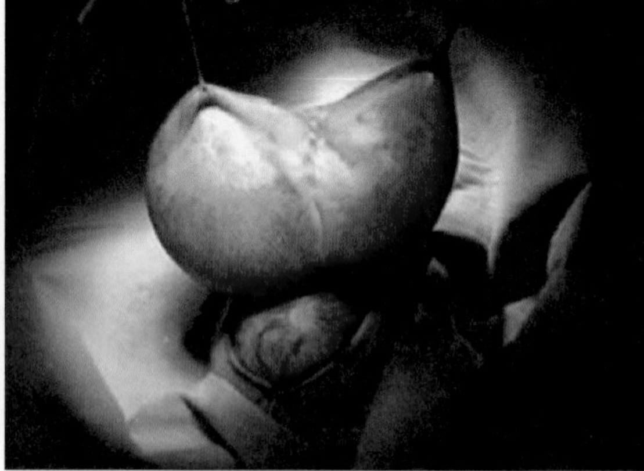

FIGURE 48-3

dura mater and skin is defined with dissection. The encephalocele mass is then opened, allowing egress of cerebrospinal fluid and exploration of the contents of the encephalocele sac. If the contents contain nonfunctional tissue (e.g., fibrous, gliotic), the sac can safely be transected at the level of the skull.

- **Figure 48-5:** If a large amount of functional herniated nervous tissue is present, an expansion cranioplasty may be attempted with titanium mesh, dural patch, or

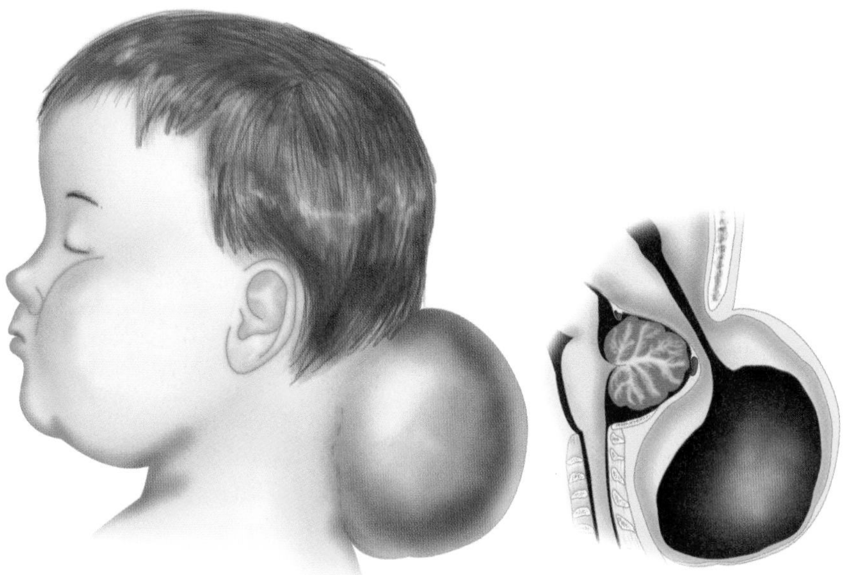

FIGURE 48-4

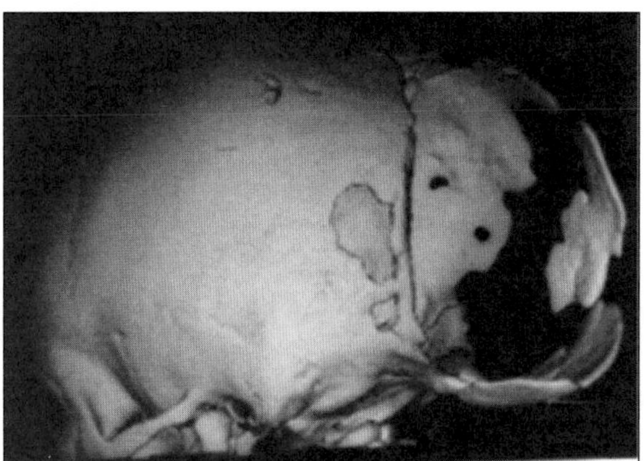

FIGURE 48-5

harvested bone. Alternatively, soft tissue can simply be closed around the neural elements, and the skull defect can be repaired at a later stage. Computed tomography (CT) scan shows a technique used by Mohanty et al using harvested calvarial graft to obtain partial bony coverage of the encephalocele.

- **Figure 48-6:** Sincipital encephaloceles require a different surgical approach. Lesions may vary in severity from occult encephaloceles to encephaloceles creating severe craniofacial deformities. The patient is positioned supine on a horseshoe headrest or in three-point fixation depending on the extent of the planned surgery.
- **Figure 48-7:** A bicoronal incision is used to achieve a cosmetic midline exposure of the defect. A midline frontal craniotomy is created. The dura is opened, and the superior sagittal sinus is ligated and divided.
- **Figure 48-8:** Frontal lobes are elevated, exposing the site of the bony defect and the herniating neural elements. The encephalocele is resected flush with the anterior cranial fossa.
- **Figure 48-9:** The dural defect is repaired with pericranium, fascia lata, or dural substitute graft.

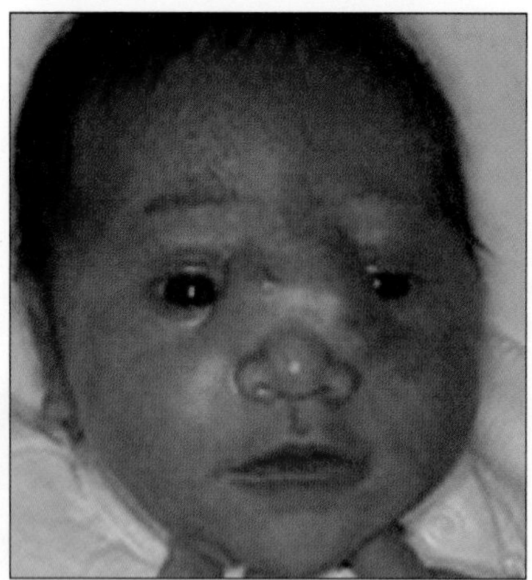

FIGURE 48-6

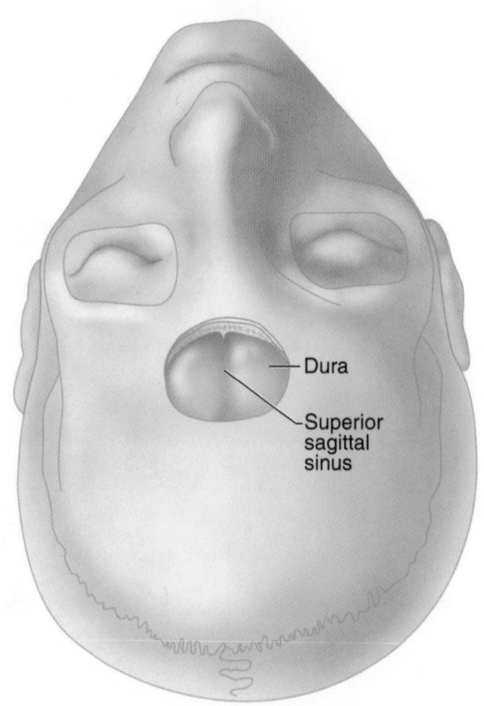

FIGURE 48-7

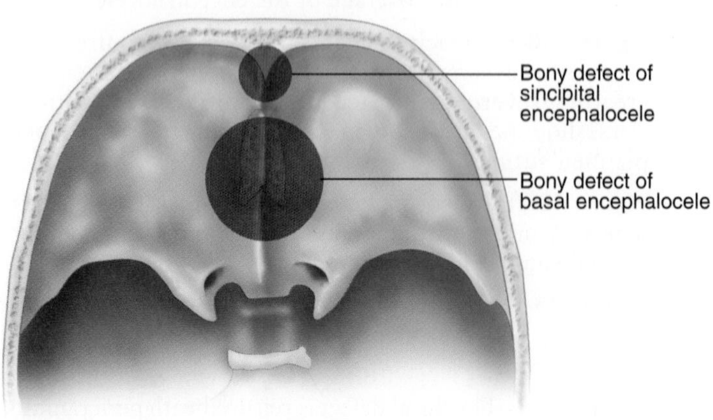

FIGURE 48-8

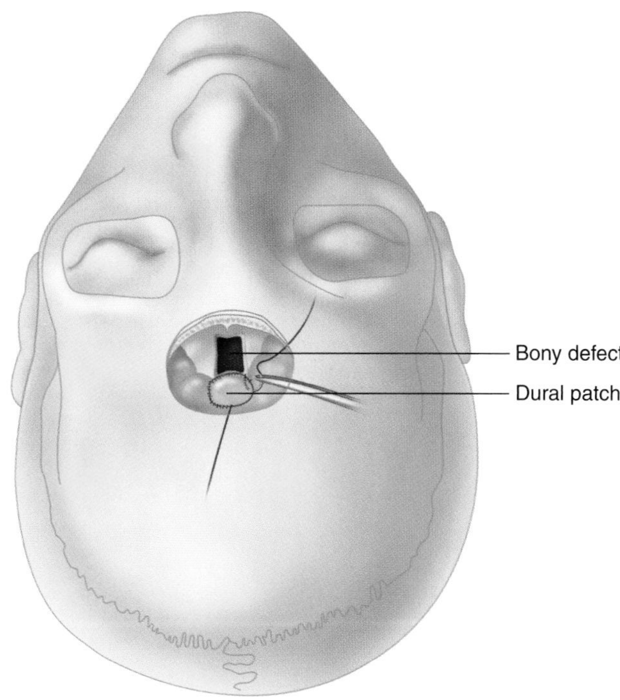

FIGURE 48-9

TIPS FROM THE MASTERS

- Intraoperative observation of the encephalocele contents can lead to a more accurate prognostic evaluation. If primitive glial tissue only is found within the encephalocele sac, the prognosis for neurologic outcome is optimistic. If functional and vital nervous tissue is found, the prognosis is less favorable.
- To prevent infection in patients who present with intact encephaloceles, every possible measure should be taken to avoid rupture. Pressure should be kept off the encephalocele sac at all times.
- Children with anterior encephaloceles benefit from a multidisciplinary craniofacial team to ensure correction of hypertelorism, obstructed nasolacrimal ducts, and other nasal deformities.

PITFALLS

Failure to identify an encephalocele in utero may lead to rupture of the encephalocele sac at the time of birth. A planned cesarean section allows for the protection of vital neural structures during delivery.

Vascular structures are frequently encountered within occipital encephaloceles. Inadequate preparation for the possible presence of these structures may lead to injury or sacrifice of critical draining veins and sinuses.

Inadequate exposure leads to incomplete resection of the encephalocele and poor postoperative results.

BAILOUT OPTIONS

- Large calvarial defects sometimes can be corrected by extending the skin incision into adjacent parietal regions and harvesting a craniotomy that can be transposed to the site of the defect. The parietal region contains osteogenic dura that ossifies and creates new bone within 6 months.

- Insufficient soft tissue or inadequate closures can result in dural defects, postoperative cerebrospinal fluid leaks, or pseudomeningocele formation. The use of dural grafts and sealants and lumbar drains helps to minimize this risk.

SUGGESTED READINGS

Bartels RH, Merx JL, Van Overbeeke JJ. Falcine sinus and occipital encephalocele: a magnetic resonance venography study. J Neurosurg 1998;89:738–41.

Mohanty A, Biswas A, Reddy M, et al. Expansile cranioplasty for massive occipital encephalocele. Childs Nerv Syst 2006;22:1170–6.

Mowafi HA, Sheikh BY, Al-Ghamdi AA. Positioning for anesthetic induction of neonates with encephalocele. Internet J Anesthesiol 2001;5(3).

Sather MD, Livingston AD, Puccioni MJ, et al. Large supra- and infra-tentorial occipital encephalocele encompassing posterior sagittal sinus and torcular Herophili. Childs Nerv Syst 2009;25:903–6.

Tubbs RS, Wellons JC, Oakes WJ. Occipital encephalocele, lipomeningomyelocele, and Chiari I malformation: case report and review of the literature. Childs Nerv Syst 2003;19:50–3.

Procedure 49

Craniosynostosis: Frontoorbital Advancement and Cranial Vault Reshaping (Open and Endoscopic)

Ryan C. Frank, Steven R. Cohen, Hal Meltzer

INDICATIONS

- The main indications for surgical intervention for craniosynostosis are the prevention of potential neurologic impairment and correction of deformity. Increased intracranial pressure, hydrocephalus, mental retardation, visual abnormalities, and learning disabilities all can be associated with craniosynostosis. Generally, the more sutures that are fused (as in the syndromic forms of craniosynostosis), the greater the likelihood of neurologic compromise. If there is any evidence of neurologic compromise, urgent surgical intervention should be performed.
- A secondary indication for surgical intervention is esthetic improvement of the skull shape, although for many patients this is the primary indication for treatment. Deformities of the skull as a result of craniosynostosis are best treated with cranial vault reshaping, preferably at an early age, before the calvarial bones have fully ossified.
- We prefer to perform open cranial vault reshaping on patients with multiple suture synostoses or severe single suture synostosis deformities, especially in older children The open approach of the affected skull via bicoronal incision provides the necessary exposure to address these deformities properly.
- We prefer to perform endoscopic cranial vault reshaping on patients with mild to moderate single suture synostoses before 4 to 6 months of age. The main benefits of this approach are diminished blood loss and limited incisions. Other benefits include decreased scarring and shorter hospital stays.
- We perform endoscopic repair for patients 3 to 6 months old with mild to moderate sagittal synostosis. We reserve the open approach for sagittal synostosis for patients with severe deformity.
- We perform endoscopic repair for patients 3 to 6 months old with mild metopic synostosis. We perform open cranial vault reshaping with frontoorbital advancement for patients with moderate to severe metopic synostosis.
- We perform endoscopic repair for patients 3 to 6 months old with mild unicoronal synostosis. We perform open cranial vault reshaping with frontoorbital advancement for patients with moderate to severe unicoronal synostosis.
- We perform open cranial vault reshaping for patients 3 to 6 months old with mild to moderate to severe lambdoid synostosis.
- We perform open cranial vault reshaping with or without frontoorbital advancement for patients with syndromic craniosynostosis or multiple suture–involved nonsyndromic craniosynostosis.
- Treatment of midface deformity and associated hypertelorbitism is beyond the scope of this chapter, but such treatments are critical aspects of care in most patients with syndromic craniosynostosis.

CONTRAINDICATIONS

- Significant medical comorbidities that would preventing a safe anesthetic should be adequately dealt with before surgical intervention.

- No cranial vault reshaping should be performed if there is questionable soft tissue coverage present over the calvaria, or if there is active infection present in any of the layers of the scalp.

PLANNING AND POSITIONING

- Preoperative evaluation includes obtaining laboratory values (complete blood count) and crossmatching for 1 to 2 U of packed red blood cells. Three-dimensional reconstruction of a computed tomography (CT) scan of the head is obtained preoperatively in all patients. Blood products usually are not required for endoscopic patients; however, most patients undergoing open vault reshaping require transfusion of blood products.
- Patients are given preoperative antibiotics immediately before skin incision.
- For anterior skull exposure, the patient is positioned supine.
- For vertex and posterior skull exposure, the patient is positioned in the sphinx position.
- **Figure 49-1:** The patient is positioned so that easy, complete access to the pathologic deformity is obtainable.
- **Figure 49-2:** Two small incisions are used for endoscopic sagittal synostosis repair. One incision is placed anterior to the fused suture, and one is placed posterior to the fused suture. Incisions are long enough to allow introduction of the necessary instruments for proper exposure and resection of suture with synostosis.
- **Figure 49-3:** Planned incisions are injected with a mixture of 0.25% bupivacaine and 1:200,000 epinephrine.

PROCEDURE

- **Figure 49-4:** Scalp incisions are made with cutting frequency on monopolar cautery. Dissection is carried out in the subgaleal plane over the fused suture and surrounding calvaria.
- **Figure 49-5:** Dissection is performed in the subpericranial plane directly around the fused suture and around the fontanelles.
- **Figure 49-6:** Dissection is performed between the inner table of the fused sagittal suture and the underlying dura.

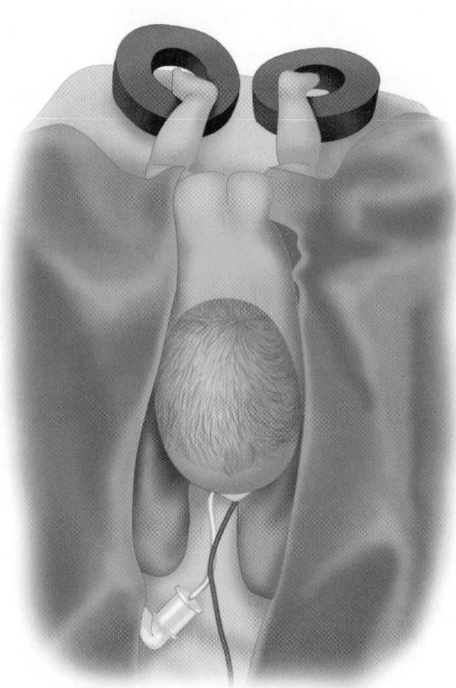

FIGURE 49-1

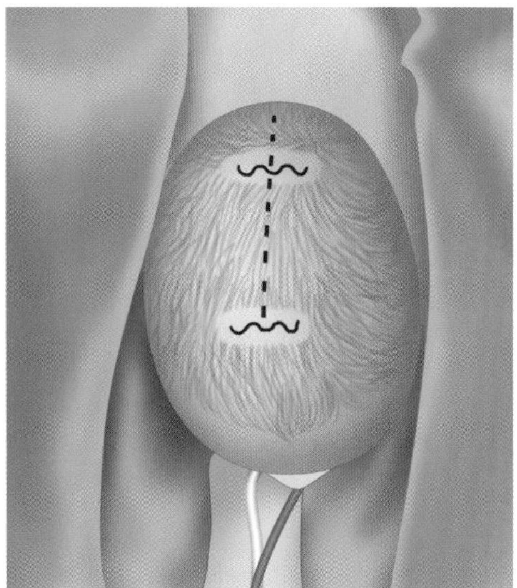

FIGURE 49-2

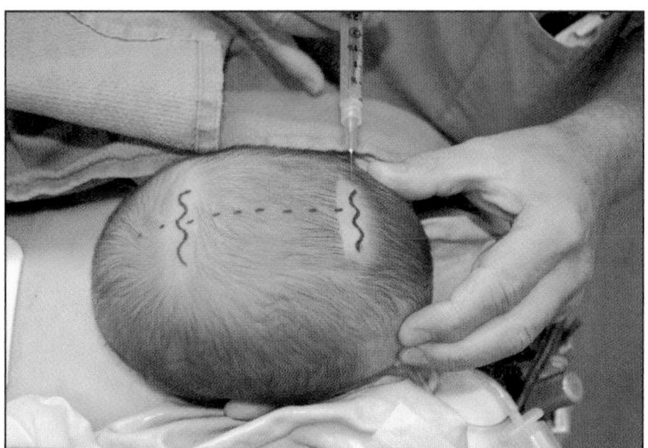

FIGURE 49-3

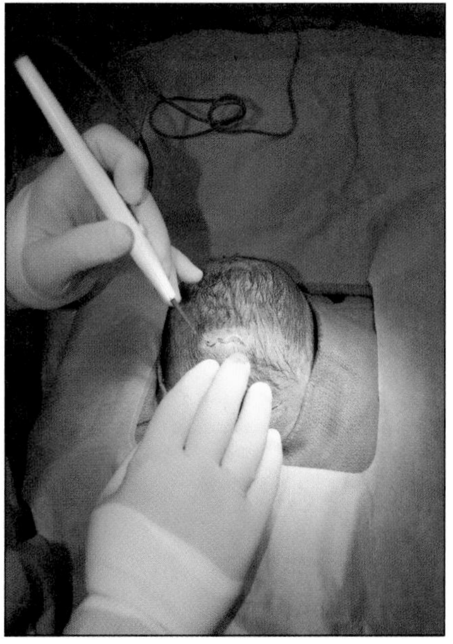

FIGURE 49-4

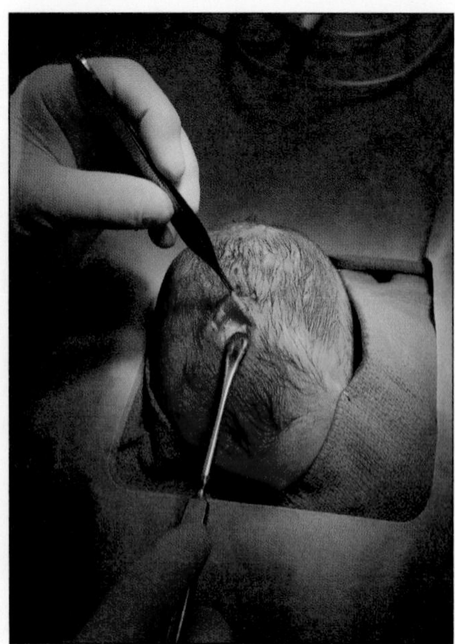

FIGURE 49-5

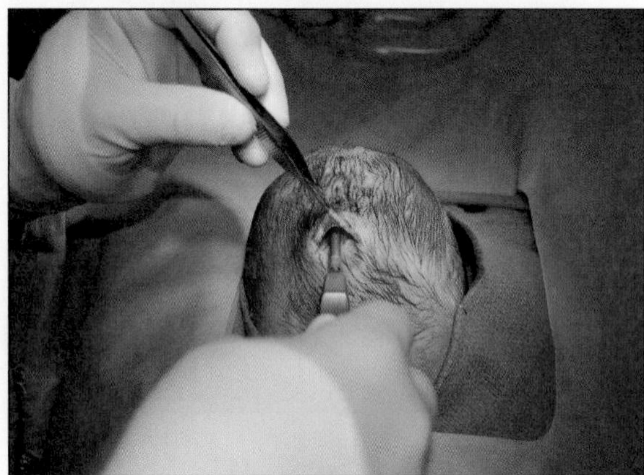

FIGURE 49-6

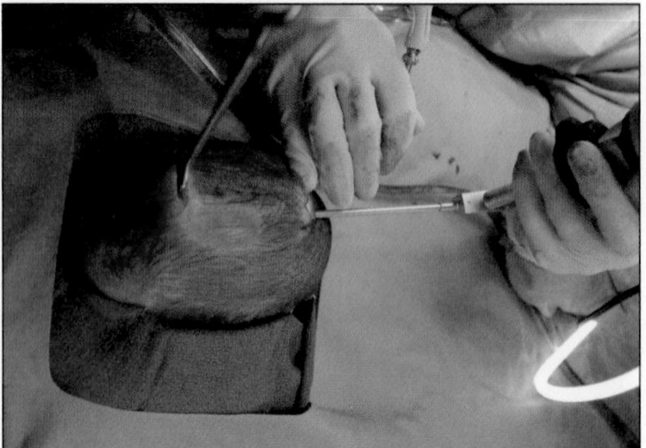

FIGURE 49-7

- **Figure 49-7:** The endoscope is introduced beneath calvarial bone on one end of the fused suture.
- **Figure 49-8:** Mayo scissors are used to cut bone on either side of the fused suture, while watching via endoscope that the scissors remain safely away from the dura. The fused suture is then removed.

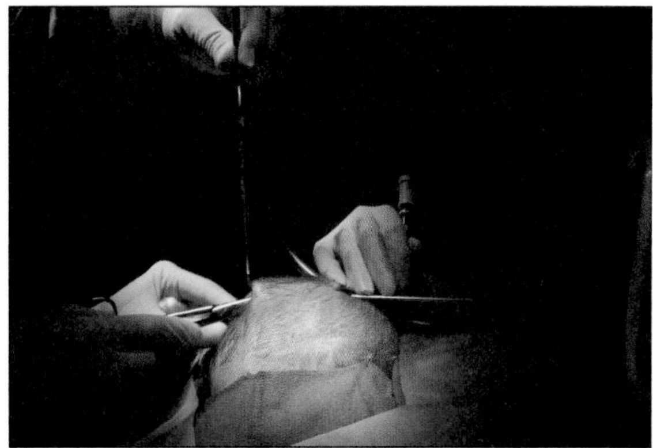

FIGURE 49-8

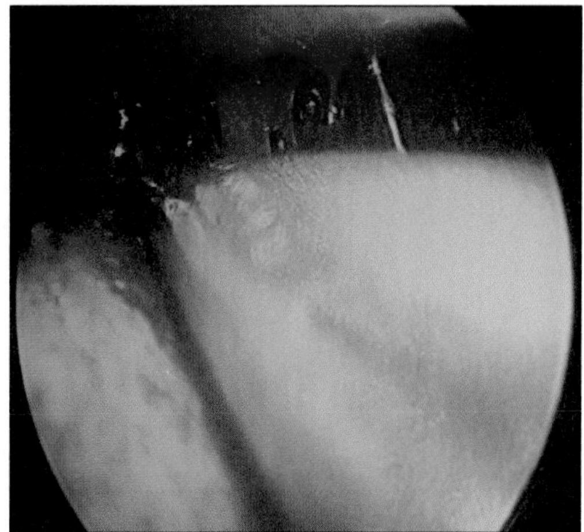

FIGURE 49-9

- **Figure 49-9:** The endoscope is used to ensure safe dissection of the dura and removal of the fused segment of the calvaria.
- **Figure 49-10:** When the fused calvaria is cut on either side of the fusion, it can be removed.
- **Figure 49-11:** Hemostasis is obtained with bipolar cautery and topical hemostatic agents.
- **Figure 49-12:** The wound is thoroughly irrigated with bacitracin saline. Suture closure of the galea aponeurotica and scalp skin is performed.

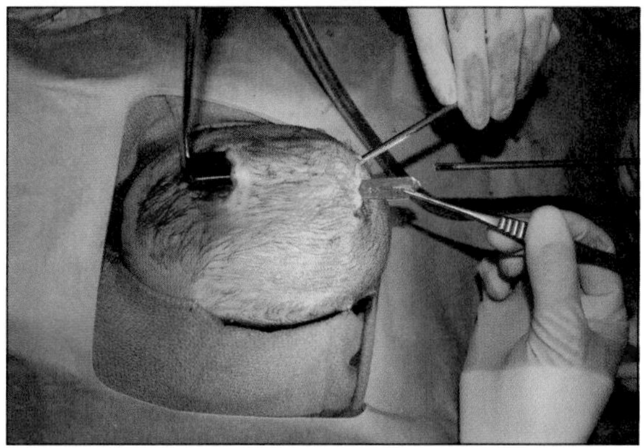

FIGURE 49-10

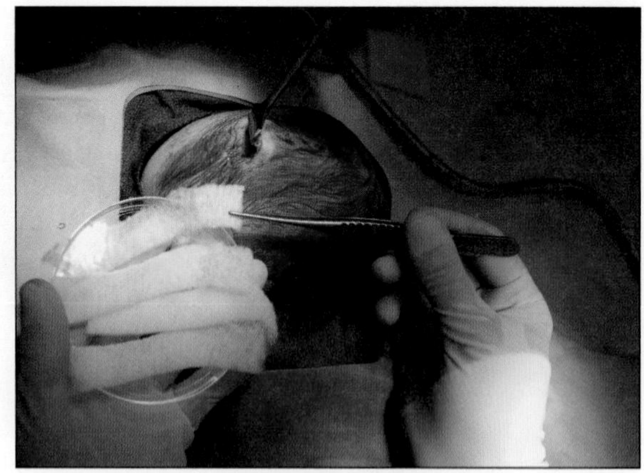

FIGURE 49-11

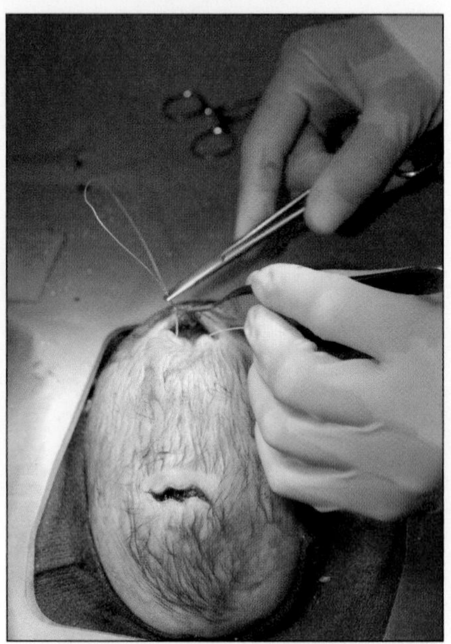

FIGURE 49-12

TIPS FROM THE MASTERS

- Endoscopic reshaping ideally should be performed by 3 to 4 months of age to optimize esthetic outcomes. We have found protracted cranial banding and suboptimal reconstructive results to be common in older children undergoing endoscopic approaches.

PITFALLS

Patients treated via endoscopic reshaping should be placed in a cranial molding helmet within 1 week of the surgery. This component of the treatment is necessary to optimize the desired postoperative cranial vault shape. Helmet therapy typically lasts 3 to 6 months after operative treatment.

BAILOUT OPTIONS

- If significant intraoperative bleeding or evidence of intravascular entrainment of air is encountered, rapid conversion to an open approach should be considered in these potentially life-threatening conditions.

SUGGESTED READINGS

Cohen SR, Holmes RE, Meltzer HS, et al. Immediate cranial vault reconstruction with bioresorbable plates following endoscopically assisted sagittal synostectomy. J Craniofac Surg 2002;13:578–82.

Cohen SR, Holmes RE, Ozgur BM, et al. Fronto-orbital and cranial osteotomies with resorbable fixation using an endoscopic approach. Clin Plast Surg 2004;31:429–42.

Hinojosa J, Esparza J, Munoz MJ. Endoscopic-assisted osteotomies for the treatment of craniosynostosis. Child Nerv Syst 2007;23:1421–30.

Stelnicki EJ. Endoscopic treatment of craniosynostosis. Atlas Oral Maxillofac Surg Clin North Am 2002;10:57–72.

Procedure 50 Arachnoid Cyst Fenestration

Lissa C. Baird, Andrew P. Thomas, Michael L. Levy

INDICATIONS

- Fenestration of arachnoid cysts is indicated in cysts that show significant increase in size or associated clinical symptoms. The size of an arachnoid cyst typically remains stable or increases over time, and associated symptoms are unlikely to resolve spontaneously. Symptoms may include headaches, craniomegaly, developmental delay, and seizures.
- Surgical treatment of arachnoid cysts that are large enough to cause mass effect but that remain asymptomatic is controversial. One option is to observe these cysts; however, many neurosurgeons believe that any arachnoid cyst causing significant mass effect should be treated to minimize the possibility of developmental adverse effects or the risk of subdural hemorrhage.
- If initial fenestration fails, or if the cyst is in an anatomic location that makes success with fenestration unlikely, a shunting procedure is indicated. Cyst-peritoneum, cyst-ventricle, or cyst-subarachnoid shunts all are possible shunting treatment options.

CONTRAINDICATIONS

- Most arachnoid cysts do not require treatment. Small and asymptomatic arachnoid cysts should be observed clinically without any intervention.
- Incidentally found cysts that remain stable in size and do not have any associated symptoms or significant mass effect on surrounding neural structures should not be treated.

PLANNING AND POSITIONING

- Treatment options include open resection of the entire cyst wall, fenestration into the ventricle or subarachnoid spaces, and shunting procedures. Our first-line treatment for middle fossa arachnoid cysts involves a keyhole craniotomy and fenestration of the cyst allowing for communication with the basal cisterns.
- Similar fenestration procedures can be performed for cerebellopontine and retrocerebellar arachnoid cysts.
- Whenever possible, the procedure should be planned to fenestrate the arachnoid cyst in two locations: at an entrance site and an exit site.
- **Figure 50-1:** Appropriate neuroimaging is obtained to show the anatomy of the arachnoid cyst and its relationship to surrounding cerebrospinal fluid (CSF) spaces and neural and bony structures. Although the diagnosis of arachnoid cyst is most commonly confirmed with computed tomography (CT), magnetic resonance imaging (MRI) is the most sensitive study for evaluating an arachnoid cyst. The appearance is typically a well-defined nonenhancing mass that is isointense to CSF on all MRI series. This appearance differentiates them from other types of cysts that contain more proteinaceous fluid.
- **Figure 50-2:** Patient positioning depends on the location of the cyst. For microsurgical keyhole fenestration of middle fossa arachnoid cysts, the patient is positioned supine and in three-point Mayfield pin fixation. The head is turned so that the side with the cyst is positioned at the uppermost aspect.
- **Figure 50-3:** A 1.5-cm vertical incision is planned superior to the zygoma and behind the hairline.

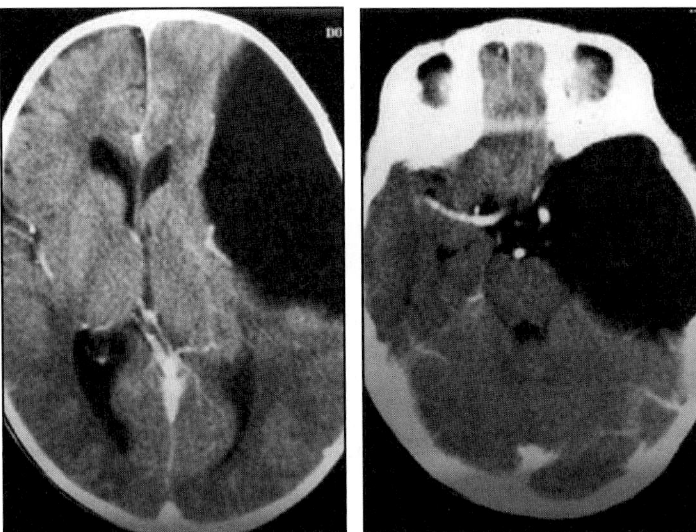

FIGURE 50-1

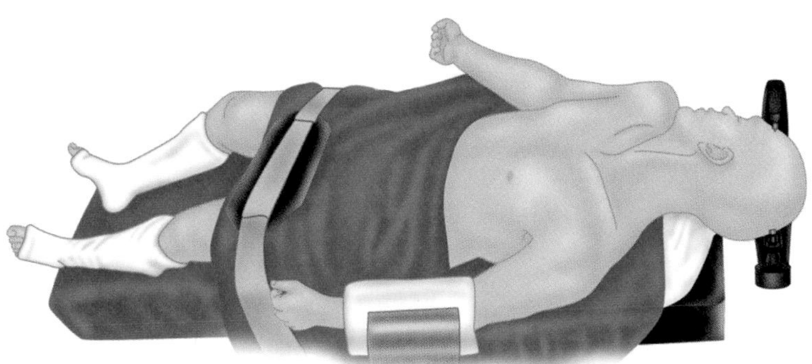

FIGURE 50-2

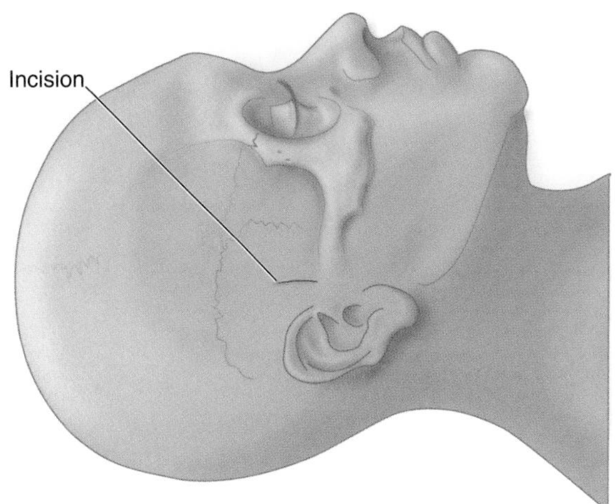

FIGURE 50-3

PROCEDURE

- **Figure 50-4:** After the incision, dissection is carried out through the temporalis muscle down to temporal bone. The soft tissue is elevated laterally with a periosteal instrument, and a small self-retaining retractor is placed.
- **Figure 50-5:** A single burr hole is placed at the inferior aspect, and a small craniotomy is created using retraction of soft tissue circumferentially as the craniotomy is turned.

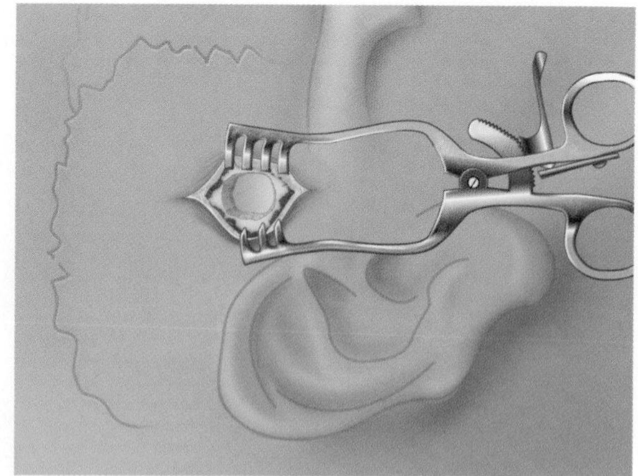

FIGURE 50-4

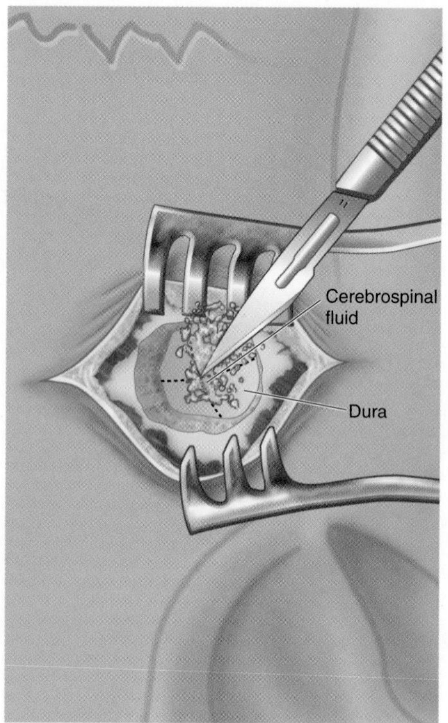

FIGURE 50-5

The diameter is approximately 1 cm. The dura is identified, coagulated, and opened in a cruciate fashion with a No. 11 blade.

- **Figure 50-6:** The dural leaflets are reflected outward. The superficial thickened arachnoid of the cyst wall can be identified at this point.
- **Figure 50-7:** Under microscopic vision, appropriate landmarks are identified. These landmarks include the temporal floor, tentorium, and cranial nerves III and IV. The deeper arachnoid wall of the cyst can be identified and typically noted to be thickened and grossly abnormal. Division of membrane allows CSF egress and identification of vascular structures, including the internal carotid artery and posterior communicating artery.
- **Figure 50-8:** The thickened arachnoid around cranial nerve III and the posterior communicating artery is fenestrated. Next, the membrane of Lillequist is identified and opened. On completion of fenestrations, wide communications should exist

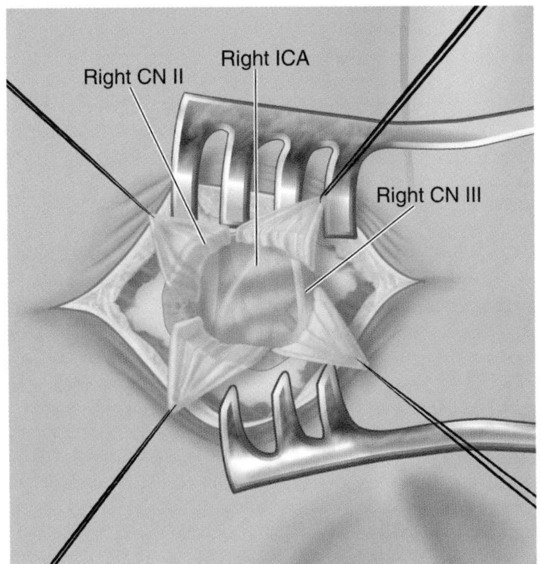

FIGURE 50-6

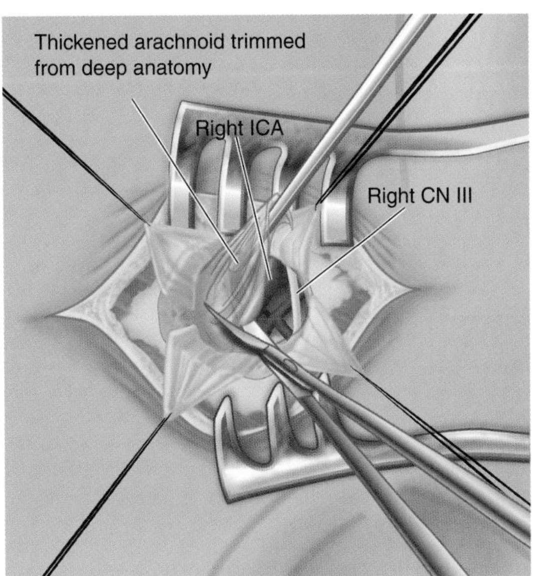

FIGURE 50-7

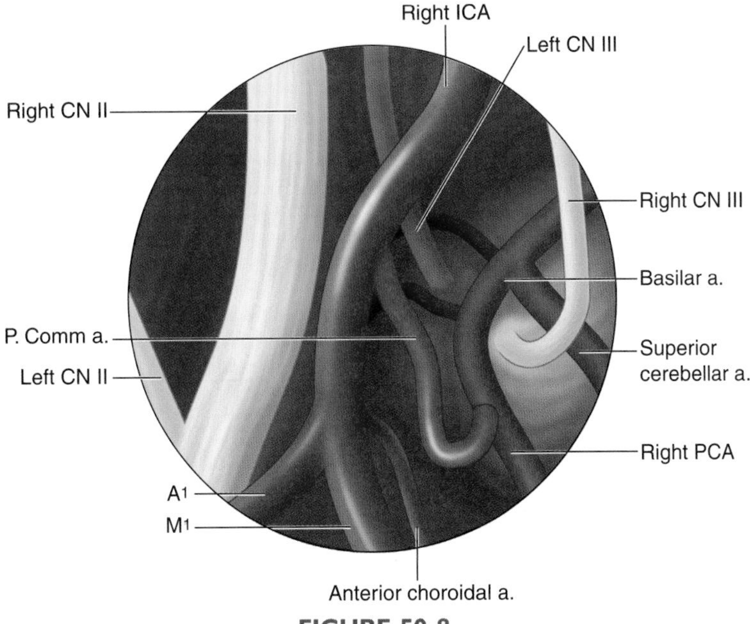

FIGURE 50-8

between the space of the arachnoid cyst and the basilar cisterns, allowing for flow of CSF between these spaces. The basilar artery, superior cerebellar artery, and posterior cerebral artery should be visualized.

Closure

- After flow of CSF through the fenestrations is verified, the dura is reapproximated with 4-0 Nurolon suture (Ethicon, Inc., Sommerville, NJ). Gelfoam is placed over the dural closure, and the bone flap is secured with titanium microplates.

TIPS FROM THE MASTERS

- Most surgically treated arachnoid cysts are not completely obliterated on follow-up neuroimaging; this does not correlate, however, with symptomatic improvement.
- Although open craniotomy and fenestration is preferable for cysts being fenestrated superficially or into basal cisterns, endoscopic fenestration for cysts within the ventricular system may be the ideal approach.

PITFALLS

Inadequate or limited fenestrations do not allow for effective communication of CSF with the basal cisterns and contribute to failure of the procedure.

The perforating vessels of the basilar artery must be protected, and great care should be taken when opening the membrane of Lillequist and creating communication pathways into the basal cisterns.

Because the incision is frequently in close approximation to a large CSF space, a watertight closure should be attempted to minimize the risk of a CSF leak.

BAILOUT OPTIONS

- Shunting of a cyst in the setting of a failed fenestration or shunting of cysts not adjacent to a cistern is the fallback procedure of choice.
- Associated hydrocephalus frequently does not improve after treatment of a symptomatic arachnoid cyst and may occasionally occur as a delayed finding from abnormal CSF circulation. These patients require treatment with a ventriculoperitoneal shunt.

SUGGESTED READINGS

Fewel M, Levy ML, McComb J. Surgical treatment of 95 children with 102 intracranial arachnoid cysts. Pediatr Neurosurg 1996;25:165–73.

Levy ML, Meltzer HS, Hughes S, et al. Hydrocephalus in children with middle fossa arachnoid cysts. J Neurosurg 2004;101(1S):25–31.

Ozgur BM, Aryan HE, Levy ML. Microsurgical keyhole middle fossa arachnoid cyst fenestration. J Clin Neurosci 2005;12:804–6.

Pradilla G, Jallo G. Arachnoid cysts: case series and review of the literature. Neurosurg Focus 2007;22:E7.

Tamburrini G, D'Angelo L, Paternoster G, et al. Endoscopic management of intra and paraventricular CSF cysts. Childs Nerv Syst 2007;23:645–51.

Figures 50-3 through 50-8 redrawn with permission from Ozgur BM, Aryan HE, Levy ML. Microsurgical keyhole middle fossa arachnoid cyst fenestration. J Clin Neurosci 2005;12:804–6.

Procedure 51 Endoscopic Third Ventriculostomy

Lissa C. Baird, Michael L. Levy

INDICATIONS

- Patients with late-onset (adolescent or adult) nontumoral obstructive hydrocephalus have the highest rate of success after endoscopic third ventriculostomy (close to 90%). The high success rate in this group is likely related to the presence of intact pathways for cerebrospinal fluid (CSF) absorption.
- Patients with obstructive hydrocephalus resulting from other etiologies also have high success rates after this procedure. These etiologies include CSF pathway obstruction from tumors, cysts, infectious or hemorrhagic processes, and congenital obstructive hydrocephalus.
- Attempts to treat other forms of hydrocephalus with endoscopic third ventriculostomy have lower rates of success and are controversial. Regardless, successful outcomes have been reported after this procedure in patients with spinal dysraphism–associated hydrocephalus, slit ventricle syndrome, shunt infection or malfunction, normal-pressure hydrocephalus, encephalocele-associated hydrocephalus, and idiopathic hydrocephalus.

CONTRAINDICATIONS

- Patients who have anatomic features that prevent them from being able to undergo endoscopic third ventriculostomy safely are not candidates for the procedure. The patient must have sufficient space between the basilar artery and the clivus under the floor of the third ventricle and a sufficiently enlarged third ventricle to allow for movement of the endoscope without injury to the lateral walls of the ventricle or surrounding structures.
- Patients with a history of prior whole-brain radiation, meningitis, or subarachnoid hemorrhage with associated subarachnoid scarring have impaired CSF absorption pathways and are highly unlikely to benefit from endoscopic third ventriculostomy.
- Relative contraindications include the presence of communicating hydrocephalus, slit-like ventricles, thin cortical mantle, history of prior shunt placement or meningitis, and age younger than 2 years. Because successful reports have been described in patients who have all of these features, the decision to offer the procedure to patients with relative contraindications is at the discretion of the treating neurosurgeon.

PLANNING AND POSITIONING

- Before surgery, standard laboratory values should be obtained, including basic metabolic profile, complete blood count, and coagulation profile. The etiology of hydrocephalus should be assessed, and the likelihood of a successful outcome and possibility for future shunting procedures should be discussed with the patient and family.
- **Figure 51-1:** Preoperative evaluation should include careful study of the patient's ventricular anatomy. Sagittal magnetic resonance imaging (MRI) should be obtained to evaluate the relationship between the floor of the third ventricle and the underlying structures in the interpeduncular cistern.
- **Figure 51-2:** After induction of anesthesia, the patient is placed in the supine position with a small roll under the shoulders. The head is placed in a doughnut-shaped head support or horseshoe headrest and elevated approximately 30 degrees to prevent excessive CSF loss. The endoscope monitor should be positioned directly opposite the surgeon for unobstructed viewing during the endoscopic portion of the procedure. A small area of the scalp is shaved, and after standard skin preparation and draping, a 2- to 3-cm vertical incision is made based at the coronal suture and in the mid-pupillary line.

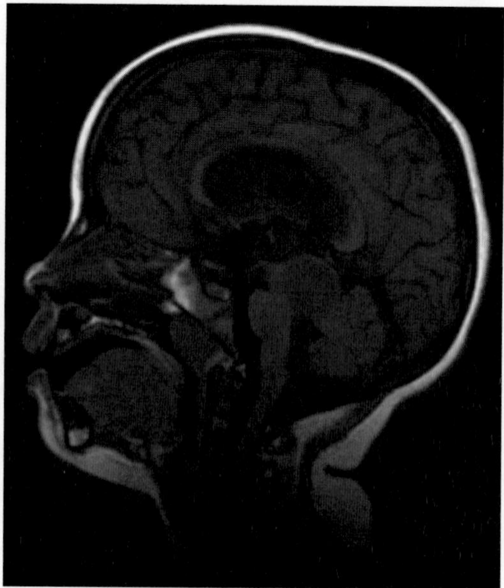

FIGURE 51-1

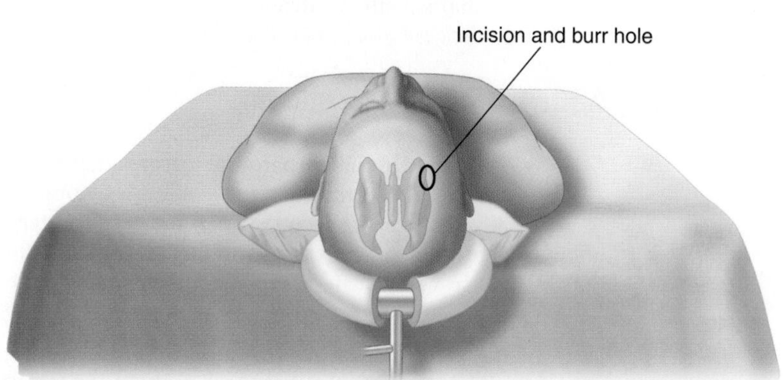

FIGURE 51-2

PROCEDURE

- **Figure 51-3:** A burr hole is placed in the skull slightly anterior to the coronal suture at the mid-pupillary line. The dura is incised and coagulated. The lateral ventricle is cannulated using a peel-away sheath with a ventricular introducer. The sheath is secured to drapes. After the stylet is withdrawn, the endoscope is inserted through the sheath into the lateral ventricle. Structures of the lateral ventricle are identified, including the fornix, choroid plexus, and septal and thalamostriate veins.
- **Figure 51-4:** The endoscope is advanced through the foramen of Monro and into the third ventricle. Mammillary bodies are identified and used as the posterior landmark. The infundibular recess is identified as the anterior landmark of the area of interest.
- **Figure 51-5:** The floor of the third ventricle is usually attenuated, and the basilar artery may be visualized. The fenestration site should be selected immediately posterior to the infundibular recess.
- **Figure 51-6:** The initial opening in the floor can be made with neuroendoscopic instruments or monopolar cautery. A small Fogarty balloon is advanced through the working channel of the endoscope and passed through the initial fenestration.
- **Figure 51-7:** The fogarty balloon is slowly inflated to dilate the opening. A small amount of bleeding is frequently seen and usually resolves with gentle irrigation.
- **Figure 51-8:** After creation of the fenestration, fluctuations in the floor of the third ventricle indicate CSF flow. The endoscope can be passed through the opening and

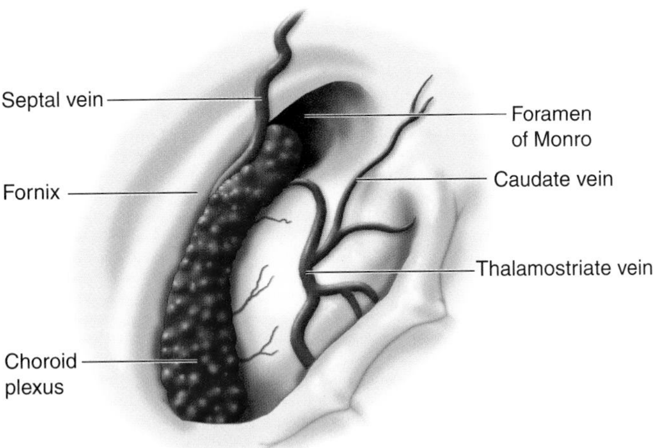

FIGURE 51-3

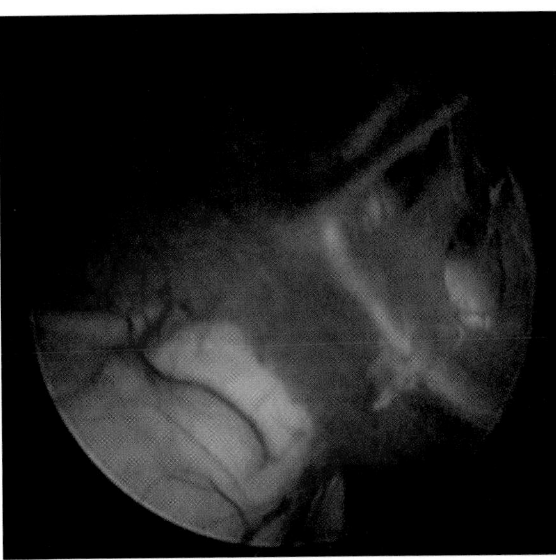

FIGURE 51-4

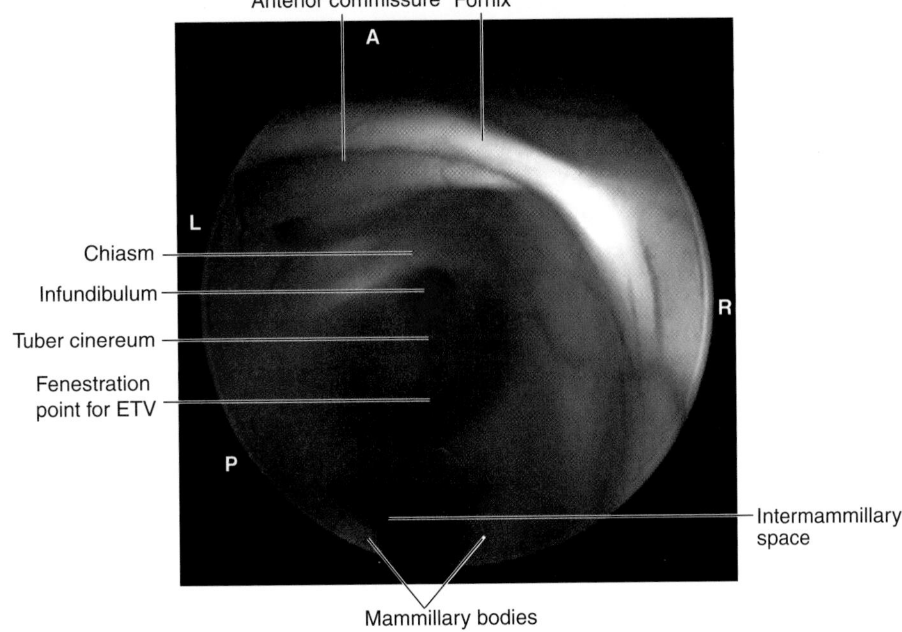

FIGURE 51-5

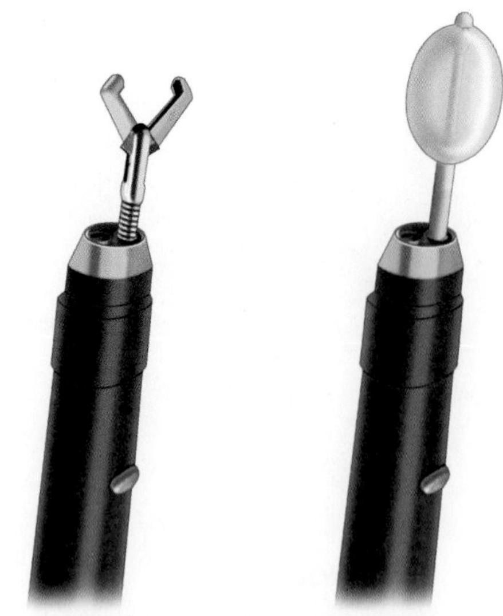

FIGURE 51-6

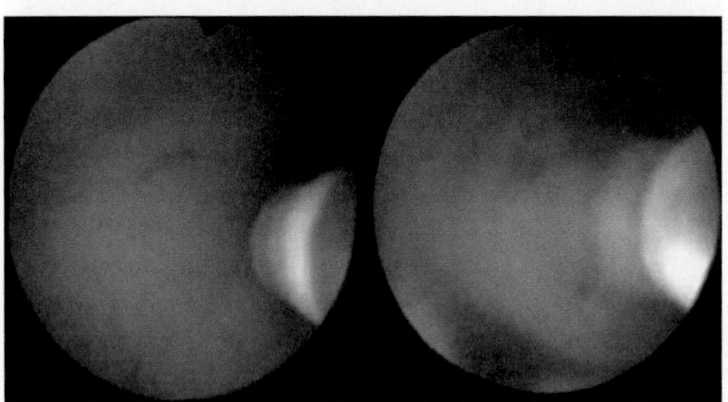

FIGURE 51-7

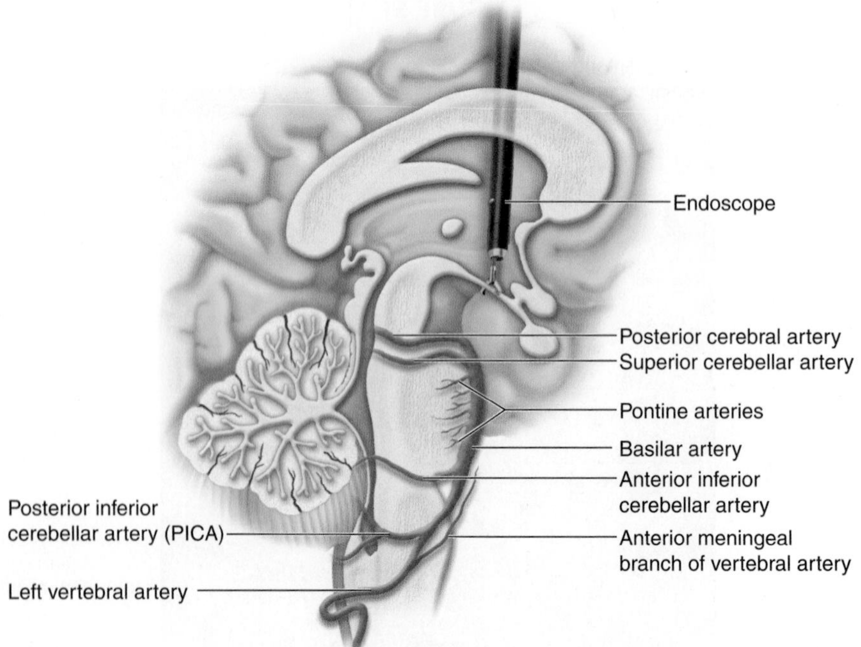

FIGURE 51-8

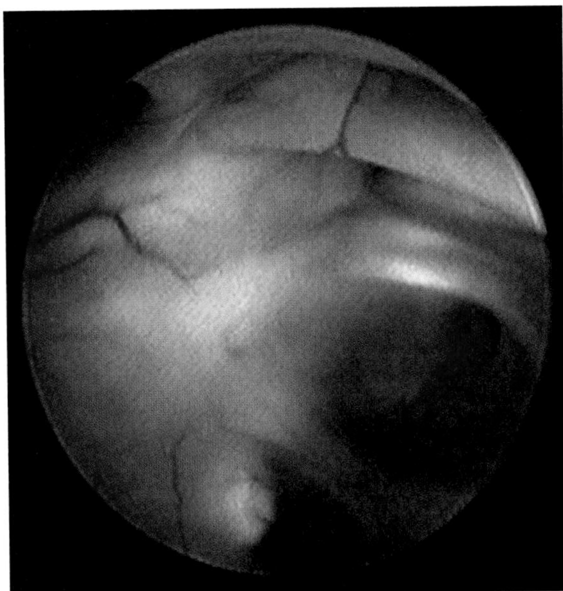

FIGURE 51-9

into the interpeduncular cistern to ensure no structures were injured and to assess for complete fenestration and opening of the membrane of Lillequist.

- **Figure 51-9:** The basilar artery and branches can be visualized during this step. The endoscope is slowly withdrawn into the lateral ventricle and through the parenchymal tract along with the sheath to inspect for hemostasis. If excessive bleeding is encountered during the procedure, or if there is concern for elevated intracranial pressure, a ventriculostomy catheter should be left in place. A Gelfoam pledget is placed in the burr hole. In larger openings, a burr hole plate can be used. The scalp is closed in anatomic fashion.

TIPS FROM THE MASTERS

- Fenestration should be performed at the most transparent portion of the third ventricular floor to minimize the risk of vascular injury.
- Using blunt instruments for the initial fenestration instead of cautery or sharp instruments minimizes the risk to underlying vascular structures that are not directly visualized.
- When endoscopic third ventriculostomy is performed before posterior fossa tumor resection, the incidence of postoperative hydrocephalus is significantly reduced.

PITFALLS

A misplaced fenestration is the primary cause of severe complications, including injury to the hypothalamus or basilar artery. A basilar injury is the most serious complication and can result in hemorrhage, stroke, or pseudoaneurysm formation.

Excessive manipulation of the endoscope while in the third ventricle can lead to damage to the structures surrounding the foramen of Monro, including the fornix. Such damage can lead to short-term memory deficits.

Blind inflation of the Fogarty balloon in the interpeduncular cistern before withdrawing the balloon into the third ventricle may inadvertently tear small perforating vessels. It is safer to inflate the balloon with the epicenter at the level of the fenestration.

An unrecognized delayed failure of endoscopic third ventriculostomy can lead to herniation and death.

BAILOUT OPTIONS

- If hemorrhage is encountered during the procedure, persistent irrigation should be used until the bleeding stops and CSF clears.
- If the presence of blood in CSF significantly compromises visibility through the endoscope, the procedure should be aborted to prevent injury to neurovascular structures that cannot be visualized clearly.
- A ventriculostomy drain can be left in place if there is blood or debris left in the ventricle to allow for postoperative drainage and intracranial pressure monitoring.

SUGGESTED READINGS

Drake JM. Ventriculostomy for the treatment of hydrocephalus. Neurosurg Clin N Am 1993;4:657–66.

Drake JM, Kulkarni AV, Kestle J. Endoscopic third ventriculostomy versus ventriculoperitoneal shunt in pediatric patients: a decision analysis. Childs Nerv Syst 2009;25:467–72.

Farin A, Aryan HE, Ozgur BM, et al. Endoscopic third ventriculostomy. J Clin Neurosci 2006;13:763–70.

Rekate HL. Selecting patients for endoscopic third ventriculostomy. Neurosurg Clin N Am 2004;15:39–49.

Teo C, Jones R. Management of hydrocephalus by endoscopic third ventriculostomy in patients with myelomeningocele. Pediatr Neurosurg 1996;25:57–63.

Procedure 52

Insertion of Ventriculoperitoneal Shunt

Hal Meltzer

INDICATIONS

- Hydrocephalus, communicating or obstructive, which is not amenable to endoscopic third ventriculostomy or treatment of primary etiology (i.e., removal of fourth ventricle neoplasm)
- Failure of previously placed shunt system

CONTRAINDICATIONS

- Fevers or any evidence of active intracranial infection
- Abnormal cerebrospinal fluid (CSF) rheology (high protein, pleocytosis, intraventricular hemorrhage)
- Body weight less than 2 kg (relative)

PLANNING AND POSITIONING

- All patients should have recent preoperative imaging with computed tomography (CT) or magnetic resonance imaging (MRI).
- The patient receives preoperative antibiotics before the skin incision. Hair clipping is minimized.
- **Figure 52-1:** The patient is positioned supine with the head turned to the left. A bump is placed under the shoulders to allow for straight trajectory from the right occiput, across the clavicle, to the abdomen.

PROCEDURE

- **Figure 52-2:** An abdominal incision is made in a horizontal fashion in the right mid-abdomen with needle electrocautery. Fascial layers are incised sharply, and muscle fiber division is minimized.

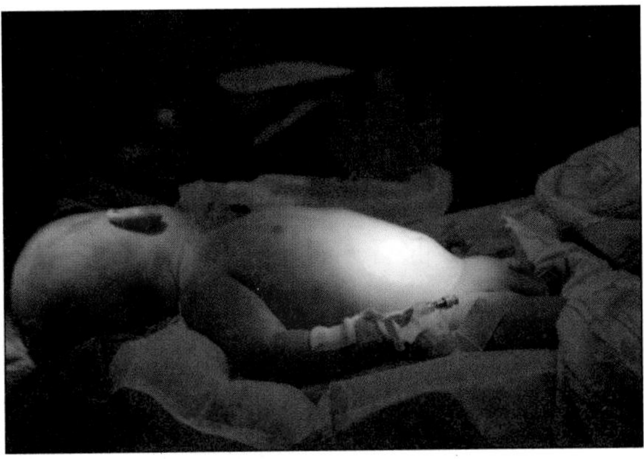

FIGURE 52-1

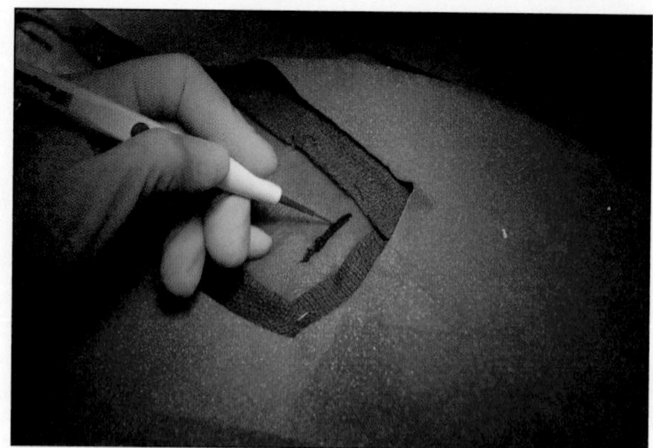

FIGURE 52-2

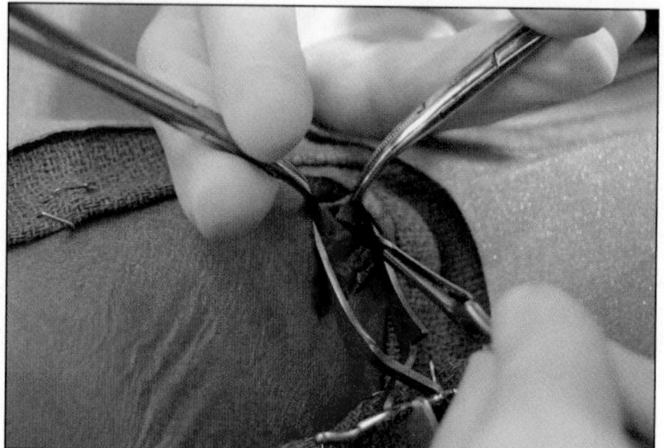

FIGURE 52-3

- **Figure 52-3:** The peritoneum is gently elevated with mosquito clamps and incised with a No. 11 blade. Care is taken to avoid bowel injury. Visual confirmation of entry into the peritoneal cavity is made.
- **Figure 52-4:** A cranial incision is made in a curvilinear fashion over the flat portion of the right parietooccipt with needle electrocautery.
- **Figure 52-5:** A small burr hole is made at the approximate horizontal level of the nasion with a high-speed drill and "matchstick" bit.
- **Figure 52-6:** After creating a subcutaneous pocket with blunt dissection to accommodate the reservoir and valve, a subcutaneous tunneler is passed from the cranial to the abdominal incision. An antibiotic-impregnated distal catheter is passed through the tunneler, and the tunneler is removed.
- **Figure 52-7:** An antisiphon valve is secured to the proximal end of the distal catheter.
- **Figure 52-8:** A small hole in the dura, slightly larger than the diameter of the ventricular catheter, is made by electrocautery applied to a blunt needle.
- **Figure 52-9:** The antibiotic-impregnated ventricular catheter is cut to an age-appropriate length and passed over a stylet into the right lateral ventricle. After egress of clear CSF is confirmed, the ventricular catheter is secured to the valve, and the valve is placed in the previously created subcutaneous scalp pocket.
- **Figure 52-10:** After confirmation of steady egress of CSF from the distal catheter, the catheter is fed into the peritoneal cavity under direct vision.

Closure

- The abdominal incision is closed in peritoneal, fascial, subcutaneous, and skin layers. The scalp incision is closed in galeal and skin layers.

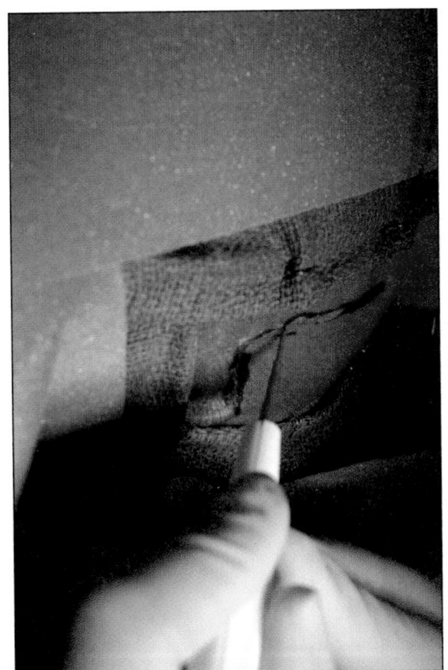

FIGURE 52-4

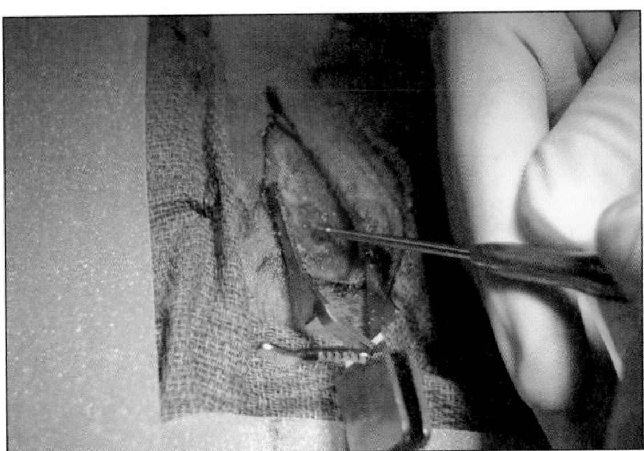

FIGURE 52-5

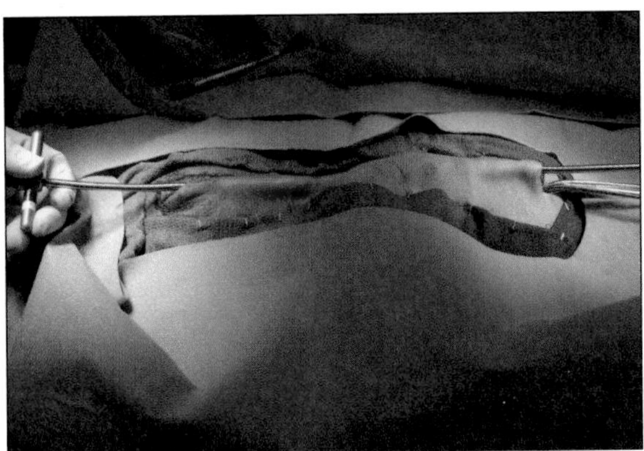

FIGURE 52-6

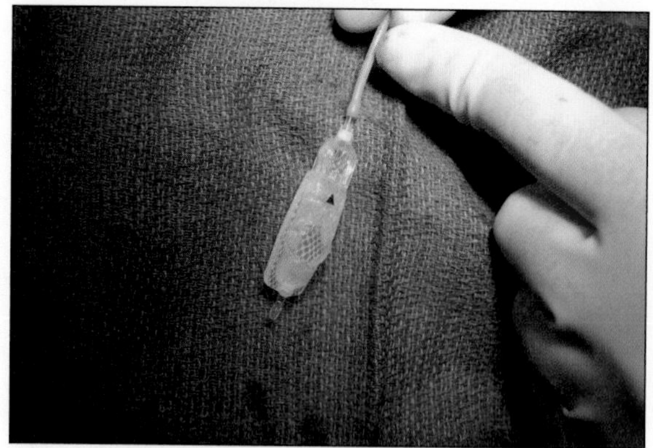

FIGURE 52-7

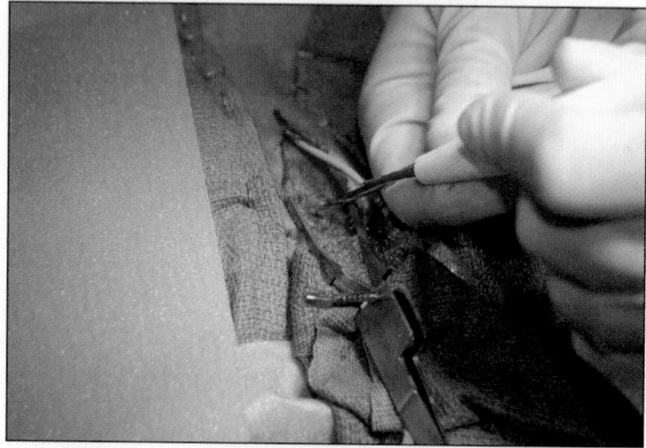

FIGURE 52-8

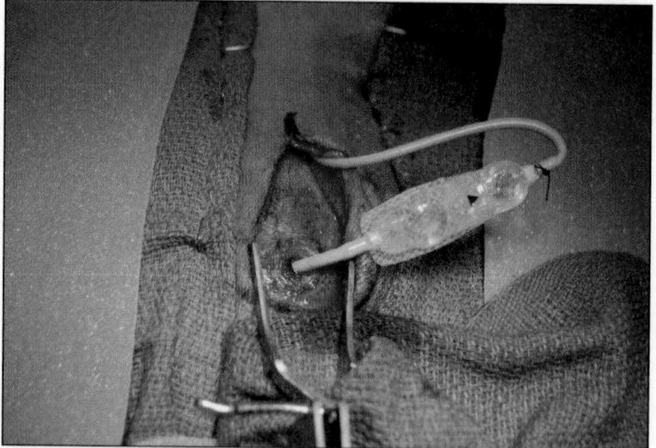

FIGURE 52-9

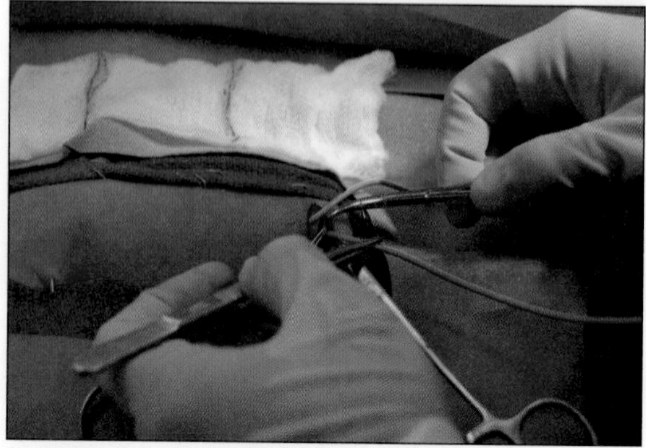

FIGURE 52-10

TIPS FROM THE MASTERS

- To minimize the infection rate, surgical sponges should be avoided, implants should not be opened from sterile packaging until immediately before use, implants should be handled with surgical instruments using a "no touch" technique, extraneous room traffic should be minimized, and care should be taken to expedite surgical time from incision to closure.
- A "perpendicular to the skull" catheter trajectory usually results in prompt entry into the ventricle, and if the catheter is advanced while removing the stylet, the tip of the catheter heads toward the frontal horn.
- Scalp closure with nonabsorbable monofilament suture in a simple running fashion minimizes wound breakdown and CSF-cutaneous fistulas, particularly in an active child.

PITFALLS

Never secure the ventricular catheter to the valve unless the CSF is clear. Gentle, patient irrigation through the catheter can usually resolve issues with blood or debris in the ventricular catheter.

Do not implant the peritoneal catheter unless continuous CSF egress is observed. Correctable issues in this regard include "air blocks" in the tubing and "kinking" of the distal tubing at the level of attachment to the valve in an insufficiently capacious subcutaneous scalp pocket.

If there is any concern regarding placement of peritoneal tubing (i.e., morbidly obese patient, patient with a prior history of laparotomy and excessive scarring), obtain a radiograph of the kidneys, ureters, and bladder before the patient leaves the operating room.

BAILOUT OPTIONS

- Intraoperative ultrasound, intracatheter endoscopy, frameless stereotaxy, and intraoperative CT or MRI can be useful adjuncts for ventricles that are difficult to cannulate.
- Admission of the patient to the intensive care unit with the hope of progressive ventricular dilation before reoperation is a potential option for ventricular cannulation failure.
- If all options have been exhausted and the patient's life is in jeopardy, it is potentially possible to place a shunt in a CT scanner suite.

SUGGESTED READINGS

Anderson RCE, Garton HJL, Kestle JRW. Treatment of hydrocephalus with shunts. In: Albright AL, Pollack IF, Adelson PD, editors. Principles and Practice of Pediatric Neurosurgery. New York: Thieme; 2008. p. 109–30.

Aryan HE, Meltzer HS, Park MS, et al. Initial experience with antibiotic-impregnated silicone catheters for shunting of cerebrospinal fluid in children. Child Nerv Syst 2005;21:56–61.

Drake JM, Sainte-Rose C. The Shunt Book. Cambridge: Blackwell Science; 1995.

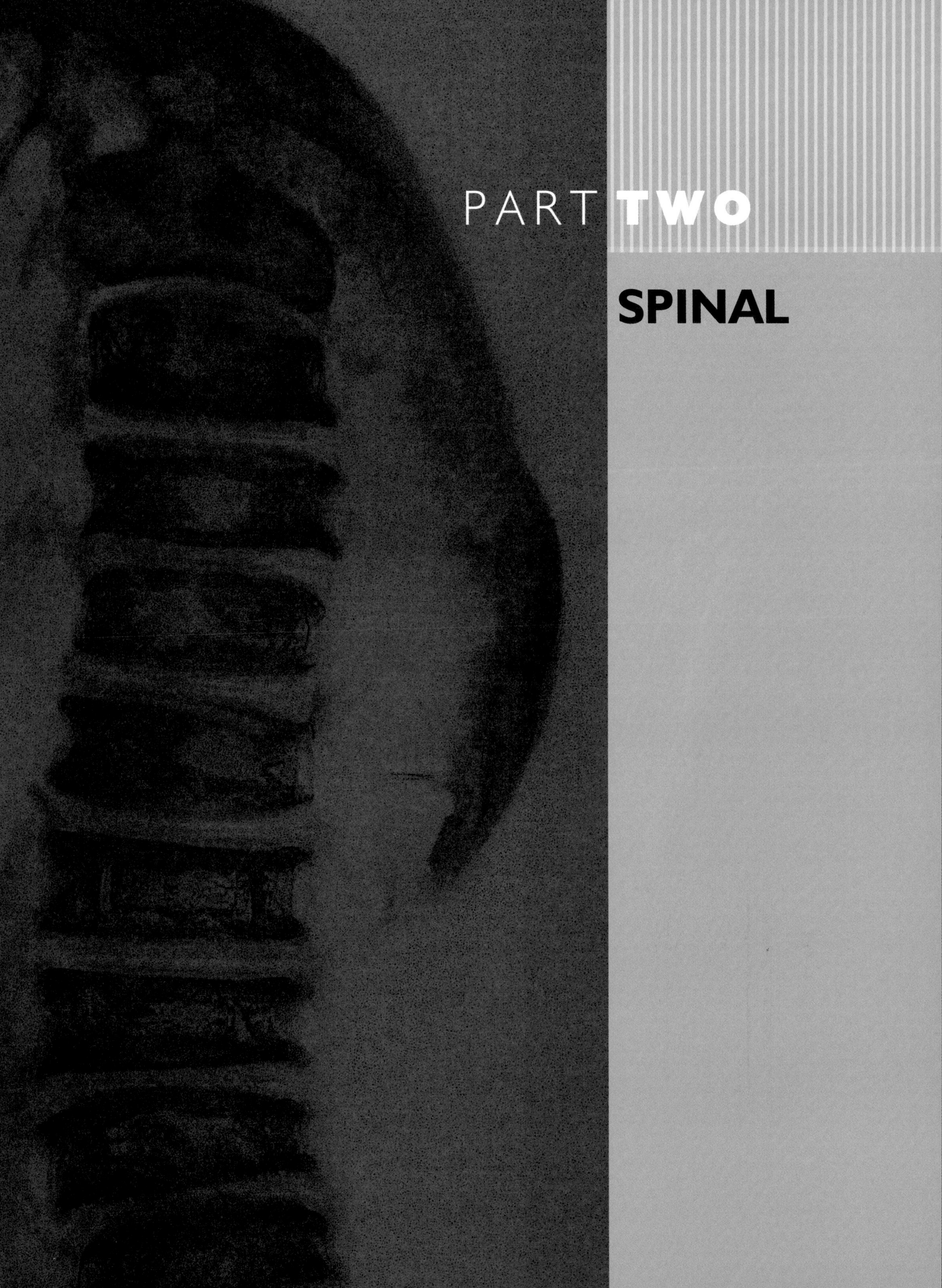

PART TWO

SPINAL

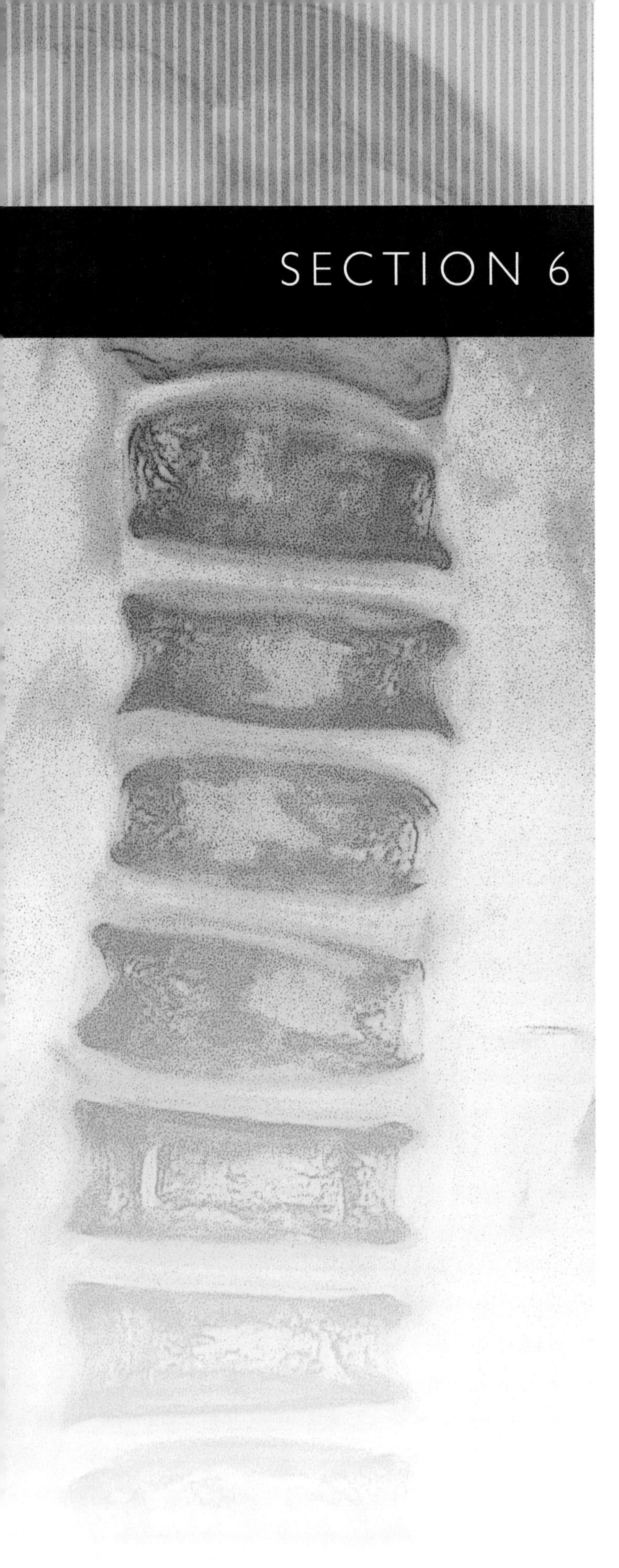

SECTION 6 Cervical

SECTION EDITOR — JON PARK,
WITH MELANIE G. HAYDEN GEPHART

Procedure 53

Anterior C1-2 Fixation

Carmina F. Angeles, Jon Park

PROCEDURE NOTES

- Instability of C1-2 may be due to trauma, infection, tumors, or rheumatoid arthritis. In deciding the appropriate management of unstable C1-2 injuries, the patient's age, medical status, and compliance and the fracture pattern and whether or not ligamentous injury is involved must be considered. One treatment modality that is widely accepted is closed reduction with halo vest placement. This treatment can cause patient dissatisfaction, however, and lack of compliance may lead to pin site infection and loss of alignment.
- Over the last decade, internal fixation has become a standard treatment for managing unstable C1-2. Posterior wiring techniques as described by Brooks and Jenkins and by Gallie have been widely used but have a significant rate of nonunion and fracture displacement. Posterior transarticular screw fixation, as later described by Magerl and Seeman, has decreased failure rates but is technically more demanding and has a high risk of inadvertent vertebral artery injury. Anterior C1-2 fixation may be used as an alternative method when posterior fusion is undesirable.

INDICATIONS

- For treatment of C1-2 instability (from trauma, infection, tumors, or rheumatoid arthritis).
- Inability to tolerate prone position surgery because of pulmonary issues and requiring C1-2 fixation.
- Unstable odontoid fracture, nonunion, or os odontoideum.
- Tumor resection involving the dens.
- Basilar impression.
- Posterior arches of C1-2 are injured and cannot hold hardware for stability.
- Dorsal bony anatomy of C1-2 precludes placement of posterior transarticular screws.

CONTRAINDICATIONS

- Short neck and barrel-shaped chest hindering operative access
- Facial fractures or temporomandibular pathology
- Injury to anterior bony architecture injury and cannot hold hardware for stability

PLANNING AND POSITIONING

- In deciding the appropriate management of unstable C1-2 injuries, the patient's age, medical status, and compliance and the fracture pattern and whether or not ligamentous injury is involved must be considered.
- Preoperative computed tomography (CT) can be reviewed to evaluate adequate bony integrity of C1 lateral masses and C2 vertebral body and to select appropriate length for screws.
- Closed reduction of C1-2 segment may be adequately achieved with halo or Gardner-Wells tong traction.

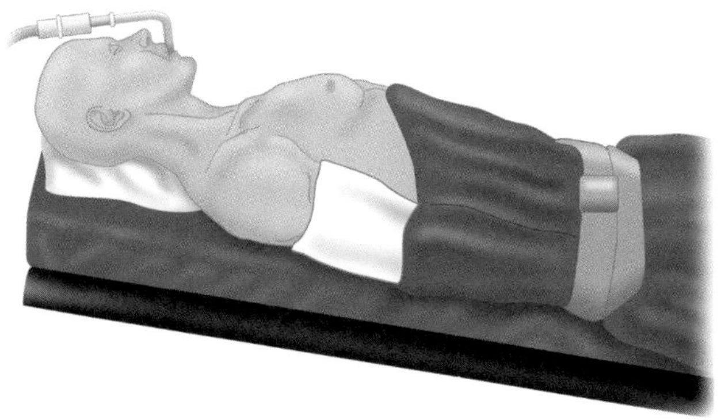

FIGURE 53-1

- The patient is positioned supine on a radiolucent table with the head slightly extended. Proper positioning should be assessed with fluoroscopic guidance. The table may need to be rotated 180 degrees on its base to allow maximum room for fluoroscopic positioning.
- The patient is intubated via awake fiberoptic technique.
- Broad-spectrum antibiotics with gram-positive and gram-negative coverage should be given 30 minutes before the incision.
- Spinal cord monitoring is highly recommended.
- A biplanar fluoroscope is brought around the operating table and covered with sterile drapes at the beginning of the case. When the fluoroscope is draped, it can be pushed toward the foot of the table and brought in to visualize adequate reduction and hardware placement.
- **Figure 53-1:** Positioning of staff and equipment in the operating room. The anesthesiologist is positioned at the head of the patient; the scrub nurse and basic table are placed at the patient's torso on the same side as the surgeon; the operating microscope comes in behind surgeon; the C-arm is draped and pushed down in between the surgeon and scrub nurse with the base located opposite from the surgeon; electrophysiology monitoring is positioned at the contralateral side of the surgeon.

PROCEDURE

Surgical Approach

Transoral Approach

- A transoral approach is superior for rheumatoid arthritis, dens tumors, basilar invagination, and fracture pattern wherein odontoid resection is required. This approach allows for C1-2 transarticular screw placement or C1-2 plate application. The main complication of this approach is infection, which can lead to sepsis.
- The patient must be able to open the mouth at least 25 mm. A Spetzler-Sonntag retractor is placed with the patient's tongue and endotracheal tube retracted downward, exposing the soft palate and posterior pharynx. The tongue retractor must be released every 30 to 45 minutes to prevent pressure necrosis. Teeth guards may be placed to protect the patient's dentition. The oropharynx and retractors are prepared with povidone-iodine (Betadine) solution, and the pharynx is packed to occlude the laryngopharynx and esophagus. The soft palate and posterior pharynx are infiltrated with local anesthetic and epinephrine to minimize use of cautery in controlling bleeding during incision.
- **Figure 53-2:** The incision is made on one side of the uvula and carried cephalad curving toward the midline of the soft palate.
- **Figure 53-3:** The soft palate is reflected laterally. The posterior pharyngeal wall is opened longitudinally at the midline. Mucosa and prevertebral muscles are elevated as one layer and retracted laterally using soft tissue retractors. Lateral dissection must not exceed 1.5 cm from the midline to avoid inadvertently injuring the vertebral artery.

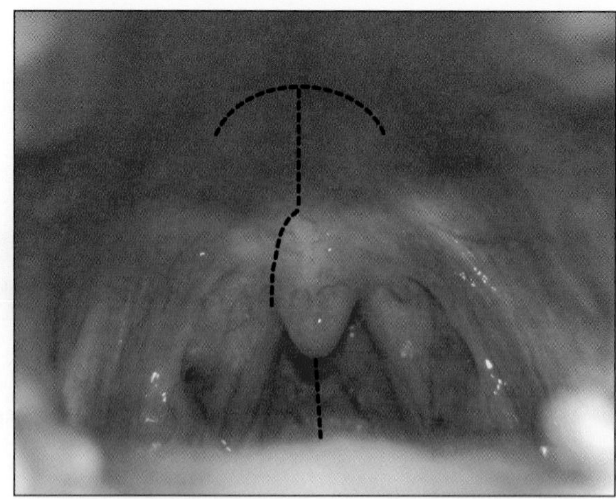

FIGURE 53-2

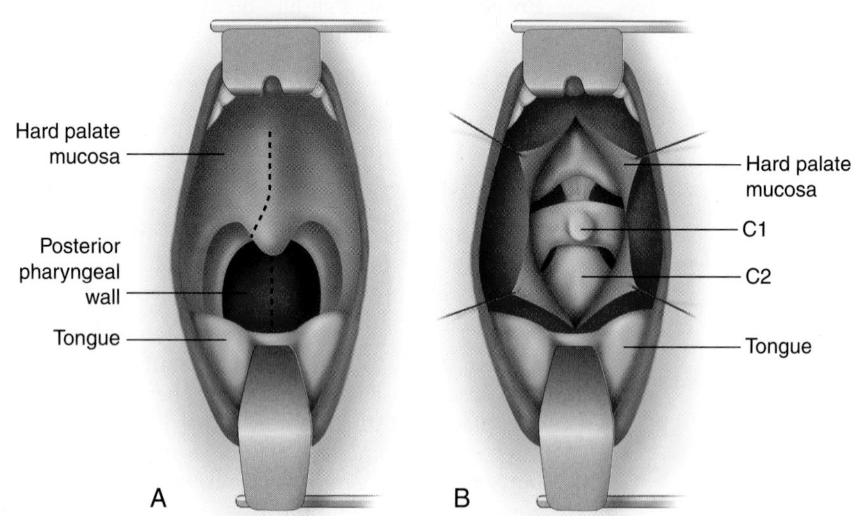

FIGURE 53-3

- Depending on the lesion, a high-speed drill may be used to perform bony decompression, whereas an ultrasonic dissector may be used for soft tissue removal in the case of a pannus or tumor. Decompression is followed by anterior C1-2 stabilization with transarticular screws or plate application as described subsequently.
- At the end of the surgery, mucosa and prevertebral muscles of the pharyngeal wall are closed as one strong layer with interrupted No. 1 polyglactin 910 (Vicryl) or other heavy absorbable suture. The soft palate is closed in a similar fashion. A nasogastric feeding tube is placed under direct vision. In case of cerebrospinal fluid leakage, all efforts must be made to achieve a watertight closure of the dura, and a lumbar drain should be placed.
- In some cases, it is necessary to extend the exposure inferiorly, and a transoral mandibular splitting approach is employed. A tracheostomy is initially performed. A midline skin incision through the lip and chin is then made. A mandibular osteotomy is made in a stepwise fashion to maximize postoperative stability. The mandibles are spread laterally, and the tongue is depressed downward exposing the posterior pharynx.

Anterior Retropharyngeal Approach

- **Figure 53-4:** The anterior retropharyngeal approach was originally described by Southwick and Robinson in 1957 to provide exposure from C3-T1. In 1969, the approach was modified by DeAndrade and McNab to include more cephalad segments. In 1999, Vaccaro et al described this approach clinically in a patient with nonunited Brooks posterior atlantoaxial fusion following a chronically displaced type II odontoid fracture with a two-part fracture of the posterior arch of C1.

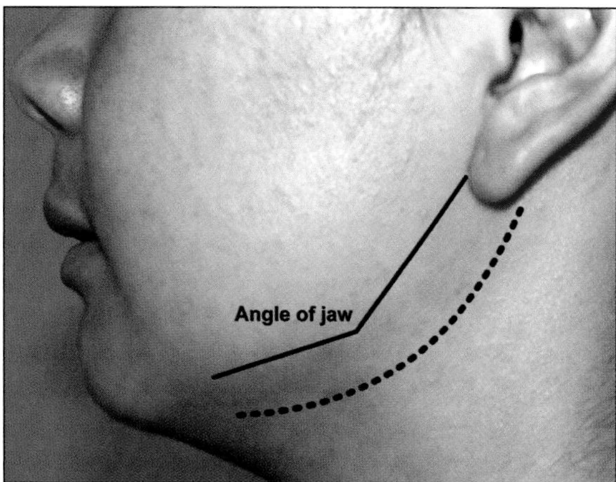

FIGURE 53-4

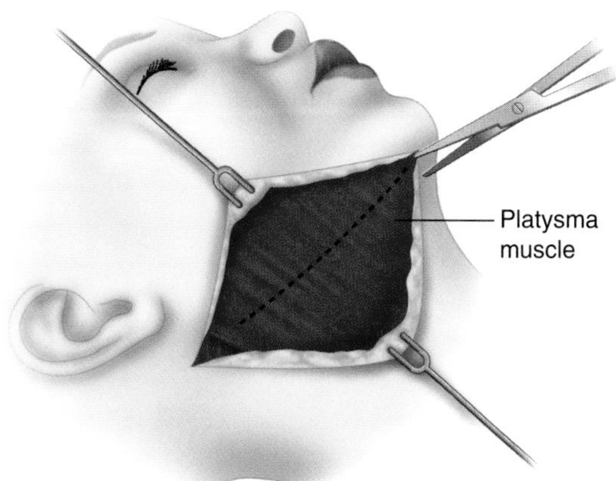

FIGURE 53-5

- A tracheostomy is typically performed to allow the jaws to close tightly.
- After infiltration with local anesthetics, a submandibular skin incision is carried out 2 cm lateral from the symphysis menti and curving around the angle of the mandible toward the mastoid process.
- **Figure 53-5:** A wide subcutaneous flap superficial to the platysma is created. The medial border of the platysma is identified, and muscle is isolated before dividing transversely using Metzenbaum scissors across its fibers.
- **Figure 53-6:** The marginal branch of the facial nerve that runs anteriorly below the angle of the mandible and lies in the upper part of the submandibular gland must be identified and preserved. The superficial cervical fascia is incised below the nerve to avoid inadvertent injury resulting in orbicularis oris paresis. The facial vein and artery can be identified lateral to the submandibular gland. The vein can be ligated and divided, whereas the artery is preserved. The inferior margin of the gland is retracted upward, and the fascia is opened exposing the digastric muscle and tendon. The hypoglossal nerve lies just deep, slightly inferior, and parallel to the digastric tendon. This nerve should be identified with the aid of a nerve stimulator and carefully preserved by retracting superiorly. Sometimes the tendon of the digastric muscle is divided and tagged for later repair.
- **Figure 53-7:** The retropharyngeal space is opened by incising the fascia overlying the hyoid bone. The carotid sheath is retracted laterally, and the strap muscles and esophagus are retracted medially. The retropharyngeal fat pad is encountered, confirming the location. Care must be taken not to injure the superior laryngeal nerve, which runs deep to the internal carotid artery and alongside the pharyngeal constrictors. This nerve is vulnerable to stretch injury from retraction—wide fascial opening helps reduce this occurrence. Sometimes it is necessary to divide the superior thyroid artery and vein, lingual artery and vein, and ascending pharyngeal artery to provide lateral mobilization of the carotid sheath.

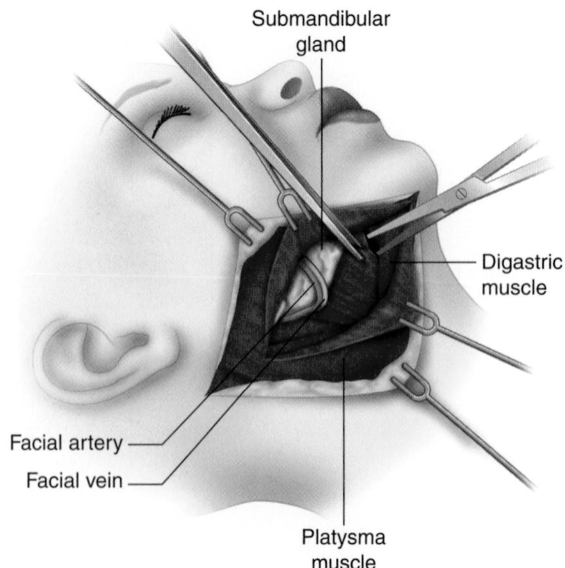

FIGURE 53-6

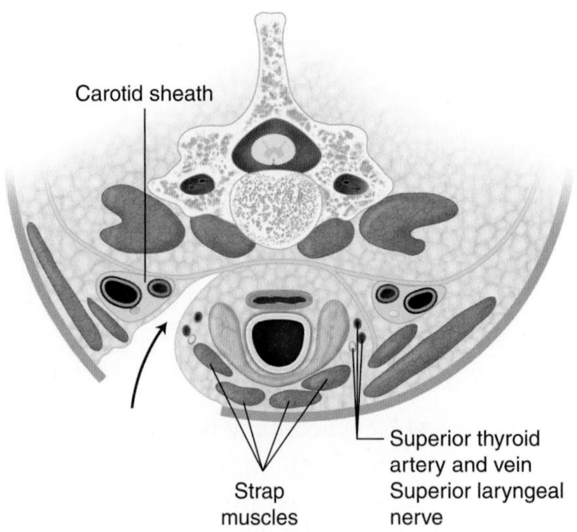

FIGURE 53-7

- Blunt finger dissection is performed down to the prevertebral fascia and longus colli muscles. The fascia is dissected with a peanut, and the longus colli muscle inserting onto the C1 anterior tubercle is elevated sharply from the anterolateral surface of C1 and C2. A similar smaller horizontal exposure is done on the contralateral side. Anterior C1-2 transarticular screw fixation or plate application can then be carried out.
- Closure includes reattachment of the digastric tendon and suction drains placed in the retropharyngeal space and in the subcutaneous region. The platysma, subcutaneous layer, and skin can be closed according to surgeon preference. The patient is placed on a hard collar, and the head of the bed is elevated 30 to 45 degrees to prevent potential hypopharyngeal hematoma and edema. Delayed extubation may be prudent.

Lateral Approach

- **Figure 53-8:** The lateral approach to the C1-2 segment was initially described by Barbour, Whitesides, and then Dutiot. This approach also requires bilateral dissection. The earlobe is temporarily reflected back by suturing to the skin anterior to the ear. The skin incision is made proximally along the anterior border of the sternocleidomastoid muscle and carried posteriorly across the mastoid process.
- **Figure 53-9:** The greater auricular nerve underneath the platysma is dissected and mobilized. The subcutaneous layer and platysma muscle are divided along the skin incision. The external jugular vein overlying the sternocleidomastoid muscle can be

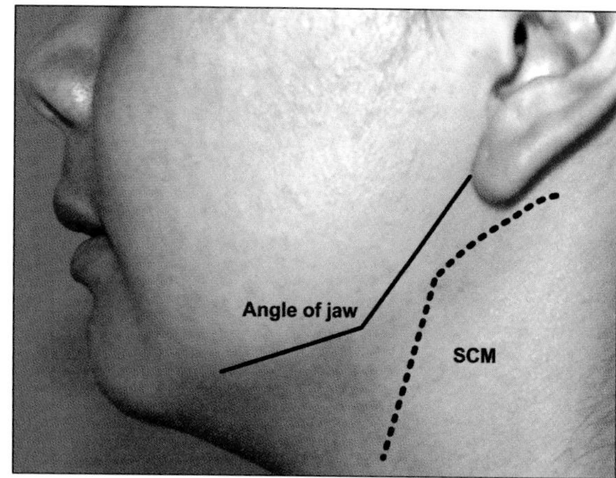

FIGURE 53-8

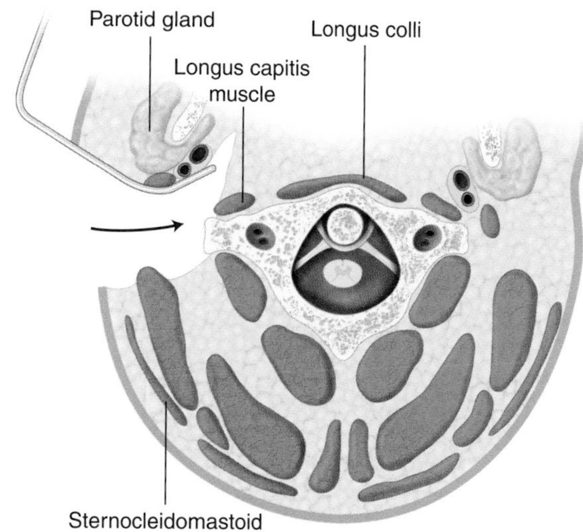

FIGURE 53-9

ligated if necessary. The posterior portion of the parotid gland can be seen on the anterior border of the sternocleidomastoid and should be protected. The sternocleidomastoid muscle is divided in its tendinous portion partially along its anterior border in a perpendicular direction. The C1 transverse process is palpated, and the spinal accessory nerve, common carotid artery, internal jugular vein, posterior belly of digastric muscle, and lymph nodes are retracted medially. Blunt finger dissection is performed between the internal jugular vein and longus capitis muscle to enter the retropharyngeal space. The lateral mass and anterior arch of C1 and C2 are exposed by elevating the longus colli and longus capitis from the transverse process of C1 and C2. Similar exposure is made on the contralateral side. Stabilization with hardware placement can then be done. The platysma, subcutaneous tissue, and skin can be closed according to surgeon preference.

Anterior C1-2 Transarticular Screw Fixation

- **Figure 53-10:** After adequate exposure, cartilage is removed from the C1-2 articulation with curets to enhance bony fusion. A Kirschner wire is placed across C1-2 articulation starting 5 mm lateral to the odontoid base directly on the undersurface of the small bony overhanging lip located on the lateral mass of C2. With 25-degree angulation from medial to lateral direction, a Kirschner wire is slowly advanced to the C1 lateral mass under fluoroscopic guidance.
- **Figure 53-11:** After tapping, a 4.0-mm cannulated screw is placed over each guidewire. The usual screw length is 15 to 20 mm. Lag screws are often preferred because this provides compression of C1-2 facets. This compression stabilizes C1-2 rigidly but sacrifices all C1-2 motion.

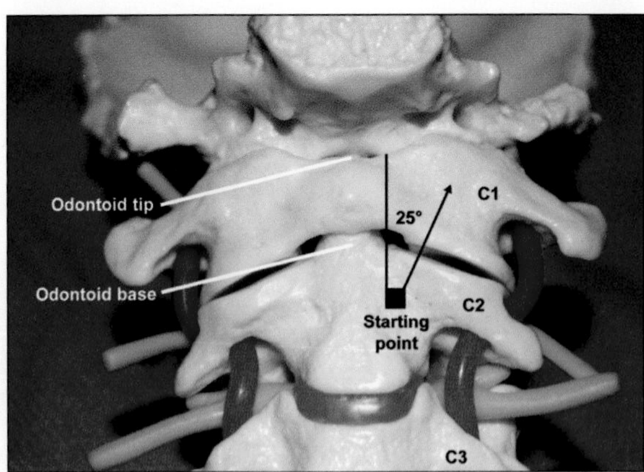

FIGURE 53-10

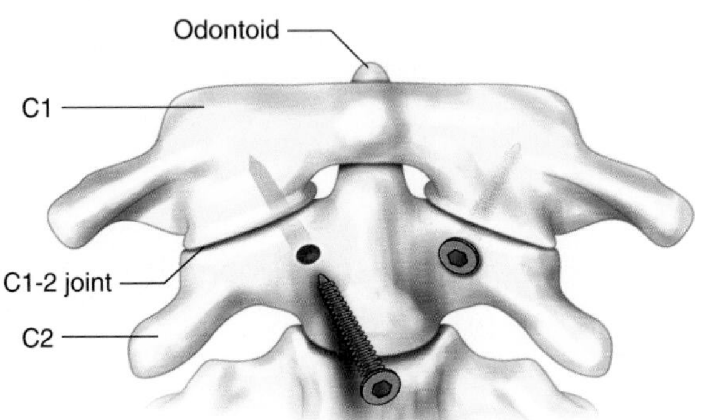

FIGURE 53-11

C1-2 Anterior Plate Fixation

- **Figure 53-12:** When adequate exposure has been achieved, decortication of C1-2 facet joints is performed using curets to enhance fusion. An appropriately sized T-shaped plate (Depuy-Acromed, Inc, Rayham, MA) is applied. Holes in the plate allow for appropriate screw placement. Under fluoroscopic guidance, screw holes can be hand drilled or drilled by power. Ideally, screws are placed into the center of the lateral masses of C1 bilaterally and into the C2 body. Lateral mass screws are angled 10 to 15 degrees in medial to lateral direction. Unicortical 3.2-mm or 3.5-mm screws are placed, followed by a locking mechanism. Lateral mass screws must not violate the posterior cortex because this poses a risk of vertebral artery injury as it courses in the vertebral artery groove along the C1 posterior arch.

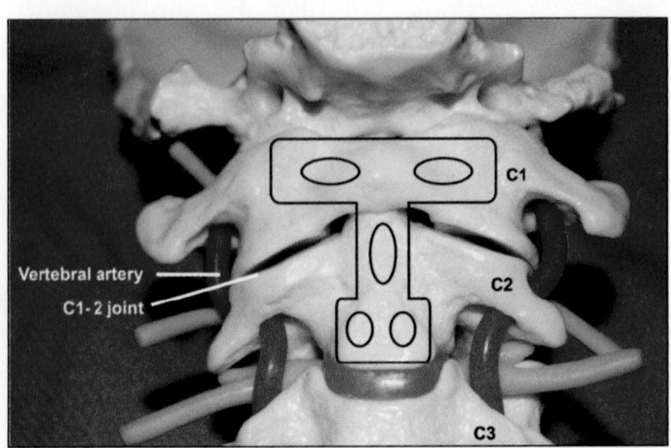

FIGURE 53-12

TIPS FROM THE MASTERS

- Use sharp technique for soft tissue dissection, and respect anatomic planes to minimize devitalized tissue and wound dehiscence.
- To help identify possible injury to the esophagus and hypopharynx, an orogastric tube is placed preoperatively, which allows intraoperative palpation and identification of the esophagus. At the end of surgery, the orogastric tube is withdrawn to the level of C1-2, and 60 mL of diluted indigo carmine is administered down the tube by anesthesia. The wound is inspected for dark blue material representing esophageal injury that requires repair.
- Tracheostomy is an option and is often necessary. Fluids and alimentation are administered through a nasogastric tube from the third postoperative day.
- A 1.5-cm portion of the anterior arch of C1 can be safely resected. The odontoid process is posterior, and no main vessels and nerves lie medial to the C1 lateral masses.
- At C1, the distance from midline to the external border to be exposed should not exceed 2.5 cm.
- At C2, the distance from midline to the external border exposed should not exceed 1.8 cm because the vertebral artery is more anterior and medial than at C1.
- Before placement of hardware, ensure that the patient's neck is in neutral position and C1-2 are aligned; otherwise, fixation may be malaligned.

PITFALLS

Infection rates are high despite use of appropriate preoperative, intraoperative, and postoperative antibiotics selective for oral flora.

Postoperative dysphagia and dysphonia are known complications and can be minimized by periodically deflating the endotracheal tube cuff and less vigorous retraction.

The recurrent laryngeal nerve or an external branch of the superior laryngeal nerve that courses with the superior thyroid artery can be inadvertently injured during the approach and cause postoperative hoarseness.

Additional injury related to the approach may include the glossopharyngeal, vagus, accessory, and hypoglossal nerves; internal carotid artery; and jugular vein.

When placing lateral mass screws to secure the anterior C1-2 plate, care must be taken not to violate the posterior cortex, which can lead to inadvertent vertebral artery injury as it courses in the vertebral artery groove along the C1 posterior arch.

BAILOUT OPTIONS

- During anterior C1-2 plate application, screws with poor purchase may be replaced with 4.0-mm to 4.5-mm screws.
- If adequate decompression at C1-2 cannot be achieved anteriorly, posterior decompression with or without posterior fusion can be performed. A posterior fusion with Harm's technique or wiring technique can be performed.
- In patients with osteoporosis, screw purchase strength can be reinforced with cement.

SUGGESTED READINGS

Kerschbaumer F, Kandziora F, Klein C, et al. Transoral decompression, anterior plate fixation, and posterior wire fusion for irreducible atlantoaxial kyphosis in rheumatoid arthritis. J Neurosurg 2002;96(3 Suppl):312–20.

Koller H, Kammermeier V, Ulbricht D, et al. Anterior retropharyngeal fixation C1-2 for stabilization of atlantoaxial stabilities: study of feasibility, technical description and preliminary results. Eur Spine J 2006;15:1326–38.

Lu J, Ebraheim NA, Yang H, et al. Anatomic consideration of anterior transarticular screw fixation for atlantoaxial instability. Spine 1998;23:1229–35.

Reindl R, Milan S, Aebi M. Anterior instrumentation for traumatic C1-C2 instability. Spine 2003;28:E329–33.

Vaccaro AR, Lehman AP, Ahlgren BD, et al. Anterior C1-C2 screw fixation and bony fusion through an anterior retropharyngeal approach. Orthopedics 1999;22:1165–70.

Procedure 54 Transarticular Screws for C1-2 Fixation

Vincent Y. Wang, Dean Chou

INDICATIONS

- Indications for C1-2 transarticular screw fixation are atlantoaxial instability, rheumatoid arthritis, congenital abnormalities, os odontoideum, tumor, and ligamentous abnormality. Trauma and rheumatoid arthritis are the two most common indications for C1-2 fixation.
- C1-2 transarticular screws can also be used in patients with atlantoaxial instability who have failed external orthosis treatment (including halo vest) and patients who develop pseudarthrosis after undergoing C1-2 fixation and fusion with other techniques such as wiring.
- Biomechanical studies in cadavers showed that C1-2 transarticular screws provide slightly better fixation than C1–lateral mass/C2 pars screws in case of rotary subluxation.

CONTRAINDICATIONS

- The anatomic relationship between the C2 foramen transversarium and the C1-2 facet joint must be studied carefully preoperatively because 18% to 23% of patients have a high-riding foramen transversarium (and vertebral artery) on at least one side that would prevent safe placement of a C1-2 transarticular screw. Thin-cut CT scans of the cervical spine with sagittal reconstruction generally offer sufficient detail to analyze the course of the vertebral artery C2.
- The procedure is relatively contraindicated in polytrauma patients with severe injury to other organ systems, elderly patients with other significant comorbidities, and patients who may be unable to tolerate a prone procedure.

PLANNING AND POSITIONING

Anesthetic Considerations

- In patients with severe canal stenosis and significant myelopathy, care must be taken to minimize flexion of the neck during intubation. Awake intubation with fiberoptic assistance should be considered in cases of difficult airway or extremely unstable spines.
- Neuromonitoring with motor evoked potentials (MEPs) or somatosensory evoked potentials (SSEPs) should be used in patients with severe myelopathy. Prepositioning baseline MEPs or SSEPs should be obtained from patients before putting the patient in the prone position to ensure positioning has not compromised the spinal cord. Anesthetic agents should be adjusted for neuromonitoring purposes in these cases.
- In cases of spinal cord injury or severe myelopathy, maintenance of blood pressure in the normotensive or slightly hypertensive (mean arterial pressure > 90 mm Hg) range may be crucial to optimize perfusion of the cord.

Positioning

- **Figure 54-1:** Patients are positioned prone for C1-2 transarticular screw placement. The patient's head is placed in a Mayfield head holder. We usually place the patient on two soft chest rolls with a regular operating table (in reverse orientation for fluoroscopy),

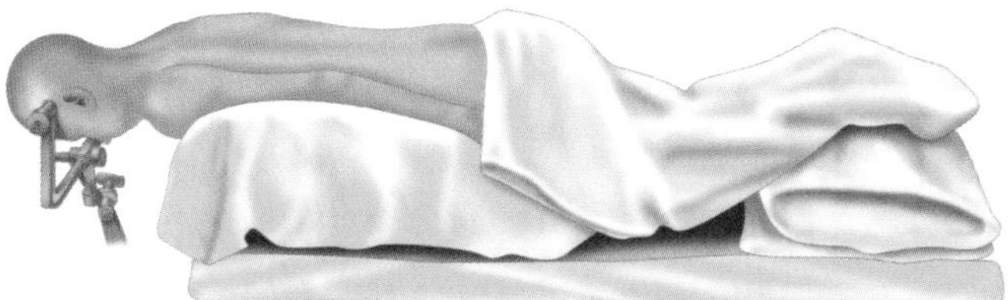

FIGURE 54-1

but it is also possible to use a Jackson table for this procedure. We usually put the operating table in a slight reverse Trendelenburg position, with the patient's legs up. The patient's arms are tucked at the sides. If iliac crest is to be used, the hip area is prepared for graft harvest.

- The head is positioned in a neutral position. Extreme care is taken to avoid forward translation and flexion of the spine, which can cause worsening spinal cord compression. Postpositioning MEPs or SSEPs are immediately checked to ensure positioning did not cause additional spinal cord compression. If significant signal changes are observed, the position of the cervical spine must be adjusted. Slight hypertension may also be used to improve perfusion of the spinal cord, and anesthetic agents should be checked. If none of these measures are able to restore MEPs or SSEPs to baseline, further repositioning should be done under fluoroscopic guidance to attempt to reduce the C1-2 subluxation as much as possible. Lateral fluoroscopy is used to confirm the positioning of the patient. Additionally, a metallic instrument can be placed along the side of the proposed C1-2 transarticular screw trajectory to ensure that the positioning does not obstruct the placement of the screw.

PROCEDURE

- **Figure 54-2:** Exposure from the occiput to the inferior aspect of C2 should be performed. The lamina of C1 and C2 and pars interarticularis of C2 should be dissected free of soft tissue. This dissection can be done using a combination of monopolar cautery and a No. 4 Penfield dissector. The facet joint of C2-3 can also be identified and used as a landmark for entry point of the screw. The interspinous ligament of C2-3 should be preserved carefully. Care should be taken during exposure of the lateral aspect of the posterior C1 ring to avoid injury to the vertebral artery.

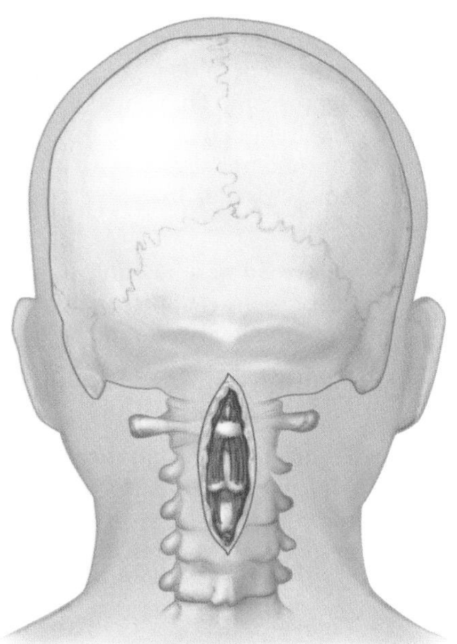

FIGURE 54-2

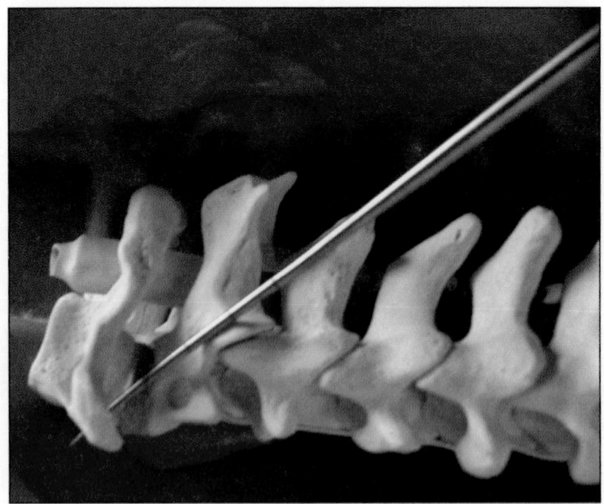

FIGURE 54-3

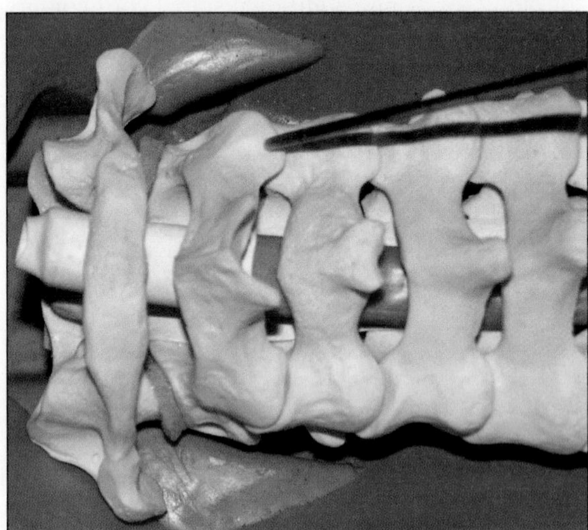

FIGURE 54-4

- If a decompression is to be done, the C1 posterior ring or the C2 lamina, or both, can be removed.
- **Figure 54-3:** The entry point of the drill guide can be identified by placing a long straight instrument along the side of the patient with the desired screw trajectory. Lateral fluoroscopy can be used to check the angle of the trajectory; this helps mark the entry site of the drill guide in the rostral-caudal dimension. The entry site is usually 1 to 2 cm lateral to the midline. Because of the angle of the transarticular screw and the location of the exposure, usually two percutaneous stab incisions further caudal in the subaxial spine must be made.
- **Figure 54-4:** The entry point of the screw is similar to the pars screw of C2. The typical entry point is approximately 2 to 3 mm superior to the C2-3 facet and 2 to 3 mm lateral to the medial edge of the C2-3 facet.
- **Figure 54-5:** After identification of the entry site, a pilot hole is made using either a high-speed "matchstick" bur or an awl.
- **Figure 54-6:** A stab incision is made in the previously identified entry site, and the fascia can be opened using scissors or a scalpel. The drill guide is placed and docked at the pilot hole. The drill guide may be inserted through a separate stab incision. Most systems use a Kirschner wire system that can be introduced after reduction of C1-2; this can be followed by the drill, tap, and screw.
- **Figure 54-7:** Under fluoroscopic guidance, the drill is advanced toward the anterior arch of atlas. The trajectory is best defined by fluoroscopy, with a typical angle between 30 and 45 degrees.

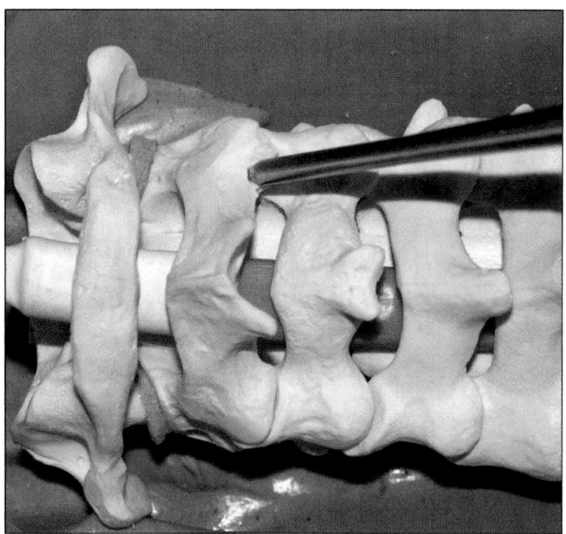

FIGURE 54-5

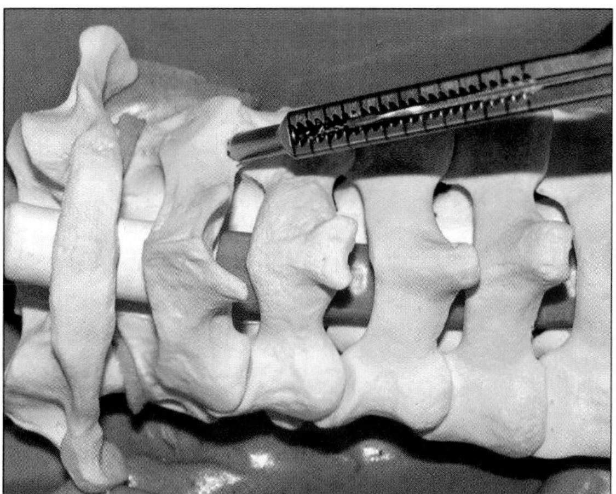

FIGURE 54-6

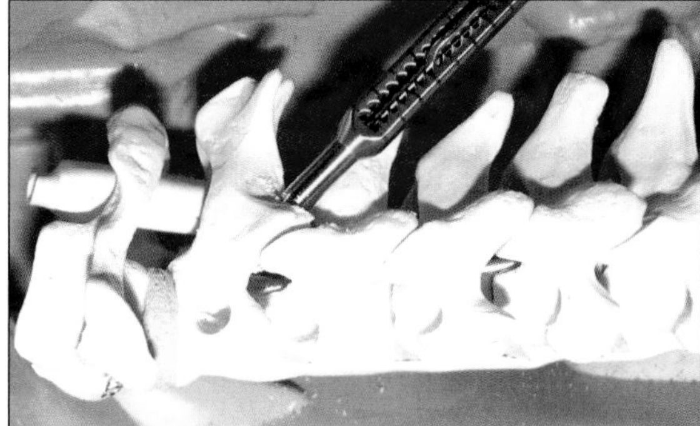

FIGURE 54-7

- **Figure 54-8:** The drill should be advanced to slightly beyond the cortical surface of the anterior arch of C1 via the C1 tubercle. The depth of the drill is used to approximate the length of the screw. A ball tip probe is used to palpate the screw track and ensure that the cortical surface of the anterior arch of C1 is drilled through.
- **Figure 54-9:** A screw of appropriate length (based on depth of the drill) is inserted slowly in the previous drill hole. We usually use a 3.5-mm titanium polyaxial screw. The medial-lateral trajectory is relatively straight.

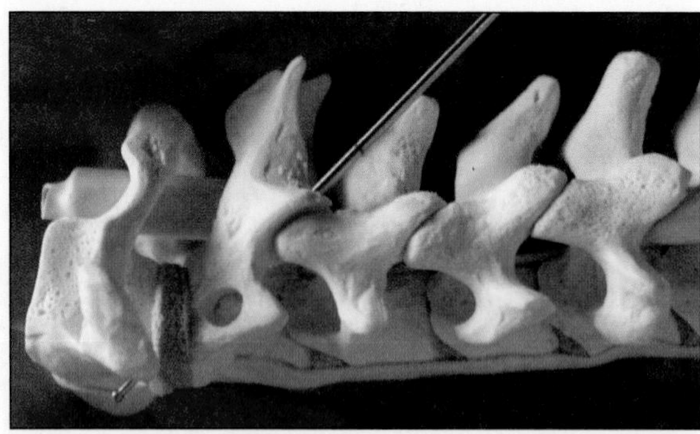

FIGURE 54-8

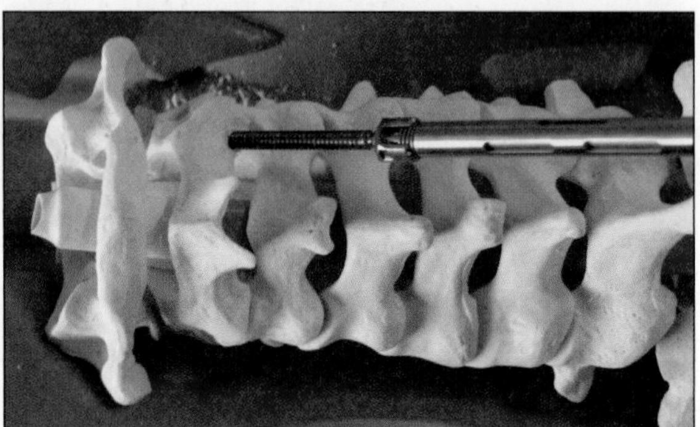

FIGURE 54-9

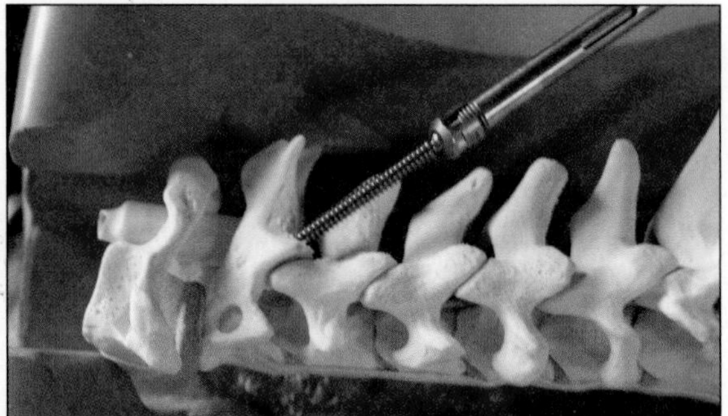

FIGURE 54-10

- **Figure 54-10:** The screw is threaded through the C1-2 facet to reach the anterior arch of C1.
- If the posterior elements have not been removed, additional stabilization and fixation can be achieved by harvesting a piece of iliac crest graft and placing it between the inferior surface of C1 and the spinous process of C2 (Sonntag technique). The graft is held in place using a cable.
- External orthosis is at the surgeon's discretion. We tend to place patients in a hard collar for 1 month. In patients with poor bone quality, a longer time may be prescribed. The patient is usually allowed to be mobilized the next day.
- **Figure 54-11:** Screws in final position.

TIPS FROM THE MASTERS

- Preoperative planning is very important for placement of transarticular screws. A high-riding vertebral artery must be recognized before the procedure to avoid injury to the artery. Injury rate to the vertebral artery is less than 5%. Patients with rheumatoid arthritis are more likely to have an abnormally located transverse foramen.

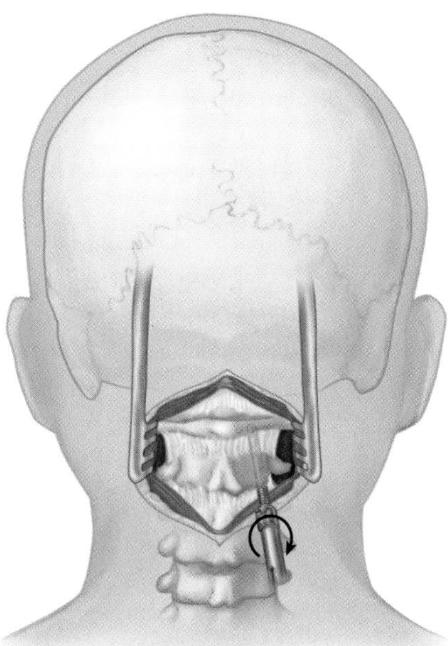

FIGURE 54-11

- Imaging guidance is helpful for placement of transarticular screws.
- In cases of severe instability (e.g., cases of trauma), it may be necessary to put the patient into a halo vest before the operation. It is recommended to position these patients in the halo vest. In such cases, the patient is rolled into the prone position with the halo vest in place. The head ring of the halo vest is secured using an adapter. Position of the cervical spine is checked with lateral fluoroscopy, and postpositioning MEPs or SSEPs are used to ensure no significant compromise of spinal cord function after positioning. After confirming the position and neuromonitoring signals, the posterior part of the vest may be removed.
- It is important to prepare and drape a wide skin area that includes the lower cervical spine and possibly the upper thoracic spine. Depending on the patient's body habitus, the skin entry point for the percutaneous drill guide may be at the lower cervical spine or the upper thoracic spine level.
- If there is significant subluxation of C1 on C2, it must be reduced before placement of the transarticular screw. Reduction is accomplished via adjustment of the Mayfield head holder. Another maneuver is to grab the spinous process of C2 with a penetrating towel clamp and reduce C2 (with C1 lamina intact) gently toward C1.
- After the C1 laminectomy is performed, anterolisthesis of C1-2 may increase significantly.
- If a vertebral artery injury is suspected, a screw should be placed as a tamponade. The contralateral screw should not be placed to avoid the risk of bilateral vertebral artery injury. Angiography should be performed postoperatively to assess for damage to the vertebral artery.

PITFALLS

Extensive venous plexus are sometimes present in the C1-2 area. They can usually be controlled with bipolar cautery, Gelfoam, or another hemostatic agent such as Surgifoam (Ethicon, Inc., Sommerville, NJ) or FloSeal (Baxter International, Inc., Deer field, IL). Care should be taken during the dissection because significant blood loss from these plexus can occur.

Failure to recognize injury to the vertebral artery can have significant clinical consequences. If a patient exhibits clinical signs of brainstem ischemia or infarct during the postoperative period, it is important to investigate the possibility of a vertebral artery injury.

If a screw is too long, it can injure the pharyngeal soft tissue.

BAILOUT OPTIONS

- If fracture of the pars interarticularis occurs, it may be necessary to extend the fusion to the occiput or C3. If the C2 lamina is of sufficient size, a rod-screw construct with C1 lateral mass screw and C2 laminar screws may be used.
- C1 lateral mass and C2 pars or C2 pedicle screws may be used to rescue the fixation if a transarticular screw cannot be safely placed.
- In cases in which only a single screw is placed because of vertebral artery injury, additional fixation may be achieved using interspinous wiring or C1 lateral mass and C2 pars/pedicle screws. If this approach is impossible, an external orthosis (including a halo vest) may be necessary, depending on the condition of the patient.

SUGGESTED READINGS

Acosta FL, Quinones-Hinojosa A, Gadkary C, et al. Frameless stereotactic image-guided C1-2 transarticular screw fixation for atlantoaxial instability. J Spinal Disord Tech 2005;18:385–91.

Dickman C, Sonntag V. Posterior C1-C2 transarticular screw fixation for atlantoaxial arthrodesis. Spine 1998;43:275–80.

Gluf W, Schmidt M, Apfelbaum R. Atlantoaxial transarticular screw: a review of surgical indications, fusion rate, complications and lessons learned in 191 adult patients. J Neurosurg Spine 2005;2:155–63.

Paramore C, Dickman C, Sonntag V. The anatomical suitability of the C1-2 complex for transarticular screw placement. J Neurosurg 1996;85:221–4.

Rocha R, Sawa A, Baek S, et al. Atlantoaxial rotary subluxation with ligamentous disruption: a biomechanical comparison of current fusion methods. Neurosurg Operative Suppl 2009;64:ONS137–44.

Procedure 55

C1-2 Posterior Cervical Fusion

Daniel C. Lu, Valli P. Mummaneni, Ramesh Teegala, Praveen V. Mummaneni

INDICATIONS

- C1-2 posterior cervical fusion is indicated in patients with odontoid fractures that cannot be repaired with an odontoid screw, including type II odontoid fractures associated with fractures of the atlantoaxial joint, type II odontoid fractures with oblique fractures in the sagittal plane that preclude odontoid screw placement, type II odontoid fractures with significant irreducible displacement that may not heal with immobilization (and are too displaced to place an odontoid screw), type II odontoid fractures with an associated Jefferson fracture, and type II odontoid fractures with a ruptured transverse ligament.
- In addition, patients with a cervicothoracic kyphosis or a very large barrel chest may be unable to be fixated with anterior odontoid screw placement (inability to achieve the trajectory required for odontoid screw placement) and are usually treated with a posterior C1-2 stabilization procedure.

Nonhealed Odontoid Fractures (Types II and III)

- Patients initially treated with immobilization who develop a pseudarthrosis are not ideal candidates for subsequent attempts at anterior odontoid screw fixation because of the material from the pseudarthrosis occupying the fracture line, which often prevents contact of the fracture surfaces.
- Type III odontoid fractures with atlantoaxial joint fracture combinations and type III odontoid fractures with associated Jefferson fracture are also unstable and may be treated with a posterior C1-2 stabilization procedure.
- Patients may also have ligamentous laxity and have resultant C1-2 instability. Ligamentous instability of C1-2 is identified with measurements of the atlantodental interval on flexion and extension views. Normally, this interval should not exceed 2 to 3 mm in adults. When the atlantodental interval exceeds 5 mm in nonrheumatoid patients and when it exceeds 7 to 8 mm in rheumatoid patients, there is instability of the C1-2 complex, and posterior C1-2 fixation is indicated.
- Atlantoaxial rotatory dislocations are also an indication for C1-2 fixation. This problem can often be treated via a posterior reduction and fusion approach (see Fig. 55-2).
- Congenital malformations of C2 (i.e., os odontoideum and odontoid agenesis), degenerative diseases, inflammatory diseases (rheumatoid arthritis), tumors, and infections (osteomyelitis) can also result in instability of the atlantoaxial complex requiring C1-2 fixation.
- Postsurgical dynamic instability relating to odontoidectomy or C1 and C2 laminectomies with or without removal of adjoining facets is another indication for posterior C1-C2 fixation.

CONTRAINDICATIONS

- Aberrant vertebral artery and inadequate bony anatomy for proper screw placement are contraindications for C1-2 posterior fixation.

PLANNING AND POSITIONING

- Preoperative magnetic resonance imaging (MRI) and computed tomography (CT) are useful to evaluate any anatomic or physical constraints that may limit the placement of C1 lateral mass screws. Preoperative imaging may reveal substantial cranial-cervical

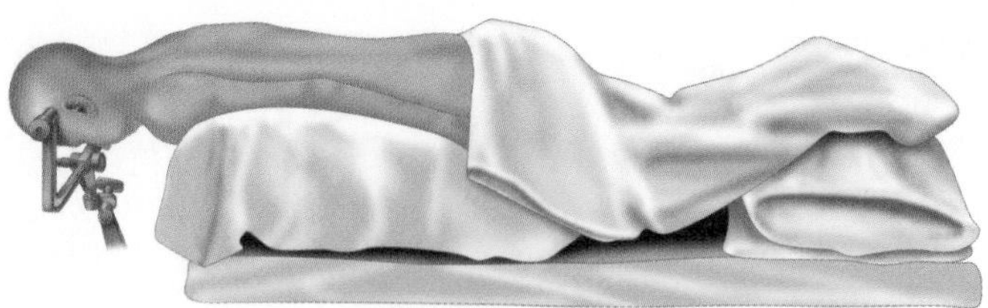

FIGURE 55-1

settling (often seen in rheumatoid patients), and the C1 ring may be partially dislocated into the foramen magnum. In such cases, traction may be needed to expose the posterior C1 lateral mass.

- MRI helps delineate the course of the vertebral arteries, and in cases with aberrant vertebral arteries, magnetic resonance angiography or CT angiography may also be ordered.
- To minimize the risk of vertebral artery injury with C1 and C2 screw placement, we routinely perform CT of the cervical spine (often with three-dimensional remodeling sequences to identify an anomalous vertebral artery course, integrity of the bone at the intended site of screw fixation, or an unacceptably small C2 pars).
- Preoperatively, patients with C1-2 pathology are often immobilized using a rigid collar or halo. In the operating room, intubation is often best performed in a neutral supine position using a fiberoptic scope. We prefer to use somatosensory evoked potentials (SSEPs) and motor evoked potentials (MEPs) during surgery to monitor neurologic function. In patients with severe myelopathy, we prefer to obtain baseline SSEP and MEP signal after intubation while the patient is still supine.
- The choice of anesthetic agents is crucial when evoked potentials are monitored. Long-acting paralytic agents cannot be used in these cases because they blunt MEPs. Likewise, nitrous oxide cannot be used because it blunts SSEPs. One minimum alveolar concentration of vapor can also blunt evoked potentials. Consequently, we prefer to induce anesthesia by using propofol (2 to 3 mg/kg) along with a short-acting or medium-acting paralytic (rocuronium), and we maintain a propofol infusion throughout the case. After induction, we prefer to use 50% of the minimum alveolar concentration of vapor (i.e., isoflurane) and remifentanil (0.1 to 0.25 mg/kg/min) as a narcotic infusion. This combination is least likely to affect SSEPs and MEPs. Large-bore intravenous lines or a central line often is inserted to assist with fluid resuscitation. In adults, we typically use an arterial line and keep the mean arterial pressure around 90 mm Hg or more to prevent spinal cord ischemia.
- **Figure 55-1:** The patient is rotated to the prone position onto chest rolls using mild manual cervical traction to maintain a neutral and reduced C1-2 relationship. The head is secured to a rigid, three-point cranial fixation system in a neutral to slightly flexed position. The abdomen is allowed to hang freely between the chest rolls, and care is taken to pad all pressure points. SSEPs and MEPs are repeated after the patient is positioned prone to ensure that the new prone position is not resulting in neurologic deterioration.

PROCEDURE

- **Figure 55-2:** A midline incision is made extending from the suboccipital area to the spinous process of C3. C2-3 facet joints are exposed (but not violated), and the dorsal arch of C1 is exposed laterally. The vertebral artery may be exposed in the vertebral groove on the superior aspect of the C1 arch (arterial sulci of C1). We review preoperative imaging to ensure that the vertebral artery does not have an aberrant course. The C2 nerve root is identified and is typically mobilized inferiorly. Bipolar cautery and hemostatic agents such as Surgifoam (Baxter, Deerfield, IL) are used to control bleeding from the venous plexus surrounding the C2 nerve root.
- **Figure 55-3:** The inferior third of the C1 lamina (which overlies the C1 lateral mass) is removed with a high-speed drill. The lateral mass of C1 inferior to the C1 arch is

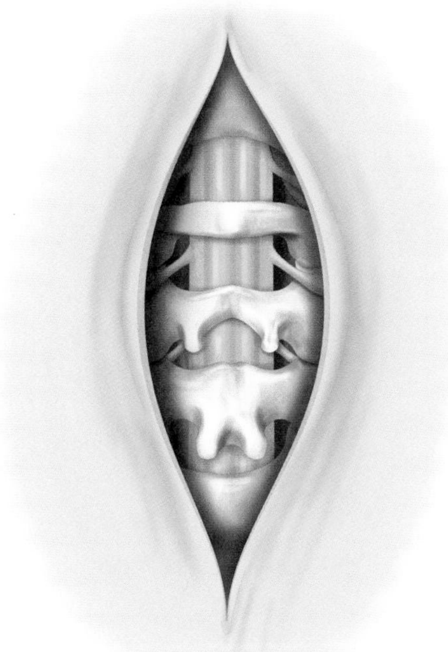

FIGURE 55-2

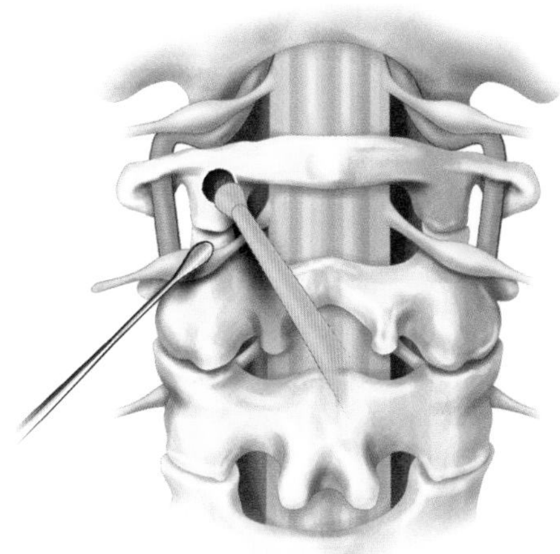

FIGURE 55-3

exposed after the C2 nerve root has been mobilized inferiorly. The medial and lateral wall of the C1 lateral mass is identified by palpation with a No. 4 Penfield dissector.

- The entry point for the C1 lateral mass screw is identified at the center of the C1 lateral mass, and this entry point is decorticated with a "matchstick" bur on a high-speed drill. Another suggested entry point is at the junction point of the midpoint of the C1 lateral mass and the inferior aspect of the C1 arch.
- A low-speed drill with a 3-mm-diameter drill bit and guide is seated into the decorticated C1 lateral mass entry point, and under fluoroscopy a pilot hole is drilled through the C1 lateral mass. The trajectory of the pilot hole is 10 degrees medial angulation in the axial plane and in parallel with the ring of C1 in the sagittal plane. The drill bit is used to penetrate the anterior cortex of C1. On lateral fluoroscopic imaging, the drill is aimed toward the center of the anterior tubercle of C1. Care is taken to avoid drilling into the posterior pharynx with the drill bit. The tip of the drill bit should not be anterior to the midpoint of the anterior tubercle of C1 on the lateral fluoroscopic image. The surgeon should take note that the anterior portion of the ring of C1 is sloped posteriorly. The tip of the drill bit has typically penetrated the anterior cortex of the ring of

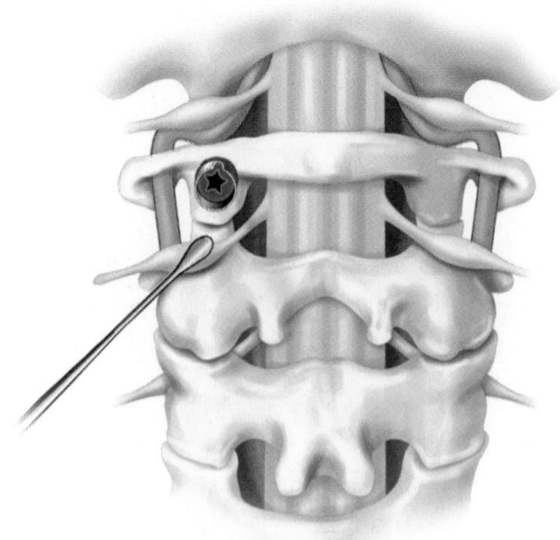

FIGURE 55-4

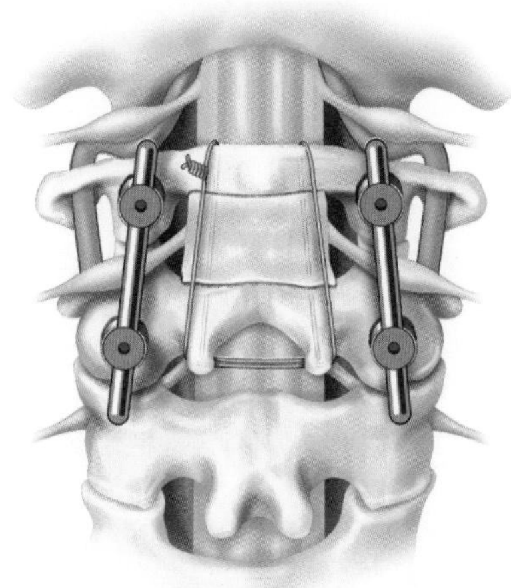

FIGURE 55-5

C1 when it is at the posterior aspect of the C1 tubercle on the lateral fluoroscopic image. Placing the drill bit anterior to the C1 anterior tubercle on a lateral fluoroscopic view is unnecessary to achieve a bicortical screw purchase.

- **Figure 55-4:** The pilot hole is tapped with a 3.5-mm tap, and a 4.0-mm diameter C1 lateral mass screw is placed. Typical dimensions for a C1 lateral mass screw are 4.0 mm wide and 36 mm long. A screw length of 36 mm allows for the polyaxial screw head to sit superficial to the C2 nerve root without causing a foraminal stenosis at C1-2. We typically do not sacrifice the C2 nerve root.
- **Figure 55-5:** A screw at C2 or C3, or both, is placed. The C2 screw can be placed in the pars of C2, in the pedicle of C2, or in the lamina of C2. We place bone graft (usually iliac crest tricortical autograft) in the interlaminar space between C1 and C2 or laterally in the facet joint of C1-2 or along the lateral lamina and pars of C1 and C2 (onlay graft).
- **Figure 55-6:** **A** and **B,** Postoperative radiographs showing C1-2 posterior cervical hardware with no movement across these segments on flexion and extension.

TIPS FROM THE MASTERS

- Preoperative CT scanning of the cervical spine can identify an anomalous vertebral artery foramina and integrity of the bone at the intended site of screw fixation.
- We ask the anesthesiologist to maintain a mean arterial pressure of 90 mm Hg for patients with myelopathy to ensure cord perfusion.

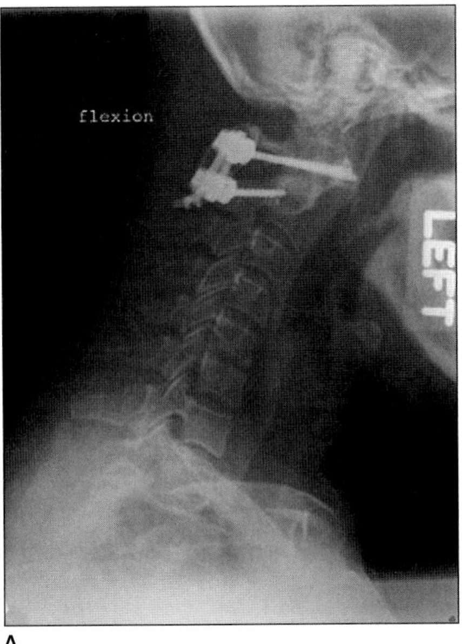

A

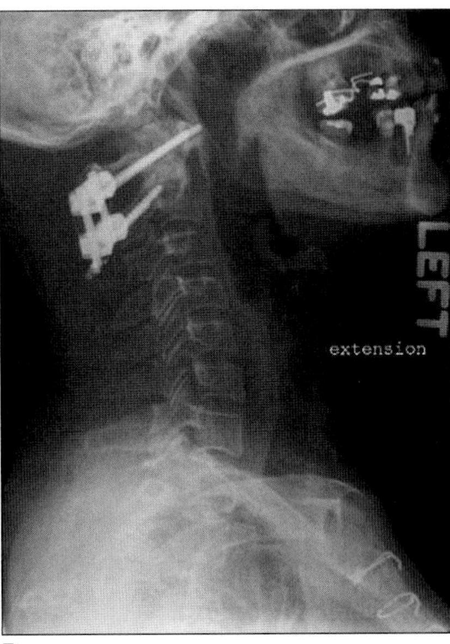

B

FIGURE 55-6

- Avoid manipulation of the thecal sac during surgery, and do not retract the cervical cord at all.
- Protect the C2 nerve root with a small dissector during drilling, tapping, and screw fixation of C1.
- If necessary, C2 rhizotomy can be performed to improve access to C1 lateral mass (leaving a residual posterior scalp numbness).

PITFALLS

Vertebral artery injury, although uncommon, is one of the most feared complications of instrumentation in the high cervical spine. When patients have anomalous anatomy in the C1-2 area, image-guided navigation may be helpful during surgery. The vertebral artery is at greatest risk of injury during the soft tissue dissection around the C1 arch and during placement of the C2 screw. If the vertebral artery is injured during screw placement, we recommend placing a short screw to tamponade the hemorrhage. If it is injured during dissection of the C1 lateral mass, packing with hemostatic agents, such as a thrombin-soaked gelatin sponge, often stops the bleeding. When a vertebral artery injury is recognized, the contralateral screw should not be placed. A patient often tolerates a single vertebral artery occlusion, but a bilateral vertebral artery occlusion is likely to lead to a significant cerebellar or brainstem stroke. When a patient with a unilateral vertebral artery injury is hemodynamically stable, he or she should be taken to interventional radiology to have the vertebral artery evaluated angiographically with embolization performed if necessary.

Injury to the upper cervical cord or C2 nerve root is possible during instrumentation of the C1-2 area. Patients with myelopathy are at increased risk of neurologic injury.

BAILOUT OPTIONS

- Place a short C2 screw for stabilization and tamponade bleeding in vertebral artery injury.
- Maintain a mean arterial pressure of 90 mm Hg in neurologic injury.
- Perform primary suture repair for cerebrospinal fluid leak or insert a lumbar subarachnoid drain.

SUGGESTED READINGS

Goel A, Desai KI, Muzumdar DP. Atlantoaxial fixation using plate and screw method: a report of 160 treated patients. Neurosurgery 2002;51:1351–6.

Gunnarsson T, Massicotte EM, Govender PV, et al. The use of C1 lateral mass screws in complex cervical spine surgery: indications, techniques, and outcome in a prospective consecutive series of 25 cases. J Spinal Disord Tech 2007;20:308–16.

Harms J, Melcher PP. Posterior C1-C2 fusion with polyaxial screw and rod fixation. Spine 2001;26:2467–71.

Mummaneni PV, Haid RW, Traynelis VC, et al. Posterior cervical fixation using a new polyaxial screw and rod system: technique and surgical results. Neurosurg Focus 2002;12:E8.

O'Brien JR, Gokaslan ZL, Riley LH, et al. Open reduction of C1-C2 subluxation with the use of C1 lateral mass and C2 translaminar screws. Neurosurgery 2008;63:ONS95–8.

Wang MY, Samudrala S. Cadaveric morphometric analysis for atlantal lateral mass screw placement. Neurosurgery 2004;54:1436–9.

Procedure 56

Occipitocervical Fusion

Nestor D. Tomycz, David O. Okonkwo

INDICATIONS

- Occipitocervical fusion is performed for craniovertebral junction (CVJ) instability resulting from various etiologies.
  - Posttraumatic: Atlantooccipital dislocation, complex fractures involving CVJ, unstable odontoid fractures with incompetence of the posterior ring of C1
  - Acquired cranial settling secondary to infectious or inflammatory disease: Rheumatoid arthritis, ankylosing spondylitis, Down syndrome, inflammatory bowel disease–associated arthropathy, pseudogout, ossification of posterior longitudinal ligament, chronic Grisel syndrome, CVJ tuberculosis, CVJ osteomyelitis
  - Neoplastic: Primary tumors of CVJ such as chordomas, chondromas, and osteoblastomas; metastatic CVJ disease
  - Congenital or developmental: Anterior and posterior bifid arches of C1, congenital basilar invagination, Chiari malformation–associated basilar invagination, absent occipital condyles or absent C1 lateral masses, os odontoideum, unilateral atlas assimilation with chronic occipitocervical rotatory subluxation
  - Iatrogenic: Unstable craniocervical junction after transoral or endonasal endoscopic CVJ decompression, C1-2 pseudarthrosis, suboccipital craniectomy for Chiari malformation, extreme lateral transcondylar approach

CONTRAINDICATIONS

- Relative contraindications include severe osteoporosis, limited life expectancy, multiple medical comorbidities in elderly patients, aberrant vertebral artery anatomy, and foramen magnum stenosis requiring suboccipital decompression.

PLANNING AND POSITIONING

- Halo vest immobilization is applied before surgery in cases of posttraumatic occipitocervical instability such as atlantooccipital dislocation and after transoral or endonasal endoscopic CVJ decompression. Halo vest immobilization is maintained through prone positioning in surgery for occipitocervical fusion.
- Preoperative evaluation includes high-resolution computed tomography (CT) of the head, cervical spine, and CVJ with sagittal and coronal reconstructions. Careful attention is paid to the thickness of the midline occipital keel for measuring appropriate occipital screw lengths. CT angiography is obtained to evaluate the course of the vertebral arteries and to assess contraindications to C1 or C2 screw placement. Magnetic resonance imaging (MRI) of the cervical spine is obtained where indicated to document the presence of spinal cord signal change, to determine whether the CVJ requires decompression, to assess for the presence of subaxial instability, and to evaluate the degree of CVJ pannus in cases of inflammatory disease such as rheumatoid arthritis. Basilar invagination can be confirmed by drawing imaginary lines on reconstructed CT of the CVJ.
- We use sagittal CT reconstructions to calculate the basion-dens interval and basion-axial interval, which have been shown to provide the most accurate assessment of atlantooccipital dislocation. Atlantooccipital dislocation should be suspected when the basion-dens interval or basion-axial interval is greater than 12 mm.

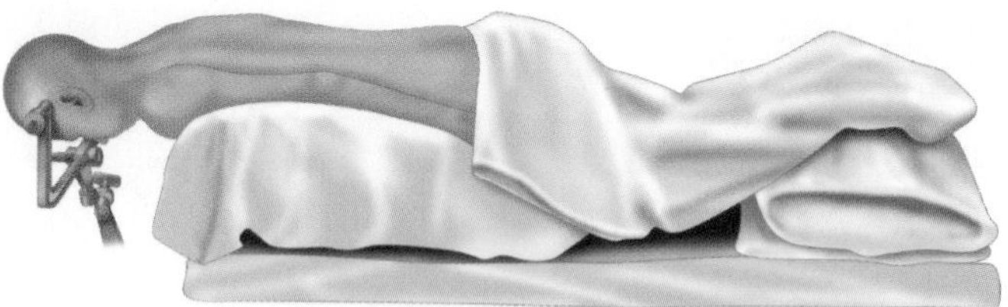

FIGURE 56-1

- Basilar invagination is present if the odontoid intersects the Wackenheim clival-canal line, which is drawn along the posterior surface of the clivus. It is also present if more than one third of the length of the odontoid lies above the Chamberlain line, which is drawn from the hard palate to the posterior margin of the foramen magnum.
- Transarticular C1-2 fixation is commonly contraindicated by aberrant vertebral artery anatomy, and a medial vertebral artery course may preclude C2 pedicle and pars screw placement.
- We perform occipitocervical fixation by connecting an occipital plate by rods to an atlantoaxial Harms construct (bilateral C1 lateral mass screws connected to C2 pars or pedicle screws). We prefer to use the Mountaineer occipitocervical instrumentation system (DePuy Spine, Inc, Raynham, MA).
- We perform continuous neurophysiologic monitoring with cortical somatosensory evoked potentials (SSEPs) and obtain prepositioning baseline SSEPs in all cases.
- An arterial line is placed, and the anesthesiologist is asked to maintain a mean arterial pressure of 90 mm Hg in all cases with preexisting myelopathy, cervical spinal cord compression, and cervical spinal cord signal abnormality on MRI. Patients are typed and crossed with red blood cells available in the operating room should a need for immediate transfusion arise.
- A persistent change in SSEPs independent of mean arterial pressure after positioning the patient prone prompts us to return the patient to a supine position and awaken the patient for neurologic examination.
- We encourage fiberoptic-assisted intubation to reduce the chance of spinal cord injury in cases with preexisting cervical cord compression and severe instability.
- **Figure 56-1:** The patient is positioned prone in Mayfield head pins with care to prevent cervical extension. If a halo vest was placed preoperatively, the patient is positioned prone with the halo connected to the Mayfield apparatus via a halo adapter. The bed is placed in reverse Trendelenburg position to elevate the head, and the patient's knees are flexed.

PROCEDURE

- **Figure 56-2:** We make a midline incision from the inion extending inferiorly to a spinous process that corresponds to a level below the desired caudal level of the fusion. Extending the incision a level inferiorly permits the upward angle necessary for lateral mass screw placement. Monopolar electrocautery is used to extend the dissection between the paraspinal muscles via the avascular midline raphe, and the occiput, posterior ring of C1, and spinous process of C2 are exposed in a subperiosteal fashion. To reduce the risk of vertebral artery injury, electrocautery is not used more than 15 mm lateral to the midline when performing the subperiosteal dissection of the superior posterior ring of C1. The bony edges of the foramen magnum and posterior ring of C1 are defined further with curets, and the posterior atlantooccipital membrane is removed with tenotomy scissors. Exposure of the surgical field is maintained with Gelpi retractors.
- **Figure 56-3:** Curets are used to define the bony margins of the inferior portion of the posterior ring of C1 out to the lateral masses of C1. Surgifoam (Ethicon, Somerville, NJ) is used to stop bleeding from the nearby vertebral venous plexus. The C1-2 joint must be exposed and denuded of soft tissue to provide a surface for bone grafting. The starting point for C1 lateral mass screws and C2 pars/pedicle screws is shown.

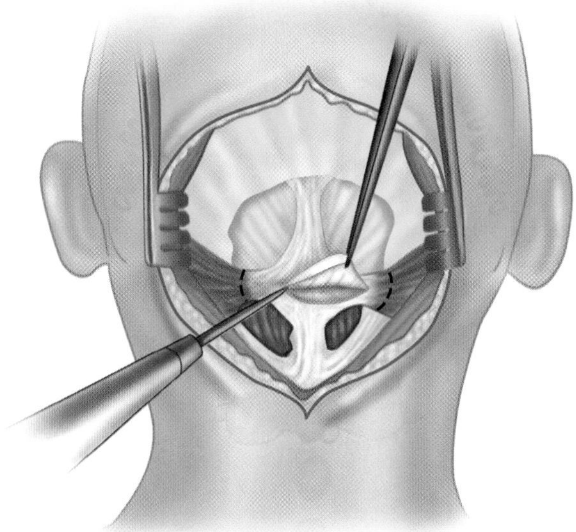

FIGURE 56-2

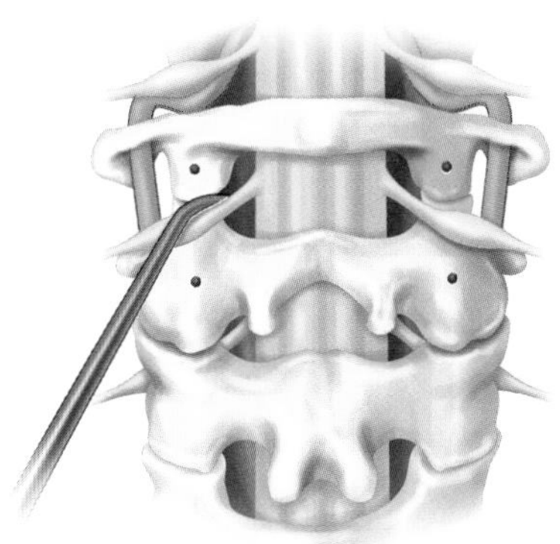

FIGURE 56-3

- **Figure 56-4:** The occiput should be exposed in a subperiosteal fashion out to the medial edge of the mastoid processes bilaterally. A high-speed drill is used to remove irregularities in the occipital bony surface that would preclude flush placement of the occipital plate. We use an inverted-Y–shaped occipital plate (Mountaineer, Depuy Spine, Raynham, MA) whose midline screws take advantage of the increased bone thickness in the midline occipital keel. A power drill with a drill stop set at 5 mm (based on measurements from the CT scan) is used to make the midline pilot holes for the occipital plate; more laterally located occipital screws are placed with the pilot hole prepared with a 4-mm drill stop. An eyeball probe is used in each hole to ensure that the dura has not been breached.
- **Figure 56-5:** We perform C1-2 fixation using lateral fluoroscopic guidance. Gentle caudal retraction on the C2 dorsal root ganglion is required to expose the C1 lateral mass screw entry point, which lies halfway between the junction of the C1 posterior arch and the inferior posterior part of the C1 lateral mass. A No. 4 Penfield dissector can be used to feel the medial border of the C1 lateral mass. A high-speed bur is used to mark the entry point. We recommend drilling some of the posterior ring of C1 that lies above the C1 lateral mass screw entry point to allow adequate room for the polyaxial head of the C1 screw. The pilot hole is drilled with the hand-held drill in a 5- to 10-degree medial trajectory along a plane parallel to the plane of the C1 posterior arch. We recommend checking the pilot hole with a blunt 1.0-mm probe and then tapping the hole. A 3.5-mm-diameter polyaxial screw whose length typically measures 18 to 30 mm is placed.

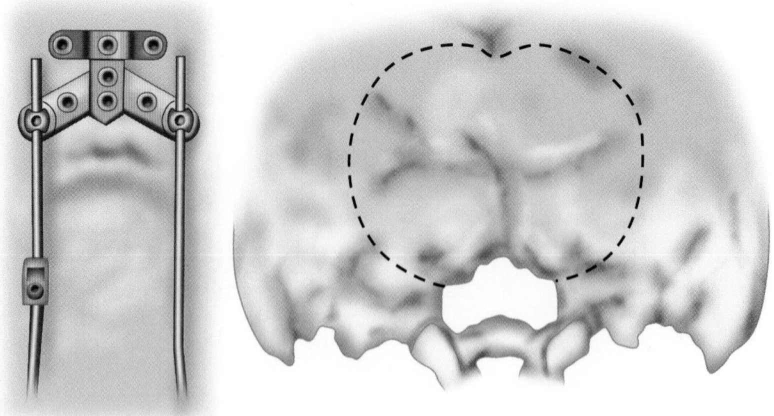

FIGURE 56-4

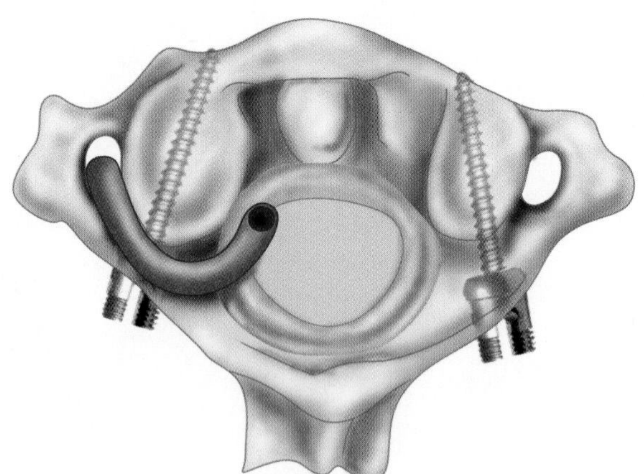

FIGURE 56-5

- **Figure 56-6:** A No. 4 Penfield dissector is likewise used to feel the medial border of the C2 pars interarticularis. The atlantoaxial membrane is detached using a blunt dissector to expose the upper surface of the C2 pedicle. The inferior articular process of C2 is divided into quadrants. The C2 pedicle screw starting point lies in the superomedial quadrant of the inferior articular process of C2 (approximately 1.75 mm caudal to the lateral mass–pars interarticularis transition zone). The pilot hole is again prepared with a high-speed bit, and the pilot hole is drilled in a trajectory oriented 20 degrees medial and 20 degrees cephalad with lateral fluoroscopic guidance. The hole is checked with a probe and tapped. A 3.5-mm screw is placed. Typical screw lengths are 30 to 35 mm.
- **Figure 56-7:** After the C1 screws, C2 screws, and occipital plate have been placed, 3.5-mm rods are placed to connect screw heads to the plate. If the fusion incorporates subaxial screws, lateral mass screws are placed in the subaxial spine using the standard Magerl technique. Locking caps are placed, and all instrumentation is finally tightened. The occiput, C1, and C2 laminae and facets are decorticated using the high-speed drill. In cases requiring decompression, removed autologous bone is mixed with demineralized bone matrix and grafted over decorticated surfaces. In cases in which decompression is unnecessary, we harvest iliac crest tricortical autograft and secure it between C1 and C2 with a Songer cable (DePuy Spine, Inc, Raynham, MA). We recommend adding bone morphogenetic protein (BMP-2; Infuse, Medtronic, Minneapolis, MN) in cases of severe osteoporosis or for patients who smoke.

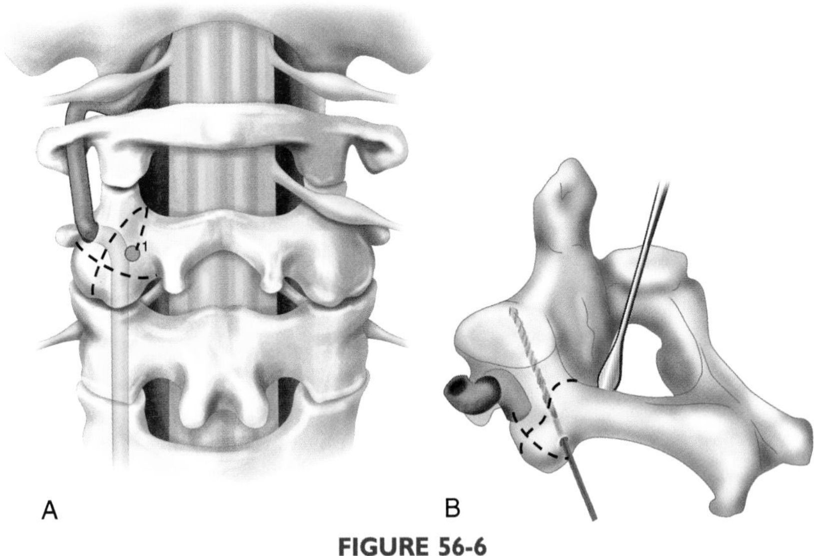

FIGURE 56-6

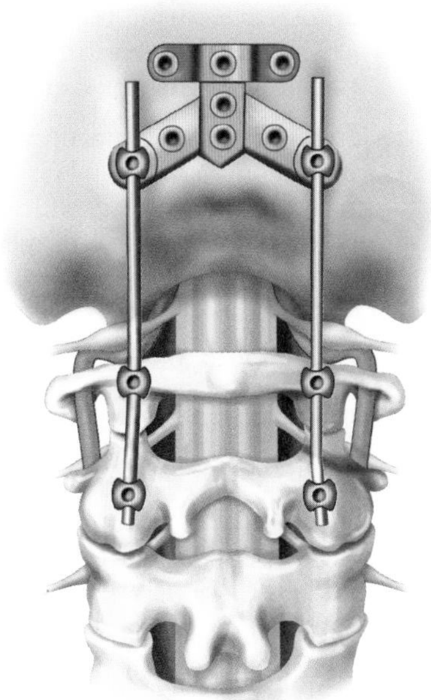

FIGURE 56-7

TIPS FROM THE MASTERS

- To prevent excessive blood loss during mobilization of the C2 nerve root, control of the vertebral venous plexus is essential. We recommend a combination of bipolar electrocautery and Surgifoam (Ethicon, Somerville, NJ).
- Although placement of C1 lateral mass screws with bicortical purchase has been described, no current data comparing the relative strength of unicortical versus bicortical C1 lateral mass screws are available. Bicortical screws place the internal carotid artery and the hypoglossal nerve, which lie over the anterior aspect of the lateral mass of C1, at risk.

PITFALLS

Visual inspection is performed to ensure that the patient's head is in a neutral position with a minimal chin tuck. Excessive cervical flexion during occipitocervical fusion may impair the patient's line of sight and swallowing function postoperatively.

In the event of injury to the vertebral artery during C1 or C2 screw placement, the anesthesia team must be immediately alerted about the threat of significant blood loss. We recommend aborting the procedure and placing hemostatic agents (Gelfoam) plus a short screw to tamponade the bleeding followed by emergent closure and angiography.

Occipital screws should be placed below the superior nuchal line to reduce the risk of venous sinus injury. If sinus bleeding results after drilling a hole for an occipital screw, the screw should be placed to tamponade the bleeding. Magnetic resonance venography should be performed, and if needed the patient can be placed on antiplatelet medications to prevent thrombosis of the sinus. Cerebrospinal fluid leakage after drilling holes for occipital screws should likewise be treated by placement of the occipital screw.

BAILOUT OPTIONS

- If satisfactory segmental screw fixation cannot be achieved at C1 or C2, we recommend a posterior wiring technique, such as a Brooks technique. In cases of wiring fixation of C1 and C2, we recommend a postoperative halo orthosis because wiring methods do not provide the same degree of immobilization.
- In salvage (reoperation) procedures or if there is a contraindication to midline keel plate placement, a lateral plate on each side of the occiput may be substituted. Screw length, screw purchase, and pullout strength all are inferior with lateral plate constructs compared with midline keel plates.

SUGGESTED READINGS

Ahn UM, Lemma MA, Anh NU, et al. Occipitocervical fusion: a review of indications, techniques of internal fixation, and results. Neurosurg Q 2001;11:77–85.

Finn MA, Bishop FS, Dailey AT. Surgical treatment of occipitocervical instability. Neurosurgery 2008;63:961–9.

Harms J, Melcher RP. Posterior C1-C2 fusion with polyaxial screw and rod fixation. Spine 2001;26:2467–71.

Harris JH, Carson GC, Wagner LK, et al. Radiologic diagnosis of traumatic occipitovertebral dissociation. 2. Comparison of three methods of detecting occipitovertebral relationships on lateral radiographs of supine subjects. AJR Am J Roentgenol 1994;162:887–92.

Rea GL, Kumar VGR. Posterior suboccipital and upper cervical exposure of the occipitocervical junction. In: Fessler RG, Sekhar L, editors. Atlas of Neurosurgical Techniques: Spine and Peripheral Nerves. New York: Thieme; 2006, p. 110–7.

Procedure 57 Transoral Odontoidectomy

Matthew J. Tormenti, Ricky Madhok, Adam S. Kanter

INDICATIONS

- Irreducible atlantoaxial subluxation with compression of cervicomedullary junction
- Ventrally located pathology of the lower clivus or atlantoaxial complex
- Unstable odontoid fractures or os odontoideum with spinal canal stenosis

CONTRAINDICATIONS

- Oral cavity or oropharyngeal infection—increases risk of postoperative infection
- Intradural lesions—better approached from a lateral approach
- Trismus
- Low-riding hard palate—requires a more extensive approach

PLANNING AND POSITIONING

- Preoperative computed tomography (CT) angiography should be performed to evaluate the level of the hard palate and position and course of the carotid arteries.
- Magnetic resonance imaging (MRI) should be considered for evaluation of the ligamentous complex and soft tissue masses.
- Dynamic radiographs are obtained to evaluate craniocervical stability.
- The patient is placed supine on the operating table with the head in a Mayfield head holder in slight extension.
- An optional preoperative tracheostomy is recommended if splitting of the mandible is required to facilitate exposure in patients unable to open their mouths.
- Disruption of the anterior osteoligamentous complex may destabilize the spine and necessitate a dorsal arthrodesis.
- Consider the use of intraoperative neuronavigation.
- Patients with spinal cord compression should have mean arterial pressure maintained intraoperatively at greater than 85 mm Hg.
- **Figure 57-1:** Special attention should be paid to vascular anatomy. Variations such as "kissing carotids" are contraindications to ventral decompression.
- **Figure 57-2:** The location of the hard palate dictates the superior border and extent of exposure and resection.
- **Figure 57-3:** Patients are positioned supine in a Mayfield head holder.

PROCEDURE

- **Figure 57-4:** A Spetzler-Sonntag retractor is placed. It is important to ensure that the tongue and endotracheal tube are behind the retractor.
- **Figure 57-5:** A linear incision is made in the pharyngeal fascia above the odontoid.
- **Figure 57-6:** The incision is opened to expose the anterior ring of C1.

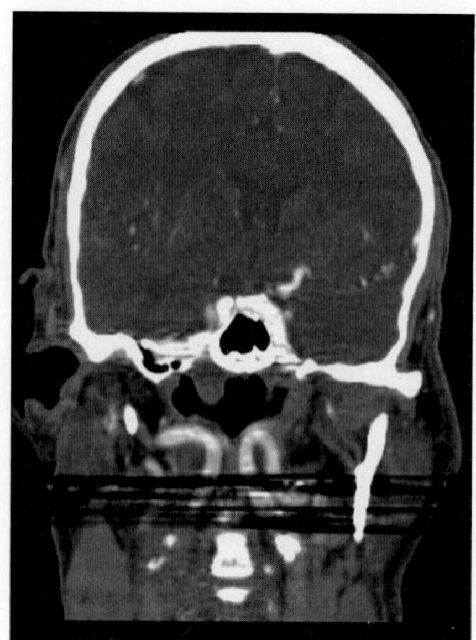

FIGURE 57-1

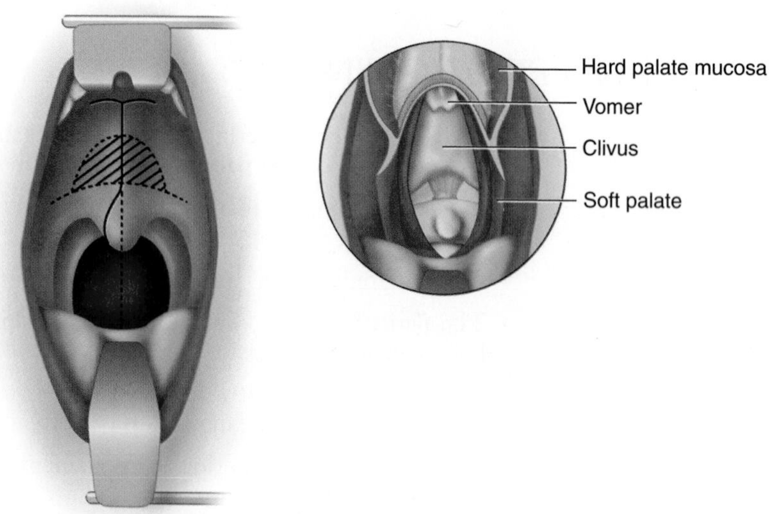

FIGURE 57-2

- **Figure 57-7:** The C1 ring is removed with a high-speed bur.
- **Figure 57-8:** The odontoid is removed using a combination of electric drills and hand tools.
- **Figure 57-9:** Decompression has been completed when the dura has been identified.

TIPS FROM THE MASTERS

- It is essential to know the location of the carotid arteries throughout the procedure; otherwise, catastrophic injury could result.
- The relationship of the hard palate dictates rostral access. The feasibility of this approach can be determined by careful scrutiny of preoperative imaging.
- To achieve successful decompression, it is important to ensure adequate lateral extension of bone removal.

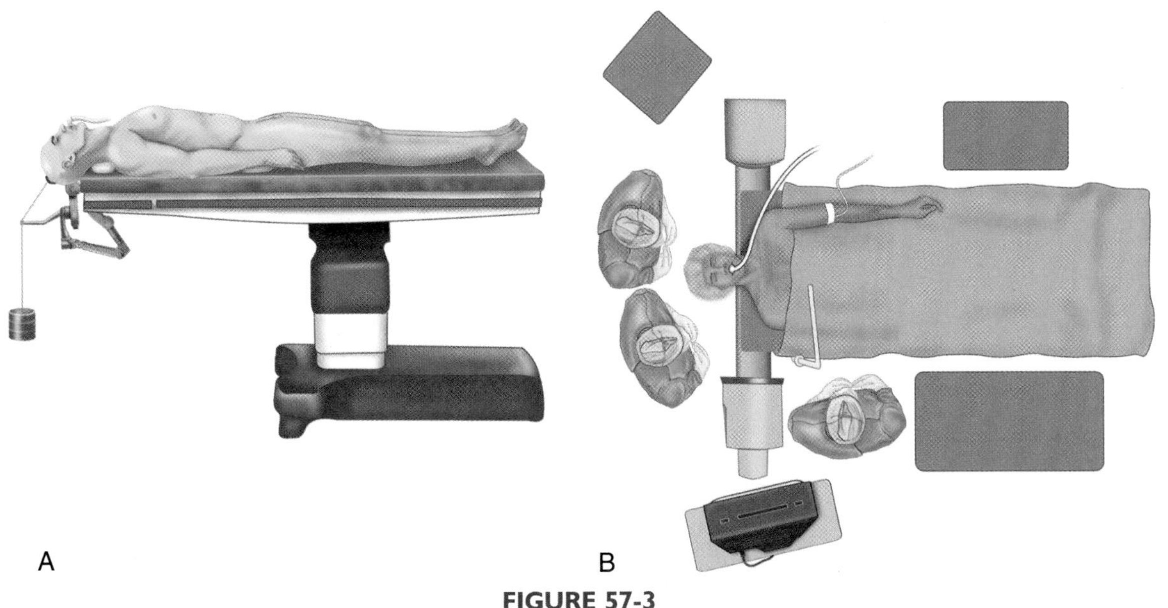

FIGURE 57-3

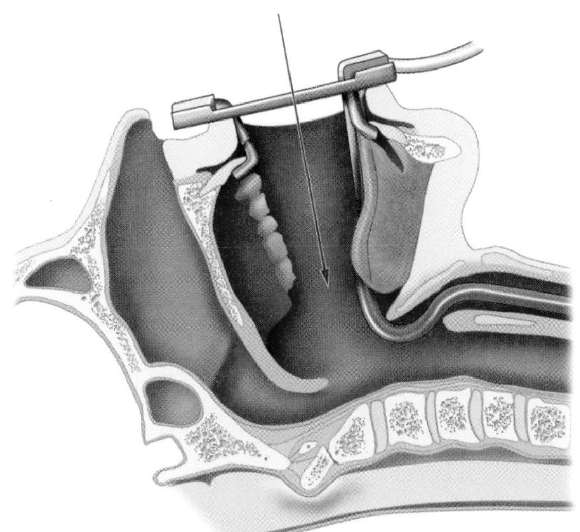

FIGURE 57-4

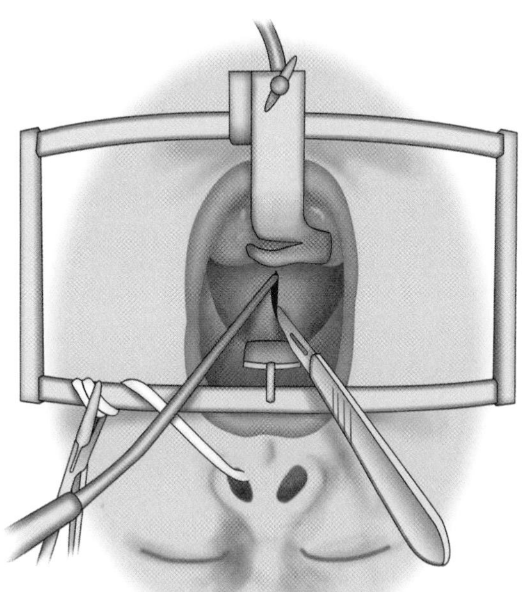

FIGURE 57-5

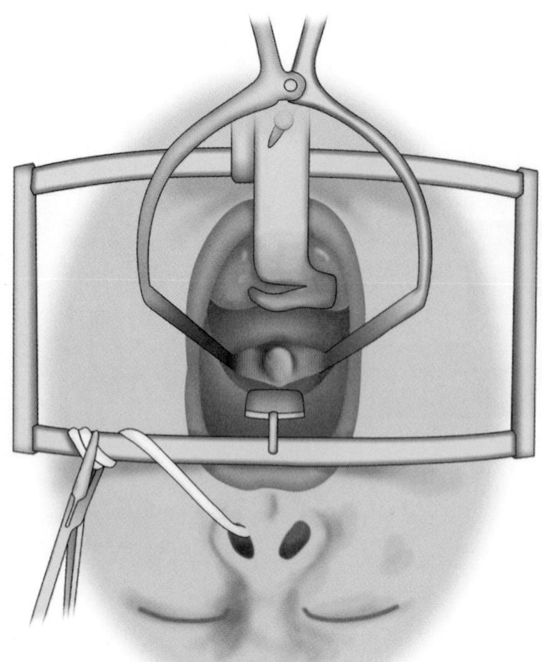

FIGURE 57-6

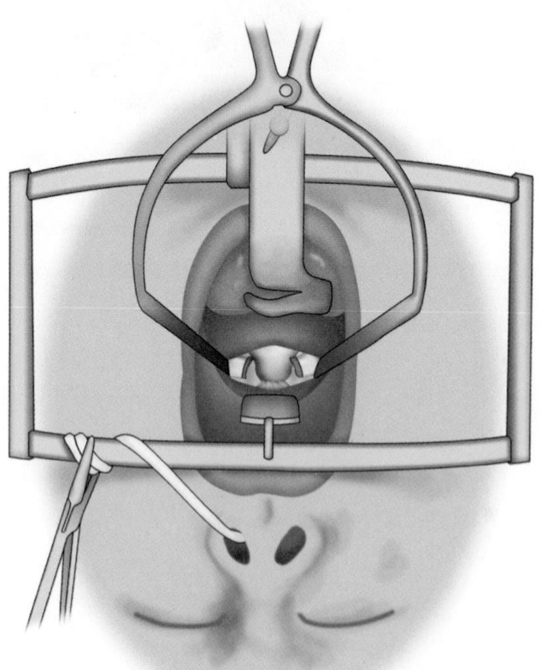

FIGURE 57-7

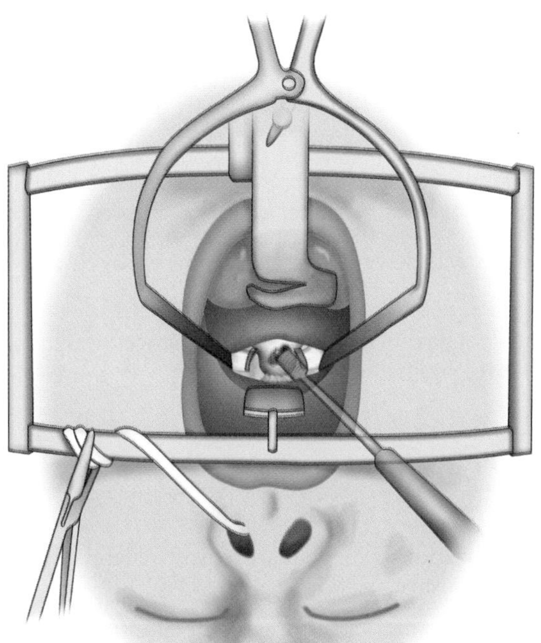

FIGURE 57-8

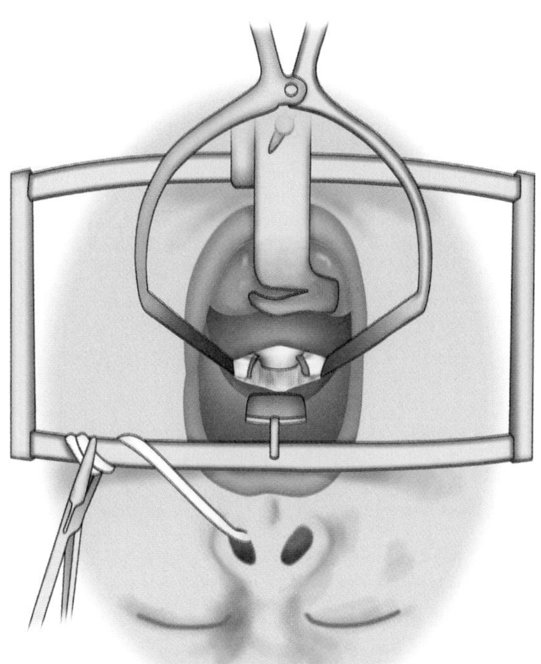

FIGURE 57-9

PITFALLS

Durotomy exposes the patient to the risk of meningitis from the spread of oropharyngeal flora.

Care must be taken during resection at the lateral margin of the exposure to avoid injury to the hypoglossal nerves, vertebral arteries, and carotid arteries.

Patients with severe canal compromise may be subject to ischemic injury during positioning or intraoperative fluctuations in mean arterial pressure.

Some patients may require an occipitocervical fusion because of disruption of the anterior osteoligamentous complex.

BAILOUT OPTIONS

- If visualization is inadequate, a soft palate split or mandibular split may provide additional exposure.
- Watertight dural closure with the addition of a fascial graft and lumbar drainage may help prevent postoperative cerebrospinal fluid fistulas.
- Pathology situated lateral to the hypoglossal nerves and vertebral arteries may be better accessed via anterolateral, lateral, or posterolateral approaches.
- An endonasal approach (independently or combined) may be appropriate in patients with compression above the hard palate. Caudal extent of lesions is a limitation to this approach.
- An endoscope can be useful to assist in visualization.

SUGGESTED READINGS

Crockard HA. The transoral approach to the base of the brain and upper cervical cord. Ann R Coll Surg Engl 1985;67:321–5.

Hadley MN, Spetzler RF, Sonntag VK. The transoral approach to the superior cervical spine: a review of 53 cases of extradural cervicomedullary compression. J Neurosurg 1989;71:16–23.

Menezes AH. Surgical approaches: postoperative care and complications "transoral-transpalatopharyngeal approach to the craniocervical junction". Childs Nerv Syst 2008;24:1187–93.

Menezes AH, VanGilder JC. Transoral-transpharyngeal approach to the anterior craniocervical junction: ten-year experience with 72 patients. J Neurosurg 1988;69:895–903.

Mummaneni PV, Haid RW. Transoral odontoidectomy. Neurosurgery 2005;56:1045–50.

Procedure 58 Odontoid Screw Fixation

Daniel S. Hutton, Kee D. Kim

INDICATIONS

- Patients with acute type II odontoid fractures (<6 months) and patients with fractures with either a transverse or an anterosuperior to posteroinferior fracture plane are the most favorable surgical candidates.
- Odontoid screw fixation is indicated for fractures with displacement of greater than 6 mm, which are unlikely to fuse with external immobilization.
- "Shallow" type III odontoid fractures, in which the fracture pattern extends only minimally into the vertebral body, can be treated with odontoid screw fixation.
- Failure to maintain reduction in halo vest or inability to tolerate halo vest immobilization is another indication.
- Elderly patients with type II odontoid fractures represent a treatment challenge because of comorbidities and varying degrees of osteopenia. Fewer treatment failures and less morbidity are associated with surgical management compared with an external orthosis.

CONTRAINDICATIONS

Absolute

- Disruption of transverse ligament—requires C1-2 fixation because repairing the odontoid fracture would not address C1-2 instability
- Irreducible odontoid fractures
- C2 body fracture
- Comminuted odontoid fracture
- Oblique odontoid fractures, specifically anteroinferior to posterosuperior plane—lead to misalignment with odontoid screw reduction
- Pathologic fracture

Relative

- A barrel chest can obstruct the needed trajectory for odontoid screw placement.
- Osteoporosis or osteopenia leads to higher rates of pseudarthrosis and screw pullout.
- Fractures more than 6 months old or with documented pseudarthrosis from nonsurgical management have been treated with odontoid screw fixation but with less favorable results. Some authors recommend curettage of the segment with pseudarthrosis and placement of two screws.
- Concomitant cervical stenosis, can lead to neurologic deficit during manipulation of fracture.

PLANNING AND POSITIONING

- Because of the highly mobile nature of type II odontoid fractures, awake fiberoptic intubation is recommended. After the airway is secured, the endotracheal tube should be secured to the side opposite to the surgical exposure. The table is turned 180 degrees away from anesthesia.

- Two fluoroscopy units are positioned for direct lateral and anteroposterior open-mouth views. A roll of gauze sponges, a radiolucent tape, or a large wooden cork is placed into the oropharynx to keep the mouth open and facilitate anterior open-mouth views. The surgeon needs to confirm true lateral and obstruction-free anteroposterior views of cervical extension; additional scapular padding or manual transoral reduction may be necessary to provide adequate alignment.
- Close attention must be paid to patient positioning, especially if intraoperative reduction is necessary. A well-positioned crack at the head of the bed may be adjusted intraoperatively to achieve more extension or flexion.
- Preoperative images such as lateral x-ray and sagittal computed tomography (CT) reconstructed view are used to obtain an approximate length of the screw to achieve bicortical purchase. Sufficient room usually exists at the craniocervical junction to accommodate up to 5 mm additional length to the screw.
- A radiopaque object should be placed in the trajectory of the odontoid screw as an approximation to the drill guide angle and working distance. Assessment of the level of skin incision and any other impediments should be addressed at this time. The typical level of skin incision is at C4-5.
- **Figure 58-1:** The operative bed is turned 180 degrees from anesthesia, with the neck carefully extended. Two fluoroscopy machines should be positioned for direct lateral view and anteroposterior open-mouth views. Monitors are placed side-by-side for surgeon's ease of viewing.
- **Figure 58-2:** Careful adjustment to cervical extension is performed to align the fracture adequately and facilitate screw placement. The positioning of the patient can often lead to reduction of the posteriorly displaced dens. For anteriorly displaced fractures, transoral manual reduction of the anteriorly displaced odontoid process is often an effective means for the placement of the odontoid screw.

PROCEDURE

- After the skin is prepared, a transverse incision is made in the typical manner for anterior cervical diskectomy. Dissection is performed to the level of the platysma, which is undermined superficial and deep to the muscle. The muscle is opened in a transverse fashion, and dissection is continued in the avascular plane medial to the carotid artery. Cloward retractors are used to retract the trachea and esophagus and carotid artery away from midline structures. With the prevertebral fascia exposed, careful blunt dissection is

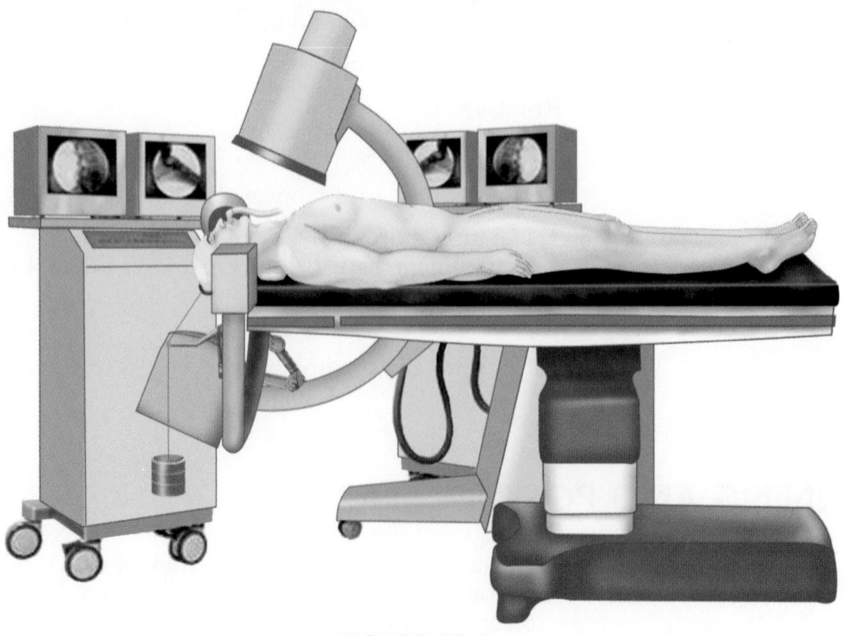

FIGURE 58-1

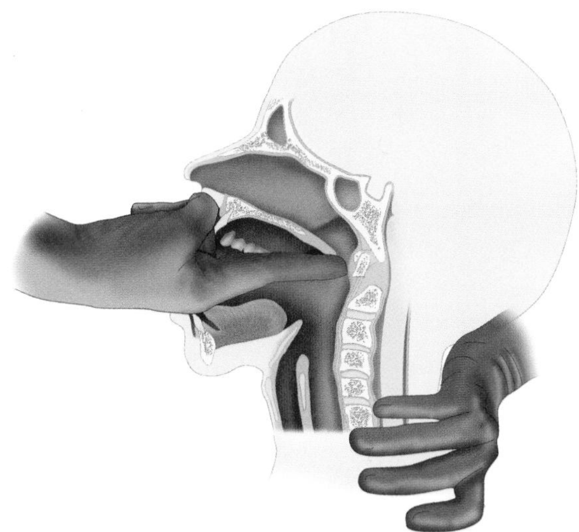

FIGURE 58-2

performed in a cephalad direction to the C2-3 disk space. A localizing lateral image is obtained for confirmation. The prevertebral fascia is opened, and longus colli muscles are reflected from its medial edge. Self-retaining retractors are placed for medial-lateral exposure. If the retractor system does not have a built-in cephalad retractor, a hand-held Cloward or Hohmann retractor may be placed for exposure superiorly. We have also used a vaginal speculum to obtain an adequate exposure in lieu of a traditional retractor.

- Typically, the anterosuperior margin of the C3 vertebral body and C2-3 disk space is hand-drilled to obtain the proper trajectory of odontoid screw. The starting point of screw placement is the anteroinferior end plate of C2, with a trajectory extending to the posterosuperior portion of the odontoid process. The single screw technique employs a midline screw starting point and trajectory. The dual screw technique starts 3 to 5 mm lateral to the midline and has slight lateral-to-medial convergence to the same endpoint.
- **Figure 58-3:** After the proper starting point and trajectory have been selected, an awl is used to gain cortical purchase at the C2 end plate. A Kirschner wire is placed at the entry point and drilled in the trajectory previously selected. This step is monitored with frequent anteroposterior and lateral images.

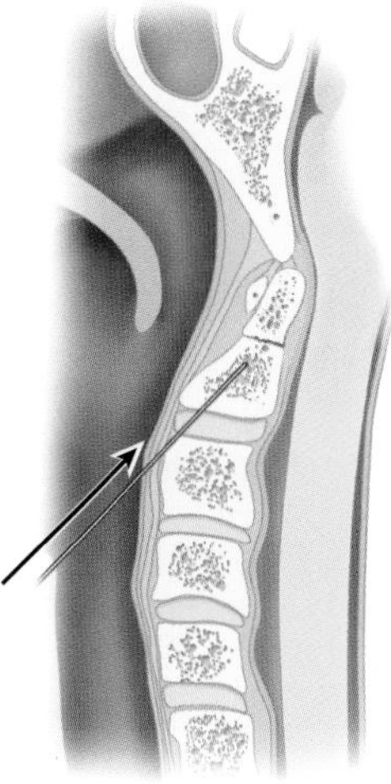

FIGURE 58-3

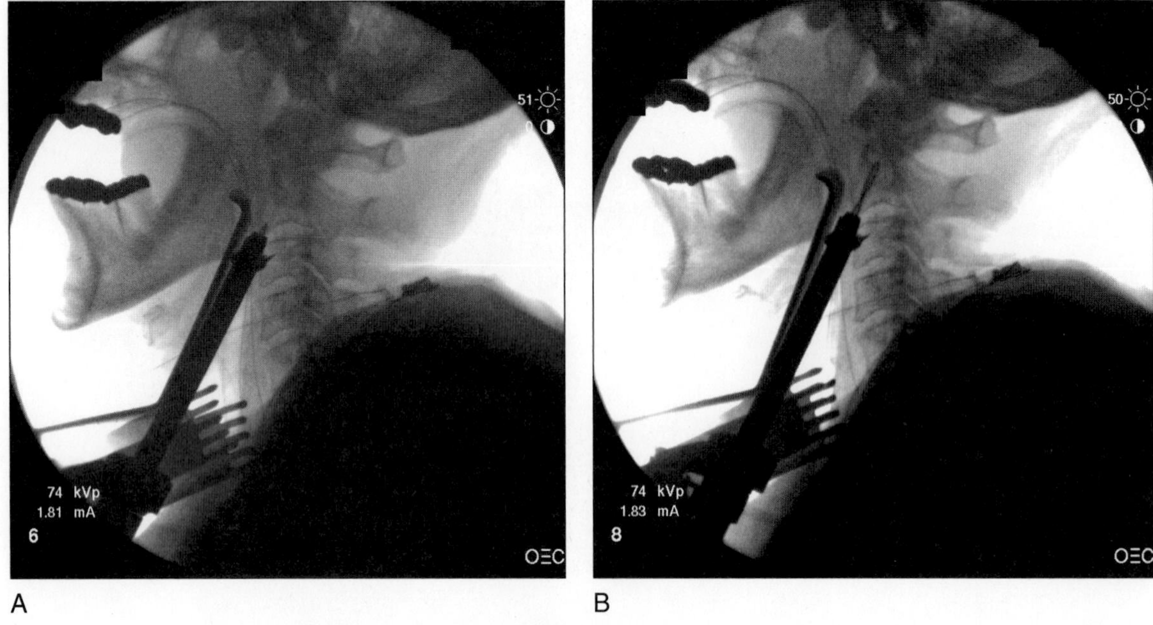

A B

FIGURE 58-4

- **Figure 58-4: A,** Lateral image depicting entry of the drill into the inferior end plate of C2 and intended trajectory. A cannulated drill bit is placed over the Kirschner wire to create a cavity for the drill bit and is secured to the C2 end plate with a spiked drill guide. The Kirschner wire and inner sleeve are removed, with the outer spiked drill guide remaining. A 2.5-mm drill is introduced through the guide, and the trajectory is confirmed again with biplanar imaging. The C2 body and fractured dens are drilled. Because of exposure limitations, a right-angled drill is often useful and more manageable than a standard drill. Frequent imaging along with tactile feel of drilling is used to monitor depth of the drill bit. The screw length is measured from the depth markers on the drill bit. **B,** Lateral imaging displaying the drill as it nears the fracture line.
- **Figure 58-5: A,** Lateral image with bicortical purchase with the drill. This is typically the optimal vantage point for bicortical purchase because anteroposterior imaging is frequently obscured by the hard palate. The length of the screw is determined by graduated marks on the drill and confirmed with biplanar fluoroscopy. **B,** Anteroposterior image confirming the coronal trajectory.

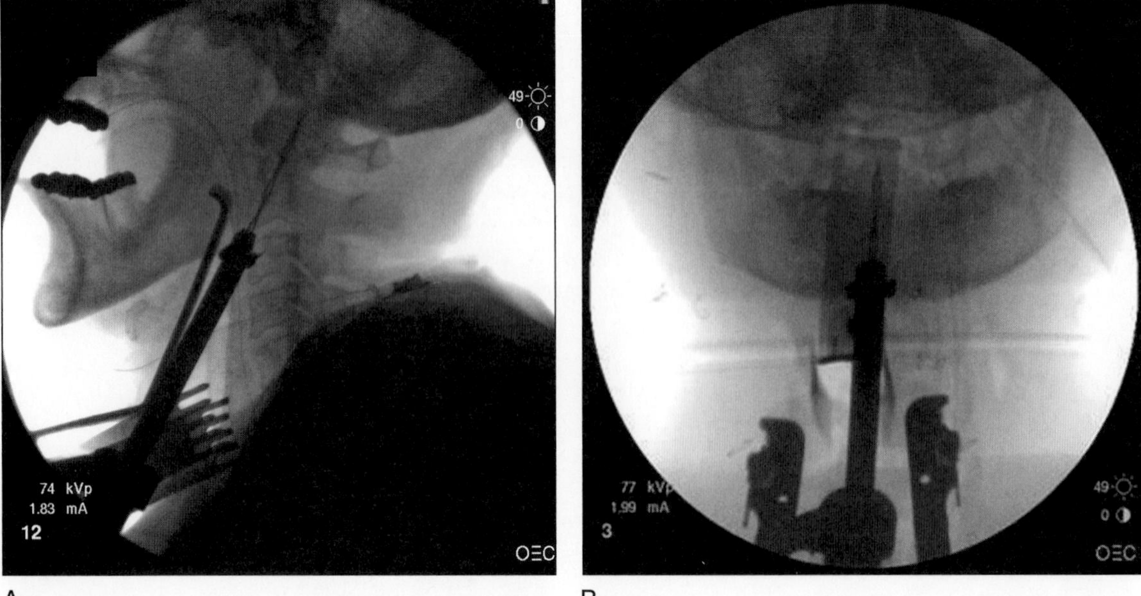

A B

FIGURE 58-5

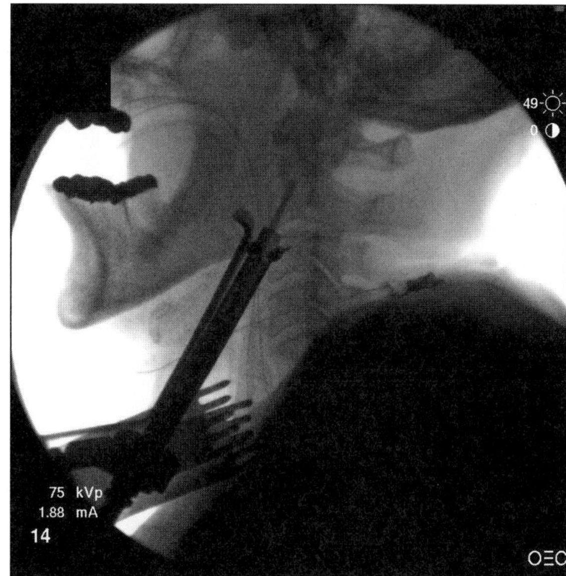

FIGURE 58-6

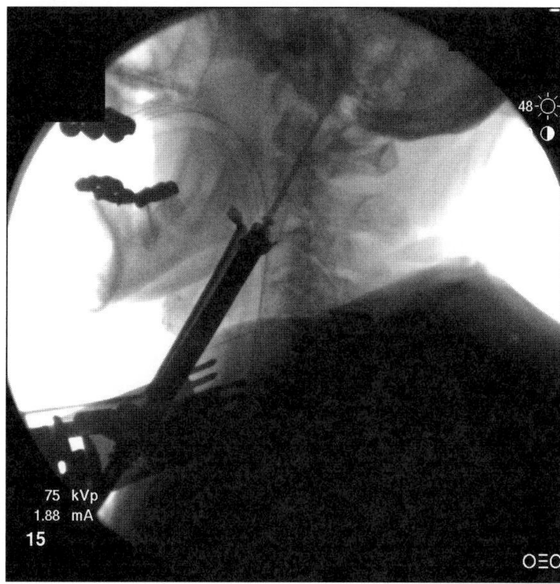

FIGURE 58-7

- **Figure 58-6:** Lateral image of odontoid screw placement. The drill is removed, and the pilot hole is tapped and the cannulated screw is placed over the Kirschner wire. The tip of the lag screw is nearing the fracture line.
- **Figure 58-7:** Lateral image of proper screw length and purchase. Objective of screw placement is bicortical purchase and close approximation of fractured dens and C2 vertebral body.
- **Figure 58-8:** Final anteroposterior **(A)** and lateral **(B)** images of screw placement. Proper trajectory and bicortical purchase are obtained.

TIPS FROM THE MASTERS

- Threaded portion of the screw should reside only in the fractured dens; otherwise, apposition of the fractured surfaces may be impossible and lead to pseudarthrosis.
- Bicortical purchase aids in proper approximation of the fracture and biomechanical strength of purchase and prevents screw backout.

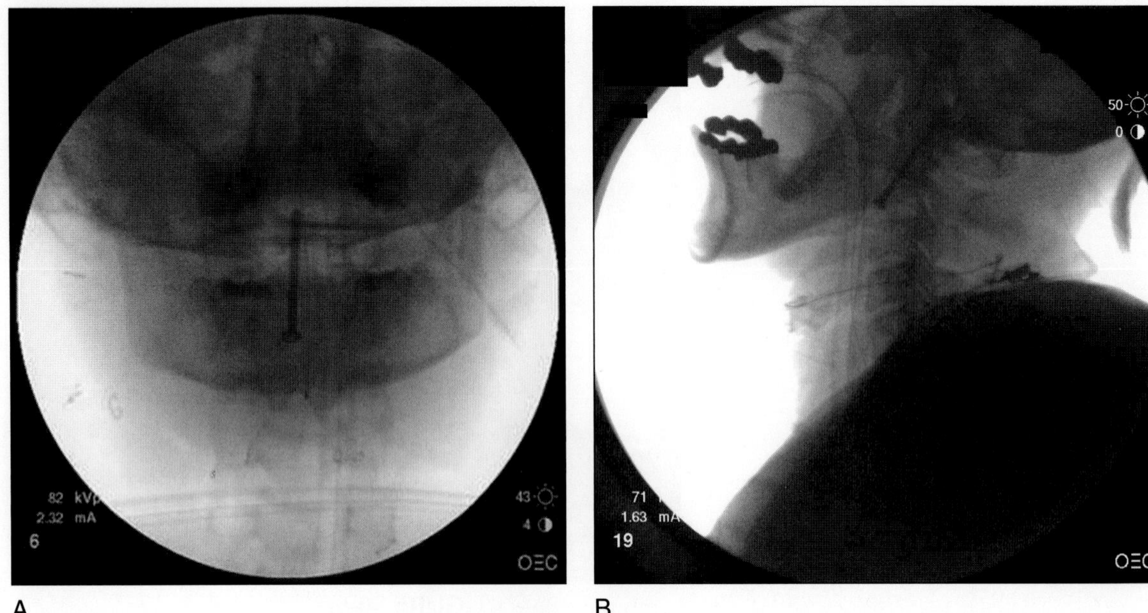

A B

FIGURE 58-8

- The odontoid screw head should be flush with the C2 body to minimize interference of normal motion at C2-3. Otherwise, accelerated degeneration, such as degenerative disk changes and osteophyte formation at C2-3, may result.
- Previously cited as a contraindication for odontoid screw placement, malalignment or angulation can be manipulated intraoperatively via posterior cervical manual pressure or direct transoral reduction for screw placement.
- The cannulated screw technique offers reliable access to a consistent surgical plane. Lack of stiffness of the Kirschner wire makes it difficult for the cannulated drill bit to follow the same course, however, if the trajectory is changed slightly. Also, mechanical strength of the cannulated screw is less than that of the noncannulated screw. More importantly, the Kirschner wire requires close observation during the procedure to prevent inadvertent removal or advancement into the foramen magnum.
- Controversies arise regarding the single screw versus dual screw for effective fixation. The single screw technique is supported in the literature as providing an excellent rate of fusion, without the postulated rotation of the odontoid process on the C2 vertebral body. The single screw versus dual screw technique largely remains the surgeon's preference.

PITFALLS
Inadequate imaging
Unable to achieve bicortical purchase
Inadequate reduction of fracture segment with lag screw
Improper screw trajectory
Aberrant hardware or Kirschner wire causing neurologic or vascular injury

BAILOUT OPTIONS

- Atlantoaxial arthrodesis can be performed if the odontoid screw cannot be successfully placed.
- When discussing placement of an odontoid screw with patients, the surgeon must always discuss the possibility of atlantoaxial arthrodesis. If the positioning of the patient or placement of the screw is inadequate or unsafe, the surgeon should proceed to atlantoaxial arthrodesis.

SUGGESTED READINGS

Apfelbaum RI, Lonser RR, Veres R, et al. Direct anterior screw fixation for recent and remote odontoid fractures. Neurosurg Focus 2000;8:1–10.

Dickman CA, Foley KT, Sonntag VH, et al. Cannulated screws for odontoid fixation and atlantoaxial transarticular screw fixation. A technical note. J Neurosurg 1995;83:1095–100.

Graziano G, Jaggers C, Lee M, et al. A comparative study of fixation techniques for type II fractures of the odontoid process. Spine 1993;18:2383–7.

Julien TD, Frankel B, Traynelis VC, et al. Evidence-based analysis of odontoid fracture management. Neurosurg Focus 2000;8:1–5.

Masciopinto JE, Kim KD, Johnson PJ. Odontoid screw fixation. In: An HS, Cotler JM, editors. Spinal Instrumentation. 2nd ed. Philadelphia: Lippincott Williams & Wilkins; 1999, pp. 221–7.

Polin RS, Szabo T, Bogaev CA, et al. Nonoperative management of types II and III odontoid fractures: the Philadelphia collar versus the halo vest. Neurosurgery 1996;38:450–7.

Procedure 59

Anterior Cervical Diskectomy

Benjamin M. Zussman, Peter G. Campbell, James S. Harrop

INDICATIONS

- Cervical disk herniation with persistent radiculopathy after conservative measures
- Cervical disk herniation with spinal cord compression
- Cervical disk herniation with significant spinal canal compromise
- Cervical spondylosis with multiple disk herniations and anterior osteophytes

CONTRAINDICATIONS

- Posterior cervical pathology is best treated with posterior approaches with or without fusion.
- Patients whose careers prohibit any risk for voice alterations may best be treated with posterior foraminotomies or laminectomies.

PLANNING AND POSITIONING

- Preoperative imaging is essential to identify pathology and verify the corresponding vertebral level.
- Useful tools include loupes and possibly an operating microscope.
- If the decision has been made for iliac crest autograft, the hip should be prepared and draped.
- **Figure 59-1:** Position the patient supine with the bed in a slight reverse Trendelenburg position. Place an inflatable cushion between the scapulae. Consider using monitoring before and after positioning if myelopathy is present.
- Wrap arms in gel pads to protect the ulnar nerve. Secure the patient to the table with tape and seat belt.

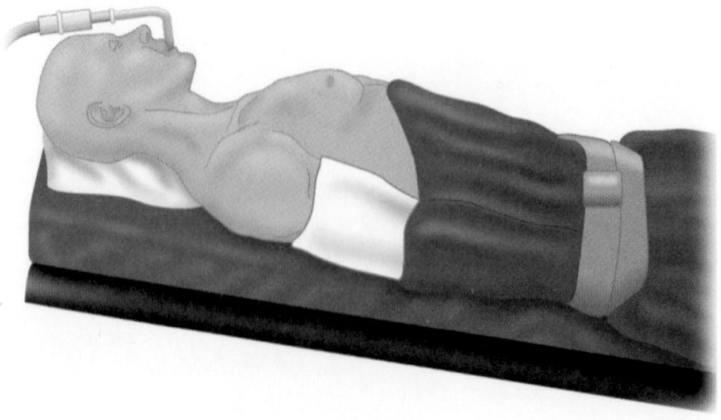

FIGURE 59-1

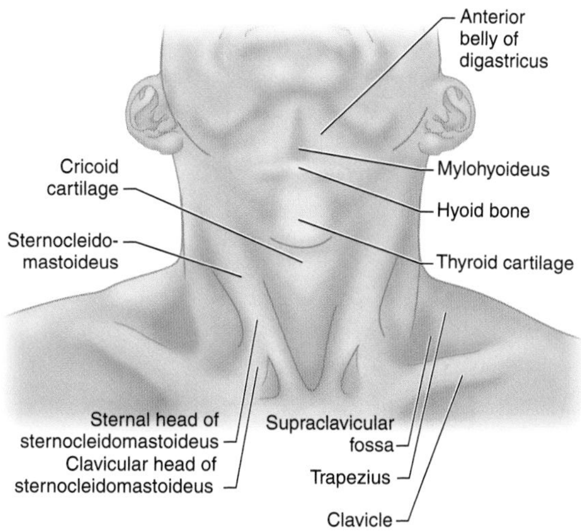

FIGURE 59-2

- **Figure 59-2:** Use anatomic landmarks to determine the cervical level; the thyroid cartilage localizes C4-5, and palpation of the carotid tubercle localizes the C6 level. If it is difficult to ascertain the level accurately, mark the incision slightly superior to the estimated level of pathology; it is easier to expose inferiorly than superiorly.

PROCEDURE

- **Figure 59-3:** Make a transverse skin incision. Incise the platysma to expose the deep cervical musculature. Use bipolar electrocautery to maintain hemostasis. Develop the avascular plane. Use blunt dissection in this plane to expose the vertebral bodies. Dissect the longus colli muscle to the prevertebral fascia laterally using blunt techniques.
- **Figure 59-4:** Place a radiopaque marker into the disk space of interest. Use an intraoperative x-ray to confirm cervical level. Attempt to use two markers in case one is removed inadvertently.
- **Figure 59-5:** Use a depth gauge to select size-appropriate retractor blades. Introduce a dull blade medially and a serrated blade laterally. Gently secure the retractors under each longus colli muscle and retract laterally to expose the bony vertebrae and disks.

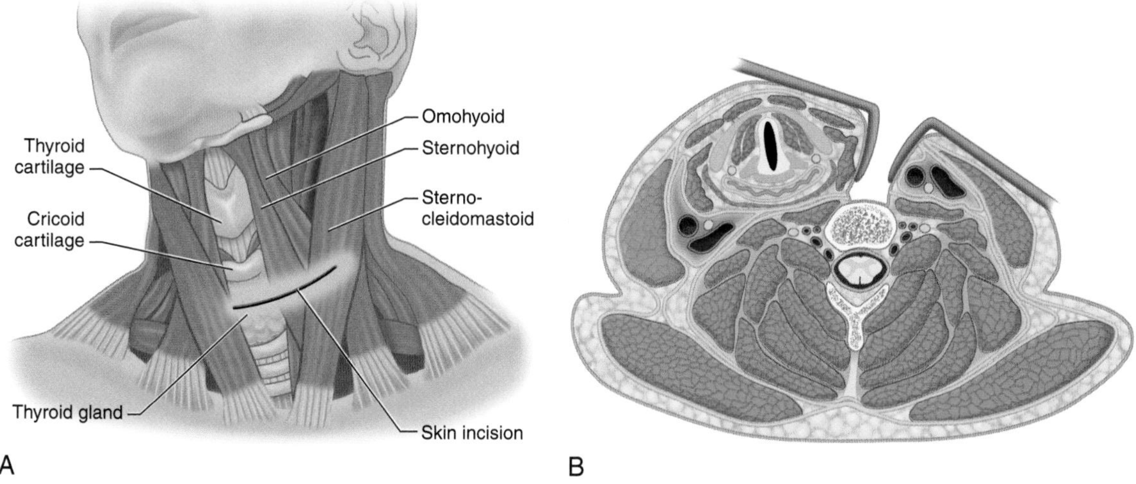

FIGURE 59-3

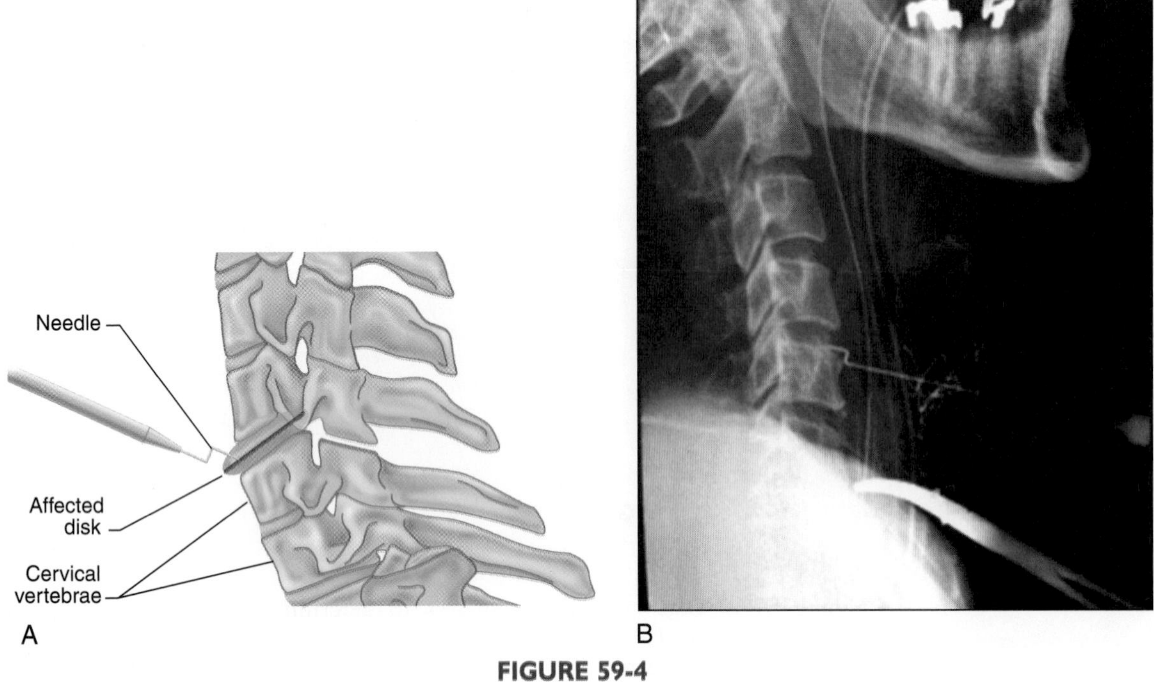

FIGURE 59-4

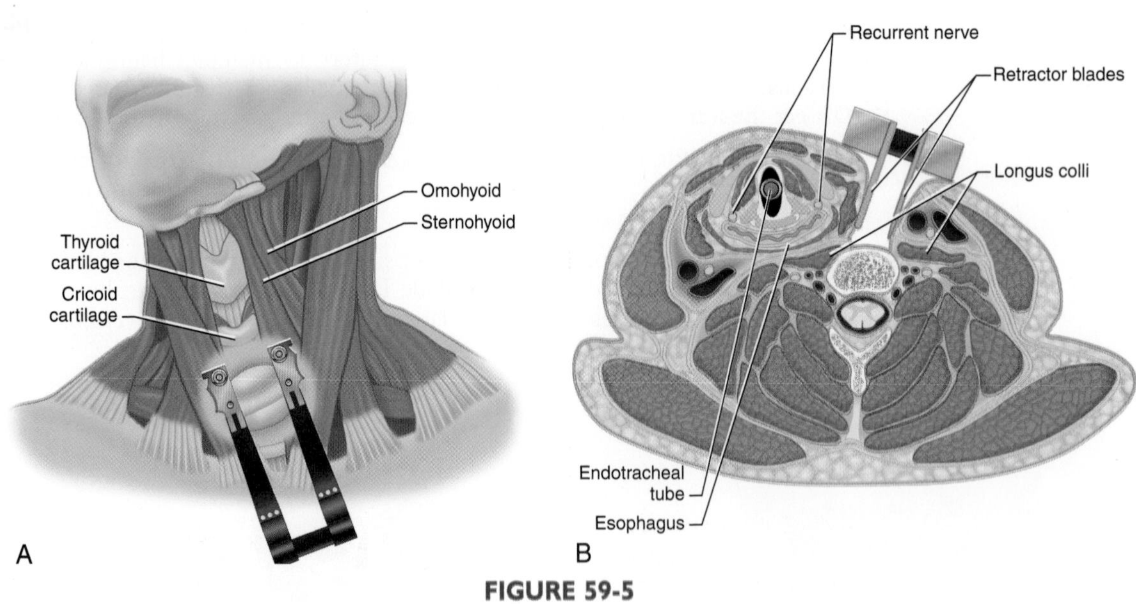

FIGURE 59-5

- **Figure 59-6:** Use Caspar distraction pins to separate the vertebrae above and below the affected disk. If a multilevel procedure is being performed, distract one disk space at a time, not several at once.
- **Figure 59-7: A,** Use the scalpel to incise the disk annulus, cutting laterally to medially in four separate cuts. **B,** Use the curet to dissect the end plate from the disk material. Remove the bulk of the disk with the pituitary rongeur. **C,** Continue to remove the disk material until the posterior longitudinal ligament is visualized.

A
B
Affected disk
Distraction pins

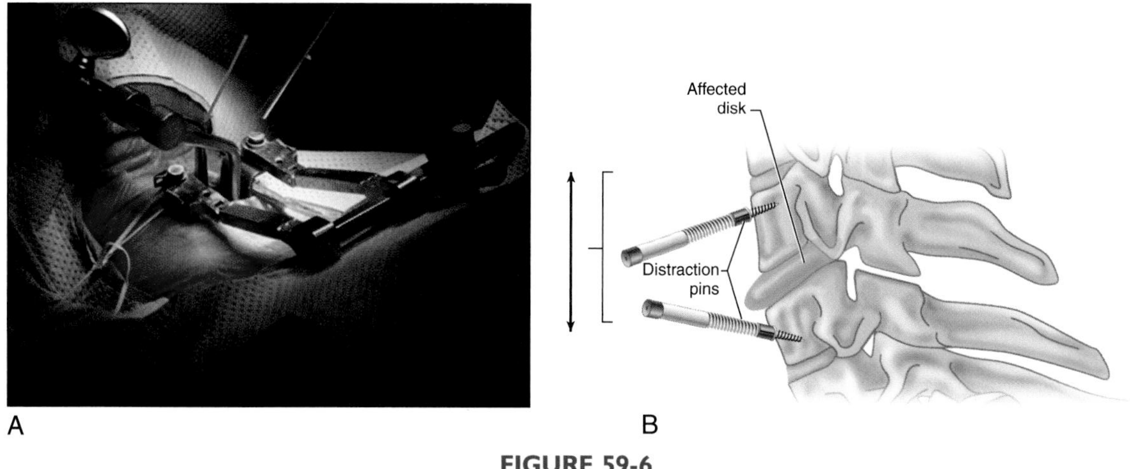

FIGURE 59-6

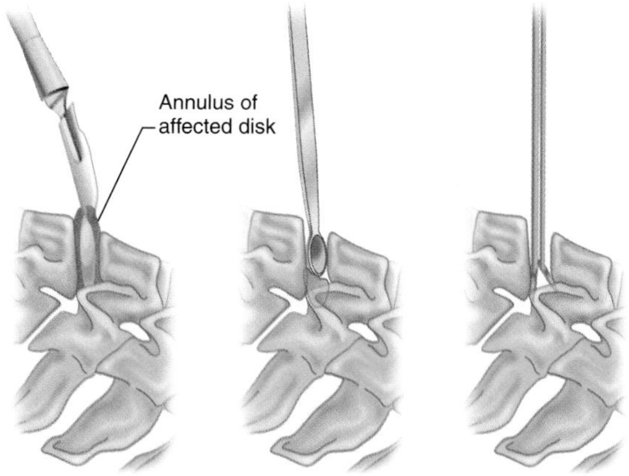

Annulus of affected disk

FIGURE 59-7

- **Figure 59-8:** Remove ventral and then dorsal osteophytes with a curet, Kerrison rongeur, or high-speed bur. Remove end plates to expose blood-rich cancellous bone.
- **Figure 59-9:** Contour a graft if necessary, and tap into the shelf space. Reinforce with metal plate; the shortest plate possible is preferred. Screw the plate into the vertebrae with superior screws angled upward and inward and inferior screws angled inward and posterior.

TIPS FROM THE MASTERS

- When the retractors are placed, deflate and then reinflate the endotracheal tube cuff. This action recenters the endotracheal tube within the larynx and may reduce the incidence of recurrent laryngeal nerve injury, by reducing the compression on the transtracheal component of the nerve.

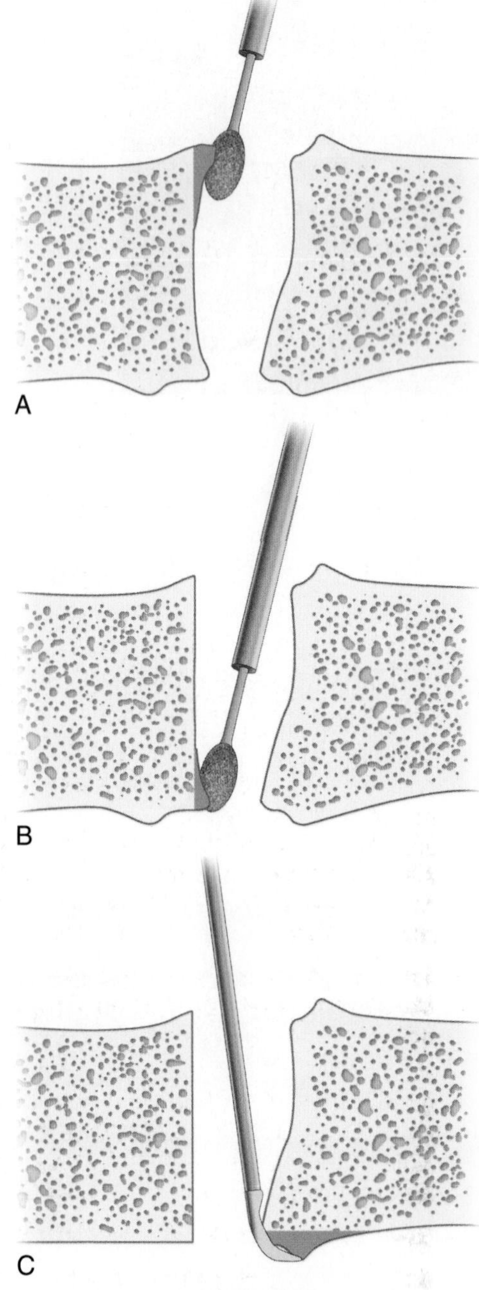

FIGURE 59-8

- When the spine is exposed, mark the sagittal plane with a pen or monopolar cautery. Later, this midline aids in positioning the graft and instrumentation.
- Surgeon preference and individual patient characteristics should be considered in determining the side of surgical approach. Right-sided versus left-sided approaches do not significantly alter outcomes.
- When significant retraction is needed, visual inspection of the esophageal undersurface can identify small tears that can be primarily repaired with absorbable sutures.
- Orogastric tube placement by the anesthesiologist before anterior cervical dissection can help with identification of the esophagus in reoperative cases.

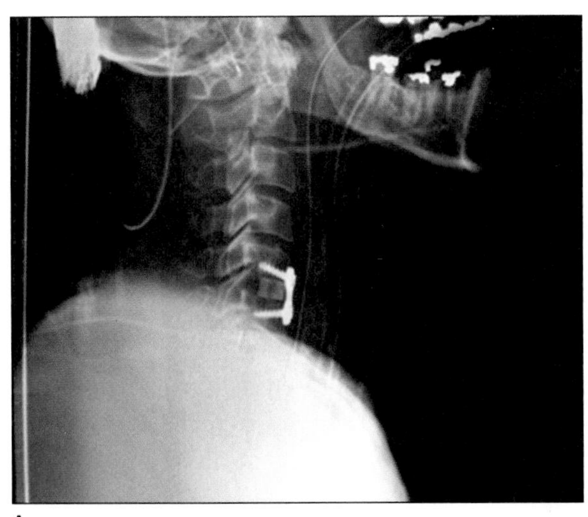
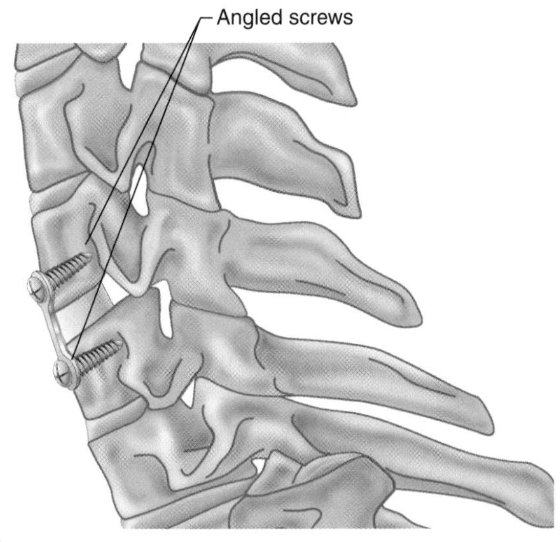

A B

FIGURE 59-9

PITFALLS

Associated morbidities include postoperative (typically transient) dysphagia in 10% of patients, postoperative wound hematoma in 6% of patients, and recurrent laryngeal nerve palsy in 3% of patients.

Neurologic vascular injuries are uncommon and may be prevented by using blunt-edged retractors conservatively. A small vertebral artery injury can be packed and followed by postoperative angiogram. Significant injury to the vertebral artery may require expanding exposure for primary control for proximal and distal arterial segments.

Dural penetration, esophageal perforation, worsening of preexisting myelopathy, Horner syndrome, instrumentation failure, and superficial wound infection are rare.

Before performing reoperative surgery on the opposite side, direct laryngoscopy should be performed to identify existing vocal cord paralysis. Bilateral vocal cord paralysis requires tracheostomy and should be avoided.

BAILOUT OPTIONS

- If perforation of the trachea, esophagus, dura, or a major blood vessel occurs, attempt to perform intraoperative repairs.
- Postoperatively, if decompression is incomplete, attempt a subsequent posterior decompression.
- If graft or instrumentation fails, collapses, or shifts, perform revision surgery with posterior instrumentation as needed.

SUGGESTED READINGS

Apfelbaum RI, Kriskovich MD, Haller JR. On the incidence, cause, and prevention of recurrent laryngeal nerve palsies during anterior cervical spine surgery. Spine 2000;25:2906–12.

Deutsch H, Haid R, Rodts G Jr, et al. The decision-making process: allograft versus autograft. Neurosurgery 2007;60(1 Suppl. 1):S98–102.

Fountas KN, Kapsalaki EZ, Nikolakakos LG, et al. Anterior cervical discectomy and fusion associated complications. Spine 2007;32:2310–7.

Harrop JS, Hanna A, Silva MT, et al. Neurological manifestations of cervical spondylosis: an overview of signs, symptoms, and pathophysiology. Neurosurgery 2007;60(1 Suppl. 1):S14–20.

Hillard VH, Apfelbaum RI. Surgical management of cervical myelopathy: indications and techniques for multilevel cervical discectomy. Spine J 2006;6(Suppl. 6):242S–51S.

Procedure 60

Anterior Cervical Corpectomy and Fusion

Carmina F. Angeles, Jon Park

INDICATIONS

- Correction of cervical kyphotic deformity
- Decompression of the cervical spinal cord in degenerative spondylotic myelopathy
- Excision of ossified posterior longitudinal ligament (PLL) that often bridges past disk spaces and cannot be adequately removed with diskectomies alone
- Treatment of osteomyelitis that fails nonoperative management
- Resection and stabilization of vertebral body tumor
- Management of traumatic fractures of the subaxial spine, such as vertebral body burst fracture, or as part of circumferential stabilization with fracture-dislocations
- Facilitation of fusion in cases with multiple contiguous levels of cervical disk herniation—a mixture of diskectomies and a corpectomy can facilitate fusion by decreasing the total number of end plates through which fusion must occur

CONTRAINDICATIONS

- Previous radiation to the anterior neck obscures dissection planes.
- Multiple prior anterior surgeries and severe anterior soft tissue injury are contraindications.
- Aberrant vertebral artery anatomy is a relative contraindication and requires attention to width of the corpectomy trough.
- Chin on chest deformity is best treated with cervicothoracic fusion and T1 osteotomy.
- Anterior bony ankylosis secondary to degenerative or inflammatory disease is a contraindication.
- This procedure cannot be done in patients with medical contraindications to general anesthesia.

PLANNING AND POSITIONING

- **Figure 60-1:** The room is set up so that the anesthesiologist is at the head of the table, the microscope and headlight are on the ipsilateral side of the incision, the fluoroscopy base is on the contralateral side, and the scrub nurse is positioned below the patient's iliac crest on the ipsilateral side as the surgeon.
- The patient is positioned supine on a radiolucent table.
- The patient is asked to extend the neck. If neck extension is adequate, general endotracheal anesthesia is administered. Often, the patient has severe myelopathy and cord compression requiring awake or fiberoptic intubation.
- A rolled sheet is placed across the shoulder to facilitate extension, and the head is supported on a foam donut. In trauma or cervical spine instability, alignment should be verified with fluoroscopy.

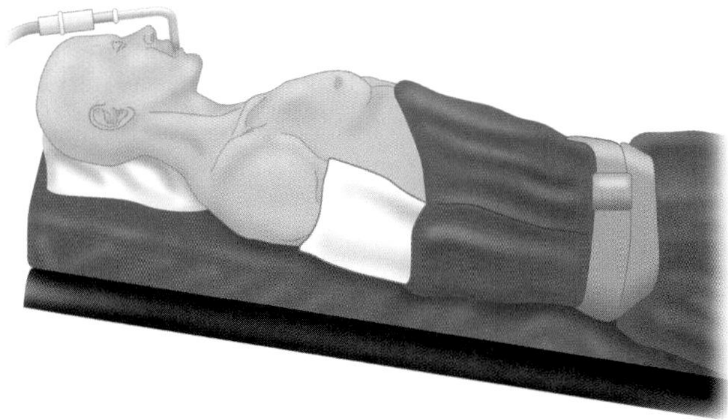

FIGURE 60-1

- Intraoperative neurophysiologic monitoring, such somatosensory evoked potentials and motor evoked potentials, may be used.
- The patient's arms are tucked to the side, and the shoulders are taped down to facilitate visualization of the lower cervical spine under fluoroscopy.
- **Figure 60-2:** The incision is planned according to the level of pathology. The incision is often made at a natural skin crease line closest to pathology to achieve a cosmetically more pleasing outcome.
- Levels of pathology are as follows:
  - C1-3—1 cm below the angle of the jaw
  - C3-4—hyoid bone
  - C4-5—top of the thyroid cartilage
  - C5-6—bottom of thyroid cartilage
  - C6-7—top of cricoid cartilage
  - C7-T1—bottom of cricoids cartilage
- The surgery can be performed from a right-sided or left-sided approach based on the surgeon's handedness (i.e., right-handed surgeons prefer a right-sided approach and vice versa), and based on the side contralateral to the arm with more severe radiculopathy.

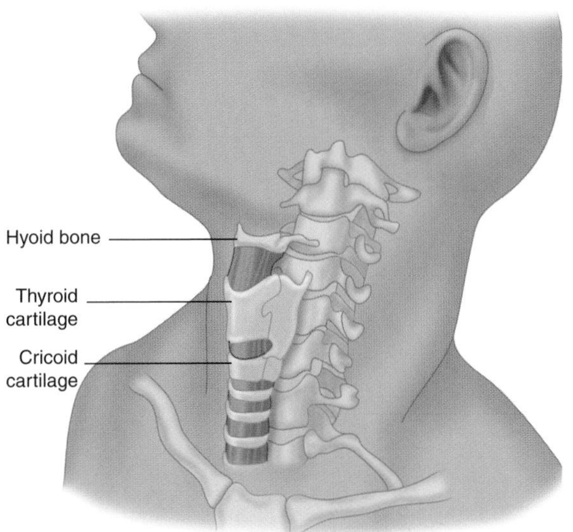

FIGURE 60-2

- If iliac crest autograft is being harvested, a pillow is placed under the buttock. The incision is planned lateral to the anterior superior iliac spine to avoid inadvertent damage to the lateral femoral cutaneous nerve.
- Draping is done in the usual manner, with the iliac crest incision site being draped separately and covered.

PROCEDURE

- **Figure 60-3:** Proposed longitudinal incision along the anterior margin of the sternocleidomastoid muscle. For a one-level cervical corpectomy, a horizontal incision can be made. For a multilevel corpectomies or in patients with short necks, cervical kyphosis, or chronic obstructive pulmonary disease, a longitudinal incision along the anterior margin of the sternocleidomastoid muscle may provide increased exposure of the cervical spine. If the lower part of C2 needs to be exposed, a horizontal incision in the submandibular area may be added at the superior end of the longitudinal incision.
- **Figure 60-4:** Schematic cross-sectional diagram showing structures encountered during exposure and layers of cervical fascia entered. A standard anterolateral approach is carried out as described by Robinson and Smith in 1955. After injecting local anesthetic, skin is incised. The platysma is encountered, elevated from the deep cervical fascia, and cut sharply with Metzenbaum scissors. The superficial layer of the deep cervical fascia is encountered as an investing layer that splits around the sternocleidomastoid muscle. The fascia is opened longitudinally along the anterior border of the sternocleidomastoid. The omohyoid muscle is encountered in the middle layer of the deep cervical fascia. Fascial

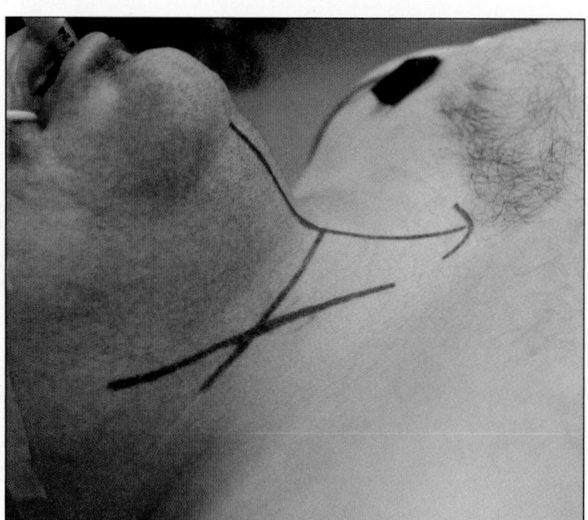

FIGURE 60-3

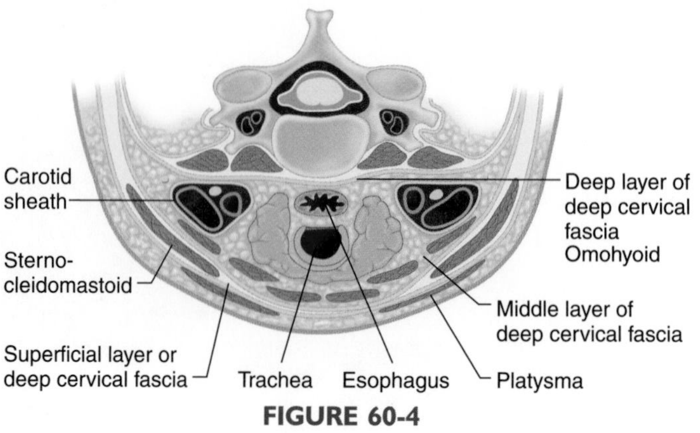

FIGURE 60-4

release and retraction is usually adequate to mobilize this muscle, but occasionally the muscle must be divided at its mid-portion. The muscle is gently retracted laterally, while the strap muscles, esophagus, and trachea are retracted medially. The carotid sheath containing the common carotid artery, vein, and vagus nerve is palpated and retracted laterally with the sternocleidomastoid muscle. This exposes the deep layer of the deep cervical fascia, which separates the trachea and esophagus from the vertebral bodies and the longus colli muscles. The longus colli muscles are elevated with pulse monopolar electrocautery creating a shelf to anchor self-retaining retractors. Retractors are secured in this shelf to prevent soft tissue injury owing to migrating retractors and may serve as a protection against the drill.

- **Figure 60-5:** Lateral radiograph showing localizing needle in disk space for confirmation of level. The needle can be contoured to prevent inadvertent, excessively deep insertion into the disk and risk of injury to the dural or spinal cord.
- **Figure 60-6:** Distraction pins need to be placed in the center of the vertebral body in cephalocaudal and medial-to-lateral directions. The midline is identified based on insertion of the longus colli muscles. The insertion of the longus colli muscles is usually equidistant from the midline and can be used to locate the midline. A No. 4 Penfield can also be used to palpate the lateral edges of the vertebral body and can help locate the midline. Identifying the disk spaces above and below the vertebral body can help locate the center. Distraction pins are inserted into the mid-portion of the vertebral bodies above and below the corpectomy level. Screws should be angled so that they are parallel to the end plates.

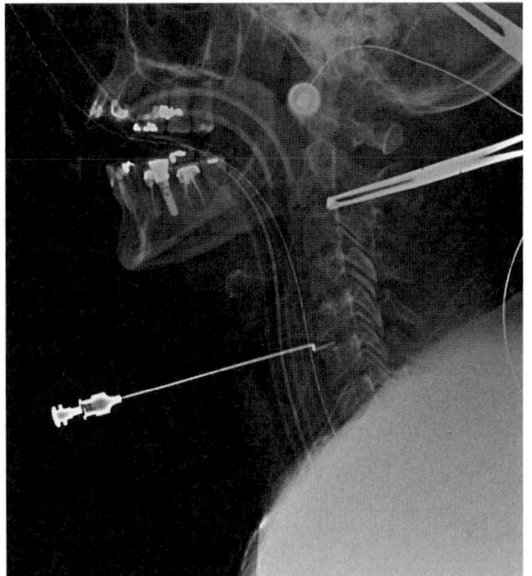

FIGURE 60-5

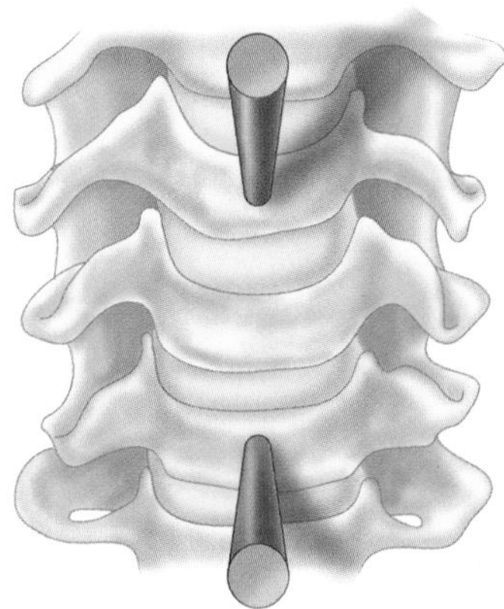

FIGURE 60-6

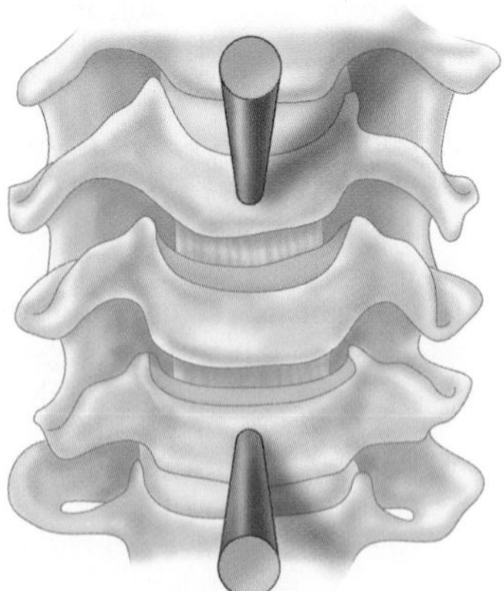

FIGURE 60-7

- **Figure 60-7:** Diskectomies are performed above and below the vertebral body to be resected. After incising the annulus, Caspar screws can be gradually distracted to provide room to use a high-speed drill to remove the disks and osteophytes. When the disk material has been cleared down to the PLL, adequate foraminotomies are also done.
- **Figure 60-8:** The corpectomy is begun by drilling a longitudinal groove 10 to 15 mm wide depending on the size of the lesion. The width of the corpectomy should not exceed 15 mm to avoid vascular injury and allow the lateral walls to help with bony fusion. The corpectomy can be completed with a high-speed drill and various rongeurs. The cartilaginous end plates are cleared away from the bony end plates with a No. 1 Penfield or curets. The PLL is elevated with a micronerve hook and removed with rongeurs. The PLL has two layers: a very tough anterior layer containing longitudinal fibers and a thin transparent posterior layer often mistaken for dura. **A,** Photograph of saw bone after corpectomy. **B,** Transverse schematic diagram showing maximum safe width of corpectomy.
- **Figure 60-9:** Photograph of saw bone with fibular graft placed in a corpectomy defect. The opposing end plates of vertebral bodies above and below the corpectomy level are prepared for fusion. Remaining cartilage is removed with a curet until bleeding surfaces are encountered. Although diligent clearing of cartilage is important for fusion, care must be taken not to be overly aggressive. Damage to cortical end plates can result in graft subsidence. A 1- to 2-mm posterior shelf of bone may be created in the superior aspect of the vertebral body below to prevent posterior migration of the graft. Distraction pins can be released slowly, compressing the graft. Alternatively, an expandable cage can be used for anterior arthrodesis.

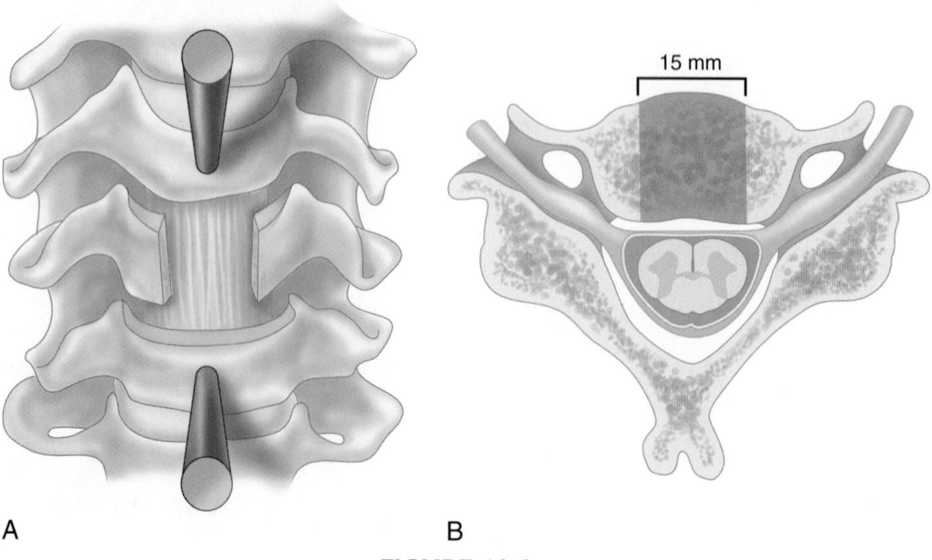

FIGURE 60-8

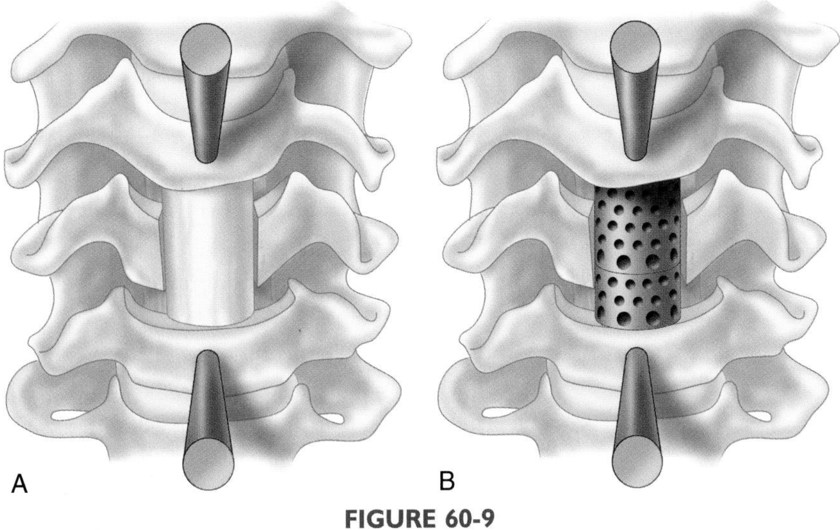

FIGURE 60-9

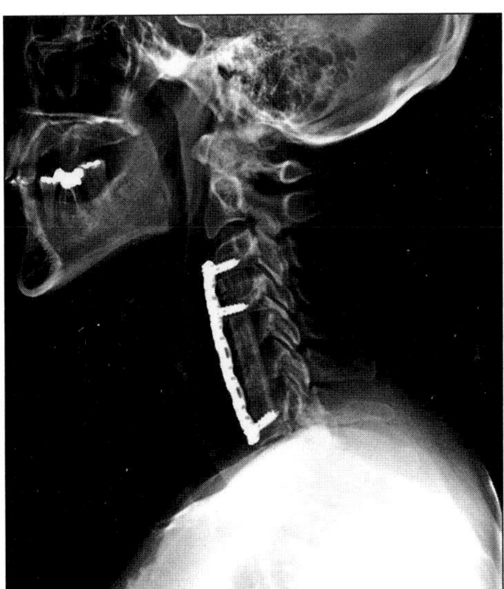

FIGURE 60-10

- **Figure 60-10:** Lateral radiograph showing two-level corpectomy (C5 and C6) with fibular strut graft and C3-4 diskectomy. Fibular allograft is frequently used to reconstruct a corpectomy defect (see Figure 60-9). Autologous bone graft can also be harvested from the iliac crest, tibia, or fibula to enhance fusion. A titanium mesh cage is occasionally used for multilevel corpectomies. An appropriate-size graft is shaped to fit bone defect and inserted while end plates are distracted. The distraction device can be slowly released, compressing the graft. Distraction pins are removed, and bleeding holes are packed with thrombin-soaked Gelfoam. The ventral surface of the vertebral bodies is flattened with a high-speed drill so that the plate seats in direct contact with the bone. An appropriate-length titanium cervical plate is selected so that the superior and inferior edges do not encroach on the disk spaces above and below, and the screw holes are located just above and below the end plates. Two holes angled 15 degrees medially and superiorly are drilled into the vertebral body above, and two holes angled 15 degrees medially and inferiorly are drilled into the vertebral body below. Self-tapping 3.5-mm-diameter screws are placed. Screws 14 to 16 mm in length are frequently used based on the premeasured anteroposterior diameter of the vertebral body so that the screw tip almost reaches the posterior vertebral cortex. The appropriate locking mechanism is applied.

TIPS FROM THE MASTERS

- It is crucial to be cognizant of the midline at all times. Drifting from the midline may cause inadvertent injury to the vertebral artery.
- The lateral aspects of the vertebral body may be identified with a No. 4 Penfield.
- Momentarily releasing the cuff pressure after placing the retractors allows the recurrent laryngeal nerve to shift its position and avoid injury from compression during its transtracheal course.
- Minimizing the use of continuous bovie electrocautery in the prevertebral area can help reduce postoperative dysphagia.
- Minimizing cautery on the bone surface can facilitate bony fusion.
- Bleeding cancellous bone can be controlled with FloSeal (Baxter International, Inc, Deerfield, IL) or thrombin-soaked Gelfoam. The use of bone wax on end plates should be avoided because this may interfere with bony fusion.
- The thoracic duct, which if injured results in chylothorax, is present only on the left side. The thoracic duct and potential injury can be altogether avoided with a right-sided approach for pathology involving the inferiormost subaxial spine.
- Before operating on the contralateral side of a previous anterior cervical surgery, direct laryngoscopy should be performed to evaluate unidentified vocal cord paralysis.
- Expandable cervical cages are a valuable alternative to strut grafting.

PITFALLS

Vocal cord paralysis can occur with retraction injury to the recurrent laryngeal nerve, superior laryngeal nerve, or vagus nerve within the carotid sheath. These structures are unlikely to be divided during the exposure, so vocal cord paralysis is usually transient.

Injury to the sympathetic chain can be avoided by taking care not to dissect lateral to the longus colli muscles and to elevate the muscle subperiosteally.

Cerebral ischemia or carotid artery thrombus or both can occur with prolonged retraction against the carotid artery.

Tissue planes must be adequately dissected and released, and the omohyoid muscle divided if necessary, to minimize retraction on the trachea and esophagus. Too much pressure on these structures can lead to postoperative edema and preclude early extubation.

Graft donor site can also be a source of complications, such as persistent drainage, hematoma formation, persistent discomfort, injury to the lateral femoral cutaneous nerve, and wound infection.

Proper strut graft length is crucial for optimal fusion. A graft that is too long can result in overdistraction. It may also create a shifting torque in either the anteroposterior or the coronal plane predisposing to graft or plate kickout. If the graft is too short, there may not be a tight opposition of bony surfaces, decreasing the chance for graft incorporation and fusion.

Proper width of the graft is also important so as to allow a nerve hook to be passed behind the graft. This nerve hook allows for any epidural or bone bleeding to escape out of the arthrodesis bed preventing epidural hematoma.

For multilevel corpectomy, incomplete gardening results in poor vertebral body purchase of screws and plate rocking. This increases the chance of plate or graft kickout.

For long plate fixation, bicortical screw purchase under fluoroscopic guidance can decrease the chance of screw pullout or plate migration.

BAILOUT OPTIONS

- If dura is torn during PLL removal, all efforts must be made to repair it primarily, followed by an onlay dural substitute placed over the defect. A lumbar drain is placed at the end of the surgery.
- If adequate decompression cannot be achieved anteriorly, or fusion failed to occur after anterior corpectomy, local foraminotomy and decompression followed by fusion can be performed posteriorly.

SUGGESTED READINGS

Acosta FL Jr, Aryan HE, Chou D, et al. Long-term biomechanical improvement after extended multilevel corpectomy and circumferential reconstruction of the cervical spine using titanium mesh cage. J Spinal Disord Tech 2008;21:165–74.

Chen Y, Chen D, Wang X, et al. Anterior corpectomy and fusion for severe ossification of posterior longitudinal ligament in the cervical spine. Int Orthop 2009;33:477–82.

Hannallah D, Lee J, Khan M, et al. Cerebrospinal fluid leaks following cervical spine surgery. J Bone Joint Surg Am 2008;90:1101–5.

Khan MH, Smith PN, Balzer JR, et al. Intraoperative somatosensory evoked potential monitoring during cervical spine corpectomy surgery: experience with 508 cases. Spine 2006;31:E105–13.

Lee MJ, Bazaz R, Furey CG, et al. Risk factors for dysphagia after anterior cervical spine surgery: a two-year prospective cohort study. Spine J 2007;7:141–7.

Procedure 61

Cervical Laminectomy and Laminoplasty

Stephen S. Scibelli, Kamal R.M. Woods, Shoshanna Vaynman, J. Patrick Johnson

INDICATIONS

- Multilevel cervical stenosis with preservation of normal lordotic curvature
- Diffuse ossification of posterior longitudinal ligament
- Posterior cord compression resulting from buckling of thickened ligamentum flavum
- Posterior exposure of intraspinal pathology, including tumor, vascular malformation, infection, and hematoma
- Factors limiting anterior neck dissection, including short neck, scarring from previous anterior neck dissection or radiation.

CONTRAINDICATIONS

- Straightening of normal cervical lordosis or kyphotic sagittal alignment
- Cervical instability resulting from trauma, tumor invasion, or connective tissue disorder
- Broad-based ventral pathology that may not be readily accessed from a posterior approach

PLANNING AND POSITIONING

- Baseline motor evoked potentials and somatosensory evoked potentials are obtained before patient positioning.
- The patient's head is secured in a Mayfield head holder.
- **Figure 61-1:** The patient is positioned prone with chest rolls, and a Mayfield head holder is fixed to the table with the head and neck slightly flexed.
- The patient's arms are tucked at the side and carefully padded at the axilla, elbow, and wrist.
- A midline skin incision if marked using palpation to identify the spinous processes. Generally, the spinous processes of C2 and C7 tend to be most prominent and easily palpated.

PROCEDURE

Laminoplasty

- **Figure 61-2:** A midline longitudinal incision is made over the operative cervical levels. Dissection is carried down to the spinous processes; this is predominantly an avascular plane. Care is taken to ensure the intraspinous ligament is left intact, ensuring the

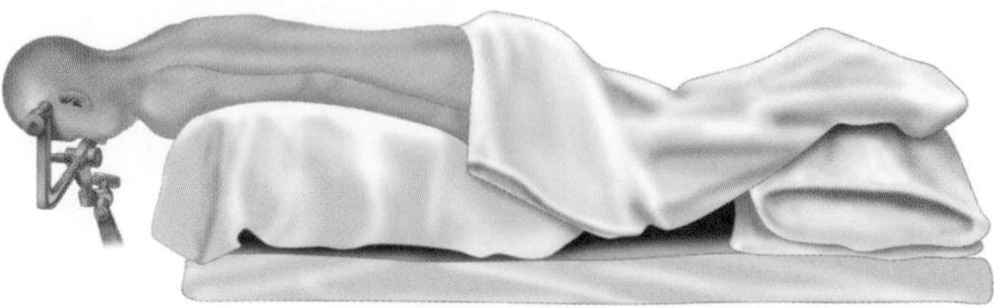

FIGURE 61-1

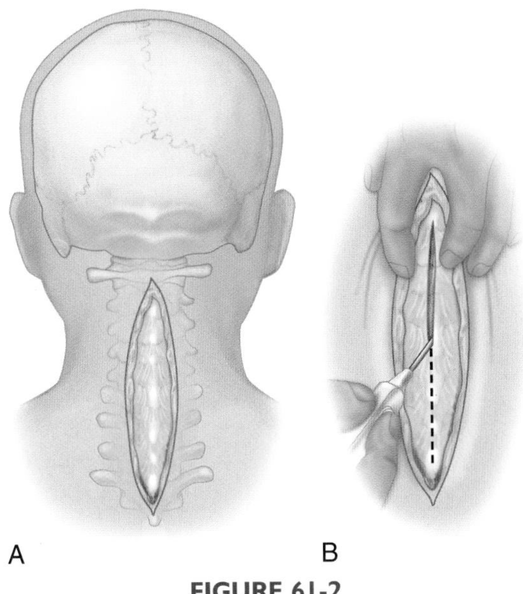

FIGURE 61-2

posture tension band is undisturbed. Exposure is continued in a bilateral subperiosteal plain. In this fashion, the paraspinous muscles are dissected and retracted laterally. Exposure is medial to the facets, which ensures the facet joint is not violated. There is no need to expose the facet because this is a motion-preserving procedure, and arthrodesis of the joints is to be avoided. Fluoroscopy or x-ray localization is used to confirm levels.

- **Figure 61-3:** When exposure is complete, cerebellar retractors are used to maintain visualization. If one side has more stenosis or is more symptomatic, this is the side on which we perform the opening. At the lamina–lateral mass junction, a 3-mm cutting bur drill bit is used to make a small laminotomy hole at the inferior aspect of the inferiormost lamina of the levels to be addressed. We use a Medtronic B-1 bit (Minneapolis, MN), a low-profile footed drill bit, to open all the levels on one side, moving in a cephalad direction. Caution is warranted at C7, when included, because of its unique angle. It is also acceptable to drill a small trough (using the 3-mm cutting bit) on the opening side and complete the opening in this fashion or with a 2-mm Kerrison punch. Any bleeding that is encountered is generally bone or venous. Both types of bleeding can be addressed with Gelfoam, FloSeal (Baxter International, Inc., Deerfield, IL), or rarely bipolar cautery. The use of bone wax is avoided if possible because the laminoplasty graft fusion is going to be formed here.

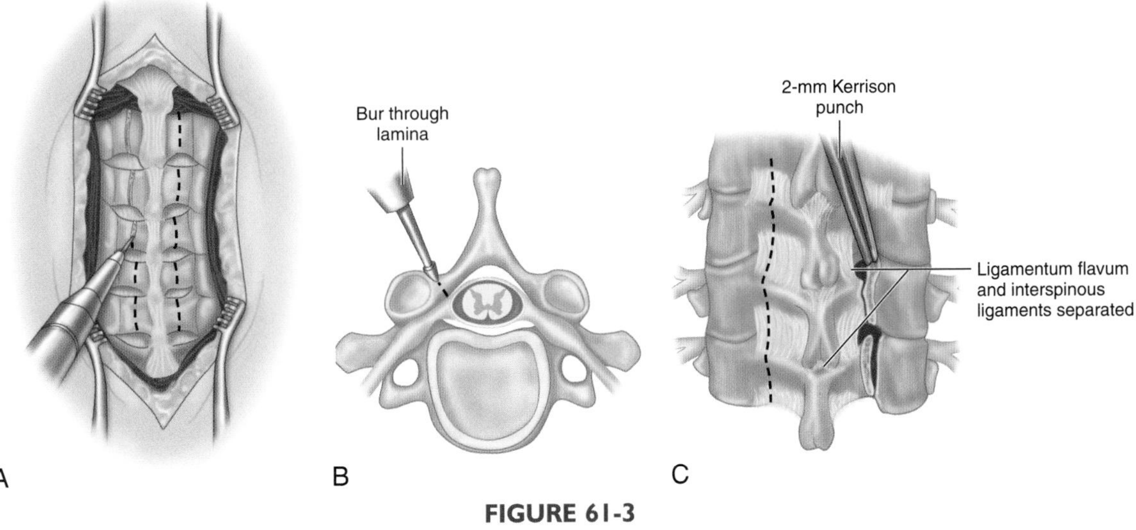

FIGURE 61-3

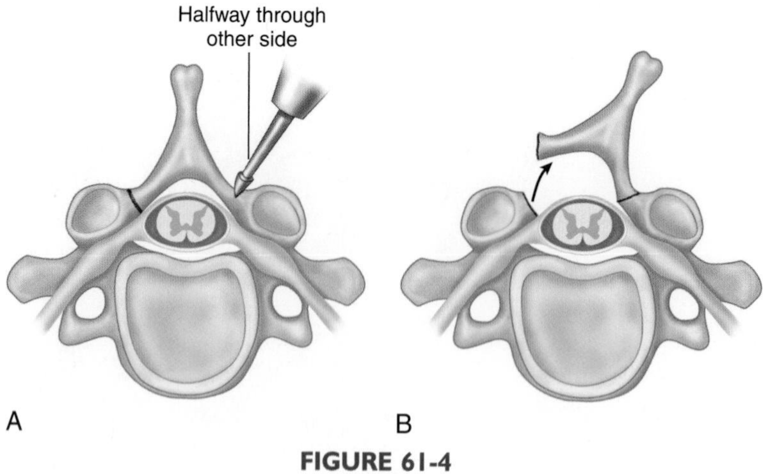

FIGURE 61-4

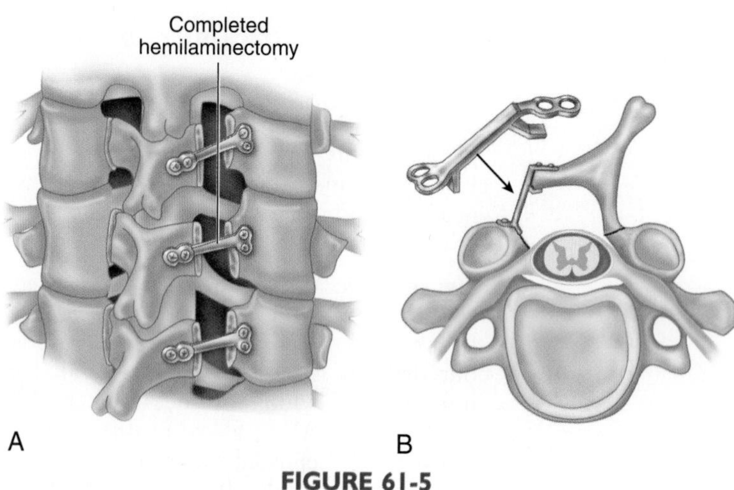

FIGURE 61-5

- **Figure 61-4:** A trough at the lamina–lateral mass junction, on the contralateral side, is drilled using a 3-mm bur. Care is taken not to breach the anterior cortical bone. Any bone bleeding on this side can be addressed with bone wax. After the hinge side trough is complete, controlled pressure is applied to the spinous process toward the hinged side to expand the opening. The ligamentum flavum is resected to complete the decompression. Sometimes one must resect ligamentum flavum, as pressure is applied to the spinous process, to open the door. Foraminotomies, if indicated, are now performed. Care is taken not to destabilize the facets. To ensure adequate decompression has been accomplished, a Woodsen is passed over and under the dura, and a large round probe is passed out each foramen.
- **Figure 61-5:** Straight craniofacial fixation plate is screwed in position connecting the lateral mass, graft, and lamina. A screw may be placed in the graft to secure it in position.

Laminectomy

- The soft tissue exposure is the same as for a laminoplasty. Care is taken to avoid exposing the facets. If the surgeon prefers not to use the B-1 technique, a 3-mm bur can be used to drill troughs at the lamina–lateral mass junction bilaterally. The bone is thinned to an eggshell thickness. A 3-mm Kerrison punch is used to complete the laminectomy. The lamina and spinous processes are removed. The ligamentum flavum is removed, and any necessary foraminotomies are performed. At completion, a Woodsen is passed under the dura, and a large round ball probe is passed out the foramen to ensure an adequate decompression has occurred.

TIPS FROM THE MASTERS

- Care is taken to avoid flexion or extension of the neck during positioning of a patient with myelopathy.
- When using the B-1 bit, the tip needs to be kept up slightly, as if performing a craniotomy, to keep the drill out of the ligament and venous plexus.
- This is a motion-preserving procedure. If one is planing on fusing the levels in question, a laminectomy and fusion is performed rather than a laminoplasty.
- Care is taken not to place any graft across the interlamina spaces to help ensure no fusion occurs across levels.
- The facets are not exposed or violated.

PITFALLS
Overexposure and entry into facet capsule—this can lead to arthrodesis
Poor patient selection

BAILOUT OPTIONS

- If the hinge side is fractured during the procedure, three simple solutions are available:
  - Often no change in operative plan is necessary because the posterior elements remain in position by wedging the graft in position and its fixation on the open side.
  - A craniofacial fixation plate can be placed across the fracture line.
  - The entire hinge side can be opened, in the same technique as the open side, and grafts can be placed.
- Bleeding from the epidural venous plexus can be brisk but is easily controlled with well-placed Gelfoam, FloSeal, or precise bipolar cautery.

SUGGESTED READINGS

Herkowitz HN. A comparison of anterior cervical fusion, cervical laminectomy, and cervical laminoplasty for the surgical management of multiple level spondylotic radiculopathy. Spine (Phila Pa 1976) 1988;13(7):774–80.

Hirabayashi K, Watanabe K, Wakano K, Suzuki N, et al. Expansive open-door laminoplasty for cervical spinal stenotic myelopathy. Spine (Phila Pa 1976) 1983;8(7):693–9.

McGirt MJ, Garcés-Ambrossi GL, Parker SL, Sciubba DM, et al. Short-term progressive spinal deformity following laminoplasty versus laminectomy for resection of intradural spinal tumors: analysis of 238 patients. Neurosurgery 2010;66(5):1005–12.

Rhee JM, Register B, Hamasaki T, Franklin B. Plate-only open door laminoplasty maintains stable spinal canal expansion with high rates of hinge union and no plate failures. Spine (Phila Pa 1976) 2011;36(1):9–14.

Woods BI, Hohl J, Lee J, Donaldson W III , Kang J. Laminoplasty versus laminectomy and fusion for multilevel cervical spondylotic myelopathy. Clin Orthop Relat Res 2010; [Epub ahead of print].

Procedure 62

Lateral Mass Fixation

Mike Yue Chen, Matthew J. Duenas, Rahul Jandial

INDICATIONS

- Cervical instability from multilevel anterior cervical diskectomies or corpectomies
- Increase in posterior tension band in patient with kyphotic cervical curve who requires an anterior procedure
- Posterior cervical laminectomy for myelopathy to reduce pathologic motion

CONTRAINDICATIONS

- Aberrant vertebral artery anatomy
- Lateral mass fracture or lateral mass of inadequate size

PLANNING AND POSITIONING

- **Figure 62-1:** The patient is positioned prone on chest rolls with Mayfield pin fixation. Preoperative fluoroscopy should be used to confirm proper cervical alignment if lateral mass fixation is part of either occipitocervical fusion or cervicothoracic fusion.

PROCEDURE

- **Figure 62-2:** Midline incision and paraspinal dissection to expose spinous processes, laminae, and lateral masses of appropriate levels.
- **Figure 62-3:** The appropriate starting point can be determined by creating an imaginary *X* over the lateral mass. The superior and inferior boundaries are the facet joints, and the medial and lateral boundaries of the lateral mass serve as the other boundaries. The ideal starting point is 1 mm medial to the middle of the imaginary *X*.
- **Figure 62-4:** A "matchstick" bur is used to penetrate the cortex and create the starting point.
- **Figure 62-5:** An up-and-out technique is used for hand drill trajectory. A medial-to-lateral trajectory at 30 degrees avoids injury to the vertebral artery, and a cephalad-caudal trajectory at 20 degrees avoids injury to the nerve root.
- **Figure 62-6:** Before the placement of screws, the facet joints of the segments included in the fusion are decorticated. The dorsal cortical surfaces are decorticated for onlay arthrodesis as well.
- **Figure 62-7:** Polyaxial screws are placed and can be measured before placement during the hand drill and feeler steps.
- **Figure 62-8:** A medial trajectory risks injury to the vertebral artery. Failing to aim cephalad places the nerve root at risk. Starting too far-lateral risks fracture of the lateral mass.

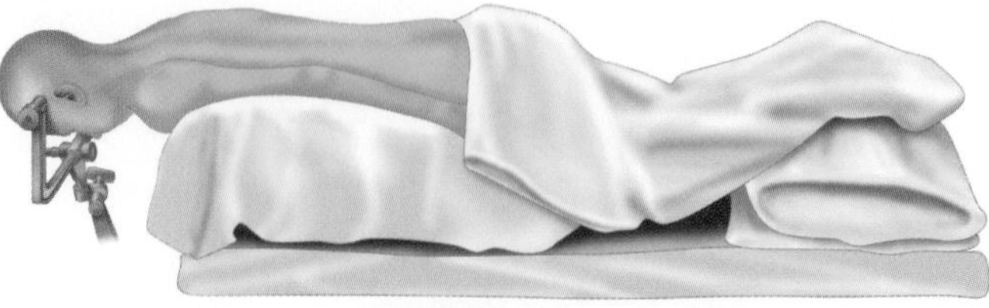

FIGURE 62-1

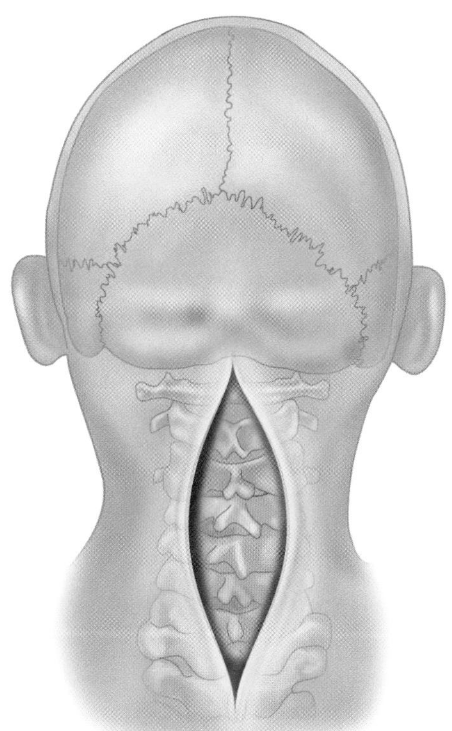

FIGURE 62-2

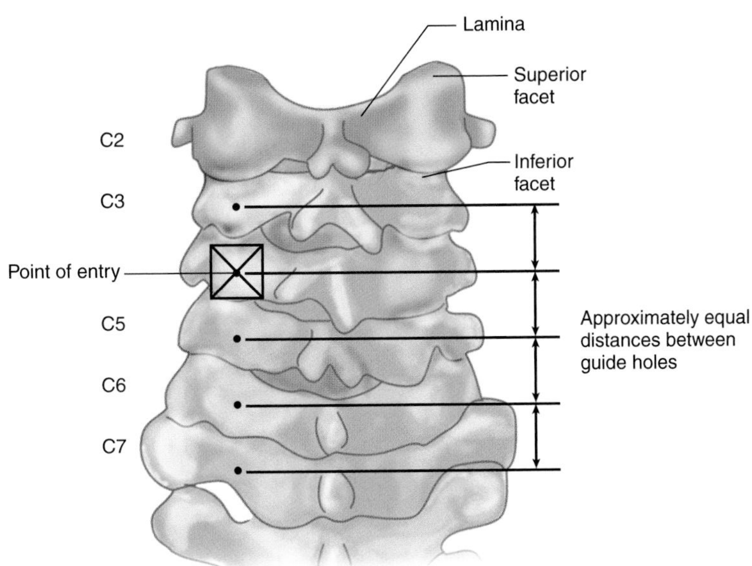

FIGURE 62-3

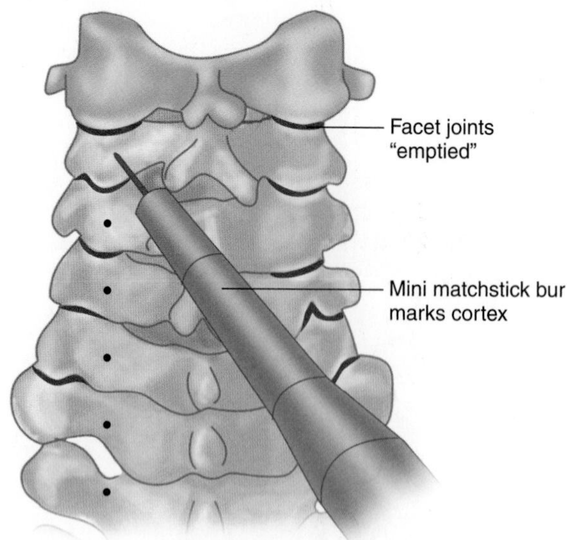

FIGURE 62-4

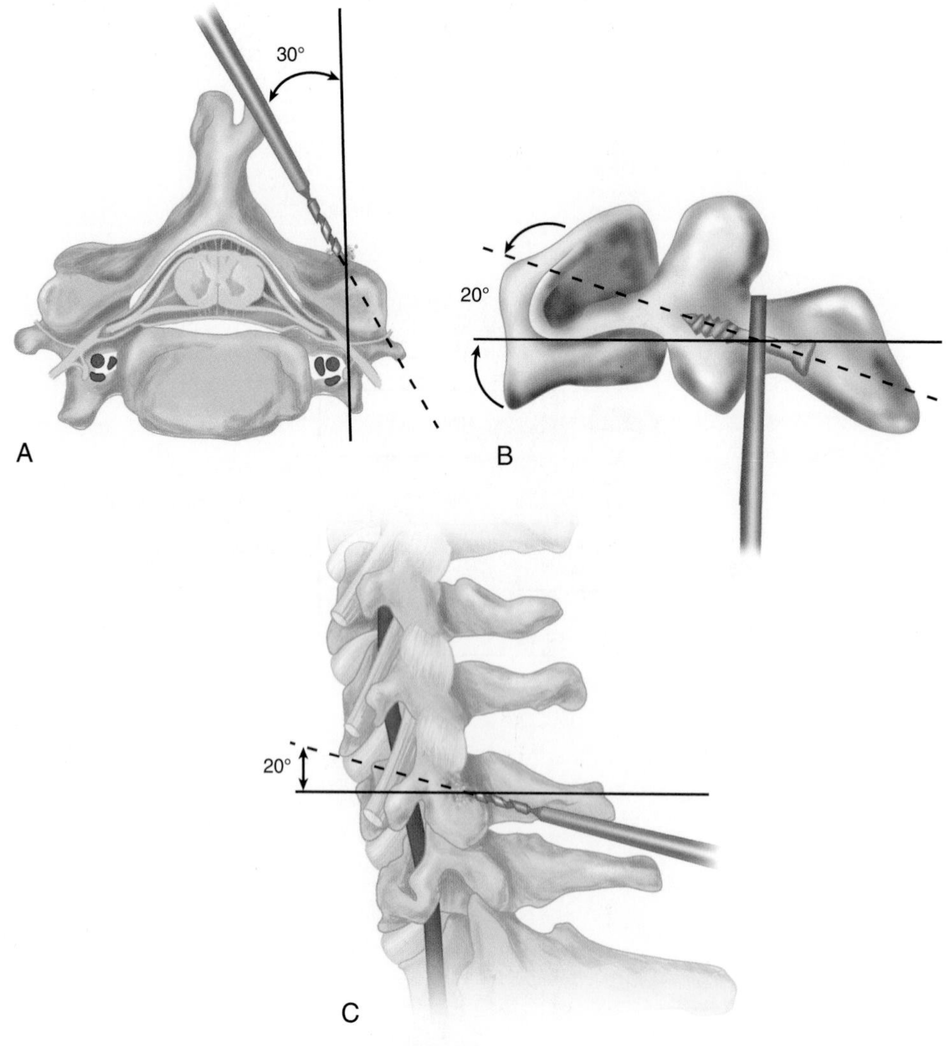

FIGURE 62-5

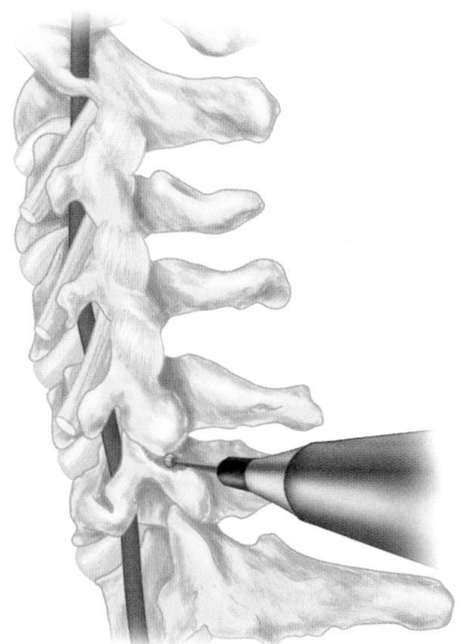

FIGURE 62-6

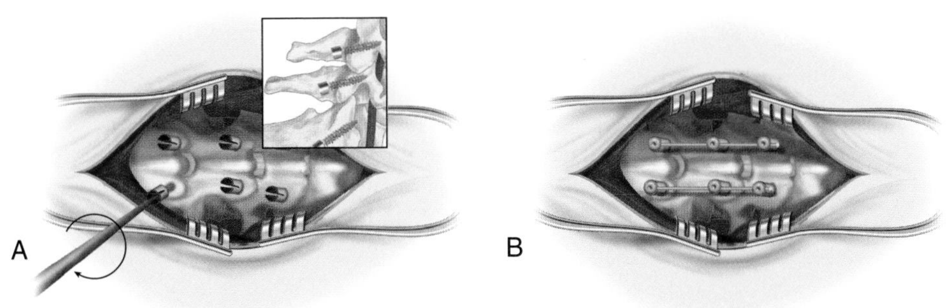

FIGURE 62-7

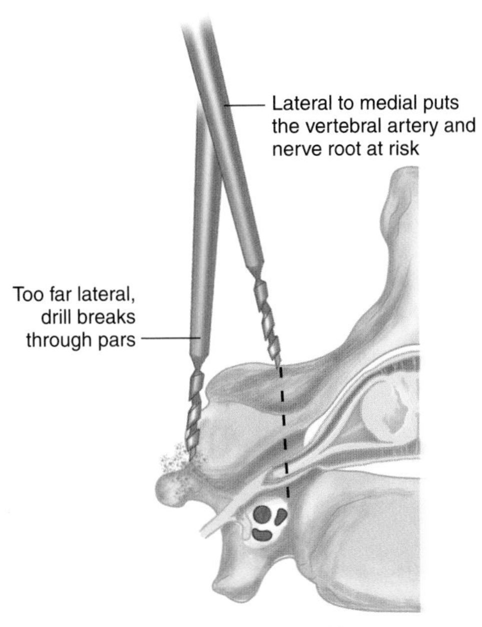

FIGURE 62-8

TIPS FROM THE MASTERS

- A No. 4 Penfield can be used to palpate the lateral edges of the lateral masses to help discern the middle starting point.
- Looking at the global starting points of posterior cervical screws, particularly in a long segment fixation incorporating the occiput, C1, or C2, can help prevent unnecessary contouring during rod placement.
- If a laminectomy is indicated as well, some surgeons prefer to place lateral mass screws first while the spinal cord is protected by posterior elements.
- Bicortical screws can be placed safely by using drill, tap, and feeler to estimate necessary size.

PITFALLS

During monopolar dissection, care should be taken to avoid inadvertent durotomy from excessive cautery in between the laminae. Some of the shingling can separate during positioning in flexion.

BAILOUT OPTIONS

- Additional fixation points can be used if lateral mass screws cannot be placed safely or successfully at any one segment.
- If the vertebral artery in the foramen transversarium is encountered, place bone wax in the hole and insert a shorter salvage screw for tamponade, and avoid placement of screws on the contralateral side. Alternative methods of fixation should be pursued if necessary, such as cervical pedicle screws.

SUGGESTED READINGS

Abumi K, Kaneda K, Shono Y, et al. One-stage posterior decompression and reconstruction of the cervical spine by using pedicle screw fixation systems. J Neurosurg 1999;90(Suppl. 1):19–26.

An HS, Gordin R, Renner K. Anatomic considerations for plate-screw fixation of the cervical spine. Spine (Phila Pa 1976) 1991;16(Suppl. 10):S548–51.

Heller JG, Carlson GD, Abitbol JJ, et al. Anatomic comparison of the Roy-Camille and Magerl techniques for screw placement in the lower cervical spine. Spine (Phila Pa 1976) 1991;16(Suppl. 10):S552–57.

Heller JG, Silcox DH III, Sutterlin CE 3rd. Complications of posterior cervical plating. Spine (Phila Pa 1976) 1995;20:2442–8.

Wellman BJ, Follett KA, Traynelis VC. Complications of posterior articular mass plate fixation of the subaxial cervical spine in 43 consecutive patients. Spine (Phila Pa 1976) 1998;23:193–200.

Procedure 63

Posterior Cervicothoracic Osteotomy

Timothy Link, Rahul Jandial, Volker Sonntag

INDICATIONS

- Severe kyphotic deformity at the cervicothoracic spine that causes radiculopathy, myelopathy, pain, restriction of gaze, or dysphagia. The deformity may arise from postlaminectomy destabilization, junctional kyphosis above a fused level, or primary diseases affecting the spine (particularly ankylosing spondylitis).
- Dorsal osteotomy allows for greater deformity correction. Mean correction angles have been cited in the literature to range from 23.3° to 53.8° based on Cobb angles (35° to 52° based on CBV angles) compared with mean correction via ventral only approach ranging from 11° to 32°.

CONTRAINDICATIONS

- Aberrant vertebral artery anatomy
- Lateral mass fracture or lateral mass of inadequate size
- Infection

PLANNING AND POSITIONING

- All patients should have preoperative computed tomography (CT), magnetic resonance imaging (MRI), and computed tomography (CT) angiography to delineate bony, soft tissue and vascular anatomy. Neuromonitoring is needed for the operation to detect neurologic injury during closure of the osteotomy and resultant stress on the spinal cord. Imaging should be used to confirm the entry of the vertebral artery into C6 segment and to identify an ossification of the anterior or posterior longitudinal ligament. Single cassette (full spine) lateral and AP radiographs in the standing position can be useful to measure the degree of desired gaze-angle and saggital (and coronal) correction.
- **Figure 63-1:** The patient is positioned prone on chest rolls with Mayfield pin fixation.

PROCEDURE

- **Figure 63-2:** Midline incision and paraspinal dissection is performed to expose the spinous processes, laminae, and lateral masses of appropriate levels from C3 to C7 in the cervical spine and then inferiorly to the T4 transverse processes.
- **Figure 63-3:** After adequate paraspinal dissection, entry sites for C3 to C6 lateral mass screws should be placed. Similarly, T1 to T4 pedicle screws should be placed.

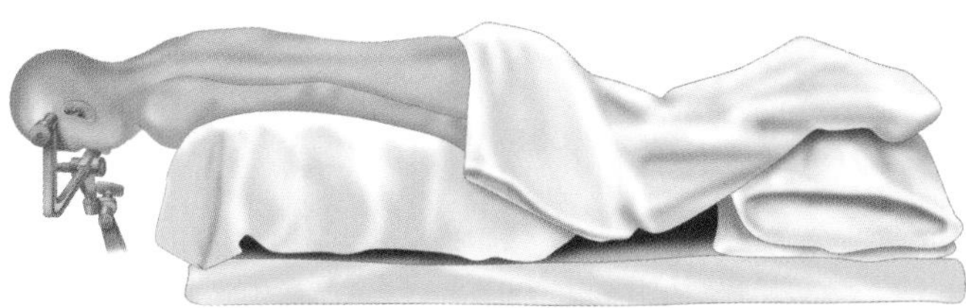

FIGURE 63-1

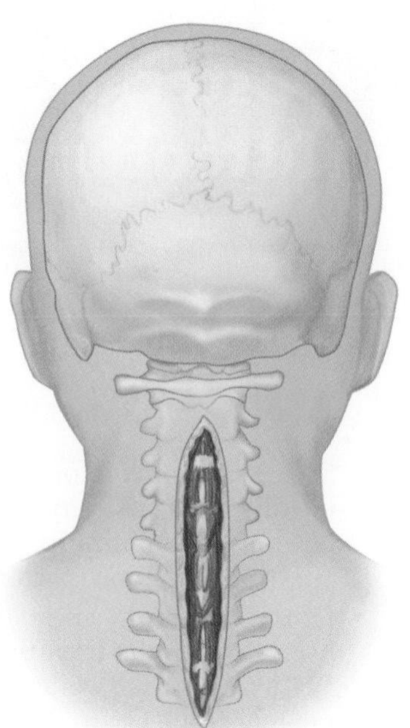

FIGURE 63-2

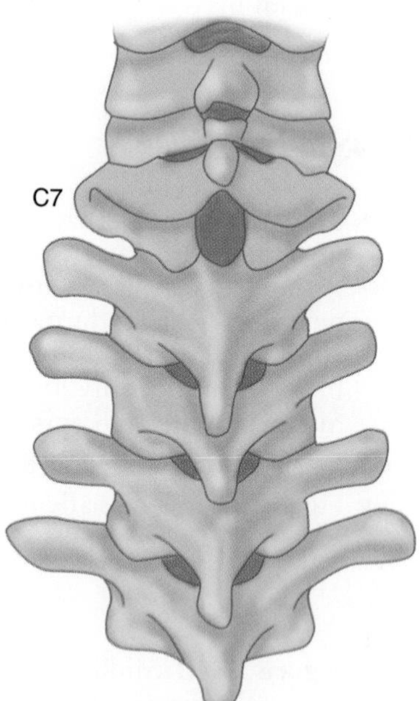

FIGURE 63-3

A transitional rod can be used ultimately to connect the lateral mass and thoracic pedicle screws to accommodate differences in screw head size.

- **Figure 63-4:** Complete laminectomy of C7 is performed, including the inferior edge of C6 and superior margin of T1. C8 nerve roots should be completely decompressed. C7 facetectomy is performed with identification of the pedicles, which are removed with a drill and rongeur.
- **Figure 63-5:** Before closure of the osteotomy, a cervical lateral mass or pedicle screw should be placed (**A**). Also, thoracic pedicle screws using establised landmarks and trajectories should be placed (**B**).

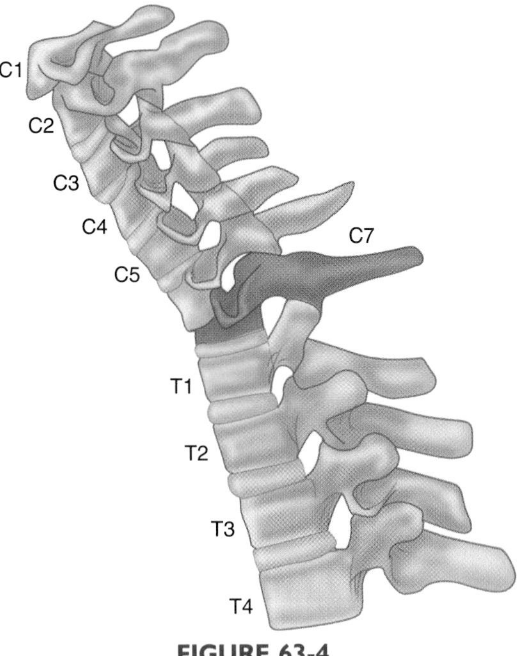

FIGURE 63-4

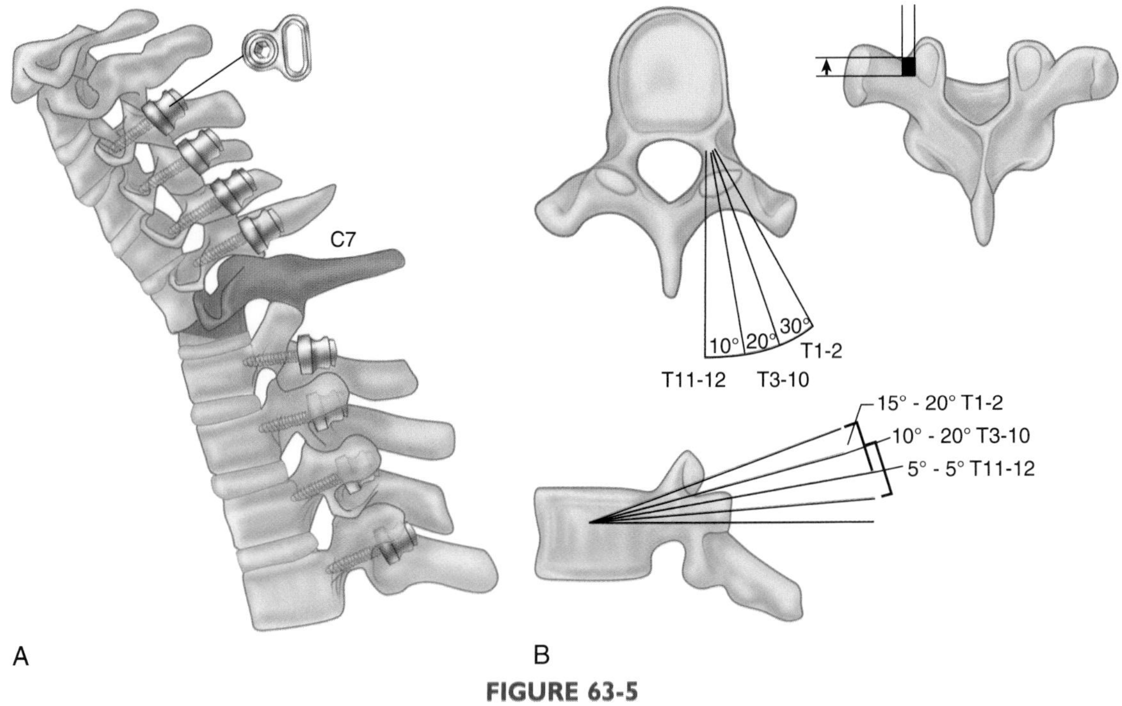

A B

FIGURE 63-5

- **Figure 63-6:** Closure of the osteotomy is best performed with an assistant who can release the cranial fixation and hyperextend the cervical spine. During this critical maneuver, the primary surgeon evaluates degree of closure and any compression on the dura and nerve roots. If correction is adequate, the head holder is locked into this position. After correction of deformity, rods are inserted and locked. Cervical facets and posterior elements of thoracic spine that are to be included into the fusion are decorticated.

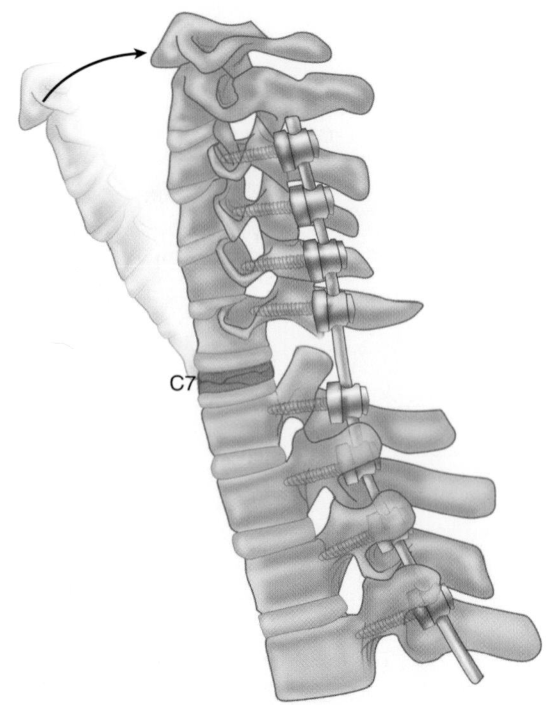

FIGURE 63-6

TIPS FROM THE MASTERS

- Fiberoptic intubation is often necessary.
- Always use intraoperative spinal cord monitoring (typically somatosensory-evoked potentials, free-running electromyography, and transcranial motor-evoked potentials).
- Ensure that the C7 laminectomy results in generous room to accommodate any dural buckling that occurs from shortening of the spine. If needed, partial laminectomies of C6 and T1 can be performed.

PITFALLS

Inadequate pediculectomy of C7 can lead to postoperative C8 radiculopathy.

BAILOUT OPTIONS

- If spinal cord injury occurs (i.e., significant, sustained intraoperative electrophysiological depressions or signal loss), the patient's cervical spine should be released and stabilized in the uncorrected preoperative position.
- If the vertebral artery in the foramen transversarium is encountered, place bone wax in the hole and insert a shorter salvage screw for tamponade, and avoid placement of screws on the contralateral side. Alternative methods of fixation should be pursued if necessary, such as cervical pedicle screws.

Figures 63-1 through 63-6 are modified with permission from Barrow Neurological Institute.

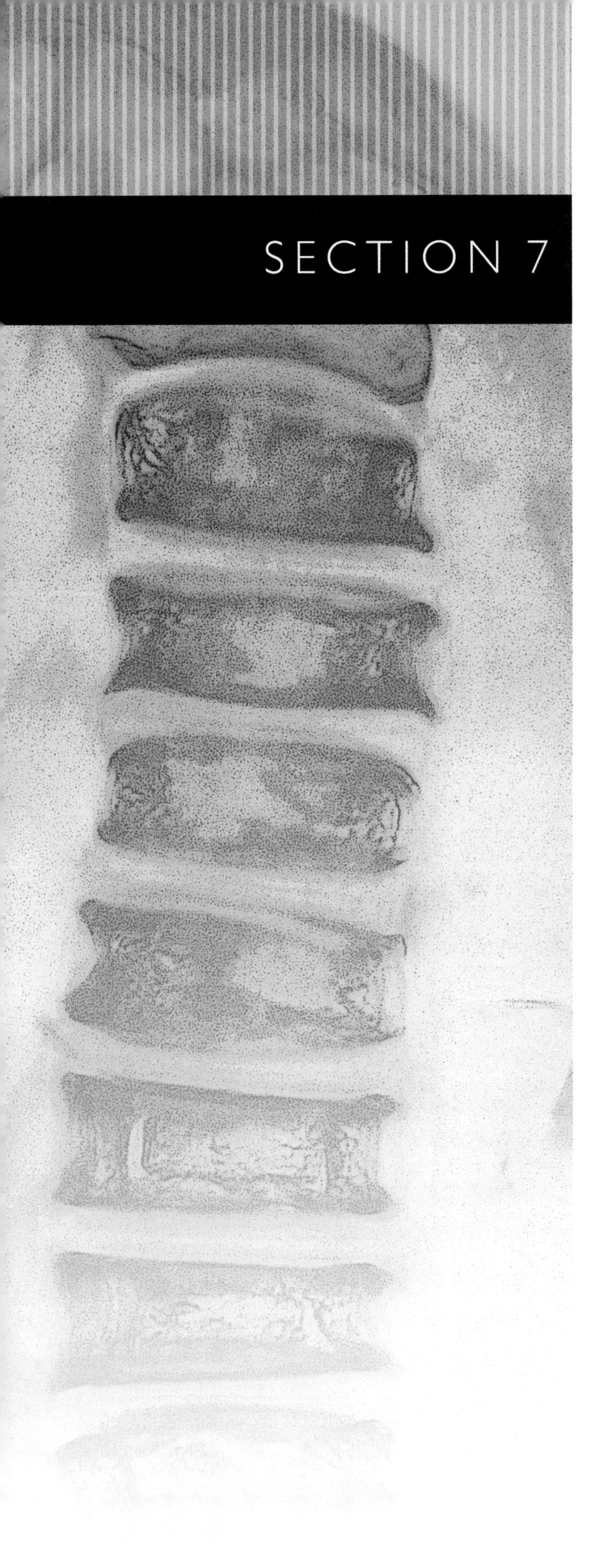

SECTION 7

Thoracic

SECTION EDITOR — CHRISTOPHER P. AMES, WITH BRIAN JIAN

Procedure 64

Thoracic Diskectomy—Transthoracic Approach

Vincent Y. Wang, Dean Chou

INDICATIONS

- Severe or progressive myelopathy caused by thoracic disk herniation
- Any spinal cord compression
- Midline disk herniation or disk osteophyte complex in the thoracic region
- Severe radicular pain unresponsive to conservative management (relative indication)

CONTRAINDICATIONS

- Patients with pulmonary pathology such that they cannot tolerate one-lung ventilation are not candidates for this approach.
- An asymptomatic or incidental thoracic disk herniation is a contraindication.

PLANNING AND POSITIONING

- Regular operating room table is positioned in reverse orientation to allow for C-arm.
- The patient is placed in lateral decubitus position for thoracotomy, usually left side up (to avoid aortic arch).
- An axillary roll is placed underneath the upper chest region to protect brachial plexus.
- The lower arm is supported on a regular arm board, and the upper arm is supported by an arm rest.
- It is important to verify the level of disk herniation on magnetic resonance imaging (MRI) or computed tomography (CT) preoperatively and to decide on the localization strategy (e.g., count from T1 down or up from T12 [verify patient has 12 ribs]; count from sacrum [evaluate for transitional vertebrae]). It is also possible to place a small metallic marker under CT guidance preoperatively to localize the level.
- A double-lumen tube should be used for intubation.
- Neuromonitoring with motor evoked potentials and somatosensory evoked potentials should be performed.
- **Figure 64-1:** The patient is placed in the lateral decubitus position and secured with tape.

PROCEDURE

- **Figure 64-2:** The incision is determined before draping using fluoroscopy and is marked out (see Figure 64-1). The incision should be two rib levels above the level of the rib corresponding to the affected level. The incision should extend from the posterior angle of the rib and follow the contour of the rib.
- **Figure 64-3:** The musculature is divided using monopolar cautery. The intercostal neurovascular bundle is dissected in a subperiosteal fashion using a periosteal elevator and Doyen elevator. Care is taken to preserve the neurovascular bundle.

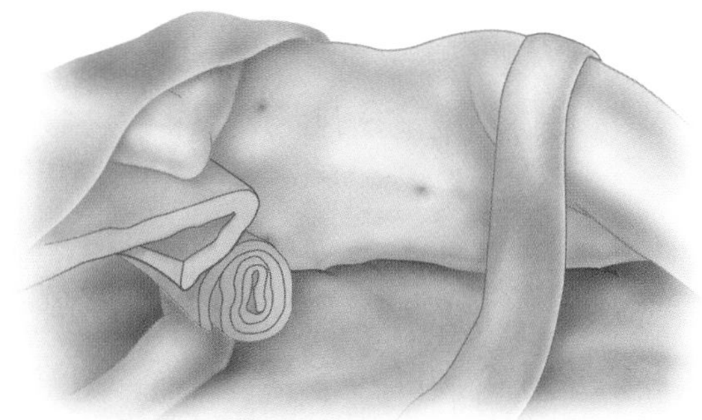

FIGURE 64-1

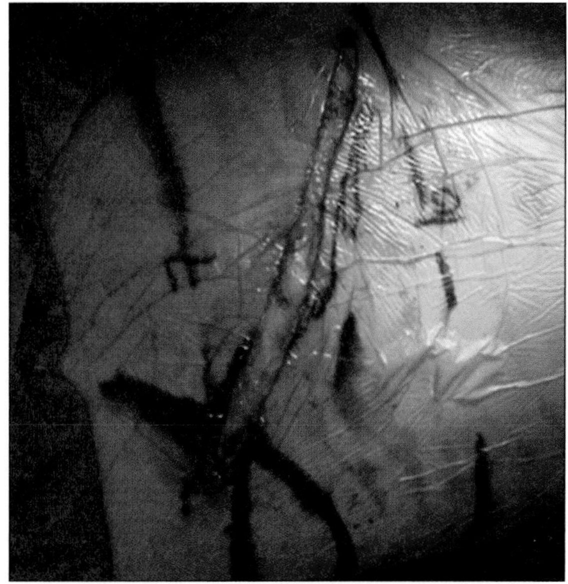

FIGURE 64-2

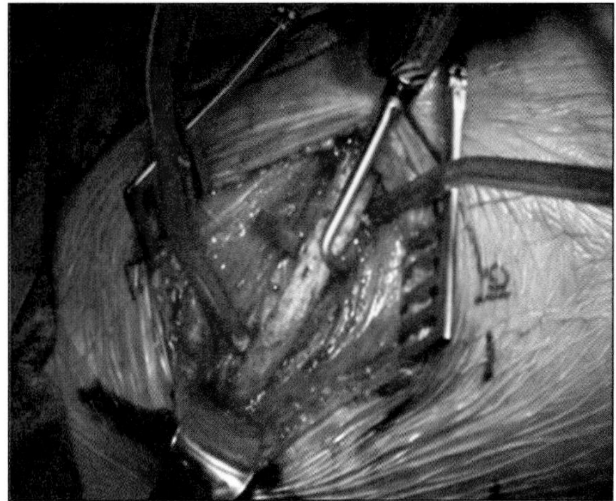

FIGURE 64-3

- **Figure 64-4:** The rib is harvested and can be saved for grafting material if needed.
- **Figure 64-5:** The parietal pleura is opened with Metzenbaum scissors.
- **Figure 64-6:** The rib spreader is used as a self-retaining retractor, and the lung is deflated.
- **Figure 64-7:** The level should be verified again with x-ray or fluoroscopy. It is also possible to count the rib levels manually, palpating the subclavian vessels and large

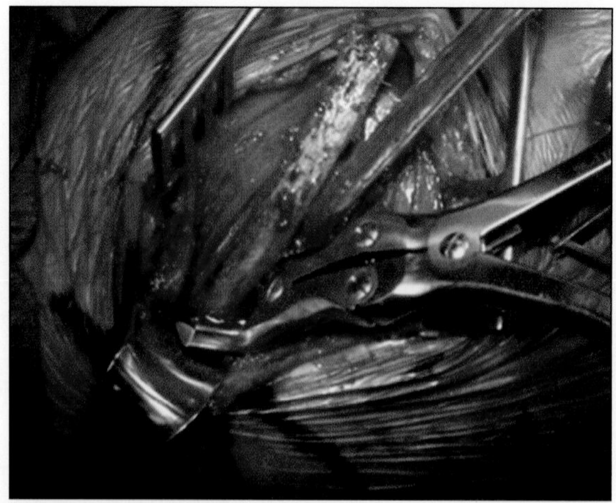

FIGURE 64-4

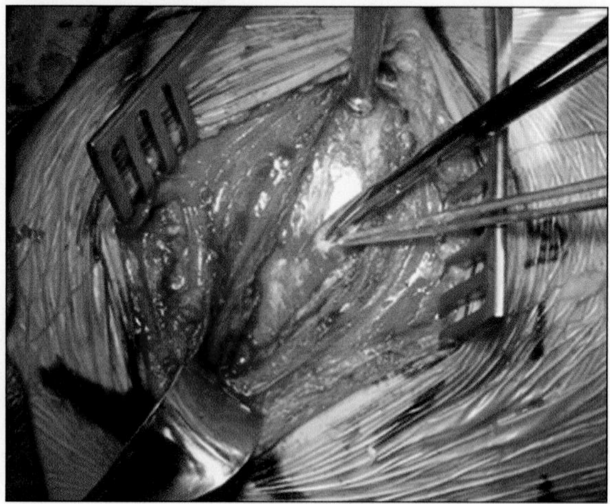

FIGURE 64-5

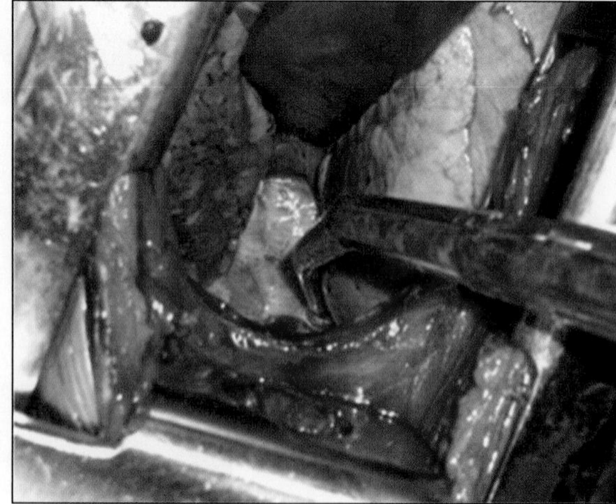

FIGURE 64-6

broad T1 rib and counting down. The rib head is identified, and the vertebral body and disk space are exposed in a subperiosteal fashion. The rib head should be removed with a high-speed drill, an osteotome, or a rongeur.

- **Figure 64-8:** Care should be taken for dissection of segmental vessels. If needed, the vessels can be ligated or cauterized.

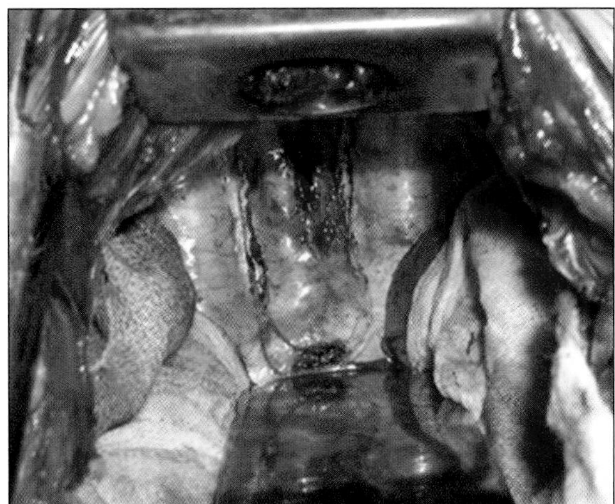

FIGURE 64-7

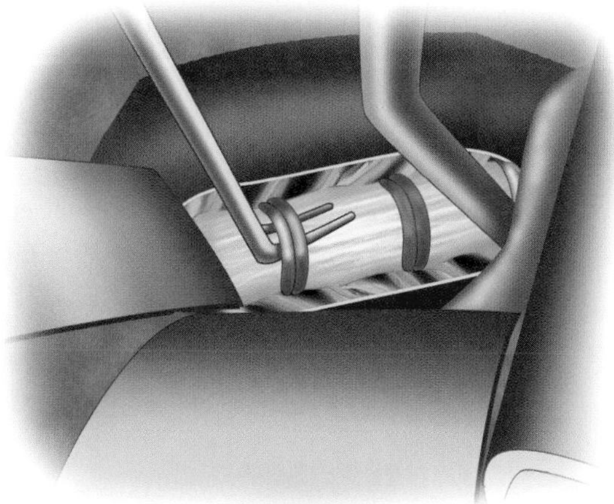

FIGURE 64-8

- **Figure 64-9:** After the adjacent vertebral bodies and disk space are exposed, the ventral margin is identified by finding the foramen and pedicle. Using a high-speed drill, the pedicle is thinned, and the spinal canal is identified. The posterolateral aspect of the vertebrae adjacent to the disk is removed using the drill.

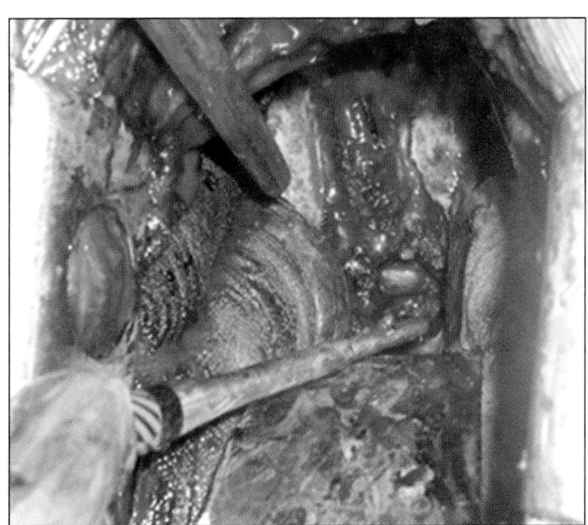

FIGURE 64-9

- The disk material is removed using a pituitary rongeur, Kerrison rongeur, or a high-speed drill.
- It is important that sufficient disk is removed to achieve thorough decompression. For a calcified central disk, the entire width of the thecal sac should be visualized to ensure thorough decompression. To ensure complete decompression to the contralateral side, the contralateral pedicle should be palpated with a blunt instrument.
- After completion of the diskectomy, hemostasis is achieved with bipolar cautery or hemostatic agents or both. One or two chest tubes are inserted (depending on bleeding during closure), and the ribs are reapproximated with heavy (No. 2 polyglactin 910 [Vicryl]) sutures. The overlying musculature can be closed in a layered fashion (with 0 Vicryl and 2-0 Vicryl sutures).

TIPS FROM THE MASTERS

- Surgeons with limited experience with thoracotomy should enlist help from a thoracic surgeon or general surgeon for access to the thoracic cavity.
- Maintenance of blood pressure is crucial in patients with severe cord compression.
- It is important to identify the correct level intraoperatively. Multiple x-rays or fluoroscopy may be needed. Also, a small screw can be placed under CT guidance preoperatively. Counting from T1 down is the most reliable method. Radiology confirmation of the level can be obtained, and long cassettes instead of fluoroscopy can be used if necessary.
- The anterior approach (transthoracic approach) can be used for all types of disk herniations. It is especially useful for central disk herniations with or without calcification. For soft, paracentral disk herniations, it is possible to use a posterior approach such as the transpedicular approach or costotransversectomy to remove the disk.
- The use of the microscope or thoracoscope may provide better visualization of the operating field during the diskectomy.

PITFALLS

The surgical level is commonly misidentified, and it is important to use all available methods to identify the correct level.

Care should be taken to avoid manipulation of the thecal sac. This manipulation is generally unnecessary for the transthoracic approach. In the case of a calcified disk that is adherent to the dura, a high-speed drill should be used to drill the disk off the thecal sac, rather than pulling it off with a rongeur.

Cerebrospinal fluid leaks can be repaired using sutures (if possible) or fibrin glue.

BAILOUT OPTIONS

- Bleeding from segmental vessels can be controlled with bipolar cautery, clips, or ligature.
- Repeat imaging and confirmatory steps help prevent wrong level surgery.

SUGGESTED READINGS

Burke TG, Caputy AJ. Treatment of thoracic disk herniation: evolution toward the minimally invasive thoracoscopic approach. Neurosurg Focus 2000;9:e9.

Chen T. Surgical outcome for thoracic disc surgery in the postlaminectomy era. Neurosurg Focus 2000;9:e12.

Krauss W, Edwards D, Cohen-Gadol A. Transthoracic discectomy without interbody fusion. Surg Neurol 2005;63:403–9.

McCormick W, Will S, Benzel E. Surgery for thoracic disc disease: complication avoidance—overview and management. Neurosurg Focus 2000;9:13.

Vollmer D, Simmons N. Transthoracic approaches to thoracic disc herniations. Neurosurg Focus 2000;9:e8.

Procedure 65

Thoracic Corpectomy—Anterior Approach

Saad B. Chaudhary, Virgilio Matheus, Edward C. Benzel

INDICATIONS

- Unstable burst fractures with anterior spinal cord compression
- Primary or metastatic vertebral tumors
- Osteomyelitis or diskitis
- Severe spinal deformities
- Sequestered thoracic disk herniation with migration dorsal to the vertebral body, leading to spinal cord impingement and neurologic deficits
- Failed previous stabilization surgery (anterior or posterior) resulting in pseudarthrosis or instability or both

CONTRAINDICATIONS

- Limited life expectancy (<3 months)—protracted recovery period and hospitalization after thoracotomy and corpectomy may not be justified for a patient with a short life span
- Medical comorbidities such as severe pulmonary or cardiac disease, which may prohibit a safe thoracotomy or prevent successful weaning from the ventilator postoperatively
- Extensive disease involving several spinal levels in which case full exposure through the anterior approach may be not feasible
- Posterior tension band injury and translational or rotational injury without the explicit intent of a concomitant posterior procedure
- Severe osteopenia or osteoporosis—should include additional posterior stabilization

PLANNING AND POSITIONING

- Preoperative work-up should include multiple imaging modalities such as x-rays and magnetic resonance imaging (MRI) that include the entire thoracic and lumbosacral spine. Radiographs must be correlated with MRI before surgery to scrutinize for transitional levels and other bony anomalies; this allows the surgeon to identify the exact level of pathology for excision or decompression intraoperatively and minimizes the risk for wrong site surgery.
- Preoperative angiography may be considered to identify the artery of Adamkiewicz and to evaluate the vascular flow to a tumor and allow for embolization when appropriate.
- The patient is usually positioned in the right lateral decubitus position, and a left-sided thoracotomy is performed for access below T5. The primary reason for this approach is the ease of mobilizing the aorta versus the vena cava and the absence of the liver on the left side. The location of the pathology and the characteristics of the surrounding vascular anatomy can alter the side of the approach, however.
- The upper thoracic spine (T1-3) is best approached through a midline sternotomy or a posterior lateral extracavitary approach. The lower thoracic spine (T11 and T12) often necessitates a combined thoracoabdominal approach.

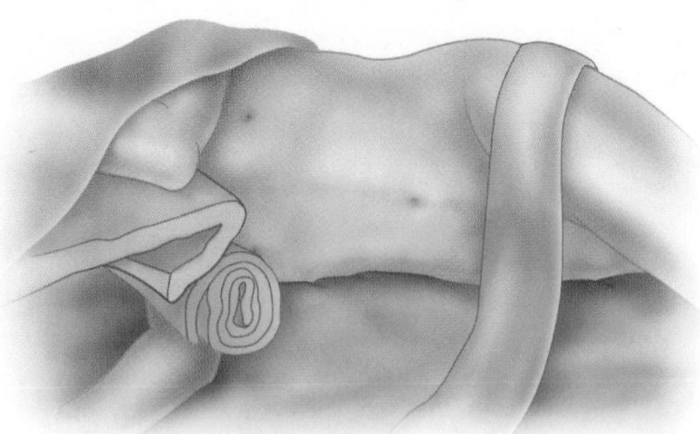

FIGURE 65-1

- Double-lumen endobronchial intubation is often preferred because it allows for selective lung ventilation. The deflated lung can be easily retracted away from the operative field.
- The patient should be placed in the lateral decubitus position by the surgeon. A beanbag can be deflated in place to help ensure that the patient remains at 90 degrees to the floor throughout the case.
- The arms can be positioned on a double arm board with an axillary role under the dependent arm to reduce the risk of a brachial plexus palsy. Both elbows must be well padded (protecting the ulnar nerve) and gently flexed up and away from the surgical field.
- The lower leg is positioned relatively straight on a pillow (protecting the peroneal nerve). The upper leg is also positioned on a pillow with the knee and the hip flexed and taped down so as to relax the ipsilateral psoas muscle for easier retraction during the case.
- The desired level should be placed on the break of the bed, and the table should be flexed for optimal access to the intercostal interval.
- **Figure 65-1:** The patient is positioned in the right lateral decubitus position with the elbows padded and slightly flexed out of the way. An axillary roll is placed one hand's-breadth caudal to the dependent axilla to minimize brachial plexus injury.

PROCEDURE

- **Figure 65-2:** The first and crucial step in this procedure is identification of the correct operative level. Standard anteroposterior x-ray or fluoroscopy can be used intraoperatively with external radiopaque markers for localization. It is of paramount importance that imaging captures the thoracolumbar junction, cervicothoracic junction, or lumbosacral junction to ensure accurate counting and identification of operative level.

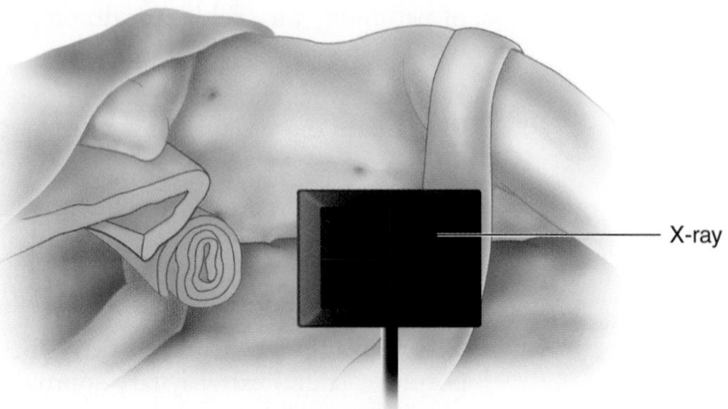

FIGURE 65-2

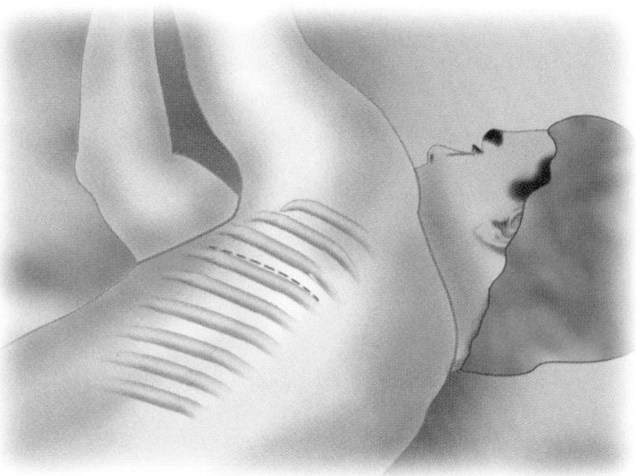

FIGURE 65-3

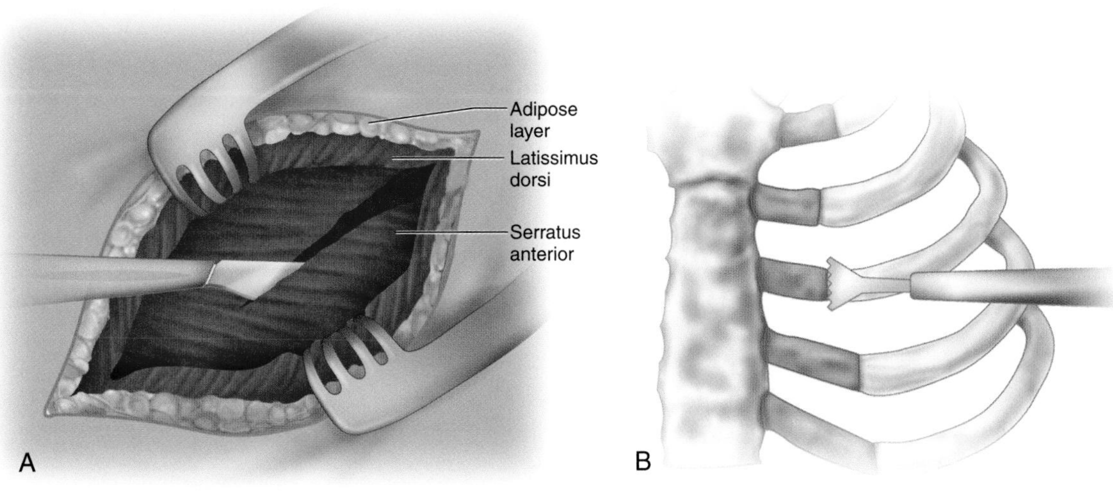

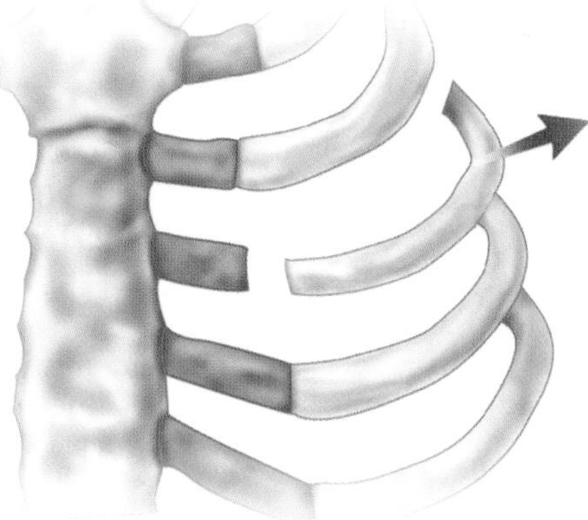

FIGURE 65-4

- **Figure 65-3:** The surgical incision is made over the rib that is one or two levels cephalad to the pathologic vertebral body. It is easier to extend the dissection and perform the corpectomy in a cephalad-to-caudad direction rather than vice versa. The incision follows the selected rib obliquely from the lateral border of paraspinal muscles posteriorly to the anterior axillary line.
- **Figure 65-4:** The incision is carried through the skin and subdermal tissue down to the muscle (latissimus dorsi and serratus anterior). Muscles are either retracted posteriorly or divided in line with the incision down to the superior aspect of the rib. Next, the rib is

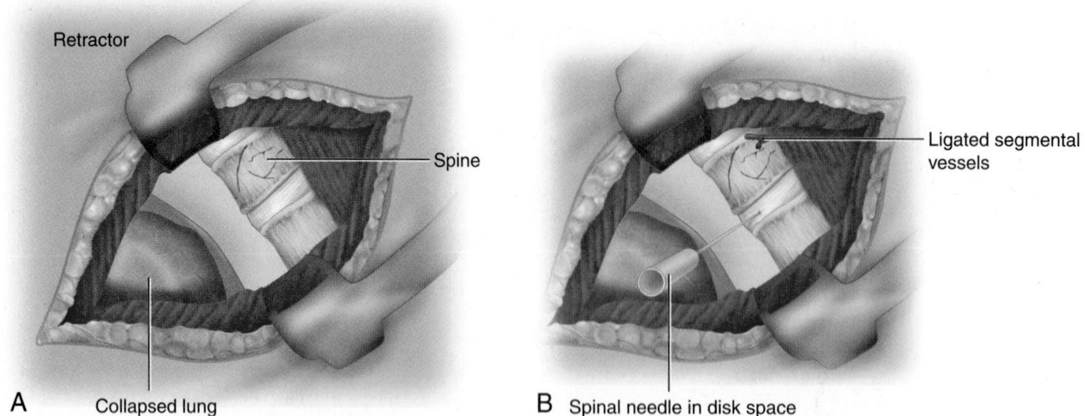

FIGURE 65-5

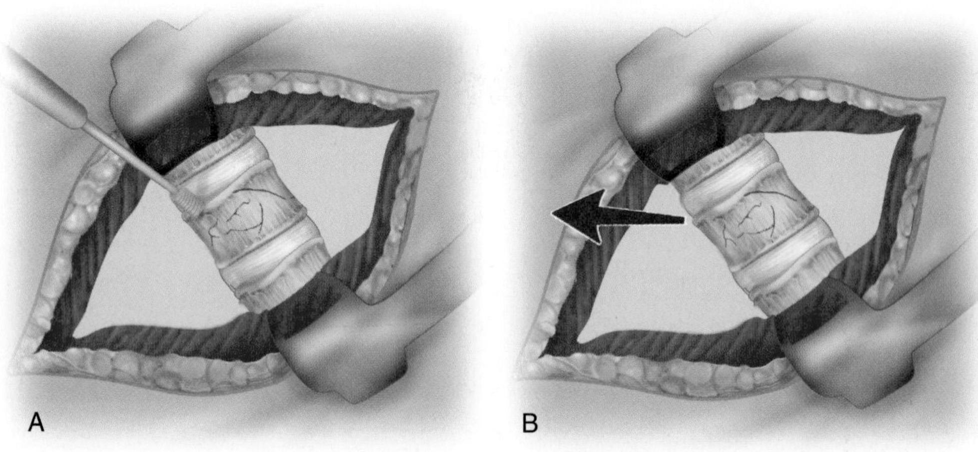

FIGURE 65-6

exposed subperiosteally from the costochondral junction to costovertebral junction and resected. Care must be taken to avoid injury of the neurovascular bundle located inferior to the rib and long thoracic nerve, which runs superficially in the surgical field.

- **Figure 65-5:** A transpleural or retropleural plane is developed bluntly through the resected rib bed down to the spine. The ipsilateral lung is collapsed, and a self-retaining rib spreader system is put into place. Next, the surgeon verifies the desired level radiographically with a spinal needle in the adjacent disk space. The parietal pleura is identified, and a rectangular piece can be incised and reflected posteriorly from the lateral border of the anterior longitudinal ligament (ALL) to the rib head. For complete exposure of the lateral wall of the vertebral body, the segmental vessels must be identified and ligated at this step.
- **Figure 65-6:** The pedicle must be isolated next. This is best done by resecting the rib head that corresponds with the vertebral body of interest. The pedicle is then thinned out and resected with a pneumatic bur and Kerrison rongeur, providing lateral access into the spinal canal and thecal sac. The surgeon now has a true understanding of the posterior limit of the corpectomy.
- **Figure 65-7:** The cranial and caudal disks are removed back to the annulus or posterior longitudinal ligament (PLL). The corpectomy is performed next with the help of rongeurs and osteotomes when preserving bone, which may be used later for autograft. A high-speed bur is essential for completing the corpectomy by drilling out the contralateral pedicle and the posterior wall back to the PLL. Alternatively, a

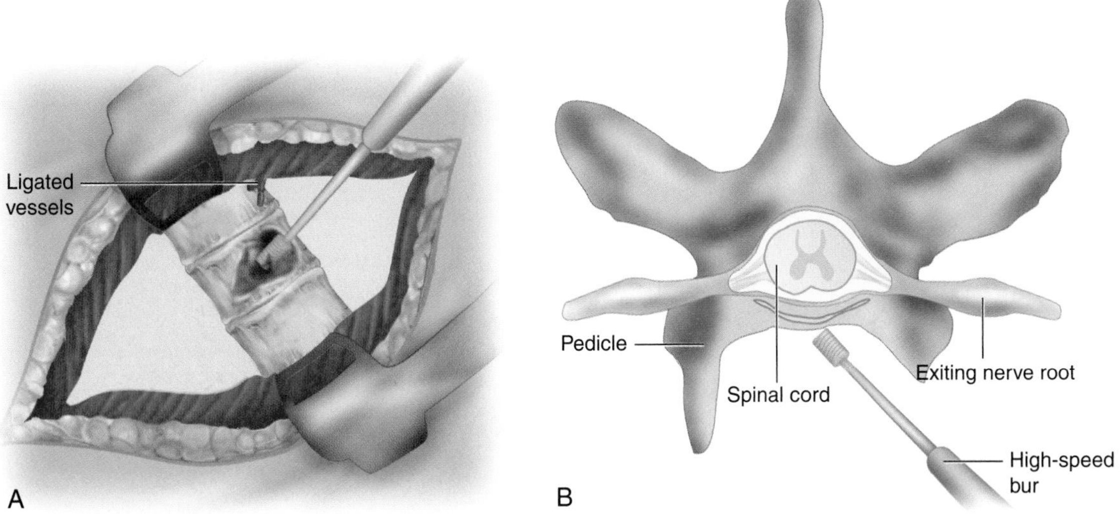

FIGURE 65-7

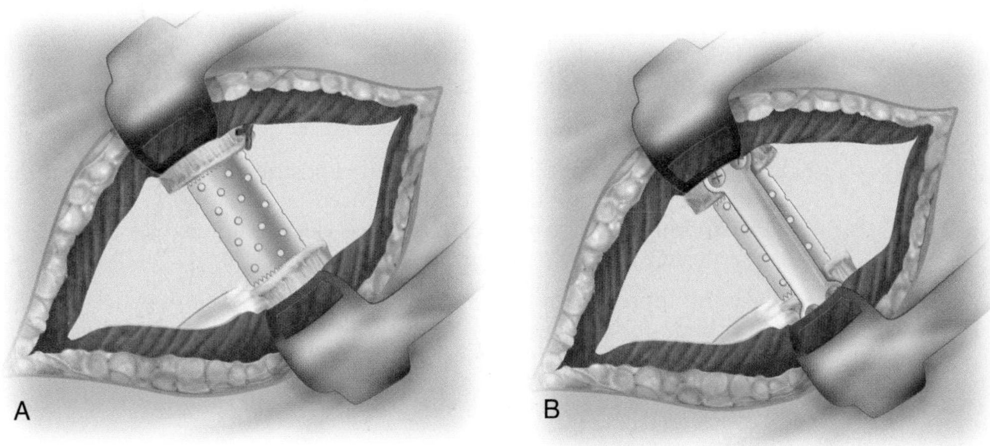

FIGURE 65-8

pneumatic bur can be used for the entire procedure if resecting pathologic bone. Finally, the PLL and any bony remnants can be removed off the dura with fine curets and Kerrison rongeurs. The ALL and a lip of bone is left behind anteriorly for stability and to prevent graft kickout, unless a tumor resection is being performed for curative purposes.

- **Figure 65-8:** Reconstruction of the corpectomy defect is the last major step, and it can be performed with various options. Tricortical iliac crest autograft, humeral or femoral allograft, and ceramic or titanium metallic cages packed with bone graft all can be used with or without instrumentation. The instrumentation can be anterior plating or posterior screw fixation for circumferential arthrodesis or both.
- **Figure 65-9:** Before closure, careful, thorough hemostasis must be obtained. If working around the diaphragm, it should be evaluated for possible tears, which must be repaired with absorbable suture before closure. A 28F to 32F chest tube is placed at the apex of the lung. If excessive bleeding is encountered or expected, a second chest tube is placed in the wound and tunneled out subcutaneously over a purse-string suture. The lung is reinflated, and the ribs are reapproximated using No. 1 polyglactin 910 (Vicryl) suture. The remainder of the wound is closed in layers, including an interrupted closure of the muscles, then subcutaneous tissue, and finally subcuticular region. Chest tubes are placed on low suction, and a postoperative chest x-ray must be performed in the recovery room.

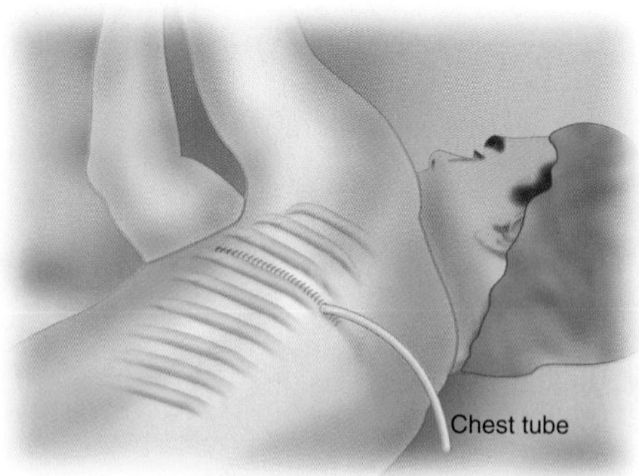

FIGURE 65-9

TIPS FROM THE MASTERS

- Perform a careful preoperative analysis of imaging studies (x-rays, MRI, with or without magnetic resonance angiography or angiography). Identify the exact level and extent of the pathology, and create a template for your reconstruction. Also, evaluate the surrounding vascular anatomy and consider preoperative embolization for vascular tumors.
- Consider using neuromonitoring.
- Secure the patient in the lateral decubitus position, and confirm that the patient remains at 90 degrees to the floor with the desired level at the break of the bed. This position allows optimal exposure when the bed is flexed and enables the surgeon to remain oriented during the entire case.
- Make the approach over the rib that is one or two levels cephalad to the pathologic vertebral body for the best working window. A position two levels cephalad is preferred because it is much easier to work down than up.
- Identify and resect the rib head and the pedicle of the involved vertebral body to gain access to the spinal canal.
- Remove the posterior vertebral body from the contralateral pedicle toward the ipsilateral side; this prevents the decompressed dura from expanding into the operative field and obscuring visualization.
- Ensure a biomechanically sound reconstruction—either all anterior or circumferential.

PITFALLS

Wrong level surgery can be performed without critical preoperative and intraoperative radiographic analysis.

Intercostal neuralgia can occur secondary to intercostal nerve injury during rib resection.

Pulmonary contusion and postoperative morbidity can occur with aggressive retraction or inadequate ventilation.

Excessive bleeding can be encountered during resection of a highly vascular tumor. If not properly identified and ligated, segmental vessels can also result in significant bleeding. Use caution when retracting the aorta or the vena cava.

Removal of the pedicle can cause inadvertent injury to the exiting nerve root.

Inadequate decompression can occur without clear identification of the contralateral pedicle.

PITFALLS—cont'd

Intraoperative spatial orientation may be a challenge and result in suboptimal screw fixation. Beware of spinal canal penetration or vascular injury with bicortical screw purchase.

Iatrogenic deformity may be introduced by locking down the construct in kyphosis or scoliosis secondary to asymmetric graft or cage placement.

BAILOUT OPTIONS

- If the anterior approach cannot be performed or completed, the surgery can be conducted through a posterior or an extracavitary approach.
- In the event of excessive bleeding despite sound surgical technique and use of hemostatic agents, consider a partial or subtotal resection or corpectomy.
- An irreparable dural injury may be encountered. Approximate the dura as best as possible with the use of sutures, facial grafts, collagen barriers, or fibrin glue. A subarachnoid drain may also be beneficial in this situation.
- A biomechanically unsound anterior reconstruction can be abandoned for or supplemented with posterior fixation.
- Consider minimally invasive techniques (video-assisted thoracic surgery, extreme lateral interbody fusion, direct lateral interbody fusion) as alternative options, especially for patients with multiple medical comorbidities who require a partial resection.

SUGGESTED READINGS

Bradford DS, McBride GG. Surgical management of thoracolumbar spine fractures with incomplete neurologic deficits. Clin Orthop 1987;218:201–16.

D'Aliberti G, Talamonti G, Villa F, et al. Anterior approach to thoracic and lumbar spine lesions: results in 145 consecutive cases. J Neurosurg Spine 2008;9:466–82.

Dickman CA, Rosenthal D, Karahalios DG, et al. Thoracic vertebrectomy and reconstruction using a microsurgical thoracoscopic approach. Neurosurgery 1996;38:279–93.

Hodgson AR, Stock FE. Anterior spinal fusion: a preliminary communication on the radical treatment of Pott's disease and Pott's paraplegia. Br J Surg 1956;44:266.

Xu R, Garces-Ambrossi GL, McGirt TF, et al. Thoracic vertebrectomy and spinal reconstruction via anterior, posterior or combined approaches: clinical outcomes in 91 consecutive patients with metastatic spinal tumors. J Neurosurg Spine 2009;11:272–84.

Procedure 66 Costotransversectomy

Timothy D. Uschold, Richard A. Lochhead, Randall W. Porter

INDICATIONS

- Costotransversectomy provides a posterolaterally directed corridor of access to the costovertebral joints, lateral spinal canal, and neural foramina and to a portion of the posterolateral vertebral body located from T1-12.
  - Lateral or paracentral soft disk herniations
  - Epidural or bony tumor debulking or removal
  - Thoracic sympathectomy
  - Osteomyelitis or diskitis with or without abscess
  - Canal decompression for trauma
  - Epidural metastasis in which palliation rather than en bloc resection is the goal
  - Intractable costovertebral joint pain associated with ankylosing spondylitis
  - Need for a thoracic approach with a relatively low rate of pulmonary and vascular morbidities

CONTRAINDICATIONS

- Anatomically, access to the midline anterior dura, epidural space, and vertebral body is most constrained; however, soft or suckable pathologies near the midline may be more readily resected in some cases, even with indirect visualization.
- Midline disk herniations (or traumatic bone fragments) via this approach—for calcified disks, including paracentral locations, an alternative approach is mandated for similar reasons.
- When spondylectomy or en bloc resection are required based on the pathology, imaging, and clinical picture.

PLANNING AND POSITIONING

- Planning begins with a thorough review of the patient's presenting neurologic symptoms, medical comorbidities, and imaging. Axial views on magnetic resonance imaging (MRI) or computed tomography (CT) are especially informative in selecting among alternative operative approaches. Myelography is particularly helpful in defining osteophytes from soft disks. For tumors, T2-weighted, fat-suppressed short tau inversion recovery (STIR) and contrasted T1 MRI sequences are useful for identifying bony infiltration. CT can additionally differentiate sclerotic from lytic lesions. Sagittal and coronal alignment of the spine can be assessed with plain x-rays.
- The key issue determining selection of an approach is the ability to visualize the lesion of interest without retraction on the already deformed spinal cord. Increased neurologic deterioration or paraplegia can occur from additional traction on an already compromised spinal cord. Preoperative imaging requires careful review, paying particular attention to the lesion of interest and its relationship to the midline, dura, disk space, pedicle, and nerve roots.
- Various patient positions accommodating numerous modifications have been described for the costotransversectomy procedure. Generally, we favor the prone position over semiprone or lateral decubitus alternatives. With the patient tightly secured to the frame, bed rotation in combination with the degree of freedom provided by the

operating microscope can typically provide adequate posterolateral visualization. The patient may be secured on a Wilson frame or gel rolls, but we typically prefer a rotating Jackson table with the arms extended upward to facilitate ease of fluoroscopy or navigation-based instrumentation. Attention to the padding of bony prominences and sites of potential neurovascular compression is essential.

- Baseline prepositioning, postpositioning, and intraoperative somatosensory and motor evoked potential monitoring is recommended in all cases.
- A common pitfall for thoracic surgery is accurate localization, and this requires careful attention to anatomy and fluoroscopic technique. Intraoperative localization usually employs fluoroscopy to count up from L5 or the last rib (assuming this is T12). This strategy can result in error. A preoperative x-ray of the whole spine should be reviewed to identify the last visualized rib and as a reference during surgery. Intraoperative confirmation of the operative level by multiple techniques in anteroposterior and lateral planes is recommended. Anatomically numbered ribs articulate with the disk space above the correspondingly numbered vertebral body. In the lowest segments of the thoracic spine, rib articulations can be found below the level of the corresponding disk space. Preoperative localization in radiology using fluoroscopy or CT can limit the chance of operating on the wrong level. We have asked the radiologist to place a localization coil or small amount of cement in the pedicle caudal to the targeted disk space.
- **Figure 66-1:** Axial views of typical thoracic vertebral body. Shaded areas correspond to approach-specific zones of bony decompression and surgical access. *Arrows* delineate the angle of approach but not location of the skin incision. Correlation with preoperative axial MRI and CT is necessary for preoperative planning. **A,** Laminectomy. Access to the vertebral body and anterior dura is precluded by excessive cord manipulation. **B,** Transpedicular or lateral gutter approach. Bony removal of the facet and pedicle to the level of the posterior vertebral body cortex facilitates the most limited access to the lateral disk, canal, and vertebral body pathology. **C,** Costotransversectomy. Disarticulation and removal of the proximal 3 to 5 cm of ribs allows greater visualization of the lateral vertebral body, disk space, and neural foramen. Anterior decompression is limited to the midline. **D,** Lateral extracavitary approach. Additional 5 to 7 cm of lateral rib removal and downward pleural retraction allows for greater exposure and a more lateral angle of entry, which translates into improved anterior decompression across the midline. **E,** Transthoracic approach. The greatest degree of access to the vertebral body is afforded through the thoracic cavity, providing access to decompress the entire anterior canal if needed. Posterior elements cannot be addressed from this approach.
- **Figure 66-2:** Posterolateral anatomic (**A**) and anteroposterior and lateral radiographic (**B**) views of mid-thoracic spine. The anatomic view depicts the relationship of the numbered rib head to corresponding disk space. Note the relationships of the sympathetic chain, rib head, transverse process, nerve root, and pedicle. The rib head and disk space are outlined and numbered again on radiographic views. Proper adjustment of fluoroscope to align the pedicles and end-plates is necessary to avoid errors in localization because of parallax.
- **Figure 66-3:** The choice of incision is determined largely by instrumentation (if needed), degree of intended exposure, and surgeon preference. Midline (**A**), paramedian (**B**), and semilunar (**C**) incisions all have been described. We favor the midline incision because of anatomic familiarity, adequacy of exposure, potential for bilateral access, and ease of subsequent instrumentation. An optional "hockey-stick" (**D**) or T in the midline incision may be added if additional rib exposure is required. Paramedian and semilunar incisions (more commonly used in lateral extracavitary approach) need not extend more laterally than the articulation of the rib head or transverse process.

PROCEDURE

- **Figure 66-4:** A midline incision is performed extending at minimum one vertebral level above the index level of interest. Dissection is continued through the thoracolumbar fascia along a strictly subperiosteal plane using monopolar cautery and Cobb periosteal elevators to expose the spinous processes, lamina, facet joints, and tips of transverse

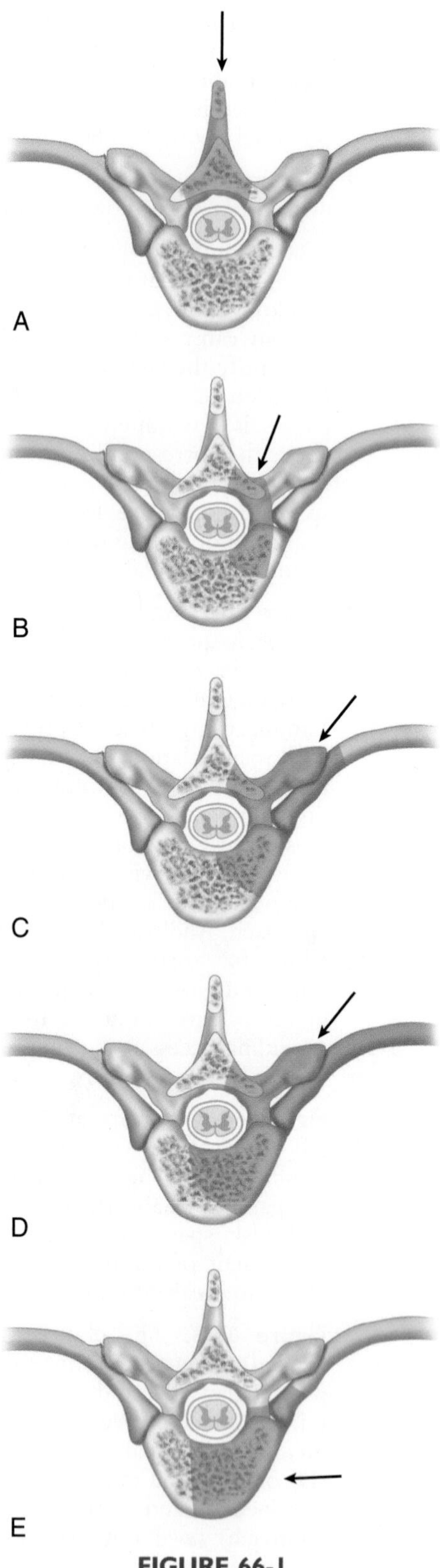

FIGURE 66-1

processes laterally. Bilateral dissection may be accomplished via the midline incision. Paramedian and curvilinear incisions proceed through the muscle and fascia using monopolar cautery in parallel alignment with the skin incision. Careful digital palpation is necessary to avoid excess laterally directed exposure and unwanted penetration through the intercostal spaces. Subperiosteal dissection may proceed medially and laterally to recapitulate unilateral exposure achieved via the midline incision.

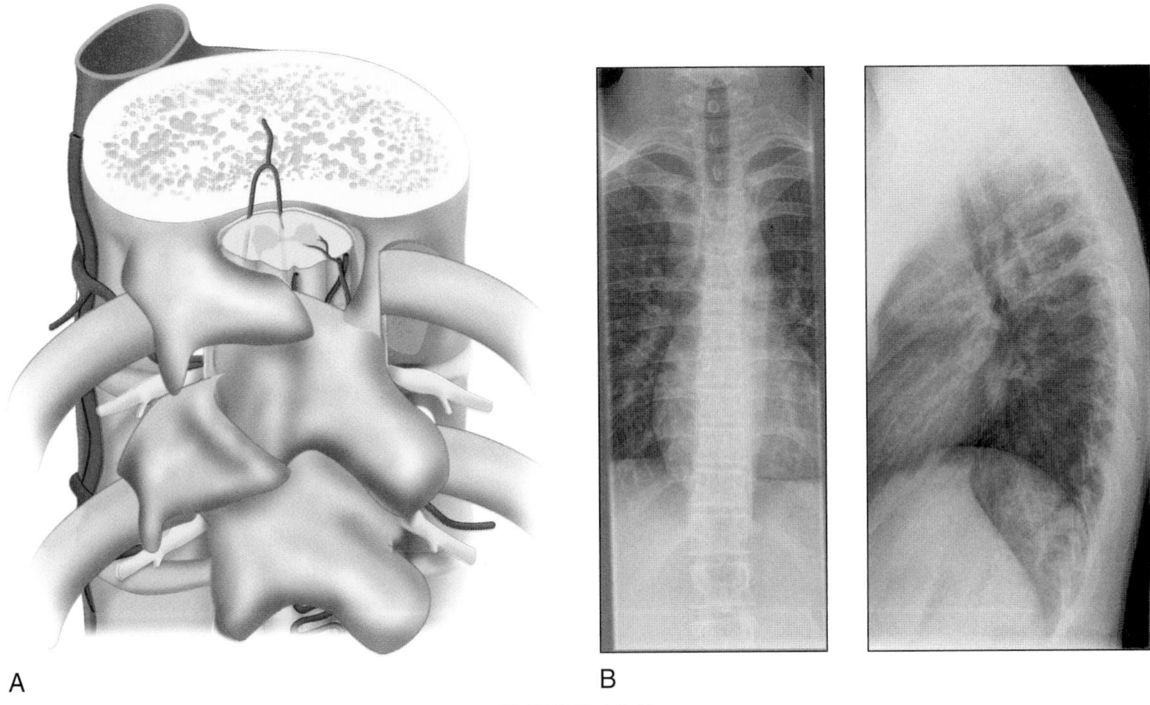

FIGURE 66-2

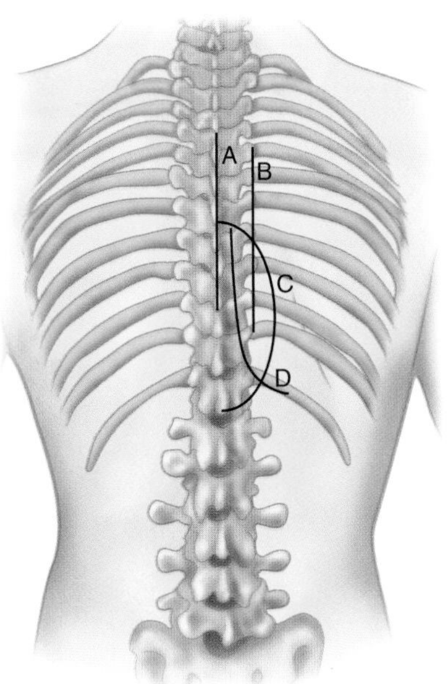

FIGURE 66-3

- **Figure 66-5:** When required for spinal cord decompression or involvement of posterior elements, laminectomy is accomplished using a Leksell rongeur, high-speed drill, and Kerrison rongeurs judiciously avoiding downward pressure on the thecal sac. Wide laminectomy facilitates medial identification of the pedicle and neural foramina. The pedicle is identified below the level of the superior facet. Unilateral facetectomy or removal of the inferior articulating process, when required for visualization, may be accomplished by osteotome or high-speed drill. Surgical (**A**) and axial (**B**) views are shown.

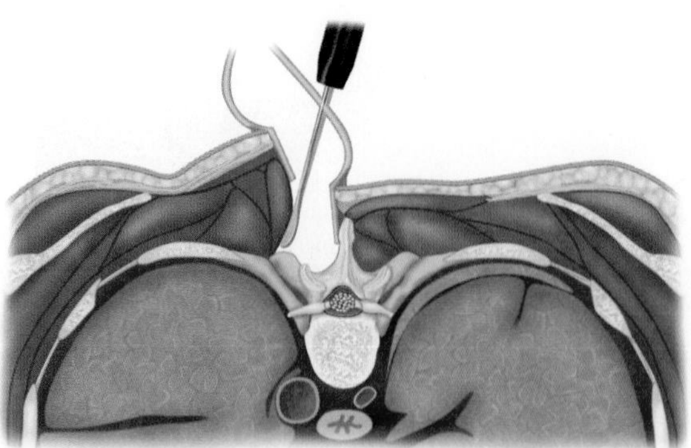

FIGURE 66-4

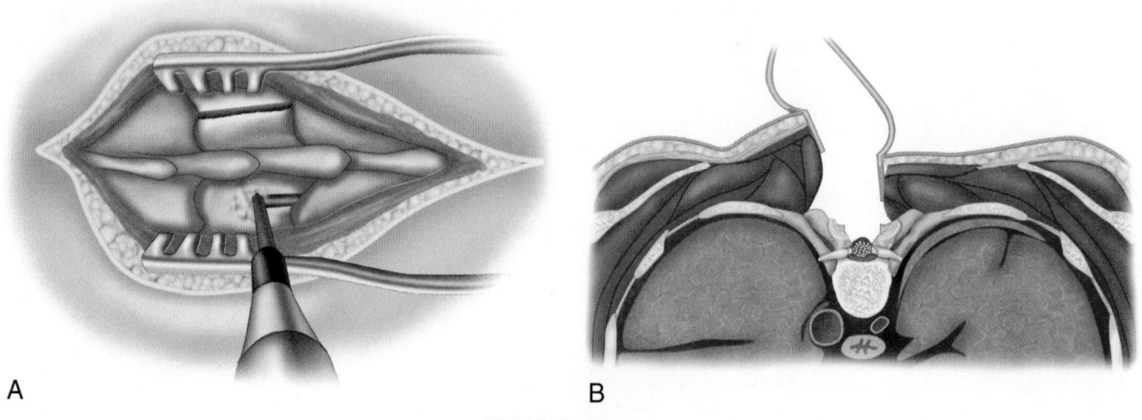

FIGURE 66-5

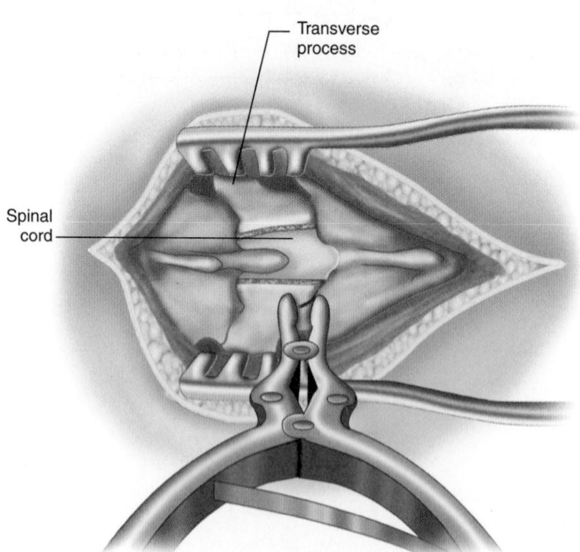

FIGURE 66-6

- **Figure 66-6:** Removal of the transverse process ensues with Leksell rongeurs. Monopolar cautery is useful to skeletonize the remaining bone and identify the costotransverse ligaments (costotransverse, lateral, and superior), which are subsequently disarticulated by Kerrison rongeurs or curved curet, or both. The rib head, costovertebral joint, lateral body, and pedicle are subsequently identified. Additional subperiosteal dissection laterally along the rib of interest may be useful to gain a superior angle for vertebral body and canal exposure.

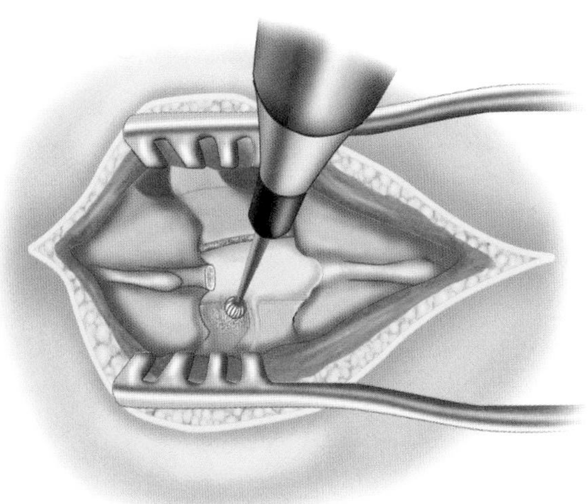

FIGURE 66-7

- **Figure 66-7:** Blunt dissection of the anterior pleura is performed with periosteal retractors, and the neurovascular bundle is identified along the costal groove at the caudal margins of the rib. The neurovascular bundle is followed medially to identify the level of the neural foramen and root. The pedicle may be drilled under magnification to the level of the posterior vertebral body cortex.
- **Figure 66-8:** After circumferential dissection from the underlying pleura, rib osteotomy may be performed distally using rib cutters, Leksell rongeur, or B-1 footplate attachment. Looking medially, the exiting nerve, foramen, and lateral canal are skeletonized further and identified during removal of the radiate ligaments and rib head at the costovertebral joint. Although the parietal pleura is typically protected by a thin layer of yellow fat, a Kerrison rongeur is preferred to a Leksell rongeur for removal of the rib head to avoid pleural violation. Alternatively, a Cobb periosteal elevator may be used to lever the head of the rib from its robust attachments to the vertebral body. After disarticulation of the rib, downward retraction on the pleura with a malleable retractor allows visualization of the lateral body. Subperiosteal dissection along the vertebral body is useful to avoid segmental vessel or sympathetic trunk transection.

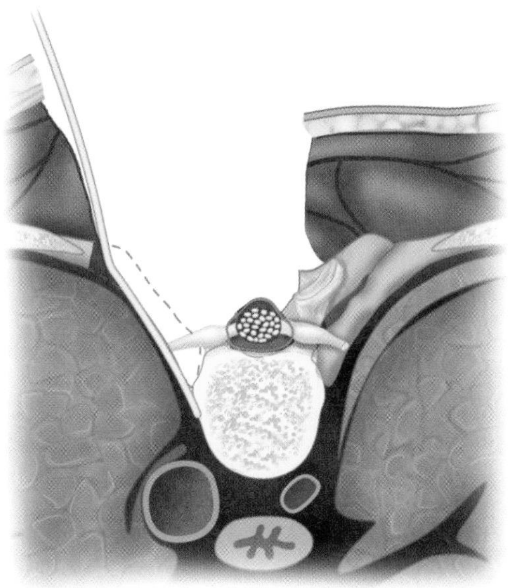

FIGURE 66-8

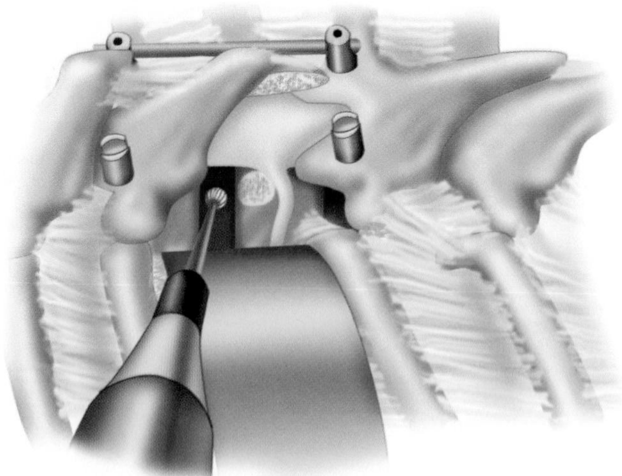

FIGURE 66-9

- **Figure 66-9:** The posterolateral annulus is identified and incised with microscopic assistance during thoracic diskectomy. Disk space is cored out posterolaterally, and a high-speed drill is used to remove a significant portion of the superior and inferior end plates. Paracentral and lateral disk herniations can be resected by downward-directed force using dental or Epstein curet into the lateral cavity described earlier. The posterior longitudinal ligament may be preserved as a useful anterior landmark to protect against dural violation. Epidural lesions including abscess or metastasis may be resected in an analogous fashion.
- **Figure 66-10:** Posterior instrumentation with or without stereotactic navigation may be accomplished before or after bony removal. Bilateral costotransversectomy is recommended for anterior graft placement so that an instrument may be passed below the posterior longitudinal ligament and anterior dura. In such circumstances, integrity of decompression and size of graft can be evaluated more adequately. Nerve root sacrifice uses silk ties before transection and is typically required to gain sufficient lateral access to accommodate an anteriorly placed graft spanning end plate to end plate. If decompression is likely to result in significant destabilization, we routinely place pedicle screws and a provisionally tightened rod on the contralateral side before removal of any bony elements.
- **Figure 66-11:** After completion of the procedure, the wound is copiously irrigated, and a Valsalva maneuver is performed under irrigation to evaluate for occult pneumothorax. This complication is indicated by effervescence from pleural violation. The presence of pleural or dural violation naturally influences the choice of chest tube placement or subfascial drainage. Muscle and fascial layers are reapproximated with 0-0 polyglactin 910 (Vicryl) suture, and the skin is closed.

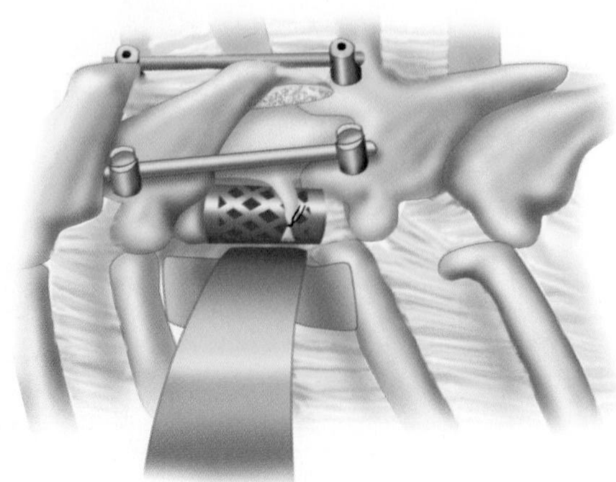

FIGURE 66-10

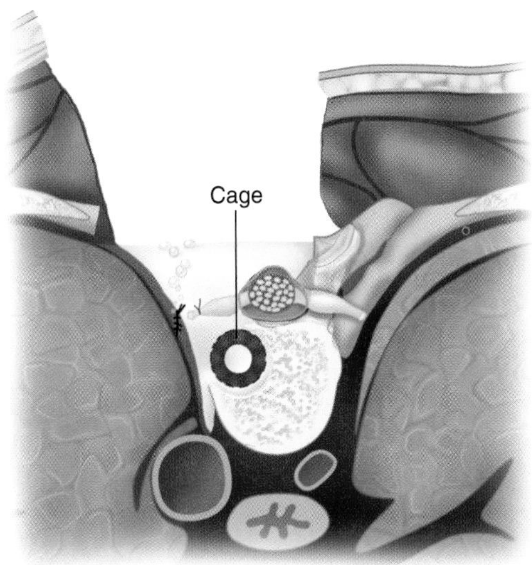

FIGURE 66-11

TIPS FROM THE MASTERS

- Optimized exposure in narrow surgical corridors is an essential component of avoiding complications, especially in the setting of distorted anatomy.
- Suboptimal or limited access to the pathology of interest may demand further maneuvers to increase the operative window. Angled dental mirrors or an angled endoscope may be valuable tools to evaluate or direct the extent of resection further.
- Radicular arteries, found intradurally along the root at the neural foramen, variably contribute to the blood supply of the thoracic cord. Vascular supply to the cord is an important consideration in the thoracic spine because of the "watershed" perfusion pattern in the mid-thoracic region and the variable location of the artery of Adamkiewicz (most commonly reported at T9-12 on the left). The value of preoperative spinal angiography to delineate the location of anterior spinal artery feeding vessels has been debated in the literature.
- Root sacrifice is sometimes necessary to facilitate anterior vertebral body reconstruction.
- When localizing the pedicle of interest, it is useful to follow the rib from lateral to medial, until one reaches the rib head where it articulates with the body below the targeted disk space. If one works superiorly and laterally to the pedicle, the disk space is readily identified.
- A small cavity can be drilled into the body so that the disk can be pushed away from the cord. At no point in the operation should one attempt to retract the cord.
- Infiltrative or extensive epidural tumor masses may be visualized early during the surgical procedure. It is advisable, however, to reserve tumor debulking until full exposure has been achieved. Early aggressive attempts at tumor resection with inadequate exposure may lead to preventable blood loss.

PITFALLS

Localization of the correct operative level requires considerable attention, particularly in the setting of diskectomy. To minimize the chance of error, we ask the radiologist to place a marker preoperatively in the pedicle of interest. Placement of a marker also minimizes the time needed for fluoroscopic localization intraoperatively. Trauma, tumors, or infiltrative lesions may become more apparent by their appearance in the operative field.

Continued

PITFALLS—cont'd

Subperiosteal dissection of the ribs, particularly at the rib heads where radiate ligamentous attachments may be more stubborn, may result in violation of the parietal pleura. Significant postoperative pneumothorax can be avoided by prompt pleural repair using 4-0 absorbable suture placed with the lung under inflation. Adequate closure is confirmed during irrigation by an airtight suture line with Valsalva maneuver. Immediate postoperative chest films should be obtained as a second confirmation. A chest tube can be placed intraoperatively or after the procedure if necessary. Routine chest x-ray may be useful if occult pleural violation or pneumothorax is considered.

Durotomy and resultant cerebrospinal fluid (CSF) leak are most commonly encountered with blind dissection or overly aggressive attempts to push the safe boundaries of midline resection. Anterior and lateral durotomies may be technically difficult to repair with suture. In such cases, layered repair with fibrin sealant and dural substitute is recommended. Lumbar CSF diversion is a second alternative. If a chest tube is required in the setting of CSF leak, it is imperative to avoid pleural suction. Drainage should be monitored for the presence of CSF because this situation may result in tentorial herniation.

BAILOUT OPTIONS

- Additional exposure is often beneficial in the case of particularly tenacious disk herniations, adherent pathology, or lesions displaced anteriorly. Extension of the incision or placement of a T over the rib of interest helps allow for greater lateral exposure.
- The approach can be expanded to the lateral extracavitary procedure with further distal rib resection, removal of multiple ribs, single-lung ventilation, and more aggressive pleural retraction to provide greater exposure of spinal cord with a more medial corridor.
- The goals of spinal stabilization should be established at the time of surgical planning. Anterior fusion may require bilateral access, extensive vertebral body resection, end plate removal, and graft preparation.
- In the case of a patient with systemic illness (e.g., palliative surgery for metastatic epidural disease), the objective of surgery may be timely decompression and early upfront fixation to facilitate mobilization. Eventual fusion may present less of a consideration. In such cases, the use of Steinmann pins alternately buttressed and seated into opposing end plates has been reported as an acceptable framework. Methyl methacrylate (MMA) may be used to fill the remaining resection cavity in the vertebral body.
- If a generous partial corpectomy is performed and anterior fusion is needed, we favor anterior cage placement when possible because of better stabilization, the potential for fusion, and the minimal investment in operative time required. Anterior cage placement is likely unnecessary when a sufficient amount of structurally adequate vertebral body remains after decompression.

SUGGESTED READINGS

Dinh DH, Tompkins J, Clark SB. Transcostovertebral approach for thoracic disc herniations. J Neurosurg 2001;94(Suppl.):38–44.

Fessler RG, Sturgill M. Review: complications of surgery for thoracic disk disease. Surg Neurol 1998;49:609–18.

Klimot P, Dailey AT, Fessler RG. Posterior surgical approaches and outcomes in metastatic spine disease. Neurosurg Clin N Am 2004;15:425–35.

McCormick WE, Will SF, Benzel EC. Surgery for thoracic disc disease: complication avoidance—overview and management. Neurosurg Focus 2000;9:1–6.

Sonntag VR, Hadley MN. Surgical approaches to the thoracolumbar spine. Clin Neurosurg 1990;36:168–85.

Figures 66-1 through 66-11 are modified with permission from Barrow Neurological Institute.

Procedure 67

Thoracic Transpedicular Corpectomy

Richard A. Lochhead, Timothy D. Uschold, Nicholas Theodore

INDICATIONS

- The decision to approach the thoracic spine with a transpedicular corpectomy depends largely on the view and angle of exposure needed. This approach provides access to the lateral spinal canal, to the neural foramina, and to a portion of the posterolateral vertebral body. A bilateral transpedicular approach can provide 270 degrees of decompression if needed. Common pathologies treated by thoracic transpedicular corpectomy include lateral disk herniations, epidural tumor, osteomyelitis or diskitis with or without abscess, and lateral canal decompression from trauma.
- Posterior segmental fixation can be performed after resection of anterior and posterior elements, for unstable lesions associated with trauma, or for deformity. An anterior graft or cage should be placed unless a minimal amount of vertebral body is removed, as in a transpedicular biopsy.
- Many approaches are available for thoracic lesions, including thoracotomy, retropleural, extensive lateral extracavitary, and costotransversectomy approaches. The appropriate procedure depends on the following factors: (1) the location of the lesion (bone, epidural, paraspinal); (2) the angle of view needed; (3) the nature of the specific lesion (hard or soft, invasive or encapsulated); (4) the goal of treatment (en bloc resection or palliative decompression); (5) the patient's comorbidities and their ability to tolerate a thoracotomy; and (6) the surgeon's familiarity with technical aspects of the procedure. Transpedicular corpectomy is often used for patients with acute neurologic decline from epidural metastasis in whom palliative decompression rather than en bloc resection is the goal.

CONTRAINDICATIONS

- Contraindications to a transpedicular corpectomy are primarily anatomic. Access to the midline anterior dura, epidural space, and vertebral body is limited. In some cases, soft or suctionable lesions near the midline may be resected without direct visualization. It is seldom possible, however, to achieve adequate or safe decompression of midline or paracentral disk herniations via this approach, especially if they are calcified. These lesions often adhere to the dura anteriorly and require sharp dissection under direct visualization to prevent spinal cord traction and injury.
- Other contraindications relate primarily to the nature of the lesion and the goals of surgery. This approach is well suited for palliative decompression from metastatic epidural compression, tumor debulking, and biopsy. When spondylectomy or en bloc resection is required, significant modifications or an alternative surgical approach are necessary.

PLANNING AND POSITIONING

- Begin with a thorough review of the patient's neurologic symptoms, medical comorbidities, and imaging characteristics. Myelography is sometimes helpful, particularly in defining osteophytes and bony anatomy. Bony tumor infiltration is best seen on magnetic resonance imaging (MRI), particularly with T1-weighted sequences with and without contrast agent and with T2-weighted sequences with fat-suppressed short-tau inversion recovery (STIR). Computed tomography (CT) can differentiate sclerotic from lytic lesions. Plain x-rays best show sagittal and coronal alignment of the spine.

- Pay particular attention to the axial views on MRI or CT to help determine the angle of view needed and the appropriate surgical approach for the case. The key issue for selection of an approach is the ability to visualize the lesion of interest without spinal cord retraction. Neurologic deterioration or paraplegia can occur from additional traction on an already compromised spinal cord. Look at the relationship between the pathologic lesion and the spinal cord, midline, dura, disk space, pedicle, and nerve root.
- The patient is positioned prone and secured tightly to the frame to allow bed rotation. We prefer a rotating Jackson table with the arms extended upward to facilitate fluoroscopy or navigation-based instrumentation, unless the lesion is in the upper thoracic spine, in which case the arms are secured downward. We use prepositioning, postpositioning, and intraoperative somatosensory evoked potential and motor evoked potential monitoring in almost all cases.
- A common pitfall for thoracic surgery is accurate localization, which requires careful attention to anatomy and fluoroscopic technique. To prevent localization errors, preoperative x-rays of the entire spine should be reviewed to identify the last visualized rib or number of lumbar vertebrae. Intraoperative counting and confirmation of the correct operative level should be done by multiple techniques in anteroposterior and lateral planes. Anatomically numbered ribs articulate with the disk space above the same numbered vertebral body. Preoperative localization with a coil or cement by interventional radiology can limit the chance of operating on the wrong level.
- **Figure 67-1:** Axial views of the typical thoracic vertebral body. *Shaded areas* correspond to approach-specific zones of bony decompression and surgical access for unilateral (**A**) or bilateral (**B**) transpedicular corpectomy. Correlation with preoperative axial MRI and CT is necessary for preoperative planning. Bony removal of the facet and pedicle to the level of the posterior vertebral body cortex facilitates access to the lateral disk, spinal canal, and vertebral body pathology. If the pathology is a soft tumor, midline anterior decompression can often be achieved.
- **Figure 67-2:** The length of the incision is determined largely by instrumentation (if needed), degree of intended exposure, and surgeon preference. If possible, anterior and posterior hardware should always be placed unless only a minimal amount of the vertebral body is removed (i.e., biopsy). If anterior hardware is needed, at least two levels above and below the corpectomy site should be exposed. We use a midline incision because of anatomic familiarity, adequacy of exposure, potential for bilateral access, and ease of instrumentation.

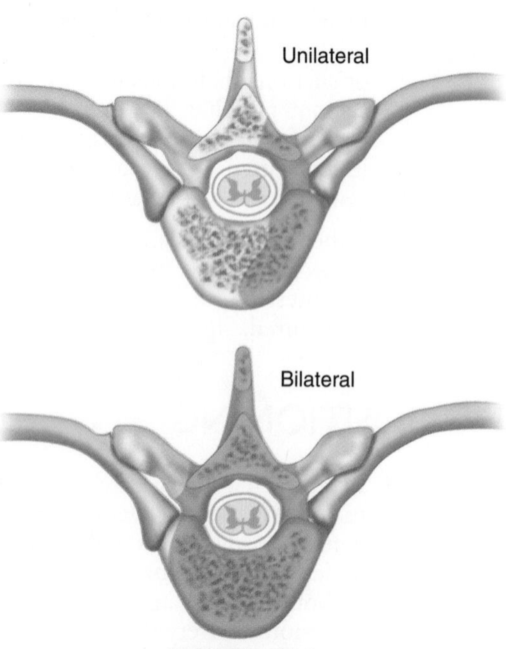

FIGURE 67-1

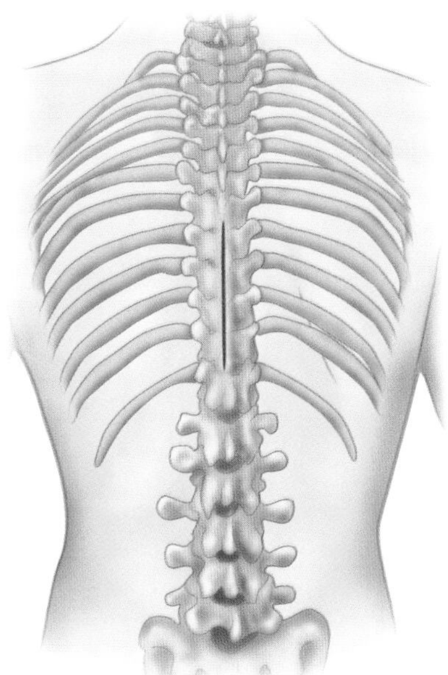

FIGURE 67-2

PROCEDURE

- **Figure 67-3:** A midline incision is performed, and dissection is continued through the thoracolumbar fascia along a strictly subperiosteal plane using monopolar cautery and Cobb periosteal retractors to expose the spinous processes, lamina, facet joints, and, if needed, tips of the transverse processes laterally. If a tumor has invaded the posterior elements, laminar strength and integrity may be compromised. Care needs to be taken during subperiosteal dissection to prevent spinal cord injury from cautery or compression. A bilateral dissection may be performed if needed.
- **Figure 67-4:** When needed for spinal cord decompression, laminectomy is accomplished with a high-speed drill and judicious use of Kerrison or Leksell rongeurs. Care must be taken to avoid downward pressure on the thecal sac and injury to already compromised spinal cord. If possible, we use a drill bit to make troughs in the lamina. While light tension is applied away from the cord, the laminectomy is finished by detaching the remaining soft tissue and bony connections with an upward curet and small Kerrison rongeurs. Wide laminectomy facilitates medial identification of the pedicle and neural foramina. Extra bone is always cleaned and morcellized for use later in the fusion if it is not involved in the pathologic process.
- **Figure 67-5:** The pedicle is identified below the level of the superior facet. With care not to compress the spinal cord, a dental instrument can be used to feel the pedicle gently and to outline the upper and lower foramina.
- **Figure 67-6:** Unilateral or bilateral facetectomy may be accomplished by a Leksell rongeur, an osteotome, a Kerrison rongeur, or a high-speed drill. A drill or narrow-tipped Leksell rongeur is useful for thinning bone over the facet.

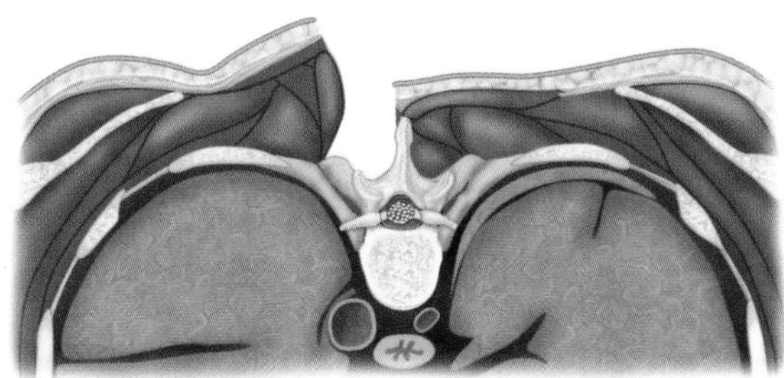

FIGURE 67-3

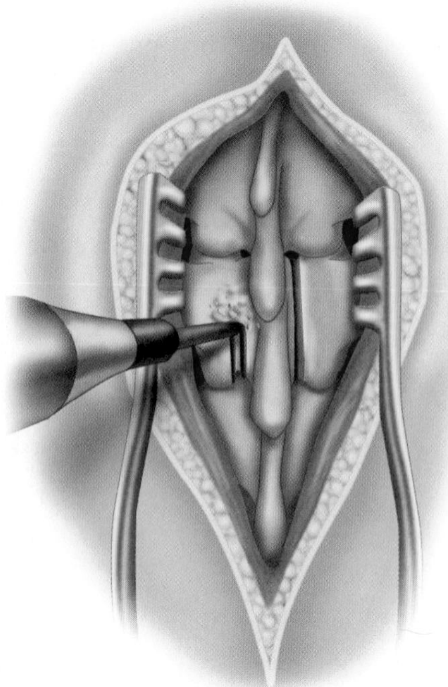

FIGURE 67-4

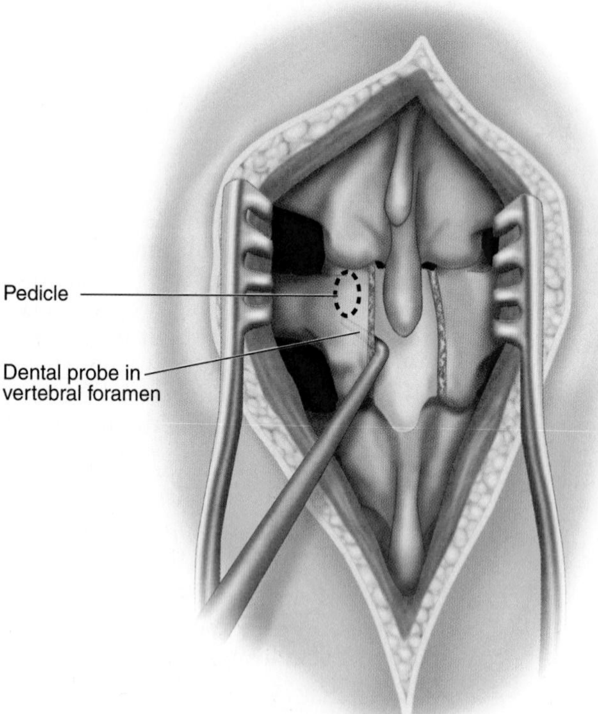

FIGURE 67-5

- **Figure 67-7:** After the facet is thinned, bony removal over the neural foramina on the caudal and rostral sides of the pedicle can be finished with a small Kerrison rongeur. This process isolates the pedicles and helps identify, preserve, and decompress the upper and lower nerve roots.
- **Figure 67-8:** The pedicle can be removed with a drill or Leksell rongeur under magnification. Tumor invasion of the pedicle can sometimes soften the bone so that suction or pituitary forceps are the only tools needed for removal.

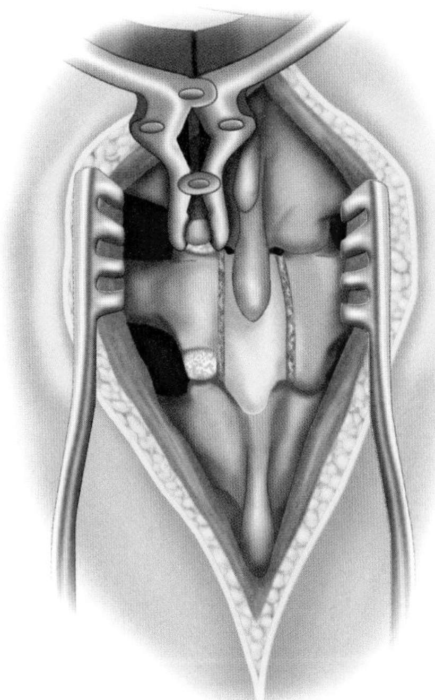

FIGURE 67-6

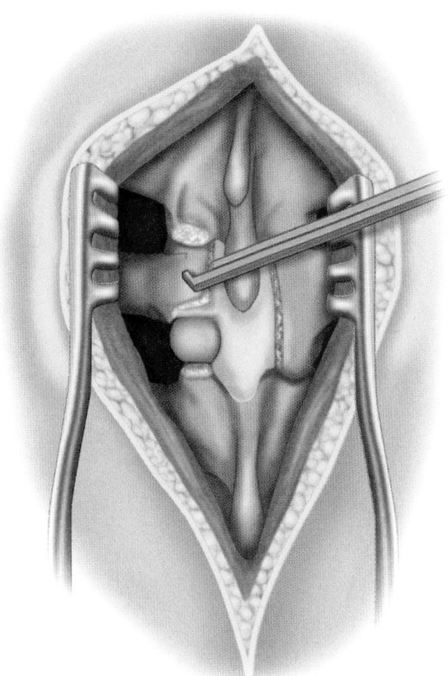

FIGURE 67-7

- **Figure 67-9:** Disk spaces adjacent to the diseased vertebral level are identified. It may be necessary to remove a portion of caudal pedicle to provide exposure to caudal disk space. With the use of an operating microscope, posterolateral annulus is incised, disk space is cored out, and end plates are exenterated.
- **Figure 67-10:** A cavity is created in the vertebral body by piecemeal resection or with a high-speed drill. Care always must be taken to avoid injury to the spinal cord. If a lateral or paracentral tumor or disk is being resected, all downward force must be directed away from the spinal cord and into the cavity created in the vertebral body.

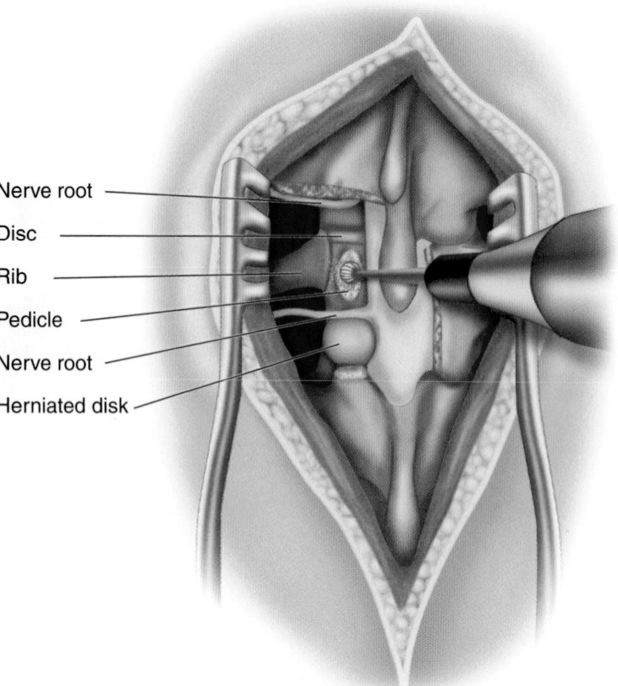

FIGURE 67-8

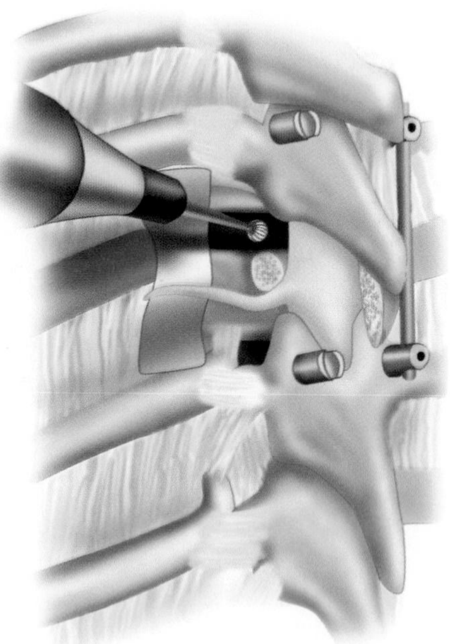

FIGURE 67-9

- **Figure 67-11:** Often a calcified disk or posterior longitudinal ligament is adherent to dura. Excessive downward pressure can injure the spinal cord. Sharp dissection can be done with tenotomy scissors and requires direct visualization. This point should be considered when the approach is planned. In tumor cases, resection of the ligament helps ensure a clean anterior dural margin.
- **Figure 67-12:** Posterior instrumentation with or without stereotactic navigation may be accomplished before or after bony removal. For cases that require a bilateral transpedicular corpectomy, contralateral screws and a temporary rod should be placed to stabilize the spine during corpectomy and cage placement.

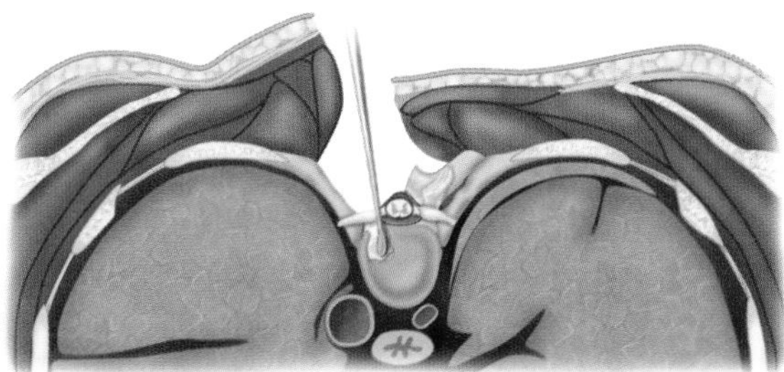

FIGURE 67-10

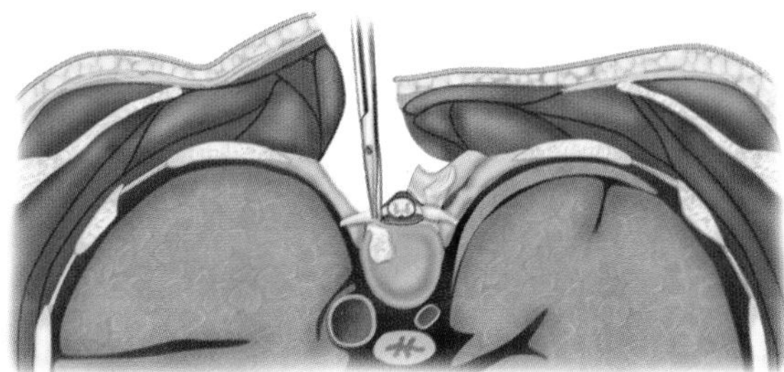

FIGURE 67-11

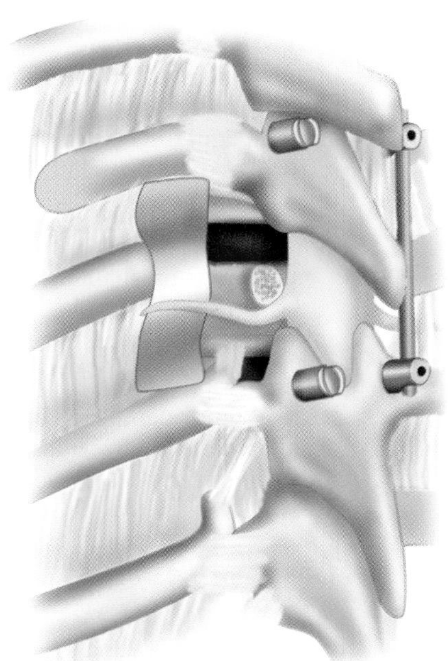

FIGURE 67-12

- **Figure 67-13:** Anterior graft placement can be done after unilateral or bilateral transpedicular corpectomy. Anterior spinal reconstruction can be done with bone graft, cages, or Steinmann pins and polymethyl methacrylate (PMMA). If possible, we prefer a static or expandable cage filled with the patient's bone, which we believe provides a solid construct with good potential for fusion. The nerve root is typically sacrificed to gain sufficient access for graft placement. After cage and screw placement, the final rods are placed, and compression is applied across the cage. Muscle and fascial layers are reapproximated with 0-0 polyglactin 910 (Vicryl) suture, and the skin is closed.

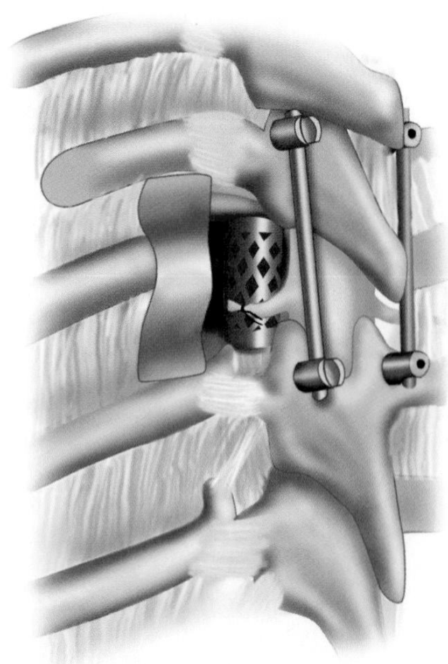

FIGURE 67-13

TIPS FROM THE MASTERS

- The major limitation of this technique is anterior midline visualization. The use of the operating microscope can improve light and surgical visualization. An angled dental mirror may help visualization and resection.
- For cases that require bilateral transpedicular corpectomy, place the screws and a temporary rod on one side after a unilateral decompression to stabilize the spine when the corpectomy is finished and while placing the cage on the other side. If changes occur in the somatosensory evoked potentials or motor evoked potentials, compression on the temporary rod may relieve tension on the spinal cord that sometimes occurs as the body settles after circumferential bony removal.
- Reserve tumor debulking until full exposure is achieved to avoid preventable blood loss. Preoperative embolization of highly vascular tumors can help minimize blood loss and can aid in intraoperative localization.

PITFALLS

Radicular arteries variably supply the thoracic cord, and watershed infarcts can occur after root sacrifice. The variable location of the artery of Adamkiewicz (most commonly on the left from T9-12) can sometimes be delineated with preoperative spinal angiography. When nerve root sacrifice is necessary, an aneurysm clip should be placed over the root sleeve for 10 to 15 minutes with electrophysiologic monitoring before suture ligation. Changes in monitoring may indicate ischemia.

Localization of the correct level in the thoracic spine requires considerable attention, particularly when treating a disk herniation. We typically ask an interventional radiologist to place a marker preoperatively in the pedicle of interest. Trauma, tumors, or infiltrative lesions are often more apparent on imaging.

Durotomy and cerebrospinal fluid leaks are often difficult to repair with suture, but layered repair with fibrin sealant and a dural substitute can be successful. Postoperatively, a lumbar drain can also be used.

BAILOUT OPTIONS

- For adherent pathology or tenacious disk herniations, additional exposure is often needed. Extension of the incision or placement of a T over the rib of interest helps increase lateral exposure and subsequent midline visualization. The approach can be converted into either a costotransversectomy or a lateral extracavitary approach if needed.
- Spinal stabilization goals should be established before surgery. When possible, anterior stabilization should be performed. The major limitation is usually not having enough space to place the cage without placing traction on the spinal cord. Increased vertebral body resection and nerve root sacrifice can help, but it is sometimes necessary to be flexible with different cage options, bone grafts, or PMMA constructs. Although not ideal, Steinmann pins inserted in opposing end plates with PMMA can provide a stable anterior construct. We favor cage or bony grafts to allow the potential for fusion, but this is not always possible.

SUGGESTED READINGS

Bilsky MH, Boland P, Lis E, et al. Single-stage posterolateral transpedicle approach for spondylectomy, epidural decompression, and circumferential fusion of spinal metastases. Spine 2000;25:2240–50.

Fessler RG, Surgill M. Review: complications of surgery for thoracic disk disease. Surg Neurol 1998;49:609–18.

Klimo P Jr, Dailey AT, Fessler RG. Posterior surgical approaches and outcomes in metastatic spine disease. Neurosurg Clin N Am 2004;15:425–35.

McCormick WE, Will SF, Benzel EC. Surgery for thoracic disc disease: complication avoidance: overview and management. Neurosurg Focus 2000;9:1–6.

Sonntag VR, Hadley MN. Surgical approaches to the thoracolumbar spine. Clin Neurosurg 1990;36:168–85.

Figures 67-1 through 67-13 are modified with permission from Barrow Neurological Institute.

Procedure 68

Smith-Petersen Osteotomy

Ram R. Vasudevan, Frank Acosta

INDICATIONS

- Correction of multiplanar spinal deformity
- Correction of fixed sagittal and coronal imbalance
- Correctable imbalance through mobile segments

CONTRAINDICATIONS

- Spinal stenosis owing to risk of exacerbating stenosis during closure of osteotomy
- Medical inability to tolerate surgery

PLANNING AND POSITIONING

- Preoperative plain radiographs and computed tomography (CT) are obtained to evaluate sagittal and coronal imbalance, bone quality, and pedicle size and angle.
- The patient is placed prone on a Jackson table to release abdominal contents from pressure, preventing epidural venous congestion and intraoperative blood loss.
- It must be possible to provide extension of the spine and hips to close osteotomy sites.
- If upper thoracic spine fixation is needed, the head must be fixed in a neutral position with a Mayfield head frame with the patient's arms secured on the sides.
- In mid-thoracic to lower thoracic spine and lumbar fixation procedures, the head does not need to be secured, and the arms are positioned at 90-degree angles above the head. The axilla is cushioned with foam pads.
- **FIGURE 68-1:** The Jackson table allows abdominal contents to hang freely, preventing epidural venous congestion and decreasing intraoperative blood loss.

PROCEDURE

- **FIGURE 68-2:** A standard midline incision is performed; the number of levels included in the osteotomy determines its length, keeping in mind that fixation points above and below osteotomy sites are needed. Subperiosteal dissection is performed using monopolar

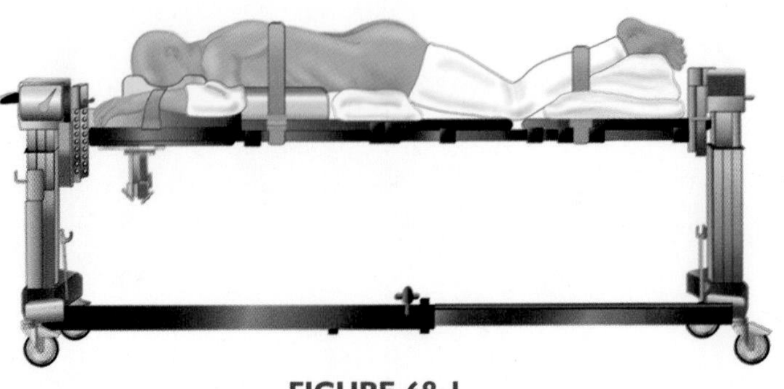

FIGURE 68-1

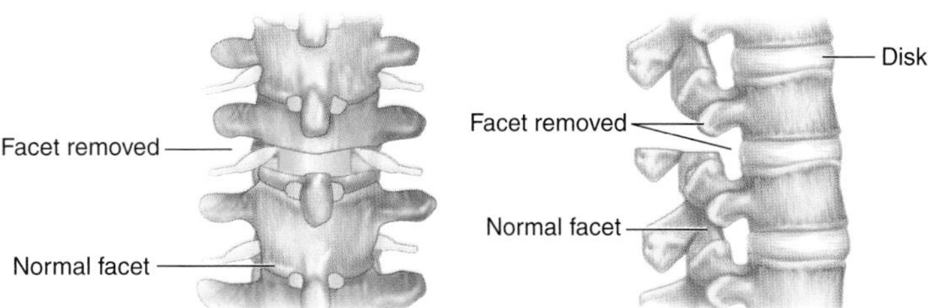

FIGURE 68-2

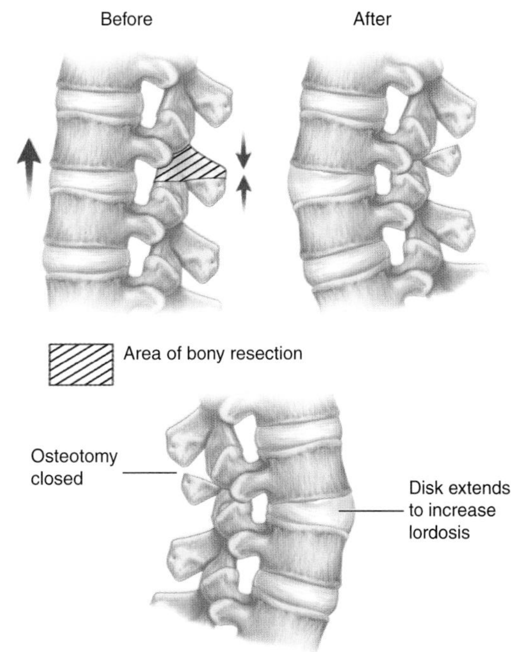

FIGURE 68-3

cautery to expose posterior elements, including the transverse processes. The posterior column including the spinous process, edges of the lamina, and ligamentum flavum are resected between the facet joints. Osteotomy is started at the interlaminar space. Resection is carried out laterally to the foraminal space, and both articular processes are excised.

- **FIGURE 68-3:** The neural foramen is undercut to prevent cord compression when osteotomies are closed. The anterior column opens through the disk space, the anterior longitudinal ligament is ruptured, and additional lordosis is achieved owing to elongation of the anterior column and shortening of the posterior column. Posterior instrumentation with pedicle screws is performed and used to fixate a shortened posterior column. When rods are placed, compression and cantilever manipulation helps close osteotomy sites. Achieving bony fusion with posterior onlay bone grafting is crucial to maintaining long-term correction.

TIPS FROM THE MASTERS

- Approximately 10 to 15 degrees of correction can be achieved with each segment. Mobile disk spaces and adequate disk height are required for this type of correction because the posterior segment of the intervertebral disk acts as the pivot point.

- There is a significant risk of pseudoarthrosis and postoperative complications with a Smith-Petersen osteotomy. Because of the risks of the procedure, a thorough preoperative medical work-up, especially in older patients, must be performed. Young patients with no significant comorbidities are the ideal candidates.
- It is important to determine spine flexibility and type of sagittal imbalance when evaluating a patient for Smith-Petersen osteotomy. Flexibility can be determined clinically or radiographically. Patients who have a sagittal imbalance on upright posture may correct when in the supine position owing to flexible segments. Obtaining a standing x-ray of the spine from the cervical to the sacral segments is important. A plumb line is dropped from the center of the seventh cervical vertebral body, and the distance from the sacrum is measured. A 2-cm margin is acceptable.
- A general rule is that patients with at least a 30-degree lumbar lordosis greater than a thoracic kyphosis are good candidates for corrective osteotomies.
- The sagittal imbalance can be classified into two types. Type 1 represents a segmental hyperlordotic or kyphotic lumbar segment in which the patient compensates for the imbalance by hyperextension of segments above and below. Type 2 represents an imbalance across a significant segment of the spine; the spine is flat, and there is segmental loss of kyphosis and lordosis. The patient is unable to compensate for this imbalance. Long sweeping kyphotic deformities are more amenable to correction with Smith-Petersen osteotomy than segmental imbalances.
- Determining the osteotomy site, number of osteotomies, fixation points, and the levels to be fused depends on the type of sagittal deformity. For a type 1 deformity, the site of the deformity determines the osteotomy site. For a type 2 deformity, correction is performed in the lower spine because there is a greater lever arm correcting the axis of view, there are fewer complications related to the thoracic viscera and vascular structures, and the correction is not hindered by the ribs.
- Care must be taken not to disrupt the most rostral and caudal segment facet capsules because these need to remain intact and are not part of the fusion segment.
- Adequate resection of underlying ligamentum flavum should be ensured before osteotomy closure.
- Adequate correction can be achieved with osteotomy width the size of the drill bit; larger osteotomies provide greater correction.

PITFALLS
Resection of pedicle
Spinal cord or nerve root compression
Aortic rupture
Blood loss and related coagulopathy
Intraoperative durotomy
Intestinal obstruction from tension on superior mesenteric artery
Monosegmental Smith-Petersen osteotomy may cause significant complications owing to kinking

BAILOUT OPTIONS

- After performing a Smith-Petersen osteotomy, if it is not feasible to close the osteotomy, one of the segments can be converted to a pedicle subtraction osteotomy.

SUGGESTED READINGS

Benzel EC. Spine Surgery: Techniques, Complication Avoidance, and Management. Philadelphia: Elsevier; 2004.

Bridwell KH. Decision making regarding Smith-Peterson vs. pedicle subtraction osteotomy vs. vertebral column resection for spinal deformity. Spine 2006;31:S171–8.

Cho KJ, Bridwell KH, Lenke LG, et al. Comparison of Smith-Peterson versus pedicle subtraction osteotomy for the correction of fixed sagittal imbalance. Spine 2005;30:2030–7.

Heary RF, Albert TJ. Spinal Deformities: The Essentials. New York: Thieme Medical Publishers; 2007.

Hsu B, Erkan S, Transfeldt E, et al. Pedicle subtraction vs. Smith-Peterson osteotomies for correction of fixed sagittal plane deformities: radiographic outcomes in 151 patients. Proceedings of the NASS 23rd Annual Meeting. Spine J 2008;97S.

Hsu B, Mehbod A, Transfeldt E, et al. Complications of pedicle subtraction and Smith-Peterson osteotomies: an analysis of 151 patients. Proceedings of the NASS 23rd Annual Meeting. Spine J 2008;89S–90S.

Smith-Petersen MN, Larson CB, Aufranc OE. Osteotomy of the spine for correction of flexion deformity in rheumatoid arthritis. J Bone Joint Surg Am 1945;27:1–11.

Procedure 69 Thoracic Pedicle Screws

Ram R. Vasudevan, Frank Acosta

INDICATIONS

- Instrumentation in the treatment of degenerative disease
- Instrumentation for acute traumatic instability
- Instrumentation for iatrogenic destabilization
- Corrective surgery for congenital and idiopathic scoliosis

CONTRAINDICATIONS

- Osteoporosis is a relative contraindication and can be managed with more extensive instrumentation and evolving screw types for poor bone quality.

PLANNING AND POSITIONING

- Preoperative plain radiographs and computed tomography (CT) should be obtained to evaluate bone quality and pedicle size and angle. The entry point for pedicle screw placement is variable in the thoracic spine, and anatomic landmarks are unreliable. Preoperative planning using CT and plain films is important. The transverse width of the pedicle can be determined using preoperative CT and is the limiting factor in screw size. Frameless stereotaxy can improve accuracy of pedicle screw placement.
- The patient is placed prone on chest bolsters, a Wilson frame, or a Jackson table to release abdominal contents from pressure, preventing epidural venous congestion and intraoperative blood loss.
- The pelvis and knees are flexed to augment normal thoracic kyphosis.
- If upper thoracic spine fixation is needed, the head must be fixed in a neutral position with a Mayfield head frame with the patient's arms secured on the sides.
- In mid-thoracic to lower thoracic spine fixation procedures, the head need not be secured, and the arms are positioned at 90-degree angles above the head. The axilla is cushioned with foam pads.
- **FIGURE 69-1:** The patient is positioned prone with chest bolsters taking pressure off the abdomen. The arms are placed at no more than 90-degree angles to prevent brachial plexus injury. A Mayfield head frame is placed in upper thoracic fusions.

PROCEDURE

- **FIGURE 69-2:** A standard posterior midline incision is made over the desired thoracic pedicles to include in the fusion. Exposure is taken as far laterally to expose the transverse processes bilaterally, staying subperiosteal to avoid excessive bleeding. Care should be taken not to disturb the facet capsule of most rostral and caudal segments to prevent instability and increased degeneration of these facet joints. Facet joints involved in the fusion construct must be thoroughly cleaned from any soft tissue. The inferior 5 mm of inferior facet joint and articular cartilage may be removed to promote intraarticular arthrodesis.
- **FIGURE 69-3:** As a general rule, the sagittal pedicle angle increases in the thoracic spine from 0 degrees at T1 to 10 degrees at T8 and decreases to 0 degrees at T12. The coronal plane angulation at T1 is 10 to 15 degrees and 5 degrees at T12. The thoracic vertebral

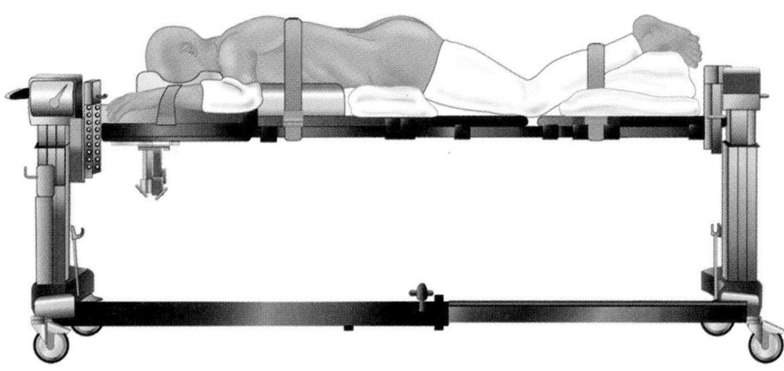

FIGURE 69-1

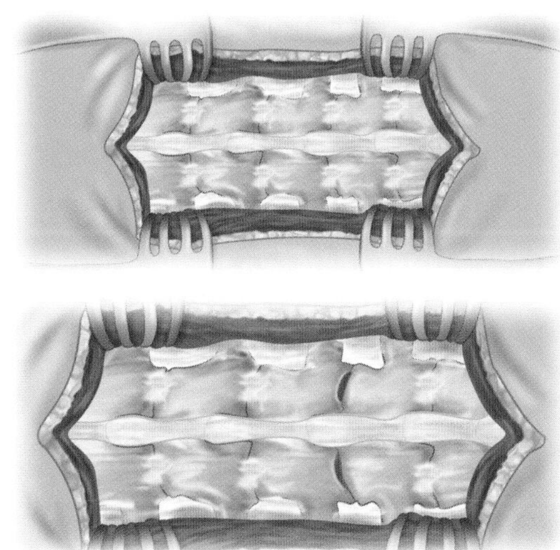

FIGURE 69-2

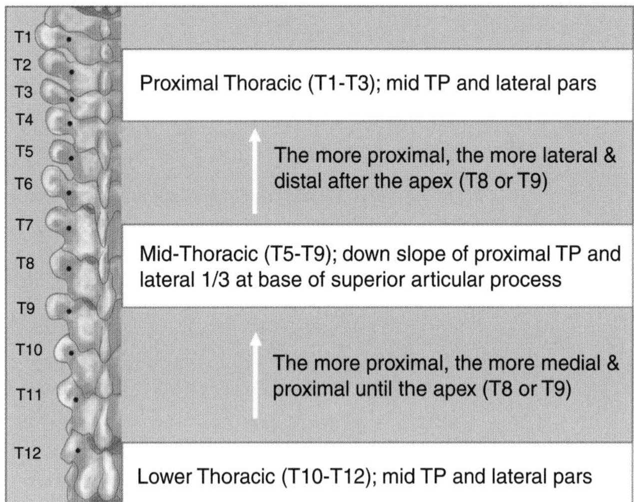

FIGURE 69-3

transverse process does not uniformly align with the pedicle in the axial plane. The transverse process is rostral to the pedicle in the upper thoracic spine and caudal to the pedicle in the lower thoracic spine, with T6-7 being the transition point. The starting point for the first thoracic vertebra is at the junction of the bisected transverse process and lamina at the lateral border of the pars. The starting point for the fourth thoracic vertebra is at the junction of the proximal one third of the transverse process and lamina just medial to the lateral border of the pars. The starting point of the mid-thoracic region is the most

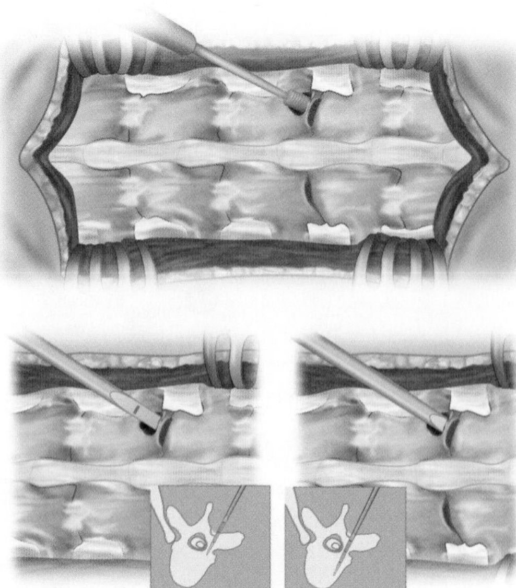

FIGURE 69-4

medially located at the junction of the proximal edge of the transverse process and just lateral to the mid-portion of the base of the superior articular process. The lower thoracic vertebra starting point is at the junction of the bisected transverse process and lamina at the lateral border of the pars.

- **FIGURE 69-4:** The entry point is decorticated using a high-speed bur or rongeur. A bur or blunt-tipped pedicle probe is placed gently into the base of the pedicle and advanced through the cancellous bone into the vertebral body. Advancement of the pedicle probe should be smooth; a sudden loss of resistance may indicate lateral or medial breach of the pedicle, and an increase in resistance may indicate abutment against the pedicle or vertebral cortical bone. When resistance is encountered, slight and smooth shifts in direction can lead the pedicle probe to return into the central cancellous region of the pedicle.
- **FIGURE 69-5:** After cannulation of the pedicle, the tract is inspected to ensure there is no pulsatile bleeding or cerebrospinal fluid leak. A flexible ball-tipped probe is inserted into the cannulated pedicle to palpate the five borders of the tract: medial border, lateral border, superior and inferior borders, and floor. Special attention is given to the first 10 to 15 mm of the tract to ensure that the spinal canal has not been entered. This is an important step to prevent malposition of screw placement and, if needed, redirection of the trajectory for accurate screw placement.
- **FIGURE 69-6:** The cannulated pedicle is tapped using a smaller-diameter tap than the pedicle screw desired. Only the length of the pedicle needs to be tapped. After tapping, the trajectory is palpated a second time ensuring intraosseous positioning, and a hemostat is used to measure pedicle screw length. Some surgeons prefer to tap to the length of the pedicle with confirmation of anterior cortex integrity with a feeler before placing.
- **FIGURE 69-7: A,** The pedicle screw is slowly placed in the same trajectory as the pedicle probe. **B,** Intraoperative fluoroscopy is performed to ensure proper positioning. On lateral fluoroscopy, the screw should be parallel to the superior end plate of the

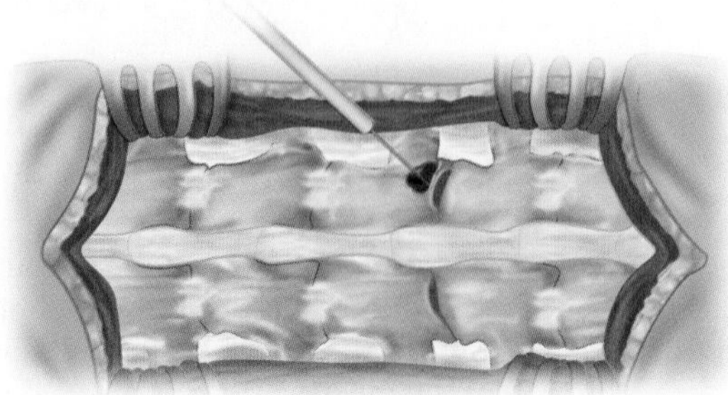

FIGURE 69-5

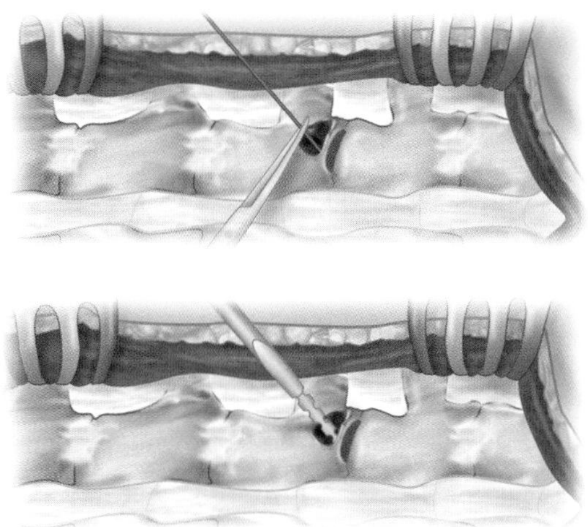

FIGURE 69-6

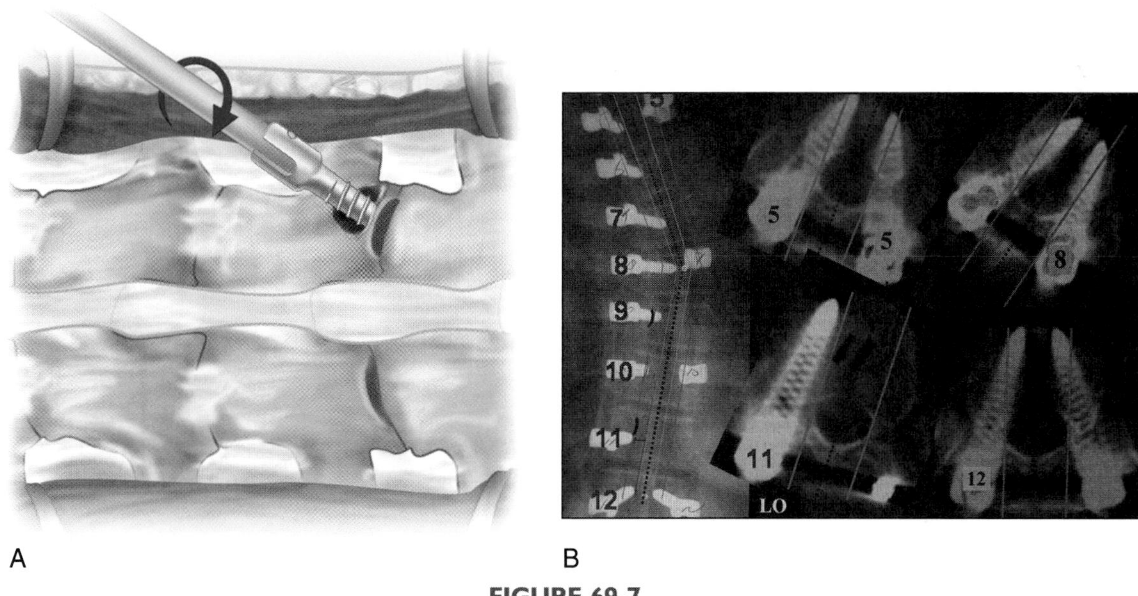

FIGURE 69-7

vertebral body and not extend past the anterior border of the vertebral body. On anteroposterior fluoroscopy, the screw trajectory should not be triangulated. Excessively vertical screws suggest lateral breech, and screw tips that cross the midline suggest medial breech. If needed, the concerning screws should be removed, and the screw tract should be palpated with a feeler to evaluate for breeches.

TIPS FROM THE MASTERS

- For upper thoracic pedicle screws, having the patient's arms secured loosely by the side of the torso facilitates fluoroscopy.
- The tip of the curved thoracic pedicle finder should be directed laterally in the pedicle for the first 20 mm to reduce risk of medial pedicle breach, then taken out of the pedicle and reinserted facing medially during passage from the pedicle into the vertebral body.
- Laminotomy or laminectomy can be used to palpate the medial pedicle border manually in cases of difficult anatomy or prior fusion mass; this is preferable to destroying a pedicle with repeated pedicle finder passes.

- A ball-tipped probe should be used to palpate the floor of the pedicle tract and passed through the soft cancellous bone to reach the hard cortical floor. This depth is measured and used to select proper screw length.
- If using neuromonitoring, triggered electromyography (EMG) stimulations are performed to ensure intraosseous screw placement. A triggered EMG threshold of less than 6.0 mA may indicate a medial breach of the pedicle wall. The screw must then be removed and the cannulated pedicle repalpated to determine if the pedicle wall has been breached. Another trajectory may be attempted, or the screw may be discarded.

PITFALLS
Intraoperative pedicle fractures, requiring further points of fixation
Misplaced screws
Screws penetrating the anterior cortex and abutting vascular structures, particularly with left-sided screws extending and penetrating or abutting the aorta
Screw tips that abut the aorta—can lead to erosion and pseudoaneurysms
Neurologic injury
Cerebrospinal fluid fistulas
Damage to retroperitoneal or intrathoracic structures
Radiographic fusion failure

BAILOUT OPTIONS

- A Kirschner wire can be used to direct the pedicle tap along the correct path after multiple passes of the pedicle finder.
- An "in-out-in" technique can be used to salvage a fractured or medially violated pedicle.
- A pedicle hook can be used to secure fixation to very small or narrow pedicles.
- For difficult to place pedicle screws, a small hemilaminotomy can be made to allow palpation of the pedicle.

SUGGESTED READINGS

Benzel EC. Spine Surgery: Techniques, Complication Avoidance, and Management. Philadelphia: Elsevier; 2004.

Heary RF, Albert TJ. Spinal Deformities: The Essentials. New York: Thieme Medical Publishers; 2007.

Kim YJ, Lanke LG, Bridwell KH, et al. Free hand pedicle screw placement in the thoracic spine: is it safe? Spine 2004;29:333–42.

Suk S, Kim W, Lee S, et al. Thoracic pedicle screw fixation in spinal deformities: are they really safe? Spine 2001;26:2049–57.

Vaccaro AR, Rizzolo J, Allardyce TJ, et al. Placement of pedicle screws in the thoracic spine. Part I: morphometric analysis of the thoracic vertebrae. J Bone Joint Surg Am 1995;77:1193–9.

Vaccaro AR, Rizzolo SJ, Balderston RA, et al. Placement of pedicle screws in the thoracic spine. Part II: an anatomical and radiographic assessment. J Bone Joint Surg Am 1995;77A:1200–6.

Youkilis AS, Quint DJ, McGillicuddy JE, et al. Stereotactic navigation for placement of pedicle screws in the thoracic spine. Neurosurgery 2001;48:771–9.

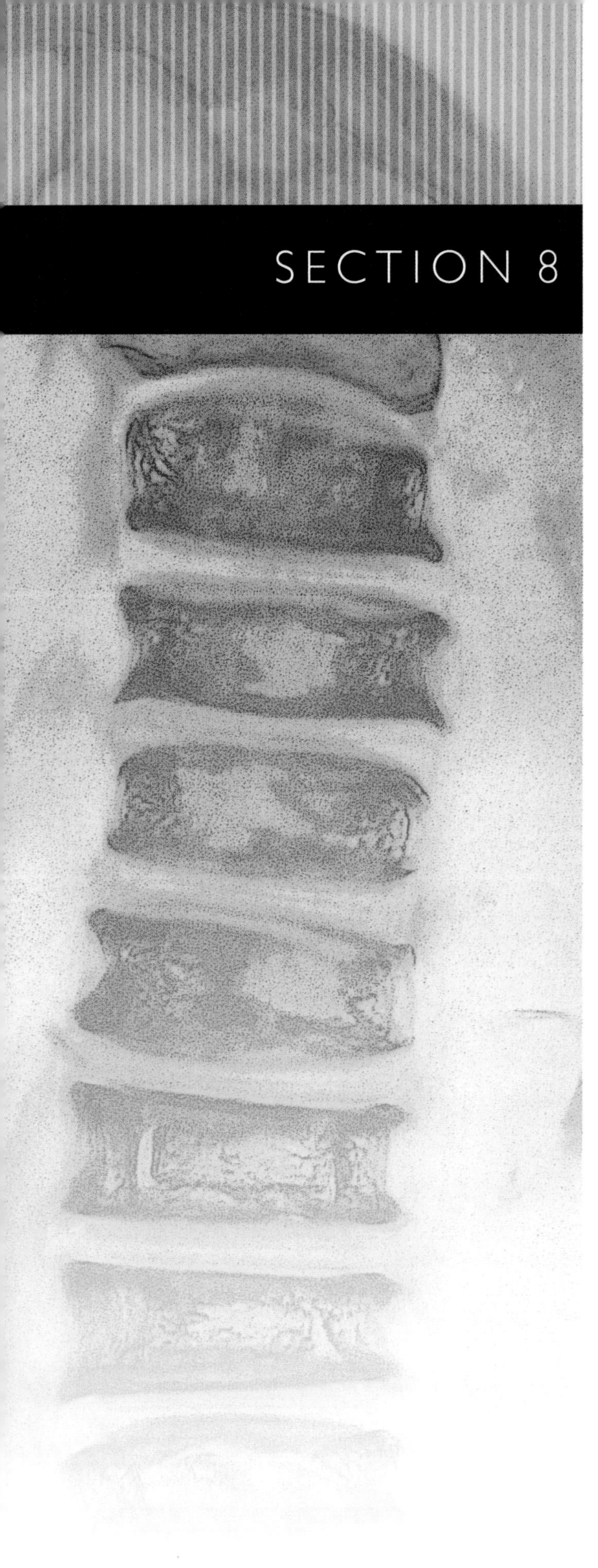

SECTION 8

Lumbosacral

SECTION EDITOR — JOSEPH D. CIACCI,
WITH JAYANT P. MENON

Procedure 70 Lumbar Laminectomy

Jayant P. Menon, Allen Ho, Joseph D. Ciacci

INDICATIONS

- Patients with spinal stenosis
- Patients with contraindications or medical comorbidities that may make it difficult to pursue an anterior approach or who cannot be under general anesthesia for an extended fusion because of increased cardiac risk

CONTRAINDICATIONS

- Laminectomy can be used to treat patients with radiculopathy. However, MRI findings of herniated disk fragments will prompt consideration of additional diskectomy and foraminotomy to further decompress the affected nerve roots
- Relatively contraindicated in patients with congenital or acquired pars defects—fusion is required to prevent dynamic instability and spondylolisthesis

PLANNING AND POSITIONING

- Preoperative evaluation includes a thorough neurologic history and examination with assessment of strength. A sensory examination should be conducted to rule out any dermatomal distribution of loss. Routine plain lateral and flexion and extension lumbar spine films can show dynamic instability that would be better treated with lumbar fusion rather than laminectomy alone. Magnetic resonance imaging (MRI) without contrast enhancement of the lumbar spine can show focal neural foraminal stenosis that may be better addressed with focused diskectomy and foraminotomy.
- After being placed prone, the patient is given a dose of preoperative antibiotics before the skin incision. Antibiotics and an intramuscular dose of ketorolac (Toradol) can be instilled at the end of the case.
- **FIGURE 70-1:** The patient is positioned prone on chest rolls on a Wilson frame to hold the spine in extension.

PROCEDURE

Skin Incision

- **FIGURE 70-2:** By palpating the anterior superior iliac crest, the L4-5 interspace can be localized for a rough estimation of the level. Some authors advocate use of preincision needle localization film to determine the correct size of the exposure. A small incision should be made at first and then extended as needed using a No. 10 blade.

Fascial and Subfascial Dissection

- Bovie electrocautery can be used for subcutaneous dissection and for achieving hemostasis. The thoracolumbar fascia is identified after dissection through the subcutaneous fat. A dry sponge raked along the fascia identifies the white tissue easily, and a periosteal elevator can be used to dissect off the subcutaneous fat from the fascia beneath. After placing a self-retaining retractor, such as a Gelpi retractor, palpation to find the midline can be done.

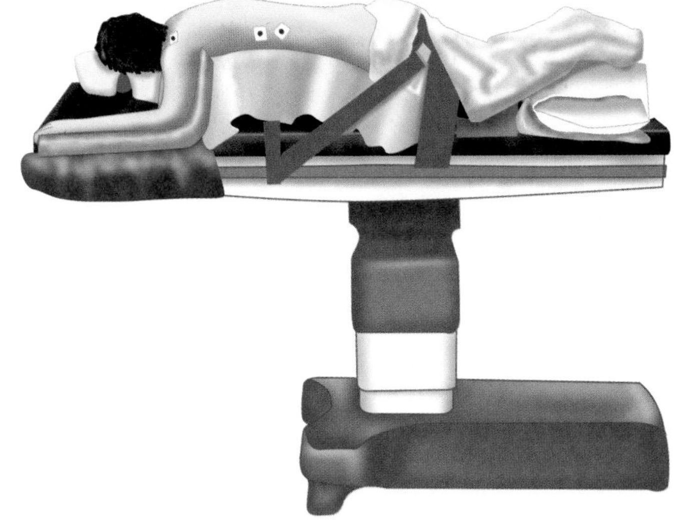

FIGURE 70-1

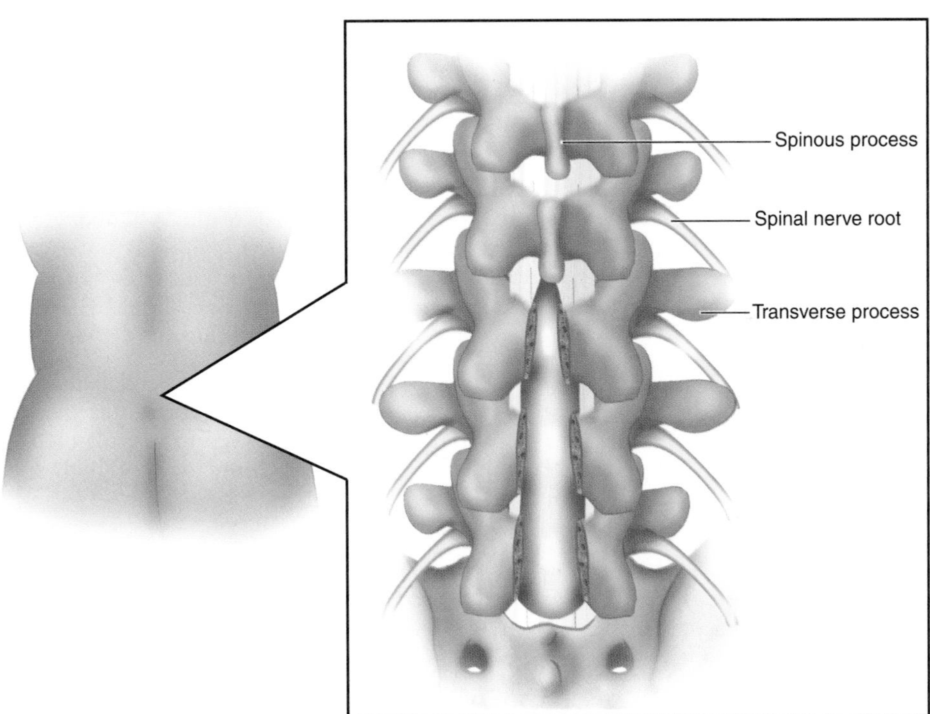

FIGURE 70-2

Subperiosteal Dissection

- Bovie electrocautery on cut function can be used to cut through the fascia. (For microdiskectomy, a paramedian fascial incision ensures the midline ligamentous structures are not damaged by dissection.) After minimal one-sided exposure is completed rapidly, a localizing film should be obtained to assess the correct level.
- Subperiosteal dissection can also be done rapidly with an open dry sponge raked ventrally and laterally along the spinous process and lamina with a large periosteal dissector, such as a Cobb elevator. This dissection can be done very rapidly and in the case of in situ lumbar fusion can be carried out to the lateral gutters to rest atop the transverse processes of the lumbar vertebrae.

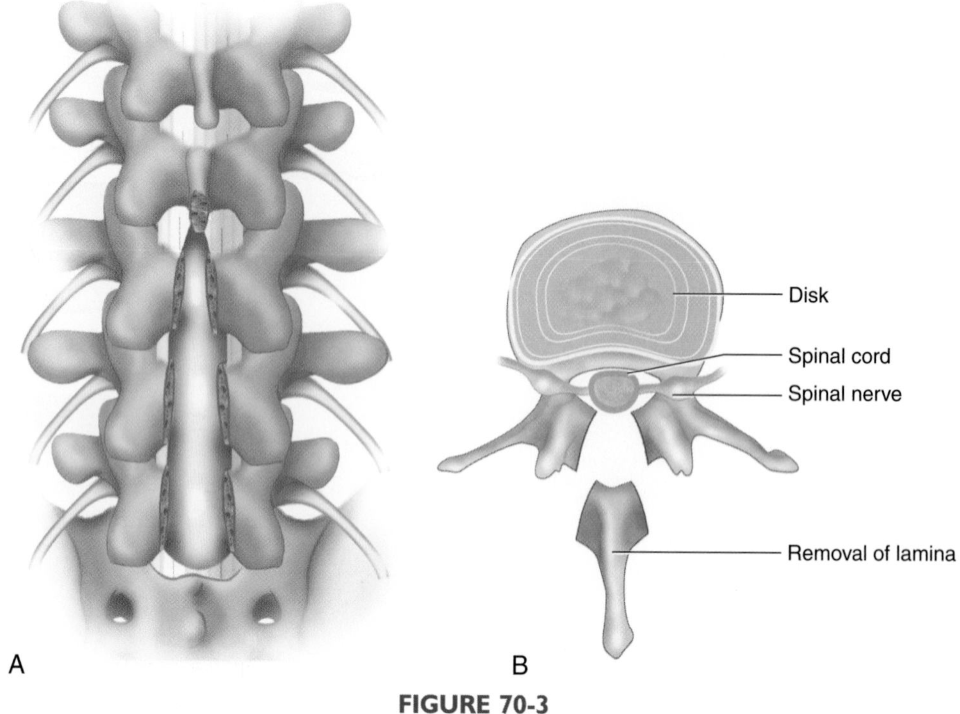

FIGURE 70-3

Beginning of Laminectomy

- **FIGURE 70-3:** When the spinous process out to the facet is dissected and hemostasis is achieved, bony dissection can begin. A Horsley bone cutter and double-action rongeur can be used to remove the spinous process. Bone can be saved and used for posterolateral in situ fusion if needed. Cortical bone at the base of the spinous process may bleed easily, and one should be prepared with bone wax. Irrigation can be used to identify further bleeding sites.
- The bone should be removed from caudal to rostral because the top of the lamina is closed to the dura, and one may encounter the dura easily in this location. When all the spinous processes are removed for the planned laminectomy, attention can be turned to completing the laminectomy with a high-speed drill or with various Kerrison rongeurs.

Laminectomy

- A 2-mm side-cutting drill can be used to thin the remaining lamina and bone to identify the yellow ligamentum flavum without violating the dura. While drilling laterally, one can create a trough to assist in subsequent completion of the laminectomy.

Removal of Lamina and of Ligamentum Flavum

- After thinning the lamina sufficiently, 2- to 4-mm up-biting Kerrison rongeurs can be used to remove the remaining bone exposing the yellow ligamentum flavum. A sharp right-angled instrument can be inserted into the ligamentum flavum and used to pull dorsally away from the thecal sac while cutting along the instrument using a No. 15 blade. The dissection can be carefully continued until the whitish blue thecal sac is identified. Careful removal of a window of ligamentum flavum can be done with a pituitary rongeur.

Completion of Wide Laminectomy

- **FIGURE 70-4:** After the ligamentum flavum is removed, attention can be turned to making the laminectomy widened to the medial edge of the pedicles. Thecal sac should appear relaxed and more pliant on palpation after laminectomy. Lateral gutters contain a venous plexus that bleeds quite easily, and various techniques can be employed to maintain hemostasis. Thrombin-soaked Gelfoam is placed, and wet ½ × ½ cottonoid can be used

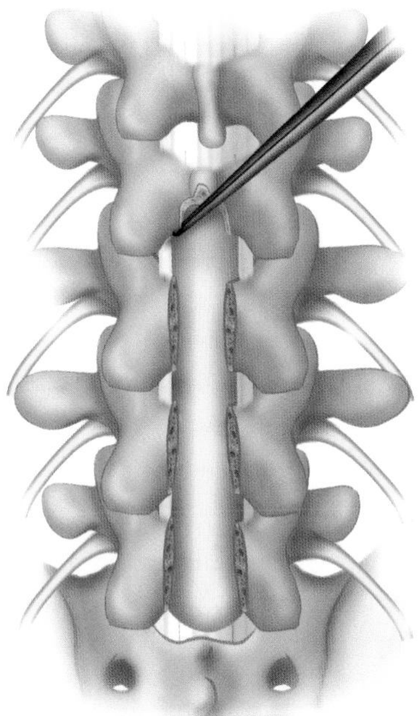

FIGURE 70-4

to impress Gelfoam in place. By irrigating on the cottonoid and holding suction, Gelfoam shrinks and fits into the desired dimensions. Alternatively, Avitene Hemostat can be placed over the bleeding venous plexus, *dry* ½ × ½ cottonoid can be placed over Avitene Hemostat, and bayonet forceps can be used to hold the clot in place.

- **FIGURE 70-5:** After successful decompression, the probe should be used to palpate the medial edges of the pedicles and foramen. Any constricted areas, particularly over the nerve roots, should be decompressed further.
- When the laminectomy is completed and wide enough, the surgeon is ready to close. The surgeon may now pursue an in situ posterolateral fusion.

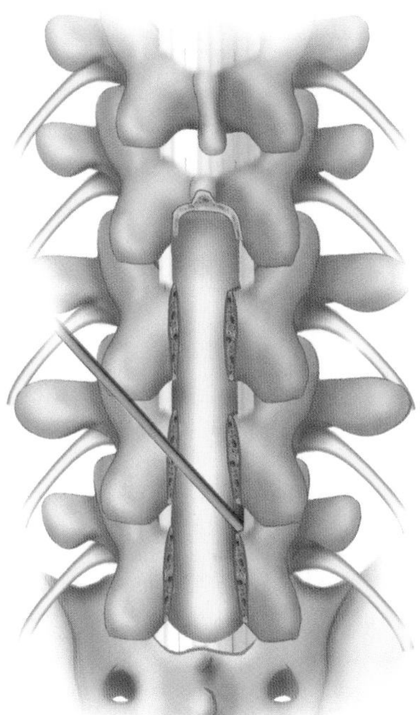

FIGURE 70-5

Closure of Operative Site

- Copious irrigation should be done, and any bleeding source should be identified and controlled until irrigation is clear. Closure should be done meticulously to prevent cerebrospinal fluid leak in the event of a subclinical violation and to allow for a quick and less painful recovery. The use of interrupted, figure-eight, 0-sized absorbable sutures to close the deep muscle layer is controversial. An absolutely watertight 0-size interrupted, noninverted layer of sutures at narrow 5- to 8-mm intervals should be completed to achieve completely dry closure.
- Superficial fascial closure is done with 2-0 inverted, interrupted sutures at equally narrow intervals to ensure adequate strength of the closure. The skin is reapproximated and closed with either staples or a running 4-0 subcuticular stitch.

TIPS FROM THE MASTERS

- Bovie electrocautery done just subperiosteally can greatly reduce the amount of muscle bleeding encountered during the operation.
- Cautery from caudal to rostral removes the paraspinal muscular attachments most efficiently and with the least blood loss. Bipolar electrocautery can be used for point source bleeding.
- Rather than attempting to place bone wax on a bleeding lamina using a Freer elevator, a small ball of wax can be placed over the bleeding site, and a dry ½ × ½ cottonoid can be used with a bayoneted pickup to compress and mold the wax into the bleeding sites.
- The thecal sac may be under pressure; to avoid a cerebrospinal fluid leak, a small ½ × ½ cottonoid can be inserted through the window of ligamentum flavum between the thecal sac and the ligamentum flavum and advanced before each bite with the Kerrison rongeur. The Kerrison rongeur bites the cottonoid rather than the thecal sac. To avoid inadvertent cerebrospinal fluid leaks from sharply angled bony spurs, bites with the Kerrison rongeur should be kept continuous and overlapping.
- To ensure deep facial closure is dry and adequate hemostasis is achieved, before placing the last facial stitch, the surgeon can irrigate into the deep space and suction out the irrigation; this should be clear in color.

PITFALLS

For revision laminectomies, one must be careful with this technique because the lamina and all the posterior ligamentous structures protecting the thecal sac are absent.

In sufficient foraminotomies can lead to persistent radiculopathy.

BAILOUT OPTIONS

- Dural violation requires primary closure under microscopy. Placement of 6-0 nylon suture using a Castro-Viejo needle driver or long Ryder needle driver may be necessary to maintain hemostasis.

SUGGESTED READINGS

Atlas SJ, Deyo RA, Keller RB, et al. The Maine Lumbar Spine Study, Part III: 1-year outcomes of surgical and nonsurgical management of lumbar spinal stenosis. Spine (Phila Pa 1976) 1996;21:1787–94.

Deyo RA, Ciol MA, Cherkin DC, et al. Lumbar spinal fusion: a cohort study of complications, reoperations, and resource use in the Medicare population. Spine (Phila Pa 1976) 1993;18:1463–70.

Fischgrund JS, Mackay M, Herkowitz HN, et al. 1997 Volvo Award winner in clinical studies. Degenerative lumbar spondylolisthesis with spinal stenosis: a prospective, randomized study comparing decompressive laminectomy and arthrodesis with and without spinal instrumentation. Spine (Phila Pa 1976) 1997;22:2807–12.

Katz JN, Lipson SJ, Lew RA, et al. Lumbar laminectomy alone or with instrumented or noninstrumented arthrodesis in degenerative lumbar spinal stenosis: patient selection, costs, and surgical outcomes. Spine (Phila Pa 1976) 1997;22:1123–31.

Procedure 71

Lumbar Microdiskectomy

Jayant P. Menon, Allen Ho, Joseph D. Ciacci

INDICATIONS

- Foraminal stenosis
- Radiculopathy that fails to improve with conservative measures
- Significant weakness

CONTRAINDICATIONS

- Large disk herniation causing central canal stenosis—a full laminectomy is indicated

PLANNING AND POSITIONING

- Preoperative evaluation includes a thorough neurologic history and examination with assessment of strength. A sensory examination should be conducted to rule out any dermatomal distribution of loss. Routine plain lateral, flexion, and extension lumbar spine films can show dynamic instability that may necessitate lumbar fusion as well as diskectomy. The diskectomy would allow for the treatment of radiculopathic leg pain but would be unable to treat mechanical back pain. Magnetic resonance imaging (MRI) without contrast enhancement of the lumbar spine can show focal neural foraminal stenosis that would allow the surgeon to focus on the level for diskectomy and foraminotomy.
- After being placed in a prone position, the patient is given a dose of preoperative antibiotics before the skin incision. Antibiotics and an intramuscular dose of ketorolac (Toradol) can be instilled at the end of the case.
- **FIGURE 71-1:** The patient is placed prone on chest rolls and a Wilson frame to hold the spine in flexion.

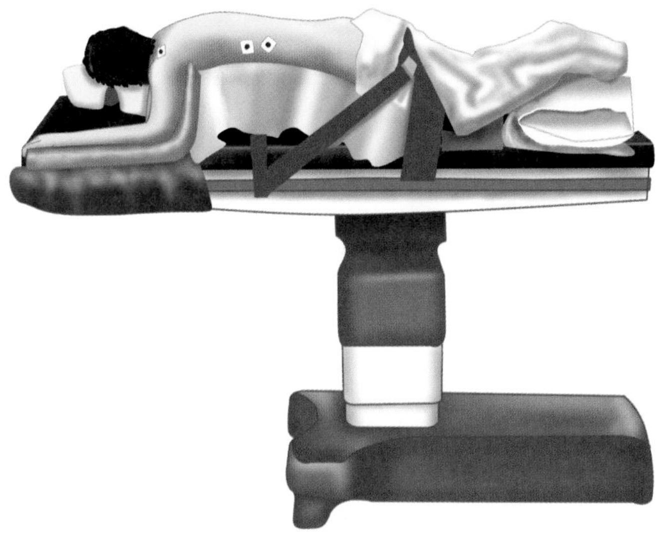

FIGURE 71-1

PROCEDURE

Skin Incision

- **FIGURE 71-2:** By palpating the anterior superior iliac crest, the L4-5 interspace can be localized for a rough estimation of the level. Some authors advocate a preincision needle localization film to determine the correct size of the exposure. After instillation of local anesthetic with epinephrine to the skin and deeper tissues, a small incision should be made at first and then extended as needed using a No. 10 blade.

Fascial and Subfascial Dissection

- Bovie electrocautery can be used for subcutaneous dissection and for achieving hemostasis. The thoracolumbar fascia is identified after dissection through subcutaneous fat. A dry sponge raked along the fascia can identify the white tissue easily, and a periosteal elevator can be used to dissect off the subcutaneous fat from the fascia beneath. After placing a self-retaining retractor such as a Gelpi retractor, palpation to find the midline can be done.

Subperiosteal Dissection

- Bovie electrocautery on cut function can be used to cut through the fascia. For microdiskectomy, a paramedian facial incision can be done to ensure the midline ligamentous structures are not damaged by dissection. After minimal, one-sided exposure is completed rapidly, a localizing film should be done to assess the correct level.
- Subperiosteal dissection can also be done rapidly with an open dry sponge raked ventrally and laterally along the spinous process and lamina with a large periosteal dissector such as a Cobb elevator.

Hemilaminectomy

- **FIGURE 71-3:** After the correct level has been identified, planning the hemilaminectomy can begin. First, find the soft interspace between two laminae of interest. Quickly thin the bone past the cortical bone in the lamina to the cancellous bone on the other side. An up-going curet can be used to remove the remaining bone. Semicircular or square laminectomy can be completed with 1- to 3-mm Kerrison rongeurs and an up-going curet.

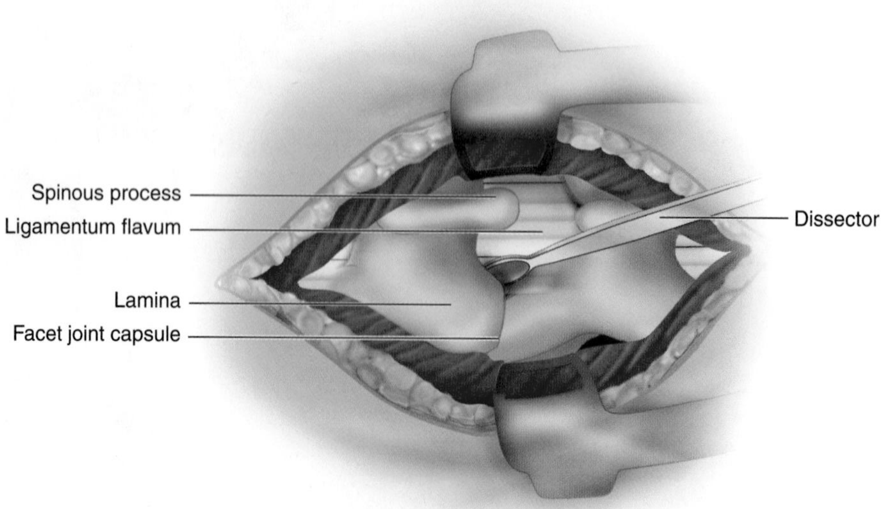

FIGURE 71-2

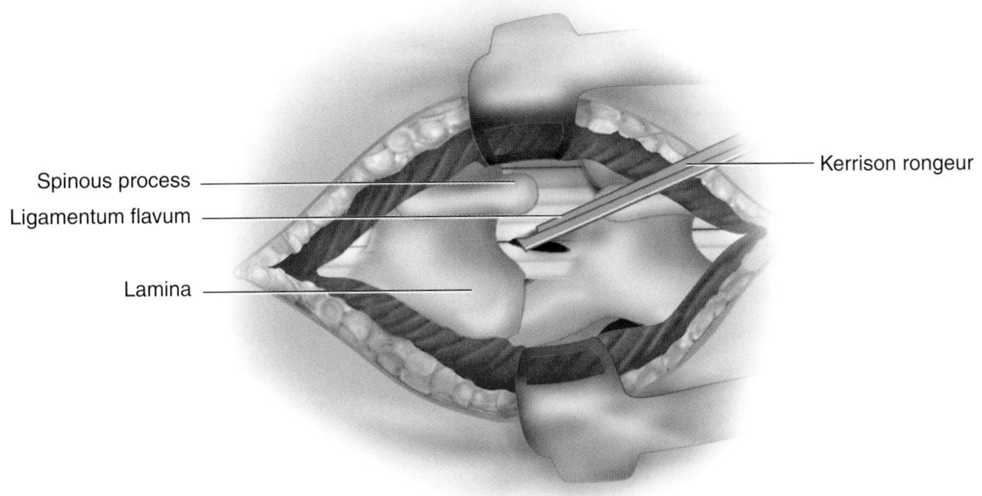

FIGURE 71-3

Removal of Ligamentum Flavum to Find Thecal Sac

- **FIGURE 71-4:** A sharp right-angled instrument can be inserted into the ligamentum flavum and used to pull dorsally away from the thecal sac while cutting along the instrument using a No. 15 blade. Dissection can be carefully continued until the whitish blue thecal sac is identified. Careful removal of the window of ligamentum flavum can be done with a pituitary rongeur. The rest of the ligamentum flavum is removed with Kerrison rongeurs to create the largest working window possible.
- **Figure 71-5:** After hemostasis is achieved, and adequate, countertension-free traction is achieved with a nerve root retractor, a No. 11 blade can be used to incise the posterior longitudinal ligament carefully. The incision is made in a medial to lateral direction to direct the sharp end of the blade away from the dura. A pituitary rongeur can be used to remove the disk material. A down-going Epstein curet or right-angled Williams instrument can be used to push down paracentral disk material into the now decompressed disk space.

Closure of Operative Site

- Copious irrigation should be done, any bleeding source should be identified and controlled until irrigation is clear. Closure should be done meticulously to prevent cerebrospinal fluid leak in the event of a subclinical violation and to allow for a quick and less painful recovery. Use of interrupted, figure-of-eight, 0-size absorbable sutures to close the deep muscle layer is controversial. An absolutely watertight 0-size interrupted, noninverted layer of sutures at narrow 5- to 8-mm intervals should be completed to achieve completely dry closure.
- Superficial fascial closure is done with 2-0 inverted, interrupted sutures at equally narrow intervals to ensure adequate strength of the closure. The skin is reapproximated and closed with either staples or a running 4-0 subcuticular stitch.

TIPS FROM THE MASTERS

- Use a straight cupped curet to remove soft tissue to find the interspinous ligament between the two laminae. When the ligament is visible, resist the temptation to dissect away under the inferior aspect of the superior lamina in the field because this would cause bleeding and ultimately interfere with the hemilaminectomy. Using a 2-mm side-cutting "matchstick" bur or a 3-mm acorn drill bit, drill medially to laterally (from the intersection of the lamina and spinous process in a lateral direction toward the facet joint).

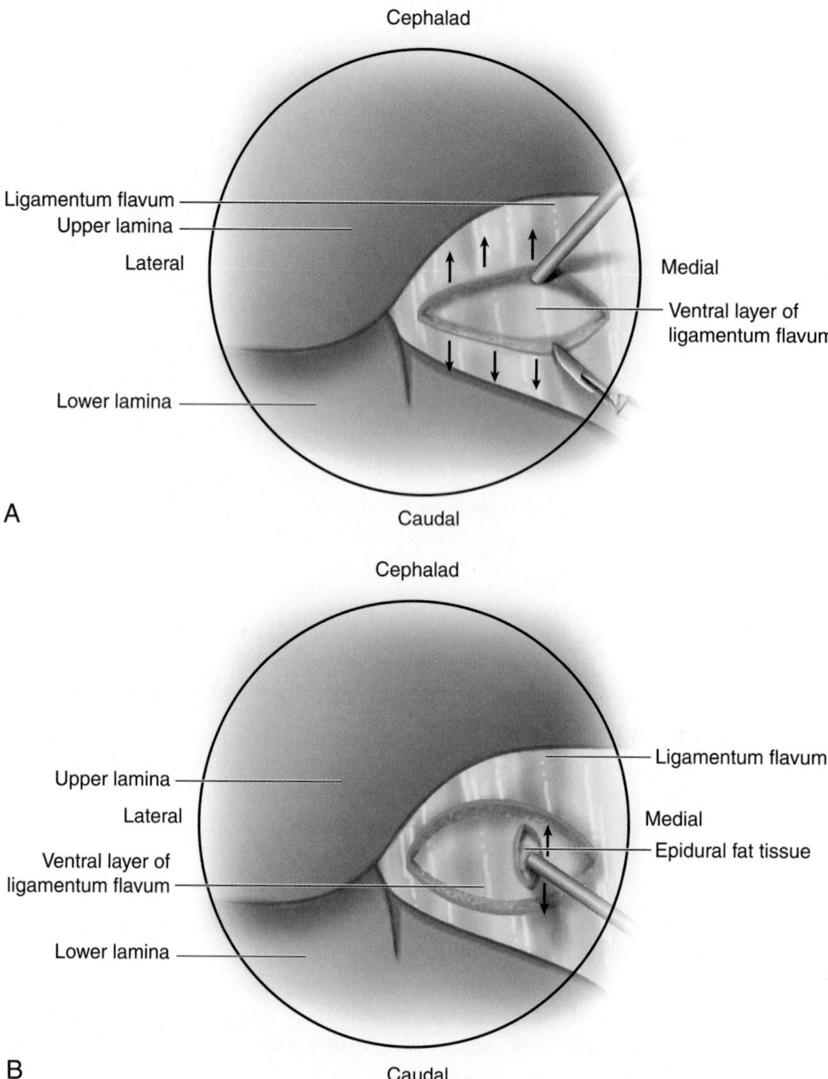

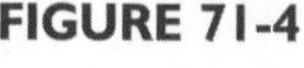
FIGURE 71-4

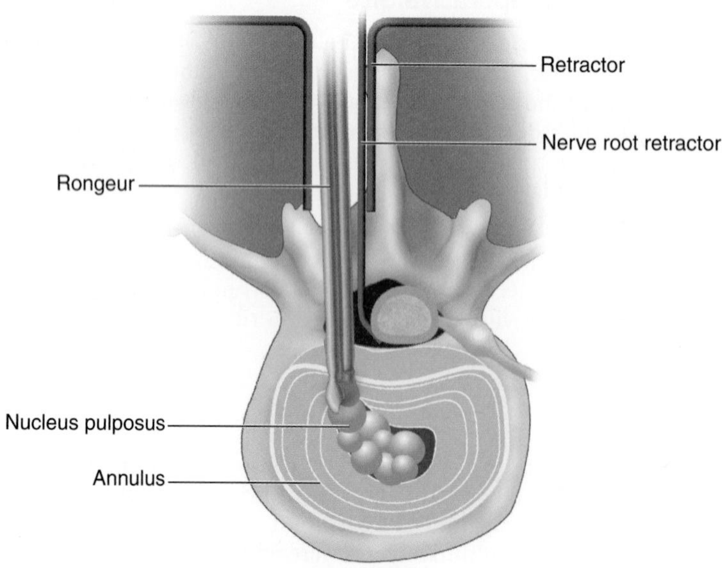

FIGURE 71-5

- Control bone bleeding with wax on a Freer elevator and mold with a ½ × ½ cottonoid and bayonet forceps.
- Cut with the blade away from the dura, and cut from medial to lateral. On the rostral-to-caudal cuts, be careful not to cut too medially.
- Performing aggressive versus limited diskectomy has been controversial; however, there is a statistical trend toward limited diskectomy so as to cause less diskogenic pain subsequently. Both approaches have the same recurrence rate. In a conservative diskectomy, the surgeon removes only the herniated disk fragment. In an aggressive diskectomy, a large open incision is made on the posterior longitudinal ligament with aggressive removal of the disk fragments and curettage of the disk space. Conservative diskectomy significantly decreased mean operative time and hospital stay. Level 3 evidence suggests that persistent back or leg pain was increased with aggressive diskectomy. There was a 2-week accelerated return to work and 1-month accelerated return to full-capacity work with conservative diskectomy. There was a statistically insignificant trend toward an increased rate of recurrent disk herniation with the conservative technique.
- A prospective, randomized clinical trial with 150 patients in each arm compared traditional open microdiskectomies with tubular diskectomy 1 year after surgery. Patients in the tubular diskectomy arm had significantly inferior patient satisfaction scores with microtubular diskectomies versus traditional open microdiskectomies.

PITFALLS

Do not drill too far laterally because entering the facet capsule can destabilize the joint and cause facet joint pain. Do not drill too far rostrally because this can create a pars defect leading to instability.

Operating on levels with associated spondylolisthesis may require upfront fusion.

BAILOUT OPTIONS

- Dural violation requires primary closure under microscopy. Placement of 6-0 nylon suture using a Castro-Viejo needle driver or long Ryder needle driver may be necessary to maintain hemostasis.
- Fibrin glue and other liquid sprayable polymers can be used. Facial closure cannot be stressed enough in these cases because this decreases postoperative cerebrospinal fluid leaks dramatically.

SUGGESTED READINGS

Arts MP, Brand R, van der Akker ME. Tubular diskectomy vs conventional microdiskectomy for sciatica: a randomized controlled trial. JAMA 2009;302:149–58.

McGirt MJ, Ambrossi GL, Datoo G, et al. Recurrent disc herniation and long-term back pain after primary lumbar diskectomy: review of outcomes reported for limited versus aggressive disc removal. Neurosurgery 2009;64:338–45.

Procedure 72

Anterior Lumbar Interbody Fusion

Joseph L. Martinez, Michael Y. Wang

INDICATIONS

- Anterior lumbar interbody fusion (ALIF) is indicated as a treatment of chronic, incapacitating low back pain secondary to degenerative disk disease or degenerative spondylolisthesis in the absence of severe neural element compression. Patients are generally not considered for operation until at least 6 months of conservative nonsurgical therapies have failed to yield adequate amelioration of symptoms. ALIF may also be used in cases of failure of previous posterior approach lumbar surgery.

CONTRAINDICATIONS

- Assuming a patient's general medical condition is adequate to undergo elective spine surgery, absolute contraindications to this procedure include conditions that limit retroperitoneal access to the lumbar spine, such as significant morbid obesity, retroperitoneal scarring from a previous surgery, or a large infrarenal aortic aneurysm and neural element compression requiring direct decompression. Direct decompression cannot be accomplished easily from an anterior approach, and in these cases a posterior procedure is required. A possible exception is radicular foraminal compression at the level of operation secondary to disk collapse, which may respond to distraction and restoration of disk height.
- Relative contraindications include congenital or iatrogenic genitourinary anatomic abnormalities, such as an ipsilateral single ureter or kidney or a history of previous retroperitoneal surgery. Many patients who are unwilling to assume the risk of retrograde ejaculation are also better treated from a dorsal access route. Severe osteoporosis also limits the feasibility of interbody fusion because of the risk of graft subsidence.

PLANNING AND POSITIONING

- **FIGURE 72-1:** For lower disk levels (L4-5, L5-S1), the patient is positioned supine on the operating table. An inflatable bladder is placed under the small of the back to increase or decrease lordosis as necessary. The surgeon can approach from the right side (patient in standard supine position). We typically use a cell saver in the event of large quantities of blood loss from vascular injury. A pulse oximeter is placed on each lower extremity to monitor for ischemia during vessel manipulation and retraction.

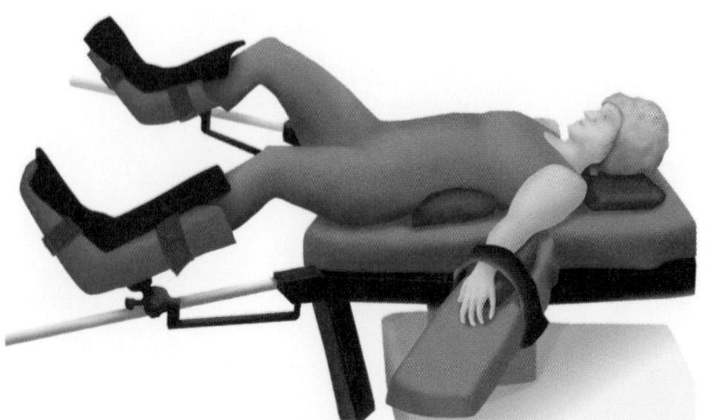

FIGURE 72-1

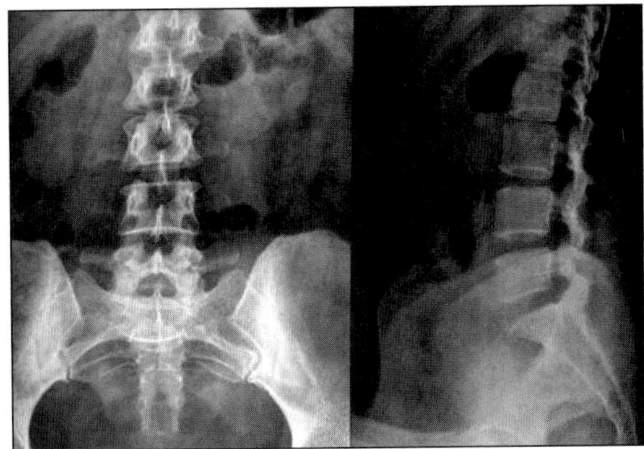

FIGURE 72-2

- **FIGURE 72-2:** Before the incision, the correct disk space is localized using anteroposterior and lateral fluoroscopy, and the skin is marked appropriately. The incision for this approach corridor is centered at this location and marked.

PROCEDURE

- **FIGURE 72-3:** Although a transperitoneal approach may be used to access L4-5 and L5-1 disk spaces, the muscle-sparing retroperitoneal approach has become more popular because of lower rates of postoperative ileus, easier control of intraperitoneal structures, and ability to sweep the sympathetic plexus bluntly to the right of the disk space. Both approaches may be performed via various incisions, including the midline, paramedian, and Pfannenstiel incisions. A horizontal incision heals with better cosmesis, whereas a vertical incision allows for easier extension in the rostral-caudal plane. An approach from the left side is generally performed because gentle manual retraction of the aorta is more safely performed than retraction of the inferior vena cava, which can be difficult to repair surgically in the event of vessel wall injury.
- When the anterior spine is visualized intraoperatively, final fluoroscopic confirmation of the correct disk level is mandatory before performing diskectomy and graft placement.

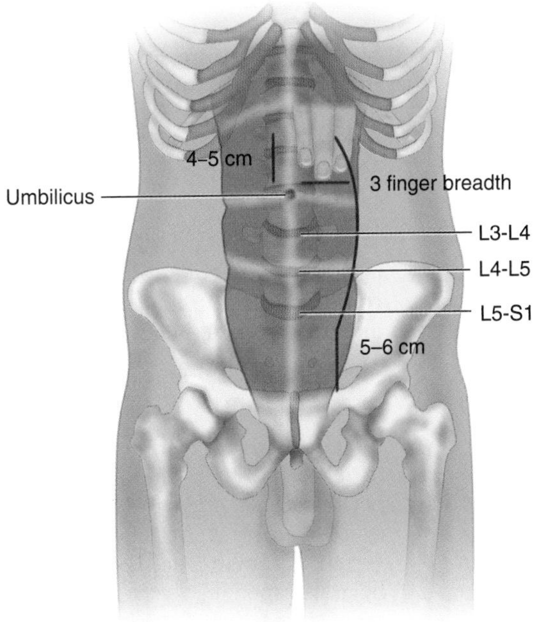

FIGURE 72-3

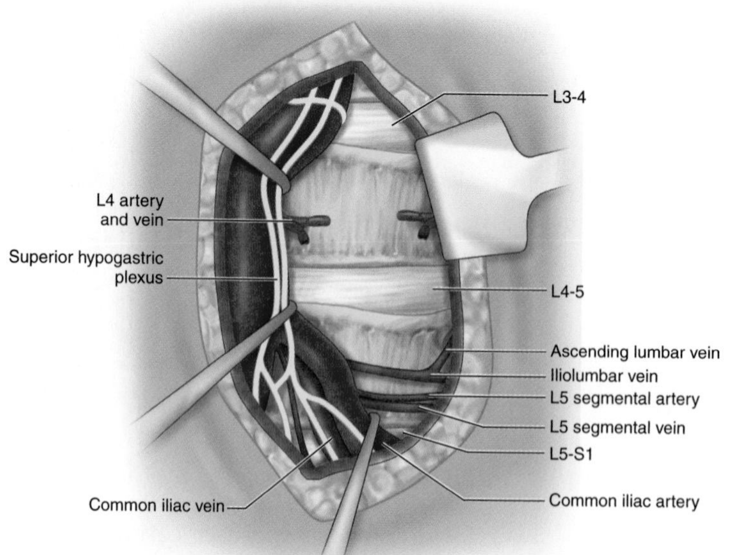

FIGURE 72-4

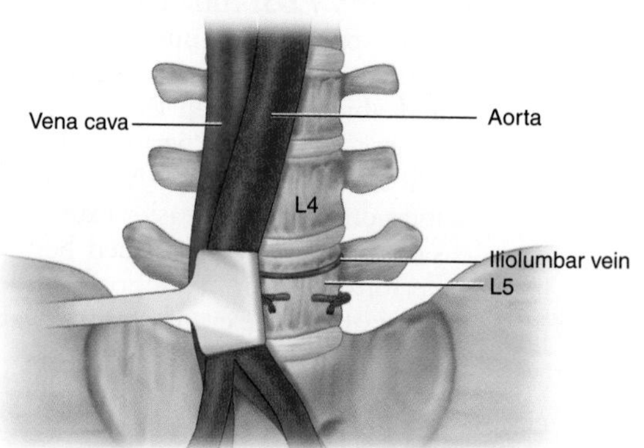

FIGURE 72-5

- **FIGURE 72-4:** Prevertebral tissue at the L5-S1 level is opened using a vertical incision. Bipolar electrocautery is used exclusively and monopolar electrocautery avoided at this level in an effort to spare injury to the autonomic nerves traversing this space. If nerve injury occurs, infertility in male patients from retrograde ejaculation may result. Mobilization of large vessels is usually unnecessary at this level because the approach can be taken through the vascular bifurcation.
- **FIGURE 72-5:** At the L4-5 level, mobilization of the left iliac vessels from left to right is performed after identification and ligation of the iliolumbar vein. This vein enters the common iliac at this level, and avulsion at this anastomosis can lead to aggressive, unnecessary bleeding.
- Access to the L3-4 disk requires more significant mobilization and retraction of the iliac vessels and aorta.
- **FIGURE 72-6:** A symmetric incision of anterior annulus of disk is performed, taking care to leave the lateral annular walls intact. Complete removal of the nucleus pulposus is performed. Caution is needed at all times from this portion of the procedure forward to avoid disruption of the posterior annulus and possible injury to contents within the vertebral spinal canal. For a large interbody graft to be placed, the diskectomy should be performed back to the posterior longitudinal ligament (PLL). For removal of a sequestered disk fragment, removal of part or all of the PLL can be performed for direct neural decompression. In these cases, enhanced illumination and magnification are necessary.

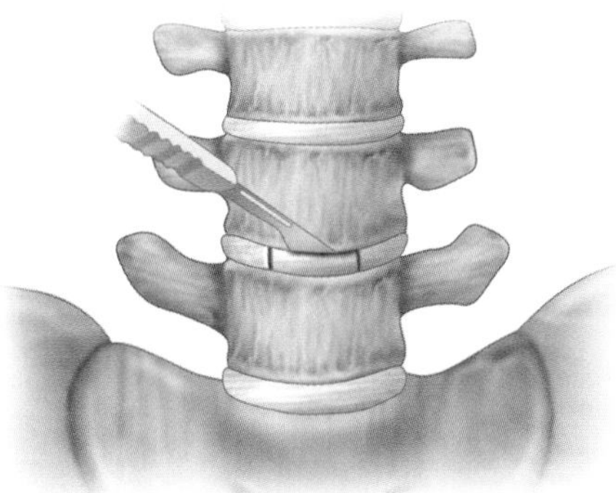

FIGURE 72-6

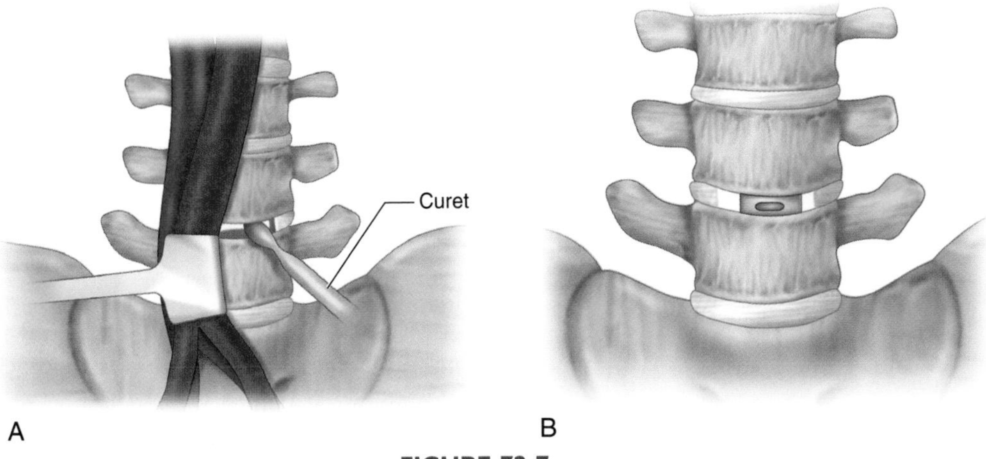

FIGURE 72-7

- **FIGURE 72-7:** Cartilage from the exposed portions of the vertebral end plates is meticulously removed to prepare the fusion bed, but the bony end plate, which is thin in the center of the disk space, should be preserved to avoid inadvertent entry into underlying cancellous bone, which can lead to cage telescoping and settling into vertebral bodies. This is accomplished with the use of curets and rongeurs.
- **FIGURE 72-8:** The disk space is distracted using various instruments of graduated size made for this purpose. At this point, inflation of the lumbar bladder can open the anterior disk space. An appropriate spacer size and depth is chosen by performing end plate measurement on preoperative axial magnetic resonance imaging (MRI) or computed tomography (CT). Fusion-promoting axial compression is attained by placement of a properly sized intervertebral spacer into the previously distracted disk space. A tightly fitted spacer also assists with immobilization of the final construct and reduces the risk of hardware failure if supplemental fixation is used. Before its placement, the spacer can be packed with bone autograft, demineralized bone matrix, commercially available bone graft extenders, or recombinant human bone morphogenetic protein (rh-BMP).
- **FIGURE 72-9: A-D,** An anterior vertebral plate can be placed as well if no supplemental posterior fixation is used. Although an anterior plate provides minimally increased biomechanical rigidity, it can be useful to prevent anterior expulsion of the intervertebral spacer in stand-alone ALIF.
- Final anteroposterior and lateral radiographs of the construct are obtained to confirm correct positioning of all implants, final hemostasis is achieved, retractors are removed, and the incision is closed in usual layered fashion. It is crucial to check the vasculature after retractor removal to ensure pulsatile iliac arteries. In addition, venous bleeding may have gone unnoticed secondary to tamponade from the retractors and be seen only after their removal.

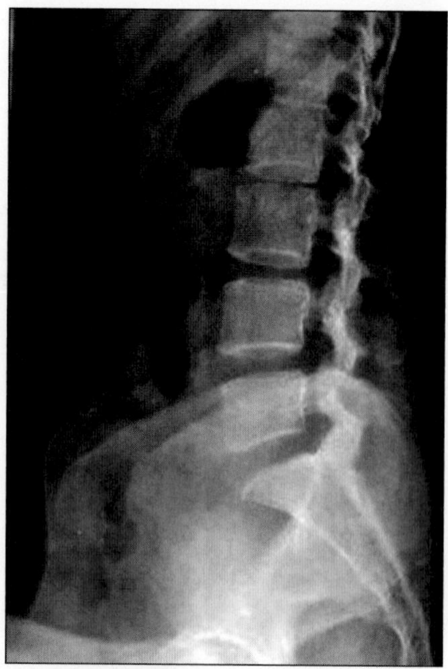

FIGURE 72-8

TIPS FROM THE MASTERS

- For male patients, it is important to discuss the risk of retrograde ejaculation, which occurs in 1% to 5% of patients. For patients who may wish to father children, banking semen remains an option so that an anterior approach can be used.
- An inflatable bladder placed under the small of the back can be useful in cases where the disk space is small. Inflation increases lordosis, allowing easier spacer placement. Deflation as the spacer is inserted allows for easier expansion of the posterior vertebral body.
- If the iliolumbar vein is likely to pose any issue, ligation is recommended. Although sacrifice of this structure is unlikely to have any clinically relevant sequelae, an inadvertent injury to this small vessel may be extremely difficult to repair and lead to several liters of blood loss.
- One advantage of ALIF over posterior lumbar interbody fusion is the ability of the anterior approach to enhance lumbar lordosis by an additional 5 to 10 degrees. For this reason, it is often beneficial to use a spacer with significant lordosis, particularly at the L5-S1 interspace. A graft with 10 to 15 degrees of lordosis would be reasonable.

PITFALLS

In select cases, access to a low L5-S1 disk space with a high sacral slope may be rendered difficult. Preincision imaging should allow the surgeon to determine the relationship of this trajectory to the pubic symphysis, which is an access-limiting structure.

Mobilization of the sympathetic plexus can result in a high rate of localized lower extremity sympathetic dysfunction. This "sympathetic effect" can be worrisome to patients and result in an asymmetric feeling of a "cold leg" or "warm leg." It is helpful to counsel patients regarding this complication preoperatively.

BAILOUT OPTIONS

- In the event that the procedure is impossible from the anterior approach, posterior interbody fusion may be pursued.

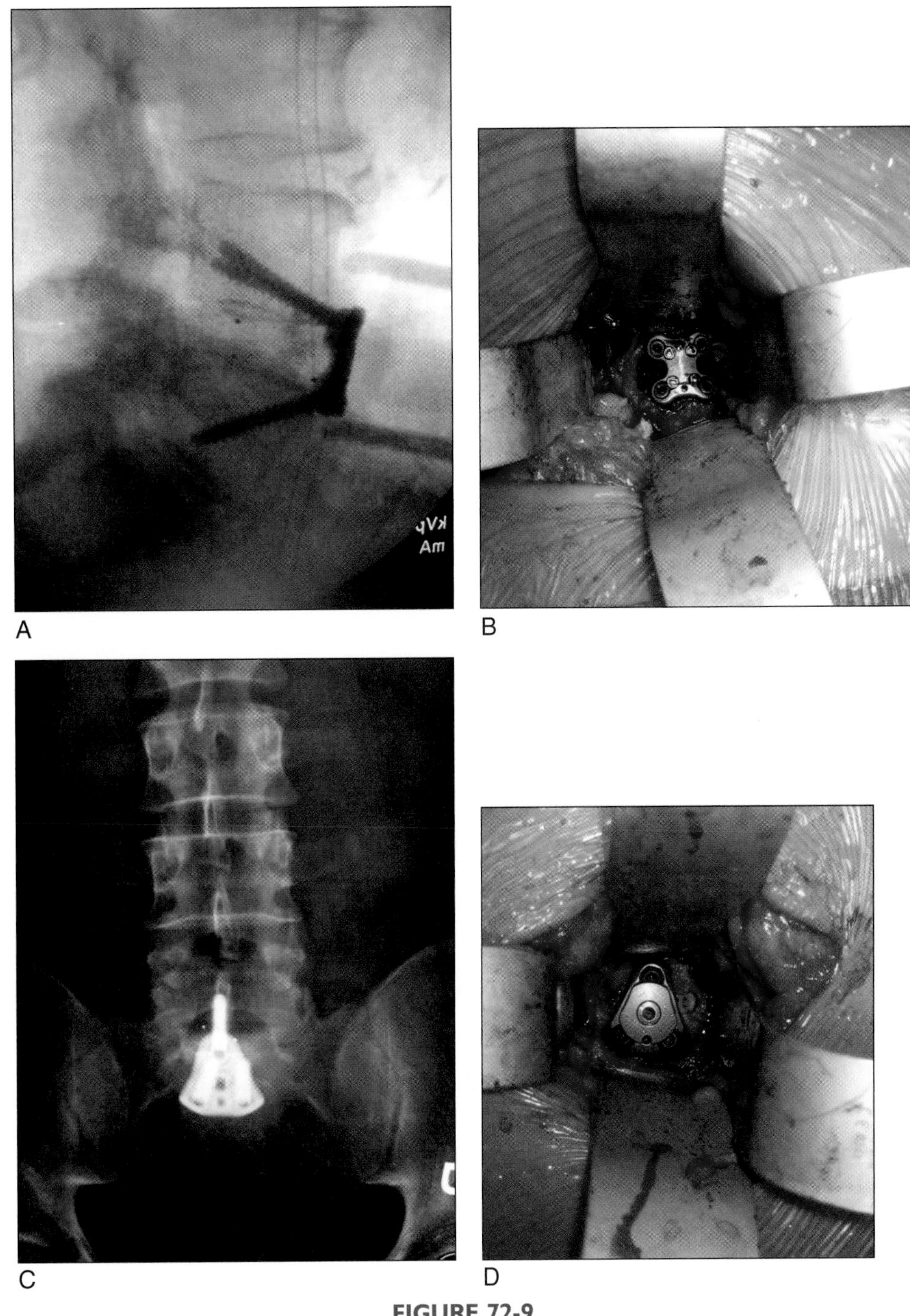

FIGURE 72-9

SUGGESTED READINGS

Brau SA. Mini-open approach to the spine for anterior lumbar interbody fusion: description of the procedure, results and complications. Spine J 2002;2:216–23.

Burkus JK, Gornet MF, Schuler TC, et al. Six-year outcomes of anterior lumbar interbody arthrodesis with use of interbody fusion cages and recombinant human bone morphogenetic protein-2. J Bone Joint Surg Am 2009;91:1181–9.

Gazzeri R, Tamorri M, Galarza M, et al. Balloon-assisted endoscopic retroperitoneal gasless approach (BERG) for lumbar interbody fusion: is it a valid alternative to the laparoscopic approach? Minim Invasive Neurosurg 2007;50:150–4.

Madan SS, Boeree NR. Comparison of instrumented anterior interbody fusion with instrumented circumferential lumbar fusion. Eur Spine J 2003;12:567–75.

Min JH, Jang JS, Lee SH. Comparison of anterior- and posterior-approach instrumented lumbar interbody fusion for spondylolisthesis. J Neurosurg Spine 2007;7:21–6.

Procedure 73 Posterior Lumbar Interbody Fusion

Matthew J. Tormenti; Edward A. Monaco, III; Adam S. Kanter

INDICATIONS

- Spondylolisthesis that is symptomatic, progressive, or requiring decompression that necessitates stabilization
- Degenerative disk disease with low back pain that can benefit from fusion at the symptomatic level or levels
- Pseudarthrosis of a previous intertransverse fusion that requires a fusion technique with higher success at achieving a solid arthrodesis
- Correction of degenerative scoliosis
- Recurrent disk herniation

CONTRAINDICATIONS

- Previous interbody graft placed at index level
- Significant epidural scar at planned level or site of operation
- Osteoporotic end plates that may not hold interbody graft, leading to subsidence
- Disease at or above the conus medullaris

PLANNING AND POSITIONING

- **FIGURE 73-1:** Patients are placed prone on an Andrews frame or a Jackson table.
- Neurophysiologic monitoring including somatosensory evoked potentials and electromyography is routinely used.
- The operative table should be positioned to enable fluoroscopy access and visualization of the surgical levels.
- Preoperative imaging should include anteroposterior and lateral radiographs or computed tomography (CT) for defining bony anatomy and magnetic resonance imaging (MRI) for defining neural elements and soft tissue structures.

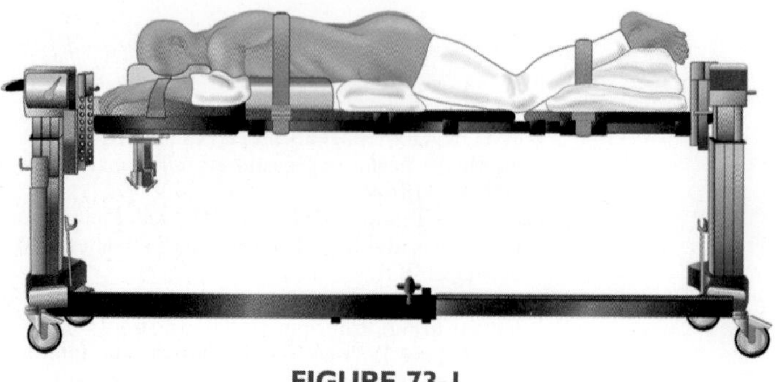

FIGURE 73-1

PROCEDURE

- **FIGURE 73-2:** A midline incision and fascial opening are followed by subperiosteal exposure of all levels involved. Dissection should be carried out laterally to the medial margin of the transverse processes.
- **FIGURE 73-3:** An appropriate operative level should be confirmed before beginning any bony decompression.
- **FIGURE 73-4:** Complete laminectomy and partial bilateral medial facetectomies are performed using a combination of Leksell and Kerrison rongeurs or bone drill or rongeurs and bone drill together. If needed, wider laminectomy and removal of pars interarticularis can be performed for greater exposure of the nerve root and disk space.
- **FIGURE 73-5:** Foraminotomies are performed to decompress any nerve roots with significant lateral recess stenosis. The disk space is identified, and annulotomy is performed with a No. 15 blade.
- **FIGURE 73-6:** A thorough diskectomy is performed while the thecal sac is carefully retracted with a nerve root retractor. Pituitary rongeurs and curets are used to remove all disk material. The end plates are gouged and prepared for interbody cage placement.

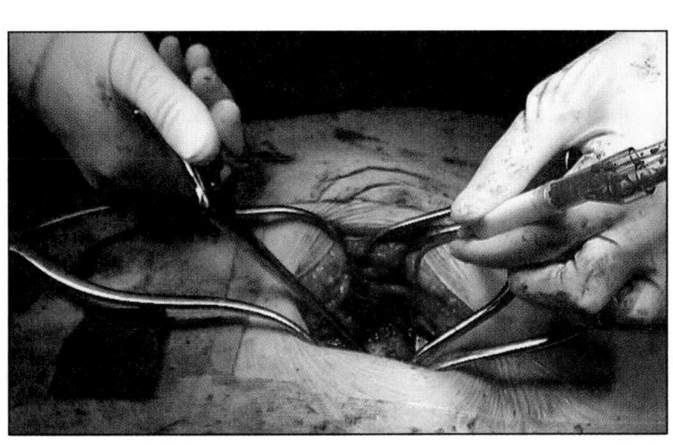

A

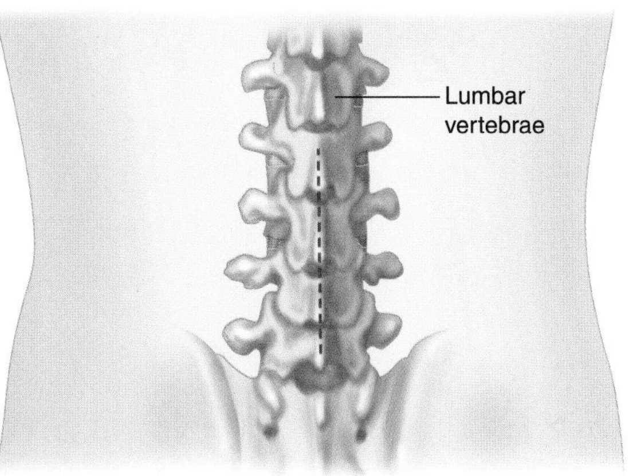

B

FIGURE 73-2

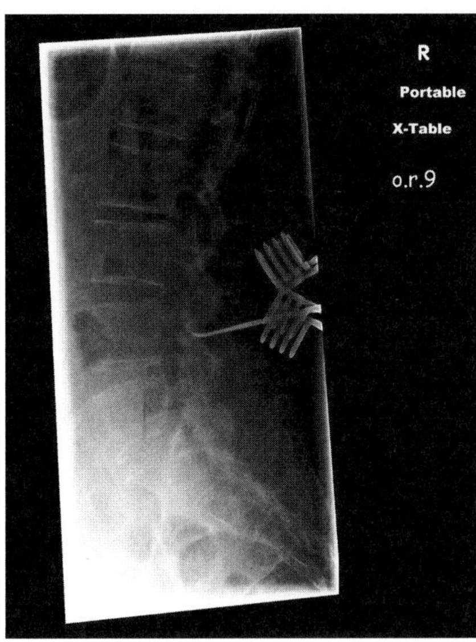

FIGURE 73-3

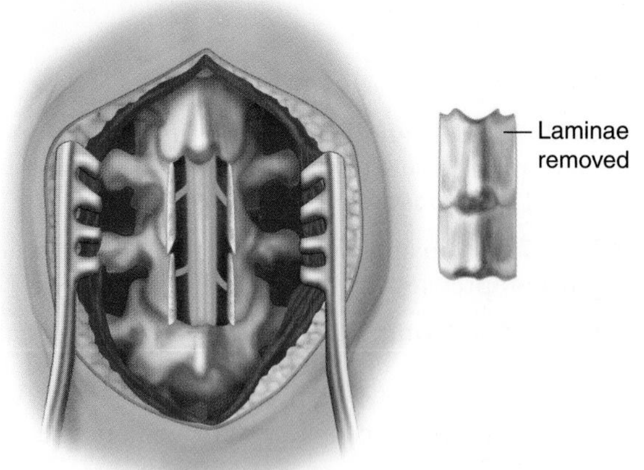

FIGURE 73-4

Diskectomies and Foraminotomies

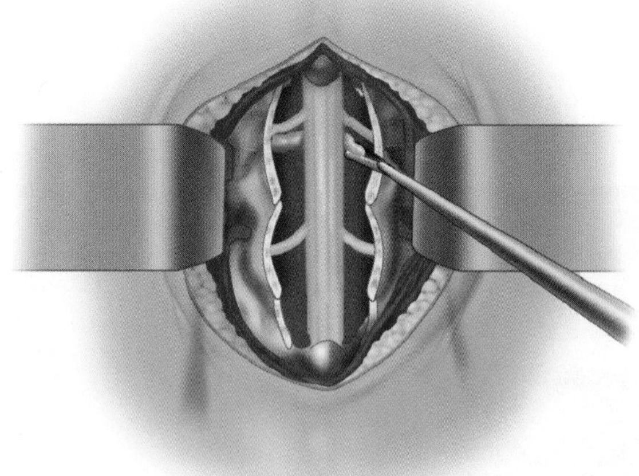

FIGURE 73-5

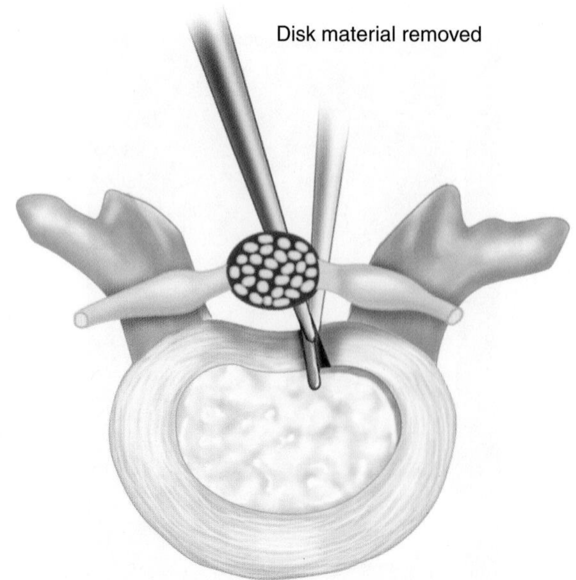

FIGURE 73-6

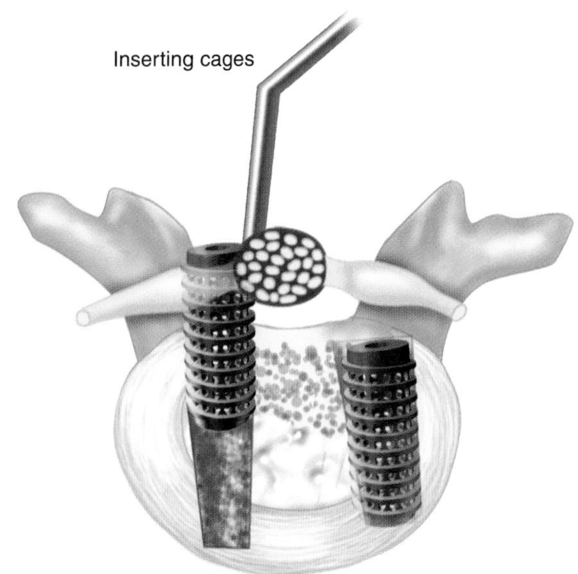

FIGURE 73-7

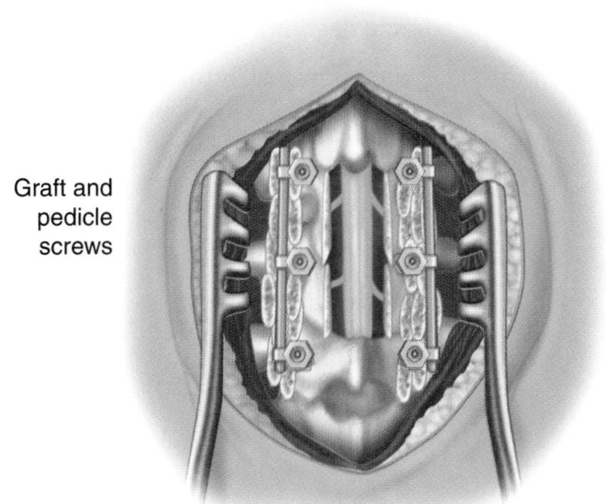

FIGURE 73-8

- **FIGURE 73-7:** Interbody grafts are placed bilaterally into the disk space. If severe collapse of the disk space is present, distraction instruments may be used to maximize interbody height and enable optimal graft size placement. During the insertion of grafts, the thecal sac can be retracted to improve exposure and reduce the risk of inadvertent durotomy.
- **FIGURE 73-8:** The interbody construct is supplemented by pedicle screws and intertransverse fusion using local bone autograft or bone graft extenders, or both, as available.

TIPS FROM THE MASTERS

- The operative level should be confirmed with fluoroscopy before any bony decompression.
- A distraction device may assist in interbody distraction and graft placement.
- Judicious use of fluoroscopy assists with end plate preparation and graft sizing.

- Hemostatic agents such as thrombin and Gelfoam are useful in controlling epidural bleeding.
- Concomitant intertransverse arthrodesis and transpedicular instrumentation increase fusion success.

PITFALLS
Durotomy
Nerve root injury during graft placement
Profuse epidural bleeding
Injury to intraabdominal structures from disruption of anterior longitudinal ligament and anterior graft placement

BAILOUT OPTIONS

- If grafts cannot be placed, bone autograft, allograft, or osteoinductive materials may be placed into the disk space instead.
- Severe epidural scarring may be reduced by a single graft placed transforaminally. Necessary decompression of symptomatic nerve roots should still be performed.
- Transforaminal lumbar interbody fusion should be considered for lesions at or above the conus medullaris because retraction of the thecal sac is not an option.

SUGGESTED READINGS

Barnes B, Rodts GE, McLaughlin MR, et al. Threaded cortical bone dowels for lumbar interbody fusion: over 1-year mean follow up in 28 patients. J Neurosurg 2001;95(Suppl. 1):1–4.

Cloward R. The treatment of ruptured lumbar intervertebral discs by vertebral fusion: indications, operative technique and aftercare. J Neurosurg 1953;10:154–66.

Madan SS, Harley JM, Boeree NR. Circumferential and posterolateral fusion for degenerative disc disease. Clin Orthop 2003;(409):114–23.

Rish BL. A critique of posterior lumbar interbody fusion: 12 years' experience with 250 patients. Surg Neurol 1989;31:281–9.

Suk SI, Lee CK, Kim WJ, et al. Adding posterior lumbar interbody fusion to pedicle screw fixation and posterolateral fusion after decompression in spondylolytic spondylolisthesis. Spine 1997;22:210–9.

Procedure 74

Transforaminal Lumbar Interbody Fusion

Edward A. Monaco, III; Matthew J. Tormenti; Adam S. Kanter

INDICATIONS

- Segmental instability requiring fusion for stabilization
- Recurrent disk herniation
- Symptomatic spinal stenosis with a significant back pain component that would benefit from fusion
- Degenerative disk disease with a significant back pain component
- Spondylolisthesis that is progressive, is symptomatic, or requires decompression with a need to fuse spondylolisthetic level
- Correction of degenerative scoliosis requiring fusion segments
- Salvage for pseudarthrosis of a previous intertransverse fusion or arthroplasty

CONTRAINDICATIONS

- Active infection
- Short life expectancy
- Severe osteoporosis
- Blood dyscrasia

PLANNING AND POSITIONING

- Anteroposterior and lateral plain films or computed tomography (CT) scan to evaluate bony anatomy
- Dynamic (flexion-extension) x-rays to evaluate degree of motion or instability
- Magnetic resonance imaging (MRI) to evaluate neural elements and soft tissue (e.g., disk)
- **FIGURE 74-1:** The patient is placed in the prone position with chest rolls on a Jackson table.
- Fluoroscopy and neuromonitoring, including somatosensory evoked potentials or electromyography or both

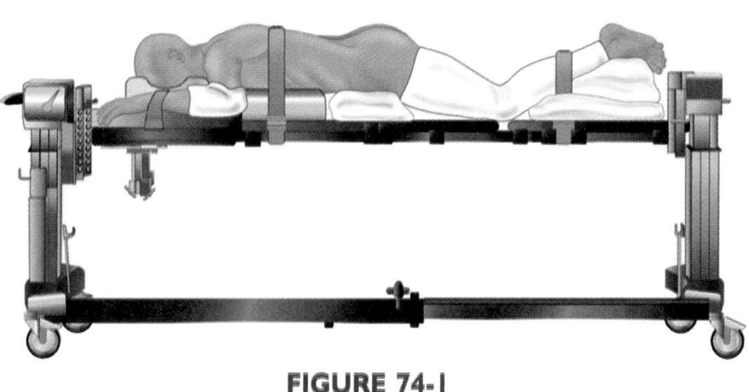

FIGURE 74-1

PROCEDURE

- **FIGURE 74-2:** Midline subperiosteal dissection of all involved levels is performed. If pedicle screws are planned, dissection should be carried out to reveal medial transverse processes.
- **FIGURE 74-3:** A full laminectomy is performed as indicated.
- **FIGURE 74-4:** Complete facetectomy and removal of the pars is performed to reveal the exiting and traversing nerve root at the identified level such that the underlying disk space is readily visualized.

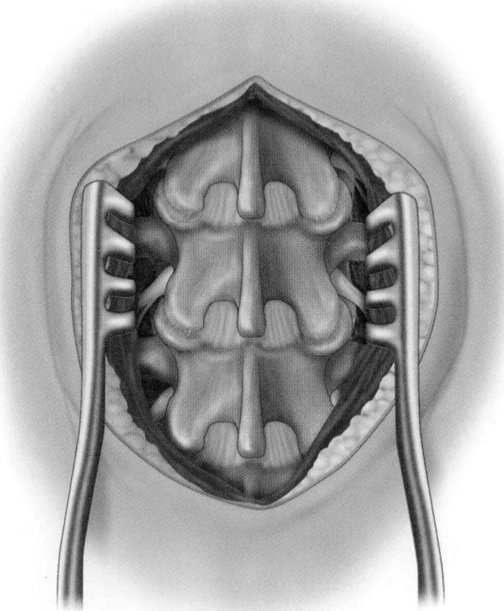

FIGURE 74-2

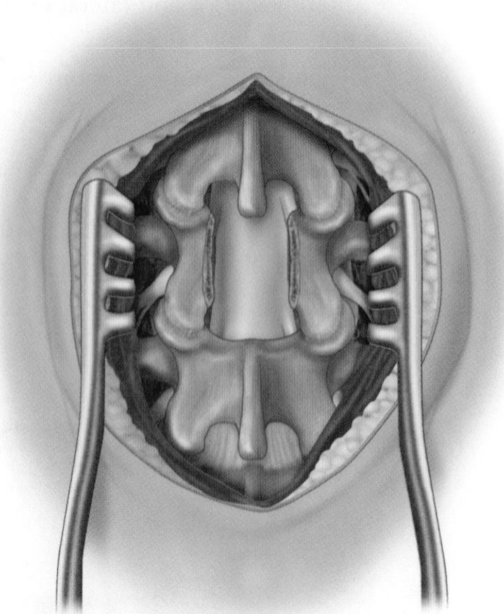

FIGURE 74-3

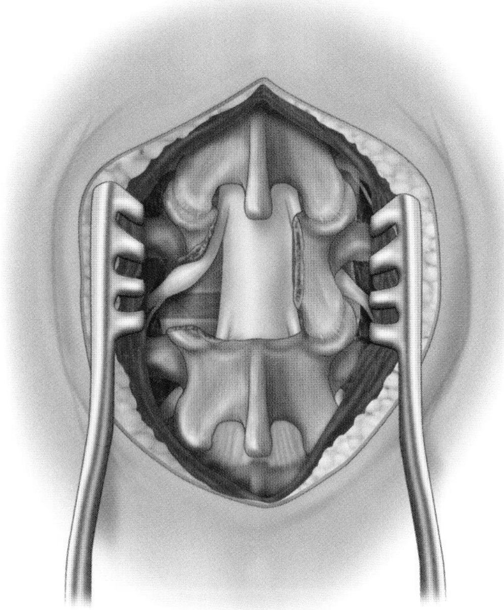

FIGURE 74-4

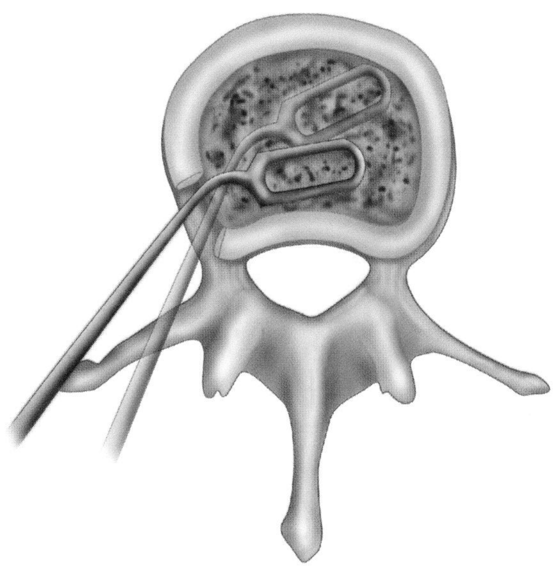

FIGURE 74-5

- **FIGURE 74-5:** After an annulotomy, a radical diskectomy is performed. It is essential to cross the midline and ensure that the contralateral disk is removed. The end plates are prepared for cage placement without violation of the annular ring. It is important to remove the cartilaginous end plate component to optimize fusion success.
- **FIGURE 74-6:** An interbody graft is placed. Various graft shapes exist for implantation (e.g., boomerang, bullet); regardless of shape, the surgeon should attempt to place the graft in the middle of the disk space. If the disk space is significantly collapsed, pedicle screws can be used with distraction retractors to heighten the interbody space and enable larger graft placement.
- **FIGURE 74-7:** Supplementation of the construct with pedicle screws and intertransverse fusion adds construct strength and increases the success of the fusion.
- **FIGURE 74-8:** A final radiograph in the anteroposterior and lateral planes should be obtained to confirm the proper placement and positioning of all hardware and grafts.

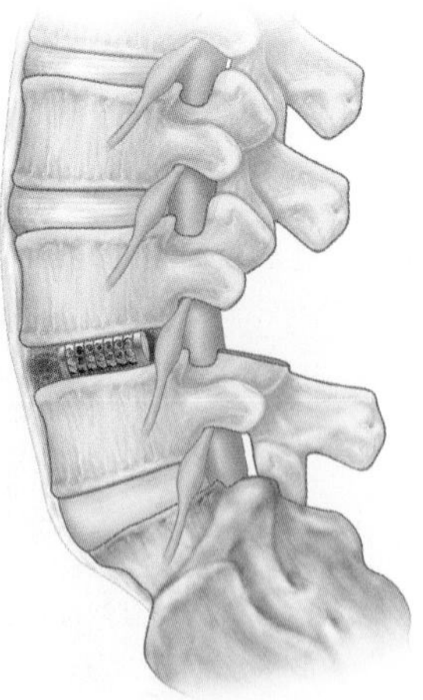

FIGURE 74-6

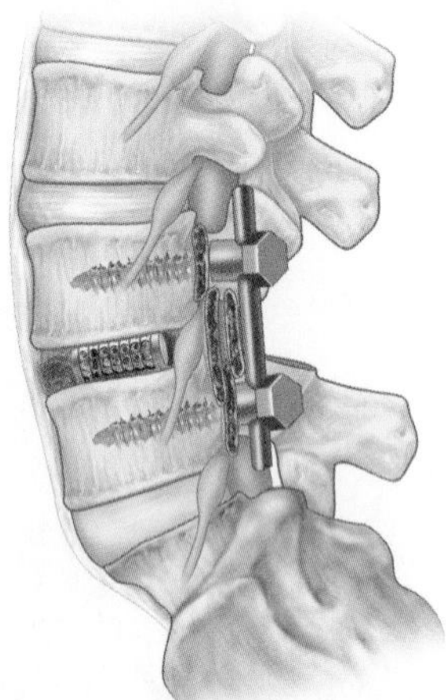

FIGURE 74-7

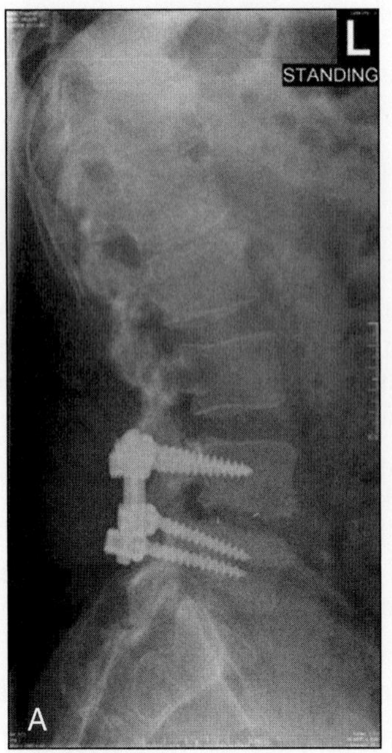

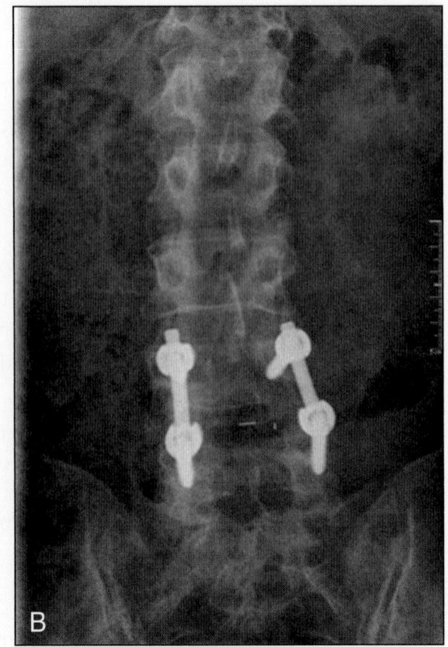

FIGURE 74-8

TIPS FROM THE MASTERS

- Confirm the operative level with intraoperative fluoroscopy.
- Distraction instruments can be used to assist with graft placement.
- Fluoroscopy can be used during graft placement for ideal positioning.
- Supplementation with pedicle screw fixation and posterolateral arthrodesis may improve long-term stability and fusion.

PITFALLS

It may be difficult to place the interbody spacer medially at L5-S1 because of the presence of the iliac crests.

The exiting and the traversing nerve roots are at risk for injury during graft placement and must be protected with nerve root retractors during graft insertion.

Grafts placed too posteriorly or grafts that are too small for the disk space may be driven back into the spinal canal.

BAILOUT OPTIONS

- If anatomic constraints inhibit transforaminal access and optimal graft placement at L5-S1, bilateral posterior lumbar interbody fusion may be used.
- If a disk space is too narrow to accept a cage, specialized distractors may be used to widen the space.
- If anatomic constraints limit the safe placement of the interbody graft (e.g., variant nerve root), an intertransverse fusion alone with pedicle screw supplementation may be performed.

SUGGESTED READINGS

Hackenberg L, Halm H, Bullmann V, et al. Transforaminal lumbar interbody fusion: a safe technique with satisfactory three to five year results. Eur Spine J 2005;14:551–8.

Harris BM, Hilibrand AS, Savas PE, et al. Transforaminal lumbar interbody fusion: the effect of various instrumentation techniques on the flexibility of the lumbar spine. Spine 2004;29:E65–E70.

Heth JA, Hitchon PW, Goel VK, et al. A biomechanical comparison between anterior and transverse interbody fusion cages. Spine 2001;26:E261–7.

Humphreys SC, Hodges SD, Patwardhan AG, et al. Comparison of posterior and transforaminal approaches to lumbar interbody fusion. Spine 2001;26:567–71.

Rosenberg WS, Mummaneni PV. Transforaminal lumbar interbody fusion: technique, complications, and early results. Neurosurgery 2001;48:569–74.

Procedure 75 Anterior Lumbar Corpectomy

J. Dawn Waters, Joseph D. Ciacci

INDICATIONS

- Tumor, fracture, tuberculosis, or other pathology of the vertebral body requiring direct decompression of the spinal canal with resection of anterior pathology
- Instability of anterior spinal elements, requiring restoration of height and stability to prevent progressive deformity and kyphosis

CONTRAINDICATIONS

- Poor quality of adjacent bone for accommodating a fusion construct because of osteoporosis, osteomyelitis, tumor, or other bone diseases
- Abdominal aortic aneurysm

PLANNING AND POSITIONING

- The focus here is on the anterolateral-retroperitoneal approach to a lumbar corpectomy and fusion. There are several options for approaching the anterior lumbar spine, including (1) anterolateral-retroperitoneal with the patient in a lateral position, (2) endoscopic anterolateral-retroperitoneal, (3) anterior-retroperitoneal with the patient supine, (4) anterior-transperitoneal with the patient supine, and (5) lateral extracavitary with the patient in a lateral position. All approaches require special consideration of the anatomy of the ribs and diaphragm for exposure of L2 and above. Lateral approaches require special consideration of the anatomy of the iliac crest for exposure of L5 and below.
- Although a left-sided approach is generally preferred, important exceptions include predominantly right-sided pathology and cases of abdominal aortic aneurysm, calcifications, or other aortic disease that impairs safe mobilization of the aorta. A right-sided approach is difficult because of retraction of the liver and the dangers of retracting the thin-walled inferior vena cava.
- The approach to the anterior spine with requisite mobilization of the great vessels is frequently performed with the aid of a general or vascular surgeon.
- Risks of this procedure include significant and brisk bleeding from the fractured vertebra, epidural veins, and major vessel injury. Ensure blood products are available, and consider use of a cell saver unless contraindicated owing to infection or tumor. Pursue a thorough preoperative medical evaluation and medical optimization for comorbid conditions.
- Consider the bony and ligamentous stability of the posterior elements of the spine, and plan appropriately for necessary adjunctive or alternative procedures for placement of instrumentation posteriorly.
- Consider preoperative embolization of particularly vascular lesions.
- Preoperative imaging should include (1) plain anteroposterior and lateral radiographs; (2) magnetic resonance imaging (MRI) for defining the neural anatomy and extent of spinal cord compression, with contrast agent to aid visualization of tumor or abscess; and (3) noncontrast computed tomography (CT) for definition of the bony anatomy for measurement and planning of instrumentation. Take care to correlate anteroposterior and lateral radiographs with other imaging modalities so that the level of pathology can be localized on intraoperative radiographs alone. Additionally, imaging of the vascular structures, such as the aorta, vena cava, and artery of Adamkiewicz, may be helpful in preoperative planning of the approach.

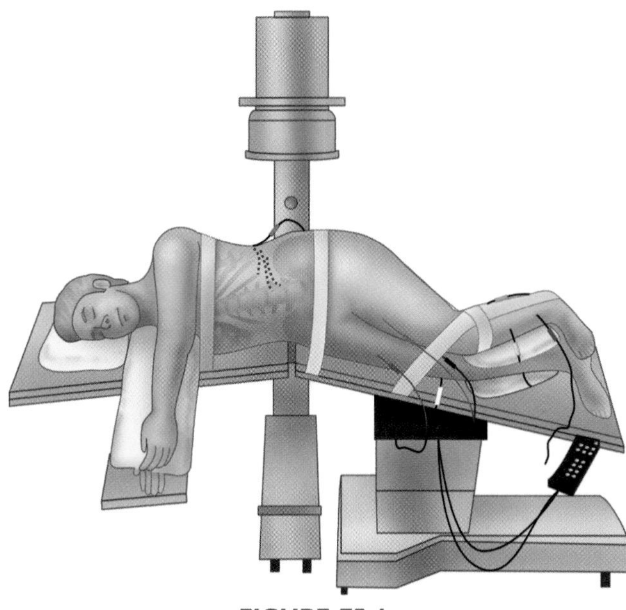

FIGURE 75-1

- Intraoperative fluoroscopy should be used, along with a compatible operating table. Ensure the fluoroscopic machines can fit around the patient in position on the table to provide anteroposterior and lateral views of the target levels.
- **Figure 75-1:** Left-sided approach. *1*, Position the patient laterally, left side up. *2*, Place beanbag or gel rolls to support the body. *3*, Place an axillary roll. *4*, Secure the patient with padded 3-inch tape across the shoulder and greater trochanter. *5*, Flex the left hip to relax the ipsilateral psoas but not so much as to interfere with dissection. *6*, Prepare and drape the patient broadly so that the anterior to posterior midline is within the field. Prepare the iliac crest if it is to be harvested.
- Plan the incision with fluoroscopy. The level of incision varies depending on the level of pathology and planned instrumentation. Fluoroscopy should be used to aid in localization and planning before incision, with the planned incision centered lateral to the vertebrae to be exposed. For levels at the thoracolumbar junction, in principle, a rib directly lateral in the midaxillary line to the pathologic vertebra is the best rib to resect for optimal exposure. In the exposure of L1, incision may extend to the level of the 10th rib.
- At the appropriate level, incise obliquely from the lateral border of the rectus muscle to the lateral border of the paravertebral musculature.

PROCEDURE

- **Figure 75-2:** Axial view of retroperitoneal dissection. The peritoneum and its contents are swept anteriorly by blunt dissection. The kidney and ureter are retracted anteriorly as well. A self-retaining retractor system, such as the Omni-Tract (Saint Paul, MN), aids in maintaining the exposure.
- **Figure 75-3:** Accessing the surface of the vertebral body. The segmental vessels coursing over the mid-vertebral bodies may be ligated about 1 cm away from the aorta for exposure of the underlying body. The iliolumbar vein may tether the aorta at the L4-5 level and may be identified and ligated as it courses from the inferior vena cava over L5. When freed, the aorta and iliac artery may be gently swept from left to right. The left iliac vein may be stretched and flattened across the L5 body or L5-S1 disk space as it courses inferiorly from the aortic bifurcation, and it may bleed profusely if it is mistaken for nonvascular tissue and cut.
- **Figure 75-4:** Diskectomy. Verify the level with fluoroscopy as needed by inserting a radiopaque marker into the disk. Identify the neural foramina above and below the planned corpectomy with a No. 4 Penfield to define the posterior border of the

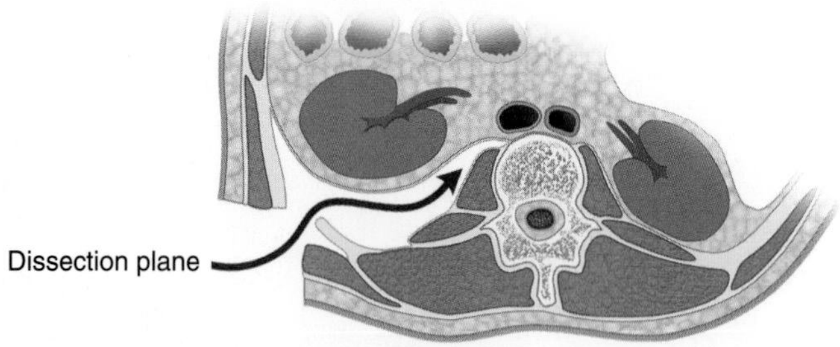

FIGURE 75-2

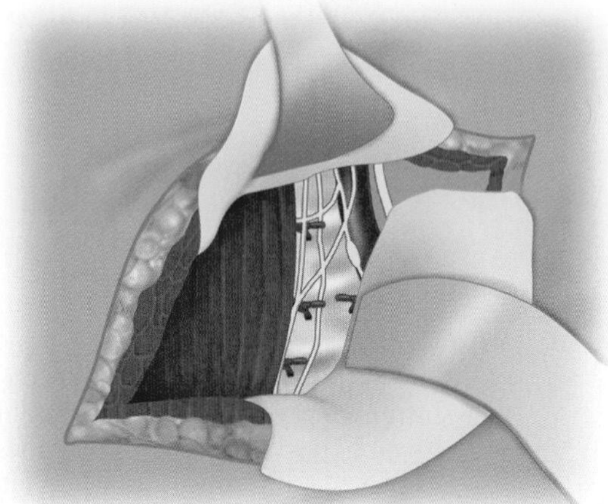

FIGURE 75-3

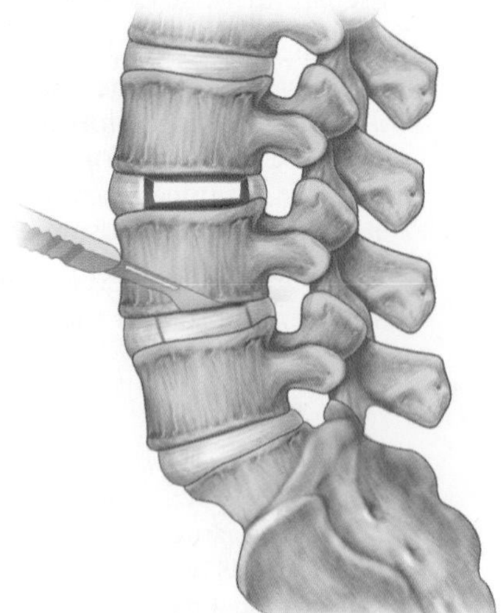

FIGURE 75-4

vertebral body and spinal canal. When the level of surgery and protected location of neural elements is established, perform the diskectomy above and below the planned corpectomy. Remove the cartilaginous end plates while preserving the bony end plates. Bleeding can be controlled with Gelfoam or similar hemostatic agent. Use of bone wax should be avoided because it interferes with subsequent fusion.

- **Figure 75-5:** Corpectomy. Remove the vertebra between the removed disks. Rongeurs and a drill with cutting burs may be used (**A**). Cancellous bone can bleed profusely, in contrast to cortical bone. Hemostasis can be maintained by timely resection of

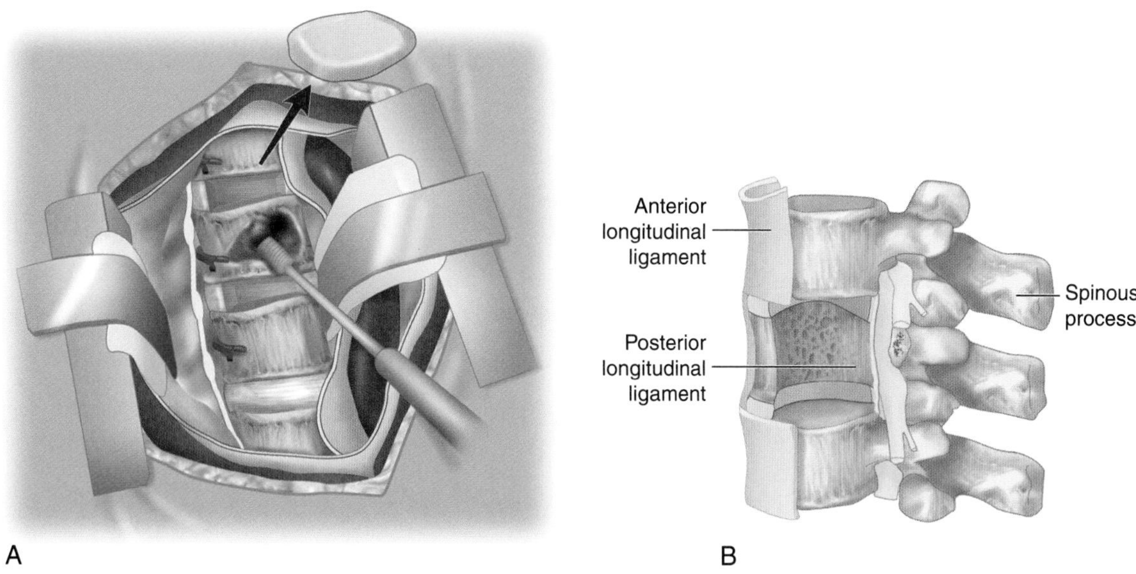

FIGURE 75-5

cancellous bone out to cortical bone, Gelfoam, or bone wax. Unless contraindicated (e.g., owing to tumor or infection), leave the anterior and contralateral bony cortex intact, and save any resected bone for later grafting. An intact anterior longitudinal ligament and anterior and contralateral cortex help protect great vessels. Decompress the spinal canal carefully to avoid tearing the dura mater, and repair any dural tears primarily if possible (**B**).

- **Figure 75-6: A-C,** Instrumentation. Anterior reconstruction generally includes an interbody cage or autograft or allograft for anterior and middle column support, along with a plate or rods affixed to the adjacent vertebral bodies to limit motion at the fusion site. The specific technique for instrumentation varies by manufacturer. General considerations are listed subsequently. Refer to the manufacturers guidelines for details of each device. Constructs designed by various manufacturers are illustrated.
- **Figure 75-7:** Anterior plate or rod placement, with placement of screws into the vertebral body. **A,** Remove any distraction applied to the vertebral construct, and adjust the table and patient positioning to restore anatomic alignment before instrumented fusion. Avoid placement of instrumentation that may cause friction against and subsequent erosion of pulsatile vessels such as the aorta. Measure the appropriate length of plate to provide adequate overlap of the vertebral body to avoid disruption of the end plate with screw placement and prevent overriding adjacent, nonfused motion segments. Using measurements of sizes of vertebral bodies from preoperative imaging, select vertebral body screw sizes accordingly. **B,** Angle screws in a triangular trajectory (not parallel) to resist screw pullout forces. The posterior screw should be angled anterior to avoid inadvertent placement near or in the spinal canal. Verify correct placement fluoroscopically before closure.
- Closure may proceed after obtaining hemostasis and verifying lack of injury to structures such as the bowel, peritoneum, and thoracic duct. If the diaphragm was dissected, reapproximate it to prevent diaphragmatic herniation. Place chest tubes and drains as needed. The layers of muscular fascia of the abdominal wall are individually reapproximated. Skin is closed in a standard fashion.

TIPS FROM THE MASTERS

- Preoperative ureteral stenting may be helpful in intraoperative identification of the ureters in especially difficult circumstances, such as retroperitoneal fibrosis or malignancy involving the ureters.
- Use of a partially radiolucent self-retaining retractor system, such as the Omni-Tract, aids in maintaining exposure and saves time because it does not need to be repositioned during fluoroscopy.

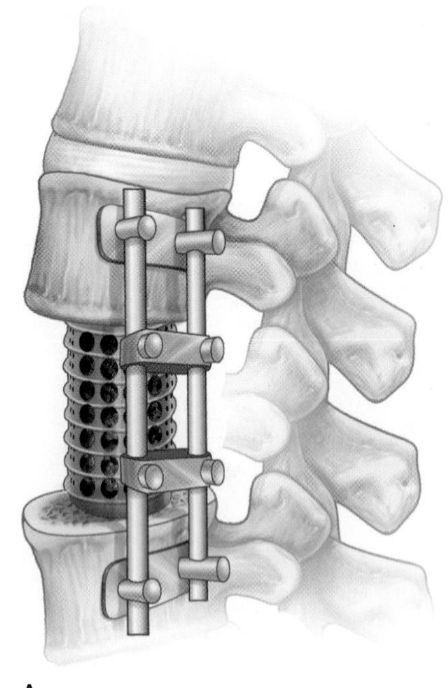

A

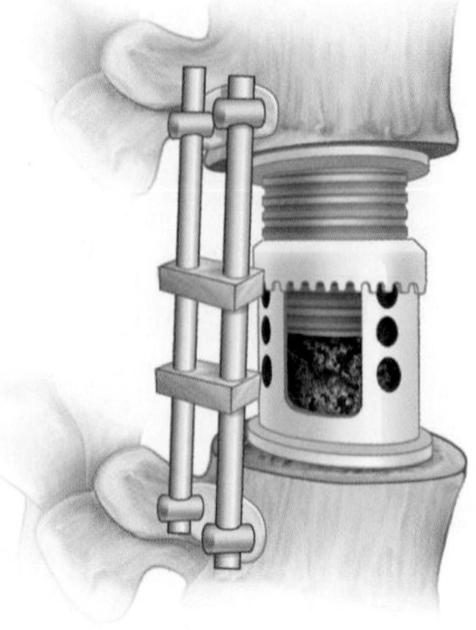

B

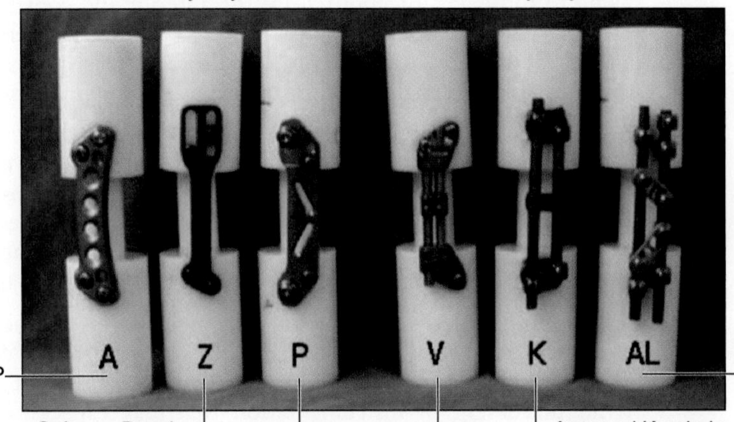

C

FIGURE 75-6

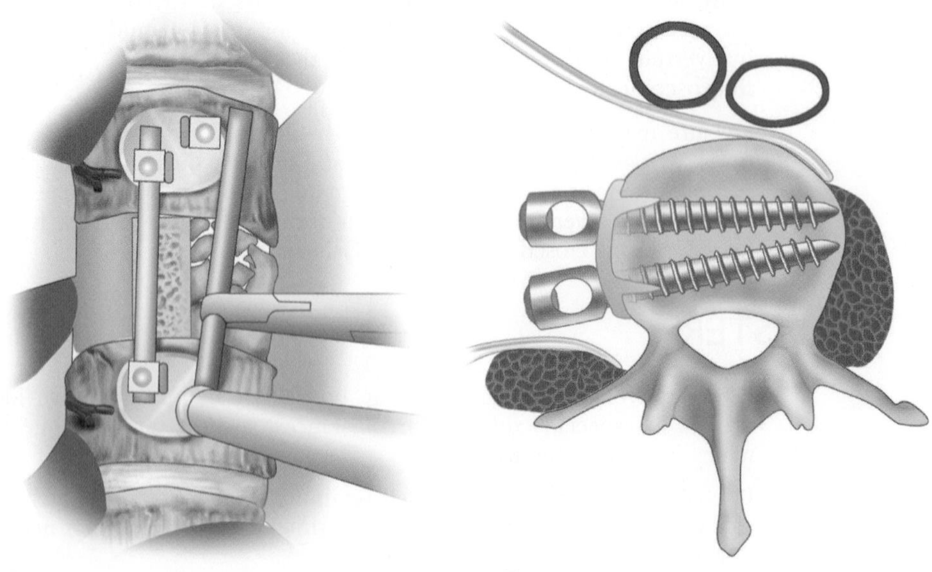

A B

FIGURE 75-7

PITFALLS

Surgery performed at the wrong level is a common and preventable mistake. Wrong-level surgery is particularly common if the patient has an abnormal number of ribs or vertebrae that makes counting more complicated. Study preoperative images carefully, correlate plain films with other imaging modalities, and employ intraoperative fluoroscopy.

Injury to the great vessels, thoracic duct, or the ureters may cause significant morbidity and mortality.

Instrumentation overhanging in contact with pulsatile arteries such as the aorta may erode the artery over time owing to friction.

Complications include deep vein thrombosis and pulmonary embolism from retraction of abdominal veins.

The left iliac vein may be stretched and flattened across the L5 body or L5-S1 disk space as it courses inferiorly within the aortic bifurcation and may bleed profusely if it is mistaken for nonvascular tissue and cut.

Do not use different types of metals or alloys within the same construct because this may result in galvanic corrosion of the more active, less noble metal.

BAILOUT OPTIONS

- If one of the great vessels is injured, compress proximally and distally to control bleeding. Temporary vascular clamps may be placed while the vessel is repaired.
- If anterior instrumentation cannot be accomplished safely, consider posterior instrumentation for stabilization.

SUGGESTED READINGS

Baker JK, Reardon PR, Reardon MJ, et al. Vascular injury in anterior lumbar surgery. Spine 1993;18:2227–30.

Barone GW, Pait TG, Eidt JF, et al. "General surgical pearls" for the anterior exposure of vertebral fractures. Am Surg 2001;67:939–42.

Brodke DS, Gollogly S, Bachus KN, et al. Anterior thoracolumbar instrumentation: stiffness and load sharing characteristics of plate and rod systems. Spine 2003;28:1794–801.

Faro FD, White KK, Ahn JS, et al. Biomechanical analysis of anterior instrumentation for lumbar corpectomy. Spine 2003;28:E468–71.

Hovorka I, de Peretti F, Damon F, et al. Five years' experience of retroperitoneal lumbar and thoracolumbar surgery. Eur Spine J 2000;9(Suppl 1):S30–4.

Westfall SH, Akbarnia BA, Merenda JT, et al. Exposure of the anterior spine: technique, complications, and results in 85 patients. Am J Surg 1987;154:700–4.

Figure 75-7C is modified with permission from Brodke DS, Gollogly S, Bachus KN, et al. Anterior thoracolumbar instrumentation: stiffness and load sharing characteristics of plate and rod systems. Spine 2003;28:1794–801.

Procedure 76

Pedicle Subtraction Osteotomy

Sassan Keshavarzi, Dzenan Lulic, Pawel Jankowski, Henry E. Aryan

INDICATIONS

- Fixed sagittal deformity secondary to previous surgery with an anterior fusion mass, traumatic deformity, neoplastic disease, or congenital anomalies
- The need to introduce up to 35 degrees of lumbar lordosis, the need to introduce 10 cm of posterior trunk translation, or correction of a sharp angular kyphosis or flat back syndrome
- Symptoms including inability to maintain horizontal gaze, severe fatigue on standing and ambulation, intractable back pain, disfigurement, generalized decreased functional capacity, and radicular symptoms
- Failure of conservative nonsurgical treatment and documented progression of deformity
- Progression of deformity after a previous surgery either secondary to pseudarthrosis or adjacent to a previous fusion

CONTRAINDICATIONS

- Medical contraindications
- Poor bone quality, which may result in failure to close or fuse across osteotomy site

PLANNING AND POSITIONING

- Standing 36-inch anteroposterior and lateral x-ray projections are obtained to assess global and regional alignment of the spine. For the lateral x-ray, the spinal deformity is most accurately represented with the knees and hips fully extended.
- Flexion and extension x-rays allow assessment of the flexibility of the deformity. The flexibility of the deformity plays a significant role in surgical planning.
- Anteroposterior images are obtained to evaluate scoliotic abnormalities.
- Magnetic resonance imaging (MRI) is performed to assess the full dimensions of the spinal canal and the degree of foraminal and central canal stenosis. This assessment is particularly important because manipulation of the spine into lordosis may significantly advance the level of stenosis leading compression of the neural elements. Under these circumstances, the surgeon may consider a decompression of the neural elements before correction of sagittal deformity.
- Patients should be examined for a hip flexion contracture, which may be the cause of sagittal plane malalignment. Using the Thomas test, patients may be evaluated for flexion contracture of the hip. The modified Thomas test can differentiate between tightness of the iliopsoas versus the rectus femoris.
- In patients with a sagittal deformity localized to the spine, it is imperative to localize the deformity to the cervical, thoracic, or lumbar spine. In patients whose deformity is localized to the cervical spine, as the patients lay in the supine position, their heads and upper thoracic spines remain elevated from the table.
- **Figure 76-1:** The patient is positioned prone on a spinal Jackson table.

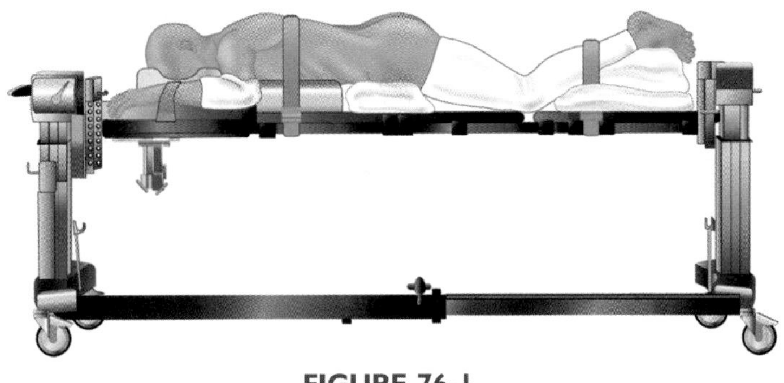

FIGURE 76-1

PROCEDURE

- **Figure 76-2:** The thoracolumbar spine has been exposed, and the psoas muscle has been dissected off the vertebral body. Pedicle screws have been placed at the adjacent levels, typically two levels above and below the level of the osteotomy. Placing the instrumentation before exposing the neural elements can limit the risk of injury to the spinal cord and thecal sac. Laminectomy and bilateral facetectomies have exposed the pedicles. Initiate removal of the pedicle by using a high-speed bur to remove the center of the pedicle, and extend drilling 1 cm into the body. This facilitates removal of the remainder of the pedicle with a narrow rongeur.
- **Figure 76-3:** Using a drill, the remainder of the pedicle can be removed, exposing and allowing access to the vertebral body. It is essential to use nerve root retractors to protect the neural elements—the nerve root and the thecal sac and spinal cord.
- **Figure 76-4:** The vertebral body is decancellated, creating a wedge resection. This may be done using a high-speed drill or 10-mm osteotome or both.
- **Figure 76-5:** The area directly under the posterior longitudinal ligament can be collapsed and removed using a curet. This is crucial because any remaining bone would prevent the closing of the osteotomy. The nerve root below the resected pedicle would limit the extent of vertebral body decancellation and the inferior margin of the wedge resection.
- **Figure 76-6:** Placement of a temporary rod prevents translation by providing vertical control as the surgeon completes any further removal of the posterior elements (e.g., advancing the laminectomy rostral and caudad).
- **Figure 76-7:** It is especially important to avoid leaving any scar tissue from a previous surgery or bony or ligamentous substance that may cause compression of the thecal sac or spinal cord after the osteotomy is closed.

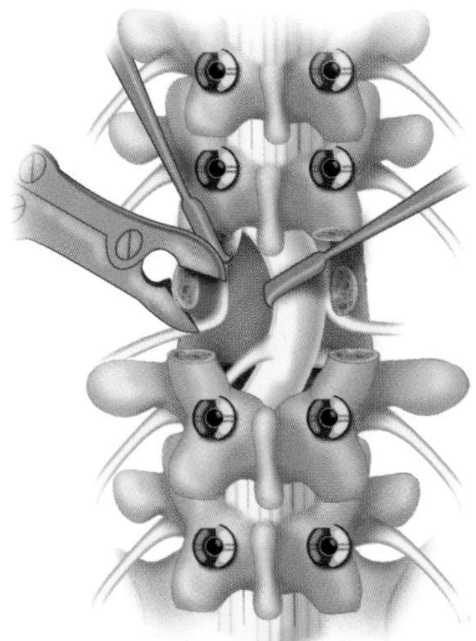

FIGURE 76-2

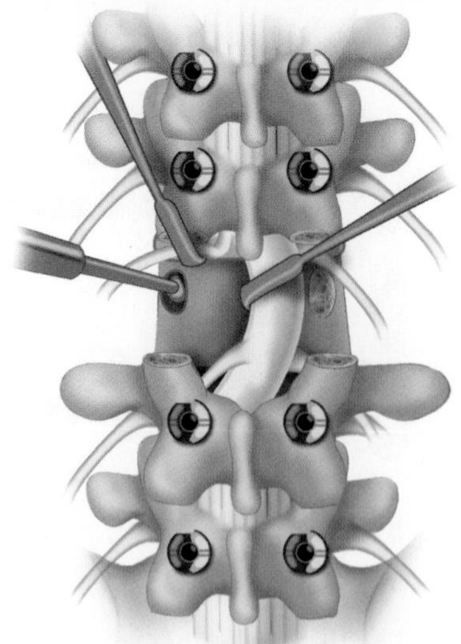

FIGURE 76-3

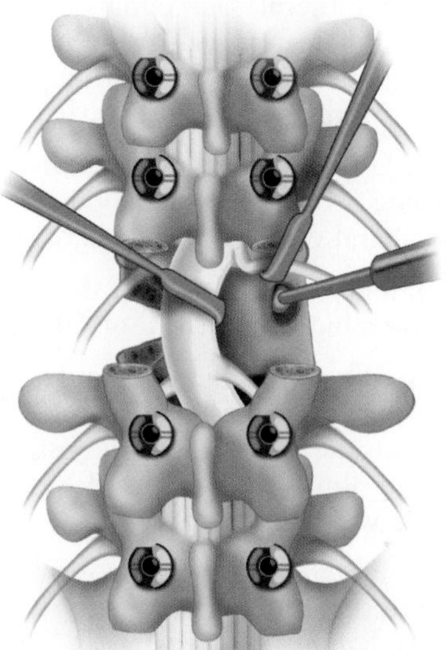

FIGURE 76-4

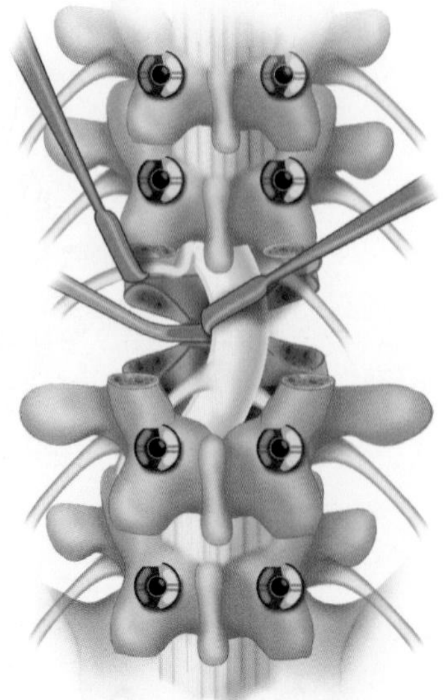

FIGURE 76-5

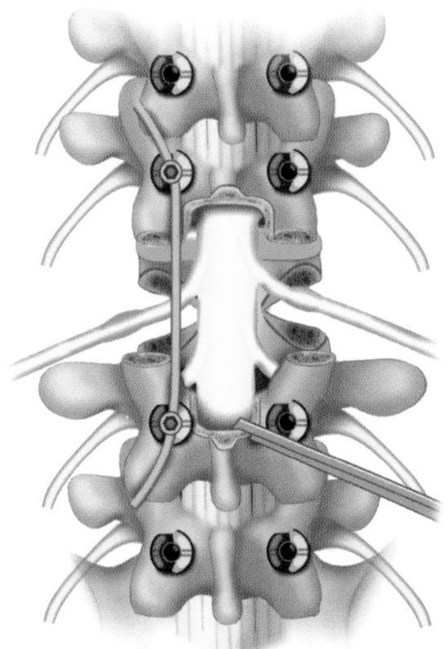

FIGURE 76-6

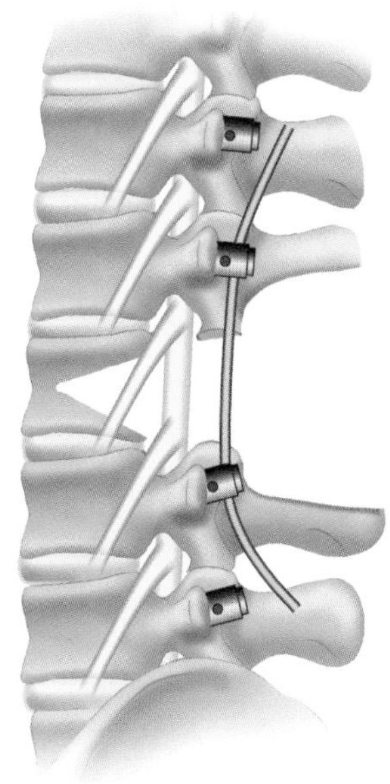

FIGURE 76-7

- **Figure 76-8:** The osteotomy is closed and secured with permanent rods, with the surgeon using compression on the pedicle screws to accomplish the degree of lordosis necessary.
- **Figure 76-9:** A 72-year-old man 30 years after a noninstrumented lumbar fusion developed iatrogenic flat back syndrome with a progressive sagittal imbalance that limited his ambulation. He underwent L3 pedicle subtraction osteotomy and posterior instrumented fusion for correction of his sagittal balance.

TIPS FROM THE MASTERS

- While creating the wedge resection via the transpedicular approach, significant blood loss can occur. Working back and forth between the two sides while tamponading with hemostatic agents and patties can help reduce this blood loss.
- It is imperative to avoid entry into the disk space above the osteotomy.

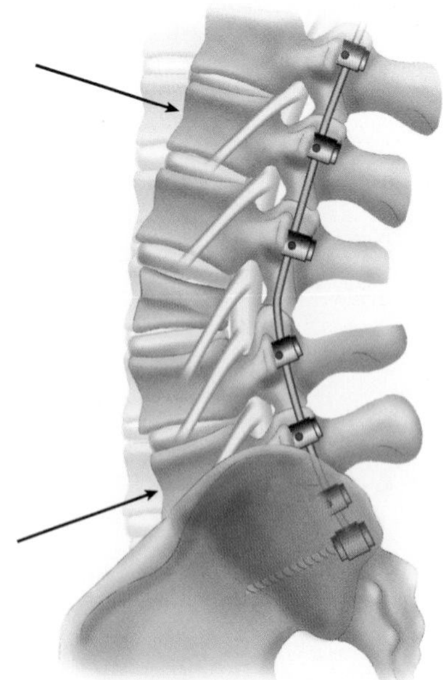

FIGURE 76-8

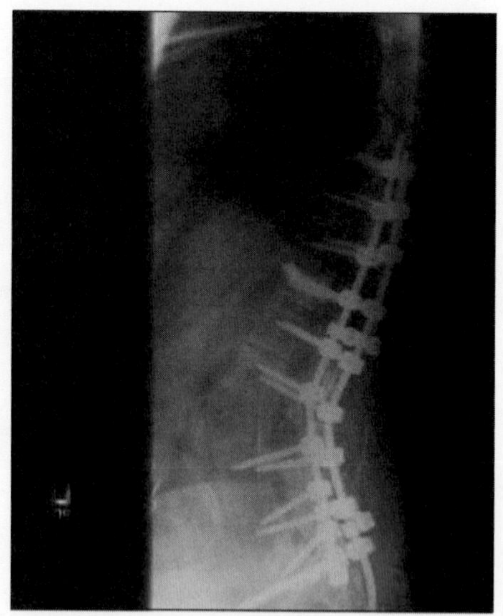

FIGURE 76-9

PITFALLS

Significant blood loss can occur. In the event of blood loss, the patient should be aggressively resuscitated.

During closure of the osteotomy, if spinal canal stenosis occurs above and below, it must be decompressed. Otherwise, compression may worsen after osteotomy closure from the angulation created.

If the osteotomy cannot be completely closed with apposition of bony surfaces, consider adding bone or bone morphogenetic protein, or both, to facilitate fusion.

BAILOUT OPTIONS

- Entering the disk space above or below may require a fusion or conversion to total vertebral column resection.

SUGGESTED READINGS

Booth KC, Bridwell KH, Lenke LG, et al. Complications and predictive factors for the successful treatment of flatback deformity (fixed sagittal imbalance). Spine 1999;24:1712–20.

Bridwell KH. Decision making regarding Smith-Petersen vs. pedicle subtraction osteotomy vs. vertebral column resection for spinal deformity. Spine 2006;31(Suppl. 19):S171–8.

Bridwell KH, Lenke LG, Lewis SJ. Treatment of spinal stenosis and fixed sagittal imbalance. Clin Orthop Relat Res 2001;384:35–44.

Bridwell KH, Lewis SJ, Rinella A, et al. Pedicle subtraction osteotomy for the treatment of fixed sagittal imbalance: surgical technique. J Bone Joint Surg Am 2004;86(Suppl. 1):44–50.

Kim YJ, Bridwell KH, Lenke LG, et al. Pseudarthrosis in long adult spinal deformity instrumentation and fusion to the sacrum: prevalence and risk factor analysis of 144 cases. Spine 2006;31:2329–36.

Vedantam R, Lenke LG, Bridwell KH, et al. The effect of variation in arm position on sagittal spinal alignment. Spine 2000;25:2204–9.

Procedure 77 Lumbar Disk Arthroplasty

Joseph L. Martinez, Michael Y. Wang

INDICATIONS

- Lumbar disk arthroplasty (LDA) is indicated as a treatment of chronic, incapacitating low back pain that is diskogenic in origin at the L4-5 or L5-S1 level and not accompanied by neural element compression resulting in claudication or radiculopathy. Diagnosis should be documented with magnetic resonance imaging (MRI), plain lumbar spine x-rays, and positive results of provocative diskography of the pathologic level.
- To be considered for surgery, patients should have failed at least 6 months of conservative nonsurgical therapies and ideally be 18 to 50 years old. Patients who have previously undergone posterior disk interventions, such as diskectomy or nucleolysis, may be candidates for LDA as long as no acute neural compression is present, and the remaining facet anatomy is sufficient to prevent distraction of the disk space and provide stability of the segment to be operated.

CONTRAINDICATIONS

- Assuming a patient's general medical condition is adequate to undergo elective spine surgery, contraindications to this procedure are active diskitis, previous (failed) fusion surgery at the pathologic level, malignancy, fracture or spondylolysis of the adjacent vertebrae, spondylolisthesis of the pathologic segment, osteopenia insufficient to support the disk prosthesis, and advanced facet arthrosis.
- As with other anterior lumbar spine procedures, relative contraindications to this approach include the presence of an infrarenal aortic aneurysm, congenital or iatrogenic genitourinary anatomic abnormalities such as an ipsilateral single ureter or kidney, or a history of previous retroperitoneal surgery.

PLANNING AND POSITIONING

- **Figure 77-1:** The patient is positioned supine on the operating table. The lumbar spine is placed in extension; the patient's legs are abducted if a lithotomy position is used. The surgeon performs the procedure standing between the legs of the patient if the lithotomy position is used. This position gives the surgeon a slightly more centered approach during prosthesis placement, which can be crucial to the success of the device.
- **Figure 77-2:** Before incision, the correct disk space is localized using anteroposterior and lateral fluoroscopy, and the skin is marked appropriately. The incision for this approach corridor is centered at this location and marked.

PROCEDURE

- **Figure 77-3:** Transperitoneal or retroperitoneal approaches may be used to access the L4-5 and L5-1 disk spaces. Both approaches may be performed via various incisions, including midline, paramedian, and Pfannenstiel incisions. An approach from the left side is generally performed because gentle manual retraction of the aorta is more safely performed than retraction of the inferior vena cava. Most surgeons prefer to use the retroperitoneal mini-open approach because of lower rates of hollow viscus injury, retrograde ejaculation, and postoperative ileus. Final fluoroscopic confirmation of the correct disk level is mandatory when the anterior spine is visualized intraoperatively.

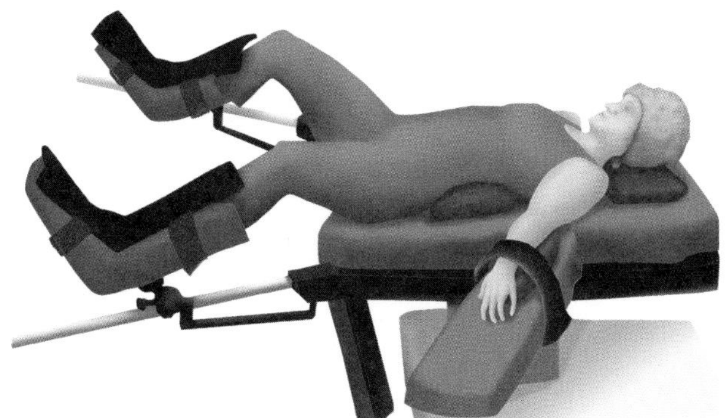

FIGURE 77-1

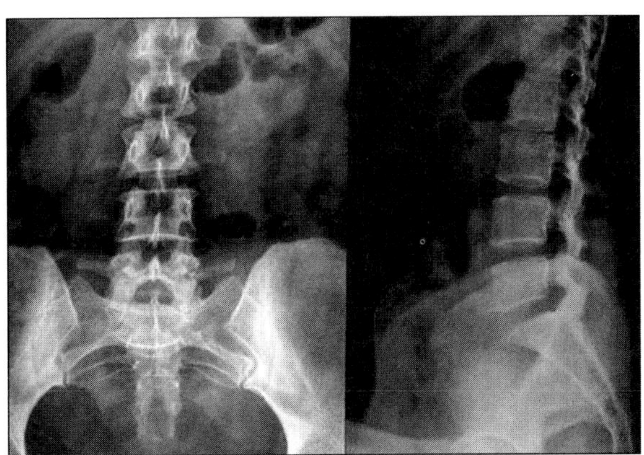

FIGURE 77-2

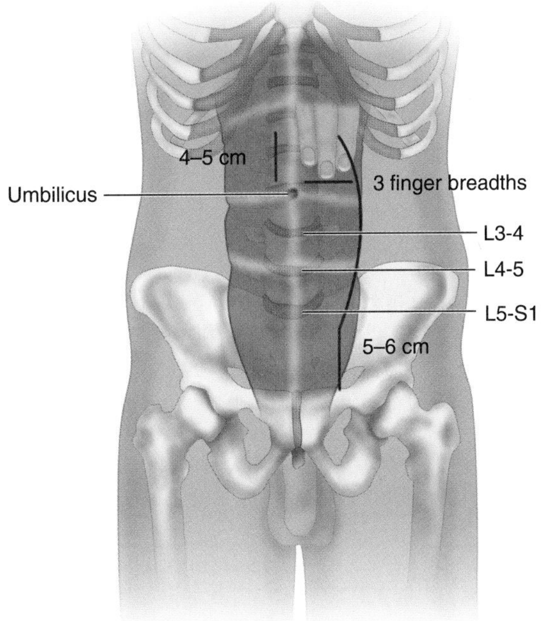

FIGUR7E 77-3

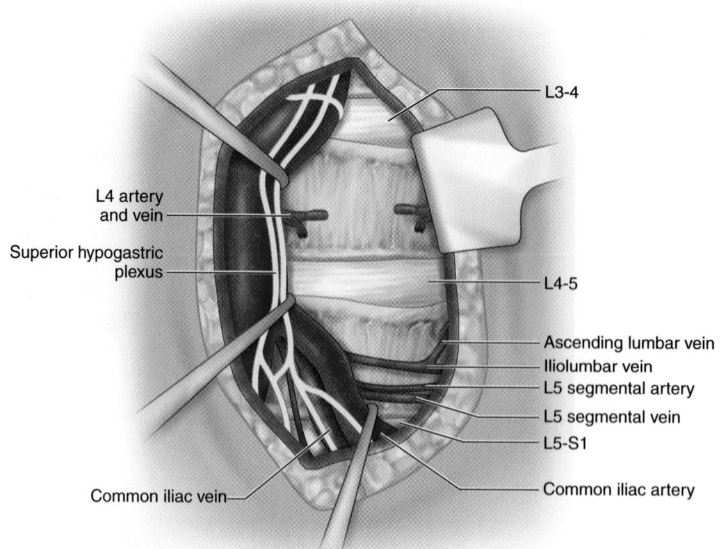

FIGURE 77-4

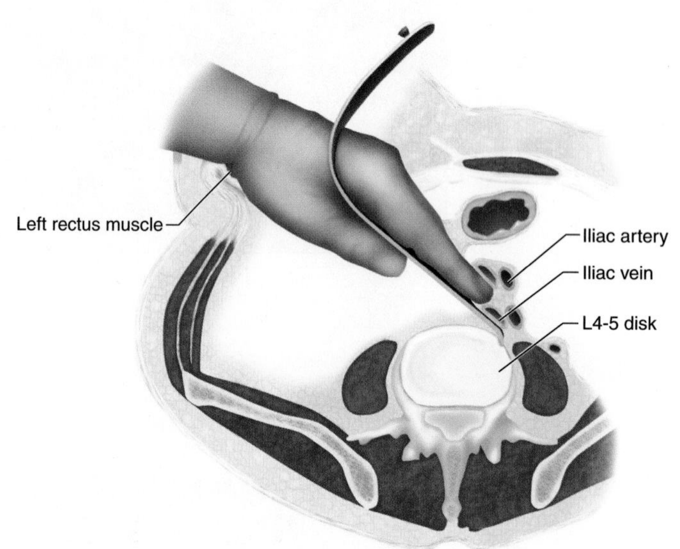

FIGURE 77-5

The anatomic midline is determined with anteroposterior fluoroscopy and marked with a screw above the disk to be removed.

- **Figure 77-4:** Prevertebral tissue at the L5-S1 level is opened using a vertical incision. Bipolar electrocautery is used exclusively; monopolar electrocautery is avoided at this level in an effort to spare injury to the autonomic nerves traversing this space. If these nerves are injured, impotence and infertility secondary to retrograde ejaculation in men may result. Mobilization of the large vessels is not commonly necessary at this level.
- **Figure 77-5:** At the L4-5 level, mobilization of the left iliac vessels from left to right is performed after identification and ligation of the iliolumbar vein. This vein enters the common iliac at this level, and avulsion at this anastomosis can lead to aggressive, unnecessary bleeding. Disk replacement devices typically require a large footprint for proper biomechanical function, contact with the outer bony vertebral rim (where

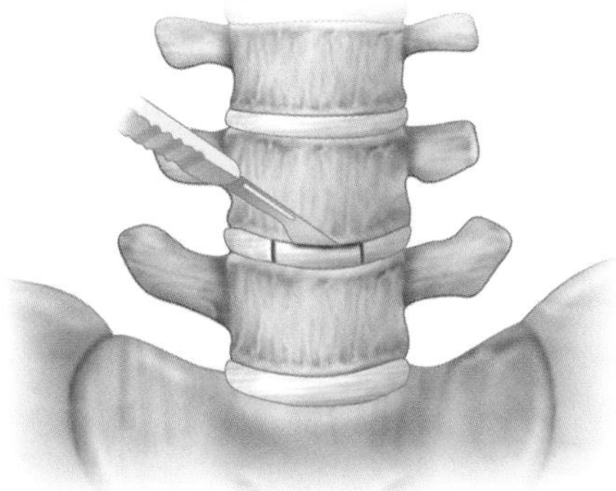

FIGURE 77-6

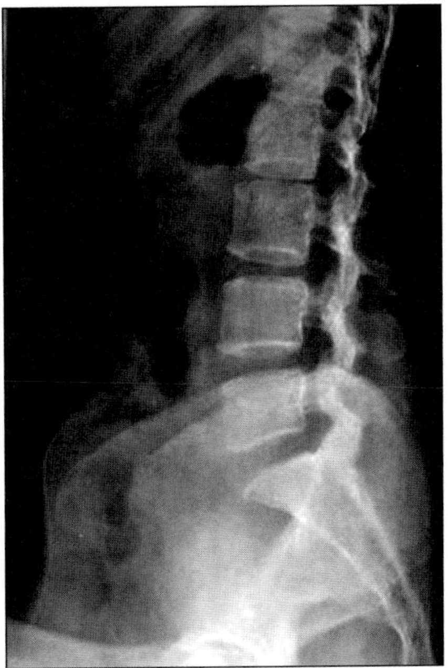

FIGURE 77-7

bone is stronger), and prevention of subsidence. Lateral vessel retraction is frequently necessary. This retraction can be achieved manually using vein retractors or with Hohmann retractors anchored into the vertebrae. Table-mounted retractors allow the surgeon to work without an assistant, and Kirschner wires drilled into the vertebral bodies can be used for gentle vessel retraction where more forceful retraction of the retroperitoneal structures is unnecessary.

- **Figure 77-6:** Incision of the anterior annulus of the disk is performed, taking care to leave the lateral annular walls intact. The nucleus pulposus and all disk tissues except for the lateral annular walls are completely removed. Both vertebral end plates are left intact. Careful attention is needed to ensure adequate removal and release of the posterior disk to allow parallel intervertebral distraction.
- The intervertebral disk height is restored by distracting the space with a central spreader and distracting chisels of graduated sizes.
- **Figure 77-7:** Optimal coverage of the cross-sectional area of the vertebral end plates is performed by placing various sizing templates within the disk space and confirming the appropriate fit with intraoperative fluoroscopy. Marking the center of the disk space can be useful to ensure proper centering of the implant because its position determines the instantaneous axis of rotation of that spinal segment.

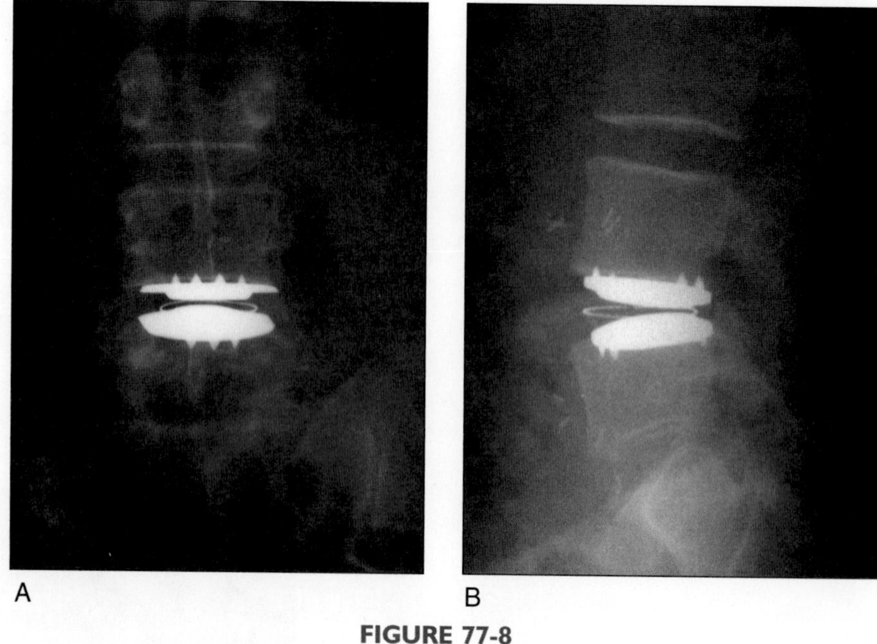

A B

FIGURE 77-8

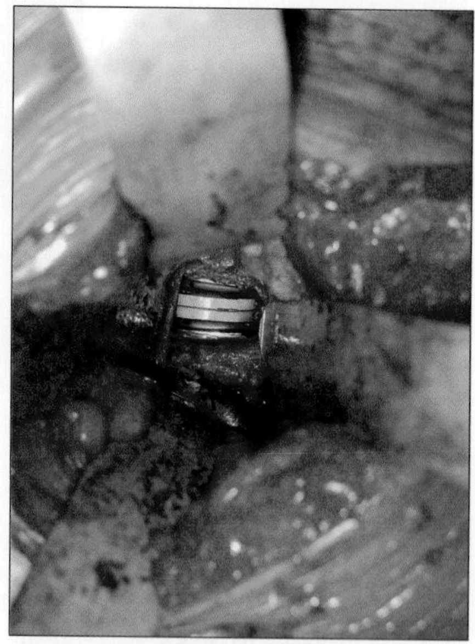

FIGURE 77-9

- **Figure 77-8:** The disk prosthesis is put into place. Most devices require use of a specialized chisel to crease end plate troughs to accommodate a stabilizing keel or teeth on the total disk replacement end plates. Careful attention is paid to positioning within the disk space. In the coronal plane (anteroposterior fluoroscopy) (**A**), it is centered in the midline, but in the sagittal plane (lateral fluoroscopy) (**B**), it is centered 2 mm posterior to midline. This location recapitulates the physiologic instantaneous axis of rotation throughout the flexion-extension arc of the normal disk as documented by Gertzbein and colleagues.
- Hemostasis is achieved, and the incision is closed in usual layered fashion.
- **Figure 77-9:** Photograph of LDA seen in Figure 77-8 in place in the patient.

TIPS FROM THE MASTERS

- Exposure of the lateral margins of the disk space is greater than that needed for anterior lumbar interbody fusion. It is useful to work with a vascular or exposure surgeon who can obtain this lateral dissection of the major vessels safely.
- Consent should be obtained in every case for the possibility of intraoperative conversion to a fusion procedure if prosthesis fit or bone quality is found to be suboptimal.
- A bowel preparation should be employed before surgery to make exposure easier and reduce constipation postoperatively.
- The largest prosthesis that can be accommodated should be used to improve disk mechanics and reduce the risk of subsidence.
- Hybrid constructs (L5-S1 anterior lumbar interbody fusion and L4-5 total disk replacement) can be used to treat two-level disease if it is undesirable to perform a two-level LDA.

PITFALLS

Avoid overdistraction of the disk space because this can lead to postoperative sciatic pain.

In patients in whom a previous laminotomy or microdiskectomy has been performed at the index level, exacerbation of sciatic pain can occur during disk mobilization, but this is typically transient.

Patients with facet joint arthrosis should not undergo LDA. Arthrosis can be identified by high T2 signal on axial MRI, test injections into the joints, or single photon emission computed tomography nuclear medicine scans.

BAILOUT OPTIONS

- In rare cases where placement of the disk prosthesis is impossible after disk removal, either anterior or posterior interbody fusion may be necessary.

SUGGESTED READINGS

Brau SA. Mini-open approach to the spine for anterior lumbar interbody fusion: description of the procedure, results and complications. Spine J 2002;2:216–23.

Burkus JK, Gornet MF, Schuler TC, et al. Six-year outcomes of anterior lumbar interbody arthrodesis with use of interbody fusion cages and recombinant human bone morphogenetic protein-2. J Bone Joint Surg Am 2009;91:1181–9.

Gazzeri R, Tamorri M, Galarza M, et al. Balloon-assisted endoscopic retroperitoneal gasless approach (BERG) for lumbar interbody fusion: is it a valid alternative to the laparoscopic approach? Minim Invasive Neurosurg 2007;50:150–4.

Gertzbein SD, Seligman J, Holtby R, et al. Centrode characteristics of the lumbar spine as a function of segmental instability. Clin Orthop Rel Res 1986;(208):48–51.

Madan SS, Boeree NR. Comparison of instrumented anterior interbody fusion with instrumented circumferential lumbar fusion. Eur Spine J 2003;12:567–75.

Min JH, Jang JS, Lee SH. Comparison of anterior- and posterior-approach instrumented lumbar interbody fusion for spondylolisthesis. J Neurosurg Spine 2007;7:21–6.

Procedure 78 Pelvic Fixation

Neil Badlani, R. Todd Allen

PROCEDURE NOTES

Fusion to the pelvis in spine surgery can be difficult because of the complex anatomy of the lumbosacral region, the decreased bone density of the sacrum, and the large biomechanical stress placed on fixation at this transitional zone between the mobile lumbar spine and the far less mobile sacrum. Nevertheless, rigid fixation to the pelvis is crucial in many situations, particularly when maintaining sagittal alignment, and minimizing the risk of pseudarthrosis and hardware failure is of utmost importance.

Pelvic fixation has evolved over the years from its beginnings in the early 20th century with spinous process and sublaminar wiring to Harrington rods and hooks via sacral bars to the more recent Galveston technique, which first used the ilium for fixation. Although sacral pedicle screws are becoming more commonplace, the workhorses of spinopelvic fixation are iliac screws and bolts, which are the focus of this chapter. These principles of fixation and fixation techniques can also be used in sacropelvic trauma.

Several biomechanical studies have shown that sacral pedicle screws alone, such as those at S1 and S2, are prone to failure under less load than when they are used in combination with additional pelvic fixation, the most effective being the iliac bolt. It has been shown that the addition of iliac screws resulted in the most significant decrease in the strain on S1 screws and significantly increased the load to failure compared with several other methods of pelvic fixation, such as any other point of additional fixation, including multiple sacral pedicle screws.

INDICATIONS

- Long segment fusions to the sacrum, particularly in patients prone to L5-S1 pseudarthrosis, such as patients with global or lumbar sagittal imbalance or bony deficiency
- Degeneration caudad to long segment fusions
- High-grade spondylolisthesis
- Correction of pelvic obliquity
- Correction of flat back syndrome requiring osteotomy

CONTRAINDICATIONS

- There are no absolute contraindications, but there are relative contraindications such as:
  - Previously harvested iliac crest bone graft, because this can make fixation more difficult
  - Severe osteoporosis
  - Prior nonunion or malunion of an iliac fracture, which can alter the anatomy and reduce the quality of bone for fixation

PLANNING AND POSITIONING

- **Figure 78-1:** Positioning is standard for surgery on the lumbar spine through a posterior midline approach. The patient is placed prone on a Jackson table.
- When the patient is positioned, adding a slight relative kyphosis in the sagittal plane allows for better access to the structures of the lower lumbar spine and pelvis.

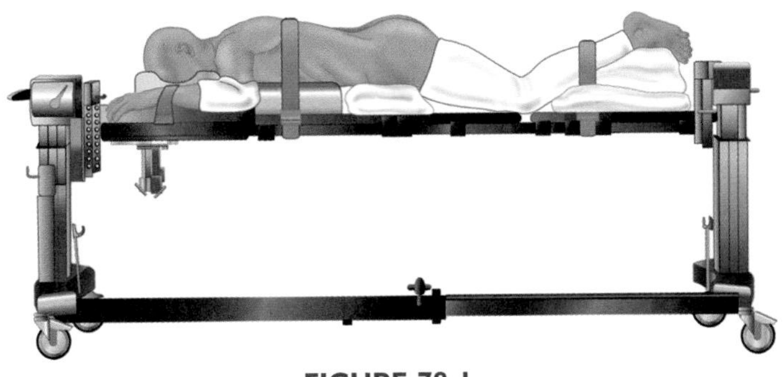

FIGURE 78-1

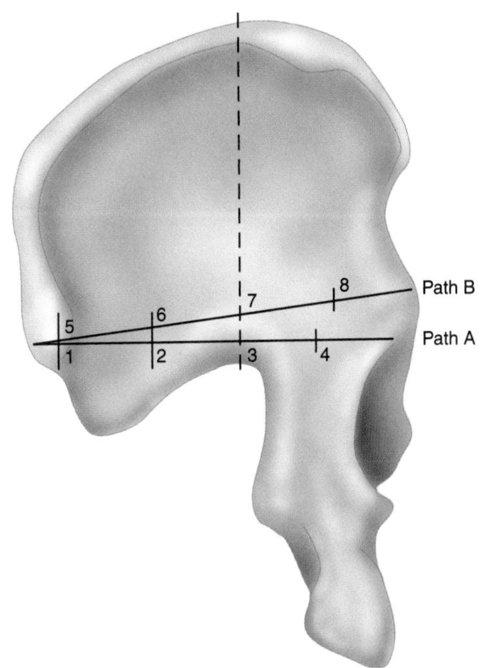

FIGURE 78-2

- Two different paths can be used for the trajectory of the iliac screws. The starting point for both is the posterior superior iliac spine (PSIS). The target for path A is the superior rim of the acetabulum, which places the hip joint at risk and is less desirable. Path B aims for the anterior inferior iliac spine (AIIS) and usually accommodates a longer screw and is safer.
- **Figure 78-2:** Paths in the pelvis for the trajectory of iliac screws.
- **Figure 78-3:** Cross section of the ilium at the level of the sciatic notch with paths indicated.
- **Figure 78-4:** Illustration of the iliac screw from the PSIS to AIIS.

PROCEDURE

- **Figure 78-5:** Palpate the PSIS, and if necessary confirm its position by intraoperative fluoroscopy. Dissect the subcutaneous tissue off this area to the level of the lumbosacral fascia. Incise the fascia over the PSIS in a longitudinal fashion, and expose the inner and outer tables of the ilium at this level using Cobb elevators and electrocautery.
- **Figure 78-6:** To prevent hardware prominence, remove a sufficient amount of bone over the PSIS with a rongeur or chisel to accommodate the screw head being used. This is usually 1 to 2 cm deep and places the starting point at or just below the level of the

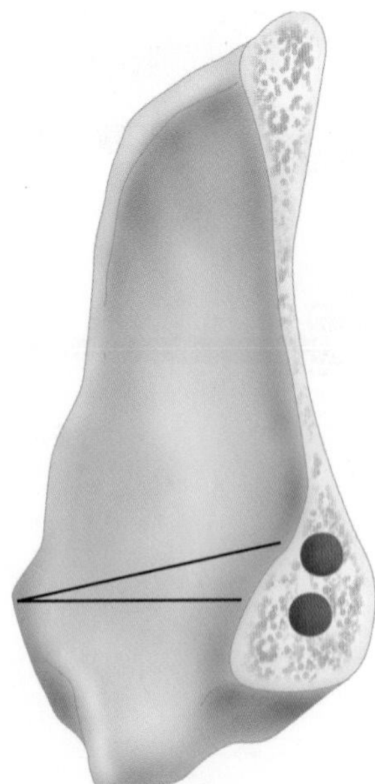

FIGURE 78-3

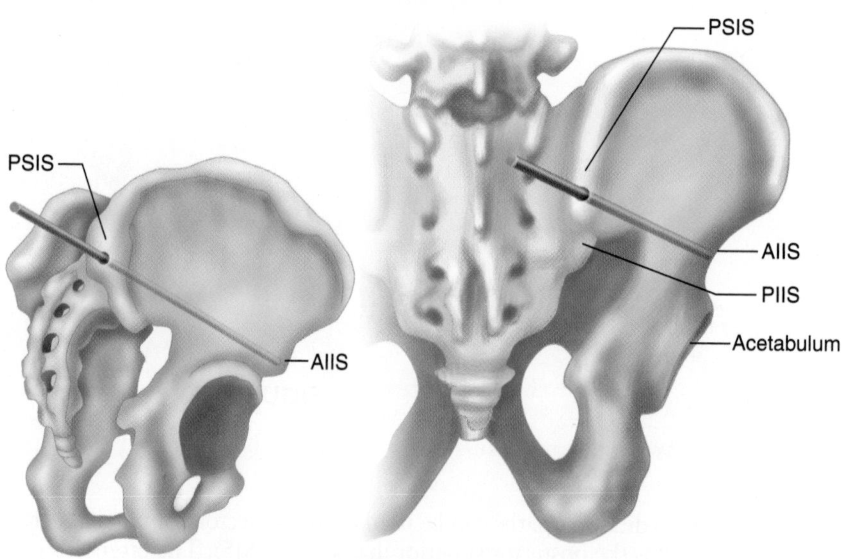

FIGURE 78-4

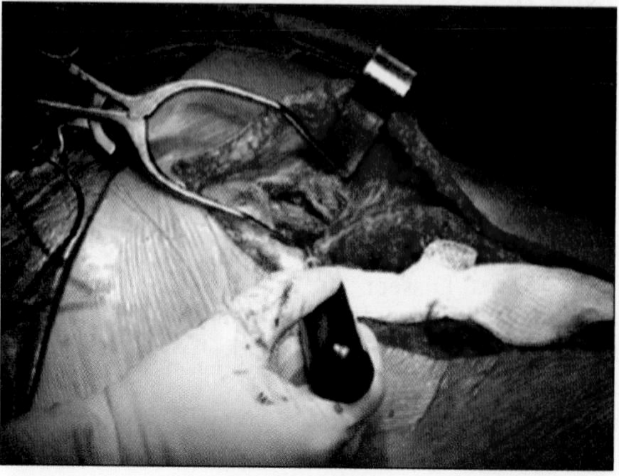

FIGURE 78-5

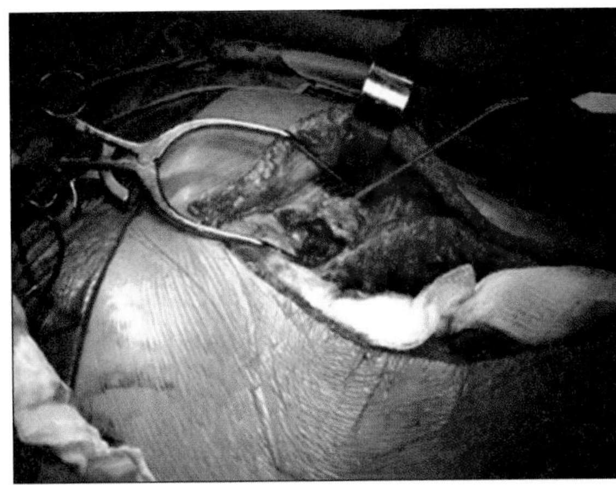

FIGURE 78-6

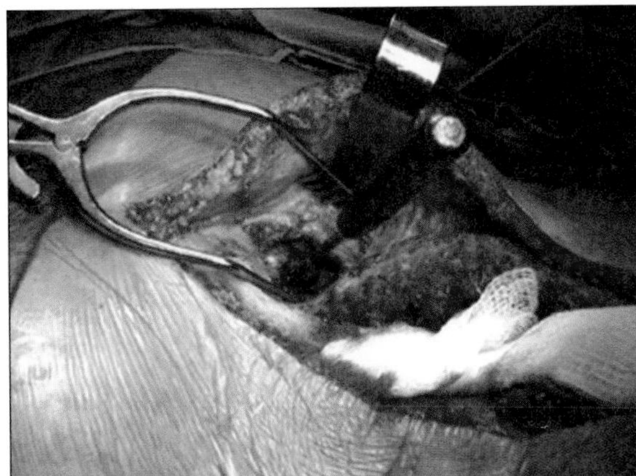

FIGURE 78-7

sacrum. Remove enough bone to accommodate the screw head and the connector that connects the screw to the longitudinal rod just anterior to the PSIS.

- **Figure 78-7:** Using a pedicle seeker, the path toward the AIIS is developed, typically aiming 25 degrees lateral from the midline and 30 degrees caudad. Fluoroscopy can aid in confirming this trajectory. The path of the screw is palpated with a ball-tipped probe to check carefully for breaches in the walls of the ilium.
- **Figure 78-8:** Screw length can be measured off the probe or during preoperative templating with axial cuts from the pelvic computed tomography (CT) scan. If necessary, the path is tapped and then the appropriate screw is placed. Typically, iliac screws measure at least 7.5 mm in diameter; we prefer to use screws 8.5 mm or greater.

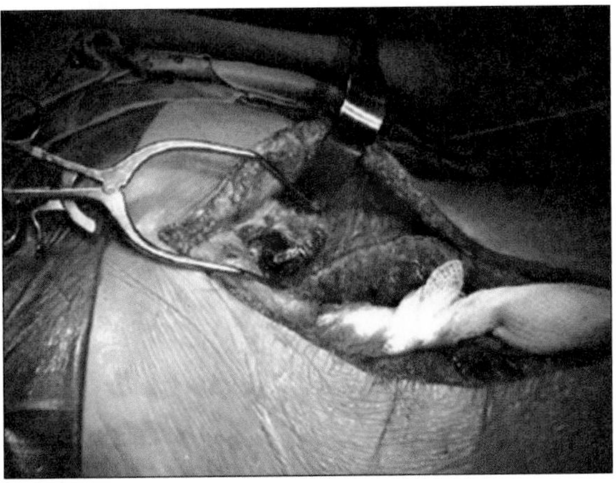

FIGURE 78-8

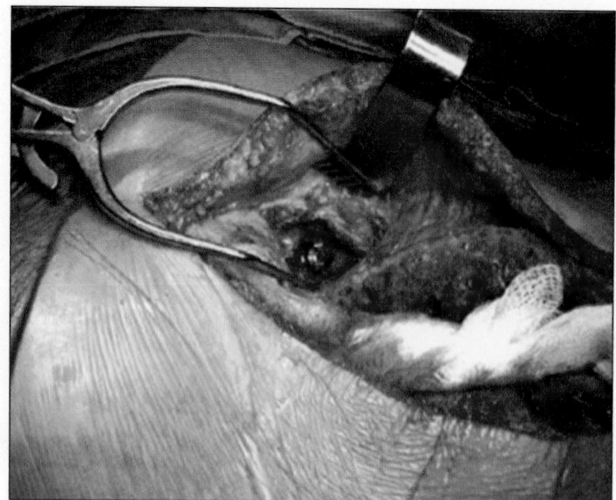

FIGURE 78-9

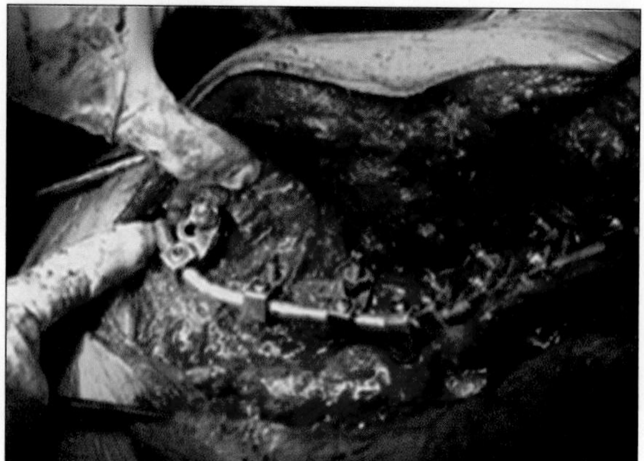

FIGURE 78-10

- **Figure 78-9:** The screw is carefully seated fully to decrease the chance of hardware prominence. The screw should be recessed more than the remaining bone anterior and posterior to the PSIS. The screw should be lined up as much as possible with more cephalad screws to facilitate ease of connection to the rod. Intraoperative fluoroscopy can be used to check proper screw placement and length.
- **Figure 78-10:** The screw is connected to the longitudinal rod using the necessary connectors. The modularity of most current systems allows relatively straightforward connection of these screws to longitudinal rods from the lumbar spine using monaxial or polyaxial connectors and offsets. Connection to the Depuy Isola system (Warsaw, IN) is depicted.
- **Figure 78-11:** Many systems are available for instrumentation of iliac screws and connection to lumbar rods. The Stryker Xia system (Kalamazoo, MI) is shown on a pelvic model.
- **Figure 78-12:** Illustration of the iliac screw as the distal anchor of the construct.

TIPS FROM THE MASTERS

- Iliac screws should be placed last, after all other pedicle screws and spinal instrumentation have been placed. Always be aware of screw alignment in longer constructs to ensure proper final screw length and height to allow connection with the cephalad screws.
- The safest trajectory for iliac screws is from the PSIS to the AIIS, and typically screws at least 80 mm can be placed to gain appropriate biomechanical advantage.

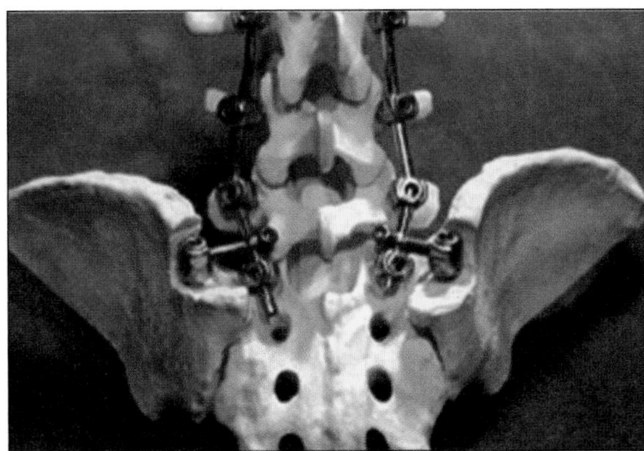

FIGURE 78-11

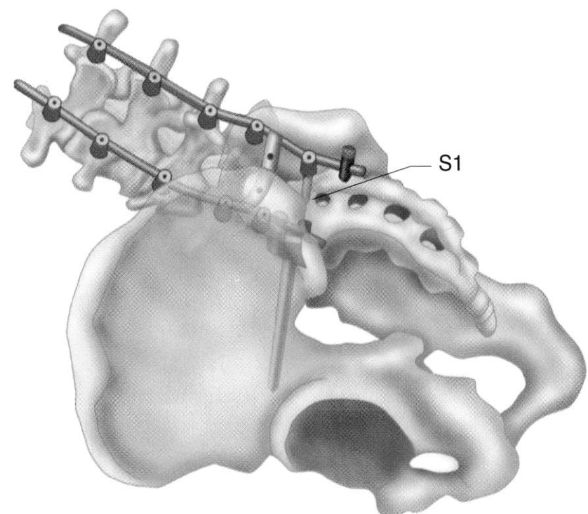

FIGURE 78-12

- If more anatomic reference is needed, expose the outer portion of the ilium to the sciatic notch before placing the screw. The notch can often be palpated with a 90-degree device.
- A subfascial approach to the PSIS provides for the easiest and most anatomic closure.
- The rod for the construct can be contoured outside the body, then placed initially to match the coronal plane curvature of the spine. In situ, the rod can be turned 90 degrees to correct the coronal plane curvature and recreate the normal lordosis of the sagittal plane.

PITFALLS

Extensive exposure is often required for this procedure, increasing the amount of blood loss and potentially the risk of infection compared with a procedure that does not extend to the pelvis.

Other pitfalls are as follows:

Vital structures in sciatic notch at risk for injury.

Acetabular violation.

Hardware prominence.

Screw loosening, indicated by development of hollows or the "windshield wiper" sign.

Rod connectivity can be difficult in longer screws if iliac screws are too far offset or of uneven height.

BAILOUT OPTIONS

- If the screws are loose, as in a revision case, it is better to replace them with bigger screws, such as 9.5-mm diameter, rather than longer screws, as shown by Akesen et al.
- In situations in which iliac crest has previously been harvested, an iliac screw on that side often has poor bite. It is still recommended to place a unilateral screw on the contralateral side because Tomlinson et al have shown that little difference exists in construct stiffness and lumbosacral motion between unilateral and bilateral iliac screws when screw length is at least 80 mm.

SUGGESTED READINGS

Akesen B, Wu C, Mehbod AA, et al. Revision of loosened iliac screws: a biomechanical study of longer and bigger screws. Spine (Phila Pa 1976) 2008;33:1423–8.

Gitelman A, Joseph Jr SA, Carrion W, et al. Results and morbidity in a consecutive series of patients undergoing spinal fusion with iliac screws for neuromuscular scoliosis. Orthopedics 2008;31(12).

Lebwohl N, Cunnighman B, Dmitriev A, et al. Biomechanical comparison of lumbosacral fixation techniques in a calf spine model. Spine (Phila Pa 1976) 2002;27:2312–20.

Peelle MW, Lenke LG, Bridwell KH, et al. Comparison of pelvic fixation techniques in neuromuscular spinal deformity correction: Galveston rod versus iliac and lumbosacral screws. Spine (Phila Pa 1976) 2006;31:2392–8.

Phillips JH, Gutheil JP, Knapp DR Jr. Iliac screw fixation in neuromuscular scoliosis. Spine 2007;32:1566–70.

Tomlinson T, Chen J, Upasani V, et al. Unilateral and bilateral sacropelvic fixation result in similar construct biomechanics. Spine (Phila Pa 1976) 2008;33:2127–33.

Tsuchiya K, Bridwell KH, Kuklo TR, et al. Minimum 5-year analysis of L5-S1 fusion using sacropelvic fixation (bilateral S1 and iliac screws) for spinal deformity. Spine (Phila Pa 1976) 2006;31:303–8.

Tumialán LM, Mummaneni PV. Long-segment spinal fixation using pelvic screws. Neurosurgery 2008;63 (3 Suppl):183–90.

Wang MY, Ludwig SC, Anderson DG, et al. Percutaneous iliac screw placement: description of a new minimally invasive technique. Neurosurg Focus 2008;25:E17.

Figures 78-8 through 78-11 are modified with permission from Moshirfar A, Rand F, Sponseller P, et al. Pelvic fixation in spine surgery: historical overview, indications, biomechanical relevance, and current techniques. J Bone Joint Surg Am 2005;87:89–106.

Procedure 79

Partial Sacrectomy

Mike Yue Chen, Julio Garcia-Aguilar

INDICATIONS

- Primary sacral tumors, many of which benefit from en bloc removal
- Locally advanced rectal cancer with sacral involvement, for which pelvic exenteration is indicated
- Nonunion of symptomatic sacral fracture

CONTRAINDICATIONS

- Patients with rectal cancer involving the sacrum must have the fat plane medial to the internal obturator preserved to be candidates for resection.
- Involvement of the S1 pedicles requires a total sacrectomy with extensive instrumented reconstruction.

PLANNING AND POSITIONING

- We prefer the prone position, but a lateral position can be used when simultaneous anterior and posterior approaches are performed.
- For the prone position, legs should be flexed at the hip and thighs should be abducted to allow for maximum exposure.

PROCEDURE

- **Figure 79-1:** Sacrectomies are often performed for pelvic tumors that extend into the sacrum. Frequently, the initial step in these operations is to use an anterior approach to dissect the tumor and associated viscera away from anterior and lateral margins. The anterior approach allows identification and ligation of the internal iliac arteries that supply the gluteal vessels, which can cause significant bleeding during dissection of the lateral sacral margin.
- **Figure 79-2:** Incision type is dictated by the need for margins. For cancer operations in which a margin is desirable, an incision that splits into a fork around the region of the interest is used. Alternatively, a midline incision can be used when margins are not required.

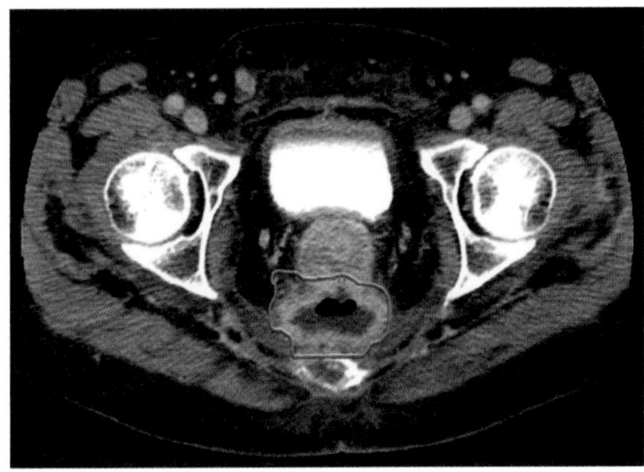

FIGURE 79-1

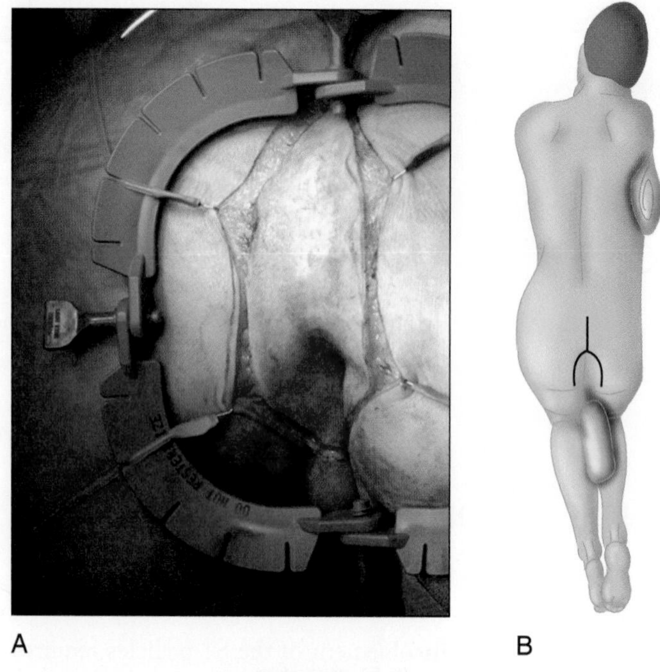

A B

FIGURE 79-2

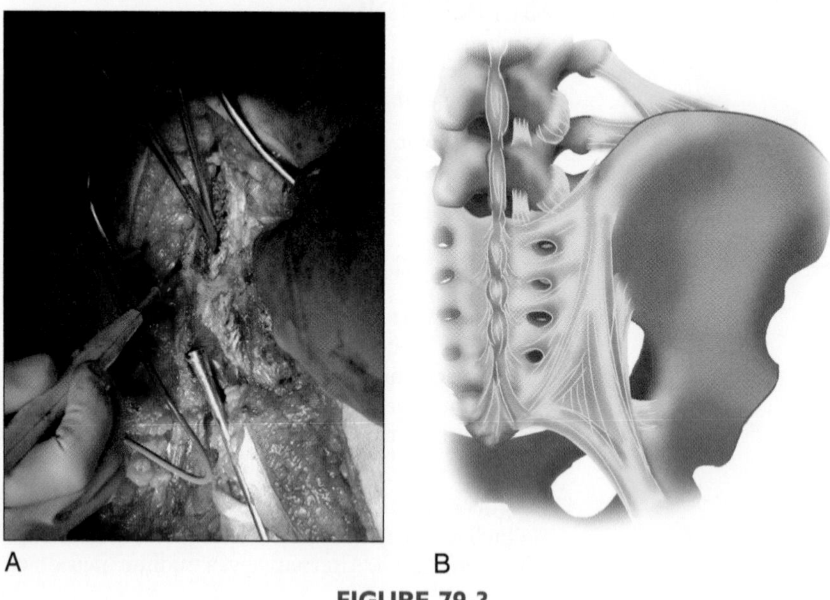

A B

FIGURE 79-3

- **Figure 79-3:** Paraspinous musculature along with the sacrotuberous and sacroiliac ligaments is reflected laterally exposing the posterior aspect of the sacrum.
- **Figure 79-4:** After exposure of the bony sacrum, count dorsal foramina starting from the hiatus to find the level at the upper margin of resection. Preoperative imaging should be used to confirm the number of foramina, which is normally four (S1-4) excluding the hiatus.
- **Figure 79-5:** Perform a sacral laminectomy starting at the dorsal foramina and working medially. Expose about 1.5 cm of the floor of the sacral canal so that you have adequate working space to perform the vertebrectomy and to ligate traversing nerves easily. Remove enough of the lamina around the dorsal foramina to follow the exiting nerve to the ventral foramen at the upper margin of resection.

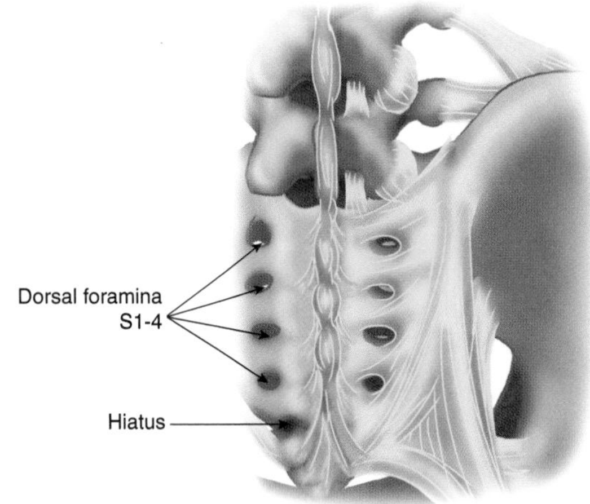

FIGURE 79-4

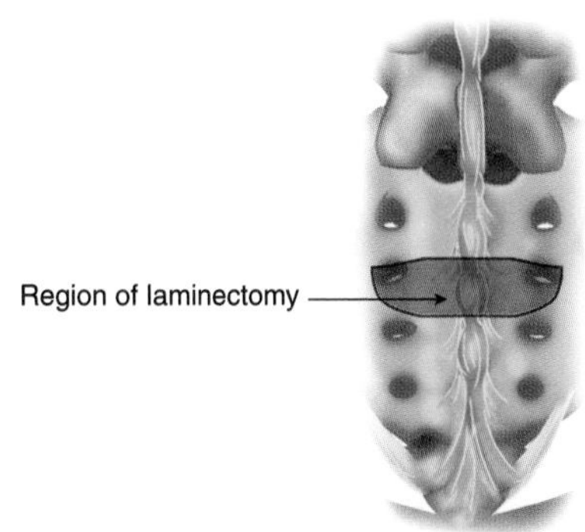

FIGURE 79-5

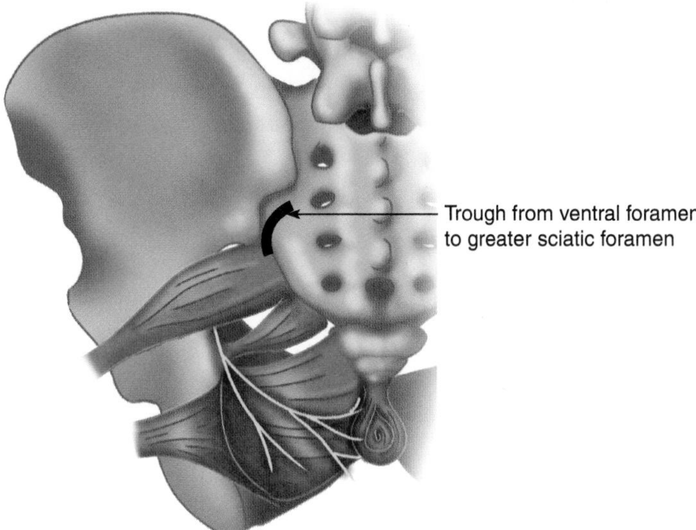

FIGURE 79-6

- **Figure 79-6:** Drill away bone lateral to the ventral foramen forming a trough to connect the ventral foramen to the medial superior angle of the greater sciatic foramen just inferior to the inferiormost part of the sacroiliac joint. Placing a No. 4 Penfield between the nerve and the bone is helpful, especially if the iliac vessels are still patent.
- **Figure 79-7:** Connect the ventral foramina in the midline by drilling from lateral to medial through the vertebral body. An osteotome can be used as well. Carefully cut the anterior longitudinal ligament.

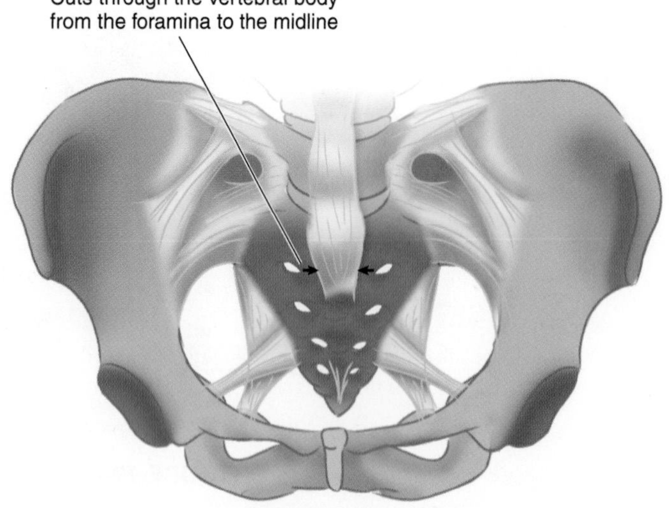

FIGURE 79-7

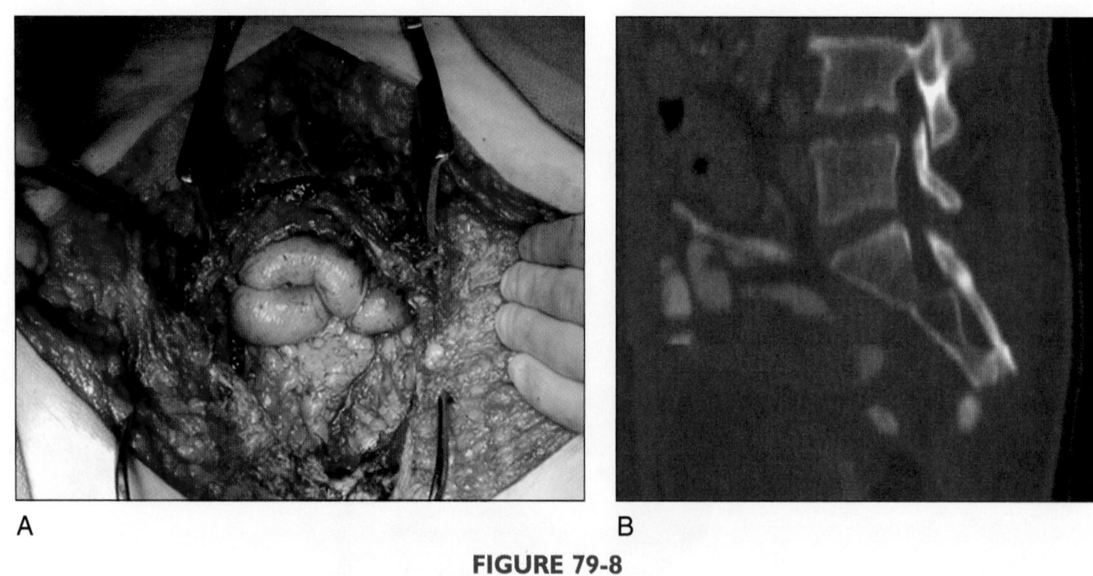

FIGURE 79-8

- **Figure 79-8:** *Left*, Exposure after radical resection of rectal cancer involving the sacrum. *Right*, Postoperative computed tomography (CT) scan shows resection of the sacrum below the S3 pedicle.

TIPS FROM THE MASTERS

- A preoperative CT scan of the sacrum with sagittal reconstruction can be obtained to indicate the superior extent of resection for planning purposes.
- Connecting the ventral foramina in the midline and forming a trough laterally to the junction of the sacroiliac is the simplest method to visualize and preserve the exiting nerve. The pedicles are not resected, however.
- To resect the entire vertebral body, perform the same exposure, but drill away the pedicle that is immediately superior to the exiting nerve until the anterior ligament is visualized. Then proceed laterally and medially as discussed.
- For surgeons unfamiliar with the surgical anatomy of this region, neuromonitoring is helpful for identifying structures anterolateral to the sacrum.
- A gluteus myocutaneous flap can be used to close large defects.

PITFALLS

Preserve at least one S2 nerve root for continence. Preservation of S3 roots ensures continence.

Avoid sciatic nerve injury by remaining medial to the sacroiliac joint during bony resection.

The superior gluteal artery exits the greater sacral foramen near the inferior portion of the sacroiliac joint. If the internal iliac is patent, care must be taken to avoid injuring this vessel or to identify and ligate it.

Incontinence from this operation can result from damage to the pudendal nerves during lateral soft tissue dissection.

Wound healing is often a problem. Meticulous closure is advised.

BAILOUT OPTIONS

- Complex reconstruction of the sacrum for stability is necessary if the S1 pedicles are compromised.
- We prefer creating a trough in the bone using a drill and Kerrison punches because this technique enhances visualization. Alternatively, osteotomes can be used.

SUGGESTED READINGS

Dickey ID, Hugate RR Jr, Fuchs B, et al. Reconstruction after total sacrectomy: early experience with a new surgical technique. Clin Orthop Relat Res 2005;438:42–50.

Guo Y, Palmer JL, Shen L, et al. Bowel and bladder continence, wound healing, and functional outcomes in patients who underwent sacrectomy. J Neurosurg Spine 2005;3:106–10.

Hugate RR Jr, Dickey ID, Phimolsarnti R, et al. Mechanical effects of partial sacrectomy: when is reconstruction necessary? Clin Orthop Relat Res 2006;450:82–8.

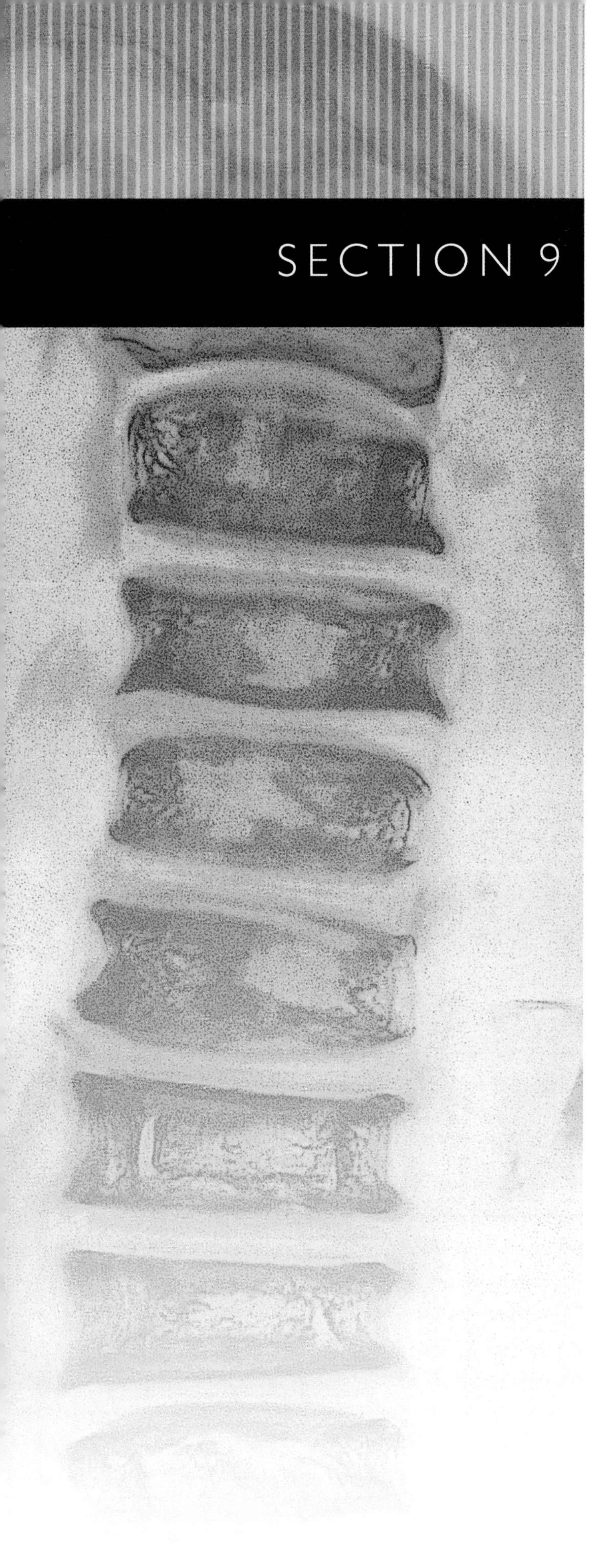

SECTION 9 Minimally Invasive Spine

SECTION EDITOR — ALFRED OGDEN

Procedure 80

Minimally Invasive C1-2 Fusion

Sathish Subbaiah, Richard G. Fessler

INDICATIONS

- Approximately 50% of the normal rotation of the cervical spine occurs at the atlantoaxial motion segment. Factors that lead to instability at the atlantoaxial junction include traumatic injury to the axis or atlas and traumatic ligamentous injury. Other pathologic processes that lead to instability at C1-2 include inflammatory conditions such as rheumatoid arthritis, congenital lesions, malignancy, and severe osteoarthritis. Because of the high degree of motion at this level, rigid internal fixation provides the most stable construct to facilitate bony fusion.

CONTRAINDICATIONS

- Absolute contraindications for surgery are related to the medical condition of the patient. The patient must be stabilized after a traumatic injury, and any coagulopathy must be corrected before proceeding with surgery.
- Preoperative imaging (computed tomography [CT] angiography) with careful attention to the bony and vascular anatomy must be reviewed. Large, tortuous, medially directed vertebral artery anatomy may preclude placement of C2 pars screws on one or both sides.

PLANNING AND POSITIONING

- After a detailed history and physical examination are completed, imaging is reviewed. Plain x-rays of the cervical spine are reviewed to evaluate for fractures or malalignment of the cervical spine.
- CT angiography of the cervical spine adds further detailed information regarding the bony integrity of C1 and C2 and vascular anatomy.
- For detailed soft tissue anatomy, magnetic resonance imaging (MRI) or magnetic resonance angiography is essential to visualize any compressive elements against the spinal cord. Analysis of MRI can also help delineate the severity of the ligamentous injury.
- Intraoperative monitoring with somatosensory evoked potentials and motor evoked potentials is often used in surgery of the upper cervical spine to identify any reversible injury to the spinal cord.
- **Figure 80-1:** The patient is placed in a Mayfield head holder while supine and is carefully rotated into the prone position on two chest rolls. Care is taken to allow for sufficient space between the patient's chin and the operative table. All dependent pressure points are carefully padded. The shoulders can be retracted with tape as needed to visualize anatomy better on fluoroscopy if necessary. Lateral

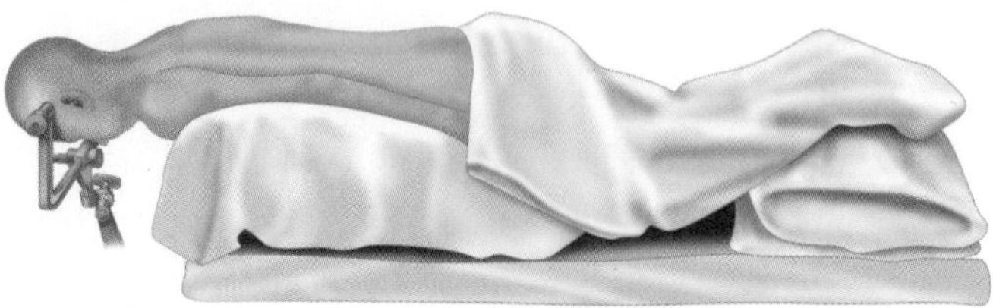

FIGURE 80-1

fluoroscopy is used to evaluate alignment of the C1-2 motion segment and to evaluate the need for any reduction. A metal indicator is placed lateral to the cervical spine to identify the correct level and angle of approach. The midline cervical spine is palpated at C2 and C7 and marked. The incision is 2.5 cm lateral to the midline and 3 cm in length.

- Preoperative antibiotics are administered before the incision, and stockings with compressive boots are placed for deep vein thrombosis prophylaxis. The patient is prepared from occiput to T1 and draped in a sterile fashion.

PROCEDURE

- **Figure 80-2:** After subcutaneous injection of the skin with local anesthetic and epinephrine, an incision is made. Bipolar cautery is used to achieve hemostasis, and monopolar cautery is used to carry the incision down to the level of the fascia. The fascia is incised with a monopolar cautery under direct vision the length of the incision. The smallest dilator is used to spread the paraspinal musculature gently. The dilator is manipulated so that it is always perpendicular to the incision and not angled medially in any way. The dilator is advanced until it rests on the lateral mass of C2.
- **Figure 80-3:** Serial dilators are sequentially placed over the initial dilator, finishing with the final dilator.
- **Figure 80-4:** Retractor is attached to the bed with the articulated arm in a manner that does not interfere with fluoroscopic images. The retractor is carefully expanded and flared open to visualize adequately from the C1 lateral mass to the C2-3 facet joint.

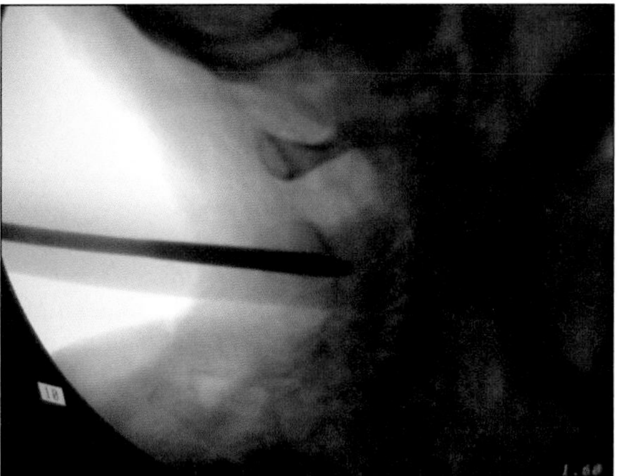

FIGURE 80-2

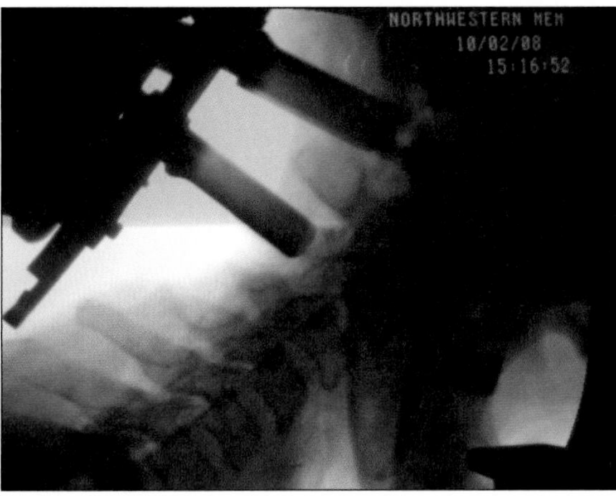

FIGURE 80-3

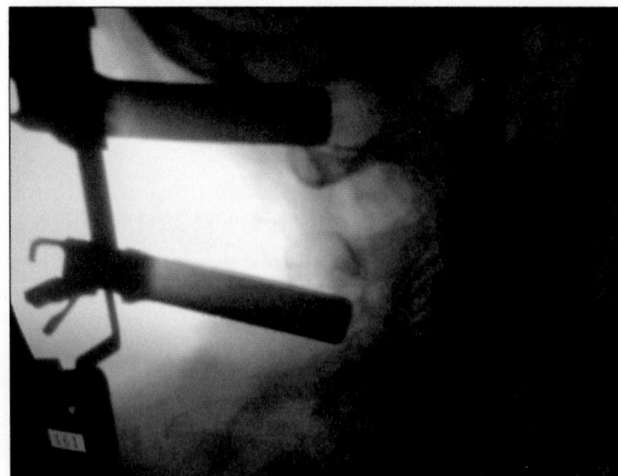

FIGURE 80-4

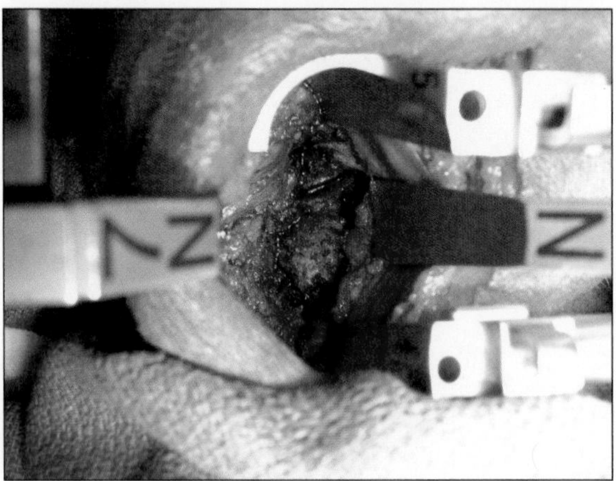

FIGURE 80-5

- **Figure 80-5:** Through the use of monopolar cautery and blunt periosteal dissectors, the C1 arch, C1 inferior lamina, and C2 lamina are exposed. The C1-2 facet joint is exposed with the use of bipolar cautery of the dense venous plexus that lies above. The C2 nerve root can be preserved and mobilized caudally. Anatomic landmarks are now clearly visualized for placement of the C1 lateral mass and C2 pars screws.
- **Figure 80-6:** A Kerrison rongeur is used to perform a small C2 laminotomy to identify the medial border of the C2 isthmus clearly. A nerve hook is placed to mark this medial border during screw placement. The entry point for the C2 screw, the midpoint of the cranial and medial quadrant of the C2 isthmus surface, is marked with a high-speed

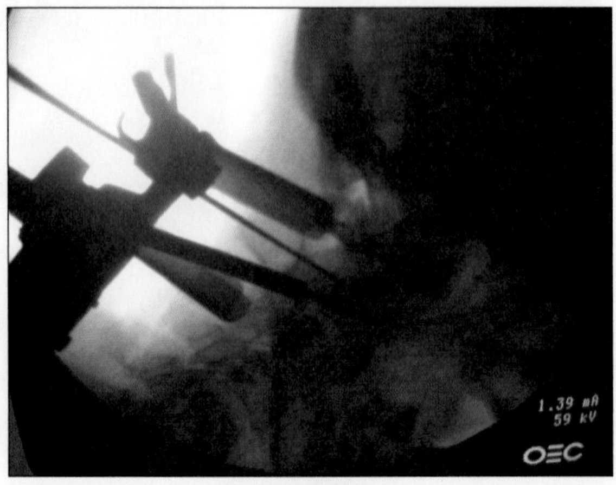

FIGURE 80-6

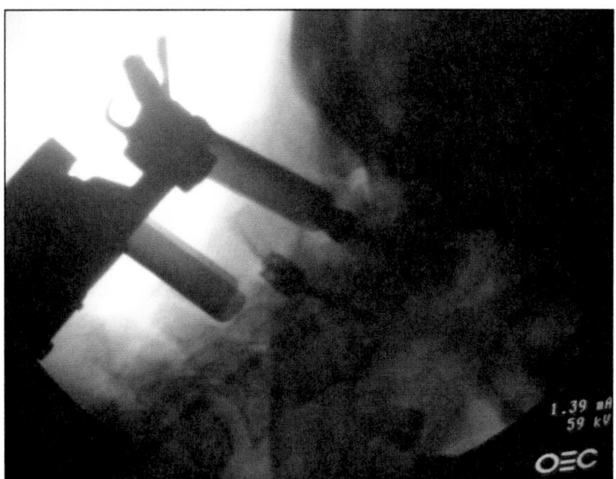

FIGURE 80-7

drill. The screw trajectory is 20 to 30 degrees medial and caudal. The pilot hole is formed with a 2-mm drill bit under live fluoroscopic guidance to visualize the superior surface of the C2 isthmus. The hole is tapped and probed to verify bony integrity, and a 3.5-mm polyaxial screw of appropriate length is inserted.

- **Figure 80-7:** For placement of C1 screws, a No. 4 Penfield dissector is positioned directly above the C1 lamina to protect the vertebral artery as it courses above. A second instrument, such as a nerve hook, is positioned at the medial border of the C1 lateral mass to protect and identify the dura and spinal cord. The entry point of the C1 screw, the junction of the posterior arch of C1 and the midpoint of the C1 lateral mass, is marked with a high-speed drill. Alternatively, if the patient possesses a large overlying C1 arch, the entry point of the C1 screw can be in the medial to lateral midpoint of the C1 lateral mass and 2 mm below the superior roof of the arch of C1. The vertebral artery is again protected by the placement of a No. 4 Penfield dissector between the vertebral artery and the roof of C1. This entry point can be beneficial in preventing the copious bleeding that often occurs during the exposure of the C1 lateral mass.
- **Figure 80-8:** The drill, tap, and screw are angled 10 to 15 degrees medially and targeted toward the anterior tubercle of C1 under lateral fluoroscopic guidance. Polyaxial 3.5-mm screws with unthreaded proximal shafts are placed to the appropriate depth.
- **Figure 80-9:** For optimal fusion of the C1-2 motion segment, the C1-2 facet joint, lamina of C1, and lamina and spinous process of C2 are aggressively decorticated with a high-speed drill. Allograft or autograft bone chips can be placed to aid in the fusion as well. Hemostasis is achieved with bipolar cautery, and a Hemovac drain is placed if necessary. The tubular retractor is carefully removed under direct visualization, and any bleeding is coagulated.

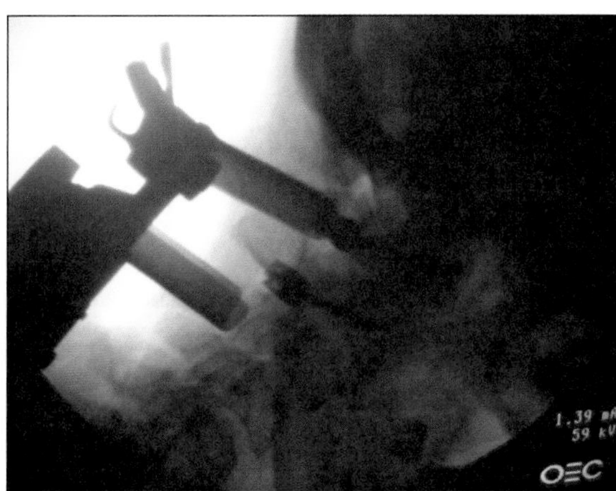

FIGURE 80-8

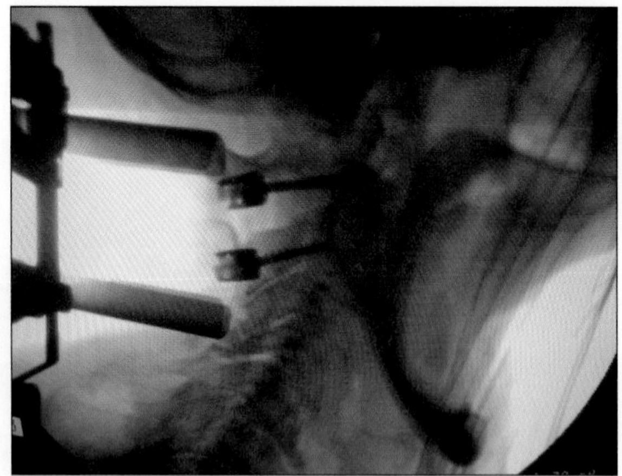

FIGURE 80-9

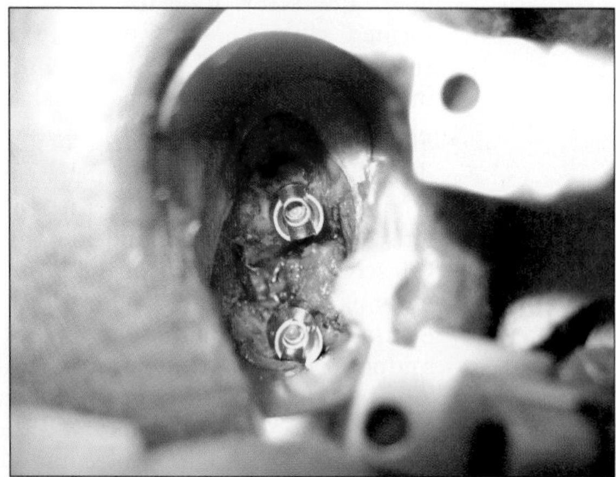

FIGURE 80-10

- **Figure 80-10:** Further reduction of the C1 and C2 segment can be performed. The rod is secured into polyaxial screw heads.
- **Figure 80-11:** The wound is copiously irrigated, hemostasis is achieved, and the tubular retractors are carefully removed paying attention to coagulate any bleeding during this process. The incision is closed in multiple layers, and the skin is closed with Dermabond (Ethicon, Langhorne, PA). This procedure is repeated on the contralateral side.

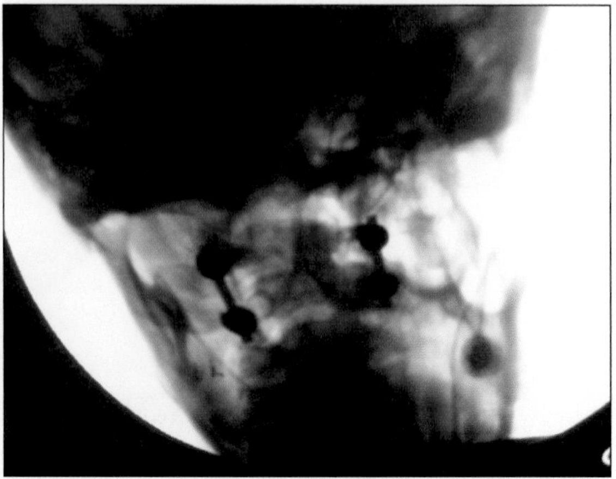

FIGURE 80-11

TIPS FROM THE MASTERS

- Precise review of the relationship of the bony and vascular anatomy on preoperative CT angiography aids in the placement of C2 pars screws. In some rare cases, this can lead to the preoperative decision not to attempt instrumentation on one side.
- The minimally invasive approach has many significant advantages over the open approach. Most importantly, it allows for preservation of the posterior tension band and prevents devascularization of posterior paraspinal musculature—both considered to be important in maintaining natural cervical lordosis.
- To facilitate the trajectory of C1 lateral mass screw placement, the adjacent posterior arch of C1 can be drilled down. Also, the C1 anterior tubercle is the anteriormost extent of the C1 anterior arch; C1 should be placed no farther than the C2 anterior tubercle.
- The minimally invasive approach also allows for potential decreased blood loss, hospital stay, and infectious risk and can possibly lead to decreased postoperative neck pain as has been seen in other posterior cervical minimally invasive approaches.
- In certain patients, a midline incision can be performed, and the subcutaneous tissue is undermined. The incision can be mobilized laterally over the facial entry site 2.5 cm lateral to the midline. The procedure can be carried out as described, and the skin incision subsequently can be mobilized to perform the procedure on the contralateral side.

PITFALLS

A Kirschner wire is not used in this procedure. It is important to open the dorsal fascia under direct vision and begin retraction with smallest dilator—spreading the muscles vertically along the direction of the fibers until the bony C2 lateral mass is encountered. It is crucial not to angle the dilator medially to prevent inadvertent entry of the dilator into the interlaminar space.

If brisk arterial bleeding is encountered after drilling the C2 pars, it is important to proceed with the screw placement on that side. Placement of the C2 pars screw is not recommended on the contralateral side, and a C2 translaminar screw can be placed. Cerebral angiography and brain MRI should be performed after the surgery is complete to evaluate for injury to the vertebral artery.

If a cerebrospinal fluid leak is encountered during the placement of either the C1 or the C2 screw, the operative microscope can be brought into the field to attempt a primary closure of the tear.

BAILOUT OPTION

- If multiple attempts of placement of instrumentation do not achieve adequate screw placement or stability, the procedure can be converted to the open interspinous fusion technique of Dickman and Sonntag. Alternatively, C1 lateral mass screws can be connected to C2 laminar screws. Rigid external fixation can also be used to augment atlantoaxial fusion.

SUGGESTED READINGS

Harms J, Melcher RP. Posterior C1-C2 fusion with polyaxial screw and rod fixation. Spine (Phila Pa 1976) 2001;26:2467–71.

Joseffer S, Post N, Cooper PR, et al. Minimally invasive atlantoaxial fixation with polyaxial screw-rod construct: technical case report. Neurosurgery 2006;58(4 Suppl. 2):ONS-E375.

Menedez JA, Wright NM. Techniques of posterior C1-C2 stabilization. Neurosurgery 2007;S1:103–11.

Payer M, Luzi M, Tessitore E. Posterior atlanto-axial fixation with polyaxial C1 lateral mass screws and C2 pars screws. Acta Neurochir 2009;151:223–9.

Santiago P, Fessler RG. Minimally invasive surgery for the management of cervical spondylosis. Neurosurgery 2007;60(1 Suppl. 1):S160–5.

Procedure 81 Lumbar Microdiskectomy

Omar N. Syed, Michael G. Kaiser

INDICATIONS

- Appropriate patient selection is an essential element when planning spine surgery to optimize patient outcome. The decision to pursue surgery is based on the history, physical examination, and radiographic findings. Radiographic evidence of a disk herniation in the absence of corresponding clinical signs or symptoms is insufficient to warrant operative intervention.
- Radiculopathy that is secondary to compression of neural structures by a herniated disk and unresponsive to a trial of conservative therapy is the primary indication for performing a lumbar microdiskectomy.
- Less common but more emergent indications include acute or progressive neurologic deterioration and cauda equina syndrome.

CONTRAINDICATIONS

- Asymptomatic herniated disk—lack of correlation between history, physical examination, and radiographic findings
- Improvement of symptoms with conservative therapy
- Segmental instability

PLANNING AND POSITIONING

- Preoperative medical clearance (including laboratory tests, chest x-ray, and electrocardiogram) should be obtained. An anesthesia evaluation may be needed if the patient has significant medical or pulmonary comorbidities. If medically appropriate, anticoagulants and antiplatelet agents should be discontinued before surgery.
- Antibiotics (gram-positive coverage) should be given at least 30 minutes before incision. Although not considered standard of care, a single dose of intravenous steroids can be administered in the presence of a neurologic deficit or sizable disk herniation.
- Following is a description of a lumbar microdiskectomy performed through a tubular retractor system.
- **Figure 81-1:** The patient is placed prone on the operative table using a Wilson frame or bolsters to promote lumbar flexion; this allows the abdomen to hang free to reduce intraabdominal pressure and reduce epidural bleeding. Appropriate padding is placed to prevent pressure neuropathies and avoid increases in intraorbital pressure. The arms are positioned no more than 90 degrees at the shoulder and the elbow joints. Lower extremity sequential compression devices are placed for venous thrombosis prophylaxis. In men, the genitalia are checked to avoid compression. A Foley catheter is generally not placed for single level diskectomy. Intraoperative imaging should be performed before skin incision to confirm the appropriate level.

PROCEDURE

- **Figure 81-2:** The skin incision is marked after localizing with fluoroscopy. A small incision (approximately 2 cm) is made in or just off the midline. A Kirschner wire is inserted through the incision, making sure it is passed on the appropriate side of the spinous processes. The Kirschner wire is passed through the lumbodorsal fascia, and imaging is

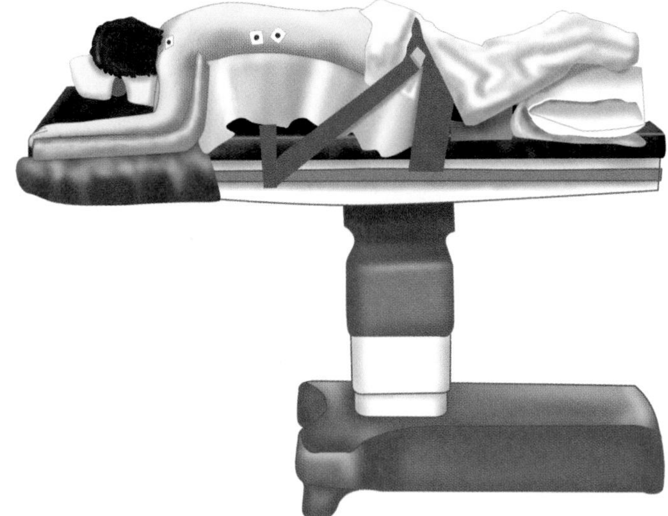

FIGURE 81-1

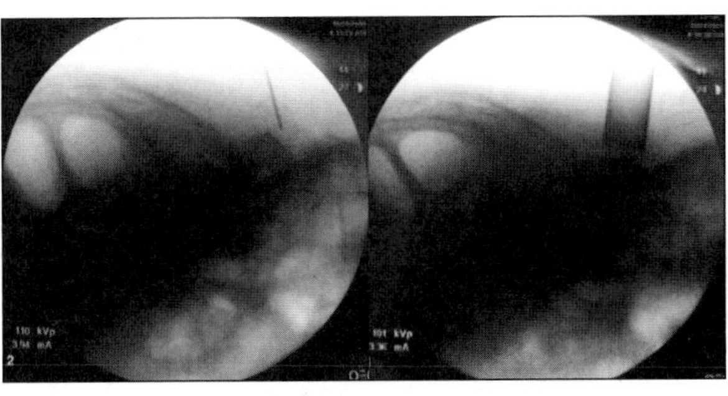

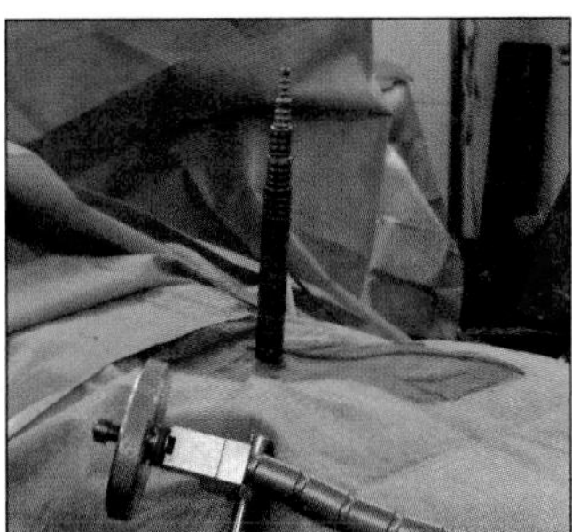

A B

FIGURE 81-2

repeated to ensure appropriate localization. The Kirschner wire is advanced until it engages the inferior aspect of the rostral lamina. Appropriate placement is confirmed with tactile feedback and repeat imaging. After the Kirschner wire is engaged, sequential dilators are passed over the wire and seated onto the lamina (**A**). It is imperative that the surgeon appreciates the tactile feedback of the Kirschner wire seated against bone to prevent incursion into the spinal canal through the interlaminar space. Subperiosteal elevation of the paraspinal muscles can be achieved by sweeping the conical dilators in a medial-lateral and cephalad-caudad motion (**B**). The depth is determined from graduated markings on the dilators, and the final tube retractor is passed and secured with a table-mounted retractor arm. The appropriate position is confirmed with intraoperative imaging. Adjustments to the final position can be achieved by angling the retractor with the final dilator inserted.

- **Figure 81-3:** The intraoperative microscope is brought into position to perform the procedure through the tube retractors. Monopolar electrocautery and a pituitary rongeur are used to define the intralaminar space and clear any residual soft tissue.
- **Figure 81-4:** After the anatomic landmarks are identified, the procedure is similar to traditional open microdiskectomy. An up-going curet can be used to free the ligamentum flavum from the undersurface of the rostral lamina. Inferior laminotomy and medial facetectomy are performed with either Kerrison rongeurs or a high-speed drill.
- **Figure 81-5:** The epidural space is entered by dissecting through and resecting the ligamentum flavum using microinstruments and Kerrison rongeurs. The caudal pedicle is the key anatomic landmark to identify before working within the epidural space. The area just rostral to the pedicle is typically considered the "safe zone" without placing the traversing nerve root at unnecessary risk. Dissection through the epidural fat reveals the lateral aspect of the thecal sac and traversing nerve root. These structures usually are displaced dorsally depending on the size and position of the herniated disk fragment.

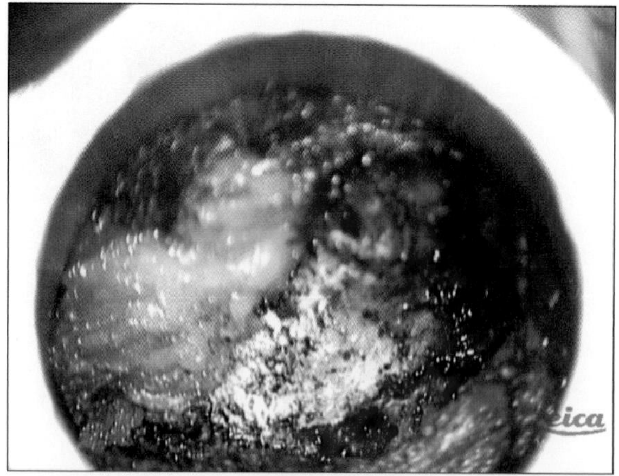

FIGURE 81-3

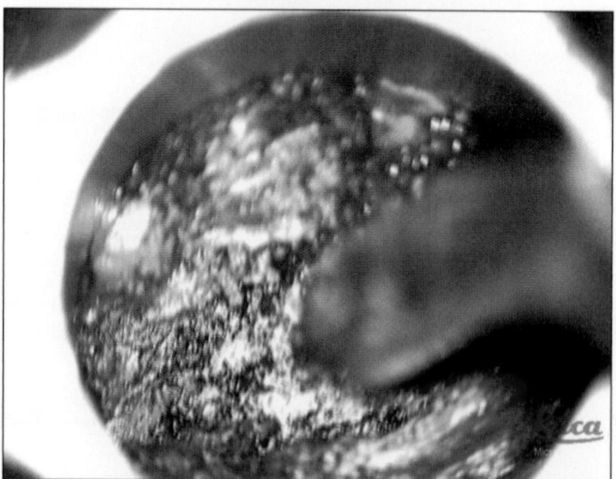

FIGURE 81-4

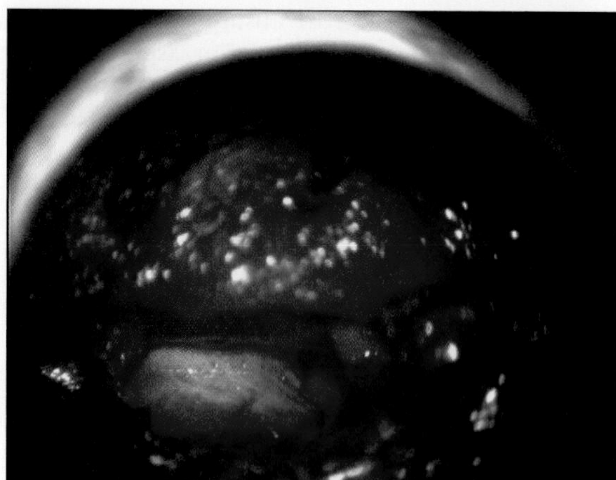

FIGURE 81-5

- **Figure 81-6:** Using a microsurgical technique, the lateral edge of the nerve root is dissected free and retracted medially to expose the herniated fragment and posterolateral aspect of the annulus. If an axillary disk is present, similar dissection techniques are used to free the material within the nerve root axilla. Epidural veins are cauterized with bipolar cautery to achieve hemostasis.
- **Figure 81-7:** Using a nerve hook, dissection ventral to the thecal sac and nerve root is performed to deliver any extruded disk fragments. A bayonetted blade is used to incise the posterior longitudinal ligament and annulus. Removal of disk material is achieved with straight and angled rongeurs. After completing the diskectomy, the uncompressed nerve root is visualized. Evidence of the thecal sac and nerve root pulsations is indicative of effective decompression.

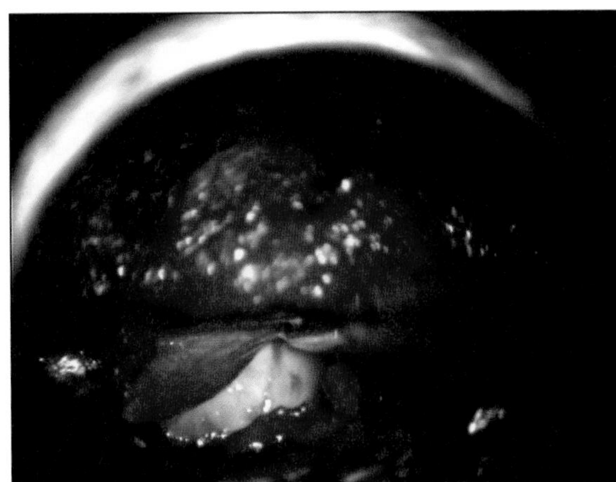

FIGURE 81-6

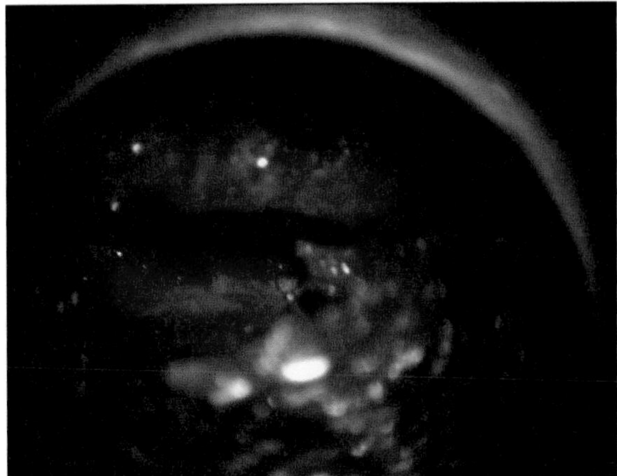

FIGURE 81-7

- Copious irrigation is used before closure. Hemostasis is achieved with a combination of bipolar cautery, bone wax, and absorbable hemostatic agent. As the retractor is removed, bipolar cautery is used to achieve hemostasis within the muscle. Bupivacaine (Marcaine) can be injected into the muscle to aid with postoperative pain relief. Typically, a single suture is placed to reapproximate the fascia, although this is unnecessary. The subcuticular layer is reapproximated in an interrupted, inverted fashion with skin glue or absorbable subcutaneous suture. If cerebrospinal fluid leakage occurs intraoperatively, locking nylon is recommended.

TIPS FROM THE MASTERS

- Appropriate evaluation of preoperative imaging is essential when performing a lumbar microdiskectomy. Determining the location and extent of the disk herniation is key to guiding the epidural exploration and optimizing patient outcome. Failure to recognize an atypical location of the herniated fragment, such as in the axilla of the nerve root, can significantly increase the surgical time, increase risk of nerve root injury, or, worse, lead to failure to locate the herniated fragment.
- The caudal pedicle is the most important anatomic landmark to identify, providing the avenue to explore the epidural space safely.
- Release of tethering epidural tissue and veins eases retraction of the traversing nerve root and decreases the risk of dural tear during exploration of the epidural space.
- The surgeon should master the open technique first before performing minimally invasive approaches.

PITFALLS

Localization may be difficult in the presence of scoliotic deformities, severe spondylotic disease, or transitional vertebrae. Appropriate evaluation of preoperative imaging and the use of real-time intraoperative imaging, such as fluoroscopy, significantly reduce the difficulties associated with these findings.

Limiting the resection of the facet joint and preserving the pars interarticularis is important to minimize the risk of postoperative instability, which can lead to clinically significant mechanical back pain that may necessitate a spine fusion.

The depth of disk space exploration should be confined to the dorsal half to avoid an anterior annulus violation and risk of injury to the intraabdominal contents, such as the iliac vein or artery.

Dural tears are best addressed during the initial procedure. If tear is extensive, a more aggressive resection of the lamina may be required to define the limits of the dural violation. Primary closure is optimal; however, if this is impossible, the dura may be reinforced with synthetic dural substitutes, a small pledget of muscle, or fibrin sealants. Placing a spinal drain for cerebrospinal fluid diversion for several days after surgery and maintaining the patient in a recumbent position may be considered.

BAILOUT OPTIONS

- If the herniated disk is not identified during epidural exploration, the surgeon should perform a checklist to ensure that an appropriate approach was performed. The images should be reevaluated to check for the correct side and spinal level and to confirm the location of the disk within the epidural space. Appropriate localization of the retractor is confirmed with intraoperative imaging. If no disk is identified despite exposing the appropriate side and level, the surgery should be completed, and repeat imaging should be performed to determine if the disk has resorbed or changed position.
- It is imperative that the surgeon master the technique of a traditional microdiskectomy before attempting the procedure through the tube retractor. Under certain circumstances, it is conceivable that the exposure provided by the tube retractor would be inadequate to achieve the surgical objective. To convert to an open procedure, the tube retractor may be removed, the incision extended, and traditional retractors placed.

SUGGESTED READINGS

Anderson PA, McCormick PC, Angevine PD. Randomized controlled trials of the treatment of lumbar disk herniation: 1983-2007. J Am Acad Orthop Surg 2008;16:566–73.

Arts MP, Brand R, van den Akker ME, et al. Tubular diskectomy vs conventional microdiskectomy for sciatica: a randomized controlled trial. JAMA 2009;302:149–58.

McCormick PC. The Spine Patient Outcomes Research Trial results for lumbar disc herniation: a critical review. J Neurosurg Spine 2007;6:513–20.

Weinstein JN, Lurie JD, Tosteson TD, et al. Surgical vs nonoperative treatment for lumbar disk herniation: the Spine Patient Outcomes Research Trial (SPORT) observational cohort. JAMA 2006;296:2451–9.

Weinstein JN, Tosteson TD, Lurie JD, et al. Surgical vs nonoperative treatment for lumbar disk herniation: the Spine Patient Outcomes Research Trial (SPORT): a randomized trial. JAMA 2006;296:2441–50.

Procedure 82

Minimally Invasive Thoracic Corpectomy

John E. O'Toole

INDICATIONS

- Conditions requiring ventral decompression of the spinal cord with removal of one to two vertebral bodies at any level of the thoracic spine
  - Extradural tumors
  - Infection (e.g., diskitis, osteomyelitis)
  - Fractures or trauma
  - Degenerative disease or focal deformity
- Patients for whom open thoracotomy or traditional open lateral extracavitary approaches may present excessive morbidity

CONTRAINDICATIONS

- Need for en bloc or marginal spondylectomy
- Greater than two-level corpectomy required
- Severe deformity requiring significant intraoperative manipulation for correction
- Patient characteristics unfavorable for surgery, such as inability to tolerate general anesthesia, uncorrected coagulopathy, life expectancy too short for palliative surgical resection (<3 months), and severe osteoporosis

PLANNING AND POSITIONING

- **Figure 82-1:** The patient is placed prone on a radiolucent Jackson table with proper padding for dependent areas. An open-frame table facilitates the use of anteroposterior and lateral fluoroscopy during the procedure. The arms can be positioned toward the head for thoracic levels as high as T6 depending on individual patient anatomy.
- **Figure 82-2:** Axial computed tomography (CT) scan from a patient with T9 lung cancer metastasis. A measurement is used to estimate the distance needed from the midline to achieve the desired approach trajectory. Analysis of preoperative imaging is crucial to determine the side of approach or need for bilateral approach (e.g., circumferential epidural tumor involvement) and to plan the distance from the midline at which to place the incision to achieve a favorable approach trajectory.

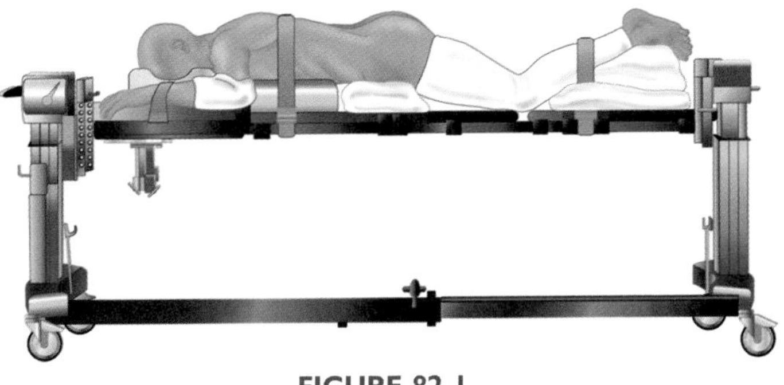

FIGURE 82-1

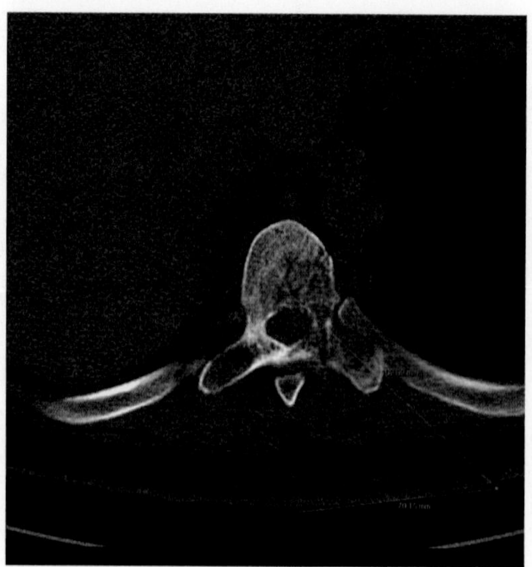

FIGURE 82-2

PROCEDURE

- **Figure 82-3:** After appropriate preparation and draping, the operative level is identified on intraoperative fluoroscopy, and a paramedian incision is marked out on the skin. The distance of the incision from the midline varies based on patient anatomy and approach trajectory desired, but on average it is approximately 6 cm off the midline. Local anesthesia is injected, and the skin is incised sharply. The thoracodorsal fascia may be incised separately if desired. Tubular dilation is performed over the transverse process using a commercially available minimally invasive surgery (MIS) retractor system (**A**). An expandable MIS retractor is placed over the dilators and fixed into place using a table-mounted arm (**B**).
- **Figure 82-4:** After removal of the dilators, the retractor is expanded to enlarge the working field. Additional retractor blades may be inserted as available. Retractors that expand in rostral-caudal and medial-lateral directions are most useful in this procedure (**A**). Position of the retractor is confirmed on lateral fluoroscopy (**B**).
- **Figure 82-5:** Residual soft tissue at the base of the retractor is removed using monopolar cautery and rongeurs to reveal the ipsilateral spinous process (*SP*), lamina (*L*), facet joint (*F*), and transverse process (*TP*). The retractor may be angled, or "wanded," to approach various parts of the relevant anatomy.

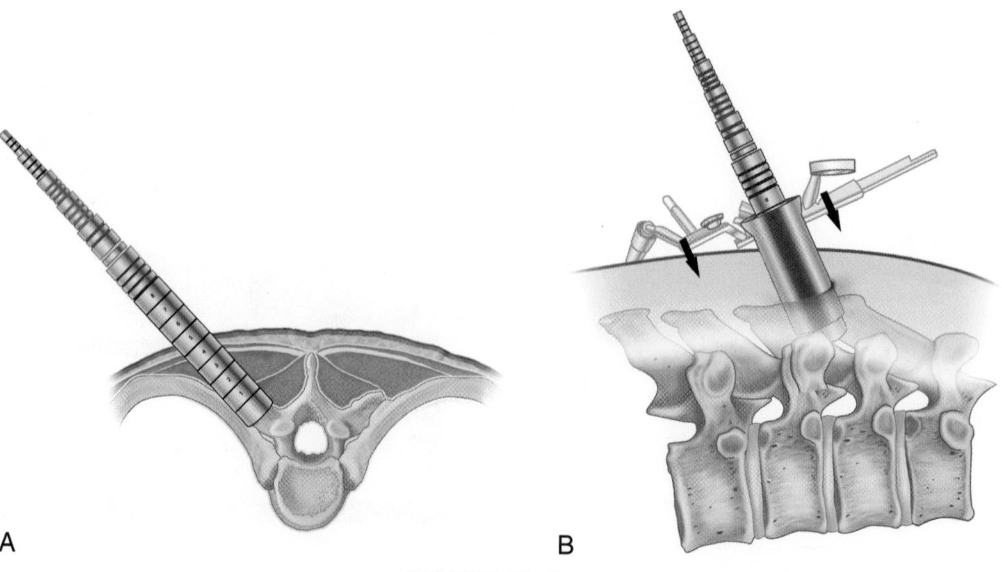

FIGURE 82-3

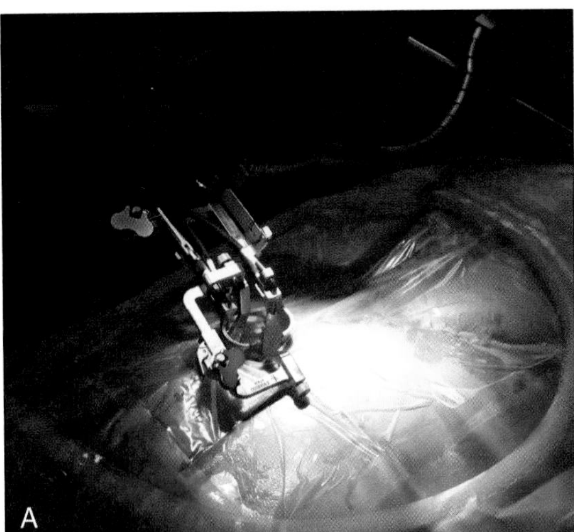

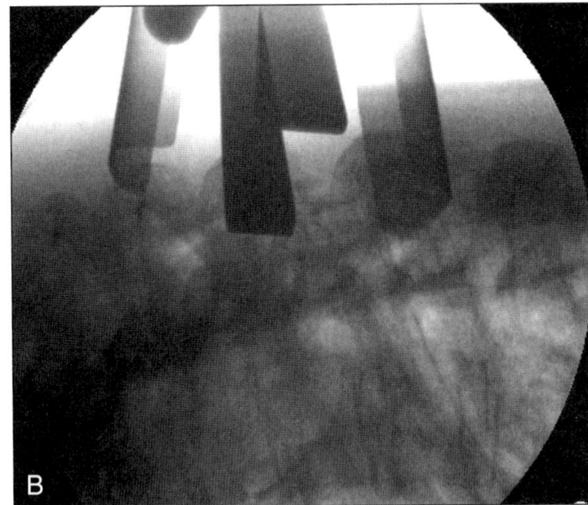

FIGURE 82-4

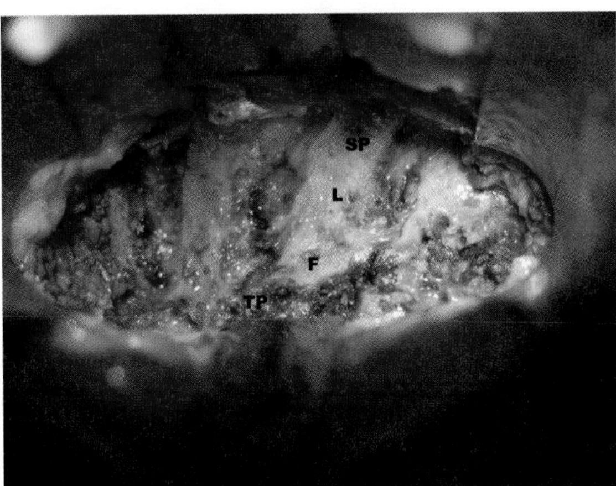

FIGURE 82-5

- **Figure 82-6:** Depending on the angle of approach and distance from the midline, this technique allows bony removal similar to that achieved during a traditional open costotransversectomy or modified lateral extracavitary approaches for corpectomy. Bony anatomy to be resected includes the proximal rib, transverse process, lamina, pedicle, and most of the vertebral body.
- **Figure 82-7:** Removal of the posterior bony structures may proceed from a lateral to medial or, as depicted here, medial to lateral direction. Photograph from cadaveric example of MIS thoracic corpectomy depicts central decompression including laminectomies and facetectomies at the affected level and at levels immediately above and below. Laminectomies should extend at least from the pedicle of the segment above to the pedicle of the segment below the desired corpectomy segment. The dura is well exposed.

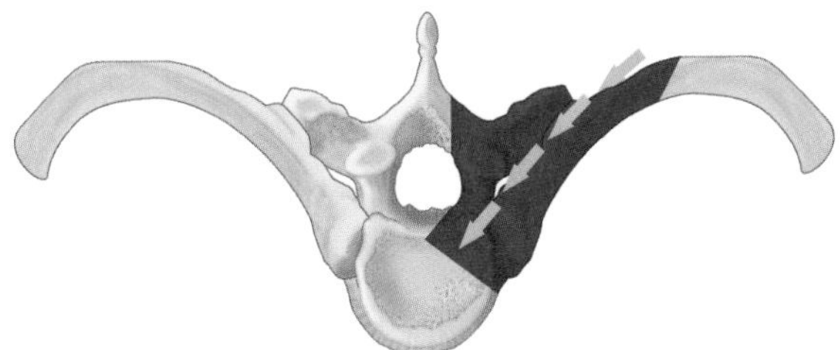

FIGURE 82-6

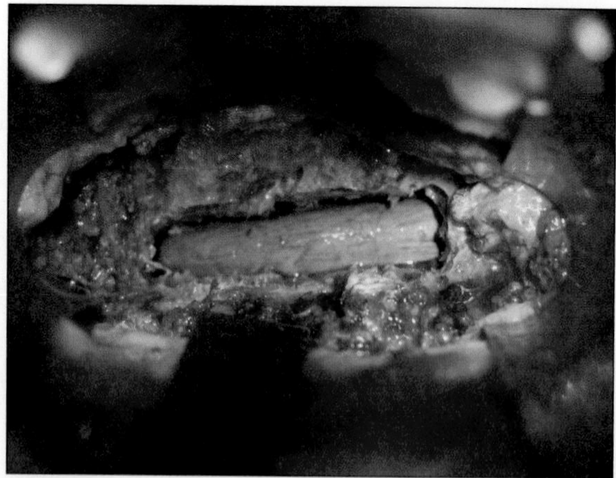

FIGURE 82-7

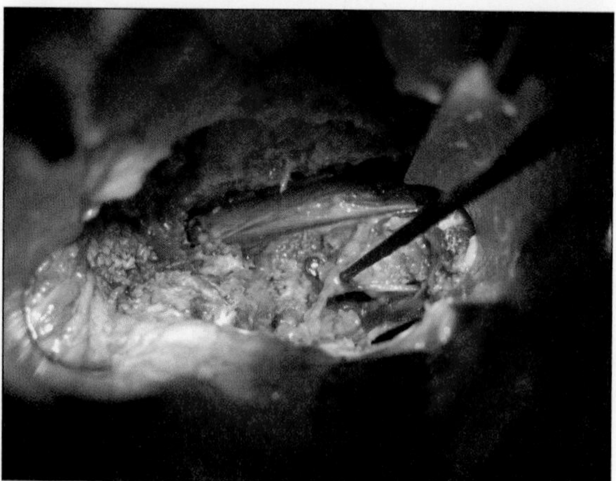

FIGURE 82-8

- **Figure 82-8:** Working more laterally, subperiosteal dissection is performed around the proximal ribs of the affected level and the level below to separate them from the parietal pleura and neurovascular bundle. About 3 to 6 cm of each rib may be removed along with the transverse processes and pedicle of the affected level, facilitating a more medial trajectory. The exiting nerve root is dissected out, and epidural veins are cauterized and divided (the instrument in the photograph from a cadaveric dissection is placed ventral to the exiting nerve root). The nerve should be ligated proximal to the dorsal root ganglion to permit greater access to the intervertebral space. Suture ligatures left on the nerve root stump may be used for gentle dural retraction during corpectomy and reconstruction.
- **Figure 82-9:** The ribs are followed to the intervertebral disks adjoining the affected vertebral body, and the rib heads are removed after dividing the costovertebral ligaments. Complete diskectomies above and below are done to define rostral-caudal boundaries of the corpectomy and to protect end plates of adjacent vertebral bodies. Corpectomy is performed in a typical posterolateral fashion using curets, bone rongeurs, and a high-speed drill. Subperiosteal dissection of the ipsilateral vertebral body wall may be performed to isolate segmental vessels and remove this cortical wall if desired. A small amount of cortical bone may be left on the contralateral and ventral aspects of the vertebral body to protect the visceral contents of the chest and to aid in containment of the intervertebral graft.
- **Figure 82-10:** The final step in bone removal is to displace the posterior vertebral body wall away from the thecal sac into the corpectomy defect using down-pushing instruments. The intraoperative anteroposterior fluoroscopic image in Figure 82-10A shows extent of complete ventral decompression achieved with the tip of the curet touching the base of the contralateral pedicle. The extent of bony resection achieved with MIS corpectomy is revealed in postoperative CT scans. An average of 80% of the volume of the vertebral body and 93% of the ventral spinal canal can routinely be removed.

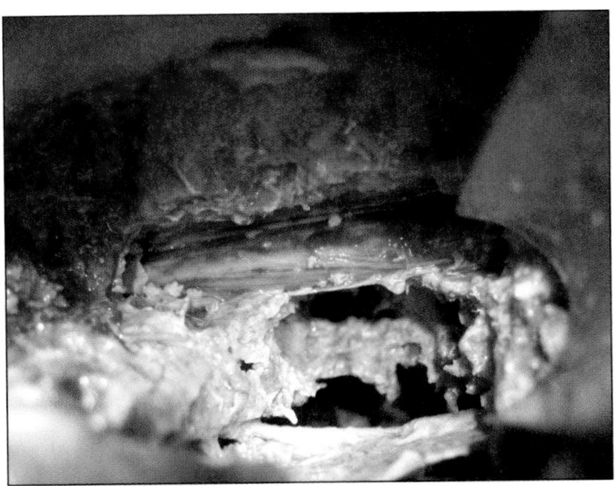

FIGURE 82-9

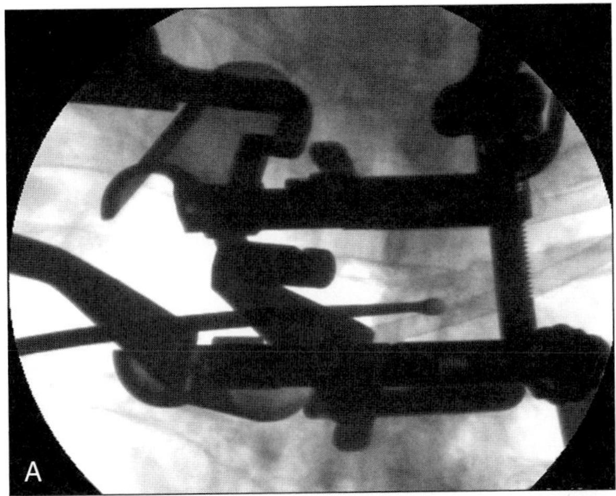

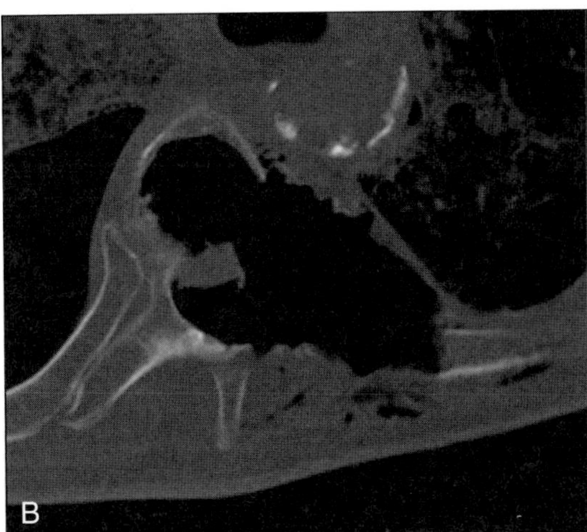

FIGURE 82-10

- **Figure 82-11:** After standard preparation of adjacent end plates for arthrodesis, an appropriate intervertebral graft may be placed. Options for reconstruction include structural allograft, titanium mesh, expandable cage, or polymethyl methacrylate.
- **Figure 82-12:** Percutaneous pedicle screw fixation under anteroposterior and lateral fluoroscopy may be performed as illustrated via standard cannulation of the pedicle with a Jamshidi needle and Kirschner wire (**A**), screw insertion over a Kirschner wire after tapping (**B**), and placement of a rod into the screw heads through the extender sleeves (**C**) followed by final tightening and extender removal.
- **Figure 82-13:** The wound is closed in multiple layer fashion with absorbable suture and skin glue.

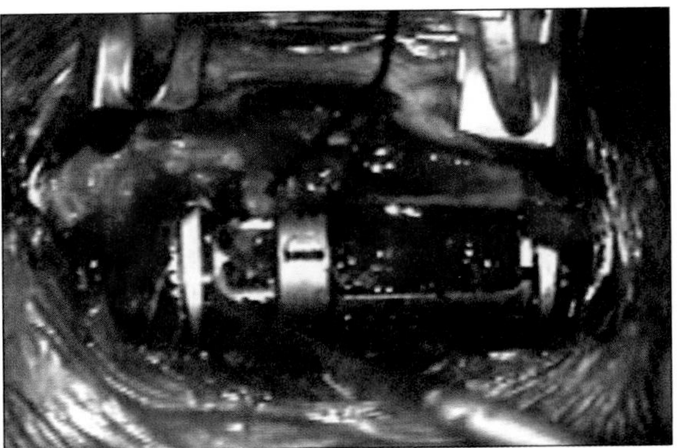

FIGURE 82-11

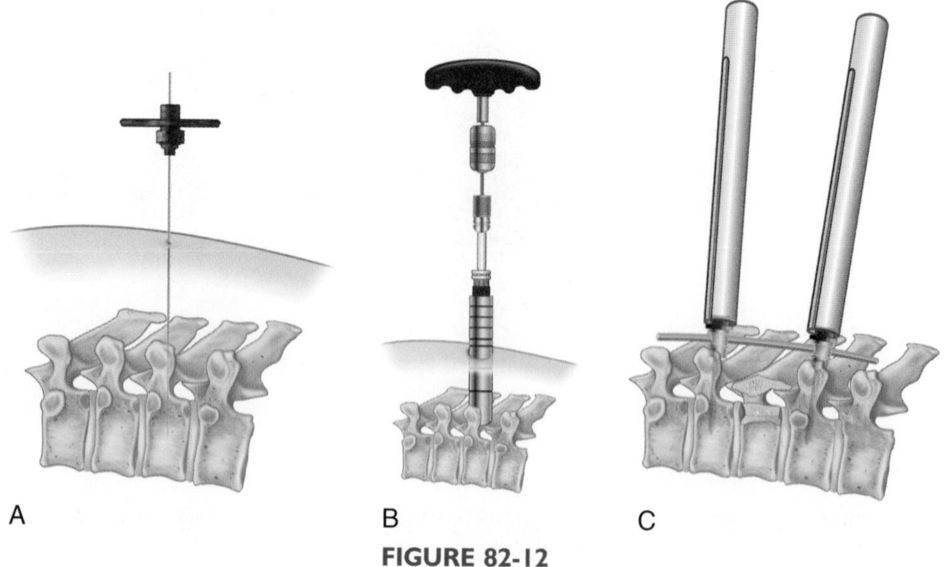

FIGURE 82-12

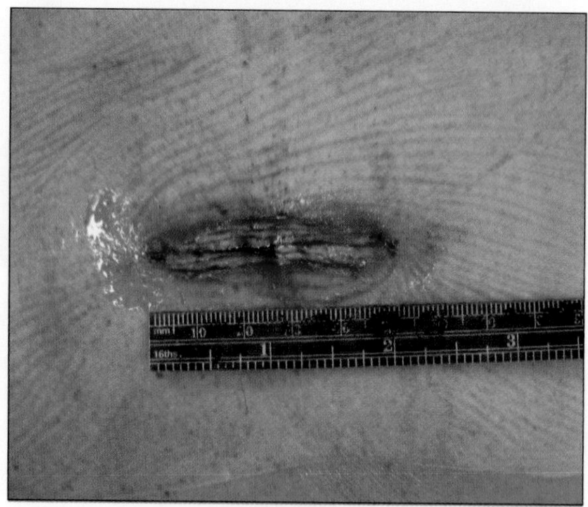

FIGURE 82-13

TIPS FROM THE MASTERS

- Depending on the approach trajectory desired, it may be helpful to resect part of the rib through the incision before inserting the retractor.
- A bilateral approach may be performed for bipedicular or circumferential disease. The contralateral incision may be made identically or more medially than the primary approach incision.
- Durotomy repair through the expandable retractor can be challenging. A primary repair is typically possible, however, using microinstruments (e.g., bayoneted microneedle drivers) and small suture (e.g., 5-0 polypropylene [Prolene]).
- Decompression of the thecal sac can be confirmed by use of a dental mirror placed ventrally below the dura.

PITFALLS

Inadequate bone removal may result when the incision is made too medially, limiting the approach angle across the midline of the vertebral body and ventral spinal canal.

Inadequate visualization because of insufficient removal of the posterior elements, ribs, or disks may result in poor decompression or reconstruction.

Inadequate spinal stabilization may similarly occur if the intervertebral construct is too small or poorly placed or if the end plates are not properly prepared for arthrodesis. Expandable cages are often easier to insert through the MIS approach than fixed length allograft struts or titanium mesh cages.

BAILOUT OPTIONS

- The procedure can be converted to a typical open posterolateral procedure, but it can be challenging to incorporate the MIS incision, and a separate incision would likely need to be made.
- Alternatively, the procedure may be converted to a standard thoracotomy approach by turning the patient to a lateral position or by staging the procedure on a separate day.
- If an intervertebral strut or cage cannot be satisfactorily inserted, polymethyl methacrylate and Steinmann pin reconstruction is a viable option, particularly in cases of malignancy.

SUGGESTED READINGS

Deutsch H, Boco T, Lobel J. Minimally invasive transpedicular vertebrectomy for metastatic disease to the thoracic spine. J Spinal Disord Tech 2008;21:101–5.

Kim DH, O'Toole JE, Ogden AT, et al. Minimally invasive posterolateral thoracic corpectomy: cadaveric feasibility study and report of four clinical cases. Neurosurgery 2009;64:746–52.

Musacchio M, Patel N, Bagan B, et al. Minimally invasive thoracolumbar costotransversectomy and corpectomy via a dual-tube technique: evaluation in a cadaver model. Surg Technol Int 2007;16:221–5.

O'Toole JE, Eichholz KM, Fessler RG. Minimally invasive approaches to vertebral column and spinal cord tumors. Neurosurg Clin N Am 2006;17:491–506.

Patchell RA, Tibbs PA, Regine WF, et al. Direct decompressive surgical resection in the treatment of spinal cord compression caused by metastatic cancer: a randomised trial. Lancet 2005;366:643–8.

Figure 82-4A is from O'Toole JE, Eichholz KM, Fessler RG. Minimally invasive approaches to vertebral column and spinal cord tumors. Neurosurg Clin N Am 2006;17:491–506.

Procedure 83

Thoracoscopic Diskectomy

Shahid M. Nimjee, Robert E. Isaacs

INDICATIONS

- Thoracoscopic diskectomy is employed for treatment of herniated disks in the thoracic spine anterior to the spinal cord using a minimally invasive anterior approach.
- Patients typically present with spinal myelopathy and cord compression.
- This approach can be used to treat thoracic radicular pain, diskitis, and other similar conditions best treated from the front of the spine.

CONTRAINDICATIONS

- A calcified disk is considered a relative contraindication to thoracoscopic diskectomy.
- The procedure is contraindicated in patients unable to undergo unilateral lung ventilation.
- A prior history of major procedures from the side of the approach is a contraindication.

PLANNING AND POSITIONING

- It is essential to confirm the pathologic level. Surgeons should have all magnetic resonance imaging (MRI) studies available in the operating room to identify relevant anatomy. Preoperative imaging must confirm the level of the operation using anatomy that can be replicated in the operating room—typically including the disk levels down to the sacrum for mid-thoracic and lower thoracic disk herniations.
- In addition to MRI, we typically obtain plain films and frequently a computed tomography (CT) scan to identify the location of the cervicothoracic or the thoracolumbar junction, the number of ribs present, and the location of the last visible rib. Imaging studies also serve to ascertain whether the disk is calcified.
- The patient is intubated with a dual lumen endotracheal tube and is given appropriate antibiotic prophylaxis.
- **Figure 83-1:** Place the patient in a standard lateral position with an axillary roll placed below the arm, which should be flexed; this helps protect the brachial plexus from injury.
- Secure the patient with three-point or four-point restraints on the patient's chest and pelvis, or tape the patient down to the surgical bed to ensure that the patient does not move during the procedure.

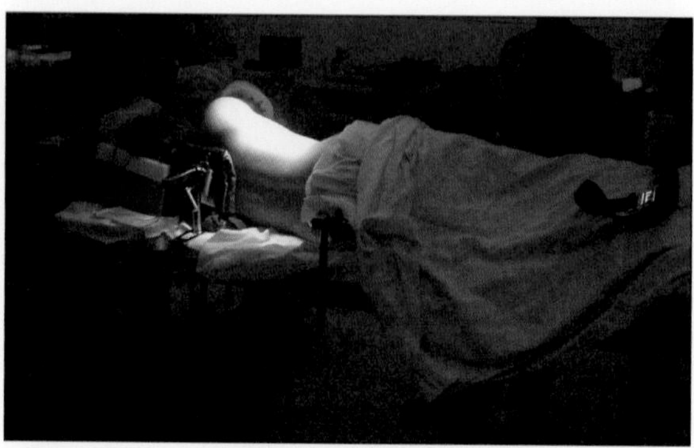

FIGURE 83-1

- Scrub the patient as if preparing to complete a true thoracotomy in case the need arises to convert to an open procedure. Scrub from dorsally around the mid-back to ventral, including the navel and axilla.

PROCEDURE

- **Figure 83-2:** Insert an 18-gauge needle through the skin and subcutaneous tissue just at the pathologic disk space as seen on anteroposterior x-ray. A second needle is placed at the thoracolumbar junction to help identify this level at the time of surgery. These serve as references during surgery.
- Place the first portal at the posterior axillary line, two disk spaces above the pathologic disk when using a 30-degree scope; when using a 0-degree scope, place it directly above the posterior aspect of the pathologic disk space. This posterior portal is an ideal initial guide because it is posterior, away from the lung, which is superior and anterior, and the diaphragm, which is anterior and inferior. Make an incision over the rib, and use a hemostat to puncture the pleura and dilate the tract. Use the trocar introducers to dilate the tract progressively to the appropriate portal size.
- **Figure 83-3:** Insert a camera into the first portal, and inspect the pleural cavity from apex to diaphragm. Count the ribs to verify the correct pathologic level. The surgeon should also use fluoroscopy or anteroposterior x-rays to verify that the localizer is in the correct place. Place a second portal in the anterior axillary line using a scalpel followed by a hemostat. The surgeon can visualize the second portal placement using the endoscope that is sitting in the first portal. The standard thoracoscopic diskectomy uses three portals: one for the endoscope, the second for a working instrument, and the third for suction. The lung can be moved out of the way by tilting the patient forward or by inserting a fourth portal and placing a fan retractor to retract away the lung or diaphragm as needed.

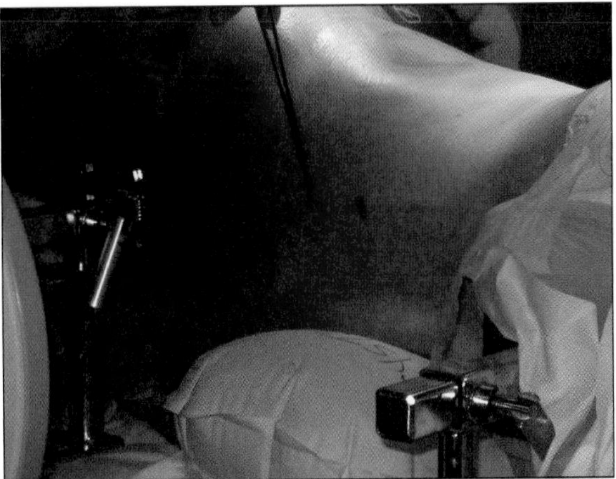

FIGURE 83-2

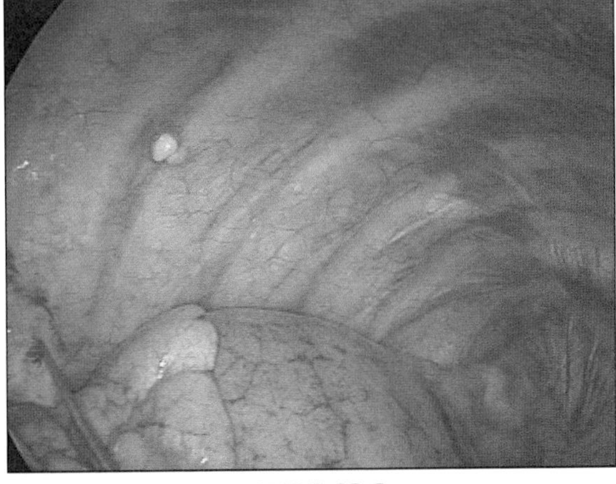

FIGURE 83-3

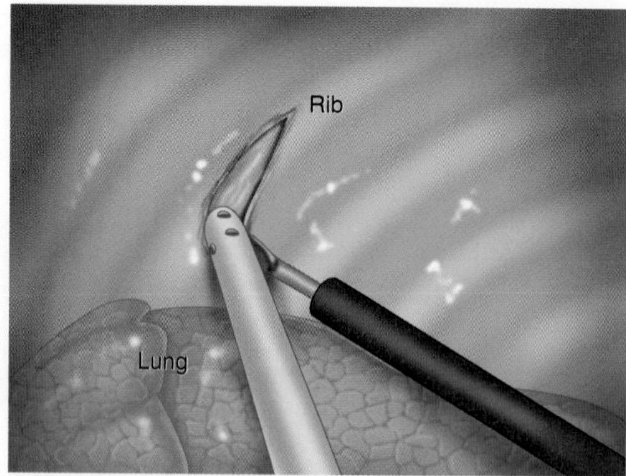

FIGURE 83-4

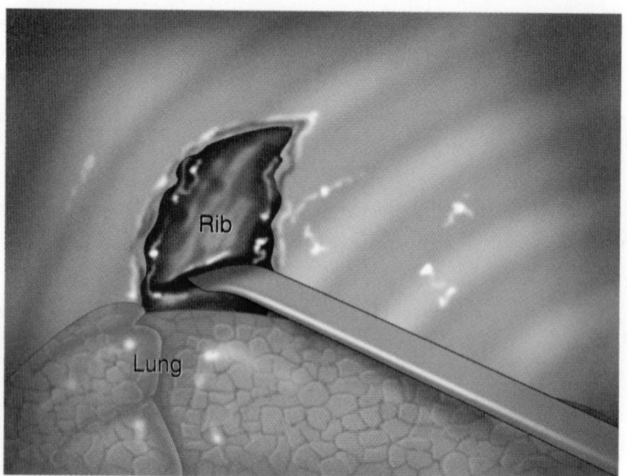

FIGURE 83-5

- **Figure 83-4:** Remove the pleura from the rib that leads to the pathologic disk and from adjacent vertebral bodies. Make a linear pleural incision along the rib, 3 to 4 cm dorsal to the rib head, and extend it over the disk space.
- **Figure 83-5:** Expose the rib using endoscopic monopolar, and cut attachments to the spine (costovertebral ligaments). These are incised with a monopolar cautery and severed with a Cobb elevator. Remove the rib head with a semicircular oscillating saw, rib cutter, or diamond bur drill bit approximately 3 cm proximal to its attachment to the spine.
- **Figure 83-6:** At this point in the operation, form a defect safely within the vertebral bodies centered around the disk space. It is then time to define the anteriormost aspect of the canal. To achieve a complete diskectomy, remove at least the superior portion of the pedicle below the level of the lesion. Thin the pedicle down using a diamond bur until just the medial cortex remains.
- **Figure 83-7:** A Kerrison rongeur can be used to define the lateral dura. Extend the pedicular resection ventrally until you cannot remove further tissue—then you have defined the ventral aspect of the canal.
- **Figure 83-8:** With the ventral canal defined, it is safe to create a pyramid-shaped defect to extract the ruptured disk. Use a diamond bur to remove remaining bone dorsal to the defect and ventral to the canal (as defined by pedicular removal). The posterior longitudinal ligament (PLL) "gives" as the dorsalmost bone is removed. Removing the PLL with the disk herniation completes the diskectomy and decompression.

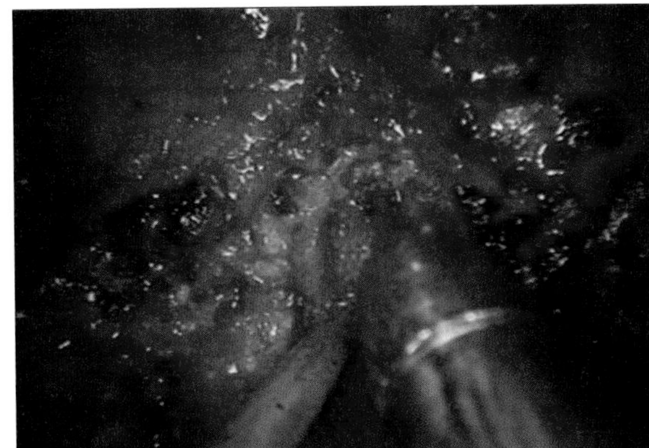

FIGURE 83-6

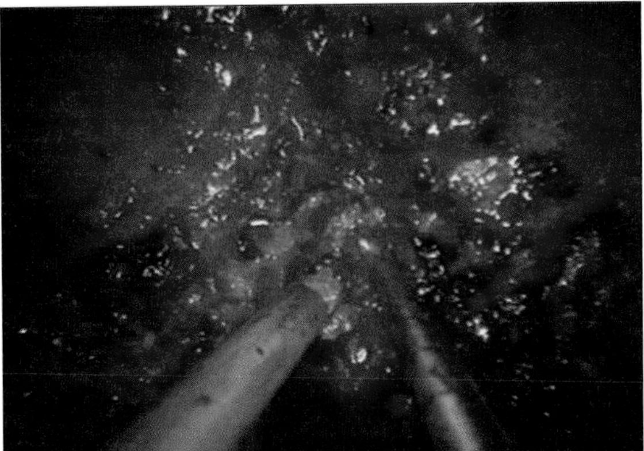

FIGURE 83-7

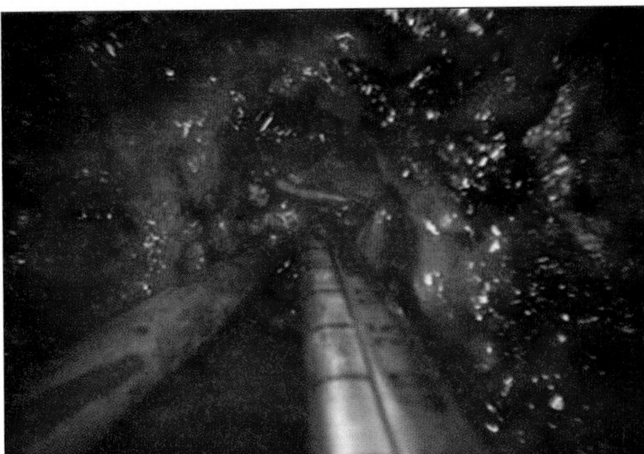

FIGURE 83-8

- **Figure 83-9:** After completing the diskectomy, ensure that the canal is completely decompressed from the pedicle above to the pedicle below the lesion and from the pedicle closest to the surgeon to the pedicle farthest away. At the end of the procedure, there should be no tissue preventing the ball probe from traveling from the ipsilateral to the contralateral pedicle.
- Verify hemostasis, and reinflate the lung under direct endoscopic guidance. Close all ports except the endoscopic port in layers with a 2-0 polyglactin 910 (Vicryl) and then a subcuticular stitch. In the remaining port, place a chest tube in the apex of the pleural cavity under direct endoscopic vision. Allow the lung to reinflate completely again

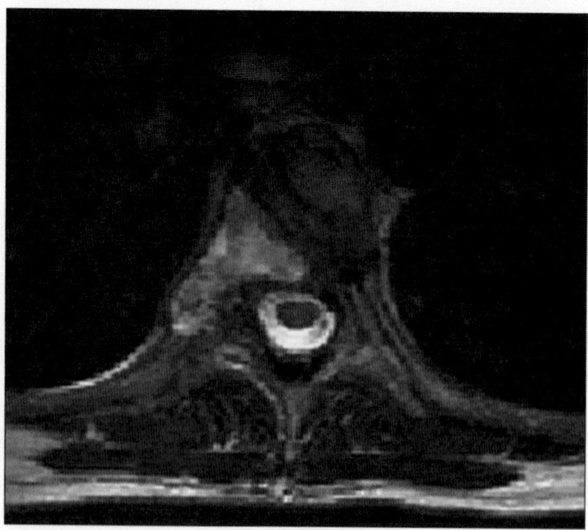

FIGURE 83-9

under endoscopic visualization. The air escapes, and once the inflation of the lung is adequate, place purse-string sutures around the chest tube. Verify that there is no air leak with a Valsalva maneuver, and (if desired) remove the chest tube and close the incision with the purse-string sutures.

TIPS FROM THE MASTERS

- During stripping of the tissue over the vertebral body, cauterize the segmental arteries to minimize bleeding; this is superior to using a hemoclip, which often comes off or is inadequate, resulting in bleeding that clouds the thoracoscopic view.
- When creating a pyramidal defect anteriorly, be generous to obtain adequate exposure to achieve complete diskectomy and adequate decompression.
- The key is to create a large defect posteriorly (the base of the pyramid) to get normal dura on each side of the herniation. For calcified herniations, this is even more critical. Make the defect fully before attempting to remove the PLL. Then, while removing the PLL bluntly, attempt to keep it intact as a single piece for as long as possible, and use it as a means to displace the disk. Severing the connections at the upper and lower aspects of the defect can facilitate disk removal substantially.

PITFALLS

Inadequate preoperative imaging to ensure correct localization of the disk herniation in the operating room

Inadequate exposure for larger disk herniations or calcified disks

BAILOUT OPTIONS

- If the disk is calcified or difficult to extract thoracoscopically, one can convert to an open procedure to achieve adequate decompression.
- Have a means to control bleeding (i.e., a cottonoid attached to a hemostat) to allow for compression of a bleeding vessel until it can be controlled thoracoscopically or, if required, to buy time until thoracotomy can be completed.
- Have spinal hardware that can be passed through portals to reconstruct the spine in cases in which spinal reconstruction is required.

SUGGESTED READINGS

Anand N, Regan JJ. Video-assisted thoracoscopic surgery for thoracic disk disease: classification and outcome study of 100 consecutive cases with a 2-year minimum follow-up period. Spine 2002;27:871–9.

Beisse R, Muckley T, Schmidt MH, et al. Surgical technique and results of endoscopic anterior spinal canal decompression. J Neurosurg 2005;2:128–36.

Han PP, Kenny K, Dickman CA. Thoracoscopic approaches to the thoracic spine: experience with 241 surgical procedures. Neurosurgery 2002;51(Suppl. 5):S88–95.

Landreneau RJ, Hazelrigg SR, Mack MJ, et al. Postoperative pain-related morbidity: video-assisted thoracic surgery versus thoracotomy. Ann Thorac Surg 1993;56:1285–9.

Regan JJ, Mack MJ, Picetti GD 3rd. A technical report on video-assisted thoracoscopy in thoracic spinal surgery: preliminary description. Spine 1995;20:831–7.

Procedure 84 Percutaneous Pedicle Screw Placement

Girish K. Hiremath, Mick Perez-Cruet

INDICATIONS

- Lumbar fusion for symptomatic isthmic, degenerative, or traumatic spondylolisthesis; intractable discogenic back pain; or correction of symptomatic degenerative scoliosis
- As an adjunct to direct lateral, transforaminal, posterior or anterior interbody fusion
- To supplement a posterolateral arthrodesis
- As a posterior adjunct to an anterior decompression or stabilization procedure for any of the following conditions:
  - Trauma (e.g., burst fracture, Chance fracture)
  - Neoplasms (resulting in instability)
  - Infection (e.g., vertebral osteomyelitis, diskitis, spinal tuberculosis)
  - Degenerative conditions (anterior lumbar interbody fusion [controversial])

CONTRAINDICATIONS

- Severe osteoporosis
- Inability to obtain adequate images even after modification of the contrast mode on fluoroscopy machine, as a result of severe osteopenia or morbid obesity
- Disease process (e.g., tumor, infection, fracture) involving or extending into pedicle of interest

PLANNING AND POSITIONING

- The following equipment is needed:
  - Fluoroscopy (needs to be draped in such a fashion as to allow anteroposterior and lateral imaging without risk of operative field contamination)
  - Radiolucent table and frame
  - Table that allows for free passage of the fluoroscopic C-arm gantry from anteroposterior to lateral position (i.e., Jackson table)
  - Kirschner wire, Kirschner wire driver, and Jamshidi needle
  - Cannulated instruments for pedicle screw placement (various systems from different manufacturers can be used)
- **Figure 84-1:** The patient is positioned prone on a radiolucent table and frame with adequate padding of all pressure points with the extremities placed outside the field of radiation.

PROCEDURE

- The spine is viewed on the fluoroscopic monitor in the same orientation as the patient is positioned on the table; this helps to prevent mental calculations when moving the pedicle targeting needle.

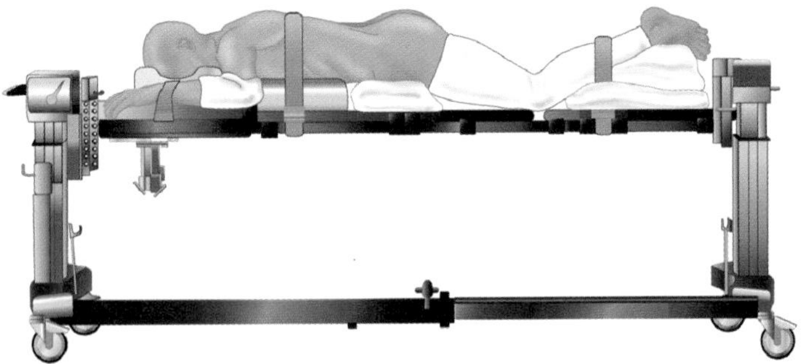

FIGURE 84-1

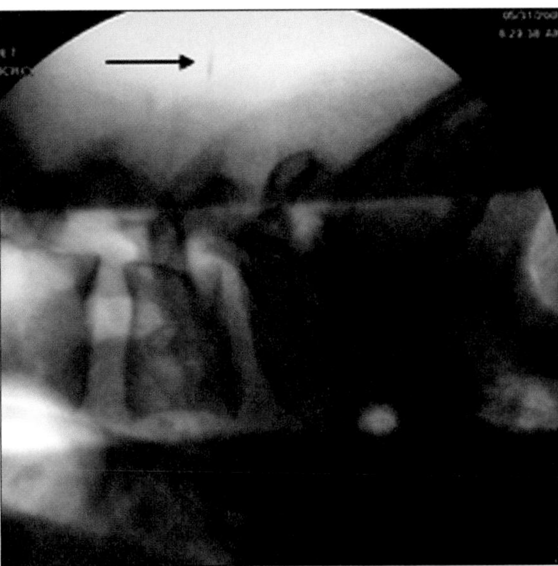

FIGURE 84-2

- **Figure 84-2:** The level is identified using a lateral fluoroscopic view and an 18-gauge spinal needle (*arrow*).
- **Figure 84-3:** **A,** The anteroposterior view can be used to identify the lateral aspect of the pedicle (*arrow*). **B,** The midline can be marked by palpation of the spinous processes or anteroposterior fluoroscopy using an overlying Kirschner wire.

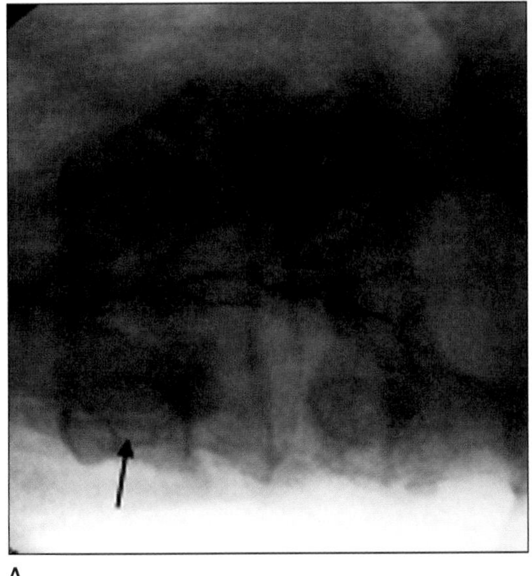

A

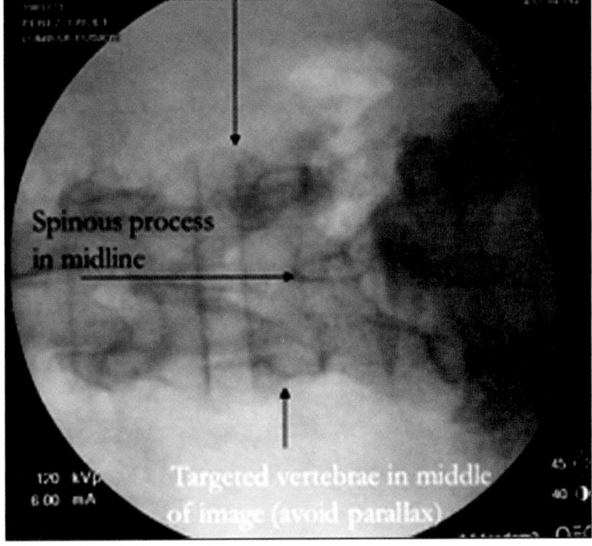

B

FIGURE 84-3

- The fluoroscopic C-arm is positioned in the anteroposterior view to target the pedicles of the desired vertebral body. To enhance the image of the targeted vertebral level, one order of magnification is used, and the image is adjusted to achieve the maximum bone visualization using the collimator mode.
- The targeted vertebral body is placed in the center of the fluoroscopic monitor to prevent parallax distortion.

- The end plate of the targeted vertebral body is viewed as a single line composed of the posterior and anterior margins of the vertebral end plate. To achieve this, the fluoroscopic C-arm gantry is moved in the proper Ferguson view plane.
  - The spinous process of the targeted vertebra is placed between the pedicles by moving the C-arm gantry in the lateral coronal projections.

Lateral-Medial Targeting of Pedicle

- A Jamshidi needle is used to identify the lateral aspect of the pedicle on the ipsilateral side (i.e., the side on which the surgeon is standing).
- An incision is made in the skin, and the fascia is incised with monopolar cautery to facilitate passage of instruments. The incision extends from pedicle to pedicle being instrumented.
- A Jamshidi needle is passed through the muscle to dock onto the junction between the lateral aspect of the facet joint and transverse process of the desired level.
- **Figure 84-4:** Anteroposterior fluoroscopy is used to target the lateral superior edge of the pedicle of interest. This is the safest point of entry into the pedicle because the exiting nerve root travels in the medial inferior aspect of the pedicle, and the traversing nerve root travels on the medial aspect of the pedicle.
- **Figure 84-5:** **A** and **B,** The Jamshidi needle is tapped with a mallet gently in a lateral-to-medial direction to pierce the lateral cortical margin and enter the cancellous core of the pedicle (*arrows*).
  - Anteroposterior fluoroscopy (see Fig. 84-5A) is used to guide the Jamshidi needle as it passes through the pedicle. The fluoroscopic C-arm is positioned in the lateral view (see Fig. 84-5B) to guide passage and angulation of the Jamshidi needle. Ideally, the tip of the Jamshidi needle should reach the junction of the pedicle and vertebral body when the tip of the Jamshidi needle is at the center of the pedicle. This positioning ensures that the needle does not penetrate the medial cortical margin of the pedicle and enter the canal possibly injuring neural elements.

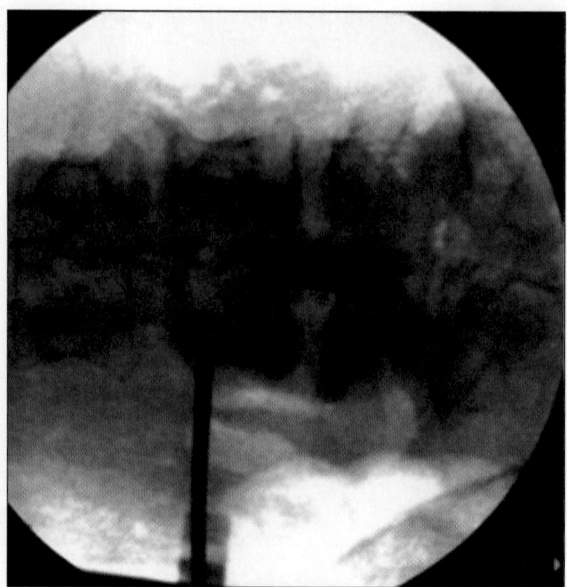

FIGURE 84-4

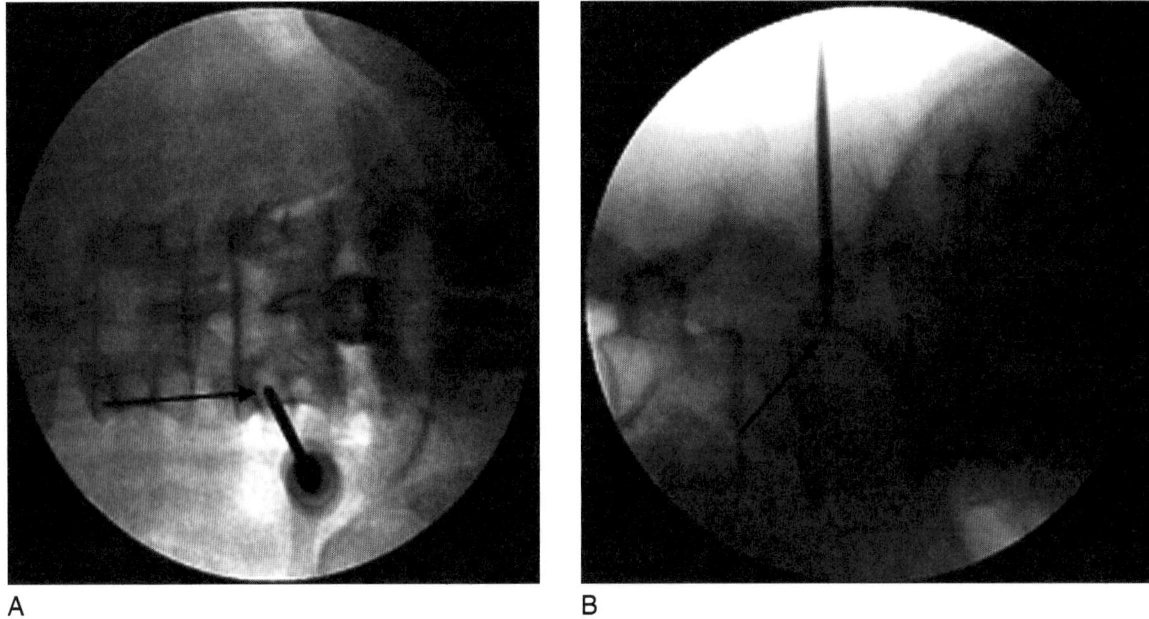

A B

FIGURE 84-5

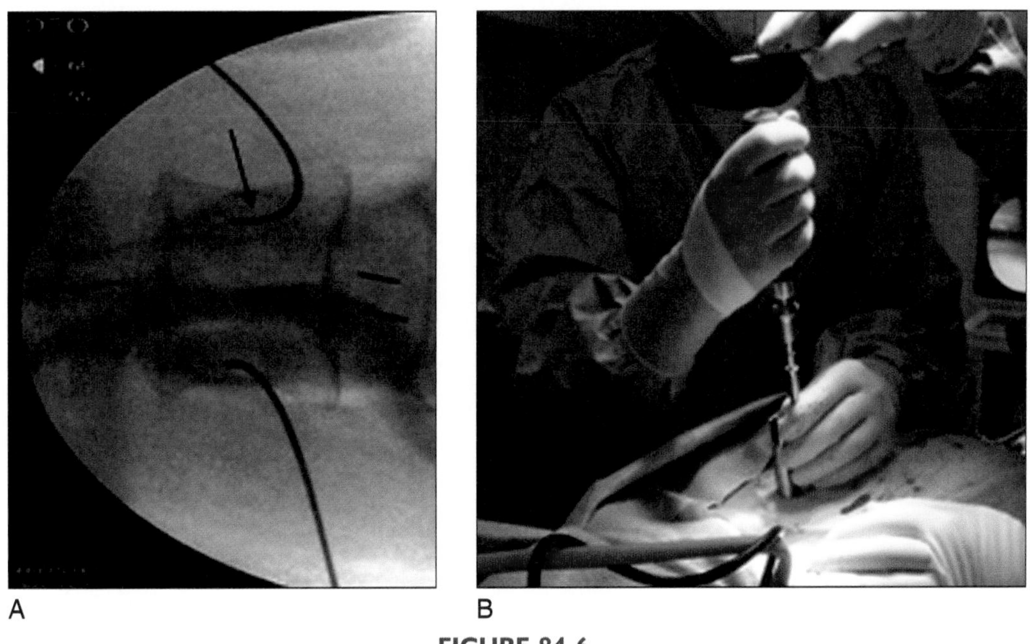

A B

FIGURE 84-6

- The Jamshidi needle can be advanced farther, approximately 1 to 2 cm into the vertebral body.

- **Figure 84-6: A,** The Kirschner wire is passed through the Jamshidi needle so that the tip lodges into the bone of the vertebral body. **B,** The Jamshidi needle is removed carefully to avoid dislodging the Kirschner wire, which is held at all times by an assistant to prevent inadvertent removal.
- We find it easier to place all of the Kirschner wires first before placing the instrumentation. To prevent inadvertent contamination of the field by a Kirschner wire perforating the C-arm drape, Kirschner wires are retracted out of the way using a towel, and an effort is made not to bend the Kirschner wires, which would make passage of cannulated instruments more difficult.

"Bull's Eye" Approach to Pedicle Targeting

- We have employed the "bull's eye" approach to target the L4, L5, and S1 pedicles but not at other levels, where pedicles are relatively small (L3 and above), or in patients with scoliosis, where the orientation of the pedicle is distorted relative to the anteroposterior and lateral projections of the vertebra.
- The advantage of this technique is less fluoroscopic exposure and movement of the C-arm gantry from the anteroposterior to lateral position, reducing time and risk for surgical field contamination.
- **Figure 84-7:** The aim is to target the superior articular facet overlying the pedicle of interest (indicated by *red oval*). The *shaded rectangle* shows the path of Jamshidi needle through the pedicle using this technique.
- **Figure 84-8:** This approach is facilitated by using the PC Pedicle Access Device (Zimmer Spine, Minneapolis, MN) but can also be done using a standard Jamshidi needle. In anteroposterior view, the tip of the PC Pedicle Access Device is placed in the center of the pedicle of interest (*arrow*).

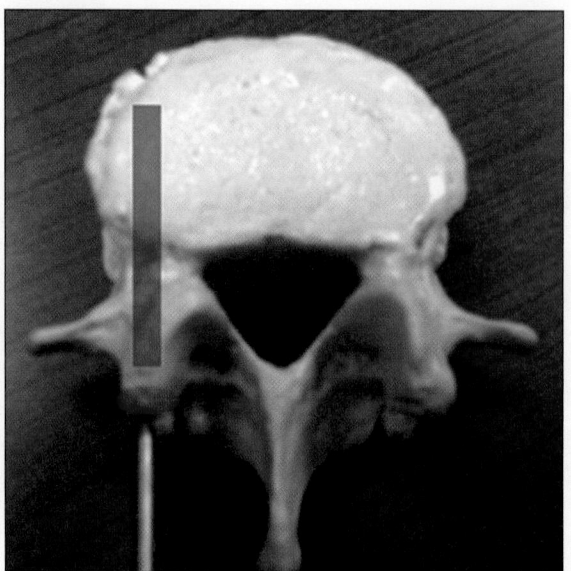

FIGURE 84-7

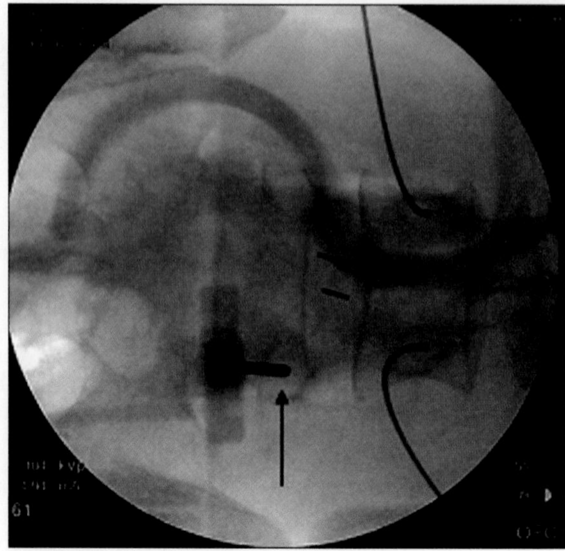

FIGURE 84-8

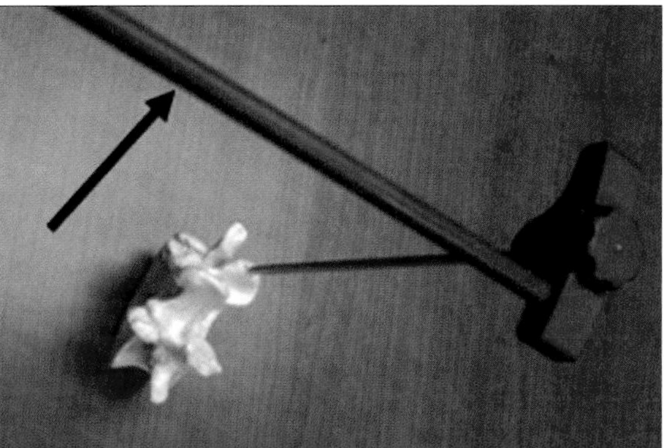

FIGURE 84-9

- **Figure 84-9:** A fluoroscopically translucent extension arm (*arrow*) allows the surgeon to hold the targeting device while limiting x-ray exposure. A few taps of the mallet seats the tip into the cortical bone.
- A Kirschner wire driver is used to pass the Kirschner wire a few millimeters into the bone to hold it in place. We typically place all Kirschner wires in the anteroposterior view first, placing the targeted vertebra in the center of the fluoroscopic image as described earlier.
- The fluoroscopic gantry is placed into a lateral projection. The PC Pedicle Access Device is placed over the Kirschner wire.
- The Kirschner wire is driven in the lateral view through the pedicle in a posterior-to-anterior direction into the vertebral body. If significant resistance is met, reevaluation in the anteroposterior view is done to ensure the Kirschner wire is not directed too medial because the resistance may imply that the Kirschner wire tip is hitting the medial cortical wall of the pedicle. Breaching this wall with the Kirschner wire can result in neural injury.
- After the Kirschner wires are placed, the pedicles are tapped, and the percutaneous pedicle screws are placed as previously described.
- **Figure 84-10:** Comparison pedicle screw insertion using the "bull's eye" approach (**A**) and the lateral-medial approach (**B**).

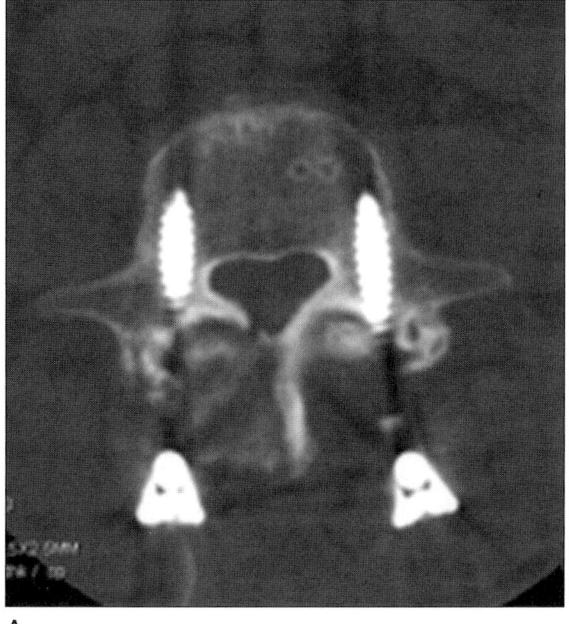

A

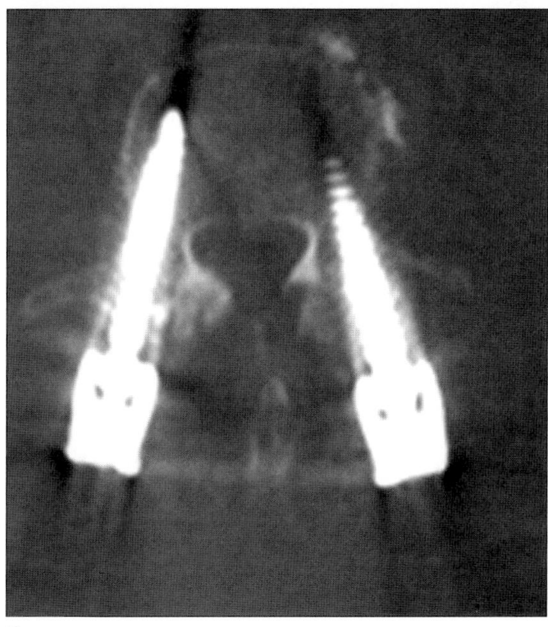

B

FIGURE 84-10

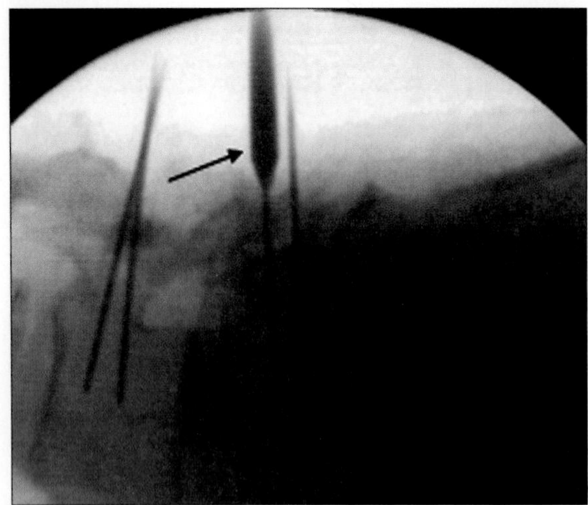

FIGURE 84-11

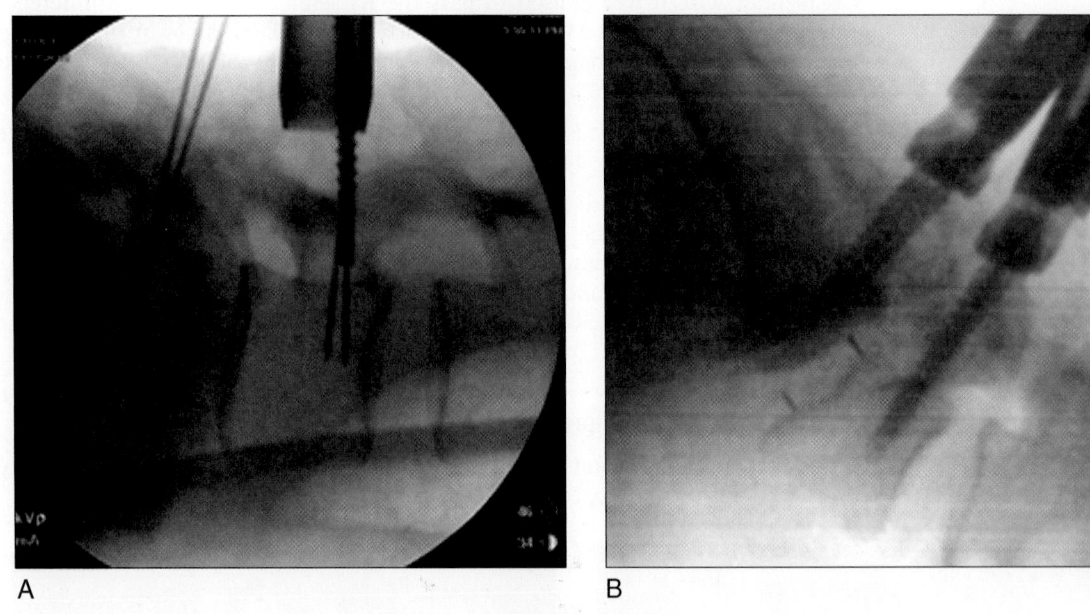

A B

FIGURE 84-12

- **Figure 84-11:** A series of muscle dilators (*arrow*) is passed over the Kirschner wire of the pedicle being instrumented. At all times during the procedure, the Kirschner wire is held with a Kocher clamp. The final working port is placed over the last muscle dilator, and the dilators are removed.
  - The cortex of the pedicle or facet is breached using an awl. Alternatively, an aggressive tap tip can be used to perform the same function.
- **Figure 84-12: A,** An appropriate percutaneous pedicle screw is placed over the Kirschner wire while using a working port and advanced into the vertebral body to allow for movement of the multiaxial head to facilitate rod placement. Multiaxial heads should be placed in subsequent targeted pedicles on a similar plane and depth to facilitate rod placement. We typically use 6.5-mm-diameter × 45-mm-long pedicle screws for L4, and 5-mm- and 6.5-mm-diameter × 40-mm-long screws for S1. We do not breach the anterior vertebral body cortex for bicortical purchase. **B,** The Kirschner wires have been removed after pedicle screw placement.
  - The above-described sequence is repeated for each pedicle. The rod can be placed on one side before proceeding to the other side.

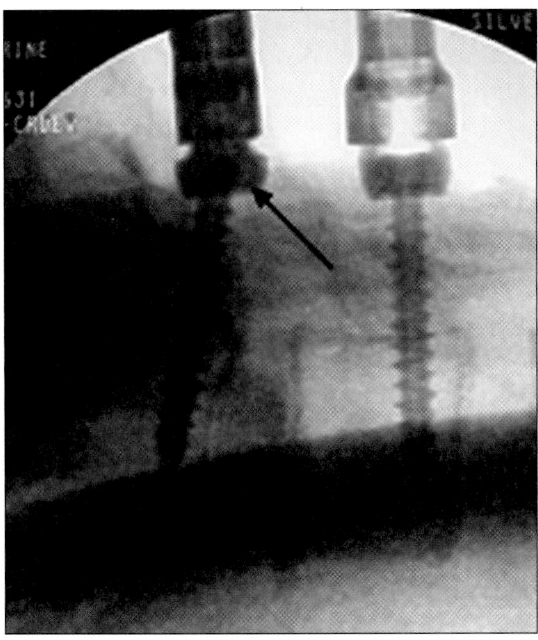

A

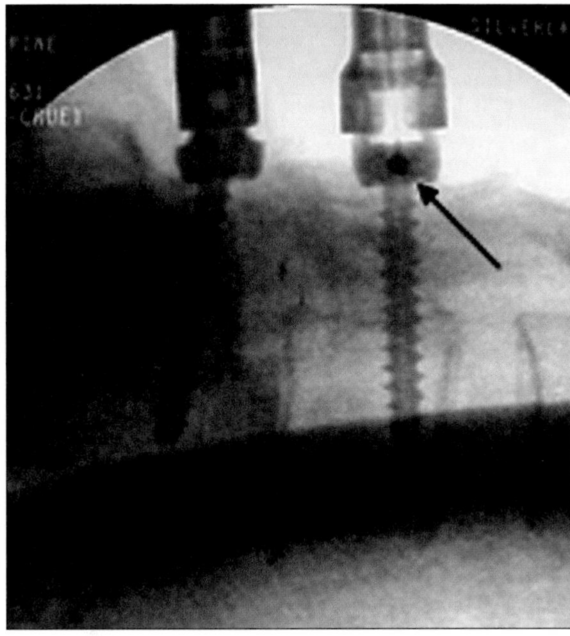

B

FIGURE 84-13

- **Figure 84-13:** We typically stimulate pedicle screw heads using an electromagnetic probe to determine if the pedicle screw is impinging neural elements. Action potentials less than 8 mA requires critical assessment of the pedicle screw location using anteroposterior and lateral fluoroscopic imaging and repositioning if necessary. **A,** Stimulation at L5. **B,** Stimulation at L4.
  - The rod is placed depending on the instrumentation used. Bolts are applied to secure the rod.

Targeting the S1 Pedicle

- The S1 pedicle can offer a challenge because the pedicle is not adequately visualized in many cases.
- **Figure 84-14:** To help define the medial border of the S1 pedicle, view the medial borders of the adjacent L4 and L5 pedicles.

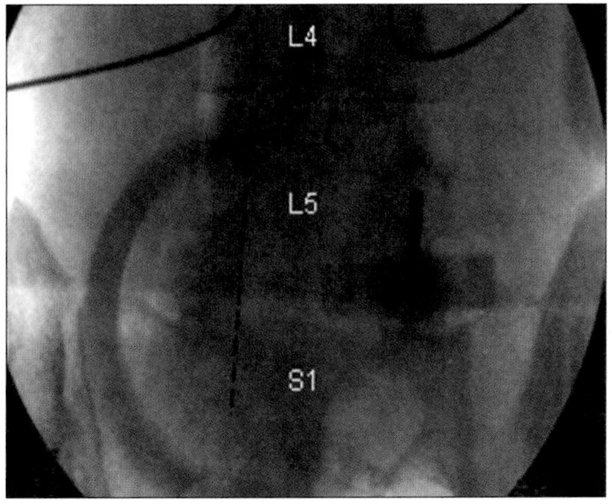

FIGURE 84-14

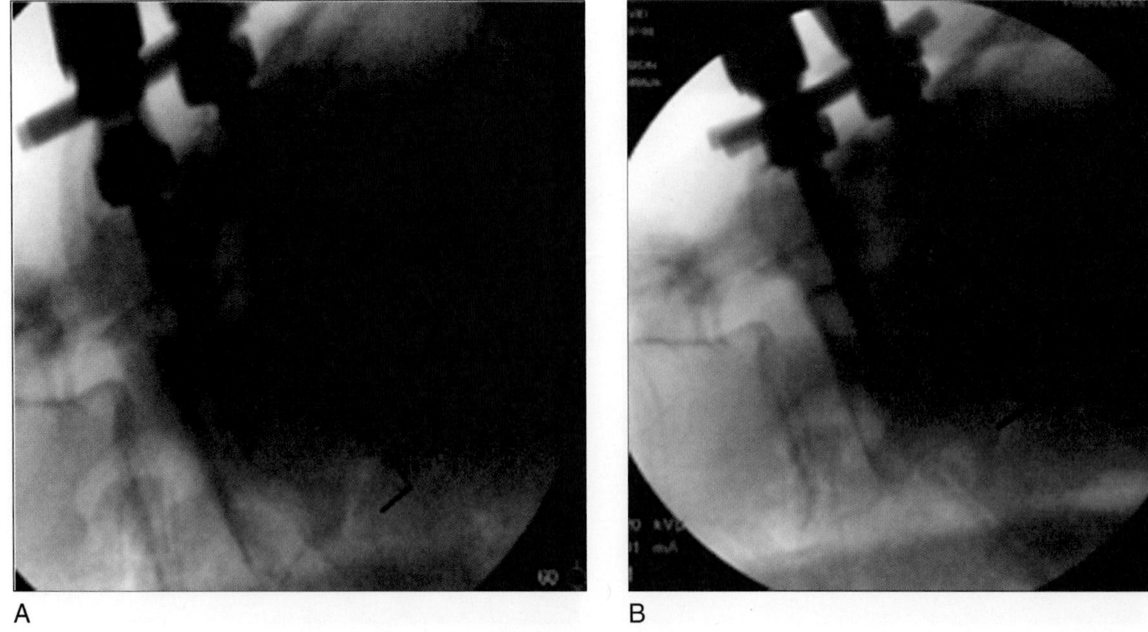

FIGURE 84-15

- The C-arm gantry needs to be placed at a Ferguson angle parallel to the end plate of the S1 vertebra; this requires that the base of the table does not interfere with the C-arm. We prefer to use a Jackson-type table.
- The Jamshidi needle or Kirschner wire needs to be advanced at a similar angle to prevent breaching the superior end plate of the S1 vertebra.
- Typically, the S1 pedicle is the largest, helping to facilitate screw placement.

Reduction Techniques

- Particular pedicle screw systems allow for minimally invasive reduction of spondylolisthesis.
- To achieve reduction, we typically place an interbody fusion device first. This allows for improved movement between adjacent facets.
- Care is taken in patients with "soft bone" because the force of reduction can cause inadvertent screw pullout.
- **Figure 84-15:** Lateral fluoroscopic images illustrating reduction of spondylolisthesis. **A,** The percutaneous pedicle screw of the more anteriorly partially dislocated vertebra is placed deeper to achieve reduction. **B,** Successful reduction.
- The reduction tools are placed, and force is applied gently to restore sagittal alignment. After reduction, the bolts are applied to hold the reduction in place.
- Wound closure is performed by reapproximating the fascial layer using interrupted 2-0 polyglactin 910 (Vicryl) suture. The soft tissue overlying the fascia is similarly closed, and a subcuticular suture is applied. The skin is closed with a skin glue adhesive. Typically, no drains are applied for a one-level or two-level instrumentation.

TIPS FROM THE MASTERS

- Fascia should be sharply incised to allow for ease of manipulation of instruments and safe passage of instrumentation toward the spine.
- Pedicle bone is cancellous and soft. If hard cortical bone is encountered during the advancement of the Jamshidi needle, the surgeon must reassess and, if needed, redirect the needle. The needle may be hitting the medial wall of the pedicle.
- Proper visualization of each individual vertebral body pedicle facilitates screw placement.

PITFALLS

Failure to obtain true anteroposterior and lateral images of the spine can result in potentially disastrous complications, such as nerve root and spinal cord injury with Jamshidi needle or Kirschner wire placement.

The guidewire must always be held by an assistant when dilators or cannulated instruments are being placed or when the Jamshidi needle is being removed. If this is not done properly, the guidewire may be removed inadvertently or inserted too far.

BAILOUT OPTIONS

- A more lateral trajectory can be attempted if the pedicle wall is breached medially. If this fails, additional cephalad and caudal levels can be used to obtain additional points of fixation.
- If the tip of the Kirschner wire gets bent and cannot be removed after placing the pedicle screw, use a mallet to tap the Kirschner wire gently out using a Kocher clamp. If still stuck, back the screw out slightly, and tap with the mallet again.

SUGGESTED READINGS

Foley KT, Gupta SK. Percutaneous pedicle screw fixation of the lumbar spine: preliminary clinical results. J Neurosurg 2002;97(Suppl. 1):7–12.

Foley KT, Gupta SK, Justis JR, et al. Percutaneous pedicle screw fixation of the lumbar spine. Neurosurg Focus 2001;10:E10.

Gepstein R, Shabat S, Reichel M, et al. Treatment of postdiscectomy low back pain by percutaneous posterior lumbar interbody fusion versus open posterior lumbar fusion with pedicle screws. Spine J 2008;8:741–6.

Kim DY, Lee SH, Chung SK, et al. Comparison of multifidus muscle atrophy and trunk extension muscle strength: percutaneous versus open pedicle screw fixation. Spine (Phila Pa 1976) 2005;30:123–9.

Perez-Cruet MJ. Percutaneous pedicle screw placement for spinal instrumentation. In: Perez-Cruet MJ, Khoo L, Fessler RG, editors. An Anatomical Approach to Minimally Invasive Spine Surgery. St. Louis: Quality Medical Publishing; 2006.

Procedure 85 TranS1 Sacral

William D. Tobler

INDICATIONS

- Symptomatic degenerative disk disease affecting L5-S1 or L4-5-S1
- Spondylolisthesis affecting L5-S1 or L4-5-S1
- Stabilization of L4-S1 segments for pathology at L5 (i.e., burst fracture, neoplasm)
- Revision fusion for pseudarthrosis at L5-S1

CONTRAINDICATIONS

- Previous surgical procedures that involved the presacral space resulting in fibrosis in this space, then rendering the rectum immobile and scarred to the anterior sacrum
- History of perirectal abscess
- Severe chronic inflammatory bowel disease
- History of pelvic radiation
- Current pregnancy
- Anomalous iliac vessels in the presacral space evaluated by magnetic resonance imaging (MRI) or computed tomography (CT) angiography
- Abnormally accentuated sacral curve that would necessitate an impossible trajectory for targeting and placement of the rod for L-5-S1 or L4-5-S1 levels (all potential patients should undergo a preoperative evaluation to assess trajectory by a lateral, standing x-ray of the lumbar spine, entire sacrum, and coccyx)
- History of pilonidal cyst or hysterectomy—not contraindications

PLANNING AND POSITIONING

- The trajectory for the procedure is evaluated with x-rays and MRI before scheduling the procedure.
- MRI or CT angiography of the presacral space is performed to evaluate for vascular anomalies or other pathology (e.g., tumor) before scheduling the surgery.
- The patient begins a clear liquid diet at noon the day before surgery and completes a bowel preparation later that day.
- The patient is positioned prone.
- Lordosis must be maintained or accentuated by placement of bolsters under the hips, thighs, or knees. Lordosis curve is checked with fluoroscopy.
- Legs must be fully abducted on the table or spine frame, specifically required for initial portion of the procedure.
- An occlusive barrier is placed just above the rectal sphincter (facilitated by placing 3-inch tape on each buttock; other end of the tape is secured laterally to the table, then retracting each buttock).

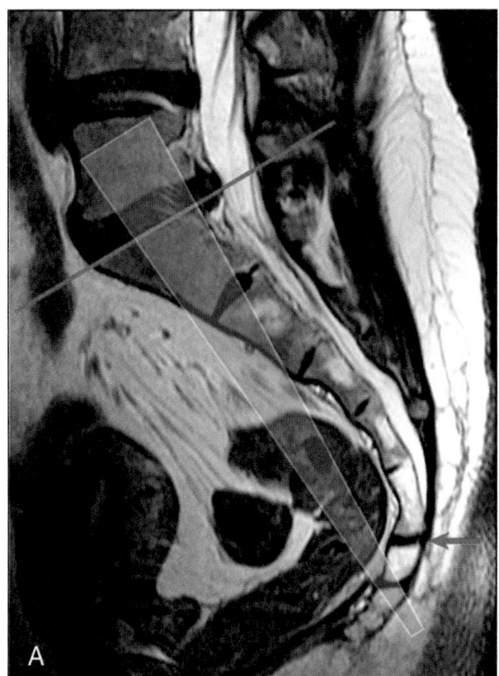

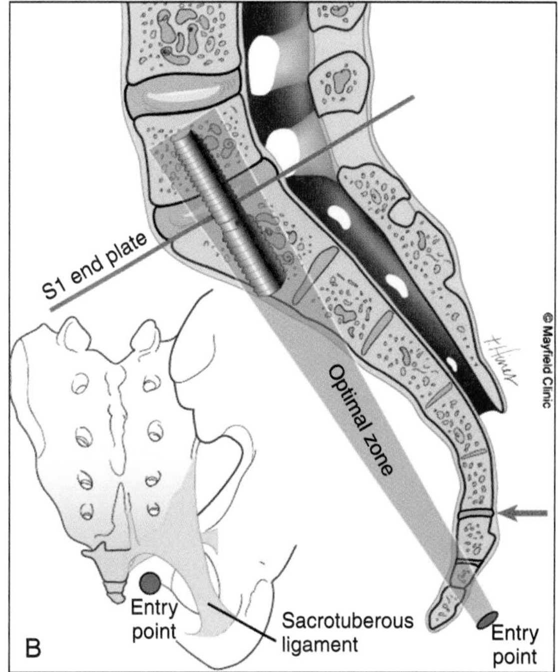

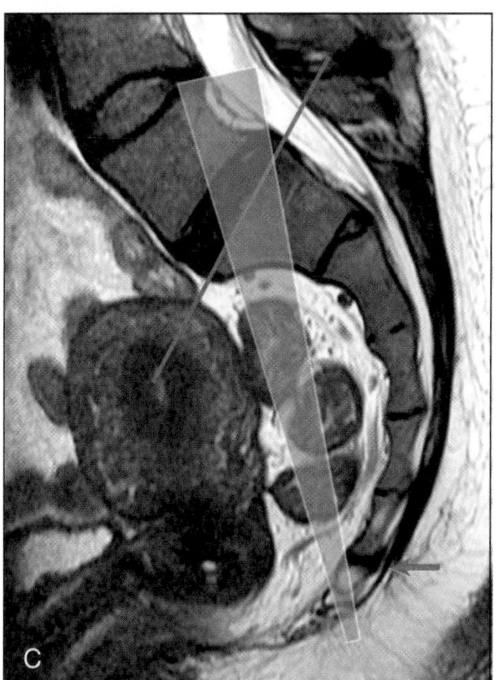

FIGURE 85-1

- A Foley catheter placed in the rectum permits injection of air to define clearly the distal portion of the rectum and its relationship to the sacrum.
- Although two fluoroscopy units are preferable, the procedure can be performed with a single fluoroscopy unit.
- **Figure 85-1:** Lumbar interbody fusion using TranS1 (Wilmington, NC) instrumentation. **A,** Typical sacrum and trajectory for the TranS1 (Wilmington, NC) approach. The rectum and presacral space are easily seen. **B,** Optimal zone for placement of the axial rod and entry point relative to the sacrococcygeal ligament and coccyx. **C,** In this example, a TranS1 (Wilmington, NC) procedure is contraindicated because the sacral curve would create a trajectory that could cause axial rod placement in the spinal canal.

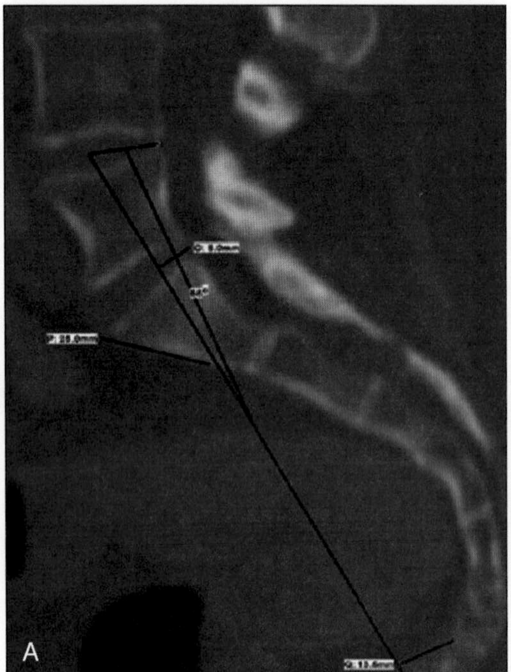

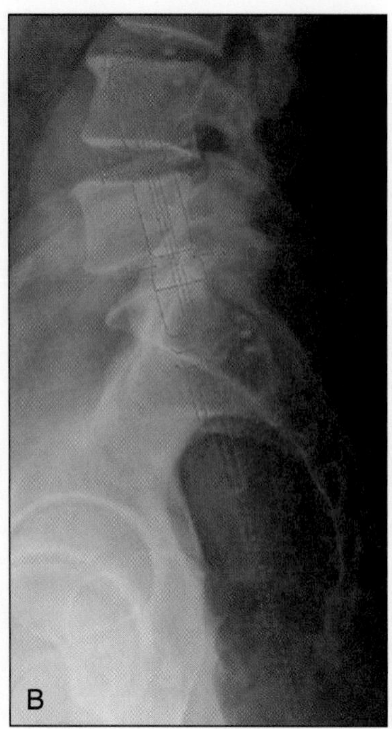

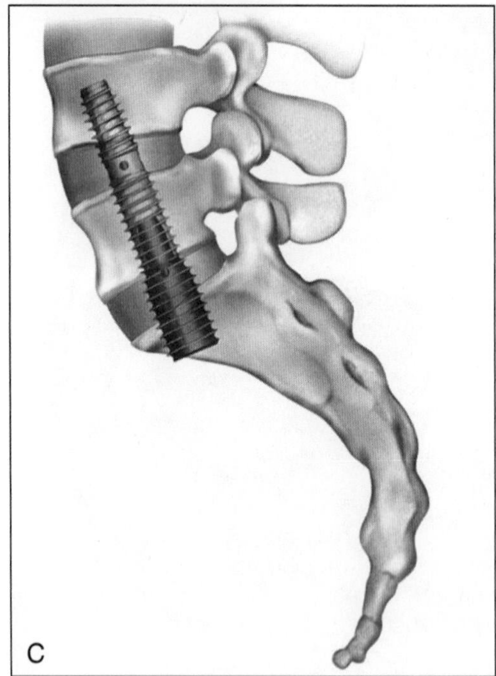

FIGURE 85-2

- **Figure 85-2:** Preoperative templating for trajectory. **A,** CT scan is used to map the trajectory for a one-level procedure. **B,** Standing lateral x-ray is preferred to map the two-level procedure because it shows the patient's preoperative lordosis. **C,** Placement of the two-level axial rod.
- **Figure 85-3:** Operating room setup for TranS1. **A,** The patient is positioned prone, with the buttocks and legs abducted. After the buttocks are retracted and secured with tape, a Foley catheter is placed in the rectum. **B,** Lateral fluoroscopy of the presacral space and the bowel after air is injected into the rectum. **C,** The occlusive drape is placed above the rectal sphincter. **D,** Two fluoroscopy units are positioned for the procedure in the lateral and anteroposterior planes.

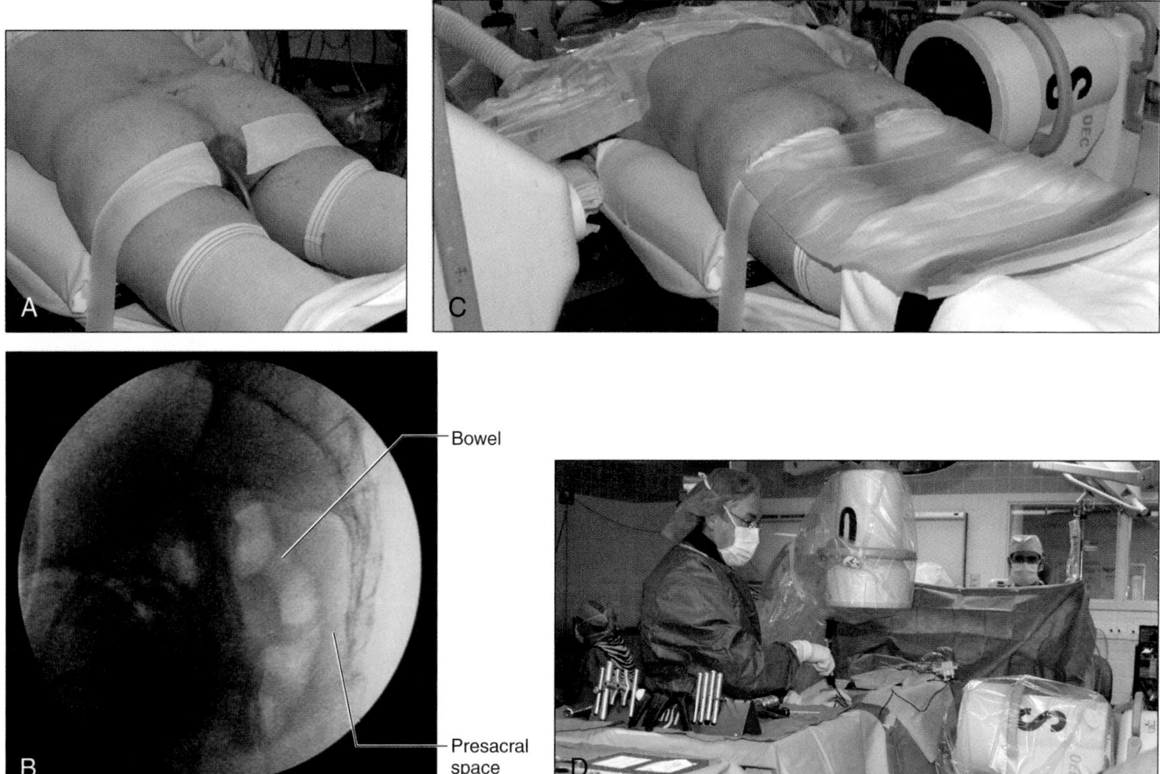

FIGURE 85-3

PROCEDURE

- **Figure 85-4:** Opening the presacral space. **A,** The surgeon uses blunt finger dissection to open the presacral space. **B,** A finger sweep displaces the rectum downward, developing the working space, even in patients with little or no presacral fat. **C,** The guide probe is advanced to the sacral entry point determined by the surgeon.
- **Figure 85-5:** Illustration (*top*) and correlative fluoroscopic (*bottom*) views. **A,** Placement of a 9-mm working cannula; the trajectory has been determined by this placement. **B,** The drill is advanced through the sacrum, past the disk space, and into the L5 vertebra.
- **Figure 85-6:** Diskectomy. **A,** Looped Nitinol cutters are placed into the disk space. Cutters come in various sizes (upcutting, downcutting, 10-mm and 15-mm lengths). **B,** The cutters are rotated circumferentially around the disk. The end plates are prepared by pushing cutting loops against the end plate.
- **Figure 85-7:** Wire-brush tissue extractors are used to extract all available disk material—photograph (**A**) and illustrative operative view (**B**). In some extractions, 10 or more brushes may be used.
- **Figure 85-8:** Filling the prepared disk space with bone graft material as per the surgeon's preference. Some autograft can be obtained from the sacral drillings. **A,** Material is delivered by a beveled cannula and can be directed circumferentially in the disk space. **B,** The channel is drilled into the L5 vertebral body. **C,** Length of the rod is calculated by placing a Steinmann pin into the drilled channel and measuring from the distal L5 vertebral body to the anterior sacral entry point.
- **Figure 85-9:** Advancement of the rod. **A,** The rod is advanced across the disk space into L5 through the exchange cannula. **B,** As the rod is placed in its final position, some distraction of the space may occur because of differential thread counts of the L5 and S1 portions of the rod. The strong purchase of the device often requires significant physical effort for insertion. **C,** Final position of the rod.

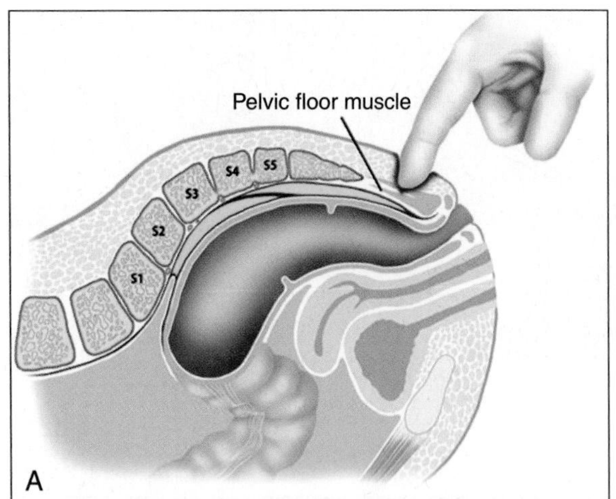

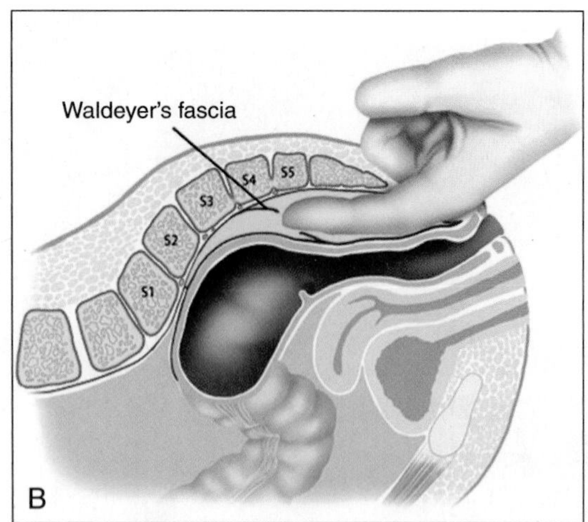

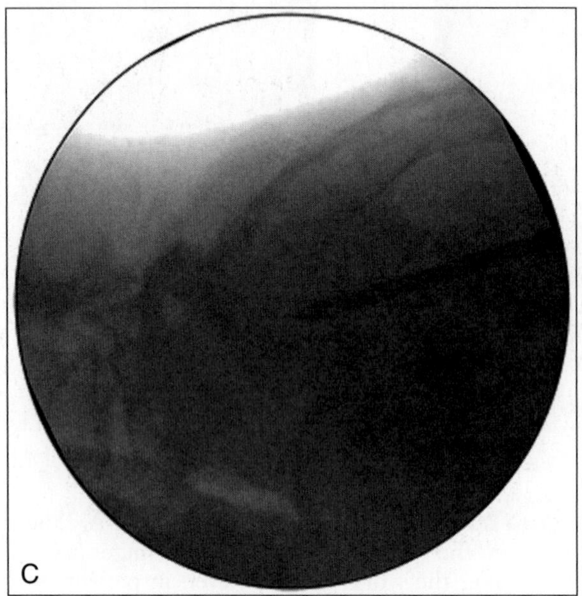

FIGURE 85-4

- **Figure 85-10:** Illustration and correlative fluoroscopic views of AxiaLIF (TranS1, Wilmington, NC) two-level procedure. **A,** After the first level is packed with graft material, instruments are advanced to the L4-5 level where the diskectomy and curettage procedure are performed. The disk space at L4-5 is packed with graft material. **B,** After measurement of rod length. A two-piece rod construct is inserted at L4-5 followed by insertion of the S1 rod. **C,** The two-level rod.
- **Figure 85-11:** Placement of facet screws. **A,** A Kirschner wire is advanced across the facet. **B,** After using the cannulated drill and tap, the surgeon advances the cannulated screw along the wire into position. **C,** Anteroposterior view of both facet screws in place. **D,** The procedure is performed through the small cannula, and an incision less than 1 cm is made at the L3-4 interspace.
- **Figure 85-12:** At 1-year follow up, CT scans show solid fusion in single-level (**A** and **B**) and two-level surgical procedures (**C**).

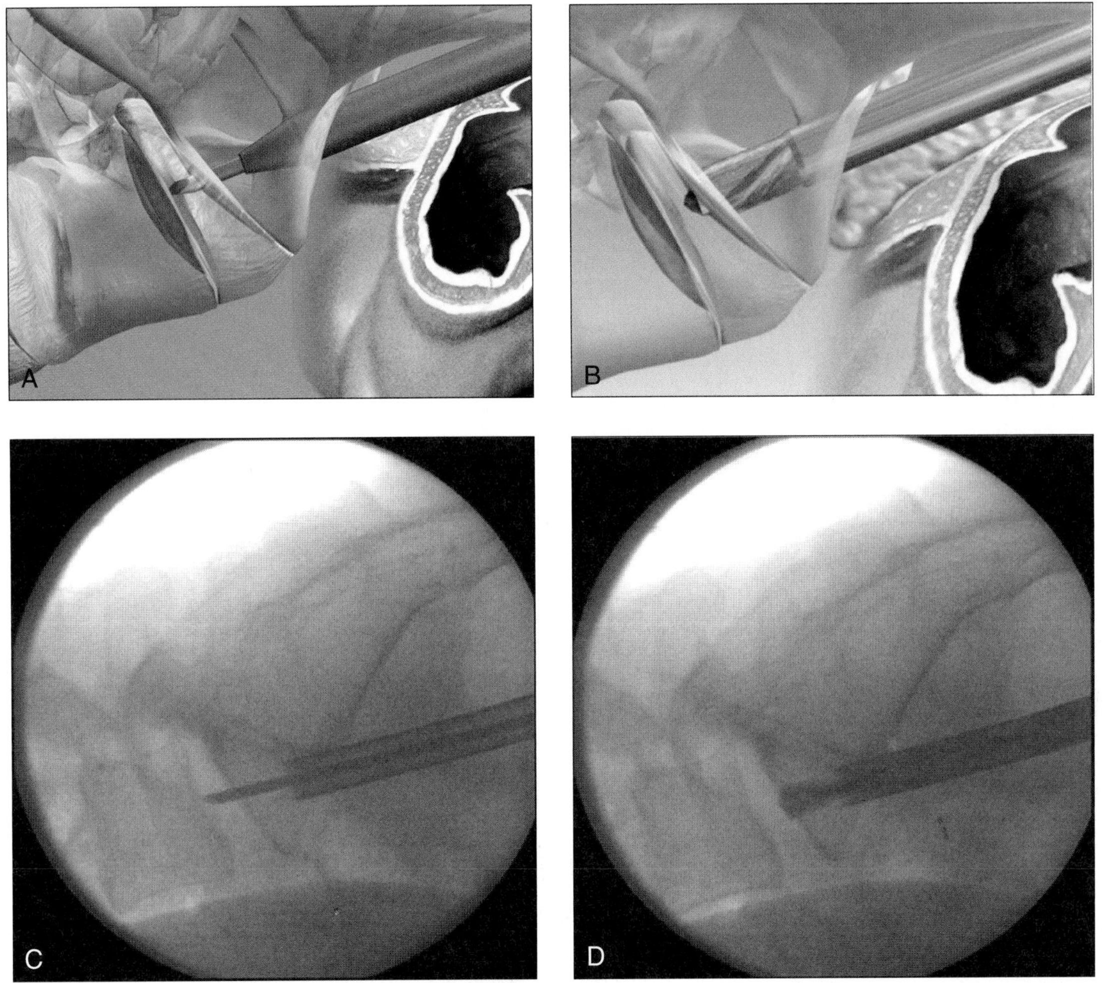

FIGURE 85-5

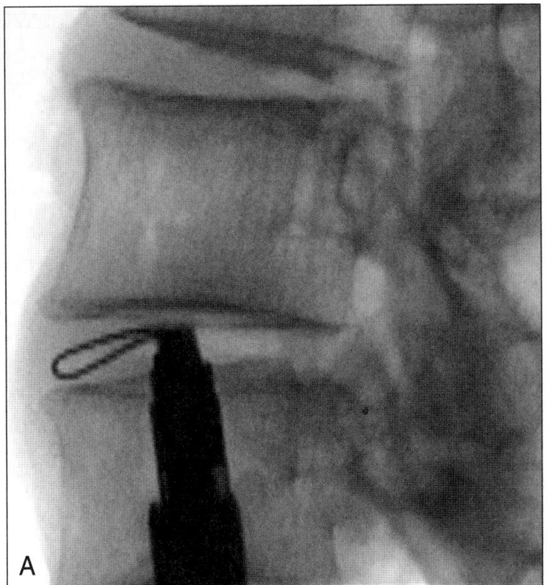

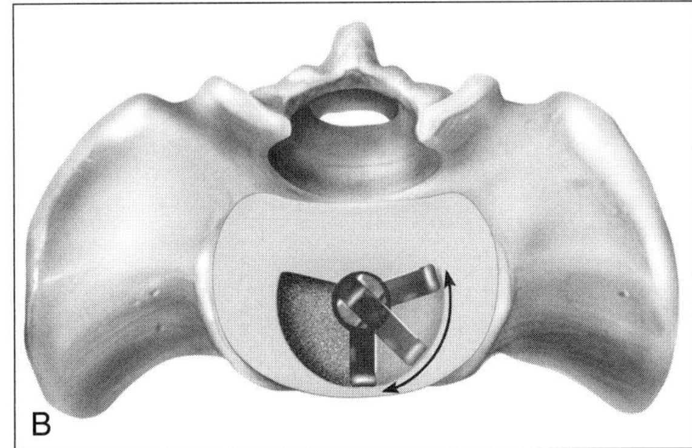

FIGURE 85-6

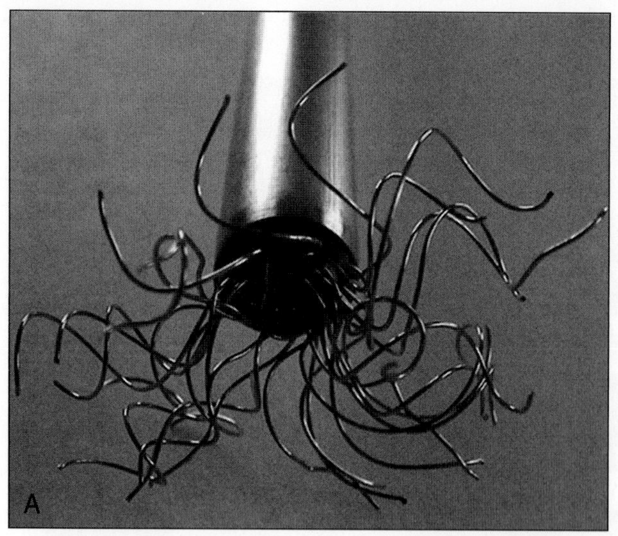

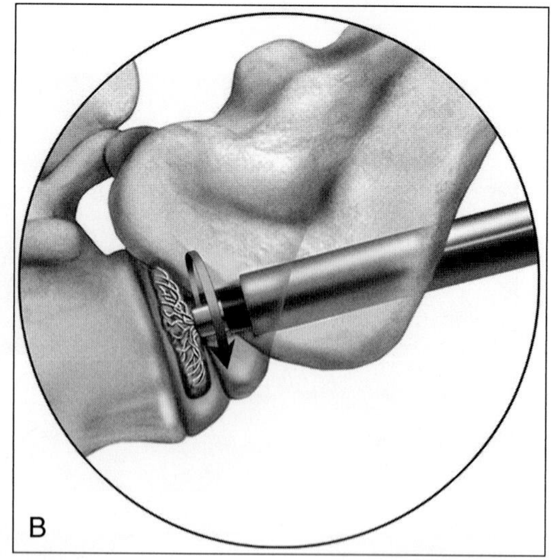

FIGURE 85-7

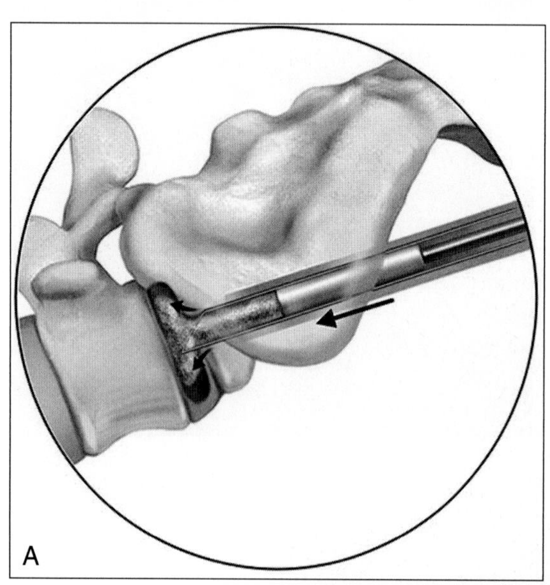

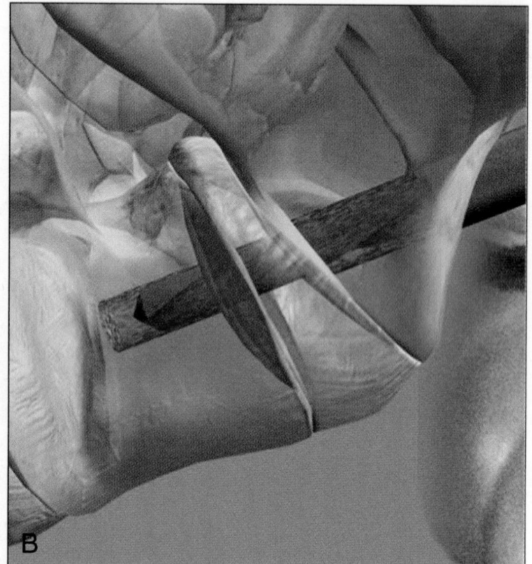

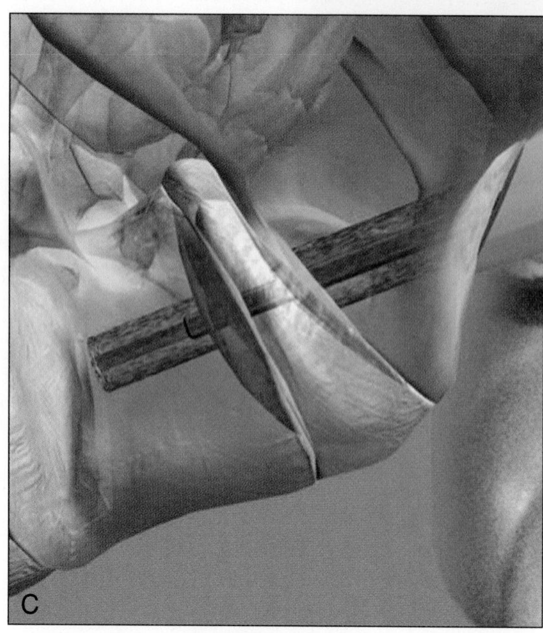

FIGURE 85-8

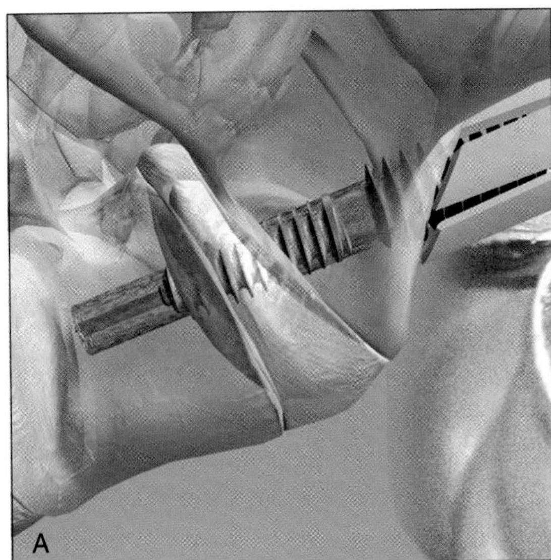

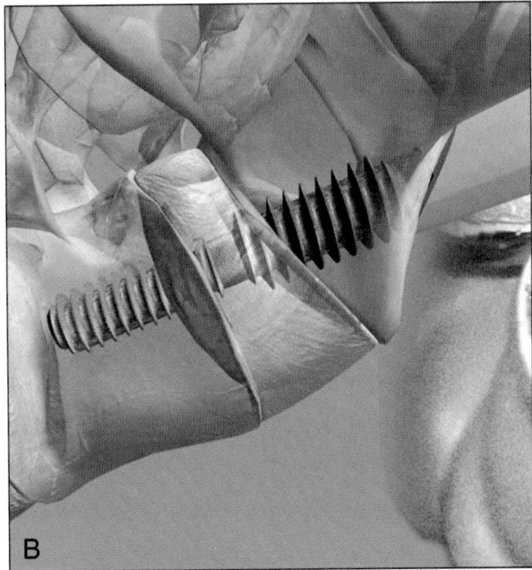

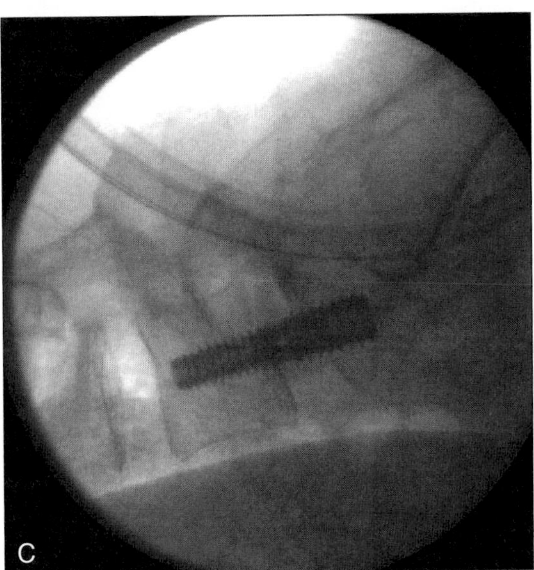

FIGURE 85-9

TIPS FROM THE MASTERS

- Always carefully template your trajectory before scheduling the procedure.
- Use a blunt finger sweep to open the presacral space.
- Use meticulous technique, with a focus on thorough aggressive disk preparation.
- The diskectomy is not complete until the brushes removed from the disk space contain no disk material.
- Always keep instrumentation in the midline and close to the sacrum.

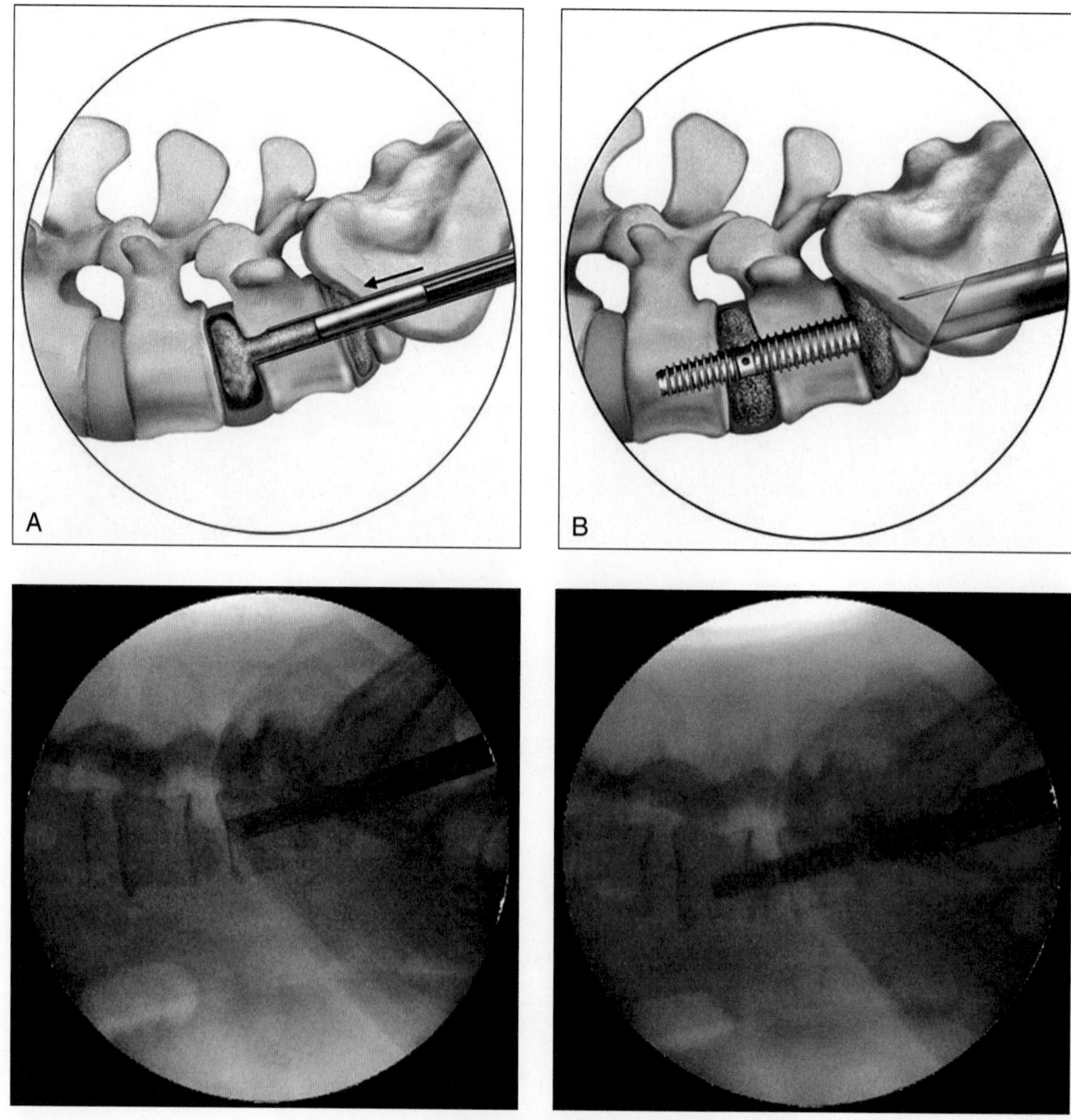

FIGURE 85-10

- Never advance any instrument without fluoroscopic guidance.
- Do not aim to place the rod perfectly straight in the coronal plane. A slightly tilted rod has better purchase and stability.
- In the sagittal plane, angling the rod with an anterior tilt, anterior to the midpoint of the vertebrae, helps to create lordosis.
- A rod placed posterior to the midpoint may distract open the posterior portion of the vertebra, resulting in a decrease in lordosis.

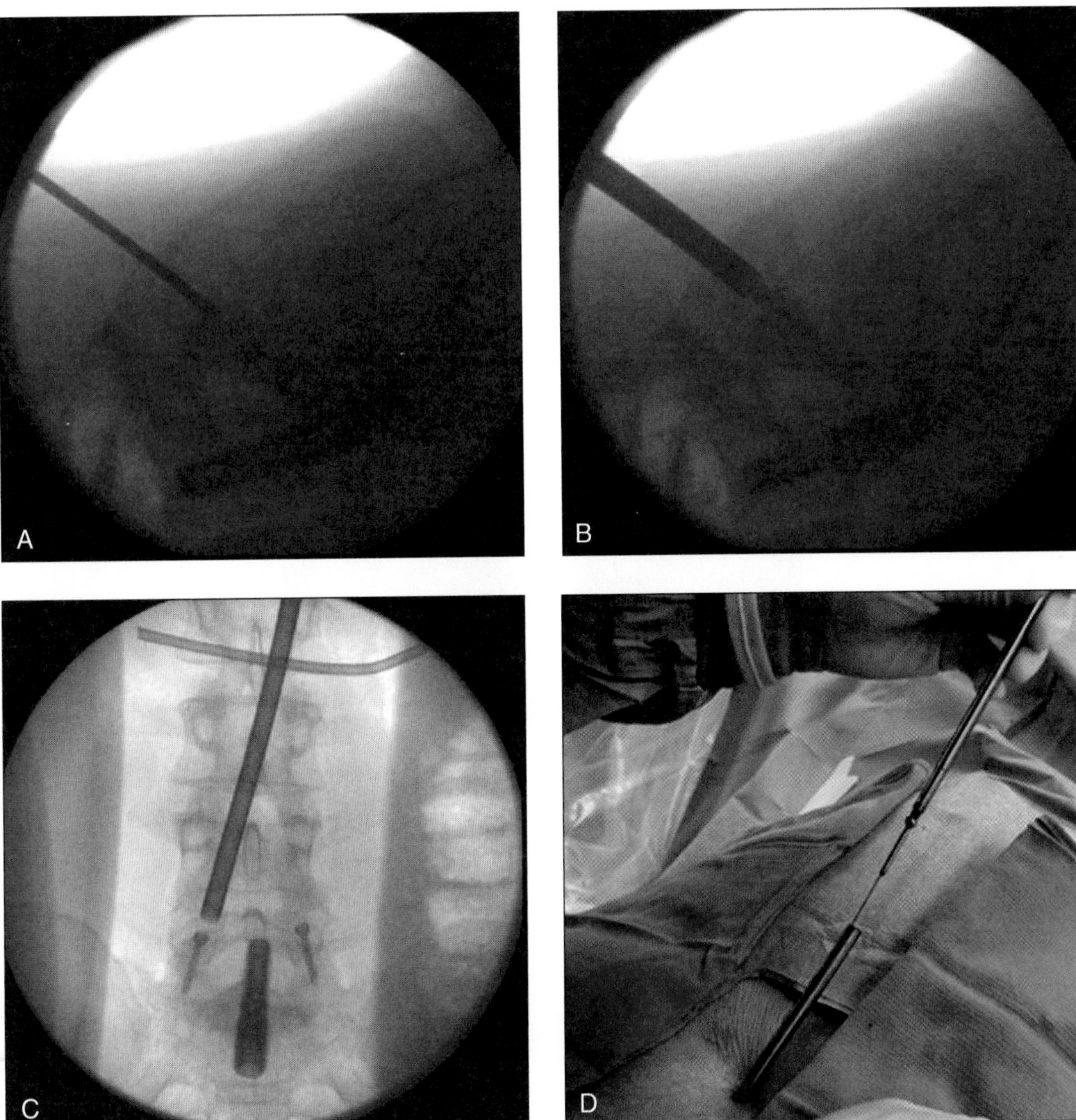

FIGURE 85-11

- Choose a rod that is long enough to protrude slightly from the anterior sacrum; this ensures that no postoperative bleeding will occur from an exposed sacral channel and that an additional point of purchase against the anterior sacrum.
- Discuss the procedure with and educate a colorectal surgeon in your institution before performing this technique.
- During surgery, a potential bowel injury can be recognized by injecting contrast agent into the rectum to identify a breach, which then can be repaired by expeditiously a colorectal surgeon. This early diagnosis can avoid an infection and colostomy.

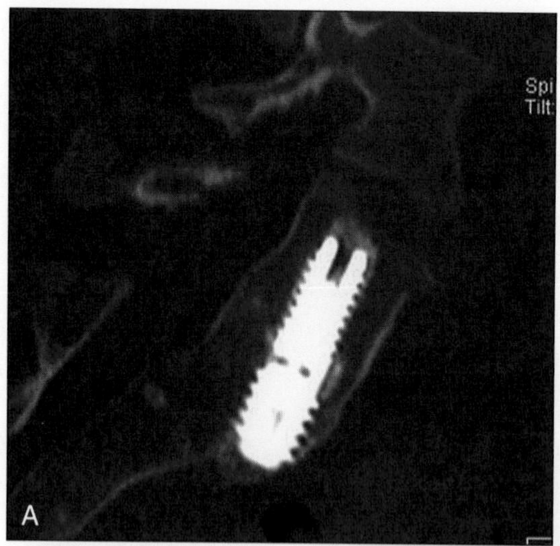

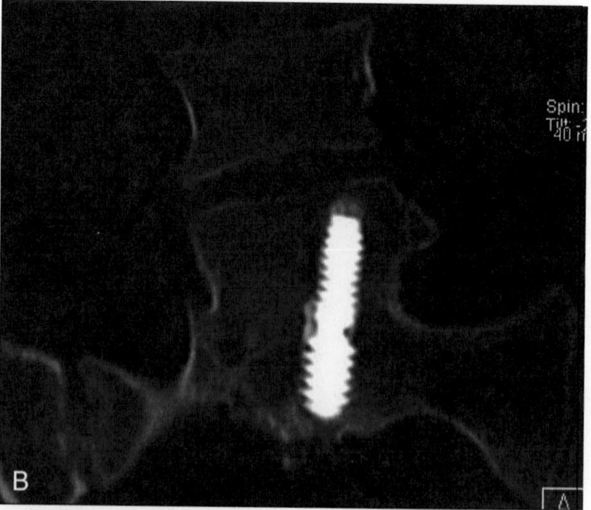

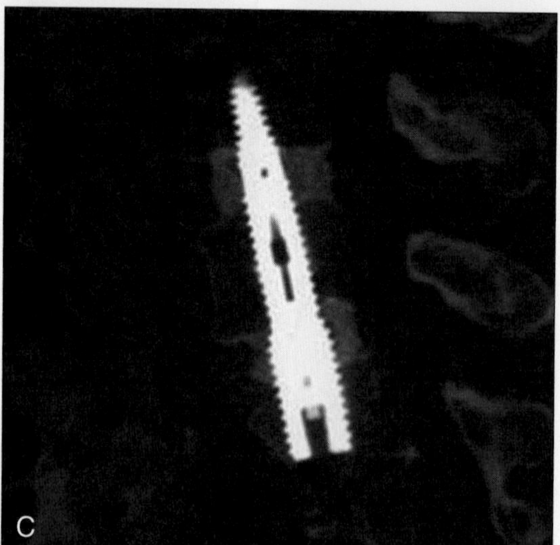

FIGURE 85-12

PITFALLS

Perfect orthogonal alignment on anteroposterior and lateral fluoroscopy is essential. A nonorthogonal view (especially in the anteroposterior view) can result in a very poor or potentially risky placement of the axial rod.

Carefully plan your trajectory: Avoid drilling a sacral channel and then decide to change trajectory. Never drill a second sacral channel.

Beware of soft bone (osteopenia), which can result in poor purchase of the rod and damage to the end plates with the Nitinol cutting loops.

PITFALLS—cont'd

Carefully evaluate the position of the loop cutters within the disk space before rotating circumferentially. Depending on their placement in the disk and the vertebral size, the cutters could sharply cut posterior into the spinal canal, resulting in damage to the neural elements. Cutting anterior beyond the confines of the anterior longitudinal ligament could result in laceration of the great vessels at L4-5.

Packing the disk with graft material in a patient who underwent a previous diskectomy (i.e., annular defect) could result in extrusion into the spinal canal, particularly if directing the material posterior toward the side of the defect.

Overly aggressive distraction can lead to delayed subsidence.

Use flat cutters for more aggressive end plate preparation and for complete loss of disk height.

Placing an oversized rod can damage the end plate above the fusion level.

BAILOUT OPTIONS

- Other fusion options include anterior lumbar interbody fusion, thoracolumbar interbody fusion, and posterior lumbar interbody fusion.
- If a two-level axial rod was planned, but its placement was deemed to be infeasible during the operation, have a plan for a thoracolumbar interbody fusion, posterior lumbar interbody fusion, or direct lateral interbody fusion as an alternative. Discuss this possibility with the patient when planning the surgery.
- Anterior lumbar interbody fusion or posterior lumbar interbody fusion cages can be placed in cases of AxiaLIF pseudarthrosis, without removing the rod.
- Removal of the axial rod using the same approach with a custom removal tool should not be difficult. This should be an extremely infrequent occurrence.

SUGGESTED READINGS

Bohinski RJ, Jain VV, Tobler WD. Presacral retroperitoneal approach to axial lumbar interbody fusion: a new, minimally invasive technique at L5-S1: Clinical outcomes, complications, and fusion rates in 50 patients at 1-year follow-up. SAS Journal 2010;4:54–62.

Carl A, Ledet E, Oliveira C. Percutaneous axial lumbar spine surgery. In: Perez-Cruet MJ, Khoo LT, Fessler RG, editors. An Anatomic Approach to Minimally Invasive Spine Surgery. St. Louis: Quality Medical Publishing; 2006, p. 654–70.

Cragg A, Carl A, Casteneda F, Dickman C, et al. New percutaneous access method for minimally invasive anterior lumbosacral surgery. J Spinal Disord Tech 2004;17:21–8.

Marotta N, Cosar M, Pimenta L, Khoo LT. A novel minimally invasive presacral approach and instrumentation technique for anterior L5-S1 intervertebral discectomy and fusion: technical description and case presentations. Neurosurg Focus 2006;20:E9.

Sandén B, Olerud C, Petrén-Mallmin M, Johansson C, et al. The significance of radiolucent zones surrounding pedicle screws. Definition of screw loosening in spinal instrumentation. J Bone Joint Surg Br 2004;86(3):457–61.

Figures 85-1, 85-3, 85-11, and 85-12 are reprinted with permission from Mayfield Clinic.

Figures 85-2 and 85-4 through 85-10 are reprinted with permission from Trans1, Wilmington, NC.

Procedure 86

Minimally Invasive Direct Lateral Transpsoas Interbody Fusion

Patrick A. Sugrue, John C. Liu

INDICATIONS

- Indications are any situation or condition requiring interbody fusion at the level of L1-2 through L4-5 including adult spinal deformity, degenerative disk disease, adjacent segment disease, low-grade spondylolisthesis, and foraminal stenosis where direct neural decompression is not required.
- The direct lateral approach can be used to correct coronal imbalance or degenerative disease by restoring alignment and providing indirect foraminal decompression.
- The patient must have favorable anatomy in terms of the ability to access the disk space via the direct lateral transpsoas approach. There must be enough space in the working channel between the 12th rib and the iliac crest. The size of the iliac crest in men may prevent access to the L4-5 disk space.

CONTRAINDICATIONS

- The direct lateral approach does not allow access to the L5-S1 disk space because of the significant risk of injury to the lumbar plexus at that level and the fact that the iliac crest prevents an appropriate working angle.
- The use of stand-alone direct lateral transpsoas interbody fusion is controversial; however, in situations in which the posterior tension band is intact without any evidence of instability, stand-alone direct lateral transpsoas interbody fusion may be appropriate. The direct lateral transpsoas technique is likely not indicated, however, at a level of high mechanical demand, such as adjacent to a previously fused segment.
- Grade II or higher spondylolisthesis is a contraindication.
- The procedure is also contraindicated in patients with prior retroperitoneal surgery or presence of a psoas abscess.

PLANNING AND POSITIONING

- Preoperative planning includes detailed study of the patient's psoas muscle (seen best on magnetic resonance imaging [MRI]) and bony anatomy including the accessibility of the appropriate disk space with regard to the working channel between the 12th rib and the iliac crest. A high iliac crest, which is more prevalent in men, may prevent access to the L4-5 disk space. The presence of long 11th or 12th ribs does not preclude access to the upper lumbar spine but may require an intercostal approach or rib resection. In scoliosis cases, the disk space can be accessed from the concavity or the convexity of the curve. Using the concavity has the disadvantages of working through a longer tube and needing to access the disk space through the collapsed side but has the advantage of rendering multiple levels accessible through a single incision. Conversely, using the convexity of the curve brings the disk space closer to the operating surgeon and takes advantage of more open disk spaces but typically requires more incisions per disk space instrumented. Likewise, abnormal vascular or muscular anatomy may determine which side provides safer or easier access.
- The use of radiography is essential in the direct lateral approach. True lateral and anteroposterior images must be obtained. Fluoroscopy (C-arm) provides real-time data and adjustable angulation but is associated with a significant risk of radiation exposure, the

need for repeatedly adjusting from anteroposterior to lateral views, and the challenge of having to work around the C-arm tube. Alternatively, intraoperative stereotactic navigation can be used to reduce radiation exposure and eliminate the obtrusive C-arm tube. The navigation images are static, however, and changes in alignment that occur after placement of even a single interbody graft can render the registration inaccurate. Likewise, the registration can be ruined by even minute alterations in the position of the reference device.

- Intraoperative neuromonitoring must be established using free running electromyography (EMG) and active or triggered EMG set at 6 to 8 mA. Free running EMG helps to identify any nerve irritation or stretch at any point during the procedure, whereas triggered EMG can identify neural structures during the dissection via direct stimulation. The genitofemoral nerve cannot be identified by neuromonitoring and must be visualized. Postoperatively, 25% of patients may experience a burning groin pain because of genitofemoral nerve irritation.
- **Figure 86-1:** The patient must be in a position to obtain true lateral and true anteroposterior imaging. The patient is placed in a lateral decubitus position with the hip over the break in the operating table with the top leg flexed to relax the ipsilateral psoas muscle. Bony prominences are padded thoroughly. The operating table is broken to increase the working distance between the 12th rib and iliac crest and to open up the disk space toward the surgeon. The use of a beanbag can aid in maintaining patient positioning, and thorough taping must be used to secure the patient fully in position on the operating table. Ultimately, the bed, not the C-arm, is moved during the procedure to obtain true anteroposterior and lateral views. The patient must also be positioned on the operating table such that the C-arm is able to move freely to visualize the area of interest.
- **Figure 86-2:** Position the C-arm before draping. The C-arm gantry should remain at 0 degrees throughout the case. Adjust the position of the bed with the patient secured to obtain true anteroposterior and lateral images. The disk space must be visualized parallel to the fluoroscopy beam so that the end plates are seen cleanly and only one pedicle is visualized in the lateral view. In the anteroposterior view, the spinous process must be in the midline with the pedicles visualized equally bilaterally. In cases involving multiple levels, the bed position must be adjusted at every level to reorient and obtain true anteroposterior and lateral views for that level. Accurate and clear fluoroscopy is key.
- **Figure 86-3:** After true anteroposterior and lateral images have been obtained with the C-arm gantry at 0 degrees, the patient can be prepared and draped. This positioning allows the surgeon to orient his or her trajectory in a direction perpendicular to the floor, accessing the disk space in a consistent fashion and at a comfortable working angle. Such orientation minimizes the risk of taking a trajectory that is too anterior, risking the aorta, inferior vena cava, or iliac vessels or placing the interbody graft off target into the foramen. The surgeon must reorient at each level by adjusting the table.

A

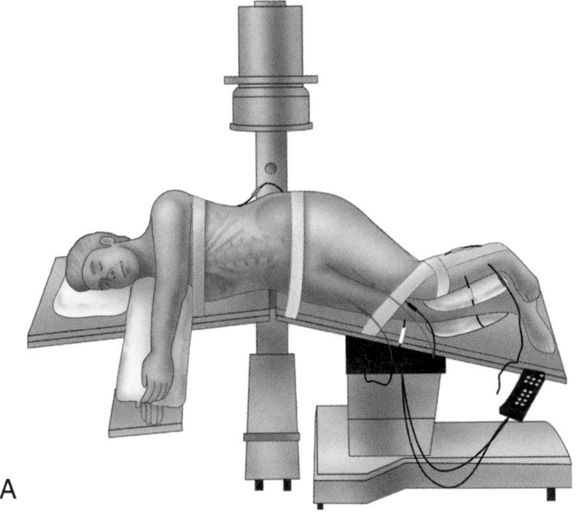

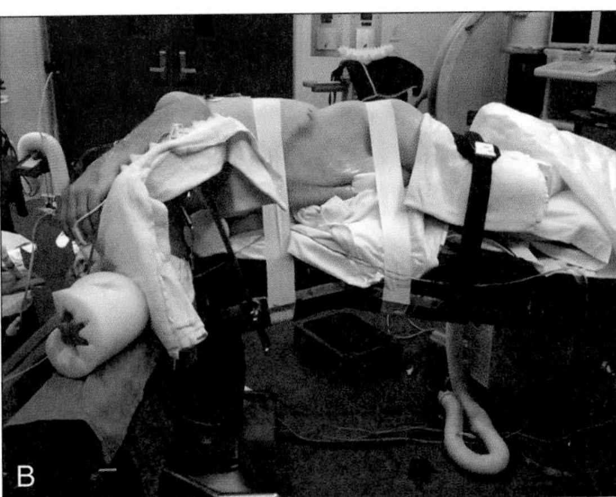

B

FIGURE 86-1

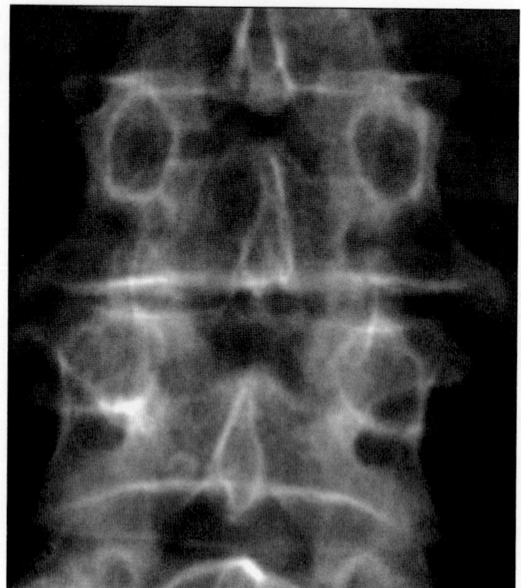

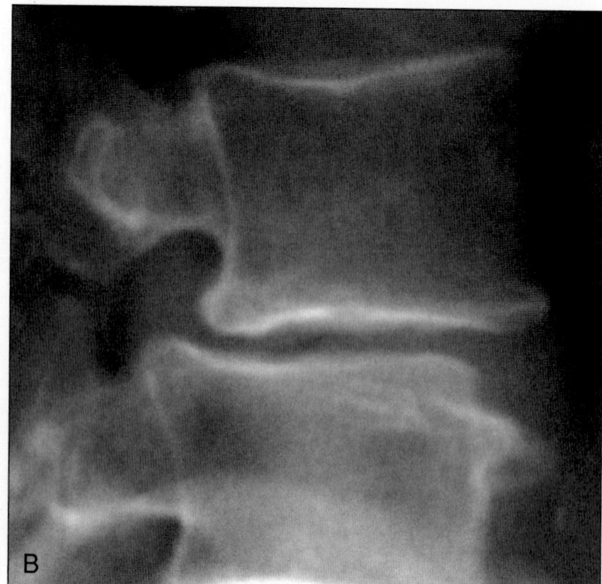

FIGURE 86-2

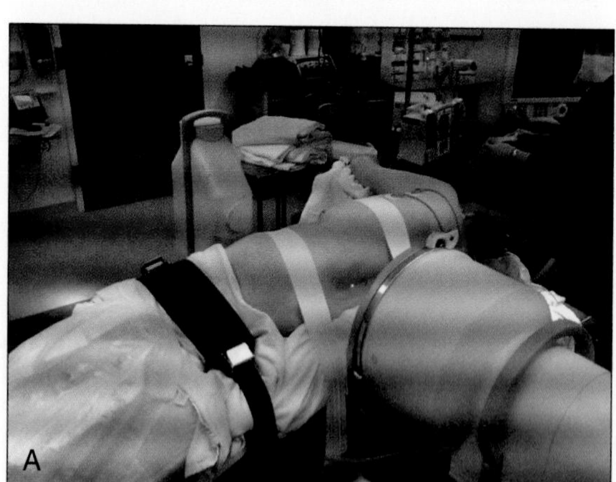

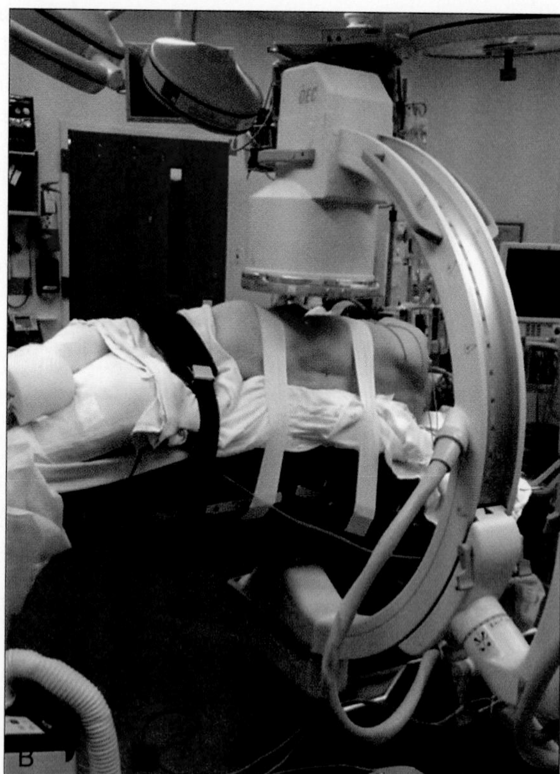

FIGURE 86-3

PROCEDURE

- **Figure 86-4:** The planned incision (2.5 to 3 cm) is typically marked with an *X* directly over the targeted disk space for a single-level case. Alternatively, a single incision can be used to access two adjacent levels, and the incision is placed at the midpoint between two adjacent levels. The incision can be transverse, horizontal, or vertical depending on the surgeon's preference. The ideal target is the anterior half of the disk space.

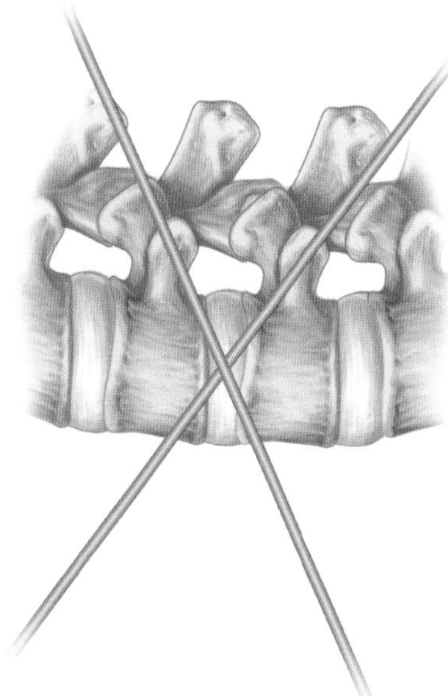

FIGURE 86-4

- **Figure 86-5:** Accessing the disk space involves a retroperitoneal dissection following the internal abdominal wall under direct visualization through the following layers in order from superficial to deep: skin, subcutaneous fat, external oblique, internal oblique, and transversus abdominis muscles. These layers can be dissected in a muscle-splitting fashion using a blunt instrument dissection. After the retroperitoneal fat is visualized, the surgeon performs a posterior-to-anterior finger sweep, feeling for the quadratus muscle and transverse process and mobilizing the fat and peritoneal contents off of the psoas muscle. This dissection should be able to be performed easily with little resistance. If there is significant resistance, the surgeon likely is in the incorrect plane. At the level of L1-2, the pleural cavity is sometimes entered, and the procedure must be performed transdiaphragmatically. A chest tube may be required.
- **Figure 86-6:** The lumbar plexus and genitofemoral nerves are at risk during the transpsoas dissection, and caution must be taken to avoid injury. The anterior one half to one third is the safest portion of the psoas muscle for dissection. More caution must be used more caudally, however, as the nerves begin to splay throughout the body of the muscle. The genitofemoral nerve originates at the level of L1 and L2 and traverses the psoas muscle from posterior to anterior between the superior aspect of the L3 vertebral body and the inferior aspect of the L4 vertebral body. It travels along the ventral aspect of the lower psoas to provide genital, perineal, and medial thigh sensation.
- **Figure 86-7:** Neuromonitoring is performed with free running and triggered EMG. Normal healthy nerve conduction should trigger at 1 to 2 mA; however, injured or chronically compressed nerve tissue may require a higher current, and the neuromonitoring probe is set at 6 to 8 mA. The probe is placed on the anterior one third to one half of the psoas muscle and passed through the psoas muscle aiming for the anterior one third to one half of the disk space. If nerve stimulation occurs, the trajectory should be verified using the C-arm to ensure that the probe is truly aimed toward the anterior aspect of the disk space. After the probe is safely passed through the muscle, the guide wire is passed and docked in the disk space, also under radiographic guidance.
- **Figure 86-8:** Over the guide wire, sequential dilators are added up to a final 22-mm-diameter tube. Free running EMG throughout the sequential dilation provides monitoring for safe muscle-splitting dissection. After the final diameter has been reached, the length of the dilator at the skin surface is noted, and the success of the muscle dilation down to the lateral aspect of the disk space is verified using anteroposterior fluoroscopy.

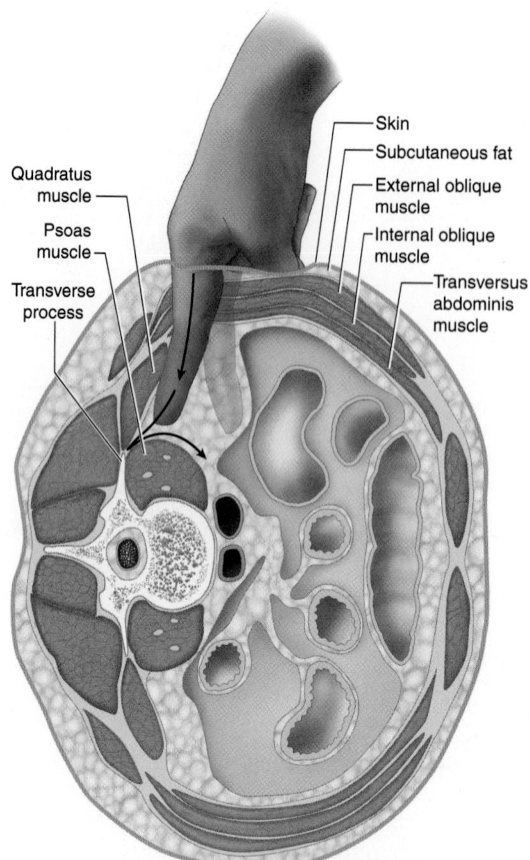

FIGURE 86-5

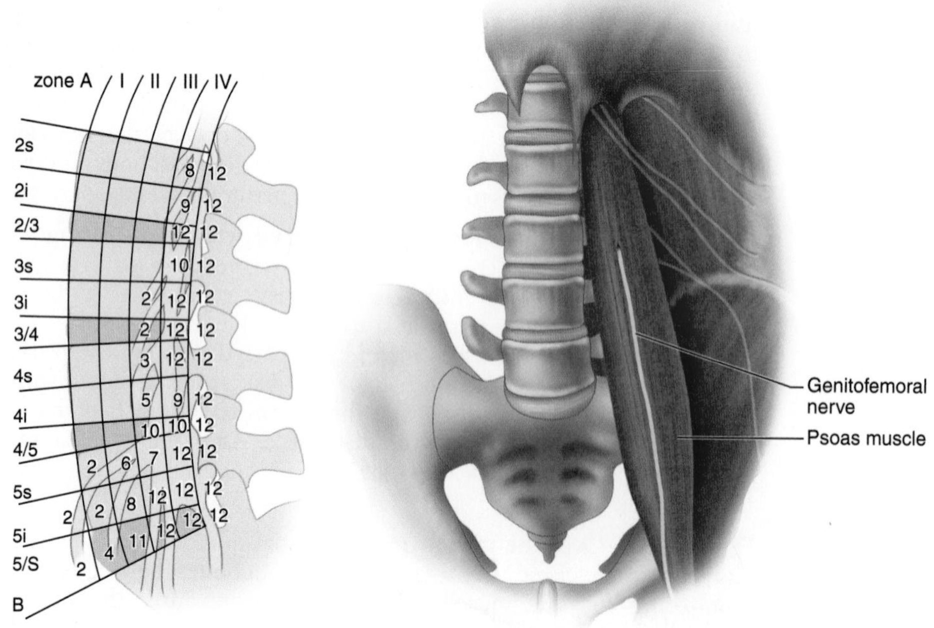

FIGURE 86-6

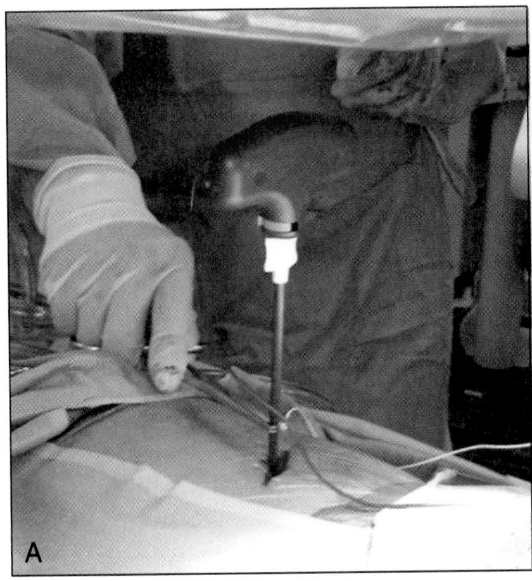

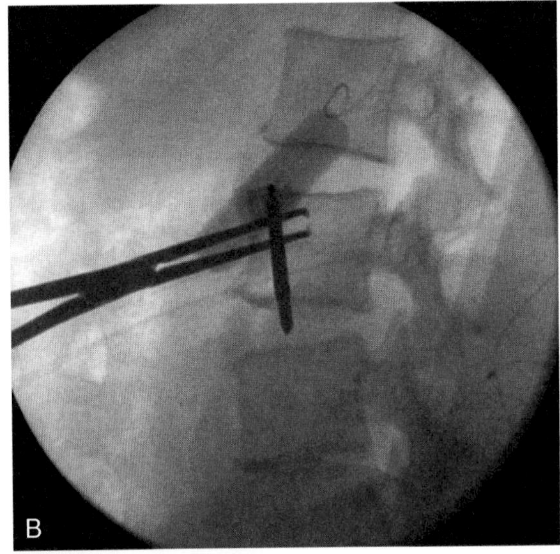

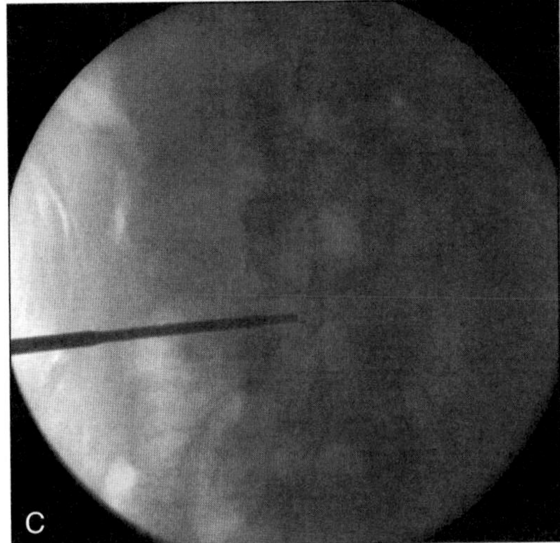

FIGURE 86-7

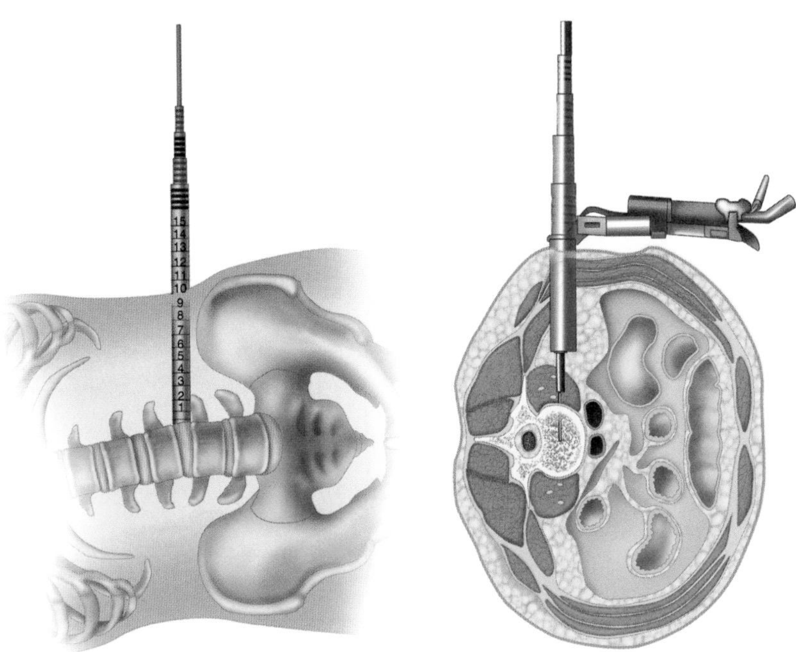

FIGURE 86-8

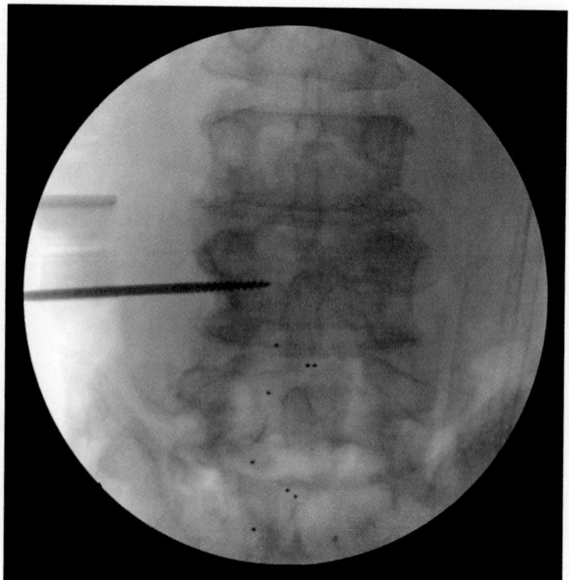

FIGURE 86-9

- **Figure 86-9:** An appropriate tubular retractor is placed over dilators and secured in place to the multiaxial arm attached to the side of the operating table. The dilators are removed while the guide wire is left in place. Additional stabilization of the tubular retractor can be achieved with either a stabilization screw or a shim depending on the retractor device. Before placing the additional stabilization device, the neuromonitoring probe and direct visualization are used to verify there are no neural structures at the site of attachment in the vertebral body. One screw or shim is typically all that is necessary to stabilize the tubular retractor, and it is important to place the stabilization device close to the end plate to avoid injury to one of the segmental arteries that tend to course over the center of the vertebral body.
- **Figure 86-10:** Before beginning the diskectomy, it is important to verify radiographically the appropriate level and trajectory in the anteroposterior and lateral planes ensuring that you are truly in the anterior aspect of the disk space. Visualization through the tube can be enhanced either with a light source attached to the retractor or with a headlight and with the aid of loupe magnification. Any remaining muscle or soft tissue first should be probed in all four quadrants for any neural structures and then bluntly dissected off the vertebral body, typically using a No. 4 Penfield dissector.
- **Figure 86-11:** Wide annulotomy is made using diskectomy knife. An efficient maneuver that aids the diskectomy and releases the contralateral annulus involves malleting a Cobb elevator along each end plate under fluoroscopic guidance. It is important to release the contralateral annulus using a Cobb elevator to ensure that the interbody

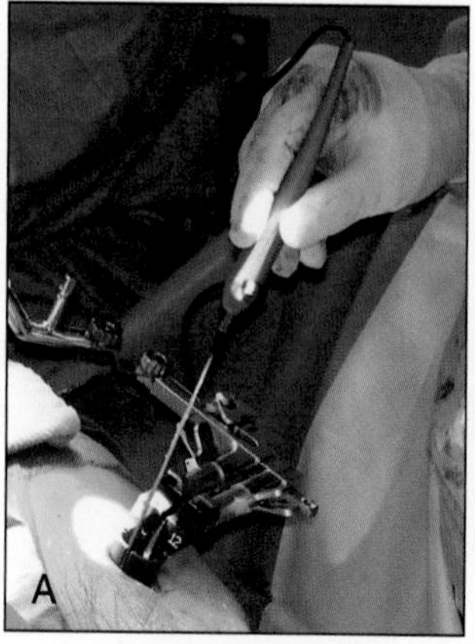

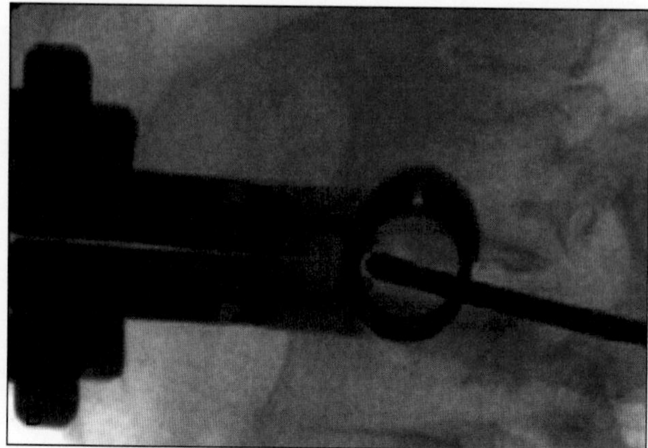

FIGURE 86-10

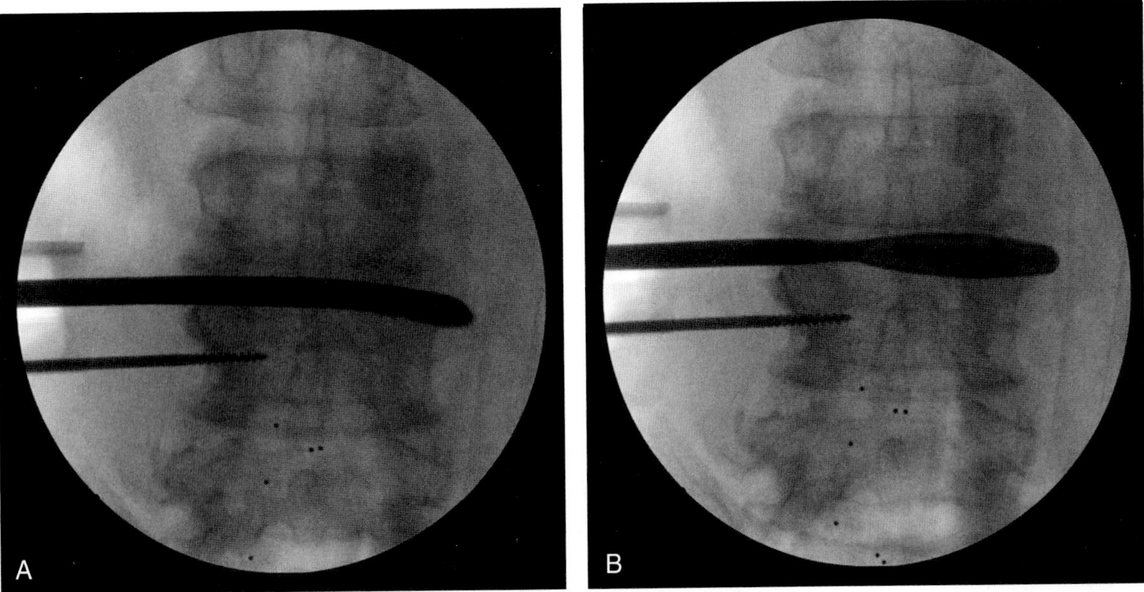

FIGURE 86-11

graft ultimately extends completely across the disk space to obtain coronal correction and indirect foraminal decompression. Diskectomy can be completed using a combination of pituitaries, shavers, and curets. Careful attention should be paid to grasp only disk or soft tissue that can be clearly visualized to minimize risk to surrounding vessels or nerves that can be adherent to the disk space. Likewise, it is important to remain perpendicular and oriented to the floor to avoid injury to the large vessels or nerves and to avoid violation of the end plate.

- **Figure 86-12:** After the diskectomy has been completed and the end plates have been prepared, it is time to select the appropriate interbody graft. The disk space is distracted with incrementally larger graft trials. It is important to ensure that the graft spans the disk space and rests ultimately on the cortical rim of the end plate to maximize strength and stability of the construct. The graft should span pedicle to pedicle in the anteroposterior plane. Various types of interbody grafts can be used depending on surgeon preference and clinical judgment. Tapered grafts may help reduce the risk of violating the end plate when placing the graft and have the advantage of a lordotic shape to the graft for placement in the lumbar spine. Likewise, the decision to use biologics is surgeon specific and must be determined based on the clinical and biomechanical data. After the graft is in place, anteroposterior and lateral radiographs can be used to verify the appropriate location. Appropriate placement of the interbody graft is essential to provide any coronal deformity correction; the ability to obtain any correction in the sagittal plane via the direct lateral transpsoas approach is controversial.
- **Figure 86-13:** Closure is performed in multiple layers: transversalis fascia, external oblique fascia, subcutaneous tissue, and skin. An UR-6 needle is helpful for the transversalis fascia layer, and the skin is ultimately closed with adhesive.

TIPS FROM THE MASTERS

- Positioning is the key to the case. It is imperative to position the hip, not the waist, over the break in the operating table. Secure the patient in place, and adjust the bed, not the fluoroscopy gantry, to obtain true lateral and true anteroposterior images.
- The use of intraoperative navigation can be very helpful by providing anatomic guidance and can be particularly useful in cases involving multiple levels by reducing overall radiation exposure and eliminating the need to work around the often cumbersome C-arm. A small amount of accuracy of navigation is lost, however, as each interbody cage is placed owing to disk space distraction. If fluoroscopy is used, it is important

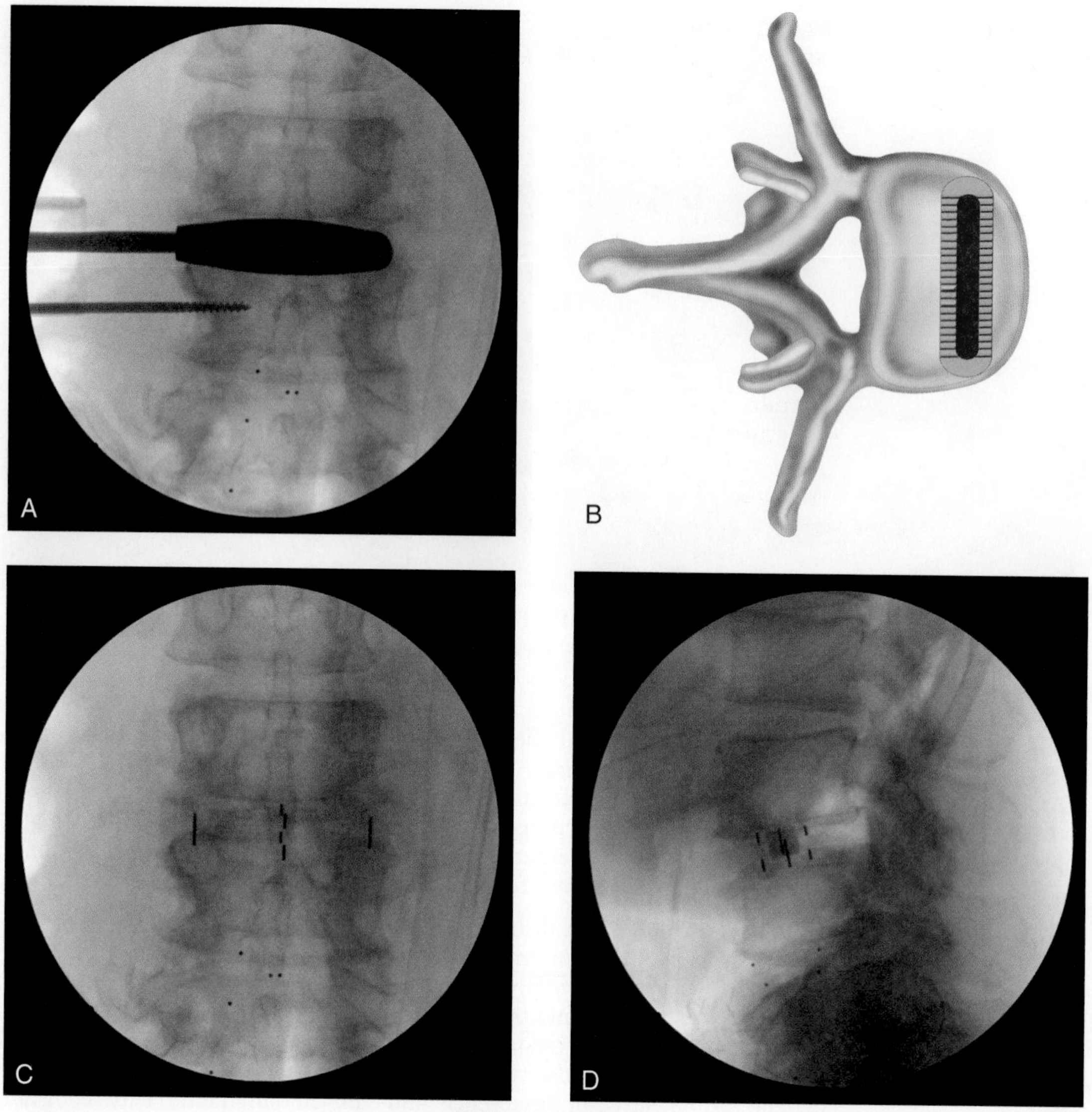

FIGURE 86-12

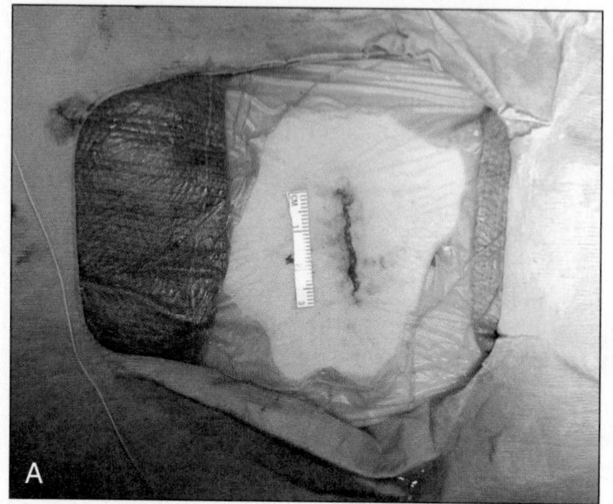

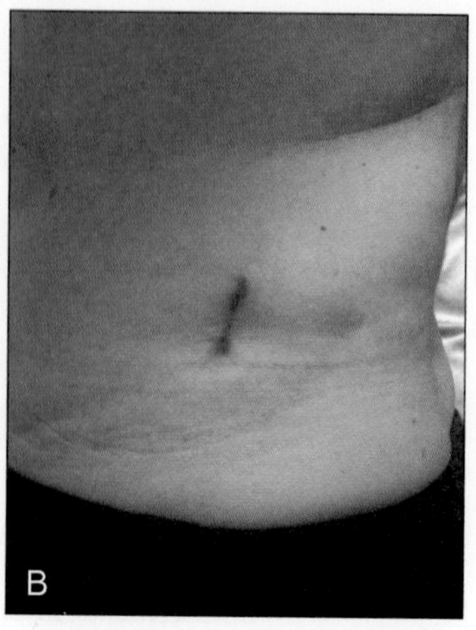

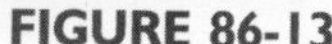

FIGURE 86-13

to adjust the patient position at each level to obtain true anteroposterior and lateral images. Ultimately, direct visualization and clinical judgment of the surgeon must guide each step.

- Understanding the anatomy and studying the imaging in the preoperative setting is essential to selecting patients who would benefit from this procedure. The L1-2 through L4-5 disk spaces can be accessed safely. The size of the psoas muscle, location of aorta, inferior vena cava, and iliac vessels must be clearly identified to minimize risk of injury. The iliac crest prohibits access to the L5-S1 disk space and in some men can make accessing the L4-5 disk space very challenging. If needed, part of the iliac crest can be resected to facilitate entry into the L4-5 disk space. The anterior half of the disk space should be targeted, and in the setting of low-grade spondylolisthesis the anterior half of the inferior end plate should be targeted.
- Intraoperatively, using neuromonitoring to identify the lumbar plexus is crucial. The genitofemoral nerve cannot be identified using neuromonitoring, and direct visualization during the dissection is essential. To reduce risk of injury to the neural structures at the level of L4-5, the tubular retractor can be docked on top of the psoas muscle so as not to injure the neural structures while passing the tubes through the muscle. It is important, however, to place the stabilization screw or shim in the vertebral body to maintain stability. The lumbar plexus and genitofemoral nerve can be visualized directly during psoas dissection.
- Postoperatively, 40% of patients may have ipsilateral iliopsoas weakness. This weakness is due to dissection through the psoas muscle and placement of the tubular retractors through the muscle down to the level of the lateral annulus. The risk of such weakness can be reduced by docking the tubular retractor anteriorly. Ipsilateral iliopsoas weakness does not represent permanent neurologic injury and typically improves over the course of 2 to 3 weeks but can persist for 8 weeks. It is important to inform the patient of this possibility preoperatively.

PITFALLS

Failing to orient properly to the floor and make all movements in the perpendicular direction increases the possibility of end plate fracture or misplacing the graft. Obtaining true anteroposterior and lateral radiographs with fluoroscopy is essential.

Both neuromonitoring and direct visualization must be used to identify the lumbar plexus and the genitofemoral nerve appropriately. Failure to do so can lead to significant morbidity. If the procedure cannot be done safely, the procedure should be aborted.

The interbody graft must be seated completely across the vertebral body spanning pedicle to pedicle in the anteroposterior plane. The interbody graft must span the disk space and rest on the cortical rim of the vertebral body to maximize the strength and stability of the construct, provide maximal foraminal decompression, and provide appropriate symmetric coronal correction.

BAILOUT OPTIONS

- If the interbody graft has violated the end plate, it is important to avoid driving the graft farther into the vertebral body and causing further damage to the vertebral body or risking retropulsion of fractured fragments into the spinal canal. If the end plate has been fractured, and the graft is positioned in cancellous bone, the construct at that level likely maintains some instability. One option would be to perform a posterolateral instrumented fusion. If there are retropulsed fragments with compression of neural elements, corpectomy from the direct lateral approach may be required with subsequent posterolateral instrumented fusion. The minimally invasive incision can be expanded—with the aid of an access surgeon if necessary—to perform the corpectomy.

- If the neuromonitoring system is not functioning, and the surgeon cannot identify the lumbar plexus, the first step is to ensure that the technical aspects of the neuromonitoring system itself are functioning properly. If needed, replace the probe or recording device, or both. There should be some nerve response at 6 to 8 mA; however, injured nerves may require higher levels, so the current can be increased until response is detected. Typically, the anterior portion of the psoas is safest; however, if nerve response cannot be detected, one must consider aborting the case because the risk of significant nerve injury is too high. Each patient should provide consent preoperatively for the possibility of posterior instrumented fusion via either open or minimally invasive techniques if the direct lateral transpsoas interbody approach cannot be performed safely.
- Injury to one of the lumbar segmental arteries must be dealt with expeditiously. Visualization through a minimal access tubular retractor can be rapidly compromised by unexpected bleeding. Typically, the bleeding can be contained through the tubular retractor and does not require converting to an open or mini-open flank incision. By first using suction and judicious hemostatic agents, the bleeding vessel must be identified and coagulated using bipolar electrocautery. Given the size of the segmental arteries, a relatively large volume of blood can be lost rapidly, and close communication with the anesthesia staff is essential and may require transfusion of blood products and close postoperative monitoring.

SUGGESTED READINGS

Benglis DM, Vanni S, Levi AD. An anatomical study of the lumbosacral plexus as related to the minimally invasive transpsoas approach to the lumbar spine. J Neurosurg Spine 2009;10:139–44.

Hsieh PC, Koski TR, Sciubba DM, et al. Maximizing the potential of minimally invasive spine surgery in complex spinal disorders. Neurosurg Focus 2008;25:E19.

Moro T, Kikuchi S, Konno S, et al. An anatomic study of the lumbar plexus with respect to retroperitoneal endoscopic surgery. Spine (Phila Pa 1976) 2003;28:423–8.

Tan JS, Bailey CS, Dvorak MF, et al. Interbody device shape and size are important to strengthen the vertebra-implant interface. Spine (Phila Pa 1976) 2005;30:638–44.

Figure 86-6 is redrawn with permission from Moro T, Kikuchi S, Konno S, et al. An anatomic study of the lumbar plexus with respect to retroperitoneal endoscopic surgery. Spine (Phila Pa 1976) 2003;28:423–8.

Figure 86-12 is from Tans JS, Bailey CS, Dvorak MF, et al. Interbody device shape and size are important to strengthen the vertebra-implant interface. Spine (Phila Pa 1976) 2005;30:638–44.

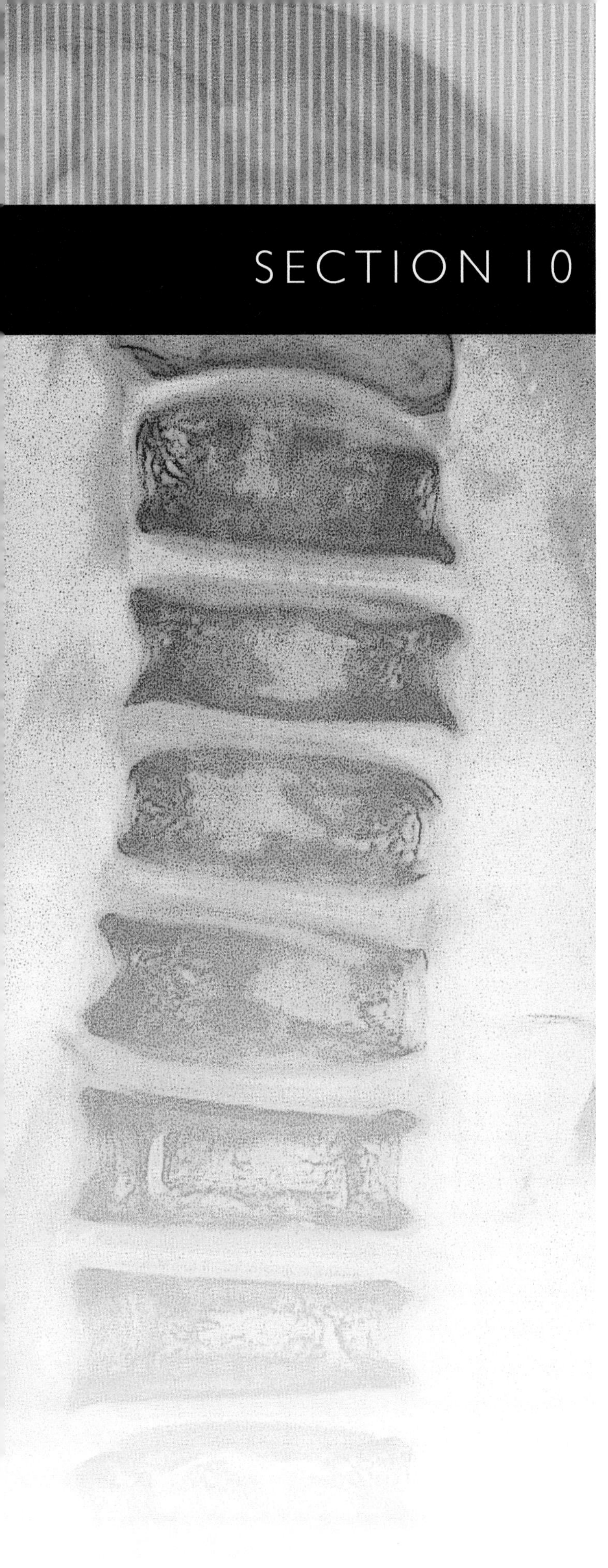

SECTION 10 Other

SECTION EDITOR — GEORGE I. JALLO

Procedure 87

Spinal Cord Arteriovenous Malformations

Anand V. Germanwala, George I. Jallo

INDICATIONS

- Spinal cord arteriovenous malformations (AVMs) causing neurologic symptoms, such as pain, neurogenic claudication, myelopathy, radiculopathy, and progressive motor and sensory dysfunction
- Spinal cord AVMs causing venous hypertension
- Spinal cord AVMs diagnosed in patients presenting with subarachnoid or intramedullary hemorrhage

CONTRAINDICATIONS

- Patients with relative contraindications to surgery include patients with serious medical comorbidities, short life expectancies, severe debilitation, and very complex, challenging intramedullary lesions (ventrally located, type 3).
- Stereotactic radiosurgery and endovascular embolization are alternatives and should be considered.

PLANNING AND POSITIONING

- A thorough history and physical examination should be performed on every patient. Screening studies such as spinal magnetic resonance imaging (MRI) (more commonly) or computed tomography (CT) myelography are initially performed. A diagnostic spinal arteriogram is performed to help determine the type of AVM, locate the fistula or nidus, allow interpretation as to the arterial supply of the malformation and spinal cord, and assess regional vascular anatomy.
- Continuous neurophysiologic monitoring, including somatosensory evoked potentials, is performed to provide feedback during surgery. A long femoral sheath is placed and attached to the lateral aspect of the patient's right thigh and draped in a sterile fashion at the beginning of the case for intraoperative spinal arteriography.
- The patient receives preoperative antibiotics and dexamethasone (Decadron).
- The patient is positioned prone, on a radiolucent operating table comprising a Wilson frame mounted onto a Jackson table permitting easy C-arm fluoroscopy access. Fluoroscopy is used at the beginning of the case for localization of the skin incision and laminectomy.
- **Figure 87-1:** MRI of the spine is a useful screening tool and helpful in the management of spinal AVMs. On sagittal T2-weighted MRI, multiple flow voids are visualized posterior to cervicothoracic cord.
- **Figure 87-2:** Preoperative spinal arteriography is crucial for precise localization of the AVM. On anteroposterior view, a type 1 AVM is shown, localized to the left T12 region.
- **Figure 87-3:** Patient positioning on a radiolucent operating table comprising a Wilson frame mounted onto a Jackson table permitting easy C-arm fluoroscopy access. The long right femoral sheath is placed before positioning to permit intraoperative spinal arteriography.

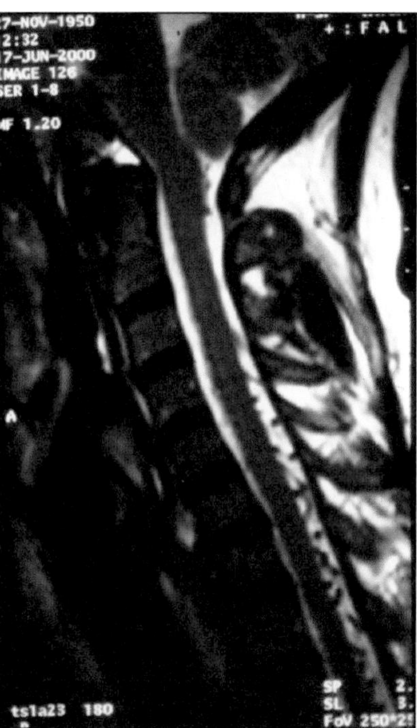

FIGURE 87-1

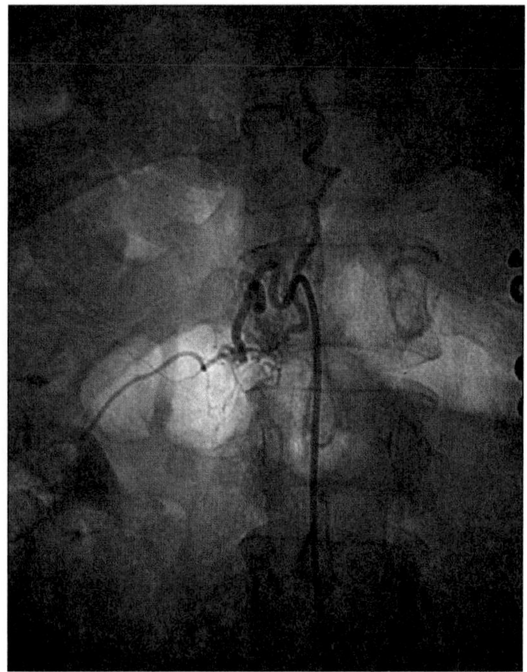

FIGURE 87-2

PROCEDURE

- **Figure 87-4:** After proper positioning and fluoroscopic localization, the patient is prepared and draped. A midline incision is made, and the paraspinal musculature is dissected subperiosteally with electrocautery exposing the posterior elements. Following this, laminectomies or laminoplasties are performed at the proper levels exposing the dura (this technique is discussed elsewhere).
- **Figure 87-5:** The dura is opened in the midline using a No. 15 blade scalpel and extended rostrally and caudally using Metzenbaum scissors. The dural opening is reflected laterally

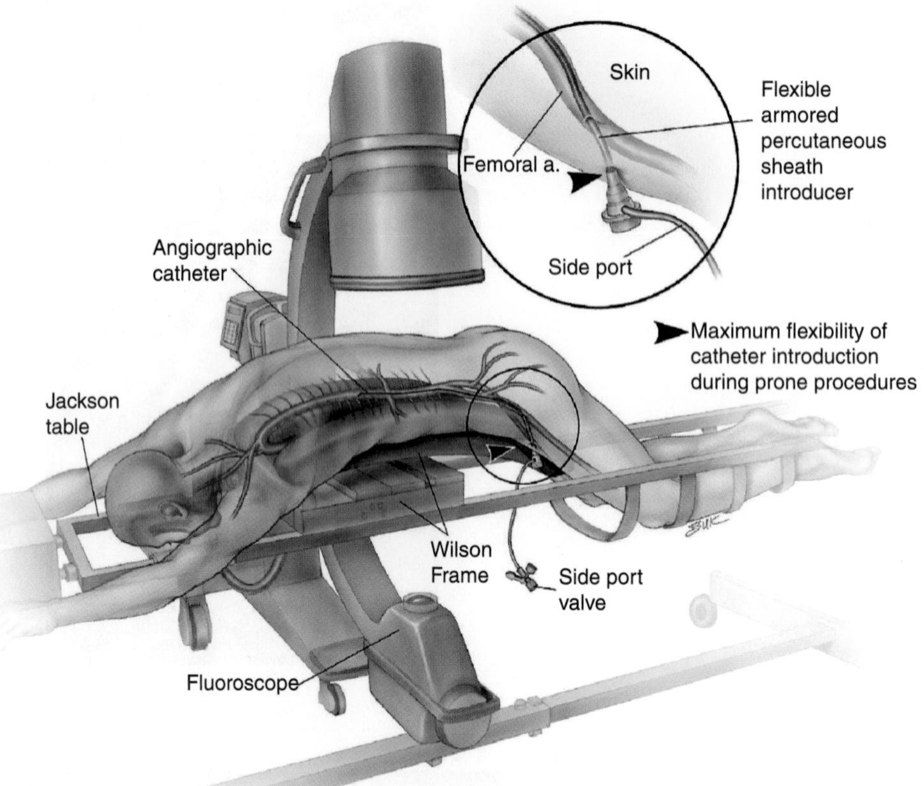

FIGURE 87-3

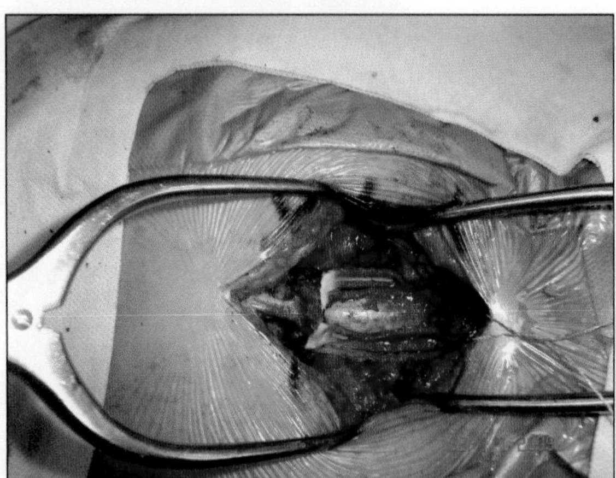

FIGURE 87-4

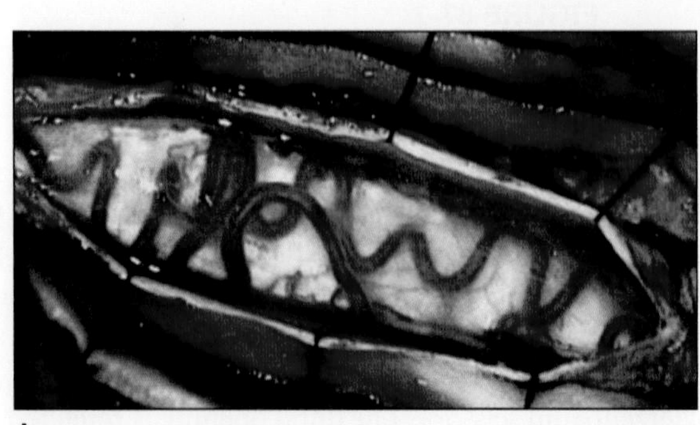

A

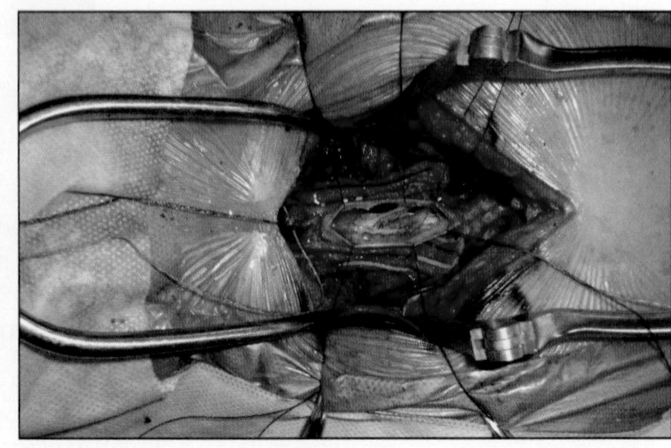

B

FIGURE 87-5

using multiple interrupted sutures placed on each side of the opening. Cottonoids are placed in the epidural spaces laterally to allow for a clean, dry surgical field with good visualization of the spinal cord and vascular malformation. The microscope is brought into the operative field. Under high magnification, the vascular malformation is addressed.

- **Figure 87-6:** Type 1 malformations (dural arteriovenous fistulas) are supplied by a dural artery and drained by a tortuous and elongated medullary vein. These are treated by locating the fistulous vein intradurally (usually adjacent to the dural penetration of the exiting nerve root) and cauterizing it with bipolar cautery or placing mini-aneurysm clips and then transecting it sharply.
- **Figure 87-7:** Type 2 malformations (intramedullary glomus AVMs) consist of a compact nidus. The pia is opened in the midline and retracted with 8-0 polypropylene (Prolene) sutures. The pial opening is extended in the rostral-caudal direction using microbipolar cautery and microscissors. The arterial supply (usually one or two vessels) and venous drainage are identified. The dissection is performed in the gliotic plane between the

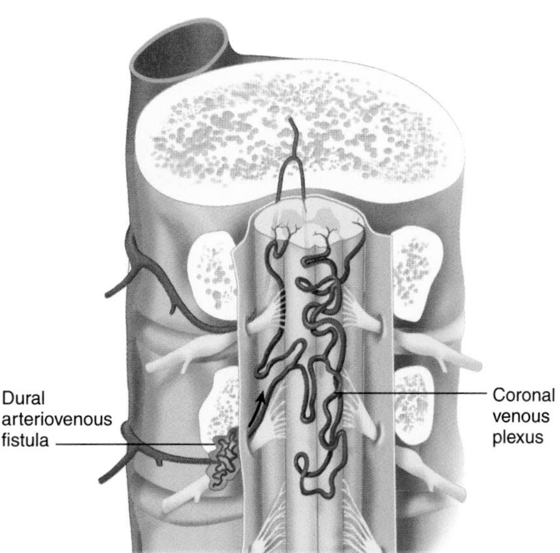

FIGURE 87-6

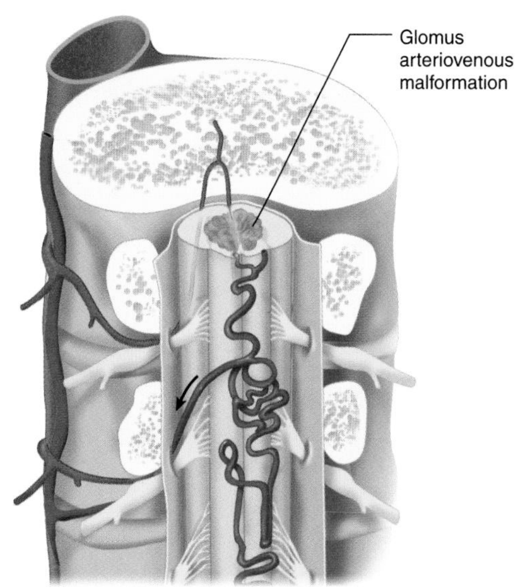

FIGURE 87-7

nidus and spinal cord using irrigating microbipolar cautery, controlled microsuction, and micropatties. The feeding vessels are obliterated with mini-aneurysm clips, and the nidus is circumferentially dissected until tethered only by the draining vein, which is clipped or cauterized and transected sharply.

- **Figure 87-8:** Type 3 malformations (intramedullary juvenile AVMs) are fed by multiple medullary arteries, and extensive, infiltrating nidus often occupies a large portion of the spinal cord. These are challenging lesions, often containing neural tissue in the interstices, and meticulous dissection must be performed to identify normal and abnormal vessels and tissue. Multiple arterial feeders are cauterized and transected (if small) or clipped (if large). The nidus is dissected, and draining veins are transected sharply at the end of dissection.

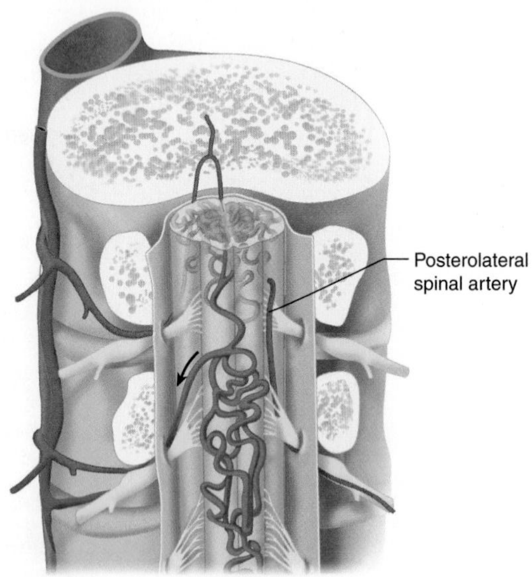

FIGURE 87-8

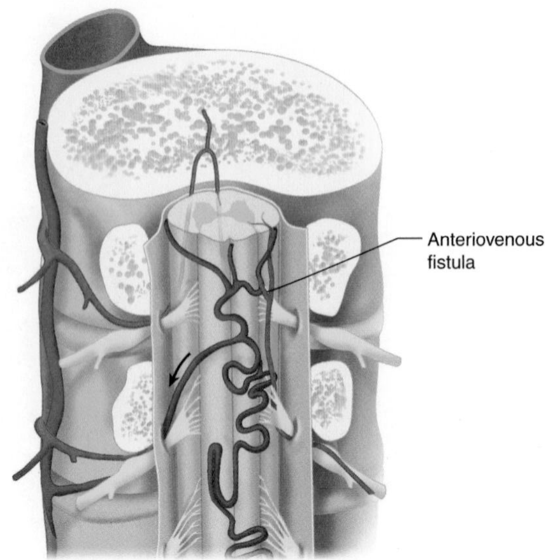

FIGURE 87-9

- **Figure 87-9:** Type 4 malformations (intradural perimedullary pial arteriovenous fistulas) are fed by medullary arteries and are often associated with small arterial or venous aneurysms. The site of the arteriovenous shunt can be multifocal and is often obscured by overlying vasculature. The site of the shunting needs to be identified, cauterized or clipped, and transected sharply. Aneurysms, if present, are usually completely excised.
- **Figure 87-10:** After resection or obliteration of the AVM, the wound is explored. Previously arterialized veins should appear dark blue and be draining completely venous blood. Complete hemostasis is obtained, and the wound is irrigated. The wound is covered with a sterile drape, and an intraoperative spinal arteriogram is performed to confirm complete resection. The surgical site needs to be reexplored if there is incomplete resection on intraoperative imaging or if arterialized veins are sill present.
- **Figure 87-11:** The dura is closed in a watertight fashion after complete resection with a running Prolene suture. The Valsalva maneuver is performed to ensure there is no cerebrospinal fluid leak. Fibrin glue is placed in the epidural space to minimize the risk of cerebrospinal fluid leak, and the laminae are reattached, if desired. The paraspinal musculature, fascia, and subcutaneous tissues are closed in the standard fashion. Skin edges are reapproximated with running nylon suture. The wound is covered with a sterile dressing. The patient is extubated and examined and taken to the neurosurgical intensive care unit for further observation and management.

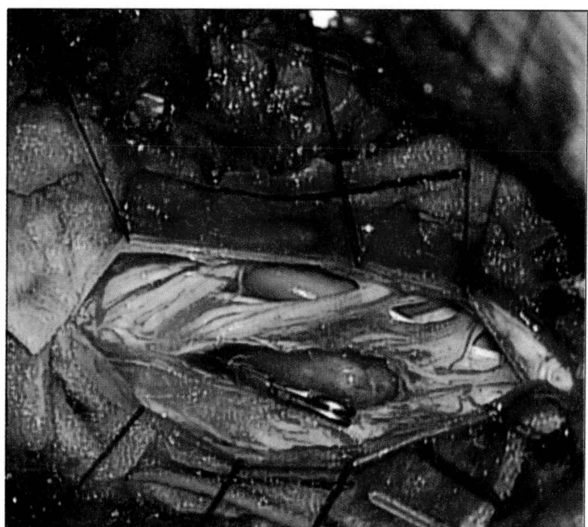

FIGURE 87-10

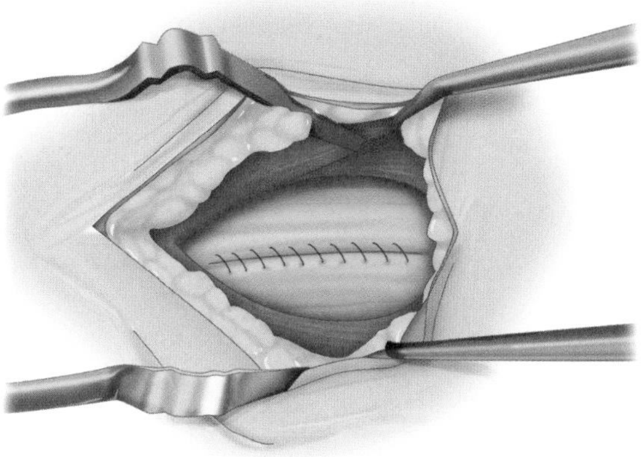

FIGURE 87-11

TIPS FROM THE MASTERS

- The goal of surgery should be complete resection or obliteration of the vascular malformation, while minimizing risk to the patient.
- Many classification systems exist for these lesions. Regardless of the nomenclature, careful attention should be paid to studying the preoperative spinal arteriogram to obtain a three-dimensional working knowledge of the supply, drainage, and location of the vascular malformation.
- Attention is required at every step, including dural and pial opening, to avoid premature injury to the venous structures.
- Embolization in a patient with acute deterioration may temporize the deficit and allow time for definitive surgical treatment.
- Postoperatively, patients are placed on short steroid tapers, and normotensive blood pressures are maintained.

PITFALLS

Retraction and manipulation should be limited to the vascular malformation because the spinal cord is often unforgiving. The dural and pial openings should be large enough so that exposure is not limited.

The intraoperative findings should correlate with findings on the preoperative studies. Surgical dissection should be deliberate, and "picking" should be avoided.

Injury to the venous structures should be prevented because this can lead to premature rupture of the malformation and severe and uncontrollable bleeding.

BAILOUT OPTIONS

- The venous drainage must remain patent in lesions that cannot be completely excised. Although suboptimal, alternative treatment options for residual spinal vascular malformations must be considered, including endovascular embolization and spinal radiosurgery.
- In the event there is damage to the spinal cord or a decrease in the neurophysiologic signals, additional steroid administration and mild elevation of the mean arterial pressures may help reduce injury.

SUGGESTED READINGS

Kim LJ, Spetzler RF. Classification and surgical management of spinal arteriovenous lesions: arteriovenous fistulae and arteriovenous malformations. Neurosurgery 2006;59(S3):195–201.

Krings T, Geibprasert S. Spinal dural arteriovenous fistulas. AJNR Am J Neuroradiol 2009;30:639–48.

Medel R, Crowley W, Dumont A. Endovascular management of spinal vascular malformations: history and literature review. Neurosurg Focus 2009;26:1–7.

Shapiro AMJ, Lakey JRT, Ryan EA, et al. Islet transplantation in seven patients with type 1 diabetes mellitus using a glucocorticoid-free immunosuppressive regimen. N Engl J Med 2000;343:230–8.

Sinclair J, Chang SD, Gibbs IC, et al. Multisession CyberKnife radiosurgery for intramedullary spinal cord arteriovenous malformations. Neurosurgery 2006;58:1081–9.

Zozulya YP, Slin'ko EI, Al-Qashqish II. Spinal arteriovenous malformations: new classification and surgical treatment. Neurosurg Focus 2006;20:E7.

Figure 87-3 courtesy of Ian Suk.

Procedure 88

Surgical Management of Spinal Dural Arteriovenous Fistulas

Kaisorn L. Chaichana, Rafael J. Tamargo

INDICATIONS

- Spinal dural arteriovenous fistulas (AVFs) are classified into two major categories. Lesions primarily associated with the nerve root are called *radicular dural AVFs*, and lesions primarily in the subarachnoid space are called *perimedullary dural AVFs*. Arteriovenous lesions that are located in the spinal cord—that is, involving the spinal pia and extending into the substance of the spinal cord—are called *spinal arteriovenous malformations*.
- Radicular dural AVFs are malformations that typically arise in the region of the dural nerve root sleeve. These lesions usually have a single arterial feeder that develops a connection or fistula to the spinal venous system. This fistula creates a high-flow, high-pressure venous drainage system that leads to venous hypertension and subsequent spinal cord hypoperfusion. Perimedullary dural AVFs are located in the subarachnoid space around the spinal cord but do not involve the pia and manifest with pathophysiology similar to radicular dural AVFs. These lesions may have more than one feeding artery.
- Symptoms of spinal dural AVFs often develop insidiously and progress over time and include weakness, sensory loss, and bowel or bladder incontinence. Dermatomal and myotomal symptoms may be distant from the actual level of the fistula. Surgery or embolization should be pursued in a timely manner to halt and potentially to reverse neurologic symptoms.

CONTRAINDICATIONS

- A medically unstable condition and active infection are relative contraindications.
- Patients unable to tolerate either endovascular or surgical procedures should be followed closely for signs of neurologic deterioration. Therapy should be pursued when patients are medically stable.

PLANNING AND POSITIONING

- The initial assessment of a patient with a suspected spinal AVF begins with a detailed history and physical examination, including bladder, bowel, and sexual function. Patients with spinal dural AVFs typically have progressive upper and lower motor neuron involvement and dorsal column involvement with sensory paresthesias, and they may have loss of vibratory and position sense. A bruit over the spine has been reported in rare cases.
- Spinal computed tomography (CT) and magnetic resonance imaging (MRI) are typically the initial imaging studies. CT and MRI typically show only prominent subarachnoid veins. Spinal angiography is the critical study for preoperative planning. Angiography is essential for identifying the precise location of the AVF, the location of all arterial feeders, venous drainage patterns, and possible venous and arterial aneurysms. CT myelography is rarely used at the present time.
- Embolization can be used as definitive treatment for most spinal dural AVFs. Alternatively, embolization can serve as a preoperative adjunct for patients with AVF. Compared

with cranial dural AVFs, spinal dural AVFs are generally more difficult to treat because of the smaller size of the feeding arteries, the low-flow nature of spinal AVFs, and the close proximity of crucial anterior and posterior spinal arteries.

- Intraoperative neurophysiologic monitoring with motor evoked potentials (MEPs) and somatosensory evoked potentials (SSEPs) is critical when operating on spinal AVFs. Because SSEPs and MEPs provide key neurologic information during surgery, the anesthetic regimen should be modified to maximize evoked potential monitoring.
- **Figure 88-1:** Preoperative MRI and angiography of a patient with a thoracic spinal dural AVF. MRI depicts signal abnormalities within the thoracic spinal canal on sagittal and axial T2-weighted images. Angiography shows AVF nidus within the left T8 nerve root sleeve. The left T8 intercostal artery fills a tortuous spinal vein early within the nerve root sleeve. These features are typical of spinal dural AVF.
- **Figure 88-2:** After intubation, a femoral catheter is placed for intraoperative angiography with the patient in supine position. The patient is then placed prone on a radiolucent Jackson table. For cervical lesions, the patient is pinned in three-point radiolucent Mayfield head fixation. For thoracic or lumbar lesions, a radiolucent Wilson frame can be used. It is critical to use radiolucent equipment to allow for intraoperative angiography. All dependent surfaces (e.g., knees, elbows) are padded to avoid peripheral nerve injury or pressure-related tissue necrosis.

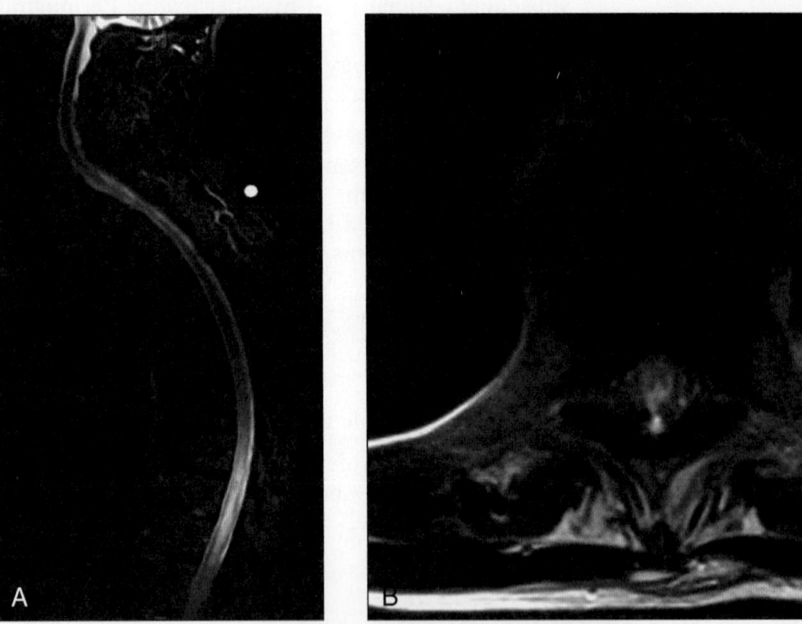

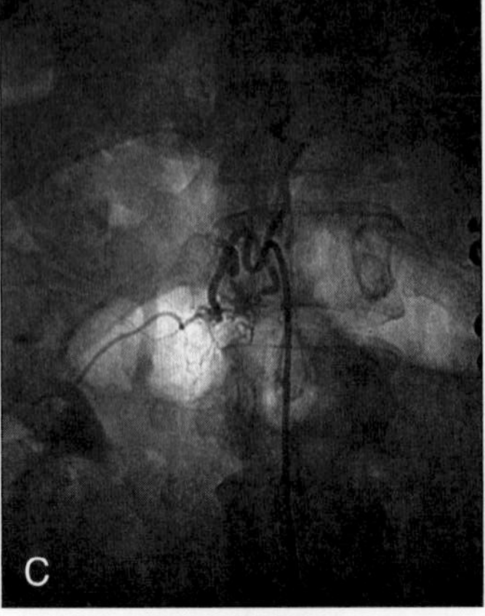

FIGURE 88-1

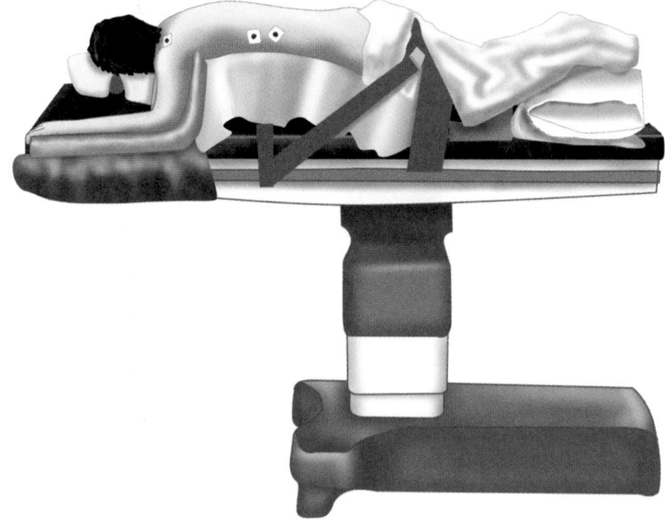

FIGURE 88-2

PROCEDURE

- **Figure 88-3: A,** Posterior spinal elements are exposed with subperiosteal dissection. During this dissection, it is important to preserve the facet joint capsules to minimize development of iatrogenic spinal instability. **B,** The dura overlying the spinal AVF is exposed with use of bilateral laminectomies. Laminectomies are performed with the use of high-speed drills, Kerrison rongeurs, and Leksell rongeurs. Adhesions between the ligamentum flavum and dura are removed with careful blunt dissection.
- **Figure 88-4:** The dural AVF is exposed by incising the dura in the midline with a No. 15 blade. The arachnoid layer should be kept intact to prevent premature egress of cerebrospinal fluid (CSF). The dura is tacked up with 4-0 Surgilon sutures (Covidien, Mansfield, MA). After opening the dura, arterialized veins can often be detected, as seen here.
- **Figure 88-5:** Under the operative microscope, the arachnoid layer is opened with an arachnoid knife. The AVF is skeletonized to identify the fistulous point, or the site at which the artery appears to communicate with the vein. Temporary clips are placed on the fistulous point, and SSEPs and MEPs are monitored for any changes.

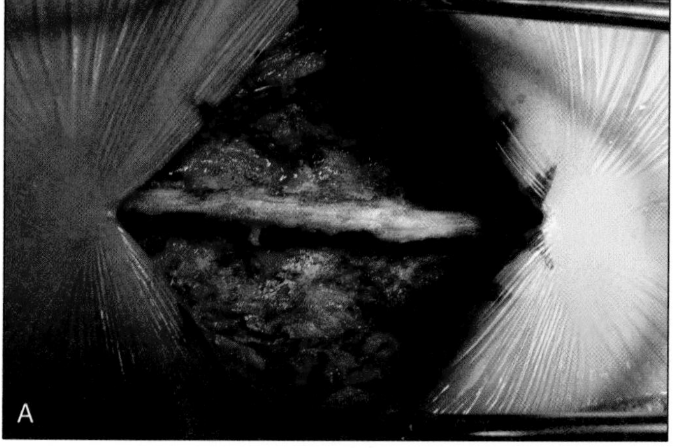

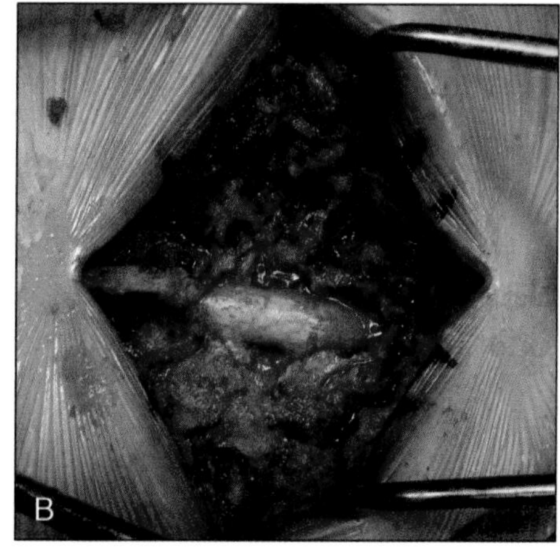

FIGURE 88-3

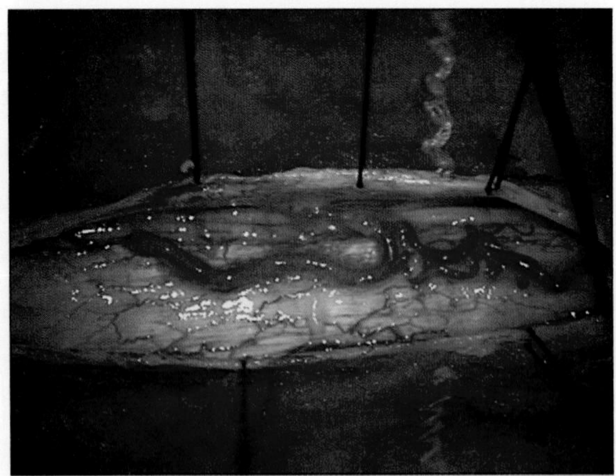

FIGURE 88-4

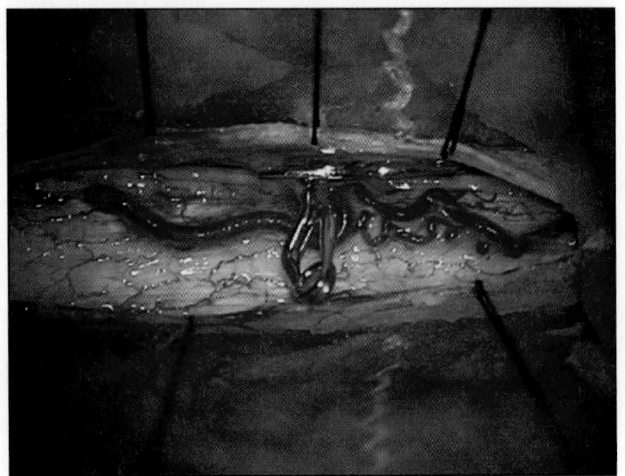

FIGURE 88-5

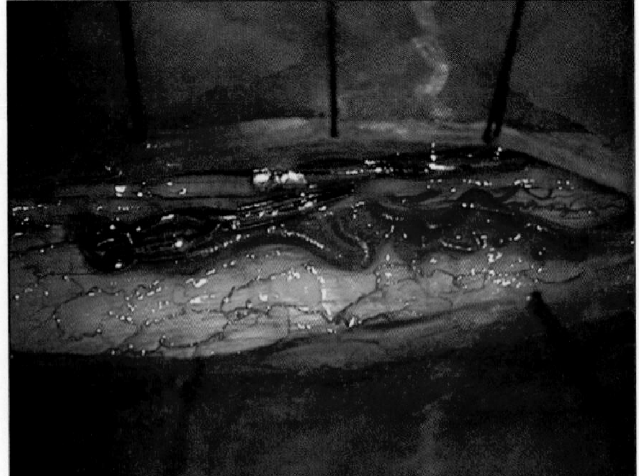

FIGURE 88-6

- **Figure 88-6:** After no SSEP and MEP changes are identified, temporary clips can be removed, and the fistulous connection can be coagulated with bipolar cautery. Permanent clips can also be applied to the fistulous connection to reinforce the ligation process.
- **Figure 88-7:** After separation of the fistulous connection, intraoperative angiography can be used to confirm closure of the fistula and absence of alternative arteriovenous connections. Indocyanine green (ICG) angiography can be used before catheter angiography.

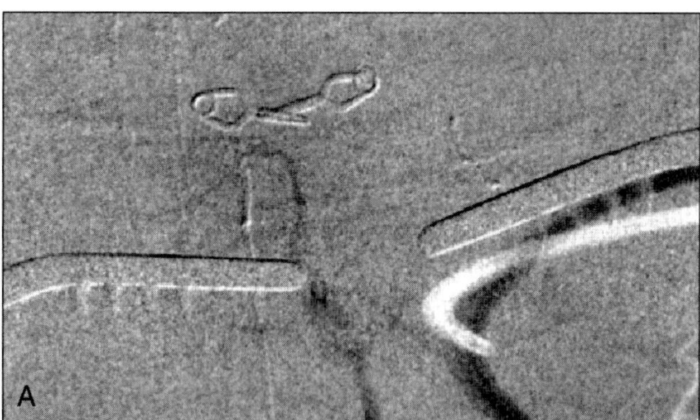

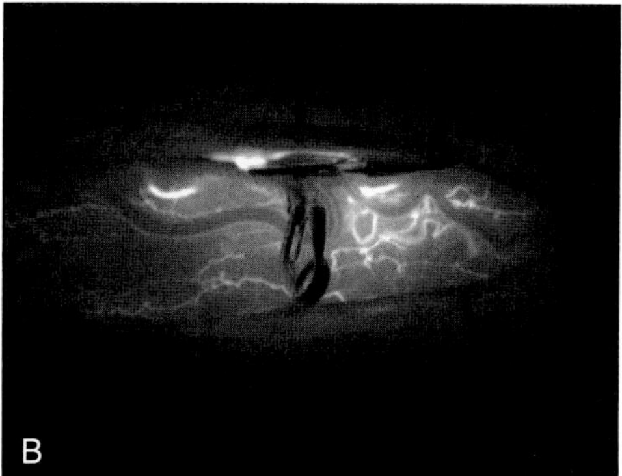

FIGURE 88-7

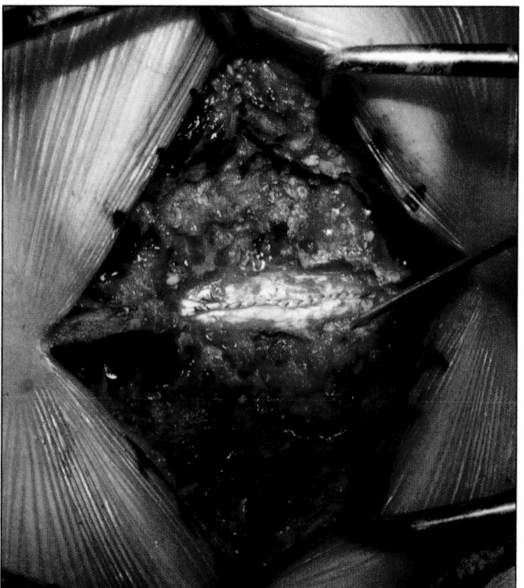

FIGURE 88-8

- **Figure 88-8:** The dura is closed in a watertight fashion with 4-0 Surgilon sutures. Fibrin glue can also be placed along the dural incision line to support the dural closure. To approximate the muscle and fascial layers, 0 polyglactin 910 (Vicryl) sutures are used. To approximate the subcuticular layer, 3-0 Vicryl sutures are used. The skin is closed with a running, locking 3-0 nylon suture.

TIPS FROM THE MASTERS

- Patients with spinal AVFs should be treated in a timely fashion because preoperative neurologic status is related to postoperative neurologic outcomes. Treatment should be pursued before a patient experiences further decline in function.
- ICG can be used intraoperatively to help confirm the extent of the contribution of an artery to an AVF. Repeat ICG injections can help elucidate normal arterial filling after elimination of the fistulous connection.
- Spinal cord rotation sometimes may be necessary to gain better access to the fistulous connection; this can be achieved by cutting and grasping the dentate ligaments to manipulate the spinal cord.
- Removal of an AVF is unnecessary. It has been shown repeatedly that interrupting the fistulous connection is all that is needed to eliminate an AVF. Removal of the venous components of the AVF is contraindicated and may compromise blood flow to the spinal cord.

PITFALLS

It is critical to obtain an intraoperative angiogram. Some spinal dural AVFs have multiple arterial sources that need to be sequentially eliminated. Some of these arterial feeders are evident only intraoperatively and after partial elimination of the fistula.

If changes in MEPs and SSEPs occur with temporary clip application, the temporary clips should be removed, and the AVF should be reassessed. Care should be taken to avoid sacrificing any arterial branches that are crucial for cord perfusion.

There is a risk for postoperative CSF leak any time the dura is opened. Intraoperatively, the surgeon should ensure the dura is closed in a watertight fashion. This closure can be supported with fibrin glue. In addition, meticulous closure of the fascia helps prevent egress of CSF.

BAILOUT OPTIONS

- If MEPs decline to less than 50% of baseline or if the latency in the MEPs is more than 2 msec, surgical manipulation should be stopped. Irrigation of the spinal cord with warm saline often results in recovery sufficient to allow for continuation of surgery.
- If the fistulous connection cannot be identified intraoperatively, intraoperative ICG or angiography may provide additional details.

SUGGESTED READINGS

Anson JA, Spetzler RF. Interventional neuroradiology of spinal pathology. Clin Neurosurg 1992;39:388–417.

Baker HL, Love JG, Layton DD. Angiographic and surgical aspects of spinal cord vascular anomalies. Radiology 1967;88:1078–85.

Oldfield EH, DiChiro G, Quindlen EA, et al. Successful treatment of a group of spinal cord arteriovenous malformations by interruption of dura fistula. J Neurosurg 1983;59:1019–30.

Rosenblum B, Oldfield EH, Doppman JL, et al. Spinal arteriovenous malformations: a comparison of dural arteriovenous fistulas and intradural AVM's in 81 patients. J Neurosurg 1987;67:795–802.

Veznedaroglu E, Nelson PK, Jabbour PM, et al. Endovascular treatment of spinal cord arteriovenous malformations. Neurosurgery 2006;595:S202–9.

Figure 88-4 is modified courtesy of Ian Suk.

Figures 88-5 through 88-7 are modified with permission from Colby G, Coon A, Sciubba D, et al. Intraoperative indocyanine green angiography for obliteration of a spinal dural arteriovenous fistula. J Neurosurg Spine 2009;11:705–9.

Procedure 89

Intramedullary Spinal Cord Cavernous Malformation

Chetan Bettegowda, Vivek Mehta, Ryan M. Kretzer, George I. Jallo

INDICATIONS

- Some experts advocate surgical resection for intramedullary spinal cord cavernous malformation only after progressive neurologic deterioration or for pain, which is often the presentation seen in adults. Others recommend surgical treatment after hemorrhage within the spinal cord, which is more commonly seen in children.
- Some neurosurgeons support early surgical intervention in symptomatic patients to halt neurologic decline.
- We recommend definitive surgical resection in all patients because untreated lesions may result in progressive neurologic decline. In addition, resection prevents potential hemorrhage, which carries with it a significant risk of neurologic compromise.

CONTRAINDICATIONS

- Asymptomatic patients with incidental cavernous malformation can undergo serial magnetic resonance imaging (MRI) with close clinical follow-up to determine if and when surgical intervention is required. In these patients, the risk of hemorrhage versus surgical risk must be weighed.
- Patients with significant medical comorbidities that make undergoing surgery difficult can be closely monitored with serial imaging and clinical examinations.

PLANNING AND POSITIONING

- The initial assessment of a patient with a suspected intramedullary spinal cord cavernous malformation begins with a detailed history and physical examination.
- MRI of the entire neuraxis is necessary to diagnose additional spinal and intracranial lesions. MRI is also needed to localize the lesion and correlate with clinical findings. In addition, imaging is useful in planning the operative approach and helps predict deficits that may result from surgical resection. Cavernous malformations are usually occult to angiography and computed tomography (CT), so these imaging modalities are of limited benefit in presurgical planning.
- MRI typically reveals a hemosiderin ring that is characteristic of cavernous malformations. The lesion does not enhance with gadolinium, and there may be minimal spinal cord expansion.
- Waiting 4 to 6 weeks before surgery may benefit patients who present with an acute hemorrhage.
- Intraoperative neurophysiologic monitoring with motor evoked potentials (MEPs) is essential when operating on spinal cord cavernous malformations. Because many anesthetic agents cause depression of MEPs, the anesthetic regimen should be coordinated with the anesthesiologist before the start of the case. Propofol, fentanyl, and etomidate are commonly used agents that do not cause a decline in MEPs.
- **Figure 89-1:** Preoperative T2 sagittal and axial MRI showing an intramedullary cavernous malformation with a hemosiderin ring and slight expansion of the spinal cord.

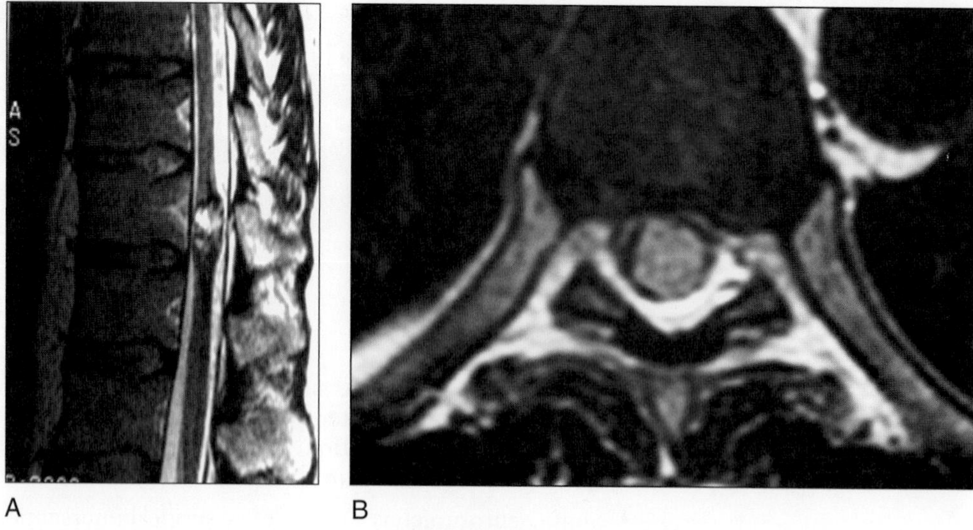

A B

FIGURE 89-1

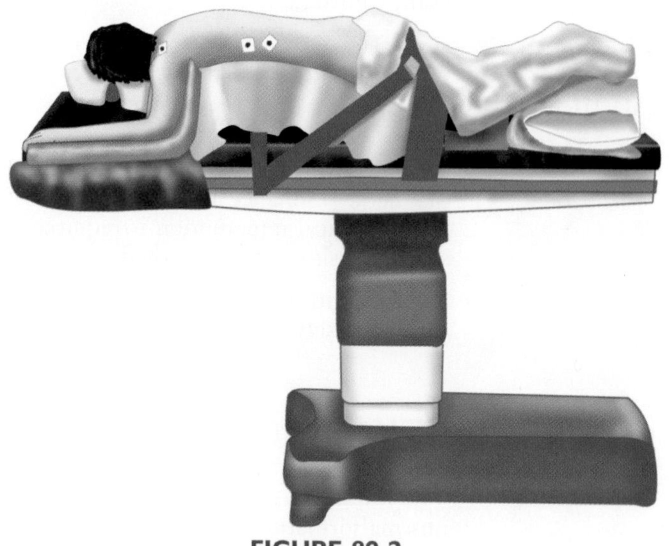

FIGURE 89-2

- **Figure 89-2:** The patient is turned prone after intubation and all neurophysiologic monitoring electrodes are placed. For cervical lesions, the patient is pinned in three-point Mayfield head fixation and positioned prone on two chest rolls. The neck is slightly flexed to aid in surgical exposure. For patients with thoracic or lumbar lesions, prone positioning can be accomplished on a Wilson frame or chest rolls without head fixation. All dependent surfaces (e.g., knees, elbows) are padded to avoid peripheral nerve injury or pressure-related tissue necrosis.

PROCEDURE

- **Figure 89-3:** Subperiosteal dissection is used to expose the posterior elements of the vertebral column, including the spinous processes and bilateral laminae. Extreme care is taken to prevent violation of the facet joint capsules, which could lead to future instability.

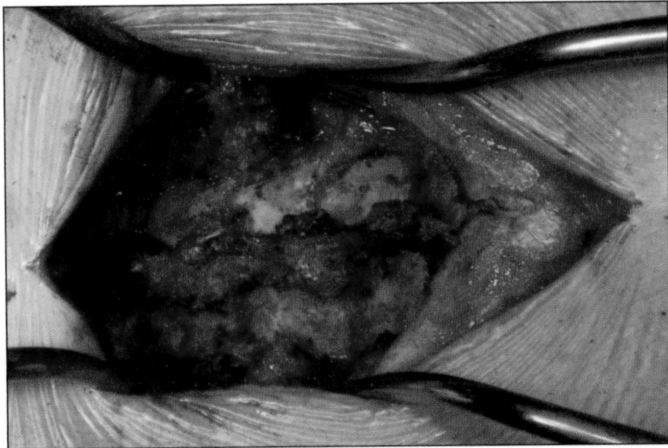

FIGURE 89-3

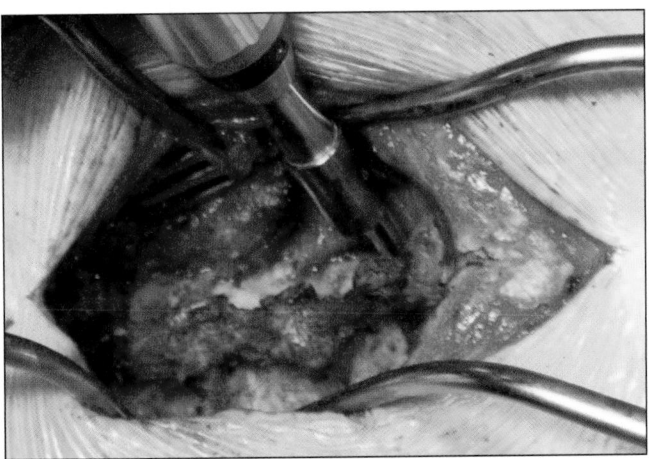

FIGURE 89-4

- **Figure 89-4:** Intraoperative x-ray is obtained to verify the location of the lesion. Bilateral laminectomies can be performed in a piecemeal fashion using Leksell rongeurs and Kerrison punches. Alternatively, we perform laminoplasty in which the laminae are removed en bloc. Initially, bilateral laminotomies are made. After dissecting away the dura from the laminotomy site, a craniotome with a footplate attachment is used to create cuts at the junction of the lamina and lateral masses bilaterally. Posterior ligaments are cut sharply, and the bone is gently lifted off the dura. Care is taken to avoid removing more than 5 mm of the pars interarticularis in the thoracic and lumbar spine during the laminoplasty to prevent future instability. The ligamentum flavum is gently removed from the dura. All epidural bleeding is controlled using bipolar electrocautery, and bleeding bone is covered with bone wax. The field must be free of active bleeding before opening the dura.
- **Figure 89-5:** The malformation is localized with intraoperative ultrasonography, often showing an echogenic focus before opening the dura.
- **Figure 89-6:** Epidural electrodes are placed at the superior and inferior aspects of the opening. Baseline recordings are performed before opening the dura.
- **Figure 89-7:** Under the operating microscope, an initial dural opening is performed using a clean No. 15 blade. Care is taken not to enter the subarachnoid space during the opening to prevent rapid egress of cerebrospinal fluid. Metzenbaum scissors are used to complete the dural opening. To maintain wide intradural exposure, 4-0 Nurolon tenting sutures (Ethicon, Somerville, NJ) are placed in the dura. Atrophic, edematous, and soft spinal cord may be seen in patients with a chronic presentation. A “mulberry” appearance, representing a collection of clots and thrombosed blood, sometimes can be appreciated.

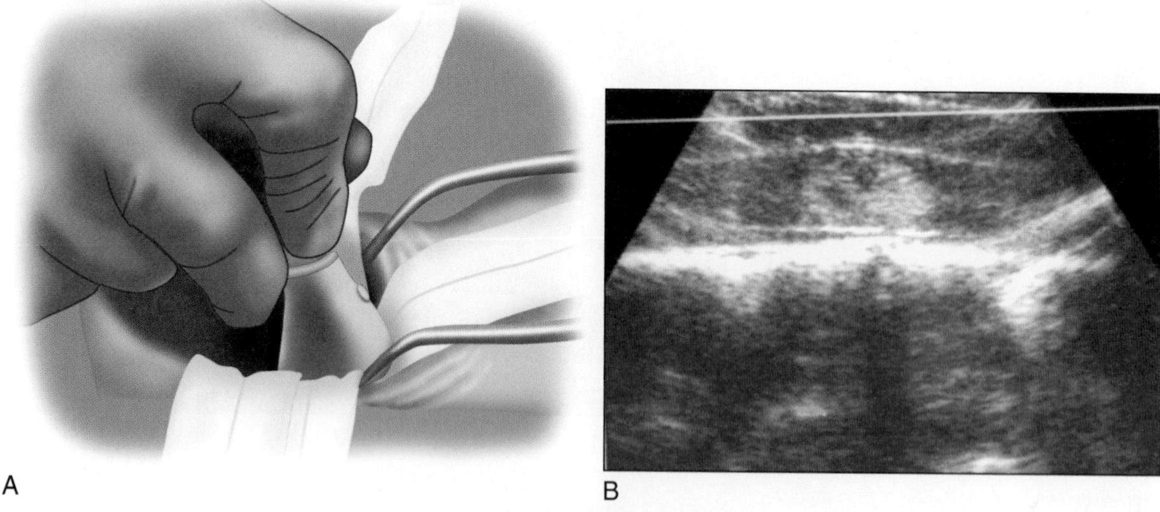

FIGURE 89-5

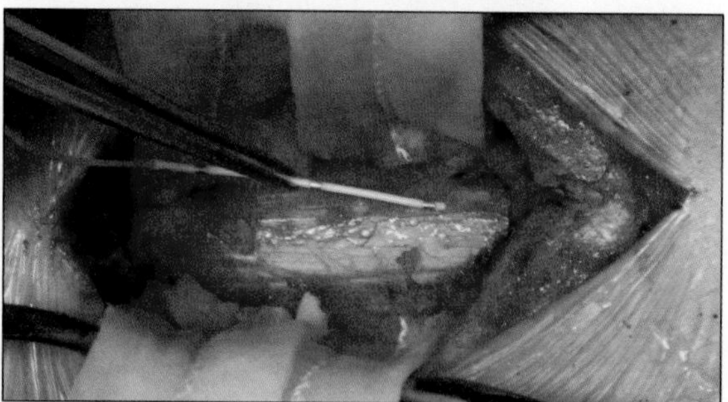

FIGURE 89-6

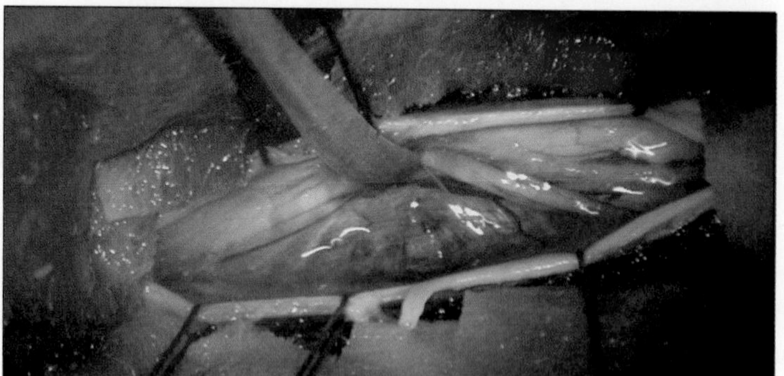

FIGURE 89-7

Midline myelotomy is performed over the area of discoloration, which usually abuts the dorsal pial surface.

- **Figure 89-8:** Plated bayonets are used to maintain the myelotomy opening. Small arteries are visualized with the microscope and avoided. Minimal capillary or venous bleeding is easily controlled with microbipolar electrocautery. Cavernous malformation is removed in an inside-out fashion, until the gliotic white matter is identified. This gliotic plane distinguishes the malformation from the normal spinal cord. Persistent bleeding that is not controlled with irrigation may be an indication of residual cavernous malformation. Complete excision is essential because residual cavernous malformations have the potential to grow, rebleed, and cause neurologic deficits. Intraoperative ultrasonography can confirm total resection of the lesion if gross or microscopic visualization is limited by a small myelotomy.

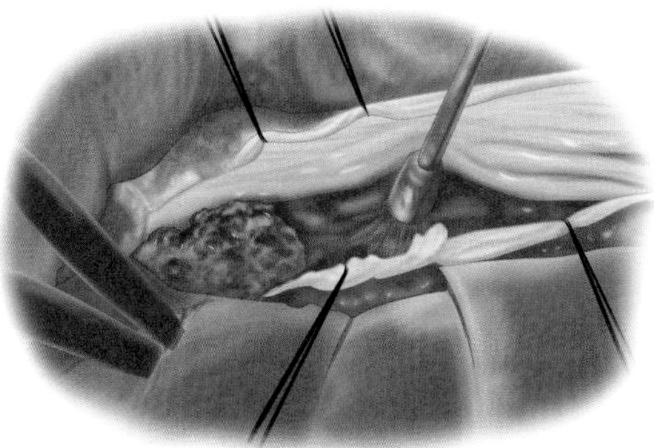

FIGURE 89-8

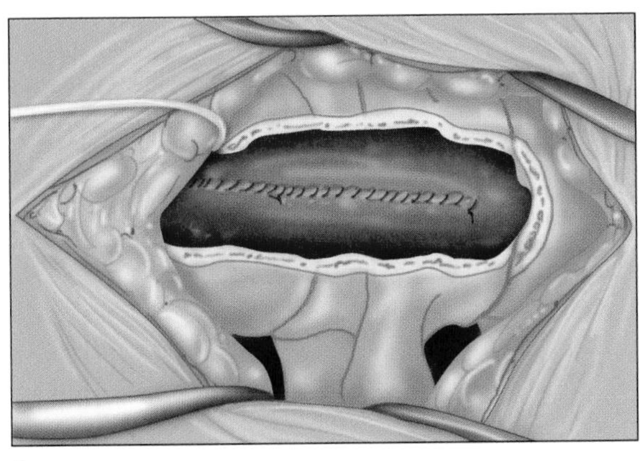

A

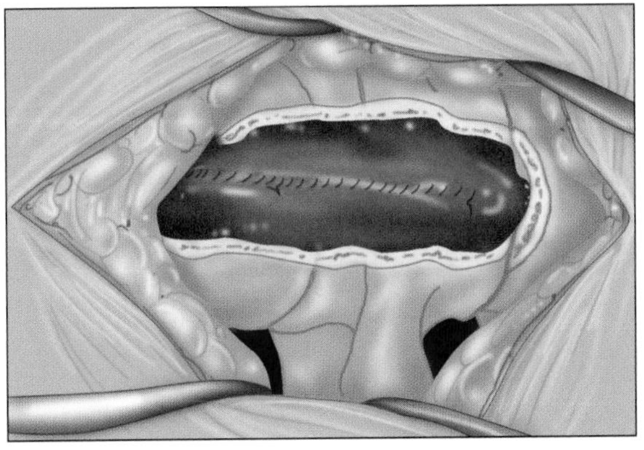

B

FIGURE 89-9

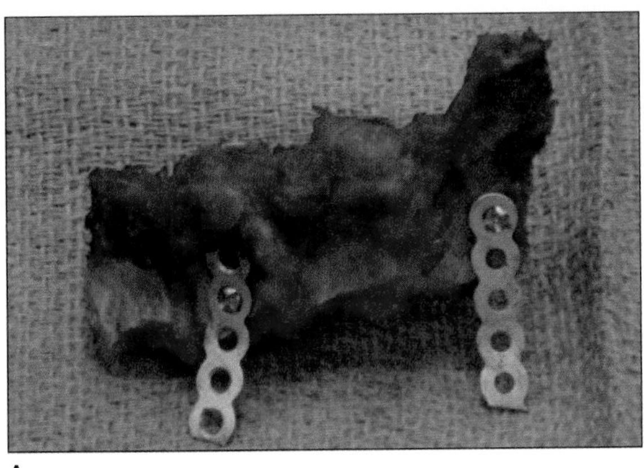

A

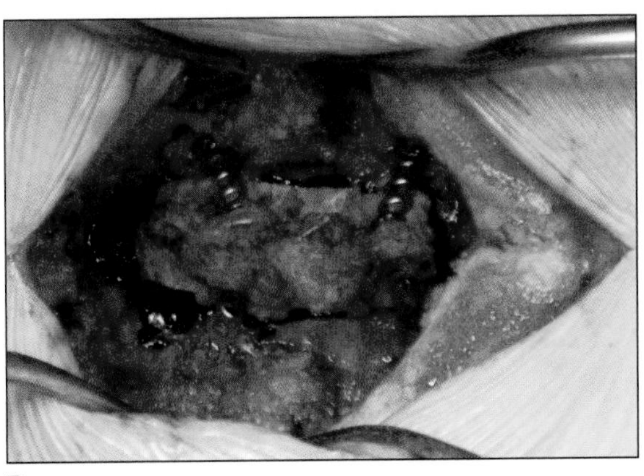

B

FIGURE 89-10

- **Figure 89-9:** After meticulous hemostasis, the dura should be closed with 5-0 Prolene (Ethicon, Somerville, NJ) sutures. Fibrin glue or DuraSeal is applied over the suture line to prevent cerebrospinal fluid leak.
- **Figure 89-10:** The laminae are plated with titanium or reabsorbable plates and screwed in place. The overlying muscle, fascia, and soft tissue are closed in the standard fashion. The skin is closed with a running 3-0 nylon suture. The patient is turned supine, a neurologic examination is performed, and the patient is extubated in the operating room and transferred to the neurologic intensive care unit.

TIPS FROM THE MASTERS

- Complete surgical resection should be the goal of surgery because subtotal resection is associated with recurrence and risk of hemorrhage.
- Although an immediate postoperative decline in neurologic status can be seen, the preoperative symptoms in most patients stabilize, and some patients experience improvements. Shorter duration of preoperative symptoms is associated with improved postoperative outcome.
- We recommend surgical resection for all symptomatic patients with spinal cavernous malformation given the high risk of neurologic injury from hemorrhage.
- Patients who present at a young age are more likely to harbor multiple cavernomas and benefit the most from MRI of the entire neuraxis.

PITFALLS

Meticulous hemostasis must be obtained before dural closure. After dural closure, ultrasonography can be performed if there is concern for bleeding. Persistent bleeding is a sign of residual cavernous malformation. If there is an unexpected decrement in the postoperative neurologic examination, emergent MRI should be obtained to evaluate for possible hemorrhage. If a blood clot is apparent on MRI, the patient should be brought back to the operating room for emergent evacuation.

The resection must begin within the lesion and extend outward toward the gliotic plane because normal spinal cord lies adjacent to this plane.

BAILOUT OPTIONS

- Surgical manipulation should be stopped if attenuation of MEPs to less than one half of the baseline occurs, or if the latency of MEPs is prolonged for more than 2 msec. Irrigation of the spinal cord with warm saline during the pause in manipulation usually results in recovery sufficient to allow for continuation of surgery.
- If subtotal resection occurs, follow-up MRI should be performed 6 to 12 months postoperatively to evaluate for growth of the cavernous malformation or recurrent hemorrhage. The use of reabsorbable, rather than titanium, plates for laminoplasty might be advised in these patients to limit MRI artifact.

SUGGESTED READINGS

Deutsch H, Jallo GI, Faktorovich A, et al. Spinal intramedullary cavernoma: clinical presentation and surgical outcome. J Neurosurg 2000;93:65–70.

Deutsch H, Shrivistava R, Epstein F, et al. Pediatric intramedullary spinal cavernous malformations. Spine (Phila Pa 1976) 2001;26:E427–31.

Jallo GI, Freed D, Zareck M, et al. Clinical presentation and optimal management for intramedullary cavernous malformations. Neurosurg Focus 2006;21:e10.

Vishteh AG, Sankhla S, Anson JA, et al. Surgical resection of intramedullary spinal cord cavernous malformations: delayed complications, long-term outcomes, and association with cryptic venous malformations. Neurosurgery 1997;41:1094–100.

Zevgaridis D, Medele RJ, Hamburger C, et al. Cavernous haemangiomas of the spinal cord: a review of 117 cases. Acta Neurochir (Wien) 1999;141:237–45.

Procedure 90

Spinal Cord Stimulator

Ryan M. Kretzer, James E. Conway, Ira M. Garonzik

INDICATIONS

- Nerve root injury with radicular pain in the absence of compressive pathology
- Nerve root injury as a complication of spine surgery, including nerve root retraction or injury secondary to interbody graft placement or pedicle screw fixation
- Painful peripheral neuropathy refractory to medical management

CONTRAINDICATIONS

- Thoracic spinal stenosis at the level of lead placement
- Reversible compressive lesion (e.g., disk herniation, synovial cyst) accounting for the patient's neurologic complaints
- Previous thoracic laminectomy with scar tissue in the epidural space at the level of lead placement
- Active systemic infection or medical contraindication to surgery

PLANNING AND POSITIONING

- The patient should have a percutaneous spinal cord stimulator trial that shows good pain coverage before permanent implantation.
- The gluteal incision for battery insertion should be placed 2 fingerbreadths below the iliac crest (i.e., below patient's belt line) and just lateral to the sacrum on the side opposite of the patient's preferred side of sleep.
- Anteroposterior fluoroscopy should be positioned so that the pedicles are symmetric and are bisected by the corresponding spinous processes, verifying that fluoroscopic images are perpendicular to the patient's spine at the operative level.
- **Figure 90-1:** In the preoperative area, the patient's back is palpated in the upright position to plan the ideal location for battery placement.
- **Figure 90-2:** The patient is intubated and positioned prone on a Jackson table with appropriate padding of all dependent surfaces to avoid pressure-related tissue necrosis or peripheral nerve injury. Fluoroscopy C-arm is used to plan the vertical midline spinal incision over the T9-10 interspace.
- **Figure 90-3:** The surgical field, including the thoracic and gluteal incisions, is prepared and draped in the standard sterile fashion. Preoperative antibiotics are given before the skin incision.

PROCEDURE

- **Figure 90-4:** The skin is incised over the T9-10 interspace, and monopolar electrocautery is used to expose the spinous processes and lamina of T9 and T10 in the subperiosteal plane, taking special care to avoid violation of adjacent facet capsules. A cerebellar retractor is used for tissue retraction, and a marker clamp is placed at the operative level.
- **Figure 90-5:** An anteroposterior fluoroscopic image is taken to confirm the appropriate spinal level.

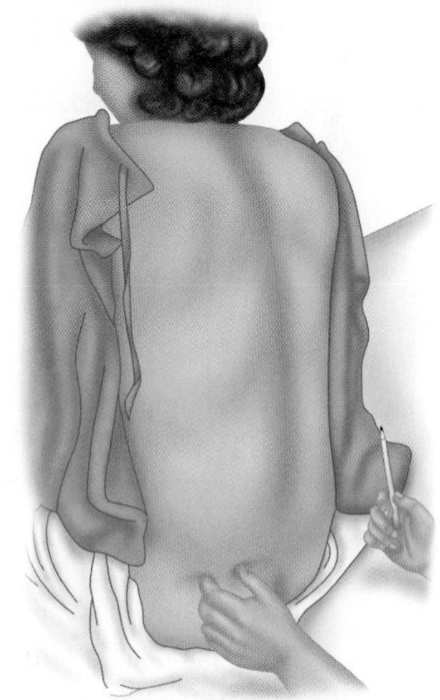

FIGURE 90-1

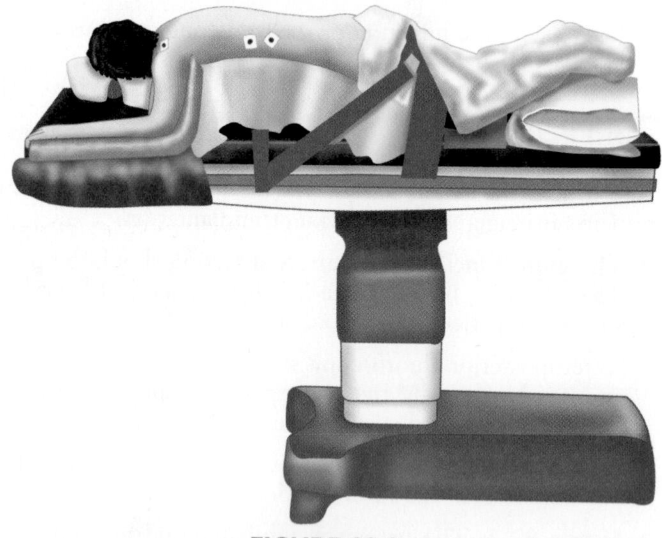

FIGURE 90-2

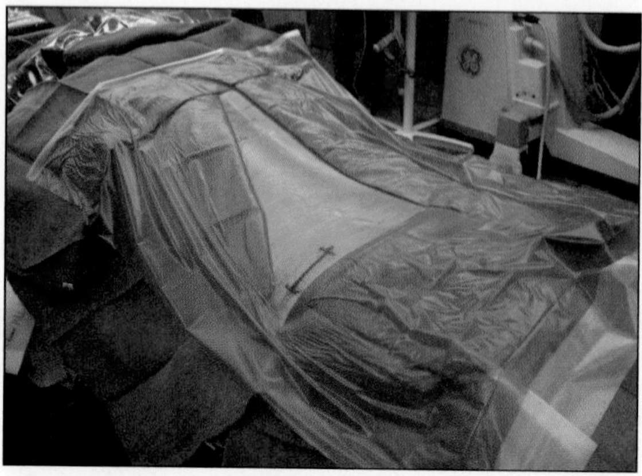

FIGURE 90-3

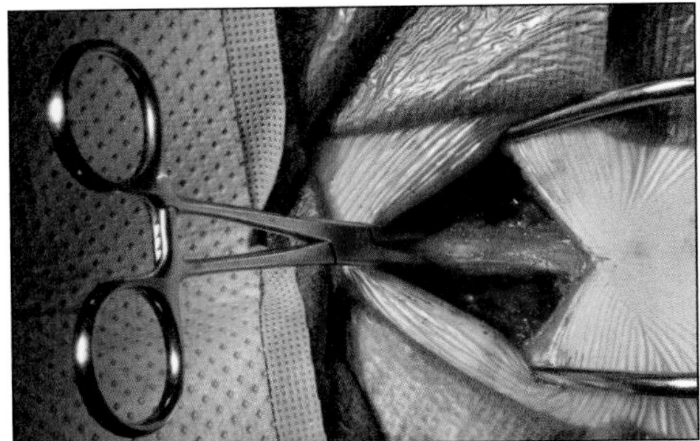

FIGURE 90-4

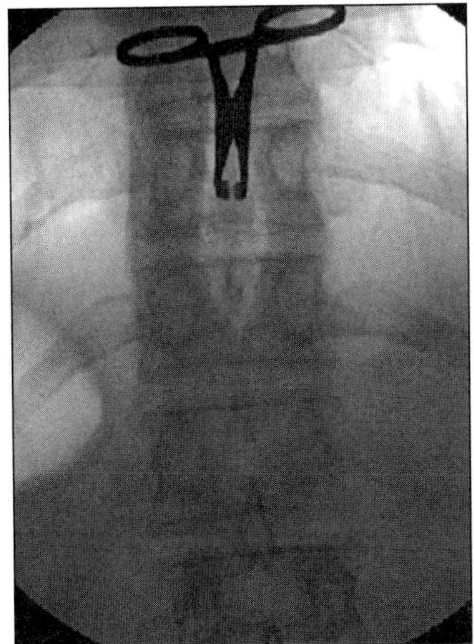

FIGURE 90-5

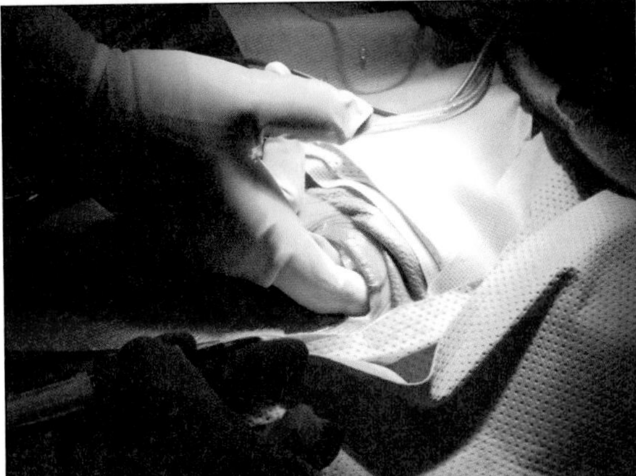

FIGURE 90-6

- **Figure 90-6:** The gluteal incision is opened sharply, and monopolar electrocautery is used to dissect to the level of the subcutaneous tissue. Blunt finger dissection allows formation of appropriate-sized pocket for battery insertion.
- **Figure 90-7:** Returning to the thoracic spinal incision, a Leksell rongeur is used to remove the T9 spinous process, the T9-10 interspinous ligament, and the superior aspect of the T10 spinous process. A hand-held drill and No. 5 diamond bur are used to create a symmetric trough to the level of the ligamentum flavum.

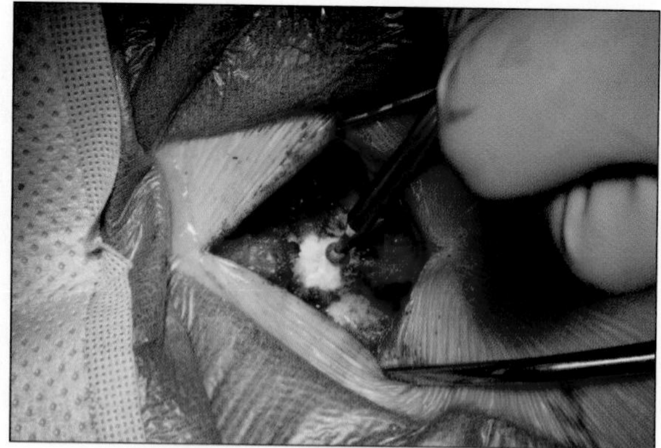

FIGURE 90-7

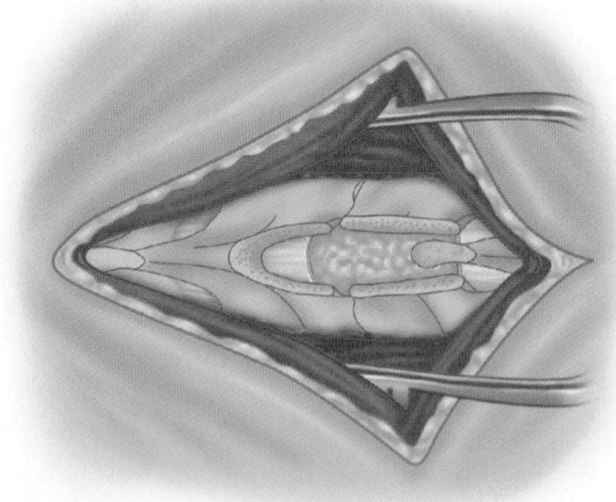

FIGURE 90-8

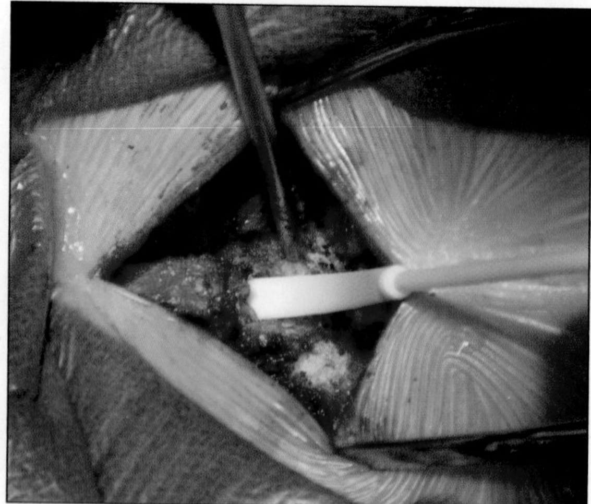

FIGURE 90-9

- **Figure 90-8:** The ligamentum flavum is removed with a 2-mm Kerrison punch, exposing the epidural fat. The laminotomy is widened with a Kerrison punch, and the dura is visualized. A small angled curet is passed under the edge of the residual T9 lamina to verify smooth access to the epidural space at T8-9.
- **Figure 90-9:** A paddle guide is passed freely and without resistance into the T8-9 epidural space.

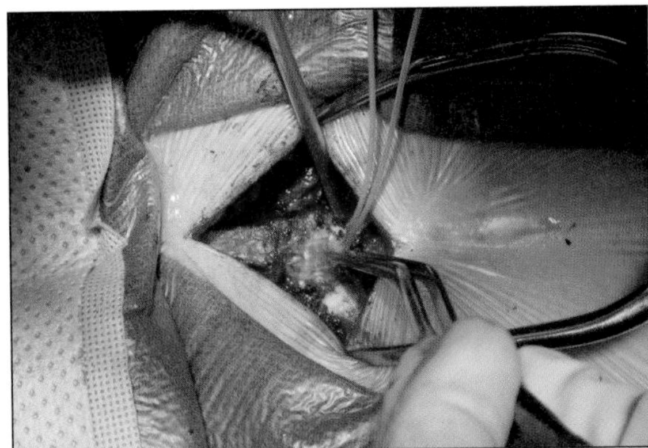

FIGURE 90-10

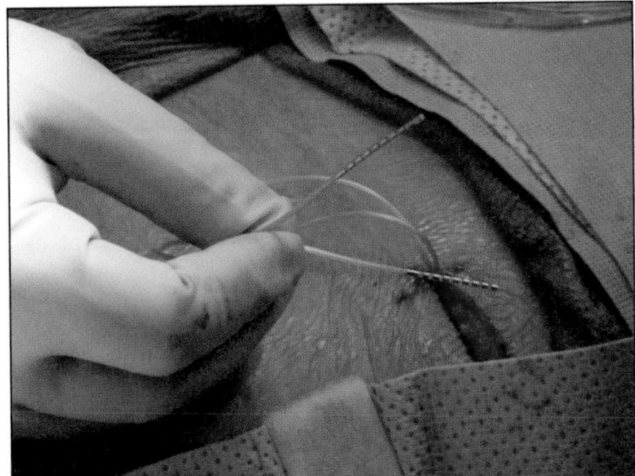

FIGURE 90-11

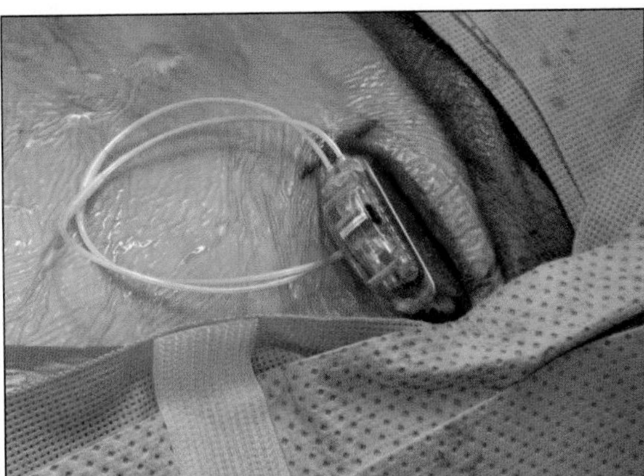

FIGURE 90-12

- **Figure 90-10:** Using bayoneted forceps, the paddle electrode is passed into the epidural space in the midline at T8-9. Anteroposterior fluoroscopy is used to verify the good position of the paddle electrode.
- **Figure 90-11:** A subcutaneous path is tunneled using a tunneling device from the thoracic spinal incision to the gluteal pocket, and the distal electrode lead is passed to the planned area of battery insertion. A strain relief loop should also be left in the thoracic wound to avoid traction and migration of the paddle electrode. The loop should be secured to the fascia with a nonabsorbable suture.
- **Figure 90-12:** The distal electrode lead is inserted into the battery, and impedances are checked. The leads are tightened into the battery ports using the screwdriver that is

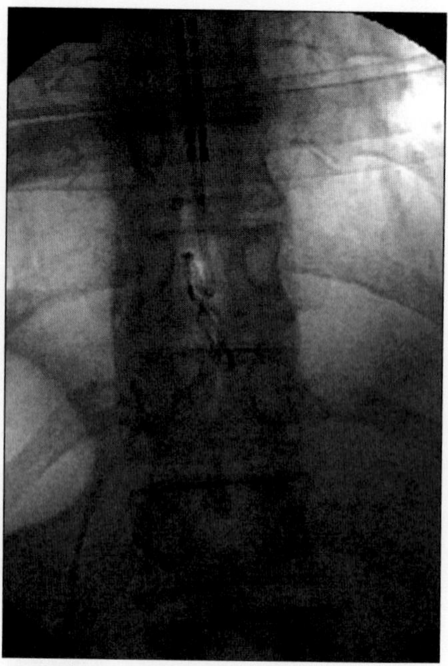

FIGURE 90-13

provided, and the battery is placed into the gluteal pocket. Excess leads are placed behind the battery in a looped fashion.

- **Figure 90-13:** Anteroposterior fluoroscopy is used to verify the final midline placement of the paddle electrode at the T8-9 level before closing the incisions.
- Both wounds are copiously irrigated and closed in layers in a standard fashion with absorbable suture. The skin is closed with a running subcuticular stitch and sealed with adhesive skin glue.

TIPS FROM THE MASTERS

- Fluoroscopic imaging of the preoperative percutaneous stimulator trial must have an identifiable spinal landmark to allow proper positioning of the permanent implant.
- A multidisciplinary approach, including close collaboration with a pain specialist, is critical to the care of patients with implantation of spinal cord stimulators.
- Accurate lead placement is crucial to postoperative outcomes, so extra time and care should be taken to ensure midline lead placement at the desired level.

PITFALLS

After permanent stimulator implantation, magnetic resonance imaging (MRI) is contraindicated. The physician should consider preoperative MRI of the spinal axis for screening purposes and to establish a baseline for continued care.

Revision of prior paddle placement carries an increased risk of spinal cord injury because of epidural scar tissue.

Centering the electrode paddle in the epidural space can be challenging. Fluoroscopic imaging should be aligned so that the pedicles are symmetric and bisected by the spinous process and the vertebral end plates are in line with the imaging plane to ensure proper lead placement.

BAILOUT OPTIONS

- The electrode paddle should be passed into the epidural space without mechanical resistance. Careful dissection with a Woodson dissector in the epidural space or removal of additional bone from the laminotomy site to aid in surgical exposure can help ensure safe lead passage.
- If difficulty is encountered at the operative level during dissection or lead passage, the physician should consider moving rostrally one spinal level or converting to percutaneous lead placement.
- To prevent lead migration, a strain relief loop should be added in the thoracic surgical site to reduce traction on the paddle electrode.

SUGGESTED READINGS

Kumar K, Taylor RS, Jacques L, et al. Spinal cord stimulation versus conventional medical management for neuropathic pain: a multicentre randomized controlled trial in patients with failed back surgery syndrome. Pain 2007;132:179–88.

Kumar K, Taylor RS, Jacques L, et al. The effects of spinal cord stimulation in neuropathic pain are sustained: a 24-month follow-up of the prospective randomized controlled multicenter trial of the effectiveness of spinal cord stimulation. Neurosurgery 2008;63:762–70.

North RB, Kidd DH, Farrokhi F, et al. Spinal cord stimulation versus repeated lumbosacral spine surgery for chronic pain: a randomized, controlled trial. Neurosurgery 2005;56:98–106.

North RB, Kidd DH, Lee MS, et al. A prospective, randomized study of spinal cord stimulation versus reoperation for failed back surgery syndrome: initial results. Stereotact Funct Neurosurg 1994;62:267–72.

North RB, Kidd DH, Petrucci L, et al. Spinal cord stimulation electrode design: a prospective randomized, controlled trial comparing percutaneous with laminectomy electrodes: part II—clinical outcomes. Neurosurgery 2005;57:990–6.

Procedure 91

Endoscopic Thoracic Sympathectomy

Bong-Soo Kim, Markus Bookland, Jack I. Jallo

INDICATIONS

- Indications for thoracoscopic sympathectomy include palmar hyperhidrosis, axillary hyperhidrosis, craniofacial hyperhidrosis and blushing, reflex sympathetic dystrophy, Raynaud disease, splanchnic pain, vascular insufficiency, angina pectoris, and heart arrhythmias such as long QT syndrome. Currently, the most common indication, and the indication for which the results are most satisfactory, is palmar hyperhidrosis.
- Patients undergoing thoracic sympathectomy should have previously completed and failed a trial of nonoperative therapy. Nonoperative options include topical therapy (primarily aluminum chloride hexahydrate [$AlCl_3$-$6H_2O$]) and iontophoresis, intradermal botulinum toxin injections, or glycopyrrolate.

CONTRAINDICATIONS

- Severe cardiocirculatory or pulmonary insufficiency and severe pleural disease (pleuritis, empyema) greatly increase the risks of thoracic endoscopic sympathectomy and are contraindications.
- Untreated hyperthyroidism, menopause, and obesity all may cause secondary hyperhidrosis. These conditions should be ruled out as etiologies for the patient's excess sweating before proceeding to surgical intervention.

PLANNING AND POSITIONING

- The anesthesiologist should be aware that double-lumen endotracheal tube placement is needed for single-lung ventilation of the contralateral lung and deflation of the ipsilateral lung. Frequent, noninvasive arterial pressure monitoring should be considered during periods of lung deflation. Invasive monitoring may be useful in patients with impaired cardiovascular function.
- **Figure 91-1:** The patient is placed in the lateral decubitus position.
- An axillary roll rests under the contralateral side, and the ipsilateral arm rests abducted at a gentle angle on an elevated arm rest.

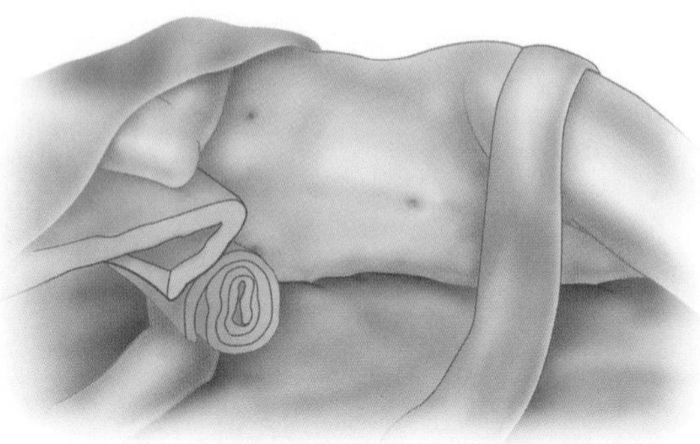

FIGURE 91-1

- Surgical preparation and exposure includes the entire thorax in the event that conversion to an open thoracotomy is necessary.
- The operating surgeon stands ventral to the patient, with the anesthesiologist at the head and the scrub nurse at the base of the field. Monitors for the endoscope should be placed opposite the operating surgeon and, if present, the assisting surgeon.
- The right side is usually operated on first because the proximity of the sympathetic chain to the hemiazygos vein can make the operation difficult, particularly if an extensive sympathectomy down to T4 is planned.

PROCEDURE

- **Figure 91-2:** After deflation of the ipsilateral lung by the anesthesiologist, the anterior axillary, midaxillary, and posterior axillary lines are identified. These mark the boundaries of the port placements.
- **Figure 91-3:** An initial 10-mm port and scope are inserted through a 1.5-cm incision in the anterior axillary line in the third or fourth intercostal space, immediately superior to the rib to avoid injury to intercostal neurovascular structures. Under endoscopic guidance, a 5-mm port is placed in midaxillary line in the fifth or sixth intercostal space. The posterior port is used to introduce the working instruments. To facilitate intraoperative exposure and dissection, the operating table is repositioned in slight reverse Trendelenburg and rotated anteriorly, allowing gravity to pull the upper lobes out of the field of dissection.
- **Figure 91-4:** Thoracic sympathetic chains run beneath the parietal pleura and usually course over the heads of the ribs, close to the costovertebral junctions and the lateral aspect of the vertebral bodies. The T2 sympathetic ganglion lies between the second and third ribs. Anatomy is shown in endoscopic (**A**) and schematic (**B**) view.
- **Figure 91-5:** By using thoracoscopic curved scissors and a Harmonic scalpel (Ethicon Endo-Surgery, Inc, Cincinnati, OH), the pleura overlying the sympathetic chain is opened. Care should be exercised to avoid damage to the underlying periosteum because this can cause severe discomfort and sunburnlike pain in the postoperative period.

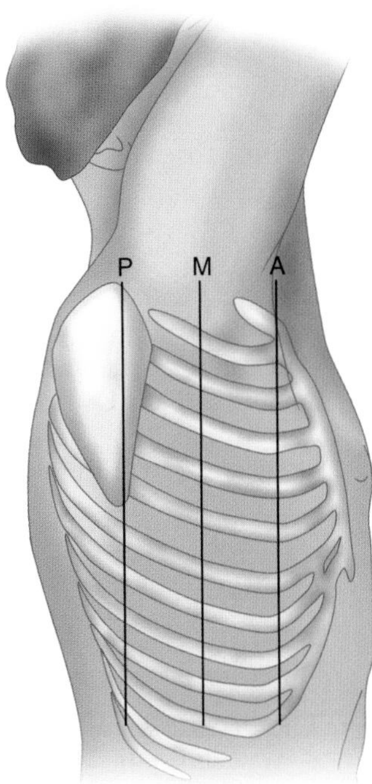

FIGURE 91-2

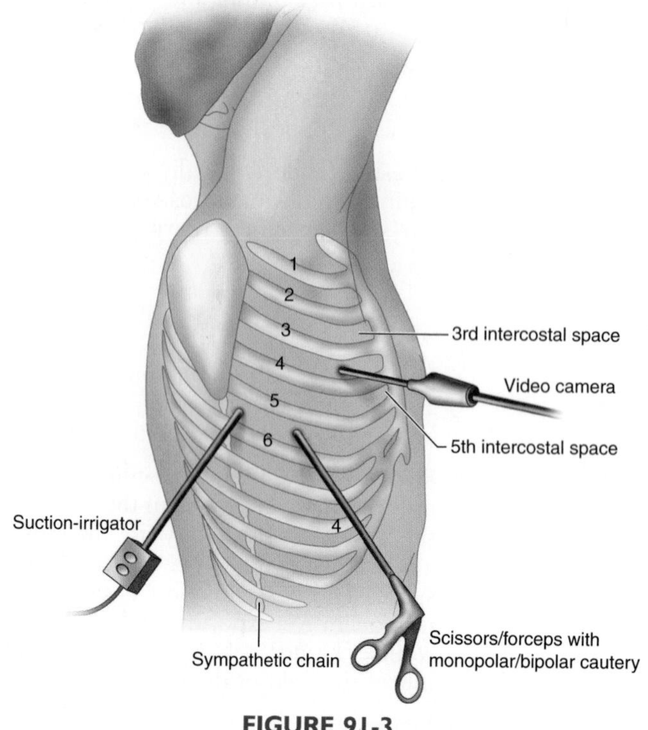

FIGURE 91-3

- **Figure 91-6:** Two clamps (5-mm endoscopic clips) are applied above the T2 ganglia, and two clamps are applied below the T3 ganglia. It is important to identify the nerve of Kuntz, which must be clamped.
- **Figure 91-7:** The dissection bed is irrigated and ensured for hemostasis, and the lung is reinflated with endoscopic confirmation. The port is removed, and the wound is closed while the anesthesiologist maintains a Valsalva maneuver to reduce the opportunity for postoperative pneumothorax.
- An 18-F chest tube is left in both chest cavities. The tube can often be removed later the same day or the next morning, when the drainage is less than 100 mL and a chest x-ray verifies absence of a pneumothorax.

TIPS FROM THE MASTERS

- Be careful of the vessels medial to the sympathetic ganglia, especially the veins at the T3 and T4 levels. These branches drain directly into the azygos arch and can cause significant bleeding if avulsed. In case of bleeding, exposure with suction and cauterization of the vessel with monopolar or bipolar current is necessary.
- A temperature probe on the palm of the hand can be used to verify adequate clip placement. Hand temperature should increase about 1° F after the sympathetic chain is clipped.
- Reverse Trendelenburg and CO_2 insufflation of the chest cavity can help move the lungs away from the working field.
- The first rib seen inside the chest cavity is the second rib. Verify the rib count with an x-ray if in doubt.
- Place the endoscope and working port in different planes to avoid interference between the working instrument and the endoscope.

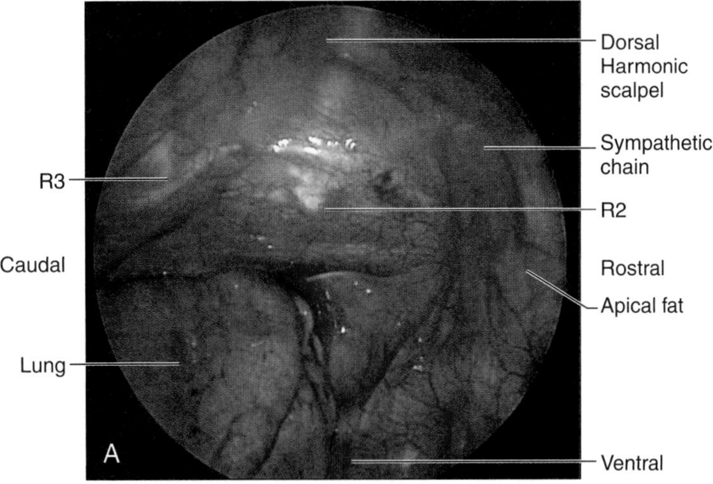

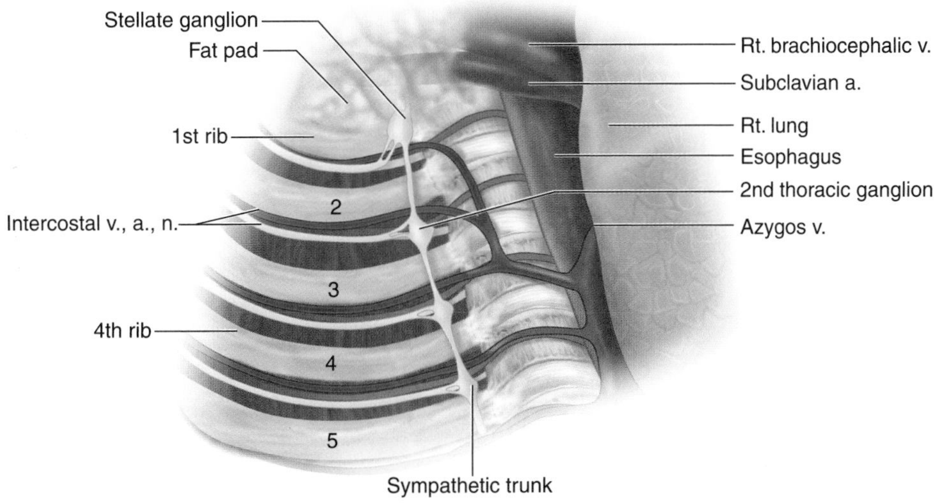

FIGURE 91-4

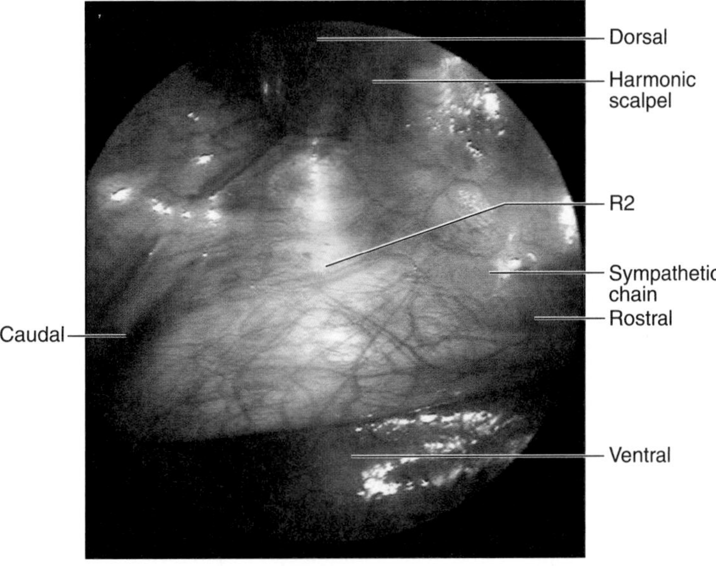

FIGURE 91-5

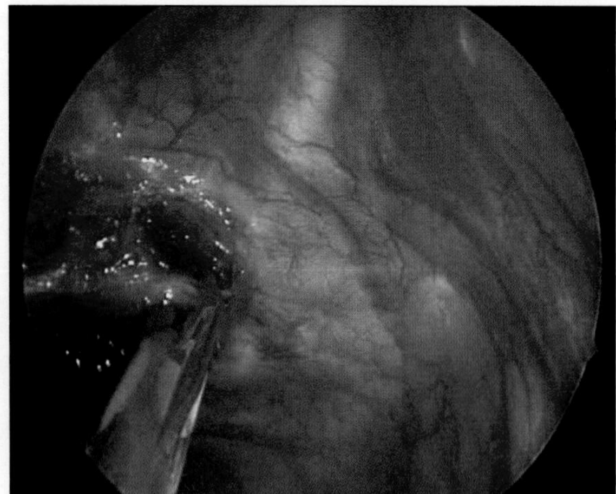

FIGURE 91-6

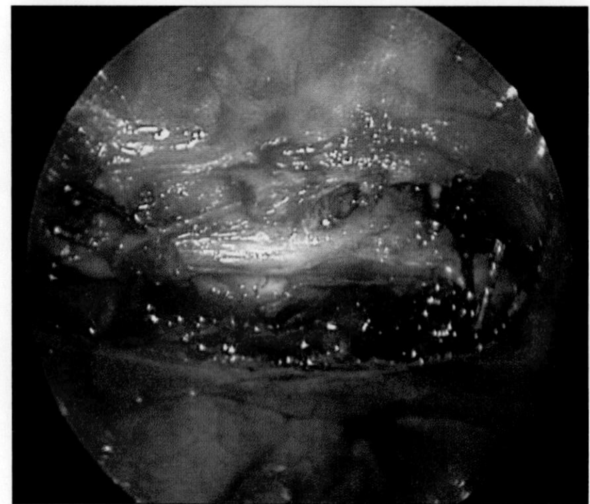

FIGURE 91-7

PITFALLS

The risk of compensatory hyperhidrosis may be minimized by limiting clipping to the second and third rib sympathetic ganglia.

Horner syndrome may result if clips are placed much above the second rib sympathetic ganglia and injure the cervical sympathetic chain.

Persistent pneumothorax can form if the lung is injured. Be aware of the lung and its location in relation to the endoscope and working instrument. Have the anesthesiologist expand the lungs before closure.

Hemothorax may be avoided with careful dissection and irrigation and tamponade and cautery of any bleeding sites.

BAILOUT OPTIONS

- Open thoracotomy is the ultimate bailout option but is rarely needed with attention to surrounding vessels.
- A clipping approach to thoracic sympathectomy has been described. If the sympathetic chain cannot be dissected free, it may always be cut to achieve a similar result.

SUGGESTED READINGS

Atkinson JL, Fealey RD. Sympathotomy instead of sympathectomy for palmar hyperhidrosis: minimizing postoperative compensatory hyperhidrosis. Mayo Clin Proc 2003;78:167–72.

Li X, Tu YR, Lin M, et al. Endoscopic thoracic sympathectomy for palmar hyperhidrosis: a randomized control trial comparing T3 and T2-4 ablation. Ann Thorac Surg 2008;85:1747–51.

Marhold F, Izay B, Zacherl J, et al. Thoracoscopic and anatomic landmarks of Kuntz's nerve: implications for sympathetic surgery. Ann Thorac Surg 2008;86:1653–8.

Sugimura H, Spratt EH, Compeau CG, et al. Thoracoscopic sympathetic clipping for hyperhidrosis: long-term results and reversibility. J Thorac Cardiovasc Surg 2009;137:1370–6.

Walles T, Somuncuoglu G, Steger V, et al. Long-term efficiency of endoscopic thoracic sympathicotomy: survey 10 years after surgery. Interact Cardiovasc Thorac Surg 2009;8:54–7.

Procedure 92 Primary Myelomeningocele Closure

Matthias Schulz, Ulrich W. Thomale

INDICATIONS

- Any newborn with an open dysraphic condition should undergo operative closure as soon as possible, preferably within the first 48 hours after delivery.

CONTRAINDICATIONS

- With an open spinal defect, there is no contraindication for closure, unless the infant is clinically unstable. In that case, closure is deferred until undergoing the procedure is possible. Severe congenital anomalies associated with overall short life expectancy should be evaluated in the respective ethical context.

PLANNING AND POSITIONING

- Clinical evaluation in a multidisciplinary approach (with clinicians in neonatology, neurology, neurosurgery, and orthopedics) should assess overall medical stability, neurologic function, and associated malformations. The presence of commonly associated conditions of hydrocephalus and Chiari malformation needs to be considered when developing a treatment plan for the newborn.
- Examination of the fontanelle and cranial ultrasound and cranial magnetic resonance imaging (MRI) should be performed to assess the degree of associated central nervous system abnormalities. The presence of hydrocephalus must be continuously monitored to plan for a timely shunt insertion. If manifest hydrocephalus exists, we plan the shunt insertion for the time of myelomeningocele closure.
- Spinal ultrasound or spinal MRI is advisable to assess anatomic conditions and to check for additional malformations (e.g., split cord, spinal lipoma).
- The infant is positioned prone with free abdomen to allow for breathing excursions. Hyperextension of the neck must be avoided in case of significant Chiari malformation. Special attention is directed to pad all pressure points and to apply appropriate warming to keep body temperature normal.
- **Figure 92-1:** Images of exemplary preoperative MRI (T2-weighted images) showing an infant with a lumbosacral myelomeningocele in the axial and sagittal planes. The laminar defect with the protruding spinal cord coursing toward its junction with the exposed placode (which is slightly rotated leftward) can be appreciated.
- **Figure 92-2:** Positioning of the infant for myelomeningocele repair. Soft gel cushions that leave the abdomen free for respiratory excursions support the chest and pelvis. A warming blanket is already placed under the infant. The arms and legs are wrapped with wadded bandages. All exposed body surfaces except the surgical field are covered with warming blankets.

PROCEDURE

- **Figure 92-3:** Incision of the intermediate zone is started cranially to the lesion and extends to the junction of dysplastic skin with the placode. Some cerebrospinal fluid (CSF) usually drains, and elevation of the edges bilaterally to the incision allows inspection of the internal anatomy of the malformation. The spinal cord emerging from the spinal canal through the defect and its junction with the cranial pole of the placode can be appreciated.

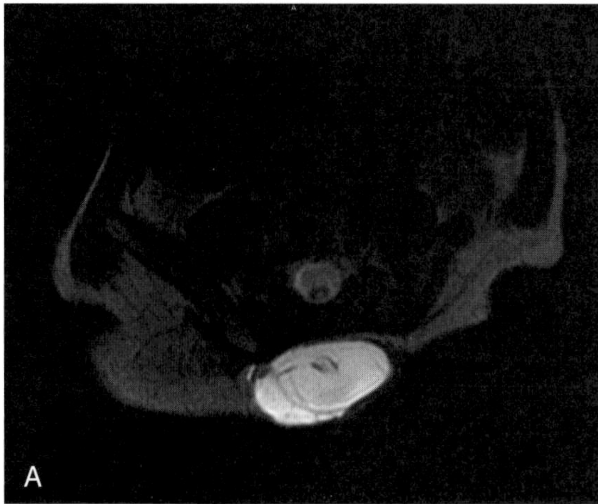

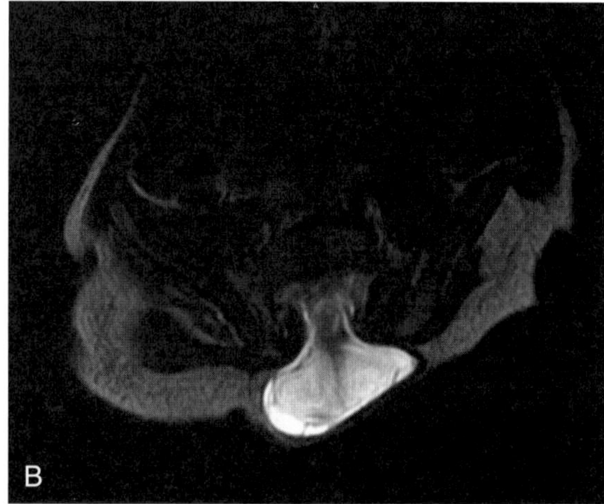

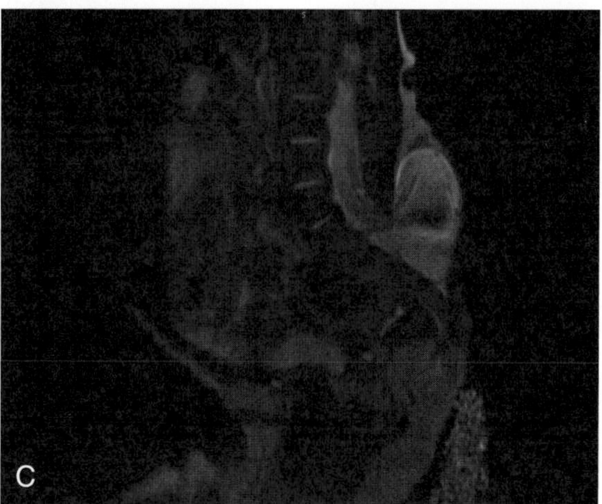

FIGURE 92-1

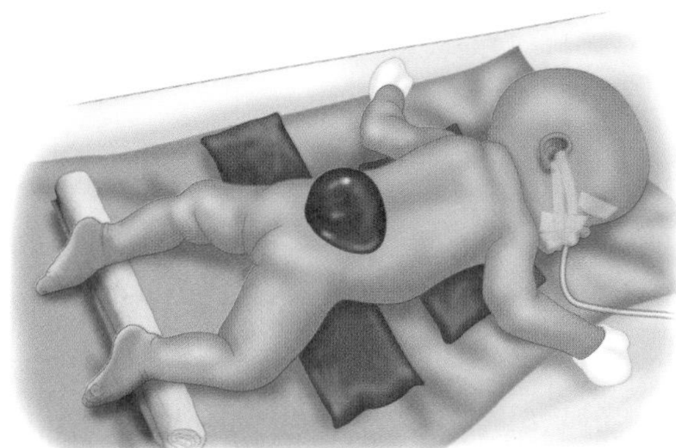

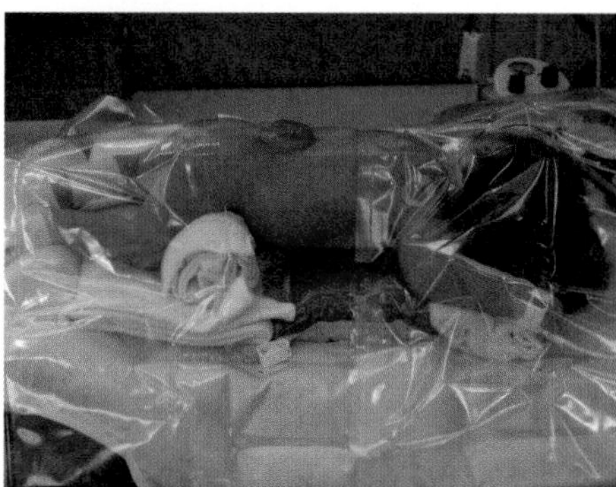

FIGURE 92-2

- **Figure 92-4:** Dissection continues laterally around the placode. Before advancement of the incision along this interface, the internal surface is inspected for laterally coursing nerve rootlets; if present, they are dissected away medially toward the placode.
- **Figure 92-5:** Care must be taken at the junction of both lateral incisions at the caudal pole of the placode. At this site, rootlets have the most variable course, and further fibrous adhesions may be encountered, which have to be divided. The terminal filum is identified and sectioned. Aberrant vessels reaching the placode at the caudal pole commonly are found and should be preserved if possible.

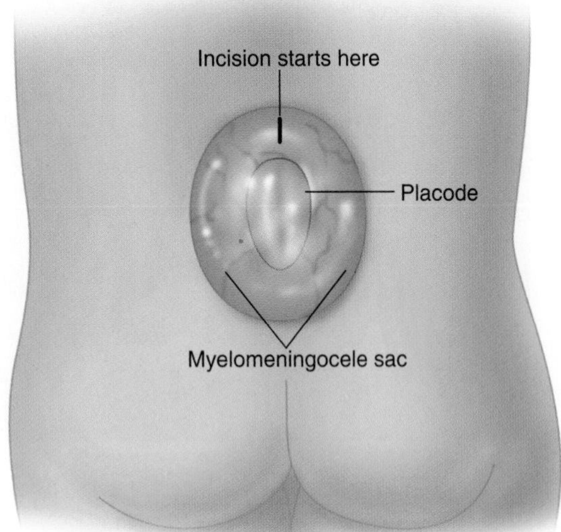

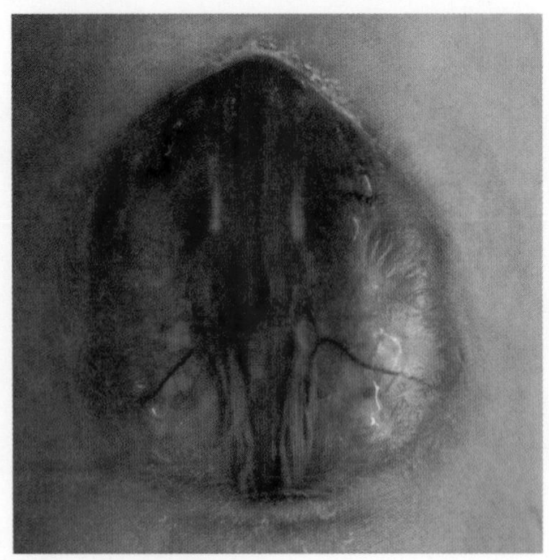

FIGURE 92-3

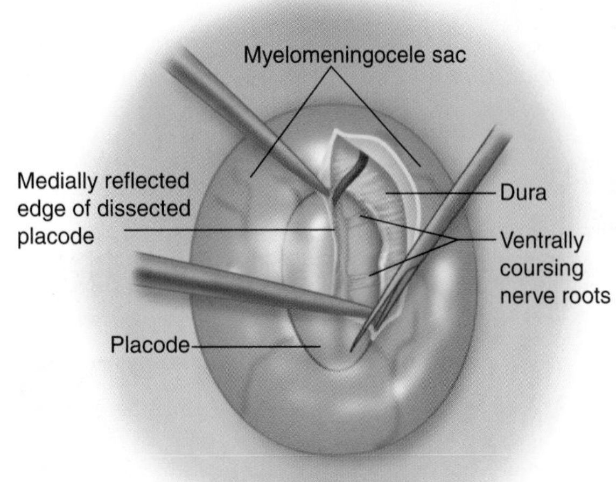

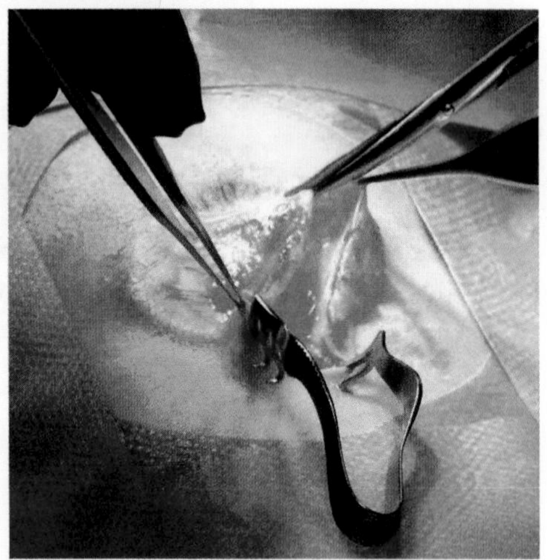

FIGURE 92-4

- **Figure 92-6:** The edges of the released placode are inspected for remaining areas of dysplastic skin. These need to be resected—verifying and preserving the course of ventrally directed rootlets.
- **Figure 92-7:** The tubular shape of the cord is reconstructed by approximating the lateral edges of placode with multiple single sutures. Fine materials such as 8-0 nonabsorbable monofilament sutures are used. The intention of this step is to create an involuted tube without any tension and to lessen the possibility for adhesion within the dural CSF space.
- **Figure 92-8:** The dural edge that blends laterally with the wall of the meningocele sac is identified at its junction with the lateral intermediate zone. Dissection starts cranially and continues bilaterally around the spinal defect. Caudally both incision lines are brought together. Vessels entering the dura and supplying placode are commonly encountered in the epidural space and should be preserved.

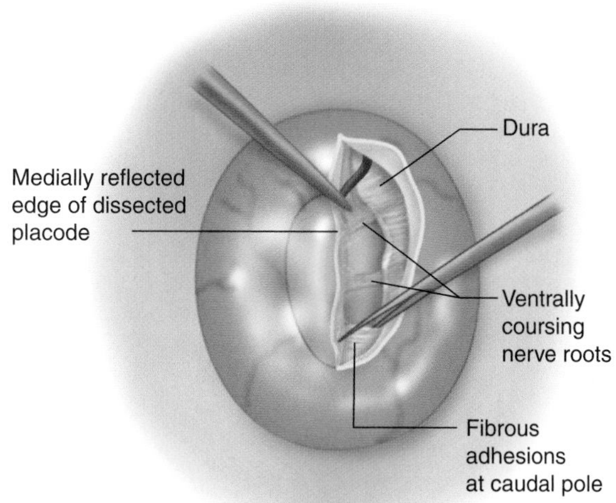

FIGURE 92-5

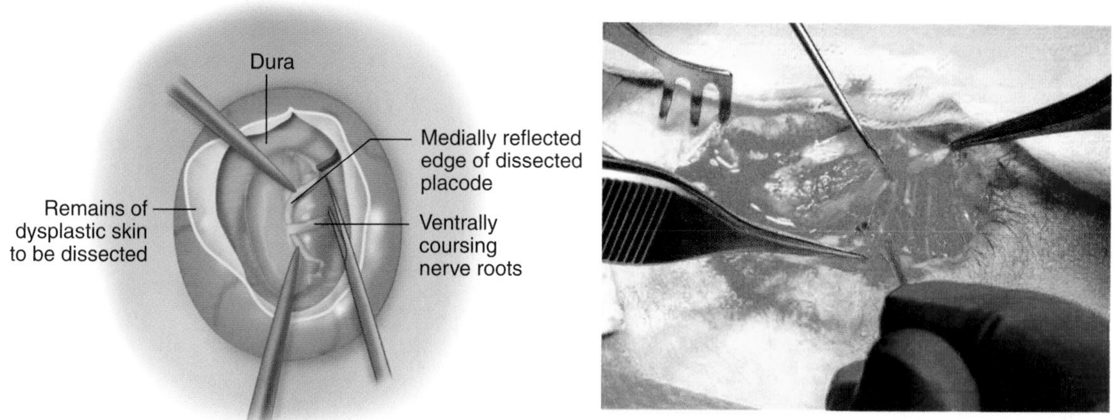

FIGURE 92-6

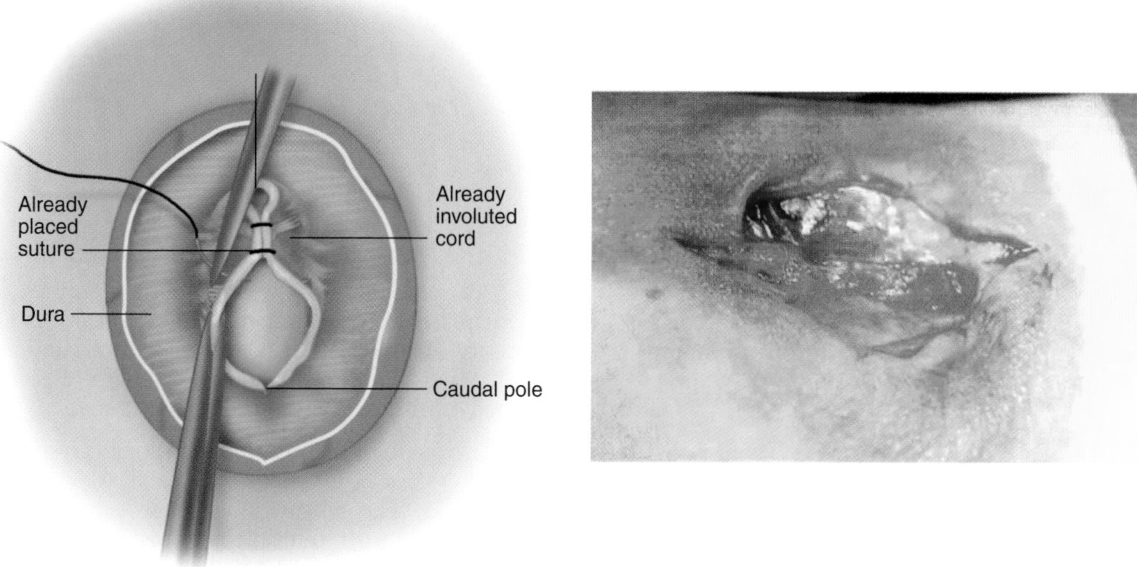

FIGURE 92-7

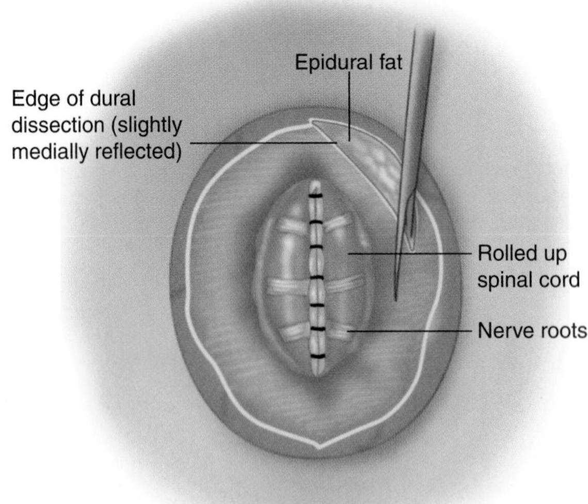

FIGURE 92-8

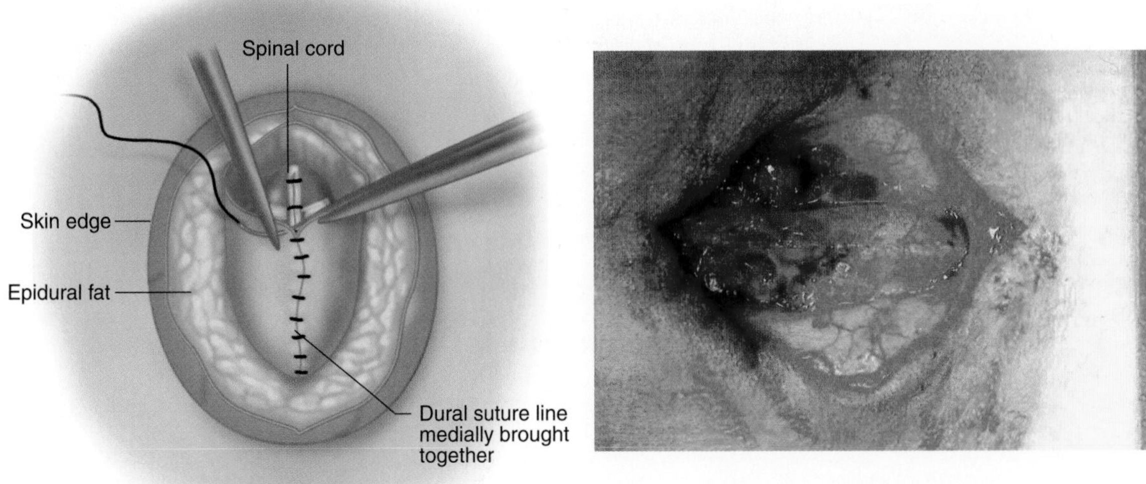

FIGURE 92-9

- **Figure 92-9:** Dural closure is obtained with a running suture line with 5-0 nonabsorbable monofilament material. If tension-free dural closure is impossible, closure with dural graft is necessary. At this step, it is crucial to avoid any pressure on neural structures within the created dural sac and to establish a wide enough compartment to allow undisturbed CSF flow around the neural tissue.
- **Figure 92-10:** All remaining dysplastic skin of the intermediate zone is resected along its junction with normal skin. The fascia is identified, and skin is mobilized circumferentially widely into the flanks. The subcutaneous layer is approximated using multiple sutures. Skin closure is done with multiple sutures using nonabsorbable monofilament material. Sterile dressings are applied. Meticulous wound care and dressing changes whenever dressings are soiled should be done.

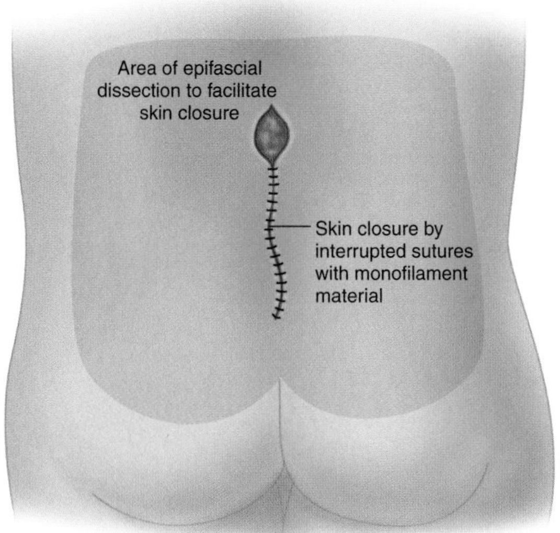

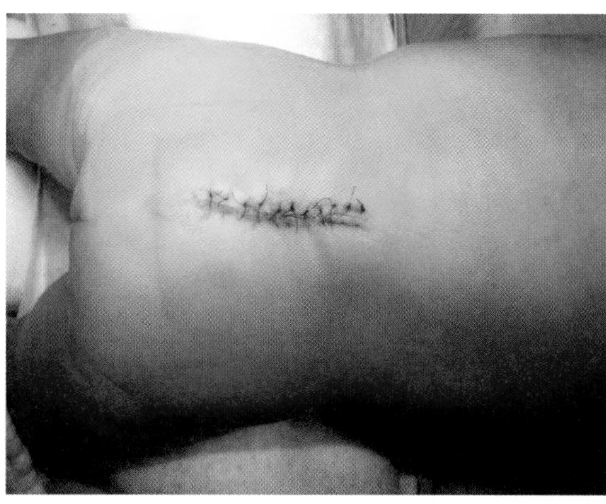

FIGURE 92-10

TIPS FROM THE MASTERS

- The initial dissection around the placode may be alleviated if a small cuff of dysplastic skin is left at the placode. Potential damage to emerging nerve rootlets is minimized. After completion of circumferential dissection, the whole edge can be reflected, and the course of the rootlets is more readily identified facilitating complete resection of the dysplastic skin remnants as the concluding step.
- Avoiding CSF leak is crucial because manifest CSF leakage increases risk of infection and results in collapse of the subarachnoid space around the neural structures, possibly promoting local tethering. Early shunt insertion when indicated and usage of dural sealants reduce the risk of CSF leak. If shunt insertion is performed at the same stage of myelomeningocele repair, the significant risk of infection must be kept in mind, and strict sterile regimens must be followed. In this context, antibiotic-impregnated catheters are beneficial.
- Longitudinal skin closure is preferred over oblique or irregular-shaped closure because it may be beneficial for a possible subsequent untethering procedure and can be accomplished in most cases by sufficient bilateral epifascial skin mobilization.

PITFALLS

Postoperative development of a subcutaneous CSF collection or transcutaneous CSF fistula might indicate manifest hydrocephalus. If initially a sufficient closure was achieved, prompt shunt insertion must be considered to lessen the risk of subsequent central nervous system infection and wound breakdown.

BAILOUT OPTIONS

- The dimensions of the dorsal defect of the vertebrae might be too small to accommodate the reconstructed spinal cord, especially if internal lipomas are involved. To allow a pressure-free positioning into the spinal canal, more width may be gained by resecting the dysplastic laminae down to the level of the pedicles. At the caudal pole of the malformation, the fascia and the caudal thecal sac may be incised to increase the longitudinal space.
- When severe vertebral anomaly is associated with a myelomeningocele, additional measures such as kyphoidectomy can be necessary.

SUGGESTED READINGS

Bowman RM, McLone DG, Grant JA, et al. Spina bifida outcome: a 25-year prospective. Pediatr Neurosurg 2001;34:114–20.

Gaskill SJ. Primary closure of open myelomeningocele. Neurosurg Focus 2004;16:E3.

McLone DG. Technique for closure of myelomeningocele. Childs Brain 1980;6:65–73.

Ozveren MF, Erol FS, Topsakal C, et al. The significance of the percentage of the defect size in spina bifida cystica in determination of the surgical technique. Childs Nerv Syst 2002;18:614–20.

Pinto FC, Matushita H, Furlan AL, et al. Surgical treatment of myelomeningocele carried out at 'time zero' immediately after birth. Pediatr Neurosurg 2009;45:114–8.

Procedure 93 Tethered Cord Release

Ulrich W. Thomale, Matthias Schulz

INDICATIONS

- Tethered cord on magnetic resonance imaging (MRI) (spinal cord adhesions, low conus medullaris, thickened fatty filum, dural sinus, lipomyelomeningocele [LMMC], split cord malformation) with progressive clinical deteriorating symptoms such as pain, sensory impairment, weakness, spasticity, urinary dysfunction, foot deformity, and scoliosis that can be correlated with the spinal cord anomaly.
- MRI diagnosis of a dermal sinus and existence of cutaneous dimpling close to the midline region associated with cerebrospinal fluid (CSF) leak or recurrent meningitis caused by atypical bacteria or both.
- MRI diagnosis without or with minor neurologic symptoms as prophylactic surgery to prevent progressive neurologic deterioration at an early stage of life, considering physical stability with a sufficient body weight at the least age of 6 months.
- Because no evidence is available to address the necessity or the optimal timing of prophylactic surgery, the individual risk to prevent any morbidity must be carefully weighed to justify surgery.

CONTRAINDICATIONS

- Severe coexisting congenital abnormalities (central nervous system, cardiac, renal) leading to instability during surgery or associated with an overall short life expectancy should be treated conservatively.
- A tethered cord that is coincidentally detected in fully grown patients with no associated clinical symptoms needs to be carefully observed in a multidisciplinary manner.

PLANNING AND POSITIONING

- Detailed physical and neurologic examinations should be performed to detect clinical findings such as subcutaneous lipomas, skin tags, hemangiomas, hypertrichosis, dimples, foot deformities, scoliosis, spasticity, and weakness. A multidisciplinary work-up (including clinicians from neurology, neurosurgery, and orthopedics; caretakers; and families) should be done to determine the indication for surgery in complex cases.
- MRI of the head and spine is used to verify any central nervous system abnormalities and to localize the lesion and characterize clearly anatomic conditions of the dysraphic spine, extension of the lipoma, condition of the spinal chord, and possible syringomyelia. X-ray or computed tomography (CT) scan or both may be necessary to characterize any spinal osseous anomalies (e.g., scoliosis, dysraphic conditions, hemivertebrae).
- Intraoperative electrophysiologic monitoring with somatosensory evoked potentials, motor evoked potentials, and motor nerve stimulation provides functional feedback of electrophysiologic integrity of the neural structures and is especially helpful if complex lipomas are involved.
- **Figure 93-1:** Patient positioning is prone with gel cushions placed under the chest and pelvis enabling free abdominal movement for regular ventilating pressure. The extremities are secured with gel or cotton wool bandages to prevent compression injury. The head is carefully tilted and positioned on a gel donut headrest.

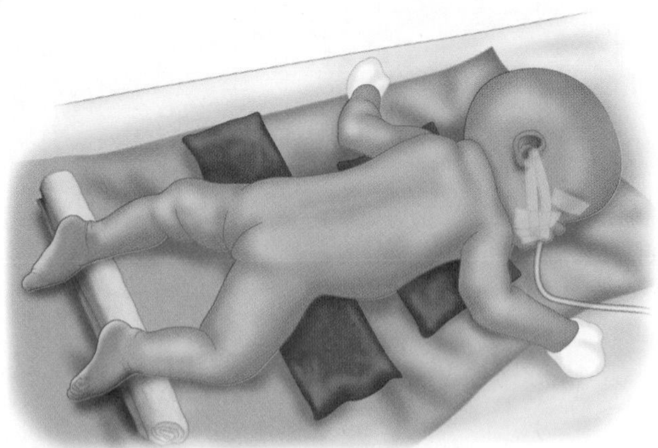

FIGURE 93-1

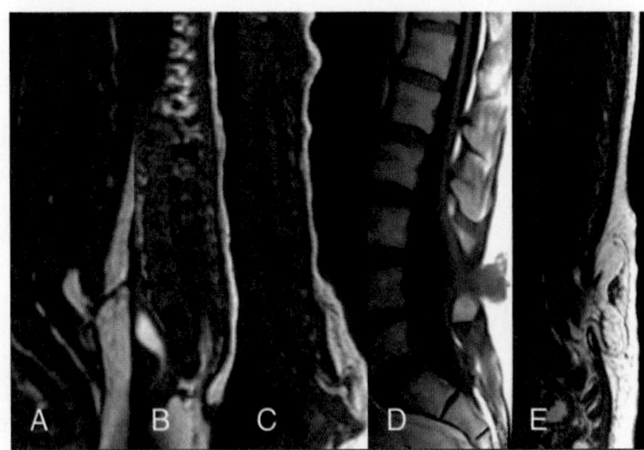

FIGURE 93-2

- **Figure 93-2:** Different congenital conditions of tethered spinal cord that represent an incomplete overview of wide variety of complex spinal malformations. **A,** Spinal lipoma with lumbar dermal sinus. **B,** Sacral dermal sinus and intraspinal lipoma with caudal regression syndrome associated with imperforated anus. **C,** Sacral LMMC. **D,** Dorsal lumbar lipomyelomeningocele associated with split spinal process malformation. **E,** Complex lipomyelomeningocele associated with dia- stematomyelia.

PROCEDURE

- **Figure 93-3:** Dorsal LMMC as shown in Figure 93-2D. After a long midline incision and exposure of the dysplastic spinal processes by bilateral paravertebral muscle retraction, a two-level laminotomy has been performed with resection of the split spinal process around the LMMC. The lipoma is exposed with its area of intersection with the dura atop intact anatomic conditions rostral and caudal to the malformation.
- **Figure 93-4:** Under microscopic view, rostral dural opening is performed with a 15-degree angled microblade for initial CSF release. The dural edges are tacked up bilaterally for continuous retraction.
- **Figure 93-5:** The dural opening is advanced toward the LMMC. Microsurgical dissection is performed with blunt microdissectors to liberate subarachnoid adhesions at the ipsilateral side of the LMMC. The intersection where the dura is merging with the lesion is identified by dissecting from inside the dural plane toward the myelon entering the malformation.

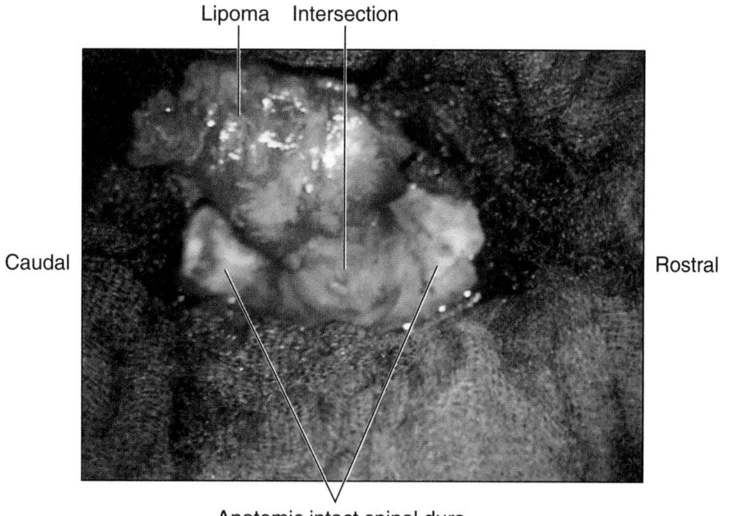

FIGURE 93-3

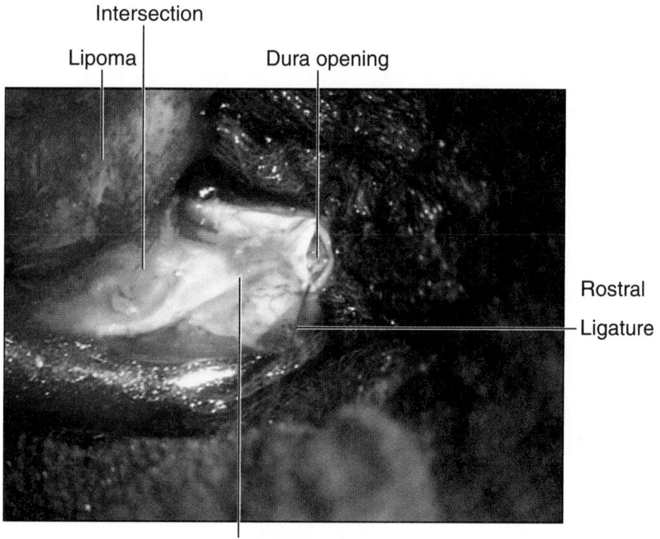

FIGURE 93-4

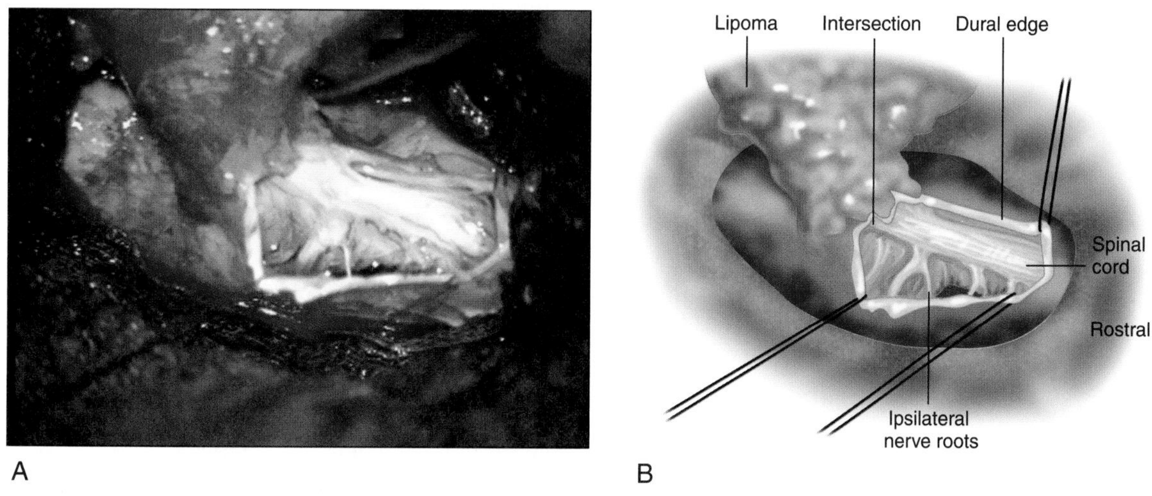

FIGURE 93-5

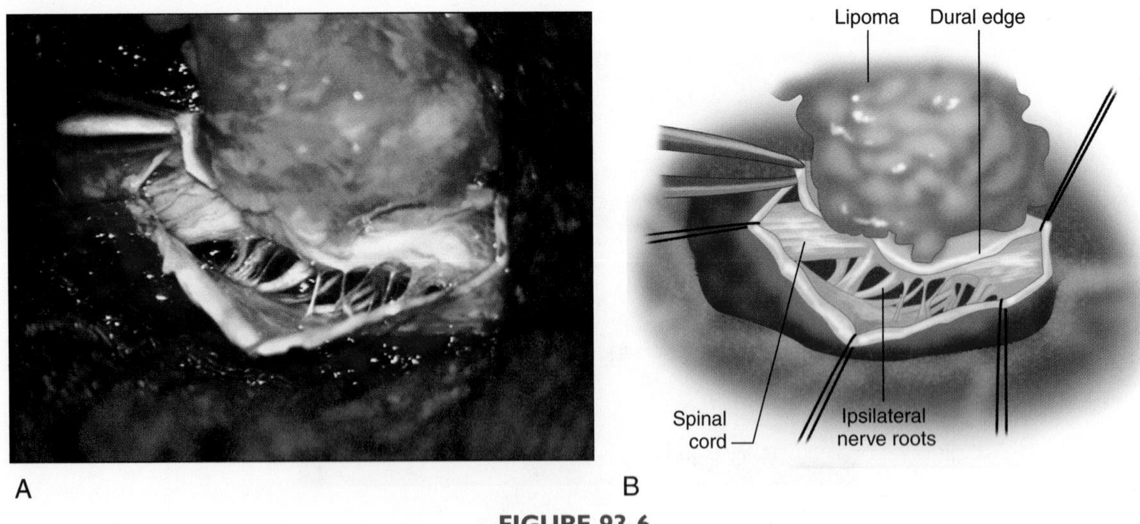

FIGURE 93-6

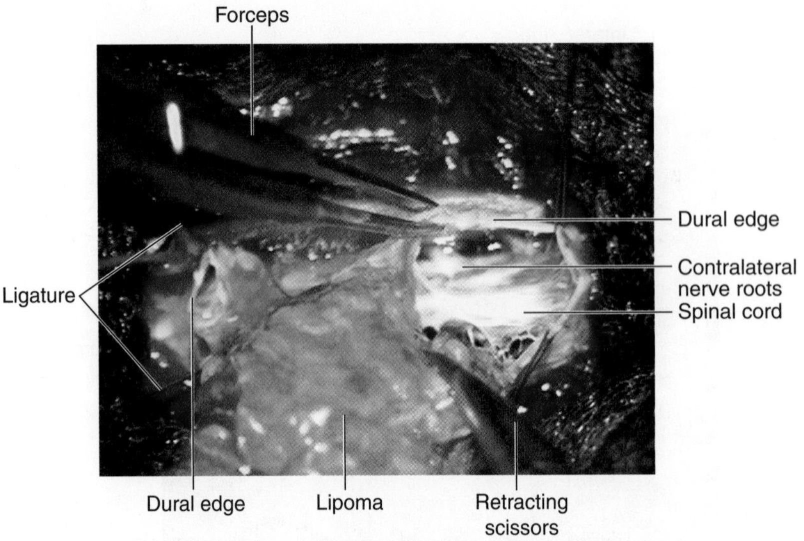

FIGURE 93-7

- **Figure 93-6:** The dura is incised slightly lateral to the area of intersection, keeping as much dura as possible intact for later closure. Within the subarachnoid space, the course of the ipsilateral nerve roots is liberated, and the LMMC lesion is medialized.
- **Figure 93-7:** After rostral and caudal bilateral ligation of the anatomic intact dura and ipsilateral dissection of the LMMC lesion, dissection is advanced to the contralateral side. In the same manner, the inside dural plane is separated from the arachnoid toward the LMMC, and the dural incision can be performed in proximity to intersection.
- **Figure 93-8:** Contralateral dural separation lateral to the LMMC is completed resulting in a circumferentially isolated midline lipoma. Liberation of the lateral nerve roots within the CSF space is warranted.
- **Figure 93-9:** At the ipsilateral side at the area of intersection, the remaining dural edge adhering to the LMMC is dissected, which shows myelon displacement outside of the dural sac toward the lipoma.
- **Figure 93-10:** The lipoma is now sharply reduced, slicing it bit by bit downward into a fibrous (intermediate) zone that covers the placode. During this action, one must be aware of the level of laterally seen myelon-lipoma interface. Functional tissue may protrude into the lipoma, so neuromonitoring is helpful to preserve functional integrity, especially in complex cases.

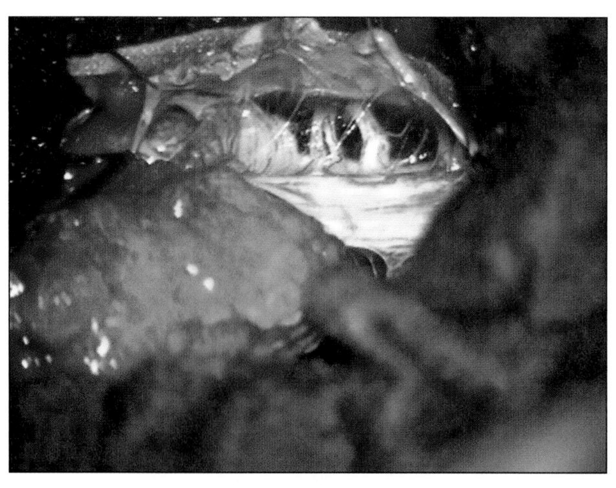

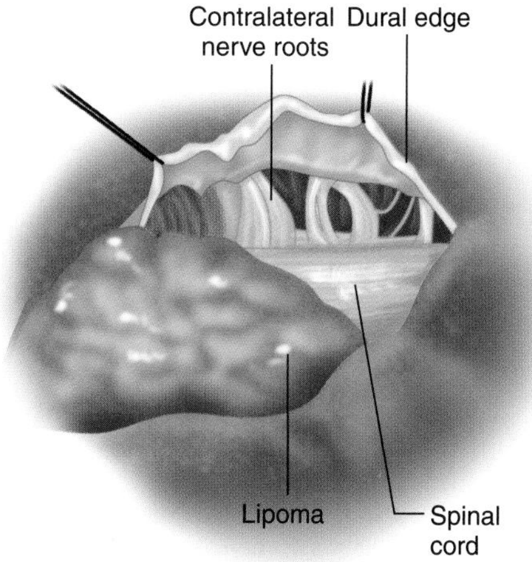

A B

FIGURE 93-8

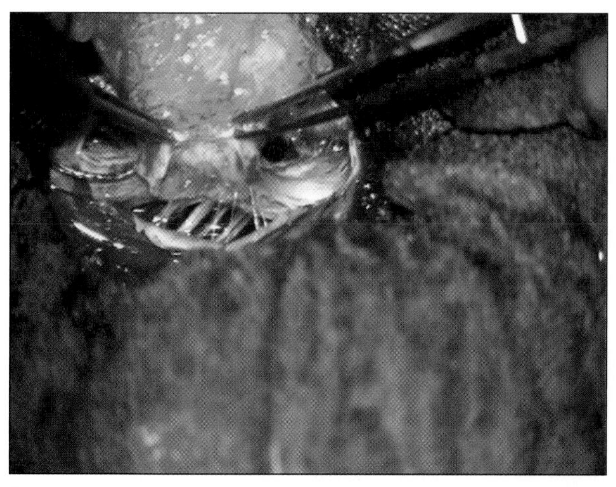

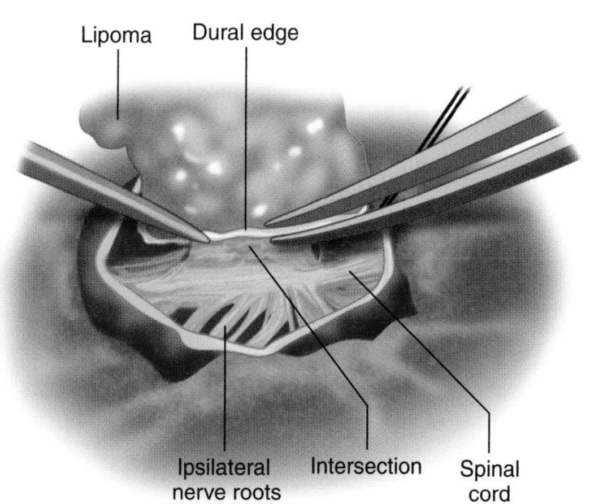

A B

FIGURE 93-9

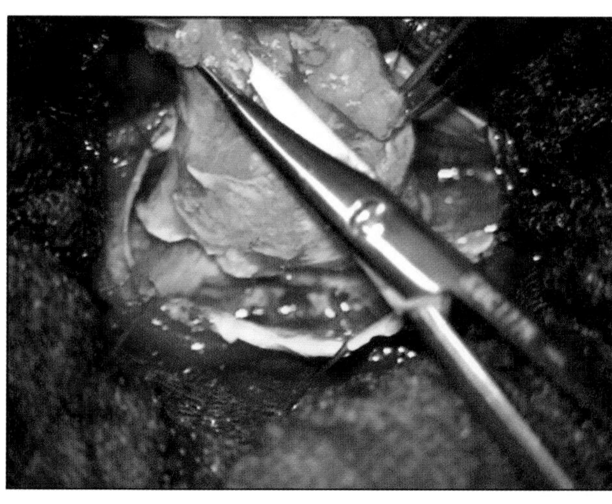

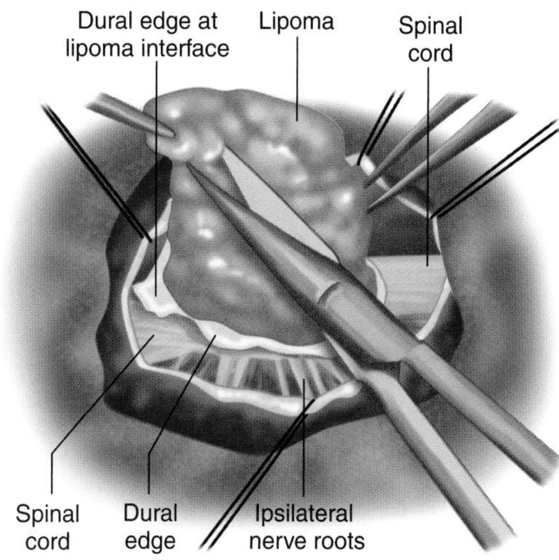

A B

FIGURE 93-10

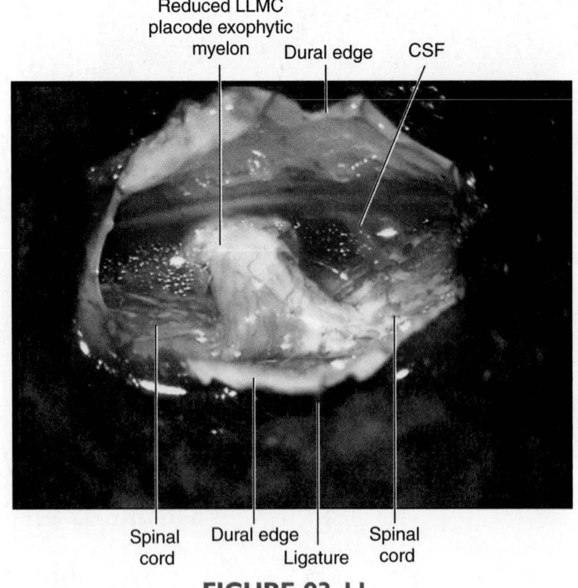

FIGURE 93-11

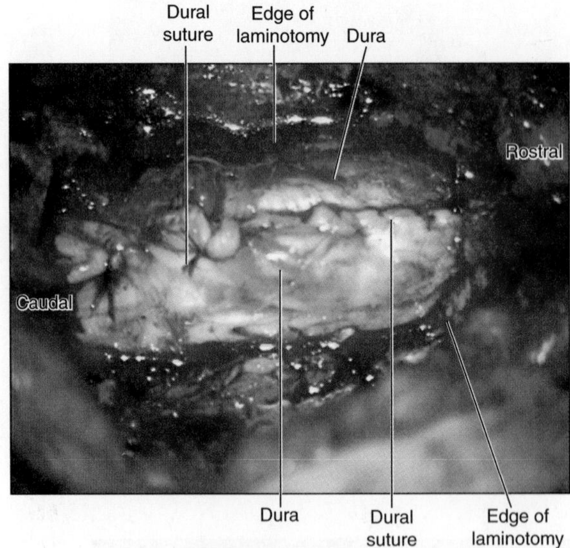

FIGURE 93-12

- **Figure 93-11:** The remaining placode covered with a safety layer of lipomatous or fibrous tissue is integrated into the dural sac, establishing free CSF flow around all neural structures and preventing retethering.
- **Figure 93-12:** The dura may be closed with a dural graft (collagen graft) or, if rarely possible, by approximation of the existing dural edges (as shown in this case) in a watertight fashion. Special attention must be drawn to ensure sufficient CSF space inside the dural sac warranting free flow of CSF at all sites. To secure the suture further, Gelfoam in combination with fibrin glue is used to cover the dural surface. If existent, removed laminae may be reinserted after the laminotomy and fixed with titanium microplates bilaterally. A tight multilayer closure of muscle tissue, fascia, and subcutaneous tissue is achieved using reasonably strong polyglactin 910 (Vicryl) sutures in close proximity. Cutaneous closure is achieved using running 4-0 monofilament sutures. Finally, a sterile dressing is applied.

TIPS FROM THE MASTERS

- Careful evaluation of anatomic conditions on preoperative MRI can help predict the risk of surgical repair, which can be taken into account for preoperative decision making of necessity for surgical repair. This is essential for caudal, transitional, and asymmetric lipomas.
- In complex lipomas, direct nerve root stimulation enables intraoperative distinction of functional and nonfunctional nerve roots to preserve function and reduce morbidity. Also, a more effective reduction of the lipoma and a more spacious reconstruction of the dural sac are feasible.
- Laser reduction of lipomatous tissue by vaporizing the fat minimizes mechanical stress for underlying neural structures.

PITFALLS

Finding the interface level of lipomas and enabling more effective reduction of intradural structures means a higher risk for neurologic deterioration.

Insufficient space for untethered intradural structures results in insufficient intradural CSF flow at the level of repair and increases the risk for recurrent adhesions and retethering.

CSF fistula is a major risk after tethered cord surgery and requires special attention to be prevented. CSF fistula possibly promotes infection, excessive scarring in the surgical site of repair, and retethering. Associated Chiari malformations might also decompensate owing to relative pressure imbalance between the spinal canal and the intracranial CSF spaces.

BAILOUT OPTIONS

- In complex cases in which the lipoma–neuronal tissue interface cannot be clearly identified or potentially functional nerve roots are involved in lipomatous tissue, neurologic deterioration may be prevented by leaving some of this tissue on the placode.
- To enable enough intradural space for effective CSF flow around the area of repair, a pouch may be formed by implanting a wide dural graft. At the site of suture, the dura and graft interface may be folded outside.
- Plastic surgical reconstruction involving muscle and skin flaps may be needed in complex cases for sufficient multilayer closure. At least as much attention must be given to closure as to anatomic dissection.

SUGGESTED READINGS

Cochrane DD, Finley C, Kestle J, et al. The pattern of late deterioration in patients with transitional lipomeningomyelocele. Eur J Pediatr Surg 2000;1(Suppl 10):13–7.

Darward NL, Scatliff JH, Hayward RD. Congenital lumbosacral lipomas: pitfalls in analyzing the results of prophylactic surgery. Childs Nerv Syst 2002;18:326–32.

Drake JM. Occult tethered cord syndrome: not an indication for surgery. J Neurosurg 2006;104(Suppl. 5):305–8.

La Marca F, Grant JA, Tomita T, et al. Spinal lipomas in children: outcome of 270 procedures. Pediatr Neurosurg 1997;26:8–16.

Samuels R, McGirt MJ, Attenello FJ, et al. Incidence of symptomatic retethering after surgical management of pediatric tethered cord syndrome with or without duraplasty. Childs Nerv Syst 2009;25:1085–9.

Procedure 94

Exploration for Injury to an Infant's Brachial Plexus

Rick Abbott

INDICATIONS

- Inability to lift hand to mouth against gravity by 5 months of age
- Plateau in recovery after 9 months of age with significant residual motor deficit

CONTRAINDICATIONS

- Medically unstable

PLANNING AND POSITIONING

- Preoperative magnetic resonance imaging (MRI) of the plexus should be done around 5 months of age.
- Preoperative electromyography and nerve conduction study can be considered.
- Intraoperative physiologic mapping should be planned for in preparation of surgery.
- **Figure 94-1:** Bipolar needle electrodes are placed in the muscles to be monitored before preparation. Electrodes to be placed in the muscles lying beneath the skin are placed sterilely after preparation. Shown are electrodes for the diaphragm, supraspinatus, deltoid, biceps, triceps, extensor carpi radialis, and flexor carpi radialis muscles.
- The infant is positioned with a roll underneath the thoracic spine. The roll extends the shoulder. The head is turned toward the opposite shoulder.

PROCEDURE

- **Figure 94-2:** Drawn skin incision. The incision extends from the level of the angle of the jaw caudally for several centimeters along the lateral border of the sternocleidomastoid muscle before turning laterally to run on a diagonal toward the shoulder. The *dotted line* shows extension into the deltoid-pectoralis groove, which is used to expose the middle and lower portions of the plexus.

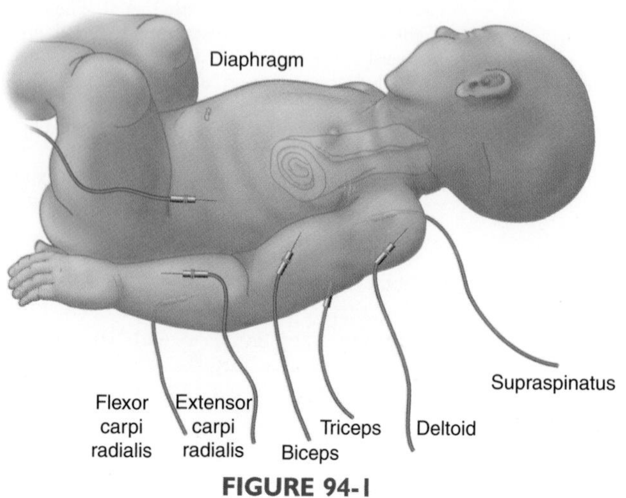

FIGURE 94-1

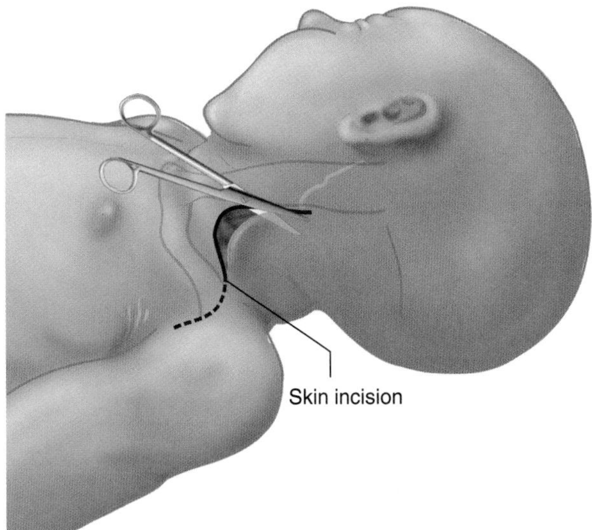

FIGURE 94-2

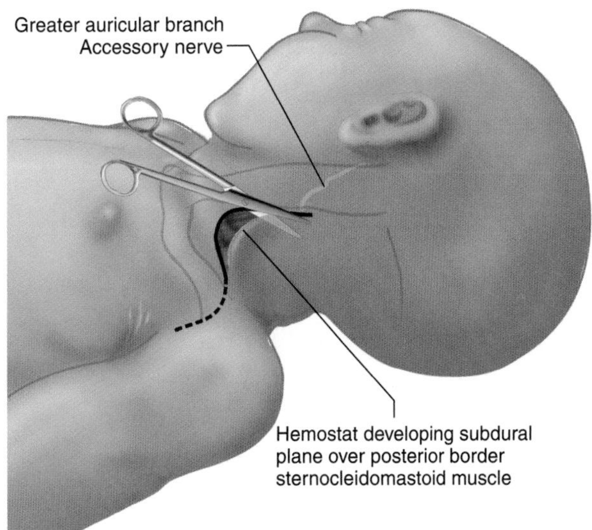

FIGURE 94-3

- **Figure 94-3:** The incision starts at the point where the line turns lateral from the posterior sternocleidomastoid muscle. Blunt dissection is done under the intended incision line rostrally in the subcutaneous fat along the lateral border of the sternocleidomastoid muscle to the level of the angle of the jaw. The overlying skin is cut while carefully looking for accessory nerve and its greater auricular branch lying on the surface of the sternocleidomastoid muscle.
- **Figure 94-4:** The incision is opened laterally to expose the posterior triangle of the neck. In infants, the platysma is not prominent and is not commonly recognized. If present, it can be split to enter the triangle. The branches of the external jugular vein can be cut to mobilize the vein either medially or laterally. The sternocleidomastoid muscle is freed from the cervical fat pad so that it can be retracted medially. The small nerve fibers off the accessory nerve and cervical plexus traveling to the skin can be cut for exposure when needed. Care is taken to identify the branches going to the trapezius muscle. The cervical fat pad is dissected off the underlying scalene muscles and retracted with the sternocleidomastoid muscle.

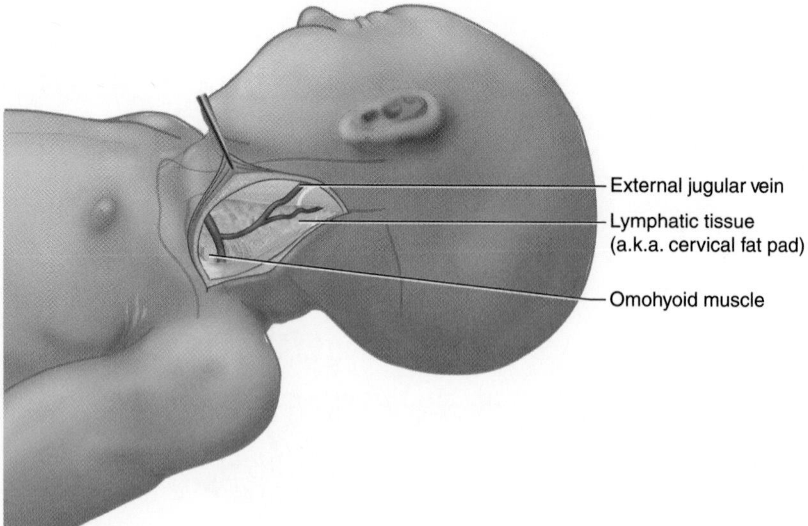

FIGURE 94-4

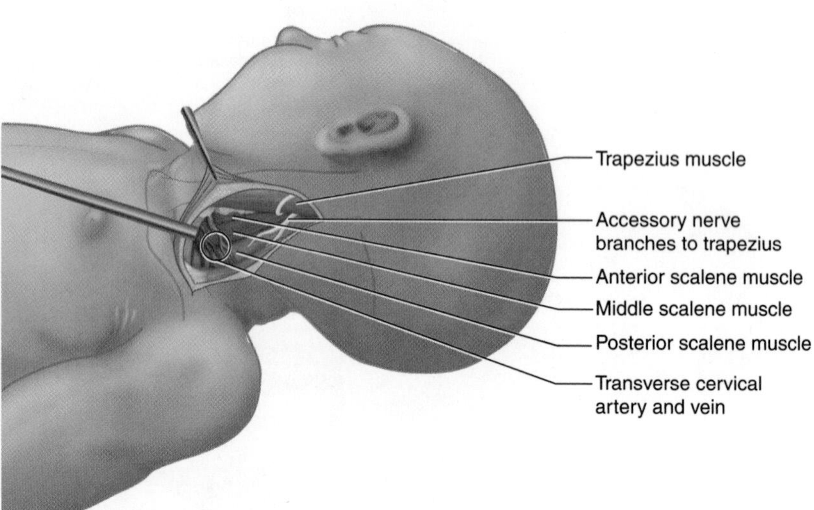

FIGURE 94-5

- **Figure 94-5:** Posterior triangle with the fat pad removed. The omohyoid muscle is retracted inferiorly. The transverse cervical artery and vein usually can be mobilized out of the way, but they may be cut if needed for exposure.
- **Figure 94-6:** After the fat pad has been lifted off the scalenes, the surgeon looks for the brachial plexus. The sternocleidomastoid muscle is retracted medially with a retraction suture placed in its ventral aspect. The upper trunk of the plexus sometimes is visible as a scar-encased bundle between the anterior and middle scalene muscles. When it is not obvious, the phrenic nerve can be located on the ventral surface of the anterior scalene. The identity of the phrenic nerve can be confirmed with stimulation while monitoring the electrodes in the chest wall placed previously to record diaphragm activity. When its identity has been confirmed, the phrenic nerve is followed proximally until its juncture with C5 is located. C5 can be followed proximally to its foramen to identify the plane between the scalenes in which tbe plexus lies.
- **Figure 94-7:** The plane between the anterior and middle scalene muscles is opened next to expose C5 through the T1 nerve roots.

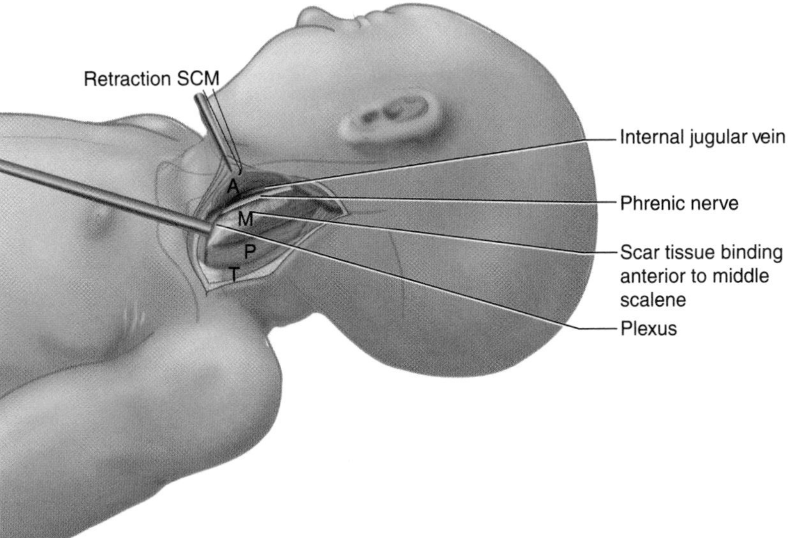

FIGURE 94-6

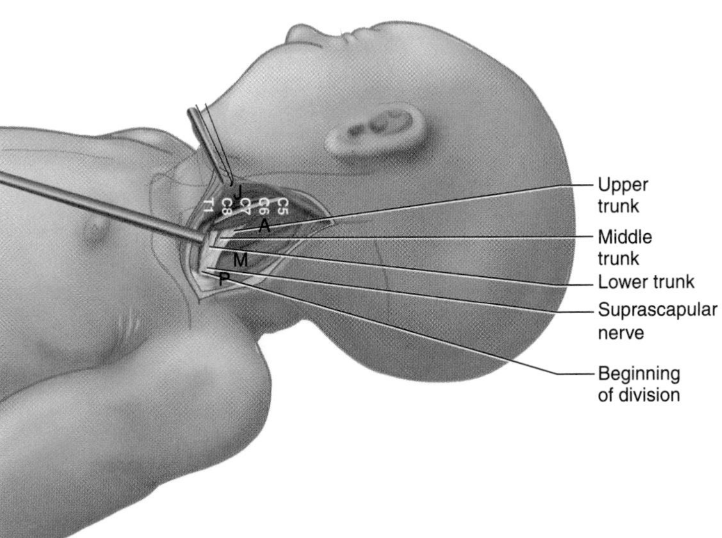

FIGURE 94-7

- **Figure 94-8:** As the plexus is exposed distally at the level of the trunks, it is frequently invested in scar tissue. This scarring can be so dense as to give the impression that the trunks are one structure. Working from the normal nerve, the trunks and distal plexus elements are separated. At some point, scarring ceases, and the normal plexus is appreciated; this is typically proximal to the clavicle. If no neuroma is found, longitudinal cuts through the perineurium (so-called neurolysis) are made for the entire length previously involved in scarring.
- **Figure 94-9:** When a neuroma is found, it is evaluated for degree of conduction. Although intraoperative stimulation of the roots proximal to the neuroma can give one some idea of continuity, it is not as accurate in predicting the ultimate return of function as preoperative motor examination. The choices for treating a neuroma are simple neurolysis, resection and grafting, or neurolysis and "jump" grafting. **A,** End-to-end graft. The plexus first is dissected to a point where it merges with the neuroma at both poles of the neuroma; then the neuroma is resected, leaving two stumps of plexus element. Next, either harvested nerve such as the sural nerve or artificial nerve conduits are used to bridge the gap. Graft can be either sewn in or glued in. **B,** When resection of the neuroma seems contraindicated, a side-to-side graft that jumps over neuroma can be considered. A linear incision is made into the plexus element proximal and distal to the neuroma, and the graft is stuck into the incision and glued or sewn to the nerve.

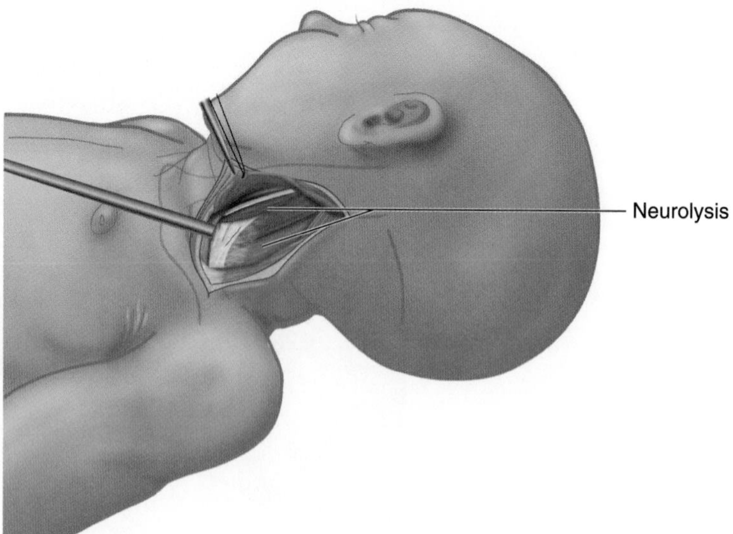

FIGURE 94-8

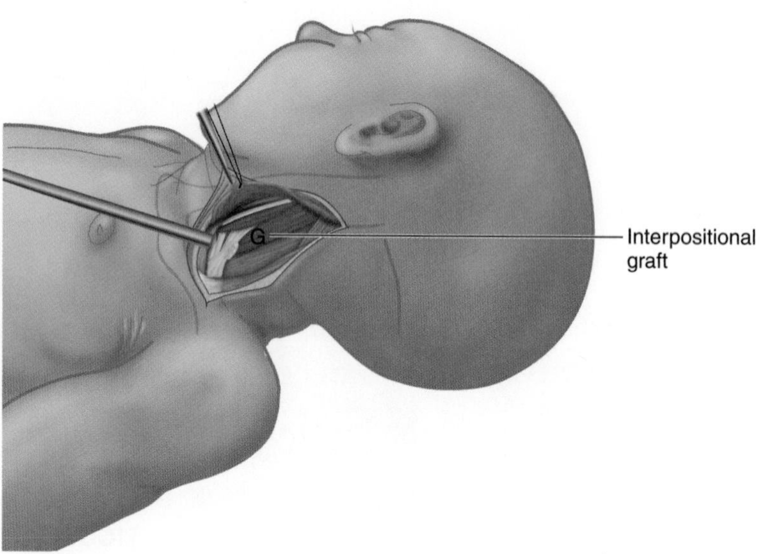

FIGURE 94-9

TIPS FROM THE MASTERS

- Careful mapping of the lateral surface of the upper trunk avoids injury to the suprascapular nerve.
- Gluing grafts is quicker and theoretically better because of growth factors present within the glue.

PITFALLS

Operating too early hampers decision making in operating room because of poor information about potential for functional recovery.

Scar tissue obscures small branches off the plexus. Liberal use of a stimulating electrode to map out these structures is of great assistance.

SUGGESTED READINGS

Ashley WW Jr, Baty JD, Hollander T, et al. Long-term motor outcome analysis using a motor score composite following surgical brachial plexus repair. J Neurosurg 2007;106:276–81.

Bain JR, Dematteo C, Gjertsen D, et al. Navigating the gray zone: a guideline for surgical decision making in obstetrical brachial plexus injuries. J Neurosurg Pediatr 2009;3:173–80.

Gilbert A, Pivato G, Kheiralla T. Long-term results of primary repair of brachial plexus lesions in children. Microsurgery 2006;26:334–42.

Piatt JH Jr. Birth injuries of the brachial plexus. Clin Perinatol 2005;32:39–59.

van Dijk JG, Pondaag W, Malessy MJ. Obstetric lesions of the brachial plexus. Muscle Nerve 2001;24:1451–61.

Procedure 95 Ulnar Nerve Release

Michael J. Dorsi, Allan J. Belzberg

INDICATIONS

- Progressive clinical symptoms of cubital tunnel syndrome include numbness and paresthesias or pain in the ulnar nerve distribution of the hand, primarily the little finger and ring finger. Sensory symptoms are usually exacerbated by activities that require prolonged elbow flexion, such as holding a telephone or prolonged pressure on the elbow. There may be weakness, stiffness, or clumsiness of the hand with difficulty writing or removing the lid from a jar.
- Clinical signs include dulled sensation or mixed hypoesthesia and hyperesthesia in the little finger or ring finger or both. Weakness of the hand intrinsic muscles, including the lumbricals to the little finger and ring finger and the abductor digiti minimi muscle, usually precedes flexor digitorum profundus weakness. Subacute ulnar neuropathy may produce marked atrophy of the hypothenar and first dorsal interosseus muscles. Chronic ulnar neuropathy results in a claw deformity. A Tinel sign is usually present in the distribution of the ulnar nerve with tapping of the olecranon notch.
- Nerve conduction slowing at the elbow should be confirmed with electrodiagnostic studies.
- A positive magnetic resonance neurogram showing increased intensity of the ulnar nerve at the level of the cubital tunnel and distally provides further diagnostic evidence.

CONTRAINDICATIONS

- Patients with mild or intermittent symptoms may benefit from a 6- to 12-week course of nonoperative therapies, including nonsteroidal antiinflammatory drugs, corticosteroid injections, education, and activity modification.
- Contraindications include other causes for the neurologic symptoms, including lower cervical radiculopathy, thoracic outlet syndrome, proximal ulnar nerve compression by the arcade of Struthers, or compression at the wrist in the Guyon canal. Amyotrophic lateral sclerosis may manifest initially with unilateral hand weakness. Spinal cord syringomyelia may produce hand symptoms but usually has a characteristic dissociated sensory loss.
- Neurolysis should not be performed if the ulnar nerve is chronically partially dislocated from the epicondylar groove or has been displaced by a soft tissue mass. Anterior subluxation is favored for revision surgery or if there is a significant posttraumatic deformity.

PLANNING AND POSITIONING

- Cubital tunnel syndrome can usually be accurately diagnosed based on clinical history and physical examination. Electrodiagnostic studies and magnetic resonance neurography serve to confirm the clinical diagnosis and evaluate the severity of nerve injury.
- Local anesthetic and minimal conscious sedation provide sufficient anesthesia for most patients. The anesthesia team should be prepared for conversion to general endotracheal intubation if intraoperative findings indicate performing anterior transposition.
- The patient is placed in the supine position. The arm is placed on an arm board with palm facing upward, and the arm is externally rotated and abducted 60 degrees.
- **Figure 95-1:** The patient is placed in the supine position with the arm externally rotated and abducted to 60 degrees. The skin is prepared and draped in the usual fashion. The incision is marked starting 3 to 4 cm proximal to the elbow on the distal medial arm, coursing between the olecranon and medial epicondyle and ending 3 to 4 cm distal to the elbow on the anterior surface of the upper forearm. The skin is infiltrated with 5 mL of 1% lidocaine with 1:100,000 epinephrine.

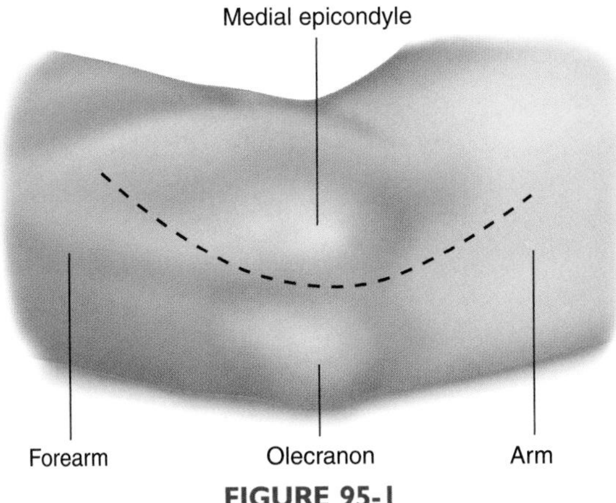

FIGURE 95-1

PROCEDURE

- **Figure 95-2:** The skin is incised, and dissection is continued through subcutaneous fat and loose connective tissue. Bipolar electrocautery is used to maintain hemostasis. A self-retaining retractor is placed to expose the underlying epicondylar fascia.
- **Figure 95-3:** Using fine scissors, the epicondylar fascia is incised to expose the ulnar nerve just proximal to its entry point into the cubital tunnel. Sectioning of the epicondylar fascia proceeds distally to the flexor carpi ulnaris muscle.

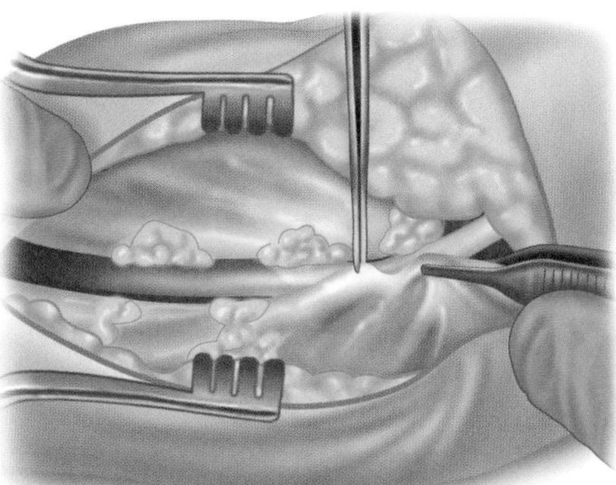

FIGURE 95-2

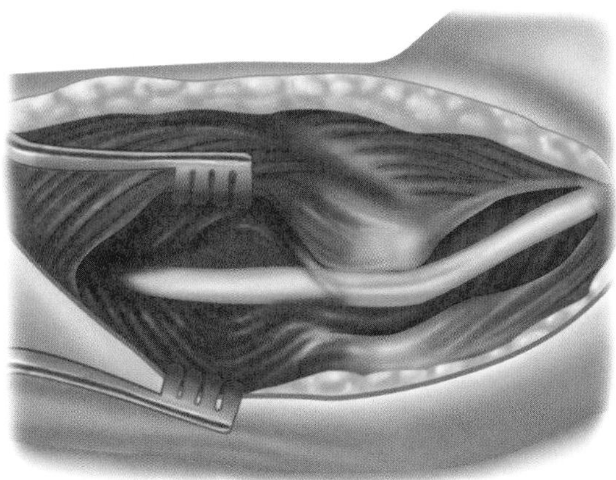

FIGURE 95-3

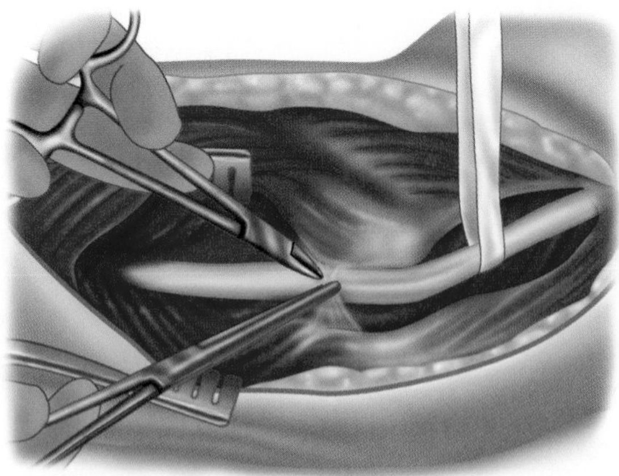

FIGURE 95-4

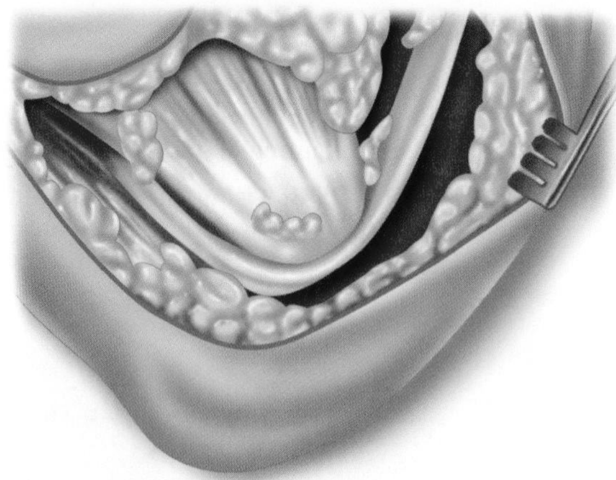

FIGURE 95-5

- **Figure 95-4:** The flexor carpi ulnaris muscle fascia is sharply incised, and the muscle fibers are separated gently to expose the underlying nerve. Dissection is continued distally to identify and divide the Osborne band. A fine-tip Crile instrument is passed proximally and distally along the ulnar nerve. Any remaining bands are sharply divided.
- **Figure 95-5:** Before closing, the elbow is flexed to inspect for subluxation of the ulnar nerve anterior to the medial epicondyle. The subcutaneous tissue is reapproximated with interrupted 3-0 polyglactin 910 (Vicryl) sutures. The skin is closed with a 3-0 running nylon suture.

TIPS FROM THE MASTERS

- The retractor may compress the medial antebrachial cutaneous nerve or median nerves in the distal arm.
- Meticulous hemostasis prevents postoperative hematomas.
- Convert to submuscular transposition if the decompressed ulnar nerve becomes partially dislocated with elbow flexion.

PITFALLS
Circumferential release may disrupt collateral blood supply of nerve.
Sensory symptoms may persist or increase for several weeks after ulnar neurolysis.
Operative failure is usually due to insufficient decompression at Osborne band.

BAILOUT OPTIONS

- Repair inadvertent nerve transections with epineurial sutures.
- Symptomatic postoperative hematomas require emergent evacuation.
- Painful postoperative medial antebrachial cutaneous neuromas may be treated by neurectomy at the midarm level.

SUGGESTED READINGS

Macadam SA, Gandhi R, Bezuhly M, et al. Simple decompression versus anterior subcutaneous and submuscular transposition of the ulnar nerve for cubital tunnel syndrome: a meta-analysis. Hand Surg Am 2008;33:1314.e1-12.

Mowlavi A, Andrews K, Lille S, et al. The management of cubital tunnel syndrome: a meta-analysis of clinical studies. Plast Reconstr Surg 2000;106:327–34.

Procedure 96

Open Carpal Tunnel Release

Michael J. Dorsi, Allan J. Belzberg

INDICATIONS

- Clinical symptoms of carpal tunnel syndrome (CTS) include numbness and paresthesias or pain in the median nerve distribution of the hand (excluding the palm) and fingers. Weakness, stiffness, or clumsiness of the hand also is seen. Atrophy of the thenar eminence may be seen with chronic CTS. Symptoms may be provoked by tapping or applying pressure over the carpal tunnel or with prolonged wrist flexion.
- Clinical signs of CTS include dulled sensation or hyperesthesia in the median innervated fingertips.
- Sensory nerve conduction slowing at the wrist should be confirmed with electrodiagnostic studies.

CONTRAINDICATIONS

- Patients with mild or intermittent symptoms may benefit from nonoperative therapies, including splinting, corticosteroid injections, and activity modification.
- Pregnancy and untreated endocrinologic conditions such as acromegaly or hypothyroidism may cause reversible thickening of the transverse carpal ligament (TCL).
- The procedure is contraindicated when there are other causes for neurologic symptoms, including cervical radiculopathy, C7 or middle trunk compression in the thoracic outlet, proximal median nerve compression by the Struthers ligament or the pronator teres muscle, and anterior interosseous nerve syndrome.

PLANNING AND POSITIONING

- CTS usually can be accurately diagnosed based on clinical history and physical examination. Electrodiagnostic studies can serve to confirm the clinical diagnosis and evaluate the severity of nerve injury.
- Local anesthetic and minimal conscious sedation provide sufficient anesthesia for most patients.
- The patient is placed in the supine position. The arm is placed on an arm board with palm facing upward, and the arm is abducted 60 degrees.

PROCEDURE

- **Figure 96-1:** The skin is incised to expose underlying loose connective tissue. Bipolar electrocautery is used to maintain hemostasis. Using a scalpel, loose connective tissue is swept laterally and medially to expose the palmar aponeurosis.
- **Figure 96-2:** The palmar aponeurosis is sharply divided to expose the TCL.
- **Figure 96-3:** The TCL is inspected for evidence of a penetrating palmar cutaneous branch. TCL is incised with the scalpel. Under direct vision, fine scissors are used to divide the TCL in the proximal to distal direction until the palmar fat pad is encountered.
- **Figure 96-4:** A fine-tip Crile instrument is passed proximally and distally along the median nerve. Any remaining bands are sharply divided.

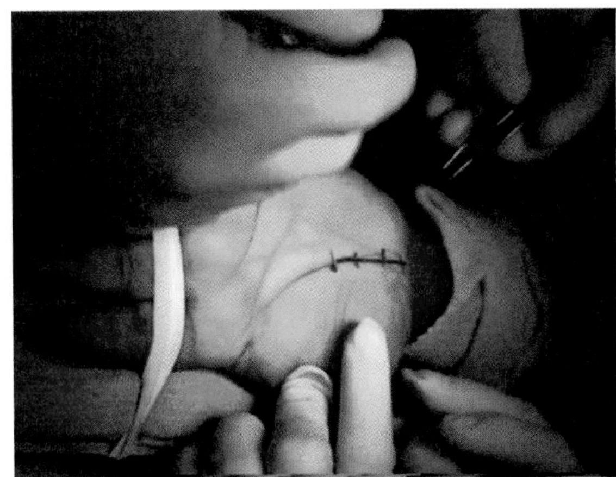

FIGURE 96-1

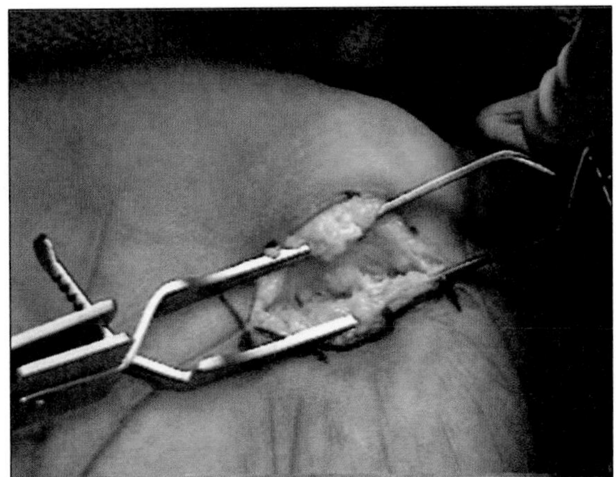

FIGURE 96-2

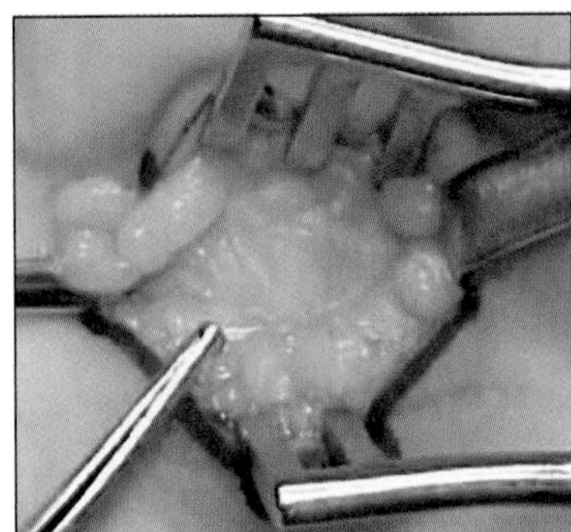

FIGURE 96-3

- **Figure 96-5:** The median nerve is inspected for changes in color or thickness and presence of adjacent tumors or masses.
- **Figure 96-6:** The palmar aponeurosis and loose connective tissue are reapproximated with 3-0 polyglactin 910 (Vicryl) sutures. Care is taken to avoid reapproximation of the TCL. The skin is closed with 3-0 nylon suture.

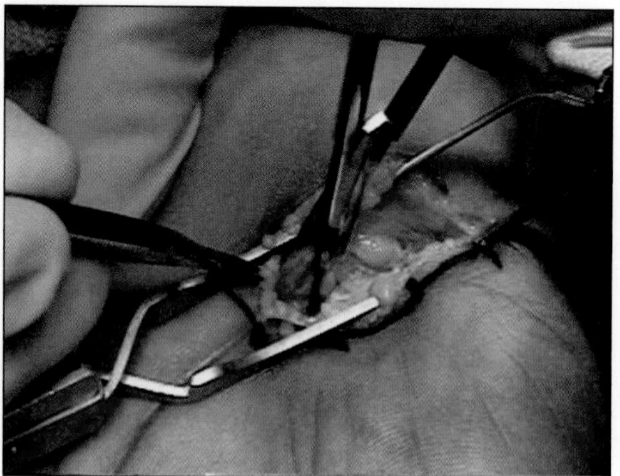

FIGURE 96-4

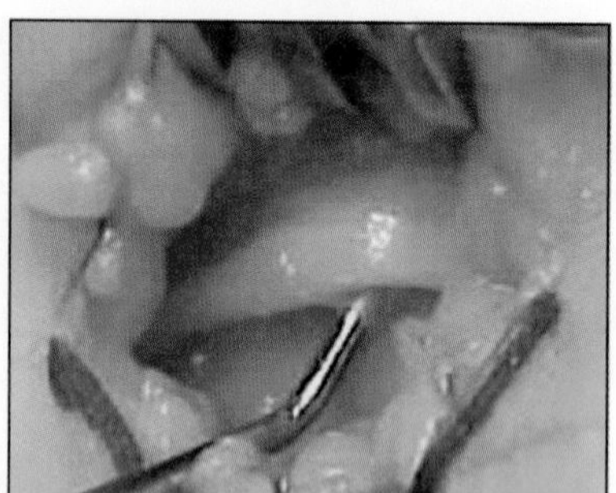

FIGURE 96-5

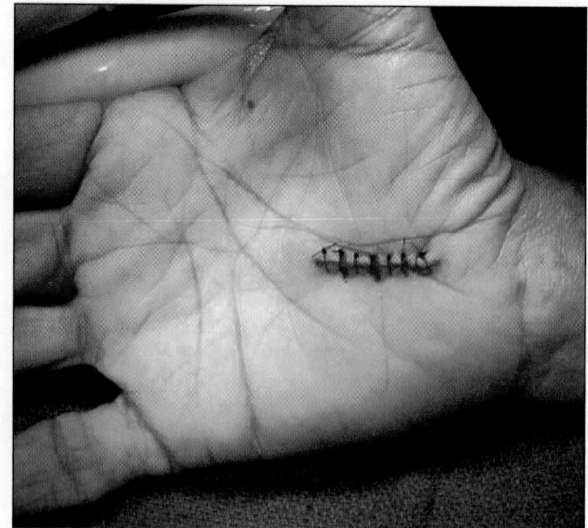

FIGURE 96-6

TIPS FROM THE MASTERS

- Inspect the carpal tunnel for tumors or cysts.
- Overretraction may compress the ulnar nerve.
- Internal neurolysis of the median nerve is usually not indicated.

PITFALLS

Sectioning the TCL on the radial side of the median nerve may injure the palmar cutaneous and thenar recurrent branches. Dissection too medial may injure structures of the Guyon canal.

BAILOUT OPTIONS

- Inadvertent transection of the median nerve or distal motor branches should be immediately repaired using epineurial sutures.
- Symptomatic postoperative hematomas require emergent evacuation.

SUGGESTED READINGS

Gerritsen AA, de Vet HC, Scholten RJ, et al. Splinting vs surgery in the treatment of carpal tunnel syndrome: a randomized controlled trial. JAMA 2002;288:1245–51.

Hui AC, Wong S, Leung CH, et al. A randomized controlled trial of surgery vs steroid injection for carpal tunnel syndrome. Neurology 2005;64:2074–8.

Jarvik JG, Comstock BA, Kliot M, et al. Surgery versus non-surgical therapy for carpal tunnel syndrome: a randomised parallel-group trial. Lancet 2009;374:1074–81.

Ly-Pen D, Andreu JL, de Blas G, et al. Surgical decompression versus local steroid injection in carpal tunnel syndrome: a one-year, prospective, randomized, open, controlled clinical trial. Arthritis Rheum 2005;52:612–9.

Verdugo RJ, Salinas RA, Castillo JL, et al. Surgical versus non-surgical treatment for carpal tunnel syndrome. Cochrane Database Syst Rev 2008;(4):CD001552.

Procedure 97 Intradural Nerve Sheath Tumors

Vivek Mehta, Chetan Bettegowda, Ryan M. Kretzer, Allan J. Belzberg, George I. Jallo

INDICATIONS

- An intradural extramedullary lesion causing neurologic symptoms, including weakness, sensory deficits, or pain, is an indication for surgery. Early and aggressive surgical resection, with the aim of gross total resection, is associated with the best outcomes.

CONTRAINDICATIONS

- Absolute contraindications include systemic infection or uncorrected coagulopathy. Patients presenting with acute and complete neurologic deficit, patients with extensive comorbidities, and patients with a short life expectancy have relative contraindications.

PLANNING AND POSITIONING

- The initial assessment of a patient with a suspected intradural nerve sheath tumor begins with a detailed history and physical examination.
- Magnetic resonance imaging (MRI) with gadolinium contrast agent for lesion localization is essential for planning the surgical approach. Schwannomas are characteristically isointense or hypointense to the spinal cord on T1-weighted images, with cystic areas represented by high T2 signal. Areas of hemorrhage or collagen are seen as low attenuation on T2 sequences. Schwannomas and neurofibromas enhance intensely in a homogeneous or heterogeneous pattern. Patients with neurofibromatosis may have multiple lesions along the entire spinal cord.
- X-rays may show enlargement of neural foramina, a classic finding associated with these lesions, and associated skeletal deformities.
- Intraoperative neurophysiologic monitoring with motor evoked potentials (MEPs) is essential when operating on intradural nerve sheath tumors. The anesthetic regimen should be coordinated with the anesthesiologist before the start of the case because many anesthetic agents cause depression of MEPs. Commonly used agents that do not cause a decline in motor potentials include propofol, fentanyl, and etomidate.
- **Figure 97-1:** Preoperative T2 sagittal and axial MRI showing a lumbar intradural nerve sheath lesion, with central T2 hyperintensity representing cystic areas.
- **Figure 97-2:** The patient is turned prone after intubation, and electrodes are placed for neurophysiologic monitoring. For cervical lesions, the patient is pinned in a three-point Mayfield head fixator and positioned prone on two chest rolls. The neck is slightly flexed to aid in surgical exposure. For patients with thoracic or lumbar lesions, prone positioning can be accomplished on a Wilson frame or chest rolls without head fixation. All dependent surfaces (e.g., knees, elbows) are padded to avoid peripheral nerve injury or pressure-related tissue damage.

PROCEDURE

- **Figure 97-3:** Skin is incised in the midline, and monopolar electrocautery is used to dissect the paraspinal muscles from posterior elements in the subperiosteal plane. Dissection should be carried out with caution at the lateral aspects of the vertebral column to prevent facet capsule disruption, which may result in postoperative instability.

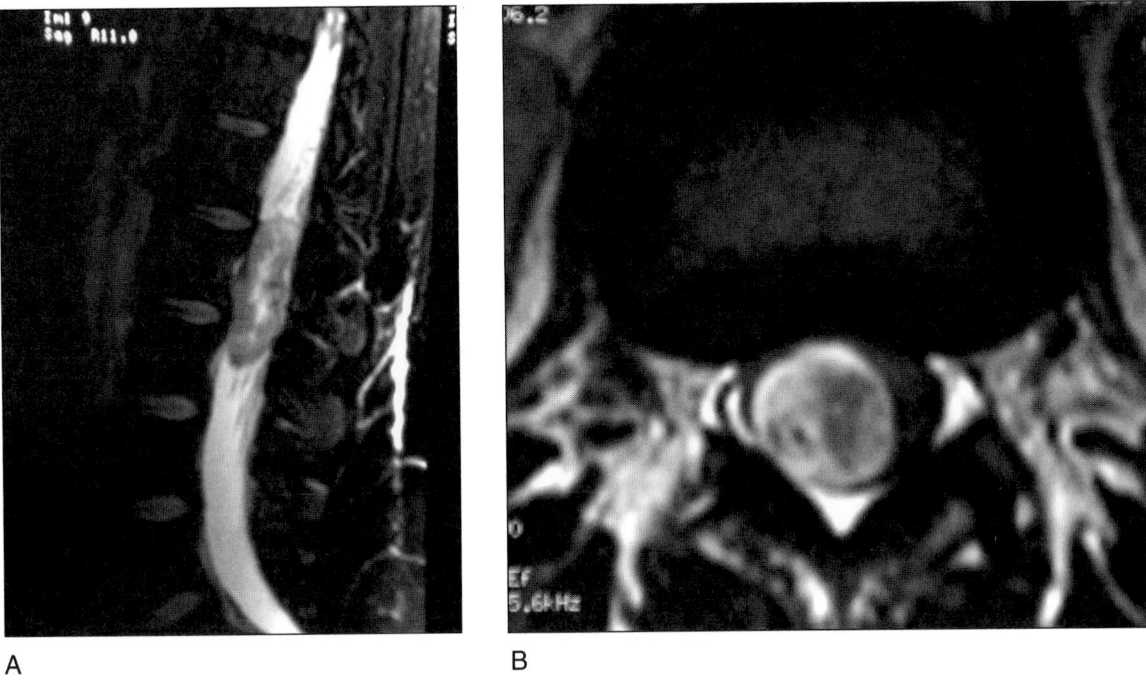

FIGURE 97-1

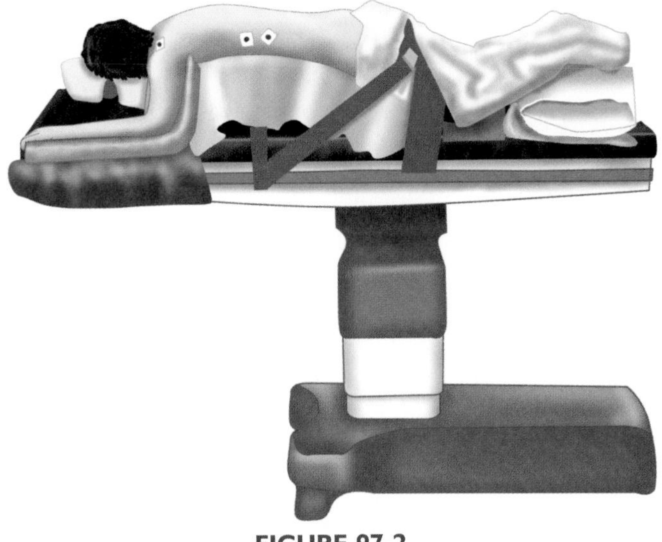

FIGURE 97-2

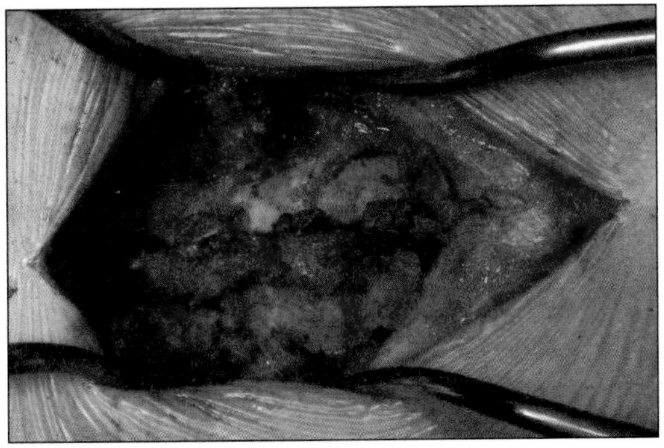

FIGURE 97-3

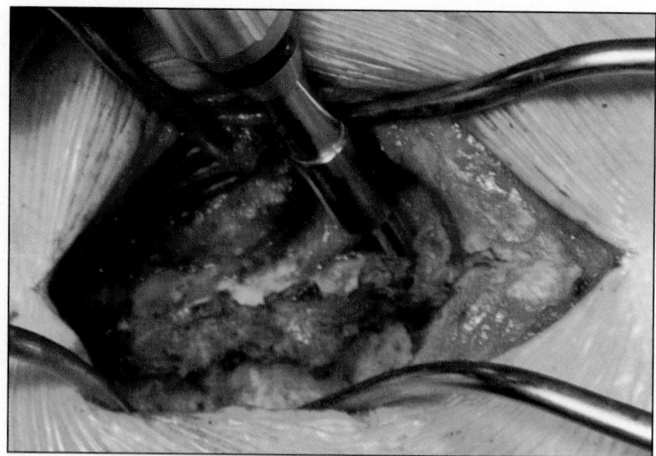

FIGURE 97-4

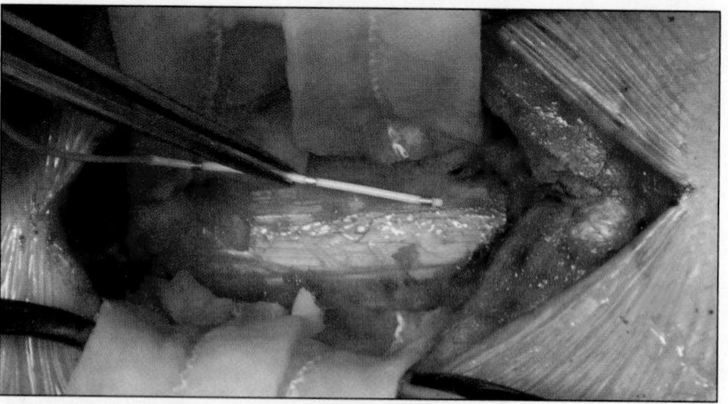

FIGURE 97-5

- **Figure 97-4:** The spinous processes and laminae are exposed, and laminotomies are performed bilaterally with a Kerrison punch. A craniotome is used to detach laminae bilaterally over the area of planned dural exposure. Transection of the rostral and caudal ligamentum flavum and interspinous ligaments allows for removal of posterior elements en bloc. An alternative approach is to use a Leksell rongeur and Kerrison punches to perform laminectomy in a piecemeal fashion. When possible, the facet joints should be preserved to prevent postoperative kyphosis. Certain tumors may require wide lateral exposure, however, necessitating removal of the facet joints. In this case, instrumented fixation may be warranted in an immediate or delayed fashion.
- **Figure 97-5:** The dura overlying the lesion is exposed. The laminectomy or laminoplasty may need to be extended to expose the entire extent of the mass before opening the dura. An epidural D-wave electrode is passed inferior to the planned area of dural exposure to monitor the function of the spinal corticospinal tract fibers.
- **Figure 97-6:** **A,** The dura is opened in the midline with a No. 15 blade scalpel and Metzenbaum scissors. The arachnoid membrane is preserved to prevent spinal herniation and bleeding from sudden cerebrospinal fluid egress. Dural tenting sutures are placed, and venous bleeding is controlled with Gelfoam, cotton surgical strips, and bipolar electrocautery. **B,** The operating microscope is brought into the field, and the arachnoid membrane is slowly incised to prevent herniation of neural elements under pressure. The tumor is localized in the intradural extramedullary compartment with lateral displacement of the spinal cord. Nerve roots are often seen running within or adjacent to the tumor.
- **Figure 97-7:** The goal of surgery is gross total resection of the lesion with minimal disruption of neural elements. **A-D,** Tumor resection is begun with careful, circumferential dissection of the tumor, aided by placement of cotton strips. Larger tumors may not be amenable to en bloc resection and may require piecemeal removal.

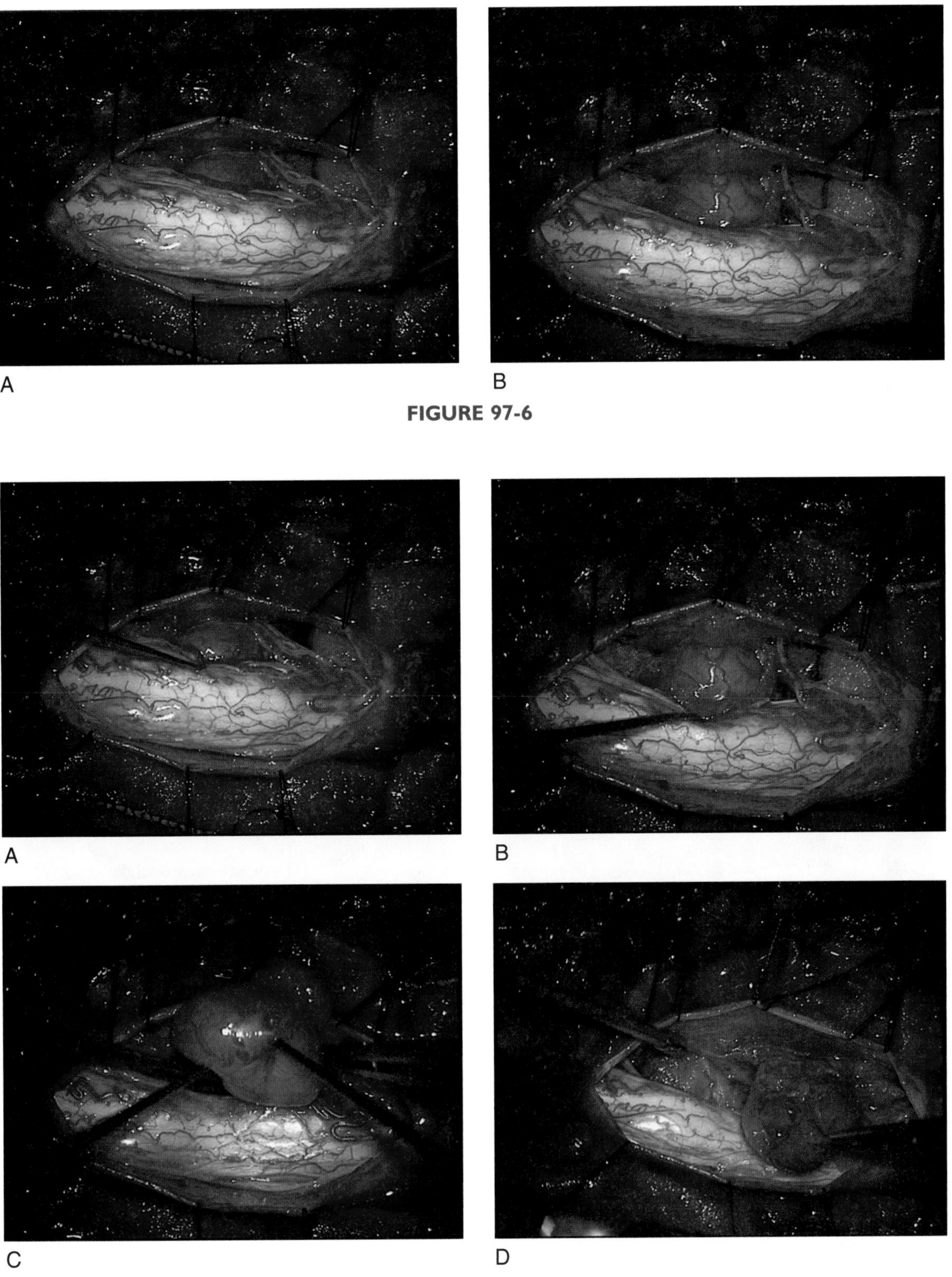

FIGURE 97-6

FIGURE 97-7

These lesions may first be decompressed internally with the ultrasonic surgical aspirator or contact laser to facilitate intraoperative manipulation. The ultrasonic aspirator allows for removal of tumor with minimal manipulation of surrounding neural tissue. The contact laser can aid in safely removing firm lesions and in preventing small capillary or arterial bleeding. These instruments are essential for safe resection of intradural nerve sheath tumors. Neurofibromas usually appear as an enlargement of a sensory nerve, and sacrifice of the nerve root is almost always necessary for complete removal. Some schwannomas have an identifiable plane between the tumor and nerve root, with only minor attachment of fascicles. This plane facilitates complete removal of the lesion without nerve root sacrifice. Resection of most nerve sheath tumors requires dorsal root resection, however, which may be carried out over several segments in the thoracic cord but over only a very few in the cervical cord where the function of arms and hands may be affected. Posterolateral or anterior tumors can be approached posteriorly by delicate rotation of the cord with a sacrificed posterior nerve root or dentate ligament. Nerve stimulation before sectioning is recommended to avoid inadvertent motor root sectioning in the rotated spinal cord. Direct traction on the cord should be avoided to minimize injury.

- **Figure 97-8:** Irrigation with warm saline and oxidized microfibrillar collagen (Avitene) aids in hemostasis after tumor removal. Before closure, normal saline irrigation is used to clear debris from the subarachnoid space to prevent postoperative aseptic meningitis. The dura is closed in a watertight fashion with running polypropylene (Prolene) or nylon suture. DuraSeal or fibrin glue is applied to the suture line.
- **Figure 97-9:** If en bloc laminoplasty was performed, titanium or resorbable plates and screws are used to secure the lamina in place. If there was disruption of joint capsules or removal of facet joints during tumor resection, spinal instrumentation should be considered to increase spinal stability. Wound healing is enhanced by ensuring that the muscle and fascial closures are not under tension. The skin is closed in several layers, with separate closure of the deep subcutaneous layer, superficial layer, and running skin sutures. At conclusion of the case, the patient is turned supine, a neurologic examination is performed, and the patient is extubated and transferred to the neurologic intensive care unit.

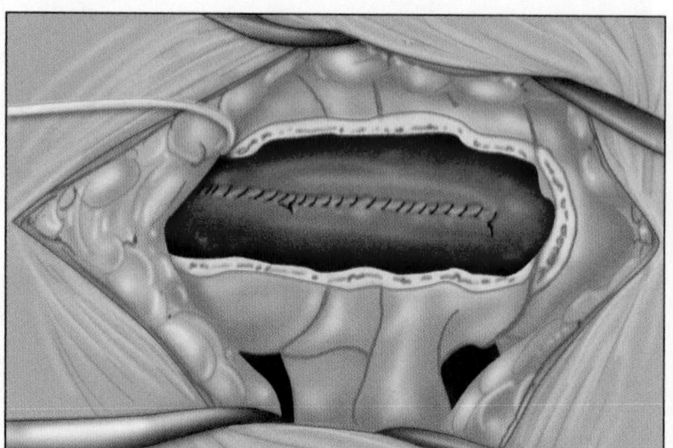
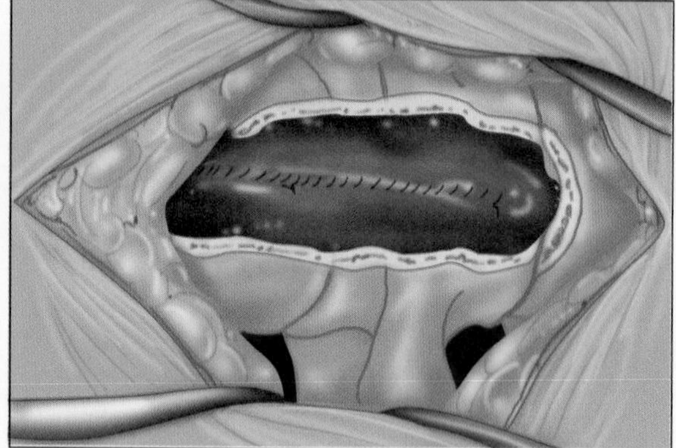

FIGURE 97-8

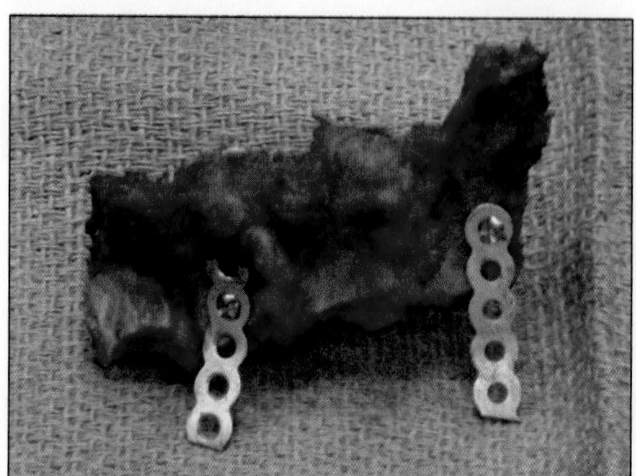
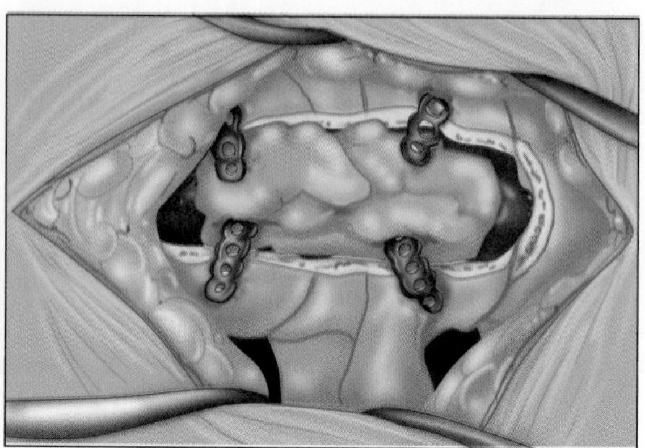

FIGURE 97-9

TIPS FROM THE MASTERS

- Muscle MEPs and epidural D-wave MEPs are essential monitoring tools in spinal cord surgery. Muscle MEPs are reported in an all-or-none fashion, whereas D-wave MEPs display a graded response. A loss of muscle MEPs is generally associated with a postoperative motor deficit, but this is likely to be transient if the D-wave amplitude is unchanged. A loss of D-wave amplitude greater than 50% is associated with long-term and often permanent motor deficits.
- Specialized instrumentation, such as ultrasonic aspiration, is essential for microsurgical resection of intradural nerve sheath tumors. These instruments allow for resection of the tumor with minimal traction on the spinal cord. Additionally, they allow a safe operative distance of 0.5 to 1 mm without injury to adjacent spinal cord tissue.
- When appropriate, bony exposure that preserves the facet joints may reduce postoperative kyphosis and instability, particularly in the cervical and cervicothoracic spine. Similarly, an osteoplastic laminoplasty may reduce the incidence of postoperative deformity in children and young adults.

PITFALLS

Postoperative spinal deformity may be avoided with an osteoplastic laminotomy, particularly in the cervical or cervicothoracic region. Instrumented fixation should be performed when facet joint disruption is required to prevent postoperative deformity. Patients should be followed closely with plain x-rays and serial orthopedic evaluations in the postsurgical setting.

Patients with prior surgery or radiation treatment are at an increased risk for wound dehiscence and cerebrospinal fluid leak, which can result in local wound infection or meningitis. This risk may be avoided with a watertight fascial closure without tension. Wound healing is promoted by the placement of a drain in the subcutaneous space for several days after surgery. Consultation with plastic surgery may be required for proper wound closure.

BAILOUT OPTIONS

- A second extraspinal resection may be necessary for nerve sheath tumors that extend through the neural foramen, into the extradural space, or into the paravertebral soft tissues.
- Malignant variants or disseminated nerve sheath tumors may require adjuvant therapy. Fractionated radiation therapy or stereotactic radiosurgery is reserved for patients in whom only partial resection is achieved or in patients who are not candidates for surgery; however, this modality has the potential to deliver toxic radiation doses to the spinal cord. Systemic chemotherapy may also be required, although no standardized protocols currently exist for these lesions.

SUGGESTED READINGS

Friedman DP, Tartaglino LM, Flanders AE. Intradural schwannomas of the spine: MR findings with emphasis on contrast-enhancement characteristics. AJR Am J Roentgenol 1992;158:1347–50.

Jallo GI, Kothbauer KF, Epstein FJ. Intraspinal tumors in infants and children. In: Winn HR, Youmans JR, editors. Youmans Neurological Surgery. 5th ed. Philadelphia: Saunders; 2004. p. 3707–16.

Levy WJ, Latchaw J, Hahn JF, et al. Spinal neurofibromas: a report of 66 cases and a comparison with meningiomas. Neurosurgery 1986;18:331–4.

McCormick PC, Post KD, Stein BM. Intradural extramedullary tumors in adults. Neurosurg Clin N Am 1990;1:591–608.

Seppala MT, Haltia MJ, Sankila RJ, et al. Long-term outcome after removal of spinal schwannoma: a clinicopathological study of 187 cases. J Neurosurg 1995;83:621–6.

Procedure 98 Intradural Tumor—Meningioma

Ryan M. Kretzer, Chetan Bettegowda, George I. Jallo

INDICATIONS

- Intradural meningioma causing pain or neurologic deficits
- Intradural meningioma causing mass effect on the spinal cord or associated nerve roots in the absence of clinical symptoms; surgery should be considered for these lesions because of the slowly progressive growth pattern and likelihood of neurologic deterioration in the future
- Intradural extramedullary lesion of unclear etiology and the need for tissue diagnosis

CONTRAINDICATIONS

- Small, asymptomatic or incidentally noted lesions can be followed with serial magnetic resonance imaging (MRI) for evidence of tumor growth before surgical resection.
- Severely debilitated patients or patients with significant medical comorbidities or short life expectancies should be considered for palliative treatment or radiation therapy.

PLANNING AND POSITIONING

- A detailed history and physical examination is important in the initial work-up of a spinal intradural meningioma. Information about the onset, duration, and distribution of symptoms and neurologic deficits helps guide surgical management.
- After initial clinical assessment, MRI is crucial for diagnosis and operative planning. Meningiomas typically appear isointense to hypointense on T1-weighted imaging, appear hyperintense on T2 sequences, and homogeneously enhance after contrast agent administration. Important MRI characteristics that distinguish meningiomas from other spinal intradural lesions include displacement of the spinal cord away from the lesion, widening of the subarachnoid space adjacent to the mass, and the presence of a "dural tail." X-ray and computed tomography (CT) scan may also be necessary to determine the need for instrumented fixation after surgical resection of the lesion. If the meningioma involves vascular structures, such as the vertebral artery in the upper cervical region or at the level of the foramen magnum, spinal angiography or noninvasive vascular imaging should be considered to determine the vascular relationship to the tumor and to assess for collateral blood flow.
- Motor evoked potential (MEP) monitoring should be used to assess for spinal cord injury during resection of intradural meningiomas. Needle electrodes should be placed in the end muscles before final prone positioning in the operating room. Propofol and fentanyl are commonly used anesthetic agents that do not affect MEP monitoring.
- **Figure 98-1:** MRI is an important diagnostic tool in the surgical management of spinal intradural meningiomas. Sagittal (*left*) and axial (*right*) T1-weighted MRI after gadolinium contrast agent administration. Note the homogeneously enhancing extraaxial mass at the T8 level involving the left side of the spinal canal and causing significant spinal cord compression.
- **Figure 98-2:** For the lesion shown in Figure 98-1, a dorsal approach is recommended, although ventral or ventrolateral tumors in the cervical or thoracic spine may be approached anteriorly. For the dorsal approach, the patient is positioned prone, either in three-point Mayfield head fixation on two chest rolls for cervical spine lesions or on a Wilson frame or chest rolls without head fixation for thoracic and lumbar tumors. All dependent surfaces (e.g., knees, elbows) should be padded to avoid pressure-related tissue necrosis or peripheral nerve injury.

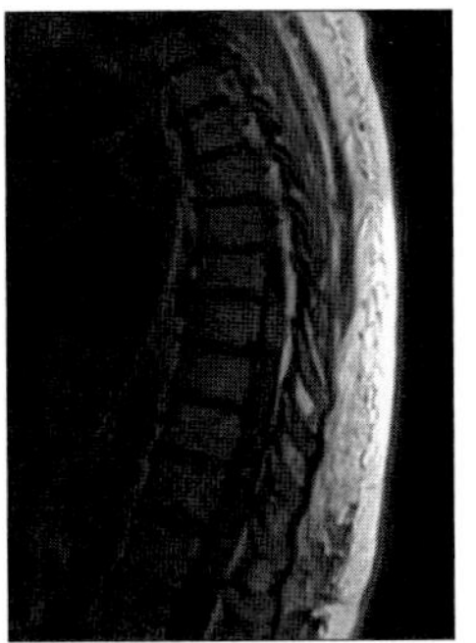
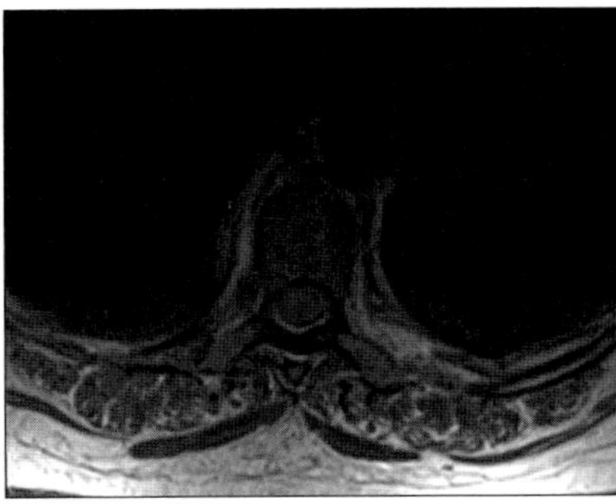

FIGURE 98-1

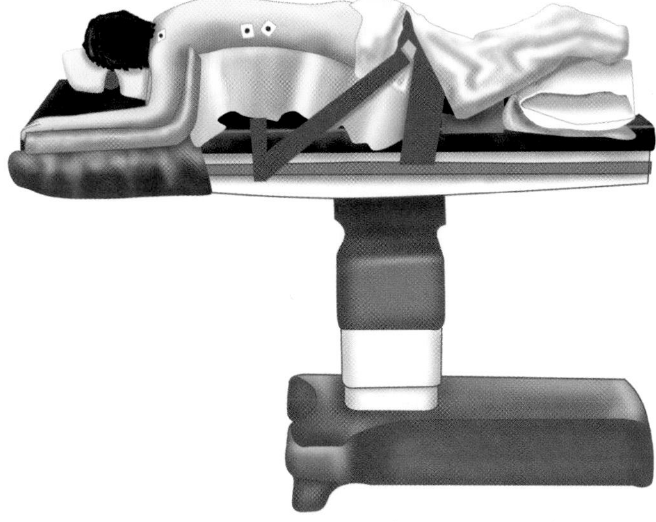

FIGURE 98-2

PROCEDURE

- **Figure 98-3:** After positioning, the incision is marked based on preoperative imaging and intraoperative x-ray localization. The skin is prepared and draped in a sterile fashion, and antibiotics are administered by the anesthesiology team. The skin incision is made, and subperiosteal dissection of posterior spinal elements is accomplished with monopolar electrocautery, taking care to leave the facet joint capsules and ligamentous structures intact to minimize iatrogenic spinal instability.

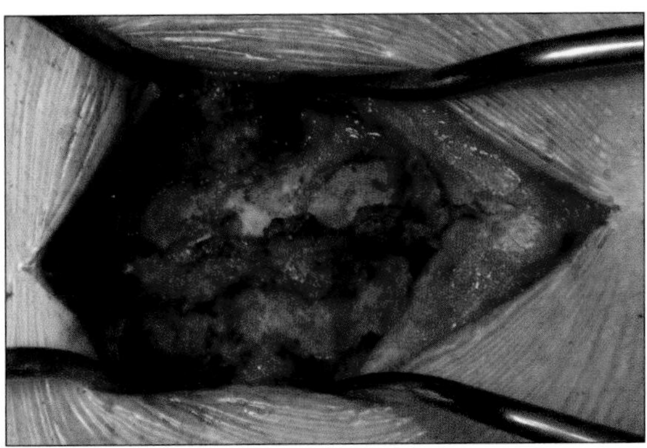

FIGURE 98-3

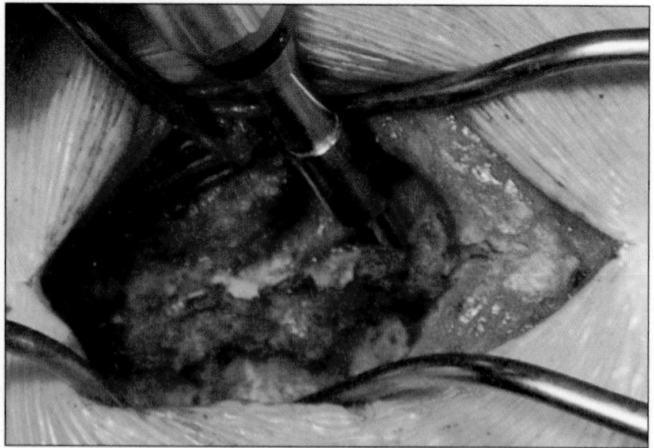

FIGURE 98-4

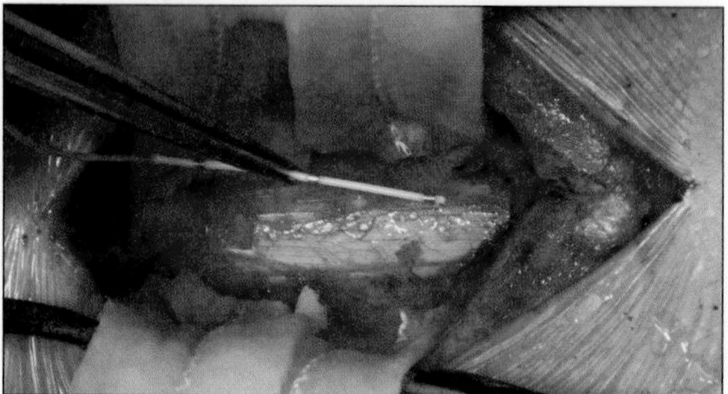

FIGURE 98-5

- **Figure 98-4:** At the caudal aspect of the planned laminoplasty, bilateral laminotomies are performed with a Kerrison punch to allow access for the craniotome footplate. The craniotome is used to detach the lamina in an en bloc fashion, followed by transection of the underlying ligamentum flavum and interspinous ligaments at the rostral and caudal extent of the dural exposure. Alternatively, the laminectomy can be performed using a Leksell rongeur and Kerrison punches. Although the laminoplasty technique may help minimize postsurgical kyphosis, the laminectomy is preferred in the setting of significant spinal canal narrowing.
- **Figure 98-5:** The dura is exposed, and epidural venous bleeding is controlled with bipolar electrocautery and cottonoids. A D-wave electrode is placed in epidural space at the caudal aspect of the dural exposure.
- **Figure 98-6:** An ultrasound probe is used to visualize the location of the meningioma before dural opening. A decision as to whether bony exposure is adequate to allow surgical resection of the lesion should also be made at this time.

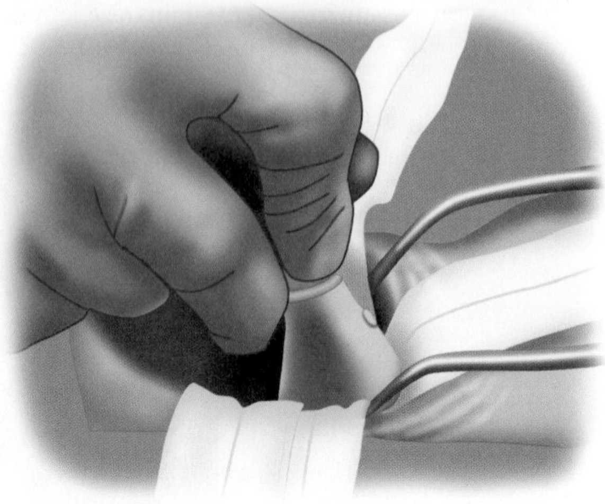

FIGURE 98-6

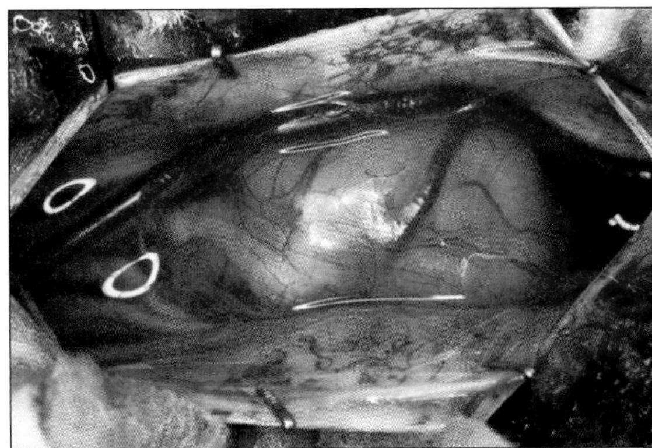

FIGURE 98-7

- **Figure 98-7:** The dural incision is made in the midline using a No. 15 blade scalpel and extended rostrally and caudally using Metzenbaum scissors. Dural tenting sutures are placed on each side of the dural opening to limit the influx of blood products into the subarachnoid space and to enhance surgical exposure of the lesion. The microscope is brought into the operative field. For ventrally located tumors treated through a posterior approach, sectioning of dentate ligaments may be required to gain access to the meningioma. When adequate exposure is obtained, the surface of the lesion is coagulated using bipolar electrocautery and incised with microscissors. Biopsy specimens are sent for pathologic diagnosis.
- **Figure 98-8:** Because of the dural attachment of meningiomas, these lesions can generally be delivered away from the spinal cord by gentle traction on the dura. For small lesions, en bloc resection may be attempted after dissection from adjacent structures. For larger lesions, internal debulking should be performed using ultrasonic aspiration or bipolar electrocautery with microsuction before dissection around the periphery of the lesion. If significant dural attachment exists, a circumferential dural incision around the dural insertion should be performed. Alternatively, if the meningioma is easily separated from the adjacent dura, the internal dural surface should be coagulated with bipolar electrocautery to minimize the risk of recurrence. For lesions that lie ventrally, dissection of the meningioma from the dura followed by cauterization of any residual tumor is preferred because of the challenges of dural reconstruction in this location. After resection of the meningioma, hemostasis is achieved in the intradural compartment before dural closure.

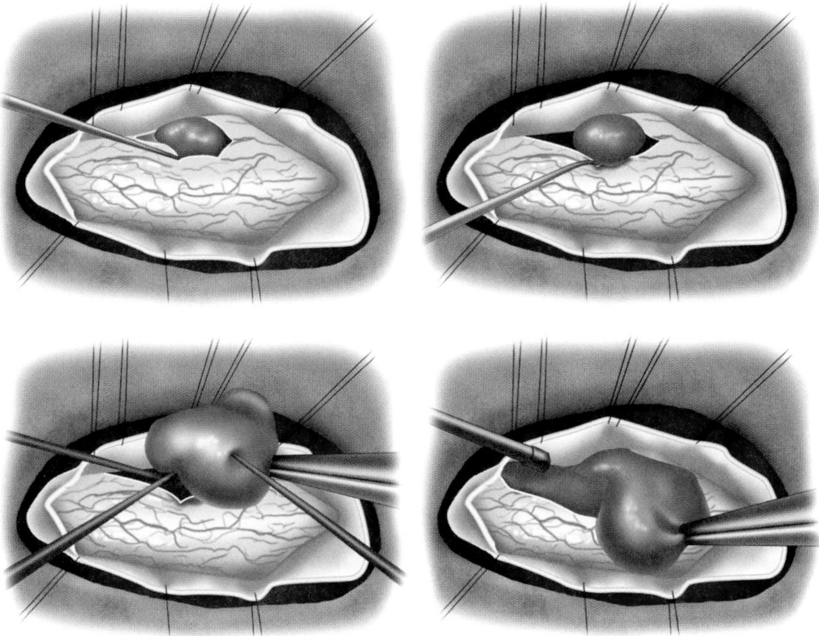

FIGURE 98-8

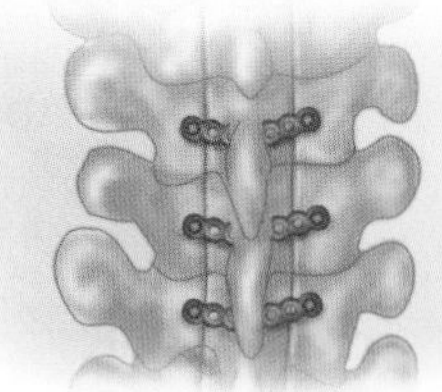

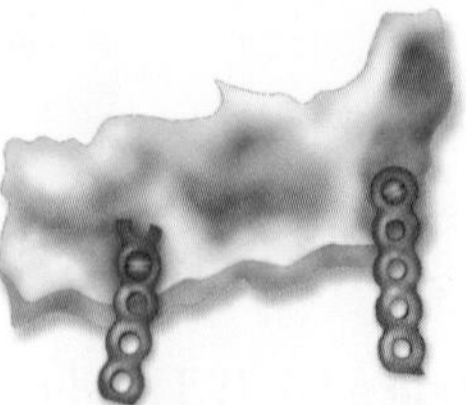

FIGURE 98-9

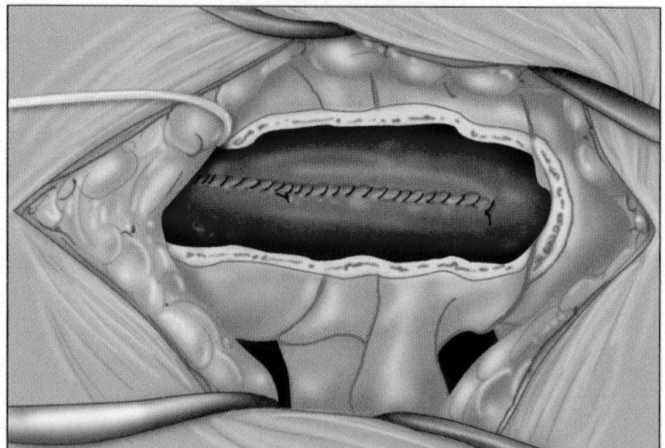

FIGURE 98-10

- **Figure 98-9:** Resected posterior elements are plated with titanium or resorbable plates and screws to allow completion of laminoplasty.
- **Figure 98-10:** If dural integrity was maintained, the midline dural incision is closed primarily with a running nylon or polypropylene (Prolene) suture. For meningiomas requiring resection of the dural attachment, a dural patch using Gore-Tex (W.L. Gore & Associates, Inc., Flagstaff, AZ) or collagen-based duraplasty materials should be used to reconstruct the thecal sac.
- **Figure 98-11:** Dura sealant or fibrin glue is used to reinforce the dural closure and minimize the risk of cerebrospinal fluid (CSF) leak in the postoperative setting.

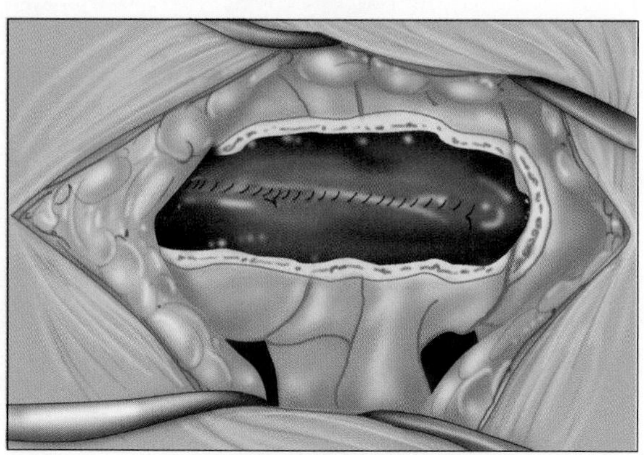

FIGURE 98-11

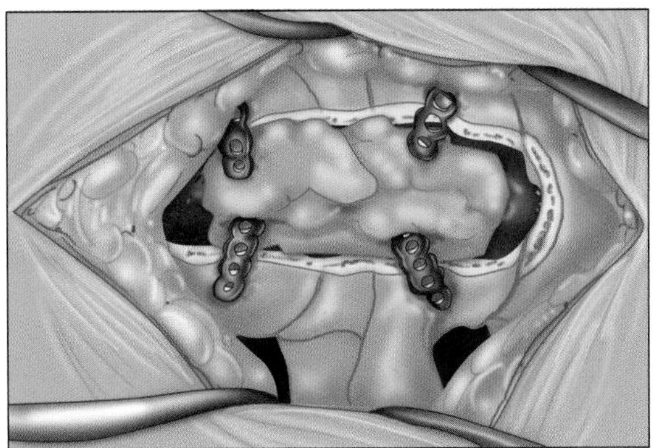

FIGURE 98-12

- **Figure 98-12:** The laminoplasty is completed by fixing the lamina to the remaining posterior elements. The overlying fascia and soft tissues are closed with absorbable suture, and the skin is reapproximated in a standard fashion. The patient is subsequently extubated, and a brief neurologic examination is performed. The patient is transferred to the neurosurgical intensive care unit for monitoring overnight.

TIPS FROM THE MASTERS

- Gross total resection should be the goal of surgery, provided that it can be achieved without causing neurologic deficits. Subtotal resection is associated with a higher recurrence rate and worse outcomes. Reoperation for recurrent meningiomas can be challenging because of arachnoid scarring, leading to a higher rate of neurologic complications.
- For small lesions, en bloc resection of the meningioma can be attempted. For larger lesions, internal debulking with either ultrasonic aspiration or bipolar electrocautery and microsuction should be performed before dissection around the margins of the tumor.
- En plaque and atypical meningiomas tend to be more invasive and are more likely to recur after surgery. Every attempt to achieve safe, complete resection of these lesions should be undertaken.

PITFALLS

Because of the dural attachment of spinal meningiomas, it may be necessary to resect a portion of the dura circumferentially to achieve gross total resection. In these cases, the risk of postoperative CSF leak is elevated, and care should be taken to reconstruct the dura in a watertight fashion to decrease the risk of CSF leak and postoperative meningitis.

For lesions located anterior to the spinal cord, gross total resection can be challenging because of the difficulty in reconstructing the thecal sac. In this case, it may be necessary to separate the meningioma from its dural attachment and cauterize the residual dural leaflet with bipolar electrocautery.

Because of the lateral or anterior location of some spinal meningiomas, extensive bone removal or disruption of ligamentous or facet structures may be necessary to achieve gross total resection; this can lead to spinal instability in the postoperative setting. The need for instrumented fixation should be assessed preoperatively, and instrumentation can be placed either at the time of initial tumor resection or in a delayed fashion if the patient develops postlaminectomy kyphosis.

BAILOUT OPTIONS

- In cases in which watertight dural closure is impossible, flat bed rest or lumbar CSF drainage or both may be necessary to decrease the hydrostatic pressure on the dural closure and allow proper wound healing.
- For meningiomas that cannot be completely resected, owing to adherence to neural or vascular structures, close surveillance for tumor progression is important. For residual unresectable lesions that have shown interval tumor growth on serial MRI, radiation therapy should be considered.

SUGGESTED READINGS

Deletis V, Sala F. Intraoperative neurophysiological monitoring of the spinal cord during spinal cord and spine surgery: a review focus on the corticospinal tracts. Clin Neurophysiol 2008;119:248–64.

Gezen F, Kahraman S, Canakci Z, et al. Review of 36 cases of spinal cord meningioma. Spine 2000;25:727–31.

Klekamp J, Samii M. Surgical results for spinal meningiomas. Surg Neurol 1999;52:552–62.

Parsa AT, Lee J, Parney IF, et al. Spinal cord and intradural-extraparenchymal spinal tumors: current best care practices and strategies. J Neurooncol 2004;69:291–318.

Setzer M, Vatter H, Marquardt G, et al. Management of spinal meningiomas: surgical results and a review of the literature. Neurosurg Focus 2007;23:E14.

Procedure 99 Intramedullary Glioma

Ryan M. Kretzer, Chetan Bettegowda, George I. Jallo

INDICATIONS

- Intramedullary spinal cord lesion on magnetic resonance imaging (MRI) in the setting of neurologic symptoms (pain, sensory disturbances, motor weakness, nonspecific complaints)
- Intramedullary spinal cord lesion on MRI or an associated cyst or syringomyelia that has progressed on serial imaging and is likely to become symptomatic in the future
- Intramedullary spinal cord lesion on MRI that is of unclear etiology despite an extensive neurology work-up, warranting a need for tissue diagnosis

CONTRAINDICATIONS

- Asymptomatic, incidentally noted lesions or lesions causing only minor symptoms can be treated conservatively with serial clinical assessments and MRI.
- Severely debilitated patients or patients with a short life expectancy because of comorbid illness or metastatic disease should be observed or treated with palliative therapy.

PLANNING AND POSITIONING

- The clinical assessment of a patient with a suspected intramedullary spinal cord tumor starts with a detailed history and physical examination.
- MRI is necessary to localize the lesion correlate with clinical findings and plan the operative approach, including establishing goals of operative intervention and considering deficits that may result from surgical resection. Other imaging modalities such as x-ray and computed tomography (CT) scan should be obtained to assess for associated scoliotic deformities and to determine the need for instrumented fixation at the time of surgery.
- Intraoperative neurophysiologic monitoring with motor evoked potentials (MEPs) provides the surgeon with real-time feedback on the integrity of the corticospinal tracts. Needle electrodes should be placed at the end muscles after the patient is asleep but before final prone positioning in the operating room. Because halogenated anesthetic agents cause depression of MEPs, the anesthetic regimen should be coordinated with the anesthesiologist. Propofol and fentanyl are commonly used agents that do not cause a decline in MEPs.
- **Figure 99-1:** Preoperative imaging, including MRI, plays a key role in surgical planning. Sagittal (*left*) and axial (*right*) T1-weighted MRI after administration of gadolinium contrast agent shows an intramedullary cervical spinal cord tumor with an associated rostral cyst.
- **Figure 99-2:** For most intramedullary spinal cord tumors, a dorsal approach is used. The patient is first intubated in the supine position, and all neurophysiologic monitors are placed. Awake fiberoptic intubation may be warranted in patients with cervical spine instability or cervical lesions causing significant canal impingement. For a cervical tumor the patient is positioned prone in Mayfield head holder. The neck is slightly flexed to aid in surgical exposure. For patients with thoracic or lumbar lesions, prone positioning can be accomplished on a Wilson frame or chest rolls without head fixation. All dependent surfaces (e.g., knees, elbows) are padded to avoid peripheral nerve injury or pressure-related tissue necrosis.

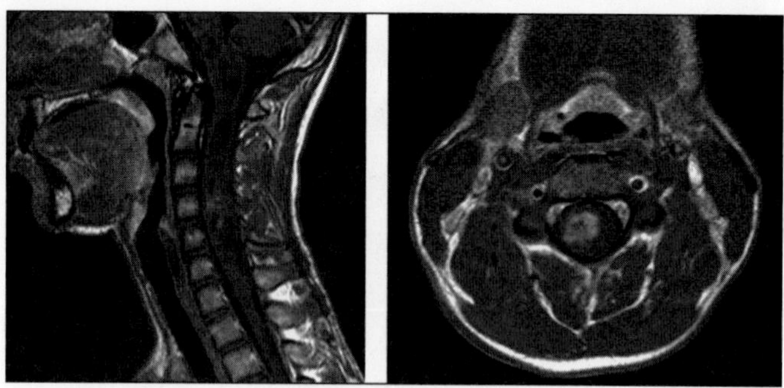

FIGURE 99-1

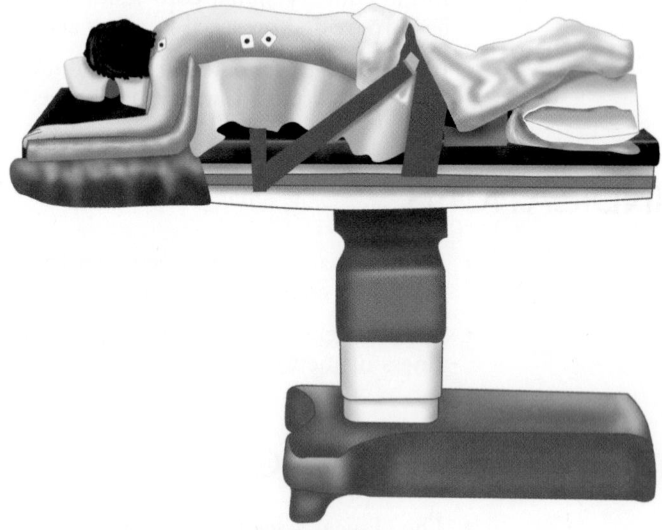

FIGURE 99-2

PROCEDURE

- **Figure 99-3:** The skin is incised in the midline, and electrocautery is used to dissect the paraspinal musculature from the posterior spinal elements in the subperiosteal plane. During dissection, it is important to avoid disruption of the facet joint capsules to decrease the risk of postlaminectomy kyphosis. After the spinous processes and laminae are exposed, bilateral laminotomies are performed at the caudal aspect of the planned laminoplasty using a Kerrison punch. A craniotome is used to detach the lamina bilaterally over the extent of the planned dural exposure, allowing the posterior elements to be removed en bloc after transection of the underlying ligamentum flavum and rostral and caudal interspinous ligaments. If significant spinal canal narrowing exists, the laminectomy can be performed in a piecemeal fashion using a Leksell rongeur and Kerrison punches.
- **Figure 99-4:** After the dura is exposed, epidural venous bleeding is controlled, and an epidural D-wave electrode is passed caudally below the planned dural opening for neurophysiologic monitoring purposes. An ultrasound probe is used to insonate the underlying tumor and to verify that adequate bony exposure has been achieved.
- **Figure 99-5:** The dura is incised in the midline using a No. 15 blade scalpel and Metzenbaum scissors. An attempt should be made to keep the arachnoid membrane intact at the time of initial dural opening. Dural tenting sutures are placed bilaterally to minimize the flow of blood products into the subarachnoid space and to aid in operative exposure.
- **Figure 99-6:** The microscope is brought into the field, and the arachnoid membrane is incised. Dorsal midline myelotomy is performed through the posterior median sulcus using a microknife or contact neodymium:yttrium-aluminum-garnet (Nd:YAG) laser.

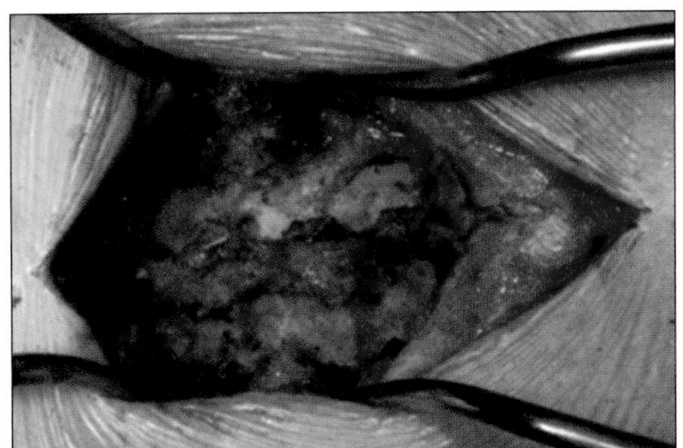

FIGURE 99-3

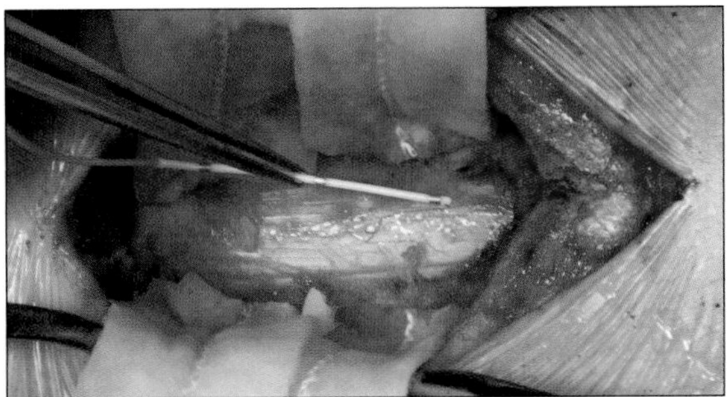

FIGURE 99-4

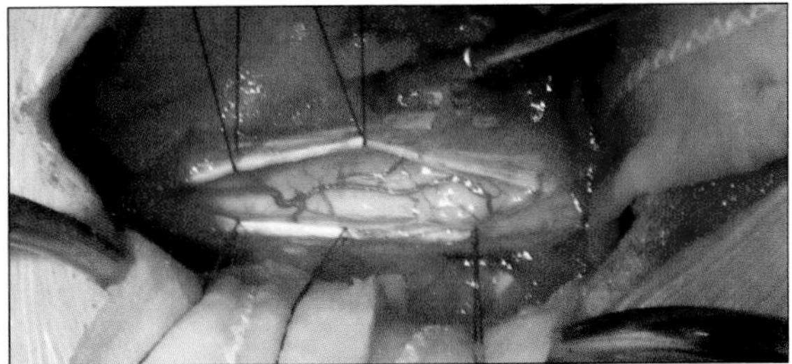

FIGURE 99-5

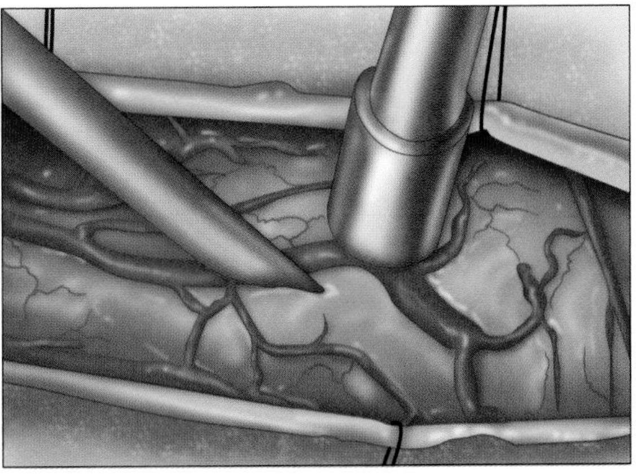

FIGURE 99-6

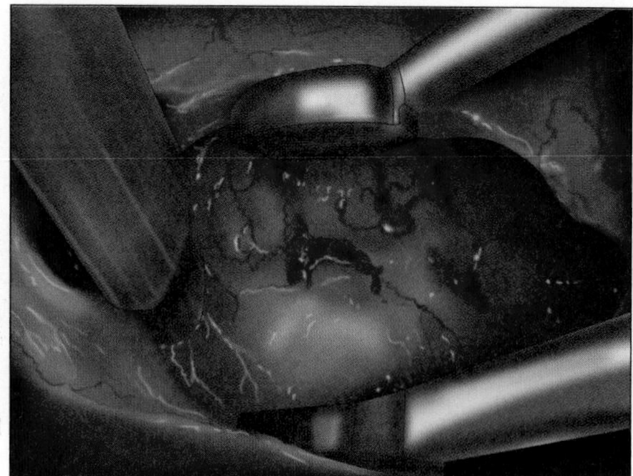

FIGURE 99-7

- **Figure 99-7:** Because intramedullary lesions typically lie several millimeters below the posterior surface of the cord, dissection is carried through the midline myelotomy until pathologic tissue is encountered. Biopsy specimens are obtained and sent for preliminary pathologic examination. Any polar cysts that are accessible should also be drained to allow relaxation of the spinal cord. The tumor is debulked internally using an ultrasonic aspirator starting in the middle of lesion; resection at the superior and inferior portions of the tumor is typically delayed because of the proximity to normal spinal cord parenchyma. Microsuction or contact laser can also be used to resect the residual tumor from the margins, with the extent of resection guided by MEP readings. Plated bayonets are used to aid in exposure of the resection cavity and can be used to develop the tumor–spinal cord interface in cases of intramedullary ependymomas.
- **Figure 99-8:** After tumor resection, hemostasis is achieved within the spinal cord.
- **Figure 99-9:** If en bloc laminoplasty was performed, the laminae are plated bilaterally with titanium or resorbable plates and screws.
- **Figure 99-10:** The dura is closed with a running nylon or polypropylene (Prolene) suture. In some cases, a dural patch of Gore-Tex (W.L. Gore & Associates, Inc., Flagstaff, AZ) or collagen-based duraplasty material may be used to expand the intrathecal space.
- **Figure 99-11:** To minimize the risk of postoperative cerebrospinal fluid leak, dural sealant or fibrin glue is typically used to reinforce the dural suture line.
- **Figure 99-12:** In en bloc laminoplasty, the posterior elements are reattached to the existing spinal column to decrease the risk of postsurgical kyphosis.

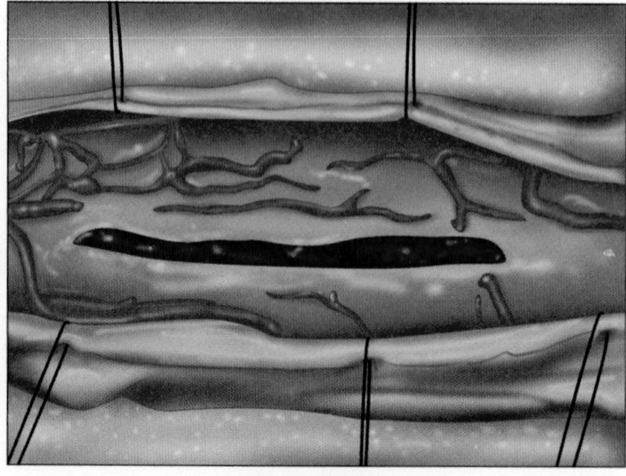

FIGURE 99-8

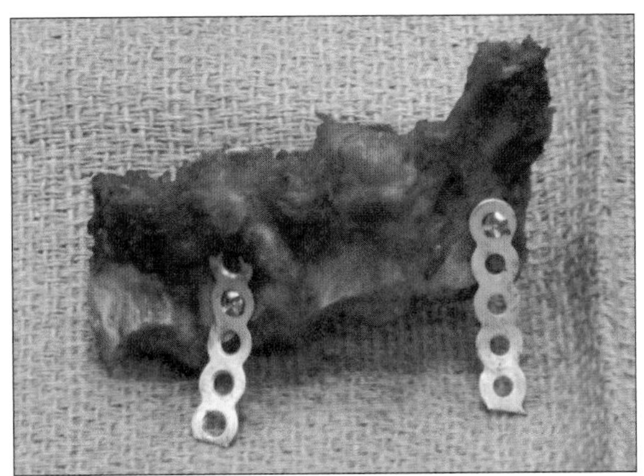

FIGURE 99-9

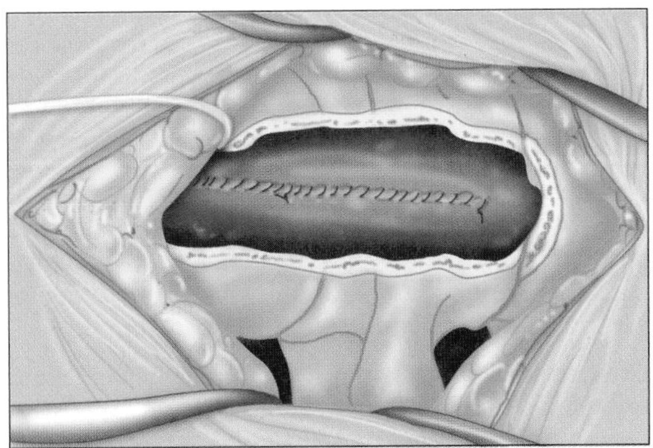

FIGURE 99-10

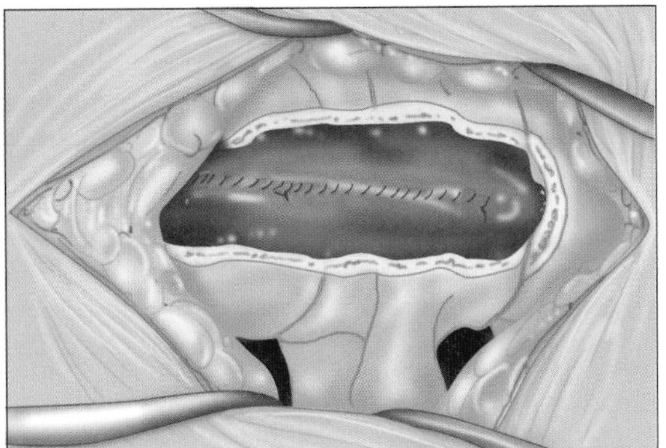

FIGURE 99-11

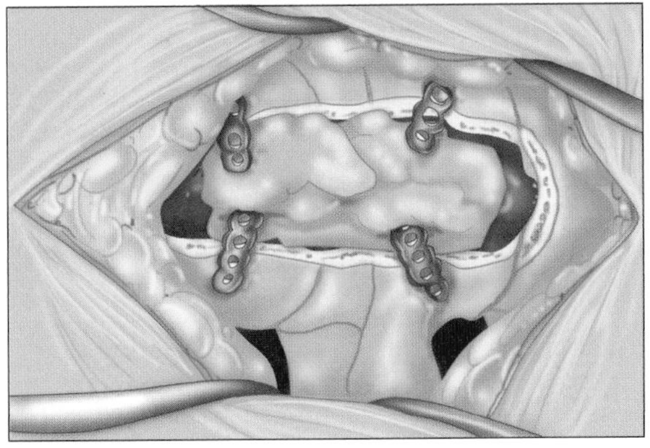

FIGURE 99-12

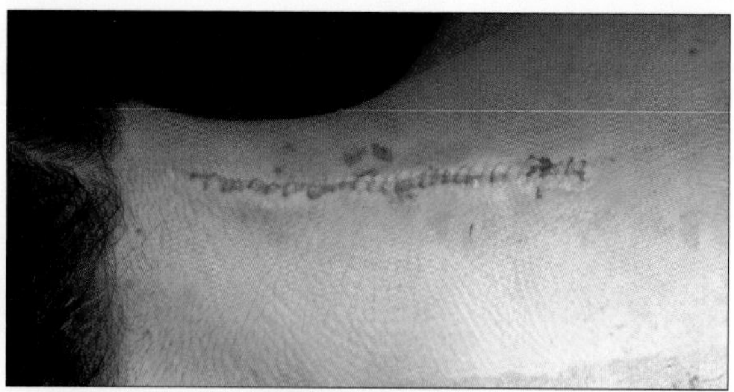

FIGURE 99-13

- **Figure 99-13:** After meticulous hemostasis, the fascia and overlying soft tissues are reapproximated with absorbable suture. The skin is closed in a standard fashion, the patient is transferred to the supine position and extubated, and a brief neurologic examination is performed before transfer to the neurosurgical intensive care unit.

TIPS FROM THE MASTERS

- Muscle MEPs and epidural D-wave MEPs should be used in combination during surgical resection of intramedullary gliomas. Muscle MEPs follow an "on-off" pattern, and the D-wave shows a graded response. As long as D-wave amplitude remains greater than 50%, any postoperative motor deficits are likely to be transient. Somatosensory evoked potentials are typically lost after the midline myelotomy and are of little use in surgical resection of intramedullary spinal cord tumors.
- Astrocytomas are infiltrating lesions, whereas ependymomas are generally well circumscribed and show a defined tumor–spinal cord interface. Although gross total resection is often difficult in the case of astrocytomas, it should be the goal for surgical resection of intramedullary ependymomas.
- When possible, performing a laminoplasty may help decrease the risk of postsurgical kyphosis, especially for tumors in the cervical or cervicothoracic spine.

PITFALLS

Care should be taken to avoid facet or ligamentous disruption during operative exposure. Such disruption may increase the risk of postsurgical kyphosis, particularly in young patients with lesions in the cervical and cervicothoracic spine. Patients should be followed for progression of spinal deformity in the postoperative setting with serial plain x-rays.

Halogenated anesthetic agents can cause depression of motor potentials and should be avoided during surgical resection of intramedullary spinal cord tumors. Propofol and fentanyl are good options that do not affect intraoperative MEP readings.

Neurologic deficits are common after surgery for intramedullary lesions, although with the judicious use of neurophysiologic monitoring, most deficits are transient and correlate with the patient's preoperative baseline level of functioning. Dysesthesias and proprioceptive difficulties are especially common as a result of the midline myelotomy that is required for tumor access. These deficits generally improve over the first 3 months after surgery with the aid of physical therapy.

BAILOUT OPTIONS

- If significant MEP changes are noted during tumor debulking, options include medications to increase the patient's mean arterial pressure, the introduction of warm saline or papaverine-soaked cotton into the resection cavity, surgical resection at a different site, or cessation of the operative procedure.

- Cerebrospinal fluid leak is a rare but potentially serious complication of surgical treatment for intramedullary gliomas. In patients who are undergoing reoperation, who have had previous radiation exposure to the operative site, or who have wound healing difficulties, the assistance of a plastic surgeon may be needed to aid in operative soft tissue closure.
- If the spinal cord remains enlarged after tumor debulking, a dural patch (Gore-Tex or collagen-based material) can be used to widen the intrathecal compartment.

SUGGESTED READINGS

Houten JK, Cooper PR. Spinal cord astrocytomas: presentation, management, and outcome. J Neurooncol 2000;47:219–24.

Jallo GI, Freed D, Epstein F. Intramedullary spinal cord tumors in children. Childs Nerv Syst 2003;19:641–9.

Miller DC. Surgical pathology of intramedullary spinal cord neoplasms. J Neurooncol 2000;47:189–94.

Morota N, Deletis V, Constantini S, et al. The role of motor evoked potentials during surgery for intramedullary spinal cord tumors. Neurosurgery 1997;41:1327–36.

Parsa AT, Lee J, Parney IF, et al. Spinal cord and intradural-extraparenchymal spinal tumors: current best care practices and strategies. J Neurooncol 2004;69:291–318.

Index

Note: Page numbers followed by "f" indicate figures; "b" boxes.

B

C

D

G

H

I

K

L

R

S

T

U

V